Springer-Verlag Italia Srl.

A. Gullo (Ed.)

Anaesthesia, Pain, Intensive Care and Emergency Medicine - A.P.I.C.E.

Proceedings of the

15th Postgraduate Course in Critical Care Medicine

Trieste, Italy - November 17-21, 2000

Springer

Prof. ANTONINO GULLO, M.D.
Head, Department of Anaesthesiology and Intensive Care
Trieste University School of Medicine
Trieste, Italy

Library of Congress Cataloging-in-Publication Data: Applied for

Originally published by Springer-Verlag Italia, Milano in 2001
ISBN 978-88-470-0136-7 ISBN 978-88-470-2903-3 (eBook)
DOI 10.1007/978-88-470-2903-3

Printed: Tipografia-Litografia «Moderna» - Trieste, Italy

SPIN 10789923

Table of Contents

NEUROLOGY

COMPUTERING

COST-EFFECTIVENESS IN ANAESTHESIA AND CRITICAL CARE

EDUCATION

Authors Index

Adembri C.
Dept. of Critical Care, Section of Anaesthesiology and Intensive Care, University of Florence, Florence (Italy)

Agrò F.
Dept. of Anaesthesia, University School of Medicine, Rome (Italy)

Allaria B.
Dept. of Intensive Care, National Institute for Cancer Research, Milan (Italy)

Antonelli M.
Dept. of Anaesthesia and Intensive Care, La Sapienza University, Rome (Italy)

Arcangeli A.
Dept. of Anaesthesia and Intensive Care, La Sapienza University, Rome (Italy)

Auler J.O.C. Jr
Dept. of Anaesthesia and Intensive Care, Heart Institute, Hospital das Clínicas, São Paulo University, São Paulo (Brazil)

Avenali S.
Dept. of Anaesthesia and Intensive Care Unit, Salesi Mother and Children's Hospital, Ancona (Italy)

Barozzi O.
Dept. of Anaesthesia and Intensive Care, Spedali Civili, Brescia (Italy)

Barzoi G.
Dept. of Anaesthesia, University School of Medicine, Rome (Italy)

Bastien O.
Dept. of Anaesthesia and Intensive Care, Louis Pradel Hospital, Lyon (France)

Biagioli B.
Dept. of Thoracic Surgery, Siena University, Siena (Italy)

Biolo G.
Dept. of Clinical, Morphological and Technological Sciences, Division of Internal Medicine, University of Trieste, Trieste (Italy)

Blanch Ll.
Intensive Care Service, Sabadell Hospital, Sabadell (Spain)

Bottino N.
Dept. of Anaesthesia and Intensive Care, Milan University, Milan (Italy)

Brandolese R.
Multidisciplinary Rehabilitation Centre, Intensive Care Unit, City Hospital of Padua, Conselve (Italy)

Brienza A.
Dept. of Emergency and Organ Transplantation, Section of Anaesthesia and Intensive Care, Bari University, Bari (Italy)

Brienza N.
Dept. of Emergency and Organ Transplantation, Section of Anaesthesia and Intensive Care, Bari University, Bari (Italy)

Busoni P.
Meyer Hospital, Florence (Italy)

Caccamo F.
La Sapienza University, Rome (Italy)

Cafiero T.
Dept. of Anaesthesia and Intensive Care, Casa Sollievo della Sofferenza, S. Giovanni Rotondo (Italy)

Caironi P.
Dept. of Anaesthesia and Intensive Care, Milan University, Milan (Italy)

Capogna G.
Dept. of Anaesthesia and Intensive Care, Fatebenefratelli Hospital, Rome (Italy)

Caricato A.
Dept. of Anaesthesiology and Intensive Care, Catholic University School of Medicine, Rome (Italy)

Caristi D.
Dept. of Clinical Sciences, Section of Anaesthesia, Intensive Care and Pain Clinic, Trieste University Medical School, Trieste (Italy)

Carli F.
Dept. of Anaesthesia, McGill University Health Centre, Montreal, Quebec (Canada)

Cataldo R.
Dept. of Anaesthesia, University School of Medicine, Rome (Italy)

Cavaliere F.
Dept. of Anaesthesia and Intensive Care, Catholic University Sacro Cuore, Rome (Italy)

Ciarlone A.
Dept. of Anaesthesia and Intensive Care, La Sapienza University, Rome (Italy)

Clementi G.
Dept. of Anaesthesia and Intensive Care, Mazzini Hospital, Teramo (Italy)

Coccia C.
Dept. of Anaesthesia and Intensive Care, University of Rome La Sapienza, Rome (Italy)

Cohen E.
Dept. of Anaesthesiology, Mount Sinai School of Medicine, New York (U.S.A.)

Conti G.
Dept. of Anaesthesia and Intensive Care, Catholic University Sacro Cuore, Rome (Italy)

Coppola M.
Dept. of Surgical, Anaesthesiological and Emergency Science, Naples University Federico II, Naples (Italy)

Costa M.G.
Dept. of Anaesthesiology and Intensive Care, University of Rome La Sapienza, Rome (Italy)

Crocè L.S.
Centre for Liver Studies, University of Trieste, Trieste (Italy)

D'Onghia N.
Dept. of Anaesthesia and Intensive Care, Bari University, Bari (Italy)

De Cillis P.
Dept. of Anaesthesia and Intensive Care, G. Rummo Hospital, Benevento (Italy)

De Gaudio A.R.
Dept. of Critical Care, Section of Anaesthesiology and Intensive Care, University of Florence, Florence (Italy)

De Robertis E.
Dept. of Surgical, Anaesthesiological and Emergency Science, Naples University Federico II, Naples (Italy)

De Vivo P.
Dept. of Anaesthesia and Intensive Care, Casa Sollievo della Sofferenza, S. Giovanni Rotondo (Italy)

Dei Poli M.
Dept. of Anaesthesia and Intensive Care, S. Donato Hospital, S. Donato (Italy)

Della Corte F.
Dept. of Anaesthesiology and Intensive Care, Catholic University School of Medicine, Rome (Italy)

Della Rocca G.
Dept. of Anaesthesiology and Intensive Care, University of Rome La Sapienza, Rome (Italy)

Diaz O.
Dept. of Respiratory Diseases, Pontificia Universitad Catolica de Chile, Santiago (Chile)

Dobb G.J.
Department of Medicine, University of Western Australia, Perth (Australia)

Estanove S.
Dept. of Anaesthesia and Intensive Care, Louis Pradel Cardiovascular Hospital, Lyon (France)

Fantoni D.
Veterinary Medicine School, São Paulo University, São Paulo (Brazil)

Farré R.
Dept. of Biophysics and Bioengineering, University of Barcelona, Barcelona (Spain)

Favaro M.
Dept. of Intensive Care, National Institute for Cancer Research, Milan (Italy)

Ferrari A.
Dept. of Surgery, University of Pisa, Pisa (Italy)

Ferrari Baliviera E.
San Filippo Neri Hospital Complex, Rome (Italy)

Ferraro P.
Dept. of Emergency Medicine, S. Paolo Hospital, Naples (Italy)

Fisher M.M.
University of Sydney Intensive Therapy Unit, Royal North Shore Hospital, St Leonards (Australia)

Forfori F.
Dept. of Surgery, University of Pisa, Pisa (Italy)

Franciosa P.
Dept. of Cardiology and Centre for the Study of Arrhythmias, Multimedica General Hospital, Sesto S. Giovanni (Italy)

Frova G.
Dept. of Anaesthesia and Intensive Care, Spedali Civili, Brescia (Italy)

Galimberti G.
Dept. of Clinical Sciences, Section of Anesthesia, Intensive Care and Pain Clinic, Trieste University Medical School, Trieste (Italy)

Gerlach H.
Dept. of Anaesthesia and Intensive Care, Charité Hospital, Campus Virchow-Klinikum, Berlin (Germany)

Giunta F.
Dept. of Surgery, University of Pisa, Pisa (Italy)

Gollo E.
Dept. of Anaesthesia and Intensive Care, S. Anna Hospital, Turin (Italy)

Grillone G.
Dept. of Anaesthesia and Intensive Care, S. Orsola Malpighi General Hospital, Bologna (Italy)

Grubbauer H.M.
Paediatric ICU, Dept. of Paediatrics, University of Graz, Graz (Austria)

Guglielmo L.
Dept. of Anaesthesia, Fatebenefratelli Hospital, Palermo (Italy)

Gullo A.
Dept. of Clinical Sciences, Section of Anaesthesia, Intensive Care and Pain Clinic, Trieste University Medical School, Trieste (Italy)

Gurman G.M.
Division of Anaesthesiology, Soroka Medical Center and Faculty of Health Sciences, Ben Gurion University of the Negev, Beer Sheva (Israel)

Haitsma J.J.
Dept. of Anaesthesiology, Erasmus University Rotterdam, Rotterdam (The Netherlands)

Hammerle A.F.
Dept. of Anaesthesia and General Intensive Care Medicine, University of Vienna, Vienna General Hospital, Vienna (Austria)

Harrison C.
Univ. Dept. of Anaesthesia and Pain Management, Leicester Royal Infirmary, Leicester (U.K.)

Hedenstierna G.
Dept. of Medical Sciences, Clinical Physiology, University Hospital, Uppsala (Sweden)

Hetz H.
Dept. of Anaesthesiology and General Intensive Care, University of Vienna Medical School, Vienna (Austria)

Inghilleri G.
Dept. of Immunohaematology and Transfusions, Gaetano Pini Orthopaedic Institute, Milan (Italy)

Jacques T.
Intensive Care Unit, The St George Hospital, Kogarah (Australia)

Josten C.
Dept. for Traumatology, University of Leipzig, Leipzig (Germany)

Jubran A.
Division of Pulmonary and Critical Care Medicine, Edward Hines Jr., Veterans Affairs Hospital and Loyola University of Chicago Stritch School of Medicine, Hines (U.S.A.)

Katscher S.
Dept. for Traumatology, University of Leipzig, Leipzig (Germany)

Kessin C.
São Paulo University School of Medicine, São Paulo (Brazil)

Kox W.J.
Dept. of Anaesthesiology and Intensive Care, University Hospital Charité Campus Mitte, Berlin (Germany)

Krenn C.G.
Dept. of Anaesthesiology and General Intensive Care, University of Vienna Medical School, Vienna (Austria)

La Mura F.
Dept. of Anaesthesiology and Intensive Care, Catholic University School of Medicine, Rome (Italy)

Lachmann B.
Dept. of Anaesthesiology, Erasmus University Rotterdam, Rotterdam (The Netherlands)

Laganà I.
Paediatric Emergency Dept., Anaesthesia and Intensive Care Unit, Salesi Mother and Children's Hospital, Ancona (Italy)

Lambert D.G.
Univ. Dept. of Anaesthesia and Pain Management, Leicester Royal Infirmary, Leicester, (U.K.)

Lanza V.
Dept. of Anaesthesia, Fatebenefratelli Hospital, Palermo (Italy)

Lehot J.J.
Dept. of Anaesthesia and Intensive Care, Louis Pradel Cardiovascular Hospital, Lyon (France)

Levi M.
Dept. of Vascular Medicine and Internal Medicine, Academic Medical Center, University of Amsterdam, Amsterdam (The Netherlands)

Locatelli M.
Institute of Radiology, University of Trieste, Trieste (Italy)

Loreto M.
Dept. of Anaesthesia and Intensive Care, Second University of Naples, Naples (Italy)

Lucangelo U.
Dept. of Clinical Sciences, Section of Anaesthesia, Intensive Care and Pain Clinic, Trieste School of Medicine, Trieste (Italy)

Lumb P.D.
Dept. of Anaesthesia, Pennsylvania State University College of Medicine, Hershey (U.S.A.)

Maffessanti M.
Dept. of Radiology, Trieste University School of Medicine, Trieste (Italy)

Mangiameli D.
Dept. of Cardiology and Centre for the Study of Arrhythmias, Multimedica General Hospital, Sesto S. Giovanni (Italy)

Manlik F.
Dept. of Anaesthesiology and General Intensive Care, University of Vienna Medical School, Vienna (Austria)

Margaria E.
Dept. of Anaesthesia and Intensive Care, S. Anna Hospital, Turin (Italy)

Mastronardi P.
Dept. of Surgical, Anaesthesiological and Emergency Science, Naples University Federico II, Naples (Italy)

Mattia C.
Dept. of Anaesthesia and Intensive Care, Umberto I General Hospital, University La Sapienza, Rome (Italy)

Maviglia R.
Dept. of Anaesthesiology and Intensive Care, Catholic University Sacro Cuore, Rome (Italy)

Melloni C.
Dept. of Anaesthesia and Intensive Care, Faenza Hospital, Faenza (Italy)

Mercuriali F.
Dept. of Immunohaematology and Transfusion, Gaetano Pini Orthopaedic Institute, Milan (Italy)

Mets B.
Dept. of Clinical Anaesthesiology, Columbia University, New York (U.S.A.)

Milic-Emili J.
Meakins-Christie Laboratories, McGill University, Montreal (Canada)

Monteferrante I.
Dept. of Anaesthesiology and Intensive Care, Catholic University Sacro Cuore, Rome (Italy)

Montenero A.S.
Dept. of Cardiology and Centre for the Study of Arrhythmias, Multimedica General Hospital, Sesto S. Giovanni (Italy)

Muchada R.
Dept. of Anaesthesia and Intensive Care, Eugène André Hospital, Lyon (France)

Muravchick S.
Dept. of Anaesthesia, University of Pennsylvania, Philadelphia (U.S.A.)

Nair P.
Intensive Care Unit, St Vincent's Hospital Darlinghurst, Sydney (Australia)

Nap R.
Health Services Research Unit, University Hospital, Groningen (The Netherlands)

Neidecker J.
Dept. of Anaesthesia and Intensive Care, Louis Pradel Cardiovascular Hospital, Lyon (France)

Nolan J.
Dept. of Anaesthesia and Intensive Care Medicine, Royal United Hospital, Bath (U.K.)

Novelli G.P.
Dept. of Critical Care, Section of Anesthesiology and Intensive Care, University of Florence, Florence (Italy)

Otsuki D.A.
Veterinary Medicine School, São Paulo University, São Paulo (Brazil)

Pagni R.
Paediatric Emergency Dept., Anaesthesia and Intensive Care Unit, Salesi Mother and Children's Hospital, Ancona (Italy)

Paladino F.
Dept. of Emergency Medicine, S. Paolo Hospital, Naples (Italy)

Parpaglioni R.
Dept. of Anaesthesia and Intensive Care, Fatebenefratelli Hospital, Rome (Italy)

Parsloe C.
Samaritano Hospital, São Paulo (Brazil)

Passariello M.
Dept. of Anaesthesia and Intensive Care, Rome University La Sapienza, Rome (Italy)

Pelosi P.
Dept. of Clinical and Biological Science, Insubria University, Varese (Italy)

Pennisi M.A.
Dept. of Anaesthesia and Intensive Care, Catholic University Sacro Cuore, Rome (Italy)

Piacevoli Q.
San Filippo Neri Hospital Complex, Rome (Italy)

Pietropaoli P.
Dept. of Anaesthesiology and Intensive Care, University of Rome La Sapienza, Rome (Italy)

Piriou V.
Dept. of Anaesthesia and Intensive Care, Louis Pradel Cardiovascular Hospital, Lyon (France)

Pozzi Mucelli F.
Institute of Radiology, University of Trieste, Trieste (Italy)

Pozzi Mucelli R.
Institute of Radiology, University of Trieste, Trieste (Italy)

Pravato M.
Institute of Radiology, University of Trieste, Trieste (Italy)

Proietti R.
Dept. of Anaesthesia and Intensive Care, Catholic University Sacro Cuore, Rome (Italy)

Ragonese P.
Institute of Neuropsychiatry, University of Palermo, Palermo (Italy)

Ranucci M.
San Donato Hospital, San Donato Milanese (Italy)

Ratti M.
Institute of Radiology, University of Trieste, Trieste (Italy)

Reis Miranda D.
Health Services Research Unit, University Hospital, Groningen (The Netherlands)

Rigato I.
Centre for Liver Studies, University of Trieste, Trieste (Italy)

Rödl S.
Dept. of Paediatrics, University of Graz, Graz (Austria)

Rogiers P.
Dept of Intensive Care, Middelheim General Hospital, Antwerpen (Belgium)

Romero P.V.
Pulmonary Function Laboratory, University Hospital Bellvitge, L'Hospitalet de Llobregat, Barcelona (Spain)

Rossi S.
Dept. of Anaesthesia and Intensive Care, Maggiore Hospital, Milan (Italy)

Rubulotta F.
Dept. of Clinical Sciences, Section of Anesthesia, Intensive Care and Pain Clinic, Trieste University Medical School, Trieste (Italy)

Rupreht J.
Dept. of Anaesthesiology, University Hospital Rotterdam, Rotterdam (The Netherlands)

Salemi G.
Institute of Neuropsychiatry, University of Palermo, Palermo (Italy)

Sanfilippo M.
Dept. of Anaesthesia and Intensive Care, Rome University La Sapienza, Rome (Italy)

Sarti A.
Dept. of Anaesthesia and Intensive Care, Research and Care Children Hospital, Trieste (Italy)

Savettieri G.
Institute of Neuropsychiatry, University of Palermo, Palermo (Italy)

Savoia G.
Dept. of Anaesthesia and Intensive Care, Fatebenefratelli Hospital, Naples (Italy)

Scheibner L.
Intensive Care Unit, University of Leipzig, Leipzig (Germany)

Schiraldi F.
Dept. of Emergency Medicine, S. Paolo Hospital, Naples (Italy)

Schneider T.
German Red Cross Emergency Medical Services, Mainz (Germany)

Schreiter D.
Intensive Care Unit, University of Leipzig, Leipzig (Germany)

Scibelli G.
Dept. of Anaesthesia and Intensive Care, Fatebenefratelli Hospital, Naples (Italy)

Servillo G.
Dept. of Surgical, Anaesthesiological and Emergency Science, Naples University Federico II, Naples (Italy)

Sinigaglia R.
Dept. of Anaesthesia and Intensive Care, S. Anna Hospital, Turin (Italy)

Sortino G.
Dept. of Anaesthesia and Intensive Care, S. Anna Hospital, Turin (Italy)

Spies C.
Dept. of Anaesthesiology and Intensive Care, University Hospital Charité Campus Mitte, Berlin (Germany)

Spinelli F.
Dept. of Anaesthesia and Intensive Care, Rome University La Sapienza, Rome (Italy)

Starikov R.
Division of Anaesthesiology, Soroka Medical Center and Faculty of Health Sciences, Ben Gurion University of the Negev, Beer Sheva (Israel)

Steltzer H.
Dept. of Anaesthesiology and General Intensive Care, University of Vienna Medical School, Vienna (Austria)

Stocchetti N.
Dept. of Anaesthesia and Intensive Care, Maggiore Hospital, Milan (Italy)

Sutcliffe A.J.
Dept. of Anaesthesia and Intensive Care, Queen Elizabeth Hospital, Birmingham (U.K.)

Tatschl C.
Dept. of Anaesthesia and General Intensive Care Medicine, University of Vienna, Vienna General Hospital, Vienna (Austria)

Tiribelli C.
Centre for Liver Studies, University of Trieste, Trieste (Italy)

Trop M.
Dept. of Paediatrics, University of Graz, Graz (Austria)

Tufano R.
Dept. of Surgical, Anaesthesiological and Emergency Science, Naples University Federico II, Naples (Italy)

Tuzzo D.
Dept. of Anaesthesia and Intensive Care, Spedali Civili, Brescia (Italy)

Valeriani V.
Dept. of Anaesthesia and Intensive Care, Maggiore Hospital, Milan (Italy)

van der Starre P.J.A.
Dept. of Cardiothoracic Anaesthesiology and Intensive Care, Isala Clinics, Weezenlanden Hospital, Zwolle (The Netherlands)

Vargas Hein O.
Dept. of Anaesthesiology and Intensive Care, University Hospital Charité Campus Mitte, Berlin (Germany)

Vatua S.
Dept. of Clinical Sciences, Section of Anaesthesia, Intensive Care and Pain Clinic, Trieste School of Medicine, Trieste (Italy)

Vilardi V.
Dept. of Anaesthesia and Intensive Care, L'Aquila University, L'Aquila (Italy)

Volpe N.G.
Dept. of Intensive Care Medicine, University Hospitals of Leicester NHS Trust, Glenfield Hospital, Leicester (U.K.)

Weksler N.
Division of Anaesthesiology, Soroka Medical Center and Faculty of Health Sciences, Ben Gurion University of the Negev, Beer Sheva (Israel)

White P.F.
Dept. of Anaesthesiology and Pain Management, University of Texas, Southwestern Medical Center, Dallas (U.S.A.)

Wolcke B.
Clinic of Anaesthesiology, Johannes Gutenberg-University Medical School, Mainz (Germany)

Zobel G.
Dept. of Paediatrics, University of Graz, Graz (Austria)

Abbreviations

5-HT, serotonin

ABA, American Board of Anesthesiology

ABF, aortic blood flow

AC, alternating current

ACGME, accreditation council for graduate medical education

ADH, antidiuretic hormone

AED, automated external defibrillator

AF, atrial fibrillation

AHA, American Heart Association

AKT, anaesthesia knowledge test

ALI, acute lung injury

ALS, advanced life support

ANZCA, Australian and New Zealand College of Anaesthetists

APACHE-II, Acute Physiology And Chronic Heart Evaluation II

APLS, advanced paediatric life support

APS, acute pain service

ARDS, acute respiratory distress syndrome

ARF, acute renal failure

ASA, American Society of Anaesthesiologists

BAL, Bioartificial liver

BAL, bronchoalveolar lavage

BB, beta-blocker

BBB, blood-brain barrer

beta TG, beta-thromboglobulin

BIS, bispectral index

BLS-D, basic life support with defibrillation

BLS, basic life support

BMI, body mass index

BP, blood pressure

BP, bodily pain

CA, combined anaesthesia

CAVH, continuous arterovenous haemofiltration

CBF, cerebral blood flow

CCISP, care of the critically ill surgical patient

CDC, Centre for Disease Control

CEGA, combined epidural-general anaesthesia

CHF, continuous haemofiltration

CME, Continuing Medical Education

$CMRO_2$, cerebral oxygen consumption

CO, cardiac output

COP, colloidosmotic pressure

COPA, Cuffed Oropharyngeal Airway

COPD, chronic obstructive pulmonary disease

CPAP, continuous positive airway pressure

CPB, cardiopulmonary bypass

CPC, cerebral performance category

CPP, cerebral perfusion pressure

CPPV, continuous positive pressure ventilation

CPR, cardiopulmonary resuscitation

CQI, Continuous Quality Improvement

CRRT, continuous renal replacement therapy

CSA, continuous spinal anaesthesia

CSE, combined spinal-epidural anaesthesia

CT, computed tomography

CVP, central venous pressure

CVVH, continuous venovenous haemofiltration

CVVHDF, continuous venovenous haemodiafiltration

DAD, diffuse alveolar damage

DBS, double-burst stimulation

DC, direct current

DEA, department of emergency and admittance

DH, dynamic hyperinflation

DIC, disseminated intravascular coagulation

DL, direct laryngoscopy

DLT, double lumen tube

DNR, do not resuscitate

DVT, deep vein thrombosis

EA, epidural anaesthesia

EBV, estimated blood volume

ECF, extracellular fluids

ECMO, extracorporeal membrane oxygenation

ED_{50}, relative median effective dose

ED, emergency department

EJR, extra-junctional receptor

EMO, estarases metabolised opioid

EMS, emergency medical service

EMST, early management of severe trauma

EMT, emergency medical technician

EPIC, European Prevalence of Infection in Intensive Care Units

ERCP, endoscopic retrograde cholangiopancreatography

$EtCO_2$, end tidal CO_2

ETT, endotracheal tube

FC, febrile convulsions

FDP, fibrin degradation product

$FECO_2$(t), capnogram versus time

$FECO_2$(v), capnogram versus volume

FEV_1, forced expiratory volume in one second

FL, flow limitation

FOB, fibreoptic bronchoscopy

FOT, forced oscillation technique

FRC, functional residual capacity

FRICE, Foundation for Research on Intensive Care in Europe

FVC, forced vital capacity

GA, general anaesthesia

GABA, gamma-amino-butyric acid

GCS, Glasgow Coma Scale

GEB, gum elastic bougie

GH, general health

GH, growth hormone

HABR, hepatic artery buffer response

HES, hydroxyethyl starch

HFO, high frequency oscillation

HMEF, heat moisture exchange filter

HPV, hypoxis pulmonary vasoconstriction

HR, heart rate

HWH, heated wire humidifiers

ICAM-1, intracellular adhesion molecules

ICD, implantable cardioverter defibrillator

ICF, intracellular fluids

ICG, indocyanine-green

ICNARC, intensive care national audit & research centre

ICP, intracranial pressure

ICU, intensive care unit

IHD, intermittent haemodialysis

IL, interleukin

ILCOR, International Liaison Committee on Resuscitation

IP, ischaemic preconditioning

IPPV, intermittent positive pressure ventilation

ITBV, intra thoracic blood volume

LMA, laryngeal mask airway

LOS, length of stay

LPS, lipopolysaccharides

LWBS, Leaving Without Being Seen

MAC, minimum alveolar concentration

MAP, mean arterial pressure

MET, medical emergency team

MH, mental health

MN, Microsoft Netmeeting

MOD, multiple organ dysfunction

MOF, multiple organ failure

MOPS, Maintenance of Professional Standards

MR, muscle relaxant

MRI, magnetic resonance imaging

MRSA, methicillin-resistant Staphylococcus aureus

NAP, nematode anticoagulant protein

NIPSV, non invasive pressure support ventilation

NIV, non invasive ventilation

NMBA, neuro-muscular blocking agents

NMBD, neuromuscular blocking drugs

NMDA, N-methyl-D-aspartate

NMJ, neuromuscular junction

NMT, neuromuscular transmission

NP, nosocomial pneumonia

NSAID, non-steroidal anti-inflammatory drugs

OLV, one-lung ventilation

OP, opioid peptide

OPALS, Ontario prehospital advanced life support

OPC, overall performance category

ORM, out-of-range measurements

OSAS, obstructive sleep apnoea syndrome

OSCE, objective structured clinical examination

PAC, pulmonary artery catheter

PACU, post anaesthesia care unit

PAD, public access defibrillation

PAF, platelet-activating factor

PAOP, pulmonary artery occlusion pressure

PART, patient-at-risk team

PBP, penicillin-binding protein

PCCO, pulse contour for continuous cardiac output

PCS, patient controlled sedation

PCT, procalcitonin

PDD, pulse dye-densitometry

PDPH, post-dural puncture headache

PEA, preemptive analgesia

PEEP, positive end expiratory pressure

PF, physical function

PHC, permissive hypercapnia

PLV, partial liquid ventilation

PMI, perioperative myocardial infarction

PMS, patient monitored sedation

PONV, post-operative nausea and vomiting

POPC, post operative pulmonary complication

PORC, post operative residual curarisation

PPF, plasma protein fraction

PTC, post-tetanic count

PVR, pulmonary vascular resistance

Q/D, quinupristin/dalfopristin

QAHCS, quality in Australian Health Care Study

QALY, quality-adjusted life years

QOL, quality of life

RACP, Royal Australasian College of Physicians

RAMP, receptor activity modifying protein

RE, role emotional

RIA, radioimmunoassay

RP, physical role

RRT, renal replacement therapy

RW, relative weight

SA, spinal anaesthesia

SaO_2, arterial oxygen saturation

SAPS, simple acute physiological score

$SatO_2$, oxygen saturation

SCARRF, severe combined acute respiratory and renal failure

SDD, selective decontamination of digestive tract

SE, status epilecticus

SEF, spectral edge frequency

SF, social function

SIP, sickness impact profile

SIRS, systemic inflammatory response syndrome

SLT, single lumen tube

SQOL, Sydney quality of life

SSSI, skin and skin structure infection

ST, single twitch

SUDEP, sudden unexplained death in epilepsy

TBW, total body water

TCI, target controlled infusion

TEE, transesophageal echocardiography

TEN, total enteral nutrition

TFPI, tissue factor pathway inhibitor

TIVA, total intravenous anaesthesia

TL, Trachlight

TLC, total lung capacity

TLV, two-lung ventilation

TNF, tumour necrosis factor

TNS, tetanic nerve stimulation

TOF, train-of-four
TPN, total parenteral nutrition
TQM, total quality management
TXB_2, thromboxane
V/Q, ventilation/perfusion
VAP, ventilator-associated pneumonia
VAS, visual analogic score
VAT, video assisted thoracoscopy
VF, ventricular fibrillation
VILI, ventilator induced lung injury
VRE, vancomycin-resistant enterococci
VT, ventricular tachycardia
VT, vitality
WPW, Wolff-Parkinson-White syndrome

ANAESTHESIA AND CRITICAL CARE: TECHNOLOGY AND STANDARDS OF CARE

Anaesthesia and Critical Care: Technology and Standards of Care

C. Parsloe

Life is short, the Art is long,
opportunity fleeting, experience
delusive, judgement difficult
Hippocrates

Anaesthesia was 100 years old when I started my residency in 1946 with Ralph Waters at the University of Wisconsin General Hospital in Madison, Wisconsin. Critical care did not exist as yet. The closest to it was the so-called stir-up regimen used in Madison for postoperative and comatose patients in attempts to prevent pulmonary complications by positional changes, incentivating breathing and promoting coughing. Technology was elementary. Standards of care were non-existing. Anaesthesia machines were built with mechanical devices and needed no electricity. No safety devices were incorporated in the machines; in fact, they had not been invented as yet. The water flowmeters measured oxygen, nitrous oxide, cyclopropane and in some machines, atavistically, carbon dioxide. The system used was carbon dioxide absorption by means of to-and-fro soda lime canisters. No ventilators existed; the hand carried out the functions of assisting or controlling ventilation. A number of small towels were kept handy in the anaesthesia machine to cope with the expected vomiting during recovery. No monitors as we understand them today existed. Nevertheless, the patient's pulse was continuously palpated and the blood pressure was faithfully measured by manual sphygmomanometry every 5 minutes. A manual anaesthesia chart was meticulously kept with the recording of heart rate and blood pressure and of usual events during anaesthesia. Metal oropharyngeal airways were commonly used but endotracheal intubation required an indication. The beginner did not use curare. In fact it was seldom used at all. Anaesthesia was very much of an art and relaxation for abdominal operations was obtained by means of deep anaesthesia. Therefore, anaesthesia signs as developed by Guedel and further by Gillespie were conscientiously observed. Essentially, that was modern anaesthesia in the late 1940s with rigorous maintenance of airway patency and normal ventilation. The cornerstones of modern anaesthesia were simple: airway patency, normal ventilation, absorption of the expired carbon dioxide and clinical signs of anaesthesia. The commonly used agent was cyclopropane, which had been introduced in Madison by Ralph Waters in 1933. The to-and-fro absorption method had also been introduced into clinical anaesthesia by Waters in 1923. Cyclopropane and the absorption system seemed to have been made one for the other, a perfect marriage. Ether was the second best agent. Most children received anaesthesia with the sequence of ethyl chloride induction to ether maintenance by open mask. Thereafter, pharyngeal insufflation with an "ether hook" was preferred for tonsillectomies with the child's head in the Rose position for drainage of blood and secretions out of the pharynx [1].

Prior to that, during my last year at medical school in 1943 and immediately after, I had occasion to administer anaesthesia with the Ombrédanne inhaler, or mask as it was generally called. Brazilian medicine and surgery were at the time very much under French influence. In fact, the Ombrédanne mask was ubiquitously used all over Latin America until practically 1945. The volatile liquid employed was a mixture of ether, chloroform and ethyl chloride, called balsoform, with added gomenol for supposed tracheal bronchial mucosa protection. That convenient, portable inhaler was far from a physiological way to administer general anaesthesia. There was no provision for carbon dioxide removal or for oxygen administration. Operations had to be of short duration or else the patient suffered progressive asphyxia. The only remedy was the periodical removal of the mask from the patient's face to allow for a few breaths of air. That was performed when incipient or frank cyanosis appeared. Under such circumstances, all that the patient received was a few breaths of air since no oxygen cylinders were available in the operating rooms. Such air breathing for alleviation of cyanosis could not be maintained for long since the patient was at the same time emerging from the plane of anaesthesia. Many times a difficult choice had to be made between the maintenance of anaesthesia with cyanosis and alleviation of cyanosis with loss of anaesthesia. Surgeons would naturally complain but there was nothing that could be done. Operative conditions were far from perfect since the accumulation of carbon dioxide caused forced diaphragmatic breathing with consequent poor abdominal relaxation. The surgeons made a distinction between abdominal relaxation and abdominal silence. The combination of both would be the ideal condition sought for but rarely, if ever, achieved. In desperation the surgeon called for full vaporization achieved by turning the inhaler knob to its highest mark, 8. This practically closed the small air intake aperture and caused full rebreathing of expired gases over the vaporizing chamber containing felt pieces imbibed with the liquid anaesthetic agent. Obviously, such a situation could not be maintained for any length of time. That was why the surgeons of the period had to be fast and worked by the clock. Their patients would not tolerate long operations on account of the disturbed respiratory physiology caused by the unphysiological inhaler. No oxygen cylinders, no suction pumps, no laryngoscopes or tracheal tubes were available [1].

No wonder that Dupuy de Frenelle stated that "Anaesthesia is that part of Surgery farthest removed from perfection" [L'anesthésie est le temps de l'acte opératoire qui est encore le plus éloigné de la perfection] [2].

Before being allowed to participate in the surgical team every young surgeon had to climb a ladder starting with the most distasteful steps: dressing wounds and giving anaesthesia. Wounds were practically universally infected and dressing required laborious time under unpleasant odours. Anaesthesia was *terra incognita*, since no one really knew anything about it. In fact, in his widely read textbook of surgery, Kirschner had strict rules for the administration of anaesthesia [3]. The anaesthetizer had to have an "anaesthesia tray" available prior to commencing anaesthesia. It contained an open mask, a bottle of ether, gauze and forceps to clean pharyngeal secretions, and several ampoules of "stimulating" drugs to combat the expected accidents during anaesthesia. He also mentioned the duties of the anesthetizer as emptying the patient's bladder before anaesthesia and passing a rectal tube and emptying the stomach before upper abdominal operations. Not a word on anaesthesia care proper since it simply was unexistent. Stertorous breathing was a "sign" of anaesthesia and not of respiratory obstruction. The worst accidents were cessation of breathing or of circulation, known respectively as "blue" and "white" syncope. Few, if any, patients recovered from those feared accidents. Surgery had to be stopped and the surgeon and his assistant performed artificial respiration by alternatively elevating the arms and compressing the chest of the patient, a manoeuvre that seemed always futile. The tongue was grasped with a pronged forceps and pulled out of the pharynx, usually with repeated movements, called the Laborde manoeuvre, which supposedly would re-start breathing. Needless to say that the efforts usually proved quite useless and that the patients died on the operating table. *In extremis*, a canvas bag containing a few litres of carbogen, a mixture of 95% oxygen and 5% carbon dioxide, was offered to the moribund or already dead patient as the ultimate treatment. This remedy was directly taken from Yandell Henderson's teaching of acapnia as the cause of anaesthetic problems and of shock. His theory took a long time to be discredited in spite of Alvaro and Miguel Osorio de Almeida, two Brasilian physiologists, having proved in 1913 that the cause of "shock" in Henderson's hyperventilated dogs was not acapnia but hypothermia caused by forceful cold air breathing. They had repeated Henderson's experiments, hyperventilating dogs with warm and humid air in Rio de Janeiro without any evidence of shock [4]. The original publication in a French journal was not read at the time. It took another article in English, published in the *Journal of the American Medical Association* in 1918 to be read and understood, among others, by Ralph Waters who then could introduce carbon dioxide absorption instead of its rebreathing as preached by Henderson and universally practised.

It could be said that there were 4 essential components of anaesthesia at the time: one patient, one anaesthetizer, usually a young aspiring surgeon to be, a catholic sister of charity or just about anyone available, one piece of equipment, either an open mask or the Ombrédanne inhaler, and one agent, ether or balsoform. Eventually, several items were added to the basic 4 but not a single one could be subtracted or else anaesthesia could not be established.

The most difficult cases were patients with intestinal obstruction arriving for operation at the terminal stages with distended abdomen, fecaloid vomitus and intense electrolyte disturbances. Patients were almost moribund before they consented to go to the hospital. There were no supportive measures. The only preventive measure against fatal vomiting at induction was the Fouchet gastric tube, a long, large diameter rubber tube, which was introduced prior to anaesthesia for gastric emptying. It was not uncommon for such patients to vomit during induction with a fatal outcome. No laryngoscopes, no endotracheal tubes and no means for positive pressure ventilation by bag and mask were available. Many times the heaving diaphragm and tight abdominal muscles prevented the abdominal closure and the surgeon resorted to wire sutures through the whole abdominal wall.

AM Dogliotti's book, "Textbook of Anesthesia-Narcosis, Local, Regional and Spinal Anesthesia" was translated into Portuguese in 1943 [5]. It proved an essential tool for learning *inter alia* the resistance test for epidural needle placement. The usual method for epidural space identification had been the hanging drop sign of Gutierrez, an Argentinian surgeon who developed epidural anaesthesia in Buenos Aires since the 1930s. Most surgeons in Brazil performed their own epidurals and proceeded to operate when anaesthesia was established. Procaine by itself or mixed with tetracaine were the usual agents. The surgeons usually worked without gloves, but after scrubbing their hands in preparation for surgery, administered epidural or spinal anaesthesia. They then proceeded to operate without the help of any anaesthesia assistant. No intravenous solutions or oxygen administration were employed. "Stimulant" drugs were mainly sparteine, digitalis, camphorated oil, cardiazol, cardiazol-ephedrine, coramine, caffeine and lobeline.

Hospitals had a distinct unpleasant odour, called the "hospital smell", which was due to a combination of ether vapour and pus. Wound infection was the natural postoperative course and required many days or weeks of hospitalization. The antibiotic era had not been invented. I witnessed the first oxygen tents installed at the emergency hospital in Rio de Janeiro in 1944. They were acquired at the request of the cardiologists. Treatment of cardiac failure and of hypertension in those days was Franciscan in comparison to the present available wide diversity of medication.

I started using anaesthesia machines in Madison. They were extremely simple with water flowmeters and a common gas outlet serving a to-and-fro carbon dioxide absorber. The usual technique was cyclopropane induction and maintenance with occasional added ether. Tracheal intubation was far from routine and most gastrectomies and cholecystectomies were anaesthetised by facemask over the nasogastric tube and the absorber balanced over a pillow. The left hand of the anaesthesiologist secured the mask over the patient's face with a finger on the facial pulse while the others supported the chin. The right hand had to perform multiple functions such as adjusting the flowmeter knobs as necessary, measuring blood pressure every 5 minutes and writing the anaesthesia record meticulously. An exercise in dexterity. The depth of anaesthesia was judged purely on clinical signs and, when required, ventilation was manually controlled. A fine distinction was made between assisted and controlled ventilation. No ventilators were ever used. Laryngoscopy was by means of straight blades since Macintosh's curved blade was still in the future. Intubations were performed in deep levels of anaesthesia without the use of muscle relaxants. Cyclopropane induction offered the possibility of tracheal intubation within a couple of minutes, a feat unattainable with any other inhalation agent. Curare was barely 4 years old and succinylcholine had not been synthesised. Occasionally, thiopental induction was preferred. Neurosurgical patients might be given rectal averting. Tonsillectomies, hare-lips and cleft palates were anaesthetised with an ethyl chloride-ether sequence by open mask followed by pharyngeal insufflation. Thyroidectomies were not necessarily intubated. Oropharyngeal airways were the usual means for avoiding and correcting upper airway obstruction.

Monitors as we know them today did not exist. Anaesthesia was controlled by clinical signs with close observation of the respiration as an indication of both depth of anaesthesia and adequate respiratory exchange. The eyes were trained to judge the synchronous or asynchronous movements of chest and abdomen in order to diagnose obstruction or depression of breathing. The electronic age had not been invented. In Madison, electrocardiographic monitoring was used only for clinical research on special anaesthesia study cases. Central venous lines and arterial lines were unheard of. Spinal anaesthesia was used especially in older urology patients but epidural anaesthesia was not. Trans-sacral block was used occasionally.

Lucien Morris was a resident somewhat my senior with whom I learned the fundamentals, including disassembling and reassembling a Foregger anaesthesia machine. We keep a long lasting friendship. He developed the "copper kettle" vaporizer for precision dosing of chloroform. Waters wanted to find out if this abandoned agent would prove worthwhile when administered with ample oxygen, carbon dioxide removal and normal ventilation. The study revealed that it was not kind to the liver although its induction and maintenance characteristics were good. Therefore, the "kettle" turned out to be used with ether.

I used all available anaesthetic agents like ether, chloroform, ethyl chloride, vinyl ether, ethylene, trichloroethylene, fluroxene, cyclopropane and nitrous oxide, before the modern era of halogenated volatile agents started in 1954. Halothane in fact destroyed the closed system and started the 5 l/min FGF fad. The first calibrated vaporizer, the Fluotec Mark 2, required a 5 l/min FGF for a constant vapour concentration output. Gone were the days of 300 ml or so of oxygen and a few millilitres of cyclopropane per minute. Electrocautery further caused the demise of cyclopropane to prevent explosions.

The closed system, or more appropriately these days, the low flow technique, is being resurrected for reasons of ecology and cost. Its use should be encouraged. Modern electronic anaesthesia machines offer such possibility without any difficulty.

Patients came to the operating room directly from their hospital rooms and returned to them after the operation. Holding or recovery areas, the modern post-anaesthesia care units, did not exist, nor did intensive care units. Those developments had to wait until Eric Nilsson from Lund, who had also been a fellow resident in Madison and a friend, changed the treatment of barbiturate coma during a sabbatical in Copenhagen by applying anaesthesia principles for the maintenance of circulation, respiration and diuresis while abandoning all "stimulant" drug treatments [6]. That experience, coupled a little later with the Copenhagen polio epidemic of 1952, marked the beginning of intensive care. The Danish colleagues having few respirators were able to keep patients alive by means of manually controlled ventilation using a to-and-fro canister in similar fashion as for anaesthesia. Teams of medical students took turns, over 24 hours, in compressing the rebreathing bags. Until then, bulbar polio patients had to be placed in expensive "iron-lungs", not widely available. The lessons learned during the early 1950s gave origin to respiratory units and subsequently to special areas with a high nursing/patient ratio. Critical care had its humble start but never ceased to improve in the intervening 40 years to the point it has now reached in terms of patient care and survival. Acid-base and pH measurements and the CO_2 electrode had their incipient start at that time. Soon after, the O_2 electrode changed the practice of following the respiratory status of patients. The names of Astrup, Sigaard-Andersen and Severinghaus became daily parts of clinical care examination, interpretation of laboratory results and prescribing. Gone were the days of the alkaline reserve measurement. Intensive care units were firmly established. Ventilators for prolonged use, tracheostomy and long-term tracheal intubation became almost synonymous with critical care medicine. A change in the indications for patient admission to intensive care was made and it became a place for recovery rather than a waiting area for the ultimate demise of patients. A whole new field of medicine and nursing started with specific knowledge, concepts, equipment and medication.

During 1949, working at the Charity Hospital in Santos, Brazil, I met my first Fallot's emaciated and cyanotic children. I had no access to literature concerning Blalock operations and anaesthesia techniques. I expected that they would not survive the ordeal. However, much to my surprise, the basic principles of airway control and ventilation maintenance with cyclopropane by means of small to-and-fro canisters worked like magic. I had a small rotameter capable of measuring fine flows of oxygen and cyclopropane for the closed system used. A series of over 20 small children with patent ductus, coartaction of the aorta and tetralogy of Fallot were successfully anaesthetised and operated upon during the next 3 years. The only monitoring consisted of clinical signs with occasional stethoscope and blood pressure measurement. The children were taken back to their rooms and kept in oxygen tents. Their guardian angels were alert and protected them. Experience was nil, judgement extremely difficult, but youth has sustaining powers. Opportunity was successfully grasped [4].

In March 1952, I returned to Madison for another almost 3-year stay. Ralph Waters had retired and Sid Orth had become chairman of the Anesthesia Department. There I was able to use in patients a Millikan ear oxymeter manufactured in Rochester, Minnesota. Finding out the saturation fall occurring during periods of respiratory obstruction in tonsillectomies without visible cyanosis was, to say the least, enlightening. The earpiece required calibration by pressurizing a thin rubber membrane. More than one membrane ruptured and required tedious replacement. Many an ear was burned since the earpiece required heating as well. When pulse oxymeters became available the lessons already learned took on new life and meaning with a great deal of operational simplicity.

During this period I visited James Elam in Saint Louis, Missouri, who was working with the early Liston Becker capnograph. His studies clarified the insidious respiratory acidosis occurring during anaesthesia with the small canisters used in the first circle filters with a capacity for only 350 g soda lime. From his studies Elam designed the first large capacity double canisters which became used thereafter in all anaesthesia machines.

The era of respiratory acidosis was fruitful in many lessons. The to-and-fro absorption system gave way to circle systems with large absorbers, which became universally employed. The water flowmeters disappeared and gave way to rotameters. In turn, these are now being replaced by electronic gas flow measurements. It seems that there is no getting back to simple mechanical anaesthesia equipment. The electronic age changed both anaesthesia and critical care. However, if one looks at the less developed areas of the world, there is as yet no place for electricity-dependent equipment. A solid argument can be raised for the use of local and regional blocks for practically all operations capable of being performed in those underprivileged areas. To insist on general anaesthesia and all its problems in noneducated hands is a call for peril. It is also a disservice to accept that general anaesthesia should be administered by non-medical personnel under less than ideal circumstances. At best it will be precarious and at worst it will abort the development of physician-administered anaesthesia.

Upon returning to Brazil in 1954 I found that Dr. Kentaro Takaoka, a Brazilian anaesthesiologist, had developed a simple portable oxygen-driven respirator. He followed it with a simple, portable, compact, universal vaporiser for ether or halothane at the time. In fact the universal vaporizer accepts any volatile liquid agent, except desflurane. That simple vaporiser-respirator combination was used in millions of patients anaesthetised with controlled respiration. It is still being used. As an example of its versatility and usefulness, it was the only anaesthesia equipment used for the first heart transplant in São Paulo over 30 years ago. Thiopental induction, Flaxedil (gallamine), intubation and halothane with controlled respiration became the usual technique in Brazil and in many countries in Latin America.

During the early 1970s the first area for postoperative recovery was installed at the Samaritano Hospital in São Paulo. It had room for 3 small transfer beds with available oxygen. It displaced the nurse's discrete coffee area. Soon after, the first properly designed anaesthesia recovery area was carved out of the space adjoining one of the operating rooms. The intensive care unit, however, was built *de novo*. It grew out of the necessity for postoperative care of the increasing numbers of cardiac operations. It soon became a routine to send patients in critical condition to the special unit. It would be an understatement to say that it proved to be a definite improvement over what we had occasionally to do practising primitive intensive care in the patient's room over 24 hours.

Witnessing the definition of standards of care and of practice parameters and the ever-innovative technological developments occurring during the 1980s onwards was a most productive learning experience. Nevertheless, in Brazil at least, by and large anaesthesiologists lost control of the critical care areas for reasons of manpower shortage.

The Brazilian Society of Anaesthesiology was founded in 1948 with 33 original members. Over the years it grew to about 7000 specialists making it today, in fact, the second largest society within the World Federation of Societies of Anaesthesiologists. From the beginning there was a definite need to increase the number of anaesthesiologists to cope with an ever growing population. For this reason the first training period was only one year. After that period, the physician had to pass an examination conducted by a special committee of the Brazilian Society of Anaesthesiology before he could be considered a specialist. At the moment the training period is 2 years with an optional third one and it is expected that soon it will be a mandatory 3 years. Meanwhile all major cities and most smaller cities in the country have been adequately covered by anaesthesiologists. Precedence had to be given to quantity before improved quality was addressed. In this context it was reassuring that in those early days the body of knowledge required for anaesthesia was considerably less than at present. Pharmacology was distinctly restricted to a few drugs, pharmacokinetics had not been developed, all general anaesthesia was by inhalation and the types of operations performed were not as challenging as today's.

Anaesthesia is considered a medical speciality in Brazil and can only be administered by physicians. Brazil is a very large country with areas of dissimilar socio-economic conditions and consequent diverse levels of development and health care availability. During its earlier years the Brazilian Society of Anaesthesiology had to generate sufficient numbers of specialists to cope with the large demand. That need was successfully fulfilled.

The *Brazilian Journal of Anaesthesiology* was started in 1950 and the yearly Brazilian Congresses of Anaesthesiology in 1954. In 1964 the Brazilian Society of Anaesthesiology organised the 3rd World Congress of Anaesthesiologists in São Paulo. There are now 80 training centres supervised by the Brazilian Society of Anaesthesiology with a yearly output of about 300 new specialists.

The treatment of postoperative pain was traditionally in the hands of surgeons. Again for lack of sufficient manpower, as well as for lack of proper emphasis, anaesthesiologists were late in paying the necessary attention to this important part of the patient's operative course. More and more anaesthesiologists are now correcting that early lack of foresight, for the benefit of increasing numbers of patients.

When the American Society of Anaesthesiologists (ASA) adopted its Standards of Monitoring, a trend was initiated and followed by most national societies of anaesthesiology. The World Federation of Societies of Anaesthesiologists has developed a set of international standards [7]. These well-defined standards are necessarily geared to inherent overall economical development, which mandates the available technology. It is difficult for less developed countries to imitate the comprehensive listing of monitors accepted by the ASA. This discrepancy in development is at the root of different descriptions of basic monitoring standards, or minimum required monitoring, to satisfy safety and good outcomes. Few countries are uniformly developed and they still exhibit islands of inequality. It is difficult to adopt a set of standards for the whole country, and even more difficult to adopt a rigid set of world-wide standards. Such a chimera will have to wait for a symmetrical world-wide development, something, which at present remains a bigger chimera. It is unrealistic to believe in unilaterally raising anaesthesia standards in the face of less than optimal overall national development. Basic human needs must be provided before anaesthesia and critical care become relevant. Populations lacking sanitation, sewage disposal, water supply, proper food and housing, education and job opportunities, faced with endemic and epidemic diseases will not consider anaesthesia and critical care as top priorities. They are right. First priority should be given to the undernourished and diseased person, not to technological paraphernalia surrounding him and the physician.

Economic development, social inclusion in the benefits of civilisation and politics are intertwined and require an ethical basis in order to offer full benefits to *Homo sapiens*. The importance of ethics has been recognised by the selection of Amartya Sen for the Nobel Prize in Economy [8]. Unfortunately, at the beginning of the new century and millennium, the world continues to be asymmetrically divided. Billions of human beings are still excluded from the benefits of adequate living conditions which are afforded to only a few millions, in some instances with an obscene over-abundance. Approximately three-fourths of the 6 billion human beings on this planet lack adequate living conditions and about one-fourth of them actually live under sub-human conditions. Potentially eradicable epidemics and endemics still abound in far too many areas of the planet. Such asymmetry with dire infra-human living conditions represents a potential bomb with more explosive force than the atomic weapon. Technology could but has not yet solved this unacceptable situation. In theory it should diminish the gap between the rich and the poor but in practice it seems to be increasing it. Technology devoid of any humanitarian counterpart produces negative effects [9].

In the quest for disseminating the ultimate technological advances to all countries some key questions must be answered before inappropriate decisions are made: Is technology needed? Is it affordable? What kind is better? How fast can it be absorbed? How should it be introduced? Can it be retained? Is there a critical mass of trained personnel and supportive infrastructure? Does the budget allow for its purchase and maintenance? The last two questions constitute a fundamental binomium without which technology cannot survive. The introduction of technology must be congruous with the overall level of existing development. It must be a consistent effort and certainly not a haphazard intermittent collage. We should seriously consider that "high tech" may have no place at all in areas without sufficient infrastructure. In fact, a sociological definition of under development could be the lack of supportive infrastructure. Under many circumstances "low tech" is the appropriate answer. Even "no tech" is far superior to "Wrong Tech". A technology-dependent anaesthesiologist is a veritable anathema in less developed areas [10-12].

Nevertheless, if we look at quality of care in anaesthesia and in hospitals in general we may find that it is not necessarily tied to technological level of development. No matter how much desired, any technology can only be applied if proper personnel and sufficient budget can maintain it. The inexistence of either or both of those preconditions destroys any ambitious motivation to follow the desired higher standards.

Dedicated physicians need little or no technological support in order to offer comfort and psychological support to their patients. Empathy is considerably better from the patient's point of view than a number of non-communicating equipment. Physicians aim to cure whenever possible, but always to offer comfort. In our attempts to use a multitude of impersonal equipment, usually called simplistically high tech, we many times lose sight of the unqualified need to listen to patients, to believe in their clinical histories and to give them sufficient time in our mutual contact. How often an extra 5 minutes of calm and reassuring conversation will do away with the need for another pill to relieve anxiety. How often patients relate an increase in pain only as a reflection of their uncertainty and anxiety over the possible outcome of their disease. How often we neglect the absolute need to inform the patient of whatever we are doing to them in order to elicit their appropriate co-operation. Medicine is not a one-way road to be travelled by a single observer. We need to travel it jointly with the patient who should be aware of and understand the curves and the hills, which may lie ahead, on the road. Anaesthesia and operation sit at a crucial time in most patients' lives. It is unrealistic to expect a smooth induction and recovery if the patient does not feel as a participant of the many pre-, peri- and postanaesthetic events which we impose on them. The more they know, the more they can cooperate. It is not a time for gentle lies. The case of children is paramount. In this particular age group it is the parents that need to be informed in order to become our allies in allaying fear risen out of ignorance and parental separation. The more the family is well structured, the less preanaesthetic medication is needed. The more the anaesthesiologist dedicates sufficient time to understand the family realm, the more the child will trust him. There simply is no medication or equipment that will substitute for loving parents and reassuring anaesthesiologists. Regrettably, those basic tenets are not always followed. Quoting Freeman

Dyson: "The thing the patient needs the most, and the thing hardest to find, is personal attention" [13].

In short, we should consider that high tech does not necessarily equate with high quality of medical care. Vice versa, low tech does not necessarily imply low quality of medical care. It is the physician, well learned and with an ethical poise and sympathetical attitude, that makes the difference. Good available equipment is strictly maintenance-dependent. The physician, in turn, needs constant and continuous education in order to keep abreast of innumerable developments. The task is Herculean but absolutely required. So far, it has proven expensive and time consuming. Time which in most instances is taken away from patient care. Hopefully, the electronic age with its information revolution promise will offer the opportunity for an ever more inclusion in the world of knowledge. And, with it, an ever increasing social inclusion in the benefits of civilisation. The means to achieve better symmetrical development exist. It is up to politicians to rise to the importance of their legislative positions and provide the necessary alleviation from sub-human living conditions wherever they exist. That should not remain a dream. As the Nobel Prize winner in Medicine, Peter Medawar, said: Politics is the art of the possible, research is the art of the soluble [14].

Genomics, proteinomics and nanotechnology are opening immense new areas for research and improvement for all mankind. What will become of their Promethean promises? It should not be an utopian desire to believe that ultimately the world asymmetry will disappear. Humanism and technology, which have been coming steadily apart over the centuries, should join hands anew [9] to achieve with the possible speed the ultimate *desideratum*, for all mankind, of *mens sana in corpore sano*. Then, and only then, we can feel proud of the outstanding innovations and the almost miraculous decrease in morbidity and mortality that our body of knowledge, technology and standards of care have achieved in anaesthesia and critical care over the past several decades.

Technology per se is nihilistic and certainly not thaumaturgic. It seems to show a tendency towards destructiveness. It can only be properly used with an ethical counterpart. Let us not forget that important *sine qua non* condition. Ethics should be a major consideration for all economic, social and technological development. Instead, profit and ideology seem to be the dominant factors. Medical care, *lato sensu*, anaesthesia and critical care, *strictu senso*, cannot improve unless the overall level of development allows for alleviation of poverty, education of all human beings and adequate living standards. The sad aspect of this unacceptable asymmetry is that the existing levels of wealth and knowledge in the world are sufficient to eradicate misery. Witness the extraordinary sums spent the world over for military reasons. Ironically, it seems that the poorer the country the higher its military budget becomes. The acquisition of literacy and of knowledge, not to mention of wisdom, is not only money- but time-dependent.

Living conditions for vast numbers of human beings have not changed as much as desired over the centuries. The French moralist La Bruyére wrote in 1688, "Il y a une espèce de honte d'être heureux à la vue de certaines misères" [15, 16]. More recently, in 1983, the Nobel Prize winner in Medicine, Pierre Changeux, stated: "Qu'a-t-il donc dans la tête cette *Homo* qui s'attribue sans vergogne l'épithète *sapiens*?" [17]. Or, as Freeman Dyson questioned in 1999: "I am looking for ways in which technology may contribute to social justice, to the alleviation of differences between rich and poor, to the preservation of the earth" [13]. Over this rather pessimistic panorama, technology has offered the means for improvement. It is up to us to make proper use of the available tools to the betterment of living conditions for those vast numbers of fellow human beings still excluded from the benesses of available technology.

Anaesthesia is now 154 years old. The first generation of anaesthesiologists gradually grasped general and regional anaesthesia from the hands of the surgeons and made it a speciality on its own right. Tied to the operating room for most of that time, anaesthesiologists have branched during the past few decades into other hospital areas of increasing importance such as critical care and more recently are assuming responsibility for the treatment of pain. It is an understatement to say that the changes have been immense. The future holds unknown advances. No matter what new developments lie in the horizon we should firmly continue to seek improvements in unison with technology and standards of care.

References

1. Parsloe CP (1999) The lifelong apprenticeship of an anesthesiologist. In: Careers in anesthesiology. Wood Library Museum of Anesthesiology
2. Dupuy de Frenelle. In: Módena V. Rachianestesia. 1932, Sociedade Impressora Paulista
3. Kirschner M (1940) Tratado de Técnica Operatoria General y Especial, 2nd edn. Editorial Labor
4. Parsloe CP (1989) The contribution of two Brazilian physiologists to the introduction of carbon dioxide absorption into clinical anesthesia. An acknowledgement by Ralph M. Waters. The History of Anaesthesia. Edited by Richard S. Atkinson and Thomas B. Boulton. Proceedings, Second International Symposium on the History of Anesthesia. Royal Society of Medicine Services. International Congress and Symposium Series Number 134
5. Dogliotti AM (1943) Tratado de Anestesia-Narcose, Anestesia Local, Regional e Espinhal. Editora Scientifica, Rio
6. Nilsson E (1951) On treatment of barbiturate poisoning. A modified clinical aspect. Acta Med Scand [Suppl]139
7. International Standards for a Safe Practice of Anaesthesia (Adopted by the World Federation of Societies of Anaesthesiologists Parsloe C) (1994) The introduction of technology in the Third World: Problems and Proposals. J Clin Monit 10(3):147-152
8. Sen A (1998) On ethics and economics. Cambridge University, Cambridge
9. Dertouzos M (1997) What will be. Harper Edge
10. Parsloe C (1994) The introduction of technology in the Third World: Problems and proposals. J Clin Monit 10(3):147-152

11. Parsloe C (2000) Anesthesia technology in our asymmetrical World. Proceedings 12th World Congress of Anaesthesiologists
12. Parsloe C (2000) Developing countries. Workstations, safety and device standards. Proceedings 12th World Congress of Anaesthesiologists
13. Dyson FJ (1999) The Sun, the genome and the Internet. Tools of Scientific Revolution. Oxford University, Oxford
14. Medawar P (1967) The art of the soluble. Oxford University, Oxford
15. La Bruyère J de (1978) Les caractéres ou les moeurs de ce siècle, 1688. In: Encyclopaedia Brittanica, 15th edn. Micropaedia V:971
16. La Bruyère J de (1985) Apud Ronai P. Dicionário universal de citações, 2nd edn Editora Nova Fronteira, Rio de Janeiro
17. Changeux JP (1983) L'homme neuronal. Librairie Arthème Fayard, Paris

CARDIOVASCULAR

Experimental Models in Hemodilution

D.T. FANTONI, D.A. OTSUKI, J.O.C. AULER JR

Despite the fact that hemodilution has been used in man for more than 4 decades, there are still many controversies related to the selection of the target hematocrit, kind of fluid to maintain normovolemia, anesthetics, and the hemodynamic responses verified in clinical studies. For these reasons, many experimental studies have been conducted in order to elucidate these factors. In this chapter we have reviewed some of these topics and the different experimental models employed and their results.

Clinical considerations

Hemodilution was introduced in the 1960s in order to avoid or reduce homologous blood transfusion requirements in patients submitted to major surgical procedures, especially cardiovascular, orthopedics, and tumor resection [1]. At that time, the principal reason was to decrease the risks of transmission of infectious diseases, especially virus transmission, and also to lessen the need for blood packs, as at the time the blood supply was limited [2]. Other benefits from hemodilution techniques have since become evident, such as the reduction of alloimmunization to blood components that could present problems in future transfusions especially for young people [2, 3], hemolytic reactions, biochemical changes that stored blood can cause, loss of coagulation factors, platelets, and 2,3-diphosphoglycerate, as well as immunosuppression with enhanced cancer recurrence [4]. Despite the fact that blood bank products are becoming much safer than ever before, the emergence of the immunodeficiency virus has had a profound impact on transfusion policy, causing a renewed interest in techniques for limiting homologous blood use.

Hemodilution considerations

Hemodilution involves the removal of one or more aliquots of whole blood from a patient, while replacing the blood withdrawn with either a colloid or a crystalloid to maintain normovolemia. After the period of major blood loss has ceased, the blood of the patient is re-transfused [5].

Hemodilution, despite its infrequent use, is often the best choice for the patient. Most of the time predonation and intraoperative salvage is employed routinely to decrease the needs for homologous blood. These two techniques have disadvantages because of preoperative preparation and the cost that can be as high as US$ 197.00/unit (predonation) and US$ 570.00/unit (intraoperative salvage) [6].

Hemodilution has the advantage of being inexpensive (US$ 9.00/unit) and of reducing red blood cell losses during surgery, since the lost blood is diluted. If additional blood is required during the perioperative period, the requirement for homologous transfusion is less in patients submitted to hemodilution [5-9].

Choice of patients

Hemodilution presents important hemodynamic repercussions. Thus, to be a safe technique selection of patients must follow some indication and exclusion criteria. The kind of surgery is the first point to be considered. Estimated perioperative blood loss has to be less than 30% of blood volume. Anemia and hemoglobin concentration < 12 g/dl, hepatic or renal disease, restrictive or obstructive lung disease, a pre-existing coagulation disorder, and infections are all contraindications for elective hemodilution. Patients for hemodilution must have a negative history of cardiac disease and normal cardiac function evaluated by clinical and laboratory assessments [4].

The rabbit, dog, and pig have mostly used for experimental studies. Nevertheless, it is important to bear in mind that many factors can alter the responses to hemodilution, which makes the comparison of different studies extremely difficult. Among these factors we can list the species, the anesthetic regimen, the hematocrit, and protocols of hemodilution, as well as the methods for determining regional organ blood flows (electromagnetic flow probes versus microspheres versus bromsulphalein versus reservoir).

When considering the different designs to study hemodilution it is very important to highlight the compensatory mechanisms. During blood removal, crystalloid or colloids are administered to maintain normovolemia, promoting a decrease in hematocrit and hemoglobin, which is accompanied by important physiological adaptations. Among the various changes that occur during hemodilution, the decrease in blood viscosity is extremely important [2]. Among the factors that explain decrease in systemic vascular resistance [10] is the release of nitric oxide. The decrease in blood viscosity causes changes in blood flow of the venous bed, causing a significant increase in venous return and preload and also of the arterial vascular bed, causing a decrease in afterload. These modifications promote an increase in systolic volume by the Starling mechanism and consequently in cardiac output, with maintenance of arterial pressure [1, 6]. Filling pressures would commonly increase during hemodilution or remain unchanged, which indicates that normovolemia is being maintained. Plewes and Fahri [11] observed maintenance of central venous pressure and pulmonary artery pressure as well as cardiac output and left ventricle end diastolic pressure during hemodilution (23%) and controlled hypotension (55 mmHg). Van der Linden et al. [12] maintained capillary wedge pressure at the baseline value, administering fluids just to ascertain normovolemia. In our previous study [13], central pressure increased but this increase was not statistically significant, which was verified by Nielsen et al. [14]. In fact, compensatory mechanisms during hemodilution, most of them adrenergic in etiology and influenced by the type of expander fluid, may interfere with the hemodynamic results.

There are many different proposed formulas to calculate the target hematocrit during hemodilution. Poli de Figueiredo et al. [15] measured hematocrit at certain fixed time intervals until reaching the hematocrit established initially. Plewes and Farhi [11] employed the following formula:

$$\text{EBV (ml)} = 80 \text{ (ml and blood/kg)} \times \text{body weight (kg)}$$

$$\text{ERCV} = \text{Hct (\%)} \times \text{EBV};\ \text{ERCV}_{(\text{control})} = \text{Hct (\%)} \times \text{EBV};\ \text{ERCV}_{(20)} = 0.2 \times \text{EBV}$$

$$\text{Red cell to remove} = \text{ERCV}_{(\text{control})} - \text{ERCV}_{(20)}$$

Blood volume to remove = 3 x red cell volume to remove where

EBV = estimated blood volume (ml)

ERCV (control) = estimated red blood cell volume during the control period

ERCV (20) = estimated red blood cell volume at hematocrit = 20%

Our group in two recent studies, and another that is still ongoing, employed the formula proposed by Gross [16]:

$$\text{EBVR} = [\text{body weigh} + \text{X } 80\ (\text{Hi} - \text{Hd})] / [(\text{Hi} + \text{Hd})/2] \text{ where}$$

EBVR = estimated blood volume to be removed

Hi = Initial hematocrit

Hd = Desired hematocrit

With this formula, the hematocrit established as the target is seldom reached. Utilizing the formula proposed by Gross [16] we frequently have encountered lower values of hematocrit than desired. For instance, if in the beginning we choose a value of 28%, at the end of blood withdrawal the hematocrit will be around 23-24%.

The value of hematocrit that should be reached during hemodilution varies largely among clinical and experimental studies. It is important to keep in mind that the target hematocrit will depend on the species chosen and the purpose of the study. For instance, the normal hematocrit of the pig is 30%, while the normal hematocrit of dogs varies between 37 and 55%. So if one wanted to analyze organ function with extreme values of hematocrit, 20% in the pig, the results obtained would not be relevant to human clinical situations. There is no consensus regarding the target or critical hematocrit in clinical practice. In man, during coronary by-pass surgery, Niinikoski et al. [17] established values of 33%, while Mathru et al. [18] established values of 15%. Monk et al. [9] had a target hematocrit of 28% and the limit value for transfusion was 25% for radical prostatectomy. In these studies no undesirable effects due to hemodilution were found. In spite of this, Nelson et al. [19] verified that a hematocrit lower than 28% was more related to ischemic events in patients with previous peripheral vascular disease.

In our studies [13], hematocrit ranged from 21 to 23%, and in a recent clinical report [20] where dogs were submitted to massive volume expansion (32 ml/kg) with physiological saline or 4 ml/kg with hypertonic saline this same range was observed. Poli de Figueiredo et al. [15] studyed the effects of hemodilution during descending thoracic aortic cross-clamping and lower torso reperfusion and established 20% as the target hematocrit. Nielsen et al. [14] evaluated three different colloid solutions and the presence of hepatic ischemia in rabbits utilizing a hematocrit of 5%. Cain [21], investigating the effects of hypoxia in dogs, obtained values of 10%. Van der Linden et al. [12] in experimental studies with dogs decreased the hematocrit to a point at which the animal could no longer maintain stable arterial pressure, and compared starch with gelatine. In these the hemoglobin had fallen to values of 6.6 ± 1.7 for the gelatine group and 3.5 ± 1.5 for the starch group. Plewes and Farhi [11] in experiments with dogs evaluated the effects of hemodilution and controlled the cardiovascular system utilizing a hematocrit of 23%. Cain [21] verified that with a hematocrit of 10% in dogs the heart showed an inability to maintain the initial increase in cardiac output. Poli de Figueiredo et al. [15] verified that although isovolemic hemodilution was associated with hemodynamic stability during descending thoracic aortic cross clamping, during lower torso reperfusion hemodynamic instability occurred. Therefore, the authors concluded that these responses might offset the potential benefits of hemodilution for surgical procedures requiring descending thoracic aortic cross clamping.

Another interesting point is the blood flow in different organs during hemodilution. Regional blood flow is among the parameters that have changed more distinctly in several investigations. Fan et al. [22] in experiments with dogs observed that in the liver, intestine, and kidney the blood flow remained unchanged from the control values. However, blood flow to the spleen decreased sharply. Nielsen et al. [14] verified in rabbits that values of hematocrit as low as 5% do not result in significant hepatic ischemia or injury as assessed by histology. In our clinical and experimental studies [13, 20], oxygen delivery was maintained as well as cardiac output. No signs of heart ischemia or reduction of urinary output were noticed during the entire period of hemodilution. Plewes and Farhi [11] in dogs submitted to hemodilution (hematocrit 23%) verified that during the first 30 min of hemodilution and controlled hypotension there were significant increases in blood flow to the brain, liver, skeletal muscles, and diaphragm. However, after this time oxygen delivery started to decrease significantly and all blood flows fell after 90 min of hemodilution, except cerebral blood flow, which returned to control levels. However, Noldge et al. [23] observed in pigs that a hematocrit of 15% was accompanied by increases in splanchnic blood flow with maintenance of this flow 2 h after the beginning of the protocol.

If hemodilution is conducted properly, oxygen transport should be preserved, unless critical levels of hematocrit and hemoblogin are to be achieved. In accordance with this, while evaluating the use of both crystalloid and colloids during blood removal, we verified that systemic oxygen transport could be preserved with hematocrits around 21% [13]. The decrease in oxygen transport during hemodilution is not uniform among regions. Noldge et al. [23] verified, for example, that for two levels of hemodilution (20 and 14%), except for hepatic arterial oxygen delivery, which was preserved during both hemodilution, all oxygen deliveries (total hepatic, portal venous, and superior mesenteric arterial) decreased progressively. Fan et al. [22] observed that with reductions of hematocrit, the oxygen transport rate to the myocardium remained essentially constant with a hematocrit as low as 12%, while in the brain, the oxygen transport rate remained the same as the control level with a hematocrit above 30%, but it declined as the hematocrit was reduced further. Plewe and Farhi [11] verified that cerebral oxygen delivery decreased 16% in relation to control values after 30 min of hemodilution and concomitant hypotension with a further decrease of 29% in oxygen delivery after 90 min of hemodilution.

There are some critical levels of hemodynamic and laboratory parameters established by different authors that should be observed during hemodilution. In accordance with Cain [21], the critical value of pvO_2 for the dog would be around 45 mmHg, while for the pig Trouwborst et al. [24] reported a value of pvO_2 of 32.3 mmHg. Van Woerkens et al. [25] established the critical value in man at 34 mmHg. With regard to oxygen saturation, no change was seen [13] in our study, while Van Der Linden et al. [12] established a value of SvO_2 of 35% in dogs, Van Woerkens et al. 56% for man [25], and Trouwborst et al. a value of 44.2% for the pig [24].

Fluids utilized during normovolemic hemodilution

With regard to the fluids employed to ascertain normovolemia during blood removal, both colloid and crystalloid solutions can be used [4-6, 26]. Usually investigators choose one or another even during experimental protocols [11, 12, 15]. Among colloid solutions, hydroxyethyl starch has been largely employed in man in recent years [27-30], as well as during experimental studies [12, 14, 15, 23]. This substance seems to cause less allergic reactions than gelatines and dextrin, and has a medium to short intravascular volume effect (plateau 3-4 h), while gelatines have a short volume effect (plateau 1-2 h) [31, 32]. Among different starches, the 450,000 molecular weight starch has more effects on the coagulation system than the 200,000 molecular weight starch [31, 32].

Beyer et al. [30] compared a 6% low molecular weight hydroxyethyl starch (HES) to a modified gelatine for volemic replacement in major orthopedic surgery. Both solutions were similar in volume replacement and effects on oncotic pressure and coagulation. Van der Linden et al. [12] compared the same solutions and found no differences in hemodynamic and oxygenation parameters. Nevertheless, Mortelmans et al. [29] observed that gelatine required infusion of extra volume, approximately 30% of the volume originally needed, due to its more-pronounced extravasation, and that the HES group presented a higher blood loss. Baron et al. [27] infused albumin or HES in a ratio of 1.2 ml of colloid for each 1 ml of blood withdrawn and performed an additional infusion of 500 ml of colloids after hemodilution [27].

Crystalloids can also be used for hemodilution, despite their weak intravascular retention. Fahmy et al. [1] employed lactate Ringer's solution exclusively for hemodilution in a ratio of 3 ml for each 1 ml of blood withdrawn in human patients and observed increases in cardiac output and oxygen delivery. Singler and Furman [33] also found satisfactory results using lactate Ringer's solution during hemodilution. Because of extravascular redistribution, the amount of crystalloid infused must exceed the quantity of blood withdrawn and additional volumes are required to maintain normovolemia [6].

Colloid solutions and crystalloid may be used together in hemodilution protocols. Fantoni et al. [13] utilized HES and lactate Ringer's solution in a ratio of 0.5 ml of starch plus 1.5 ml of lactate Ringer's solution for each 1 ml of blood in a study with dogs and observed increases in cardiac output and oxygen delivery.

Influence of anesthetics

During hemodilution, it is of paramount importance that the fall in hemoglobin and consequently of arterial oxygen must be compensated in order to preserve the delivery of oxygen to the tissues. Cardiac output is one of the parameters that increases during hemodilution and that contributes to the maintenance of oxygen delivery as previously described [1]. This increase in cardiac output is due mainly to the decrease in blood viscosity, which, with the decrease in afterload, favors blood flow and increases venous return, preload, and stroke volume [1, 6]. Nevertheless, when cardiac output does not increase, oxygen delivery can be maintained to a certain point with the augmentation of the oxygen extraction rate [6]. In accordance with some authors, the use of some anesthetic techniques could impair the increase in venous return and cardiac output in view of their negative inotropic actions [34, 28]. Biboulet et al. [34] pointed out that the different hemodynamic responses observed during several hemodilution techniques are due to the great variability of protocols and mostly due to of the anesthetic regimen employed. These authors did not observe any increase in cardiac index in ASA I patients anesthetized with enflurane and fentanyl. Rosberg and Wulff [35] in elderly patients anesthetized with droperidol, fentanyl, and nitrous oxide had the same results, which were also verified by Van Der Linden et al. [28]. These former authors have attributed the unfavorable results mainly to the use of enflurane. On the other hand, Boldt et al. [36] verified in patients submitted to myocardial revascularization and cardiac by-pass surgery and anesthetized with midazolan and fentanyl, an enhancement in cardiac index of + 1.10 l/min per m^2. Mathru et al. [18], in patients submitted to the same procedure, noticed a 73% increase in cardiac output when fentanyl was used, while Van Woerkens et al. [25] verified a 57% increase in this parameter in an elderly Jeovah's Witness patient anesthetized with enflurane and fentanyl. In animal reports the results are more comparable. With regard to inotropism, enflurane is the anesthetic that alters this parameter more markedly in dogs, followed by halothane [37, 38]. Isoflurane and sevoflurane, when used in low concentrations, are much weaker depressants. Indeed, when 1.2 MAC of isoflurane or sevoflurane are utilized in dogs, there is no change in cardiac output. On the other hand, when 2.0 MAC are employed, a 17% decrease in cardiac output is verified. Plewes and Farhi [11], in their hemodilution and hypotension model, verified an increase in cardiac output in dogs anesthetized with halothane. Doss et al. [10] evaluated the mechanism of vasodilatation during hemodilution in rats anesthetized with 1.2% halothane. They observed that the increase in cardiac output was inhibited by the administration of a nitric oxide synthesis inhibitor. Comparing the effects of halothane, isoflurane, and sevoflurane during hemodilution in dogs, we verified an 86% increase in cardiac output in the halothane group, while the increases with isoflurane and sevoflurane were 90% and 120%, respectively [39] (Fig. 1). It must be borne in mind that anemia per se does not interfere with MAC, and that the dose-response curves of cardiac output, heart rate, arterial pressure, and end diastolic left ventricle pressure are not influenced by the different values of hematocrit, at least in dogs [40]. Also in the great majority of the studies cited, the inhaled anesthetics were not used in concentrations that would surpass the value of 1 MAC for the species.

With regard to the injectable anesthetics, there are also many notable results. Van Der Linden et al. [12] utilizing ketamine (0.4 mg/kg per hour) did not verify enhancement in cardiac output during hemodilution in the dog. On the other hand, Noldge et al. [41] also employed ketamine at 4 mg/kg per hour and observed a cardiac output increase of 32%. In accordance with Traber et al. [42], ketamine increases cardiac output in many doses ranges (5, 10, and 20 mg/kg). Pagel et al. [43] verified decreases in cardiac output in dogs, but only when the autonomic nervous system was blocked. Pigs anesthetized with a continuous infusion of midazolam also presented a 40% increase in cardiac index [24]. Re-

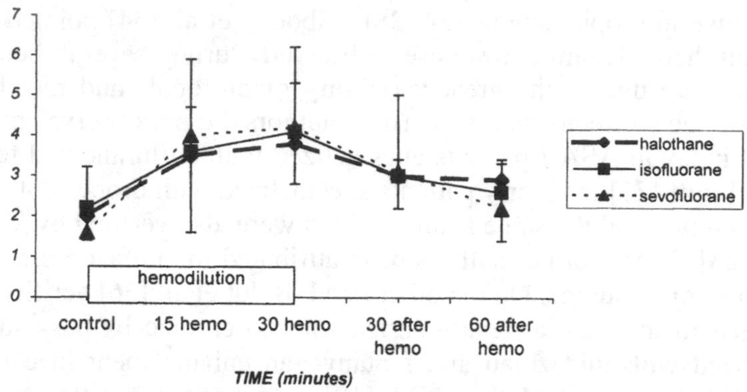

Fig. 1. Cardiac output in hemodilution comparing three different inhaled anesthetics (hemo = hemodilution)

viewing the literature it is possible to say that anesthetics play a minor role in the hemodynamic responses to hemodilution and that other factors must be responsible for some of the negative results observed. Gallagher [6] pointed out that the augmentation of filling pressures is essential for the venous return and cardiac output changes. Indeed, in many reports where the cardiac output increase was not verified, the authors did not see or did not mention the enhancement in the central venous pressure or pulmonary capillary wedge pressure. In conclusion, it is difficult to affirm the real role of anesthetics in the hemodynamic responses of hemodilution.

Experimental protocols

To conclude we will summarize the hemodilution protocols that are at present under investigation by our group.

1. Evaluation of plasma volume before and after blood removal and expansion with colloids and or crystalloid employing radioiodine-labelled human albumin in dogs.

We hypothesized that plasma expansion promoted by the colloid solution in association with Ringer's lactate would be really significant when compared to Ringer's lactate alone during hemodilution. Thus we measure the plasma volume before, at the end of blood exchange, and 60 and 120 min after hemodilution. After standard anesthesia [morphine, propofol, and isoflurane (1 MAC)], the animals were prepared for conventional hemodynamic evaluation (cardiac output, vascular pressures and resistance, hemodynamic-derived indexes). The blood volume withdrawn was calculated by the formula: blood volume = weight x 80 x (Ht – Ht target) / [(Ht + Ht target) / 2]. After previous splenectomy (1 week before) the dogs were divided into two groups, one assigned to replace half of the blood removed with lactate Ringer's at a 3:1 ratio and the second half of blood removed with HES at a 1:1 ratio. In group II blood withdrawn was replaced only with lactate Ringer's at a 3:1 ratio.

Plasma volume measurements were performed using radioiodine-labelled human serum albumin injected into the jugular vein in two different time frames. The first was given in an injection before hemodilution. Blood samples were collected by the pulmonary artery catheter 10, 20, and 30 min after the injection to calculate the control value of plasma volume. After hemodilution, blood samples was collected to calculate BG (background value) and then the second injection was given. This second injection and BG value are necessary to correct the blood withdrawn. Posterior blood samples were collected to determine plasma volume 0, 60, and 120 min after hemodilution. All blood samples had their hematocrit measured and were collected with heparin and centrifuged. Plasma radioactivity was determined after assay in a scintillation counter.

2. Progressive normovolemic hemodilution in dogs utilizing HES or lactate Ringer's: hemodynamic, echocardiographic, and biochemical evaluation. This experimental protocol evaluates the cardiovascular function during progressive hemodilution comparing two different plasma expanders. The dogs are anesthetized with etomidate and isoflurane and prepared for conventional hemodynamic evaluation (cardiac output, vascular pressures and resistance, hemodynamic-derived indexes) and transthoracic echocardiography. They are submitted to the continuous pressure driven bleeding model described by Rocha e Silva et al. [44] and blood withdrawn is replaced with HES at a 1:1 ratio (group I) or lactate Ringer's at a 3:1 ratio (group II). Bleeding is performed until the animal can no longer maintain stable hemodynamic parameters.

References

1. Fahmy NR, Chandler HP, Patel DJ et al (1980) Hemodynamics and oxygen availability during acute haemodilution in conscious man (abstract). Anaesthesiology 53[Suppl]:584
2. Martin E, Hansen E, Peter K (1987) Acute limited normovolemic hemodilution: a method for avoiding homologous transfusion. World J Surg 11:53-59
3. Brooks M (1992) Transfusion medicine. In: Murtaugh RJ, Kaplan PM (eds) Veterinary emergency and critical care medicine. Mosby Year Book, St Louis, pp 536-546
4. Kreimeier U, Messmer K (1996) Hemodilution in critical surgery: state of the art 1996. World J Surg 20:1208-1217
5. Stehling L, Zauder HL (1991) Acute normovolemic hemodilution. Transfusion 31:857-868
6. Gallagher JD (1995) Hemodilution: physiology and limits of anaemia. In: Lake CL, Moore RA (eds) Blood hemostasis, transfusion and alternatives in the perioperative period. Raven Press, New York, pp 345-380
7. Ness PM, Bourke DL, Walsh PC (1991) A randomised trial of perioperative hemodilution versus transfusion of preoperatively deposited autologous blood in elective surgery. Transfusion 32:226-230

8. Kochamba GS, Pfeffer TA, Sintek CF et al (1996) Intraoperative autotransfusion reduces blood loss after cardiopulmonary bypass. Ann Thorac Surg 61:900-903
9. Monk TGL, Goognough LT, Brecher ME et al (1997) Acute normovolemic hemodilution can replace preoperative autologous blood donation as a standard of care for autologous blood procurement in radical prostactomy. Anesth Analg 85:953-958
10. Doss DN, Estafanous FG, Ferrario CM et al (1995) Mechanism of systemic vasodilatation during normovolemic hemodilution. Anesth Analg 81:30-34
11. Plewes JL, Farhi LE (1985) Cardiovascular responses to hemodilution and controlled hypotension in the dog. Anaesthesiology 62:149-154
12. Van Der Linden P, Schmartz D, Groote FD et al (1998) Critical haemoglobin concentration in anaesthetised dogs: comparison of two plasma substitutes. Br J Anaesth 81:556-562
13. Fantoni DT, Auler JOC, Ambrosio AM et al (1998) Comparison of two different replacement methods for normovolemic acute haemodilution. In: Anaesthesia, pain, intensive care and emergency medicine. Springer-Verlag, Berlin Heidelberg New York, pp 37-39
14. Nielsen VG, Baird MS, Brix AE et al (1999) Extreme, progressive isovolemic hemodilution with 5% human albumin, pentalyte, or hextend does not cause hepatic ischemia or histologic injury in rabbits. Anaesthesiology 90:1428-1435
15. Poli de Figueiredo LF, Mathru M, Tao W et al (1997) Hemodynamic effects of isovolemic hemodilution during descending thoracic aortic cross clamping and lower torso reperfusion. Surgery 122:32-38
16. Gross JB (1983) Estimating allowable blood loss: corrected for dilution. Anaesthesiology 58:277-280
17. Niinikoski J, Laaksonen V, Meretoja O et al (1980) Oxygen transport to tissue under normovolemic moderate and extreme hemodilution during coronary bypass operation. Ann Thorac Surg 31:134-143
18. Mathru M, Kleinmam B, Blakeman B et al (1991) Cardiovascular adjustments and gas exchange during extreme hemodilution in humans. Crit Care Med 19:700-704
19. Nelson AH, Fleisher LA, Rosembaum SH (1993) Relationship between postoperative anaemia and cardiac morbidity on high-risk patients in the intensive care unit. Crit Care Med 21:860-866
20. Fantoni DT, Auler JOC, Futema F et al (1999) Intravenous administration of hypertonic sodium chloride with dextrin solution or isotonic sodium chloride solution for treatment of septic shock secondary to pyometra in dogs. JAMA 215:1283-1287
21. Cain SM (1977) Oxygen delivery and uptake in dogs during anaemia and hypoxic hypoxia. J Appl Physiol 42:228-234
22. Fan FC, Chen RYZ, Schuessler GB et al (1980) Effects of hematocrit variations on regional hemodynamics and oxygen transport in dogs. Am J Physiol 238:H545-H52
23. Noldge GFE, Priebe HJ, Geiger K (1992) Splanchnic hemodynamics and oxygen supply during acute normovolemic hemodilution alone and with isoflurane-induced hypotension in the anaesthetised pig. Anesth Analg 75:660-674
24. Trouwborst A, Van Woerkens ECMS, Tenbrinck R (1990) Blood gas analysis of mixed venous blood during normoxic acute isovolemic hemodilution in pigs. Anesth Analg 70: 523-529
25. Van Woerkens ECSM, Trouwborst A, Lanschot JJB (1992) Profound hemodiluiton: what is the critical level of hemodilution at which oxygen delivery-dependent oxygen consumption starts in an anaesthetised human? Anesth Analg 75:818-821
26. Trouwborst A, van Bommel J, Ince C et al (1998) Monitoring normovolemic haemodilution. Br J Anesth 81[Suppl]:73-78
27. Baron JF, De Kegel D, Prost AC et al (1991) Low molecular weight hydroxyethyl starch 6% compared to albumin 4% during intentional hemodilution. Intensive Care Med 17:141-148
28. Van Der Linden P, Wathieu M, Gilbart E et al (1994) Cardiovascular effects of moderate normovolaemic haemodilution during enflurane-nitrous oxide anaesthesia in man. Acta Anaesthesiol Scand 38:490-498

29. Mortelmans YJ, Vermaut G, Verbruggen AM et al (1995) Effects of 6% hydroxyethyl starch and 3% modified fluid gelatine on intravascular volume and coagulation during intraoperative hemodilution. Anesth Analg 81:1235-1242
30. Beyer R, Harmening U, Rittmeyer O et al (1997) Use of modified fluid gelatine and hydroxyethyl starch for colloidal volume replacement in major orthopaedic surgery. Br J Anaesth 78:44-50
31. Traylor RJ, Pearl RG (1996) Crystalloid versus colloid versus colloid: all colloids are not created equal. Anesth Analg 83:209-212
32. Ring J, Messmer K (1997) Incidence and severity of anaphylactic reactions to colloid volume substitutes. Lancet 1:466
33. Singler RC, Furman EB (1980) Hemodilution: how low a minimum hematocrit (abstract)? Anaesthesiology 53
34. Biboulet P, Capdevila X, Benetreau D et al (1996) Haemodynamic effects of moderate normovolemic haemodilution in conscious and anaesthetised patients. Br J Anaesth 76:81-84
35. Rosberg B, Wulff K (1981) Hemodynamics following normovolemic hemodilution in elderly patients. Acta Anesthesiol Scand 25:402-406
36. Boldt J, Bormann BV, Kling D et al (1988) Influence of acute normovolemic hemodilution on extravascular lung water in cardiac surgery. Crit Care Med 16:336-339
37. Bernard JM, Wouters PF, Doursout MF et al (1990) Effects of sevoflurane and isoflurane on cardiac and coronary dynamics in chronically instrumented dogs. Anaesthesiology 72: 659-662
38. Steffey E (1996) Inhalation anaesthetics. In: Thurmon JC, Tranquilly WJ, Benson GJ (eds) Lumb's Jones veterinary anaesthesia, 3rd edn. Williams and Wilkins, Baltimore, pp 297-304
39. Fantoni DT, Ambrosi AM, Tamura EY et al (1999) Normovolemic hemodilution in dogs anaesthetised with halothane, isoflurane or sevoflurane on acute haemorrhage. In: Anaesthesia, pain, intensive care and emergency medicine, 14. Trieste, 16-18 Nov, Moderna, Trieste, p 131 (selected papers)
40. Loarie DJ, Wilkinson P, Tyberg J et al (1979) The hemodynamic effects of halothane in anaemic dogs. Anesth Analg 58:195-200
41. Noldge GFE, Priebe HJ, Bohle W et al (1991) Effects of acute normovolemic hemodilution on splanchnic oxygen and on hepatic histology and metabolism in anaesthetised pigs. Anaesthesiology 74:908-918
42. Traber DL, Wilsno RD, Priano LL (1968) Differentiation of the cardiovascular effects of CI-581. Anesth Analg 47:769-777
43. Pagel PS, Kampine JP, Schmeling WT et al (1992) Ketamine depresses myocardial contractility as evaluated by the preload recruitable stroke work relationship in chronically instrumented dogs with autonomic nervous system blockade. Anaesthesiology 76:564-572
44. Rocha e Silva M, Negraes GA, Pontieri V et al (1986) Hypertonic resuscitation from severe hemorrhagic shock: patterns of regional circulation. Circ Shock 19:165-175

New Insight Into the Role of Microcirculation in Shock

G.P. NOVELLI

The microcirculation (MC) is the terminal region of the circulatory system that is fundamental in the pathophysiology of sepsis and septic shock. As is well known, its main components are arterioles, venules, shunts, and mostly capillaries. All the structures in the MC are capable of contraction, except capillaries which are made of endothelial cells alone, without contractile structures, except those (named "precapillary sphincters") placed at the beginning of the vessels.

However, capillaries might undergo changes of local hemodynamics during sepsis due to active constriction of sphincters, mechanical or cellular obstruction, endothelial or interstitial edema. Interstitial edema could be consequent to both hypoxic or endotoxic damage of capillaries but also, very frequently, to iatrogenic inappropriate and excessive administration of fluids. Endothelial edema is a consequence of inadequate administration of fluids.

The greatest therapeutic problem when looking at a MC devastated by sepsis or by iatrogenic maltreatment is to reverse the endothelial damage and restore the uniformity of blood flow [1]. Therefore the main goal in all shock conditions is to stabilize the MC and restore both the capillary blood flow and the uniformity of oxygen distribution.

Capillaries are the only sites where oxygen is exchanged between extravascular and intravascular spaces, due to its high solubility and diffusibility. As a consequence, tissue oxygenation strongly depends on the capillary blood flow and oxygen consumption by cells is a good indicator of the state of health of the tissue.

Models of MC

The basic organization of MC is more or less similar in every tissue, and was described many decades ago by Zweifach and Thomas [2]. Today their ancient description is still accepted and their method of visualization by transillumination microscopy of a small area of the thin mesentery is still employed. The basic method was improved by some laboratories by using different types of microscopy illumination, and perfusion of the exposed tissue, according to the needs of each research study.

To try to eliminate the effects of anesthetic drugs, a skinfold dorsal chamber, which contains striated muscles and skin, has been adopted for prolonged studies on awake rats [3]. Transparent chambers were also applied to the ears of rabbits to test a specific zone of circulation in a specific animal without anesthesia.

The functional arrangement of the MC is based on variations of the so-called Krogh's cylinder that is the cylindrical volume of tissue reached by oxygen diffusing by each single capillary. Therefore, during ischemia or occlusion only a few capillaries remain perfused and therefore the quantity of oxygen available is low.

The intravital microscopy of extensor digitorum muscle demonstrated that sepsis was accompanied by a 36% reduction of functioning capillaries, and therefore by a similar quantity of oxygen [4]. Therefore, the prognostic value of increasing oxygen delivery and consumption is obvious: it means that the microcirculatory network increase its exchange area and supplies adequate oxygen to the cells.

Astiz et al. [5] have reported a non-invasive demonstration in man of the microcirculatory problems during sepsis. In severely septic patients neutrophil aggregation, reduced red cell deformability, augmented adhesion molecules, decreased cardiac output, and reduced oxygen delivery were observed. These authors were the first to measure forearm blood flow and its reactivity. Both such parameters in the forearm were significantly modified, demonstrating the persistence of microcirculatory problems after apparent recovery in man.

How to assess the function of the MC

The above-quoted paper [5] demonstrated the relationship between the problems of MC and the evolution of sepsis. They used an atraumatic method that could provide information by simple digital compression-decompression of the nails and observation of the refilling time, but it is not currently used.

To diagnose a septic state in man a good index is the relationship between oxygen delivery and consumption [6, 7]. It is logical that a progressive increase of oxygen delivery during sepsis helps to overcome stagnation in MC. On the other hand, an increase in oxygen consumption indicates that cells are receiving blood and utilizing it.

To obtain significant data on oxygen delivery and consumption, it should be necessary to examine separately the main organs and districts. Great interest has focused on the splanchnic circulation that has an enormous importance in the pathophysiology of sepsis and septic shock due to the extension of its vascular bed, to reabsorption of toxic materials, and to bacterial translocation. Polarographic needle methods for measuring PO_2 in muscles were expensive and with many technical problems.

The idea of Fiddian-Green and Baker [7] to indirectly assess the efficacy of splanchnic perfusion with a tonometer has aroused great interest. The first tonometer was made by a special gastrointestinal catheter with a silicone balloon filled with saline. After an adequate period of equilibration the saline was aspirated and analyzed, so as to derive from PCO_2 the pH value of the mucosa. Gastric tonometry remained poorly used due to a series of questions: is gastric tonometry really indicative of splanchnic perfusion? Is pH derived from the PCO_2 of saline indicative of mucosal perfusion? Experiments demonstrated that during low flow, intestinal mucosal pH measured with the tonometer of Fiddian-Green was very similar to that measured directly [8]. A study of Gutierrez et al. [9] clearly demonstrated that intensive care patients monitored with the tonometer had a reduced hospital stay or, in other words, a better evolution.

Not withstanding the debates and some uncertainties, gastric tonometry is an interesting technique, as confirmed by attempts to develop analogous systems. Differing from the previous tonometer that was filled with saline, a new tonometer filled with air measures directly PCO_2 [10]. It is currently being produced industrially under the name Tonometrix [11].

Another apparatus is now under evaluation [12]: it consists of a optical fiber with a colorimetric sensor for CO_2 on its peripheral tip; the signal is analyzed by a specially made colorimeter. One of the many advantages is that this instrument may record all the instantaneous variations of PCO_2, to permit appropriate interpretation not only of mean values but also of acute variations in the composition of gastric content, like those induced by biliary regurgitation. The technique of gastric tonometry seems highly promising as a monitor of splanchnic perfusion and therefore as a guide to appropriate therapy (Table 1).

Table 1. Putative uses of gastric tonometer (from reference [11])

- Perioperative monitoring in major surgery
- Myocardial infarction and shock
- Heart failure
- Sepsis and septic shock
- Pulmonary embolism
- Trauma and hemorrhage
- Pericardial tamponade
- Acute pancreatitis
- Mesenteric thrombosis
- Necrotizing enterocolitis
- Ischemic colitis
- Bowel obstruction
- Chronic celiac disease
- Weaning from mechanical ventilation
- Hemodyalisis

To assess splanchnic oxidative status, an invasive system of microdialysis to assess directly the peripheral production of lactate has been suggested but not confirmed [13]. Tissue hypoxia may also be measured on the basis of biochemical markers, but unfortunately it generally needs complex biochemical analysis. For example, due to the impairment of intrinsic antioxidant defenses during hypoperfusion, it might be possible to obtain indications on the oxidative status of the organism from the decrease of reduced glutathione, an endogenous antioxidant. Leukocytes activated by ischemia produce lysosomal enzymes and oxygen radicals. Their effects on microvessels are increased permeability, mechanical obstruction, vasoconstriction, creating vicious circles [14]. Cytokines intervene in complicating the whole picture. Tumor necrosis factor (TNF) causes persistent microcirculatory vasodilatation during sepsis, which is unresponsive to noradrenaline [15].

Regulation of MC during shock and septic shock

The regulation of the MC during sepsis and septic shock is not as simple as appears, and in health involves catecholamines, acetylcholine, serotonin, endothelin vasopressin, histamine, and kinins, all co-operating together in modulating the function of arteriolar and venular vessels [16]. The motility of the MC during health is regulated by the above mediators; other agents act as regulators of permeability, whose role lies in regulating the function of the terminal circulation and mostly of the capillaries.

The main regulators of capillary function are endotoxin, hypoxia, granulocytes, oxygen radicals, and other well-known mediators that act on the permeability (and therefore on tissue water or on diffusion of intestinal content into the blood), but also on the response to catecholamines (Table 2).

The *COX inhibitors* seem to act on the MC by restoring the responsiveness to catecholamines. Increase of prostanoids, arachidonic acid intermediates, and increased defenses against oxygen radicals [16] have been taken into account to explain this phenomenon.

In conscious rats the reduced responsiveness to exogenous epinephrine is restored by the infusion of neuropeptide Y, a 36-amino acid peptide that is located in adrenal medulla, central sympathetic neurons, and in postganglionic sympathetic nerve fibers [17]. Neuropeptide Y enhances the pressor response to catecholamines, probably due to synergism with both exogenous and endogenous amines. No data are available except on rats.

An actual mediator is the transcription nuclear factor NF-kB, which is an ubiquitous DNA binding protein that is necessary for high level transcription of many proinflammatory genes [18]. Under normal conditions the NF-kB is inhibited by the factors I-kBS, but can be activated by endotoxin, by TNFs, by interleukin-6, by ischemia-reperfusion, by oxygen radicals, and by trauma [19] (Table 3).

Table 2. Putative mediators of the regulation of microcirculation

– Oxygen and oxygen radicals
– Carbon dioxide
– pH
– Nitric oxide [24]
– Catecholamines
– Acetylcholine
– Serotonin
– Histamine
– Kinins
– Granulocytes [25]
– Adhesion molecules [26]
– Neuropeptide Y
– Lysosomal enzymes [27]
– Cytokines [28]
– Prostanoids
– COX inhibitors

Table 3. Proinflammatory molecules regulated by NF-kB (from reference [19])

TNF
Interleukins-1, -2, -6, -12
Interferon
Adhesion molecules
COX_2

TNF tumor necrosis factor

Inhibition of NF-kB activation correlates with the suppression of TNF formation, reduced ICAM gene transcription and protection against endotoxin-induced liver injury [20] (Table 4). Other tissue factors have been considered in rats submitted to traumatic shock [21]. All tissue factors are reciprocally linked and tissue factor activity was accompanied by increased formation of P-selectin [19] and possibly by transmigration of activated neutrophils. Therefore, the key rheological and peroxidative mechanisms maintain their key role in the disturbances of MC and of capillary blood flow.

Acute neutrophil activation has some differences in different species and traumas, but is an early event and is implicated for leukocyte-mediated organ injury. The *adhesion molecules* are activated by endotoxin, hypoxia, and tissue factor; their presence in the MC is necessary for transmigration of granulocytes, so that their inhibition seems to be protective against sepsis and septic shock [20].

Table 4. Stimuli activating NF-kB during systemic inflammatory response syndrome, multiple organ failure syndrome, and acute respiratory distress syndrome (from reference [19])

Endotoxin
IL-1
TNF
Oxygen radicals
Hyperoxia
Trauma

Nitric oxide (NO) is one important tissue mediator with a great involvement in the pathophysiology of sepsis and septic shock. There was enthusiasm in favor of NO as a pathogenetic factor of sepsis, but recently it appeared that inhibition of NO synthesis in man is accompanied by increased adhesion of granulocytes to endothelium, exacerbating microcirculatory constriction and hypoperfusion [22, 23]. Data from our laboratory have confirmed that drugs inhibiting NO production in rats negatively affect survival after endotoxin or intestinal ischemia [24, 25].

Conclusion

New insights on the role of the MC in sepsis and septic shock have not introduced anything that could affect old and well-established concepts. The most-interesting system to be developed in future years is one of measuring oxygen consumption of the splanchnic apparatus, so to regulate fluid therapy and pharmacotherapy to the needs of the tissues avoiding both hypo- and overtherapy. Other future possibilities are those directed at modulating mediators like NF-kB and the adhesion molecules, to prevent the action of oxygen radicals on microvessels.

References

1. Intaglietta M (1989) Objectives for the treatment of the microcirculation in ischaemia, shock and reperfusion. In: Update in intensive care and emergency medicine. Springer-Verlag, Berlin Heidelberg New York
2. Zweifach BW, Thomas L (1957) The relationship between the vascular manifestations of shock produced by endotoxin, trauma and haemorrhage. J Exp Med 106:385-401
3. Menger MD, Steiner D, Messmer K (1992) Microvascular ischaemia reperfusion in striated muscle. Significance of 'no reflow'. Am J Physiol 263:H1892-H1900
4. Lam C, Tymil K, Martin C et al (1994) Microvascular perfusion is impaired in a rat model of normotensive sepsis. J Clin Invest 94:2077-2083
5. Astiz ME, De Gent GE, Lyn RY et al (1995) Microvascular function and rheologic changes in hyperdynamic sepsis. Crit Care Med 23:265-271
6. Novelli GP, De Gaudio AR, Melani AM (1995) Oxygen uptake and delivery. In: 24th Congress of Anesthesiology, Vienna 4-8 Sept 1995. Springer, Berlin Heidelberg New York, pp 337-341
7. Fiddian-Green RG, Baker S (1987) Predictive value of the stomach wall pH for complications after cardiac operations. Comparison with other monitoring. Crit Care Med 15:153-156
8. Grum CM, Fiddian-Green RG, Pittenger GL et al (1984) Adequacy of tissue oxygenation in intact dog intestine. J Appl Physiol 56:1065-1069
9. Gutierrez G, Palisaz F, Doglio G et al (1992) Gastric intramucosal pH as a therapeutic index of tissue oxygenation in critically ill patients. Lancet 339:195-199
10. Tang W, Weil MH, Sun S et al (1994) Gastric intramucosal pCO_2 as monitor of perfusion failure during haemorrhagic and anaphylactic shock. J Appl Physiol 76:752-757
11. Kolkman JJ, Otte JA, Groeneveld ABJ (2000) Gastrointestinal luminal pCO_2 tonometry: an update on physiology, methodology and clinical applications. Br J Anaesth 84:74-86
12. Brinkmann A, Calzia E, Trager K et al (1998) Monitoring the hepato-splancnic region in the critically ill patient. Intensive Care Med 24:542-556
13. Tenhunen JJ, Kosunen H, Alava E et al (1999) Intestinal luminal microdialysis. A new approach to assess gut mucosal ischaemic. Anesthesiology 91:1807-1815
14. Waxman K (1998) Shock: ischaemia, reperfusion and inflammation. New Horiz 4:158-159
15. Francdgiannis, Youker KA, Rossen RD et al (1998) Cytokines and the microcirculation in ischaemia and reperfusion. J Mol Cell Cardiol 30:2567-2576
16. Greenberg S, Curro SA, Tanaka PT (1983) Regulation of vascular smooth muscle of the microcirculation. In: Mortillaro N (ed) The physiology and pharmacology of microcirculation. Academic Press, New York, pp 39-141
17. Parratt JR (1989) Alterations in vascular reactivity in sepsis and endotoxemia. In: Vincent JL (ed) Update in intensive care and emergency medicine. Springer, Berlin Heidelberg New York, pp 27-40
18. Evequoz D, Waeber B, Corder R et al (1987) Markedly reduced blood pressure responsiveness in endotoxemic rats: reversal by neuropeptide Y. Life Sci 41:2573-2580
19. Christmas JW, Lancaster LH, Blackwell TS (1988) Nuclear factor kB: a pilotal role in the systemic inflammatory response syndrome and new target for therapy. Intensive Care Med 24: 1131-1138
20. Essani NA, Fisher MA, Jaeschke H (1997) Inhibition of NF-kB activation by dimethylsulfoxide correlates with the suppression of TNF-alpha formation, reduced ICAM gene transcription and protection against endotoxin-induced liver injury. Shock 7:90-96
21. Armstead VE, Operntanova IL, Miinchenko AG et al (1999) Tissue factor expression in vital organs during traumatic shock. Anesthesiology 91:1844-1852
22. Kirkeboen KA, Strand OA (1999) The role of nitric oxide in sepsis: an overview. Acta Anaesthiol Scand 43:275-278
23. Spain DA, Wilson MA, Bar-Natan MF et al (1994) Role of nitric oxide in the small intestinal microcirculation during bacteremia. Shock 2:41-46
24. Novelli GP, Livi P, Adembri C, Melani AM (1995) Which is the role of NO in sepsis and shock. In: Brandi MD (ed) I Orvieto Simp. On development of nitric oxide, Orvieto, pp 35-38
25. Novelli GP, Livi P, Melani AM et al (1994) Il nitrossido nell'insufficienza circolatoria. Minerva Anestiol 60[Suppl]1:201-208

The Electrocardiogram

B. ALLARIA, M. DEI POLI, M. FAVARO

In this brief chapter we will discuss the current role of the electrocardiogram in the anesthesiologist's daily practice, above all, for the assessment of perioperative myocardial oxygen levels.

The first question to be answered is whether the ECG still has a place in preoperative patient evaluation in an era in which there are numerous other noninvasive tests available whose sensitivity and specificity may exceed those of the ECG.

It should be remembered that the preoperative evaluations of the anesthesiologist and cardiologist are fundamentally different. The cardiologist's objective is to diagnose ischemic heart disease using Garber's algorithm [1] and then to prescribe either pharmacologic or surgical treatment. The anesthesiologist must decide whether or not a surgical candidate has coronary artery disease and then judge its severity. On the basis of this evaluation, a particular strategy may be adopted in order to minimize the risk of ischemic events. The use of preoperative coronary revascularization procedures to avoid intra- or postoperative ischemic events is controversial and is generally reserved for cases of unstable angina [2].

Therefore, the anesthesiologist must know whether a patient is at risk for myocardial ischemia. If so, he must try to avoid any condition which could provoke an ischemic attack such as tachycardia, hyper- or hypotension, sympathetic or vagal stimulation, hypoxemia, etc., choose the proper type of anesthesia and conduct a more rigid intraoperative and postoperative surveillance program.

It is not generally necessary to employ complex and costly tests such as PET, SPECT, thallium or technetium radionuclide scans or sonographic tolerance tests (+ dobutamine, + dipyrimadole), but it is important to know how reliable ECG based diagnostic tests are.

In the past, so-called aspecific repolarization anomalies were not considered important in the diagnosis of coronary artery disease, but this is no longer so, thanks to the study published in the Journal of the American Medical Association by Daviglus et al. [3]. These authors subjected 1673 men who were employed by the Western Electric Company of Chicago to yearly ECG's for 11 years. The objective of the study was to determine whether there was a correlation between the presence of aspecific repolarization anomalies and long term mortality due to myocardial ischemia, coronary artery disease and other causes. Aspecific repolarization anomalies included ST segment depression with a J point < 0.5 mm with a descending pattern and a negative apex < 0.5 mm under the P-R segment in either D1, D2, aVL or in V1 to V6. The following were classified as "minor" T wave anomalies: flat, negative or diphasic (±) T waves with depths of 1 mm or less in either D1, D2, V3-6 or aVL when R was 5 mm or more; positive T waves with a T/R ratio less that ½ either in D1, D2, aVL or V3-6 with an R amplitude of 10 mm or more in the same leads.

The study showed that subjects with one of these anomalies had a higher risk of death and that this risk was even greater in those subjects that presented the anomalies more than once in their yearly ECGs. There was a 38% increase in mortality for patients with anomalies in 1 ECG and a 67% increase in those with anomalies in repeated yearly tests.

These observations are certainly not sufficient to revolutionize our knowledge on the subject, and, as Goldstein pointed out in his editorial [4], further confirmation is necessary. They are, however, sufficient to launch the following message: do not underestimate the importance of so called aspecific ECG abnormalities, and, when present, especially if previously found present in past ECGs from the same patient, behave as if the patient had coronary artery disease. This message does not come from either Daviglus or Goldstein, but I believe it is appropriate in the hopes of increasing patient security.

The ECG still retains its importance in the diagnosis of the cause of chest pain. At times, it provides more information than a coronary angiogram. In 1967, Kemp [5] and Likoff [6] reported on female patients with chest pain whose exercise tolerance tests were positive in the presence of normal coronary angiograms. Kemp later coined the term "X Syndrome" to describe these cases.

The pathogenesis of this syndrome remained uncertain for many years until improvements in our knowledge on the coronary artery endothelium's response to vasodilating and vasoconstricting stimuli provided some answers. In the X syndrome, coronary microvessels have a paradoxical response to vasodilating stimuli and an exagerated response to vasoconstrictive stimuli, thereby creating a situation in which the coronary angiogram may appear completely normal in the face of ischemic events [8]. The ECG may be more sensitive and specific in these cases. However, this fact should not generate unlimited trust in the ECG. It should be remembered that the ECG may appear normal in the initial phases of an ischemic attack and in cases of unstable angina.

As Mehta and Eagle pointed out in their recent editorial in the New England Journal of Medicine [9], it is not rare to overlook ischemia caused by obstruction of the left circumflex artery on the basis of ECG findings. At times, these patients are discharged from the emergency room in spite of specific symptoms and then have an abnormally high mortality rate (24 to 33%).

Continuous, 24 h ECG recording (Holter) is an invaluable tool preoperatively for patients at risk for coronary artery disease. While this technique is obviously useful for the diagnosis of arrhythmias, whose presence should be known preoperatively, its utility has also been proven for the diagnosis of silent ischemias.

Eisenberg [10] conducted a study on high risk patients undergoing cardiac surgery and found that the 12 lead ECG and TEE offered a minimal advantage over the Holter ECG. It was concluded that the latter test is particularly indicated in the preoperative period due to its simplicity and low cost.

It should be remembered that the Holter ECG provides valuable information on the sympathetic nervous system equilibrium and RR variability. Numerous studies have shown that a low level of vagus nerve activity (as evidenced by a reduction of the high frequency HF component in the spectral analysis of RR variability) is associated with a higher incidence of ischemic events and/or ventricular arrhythmias [11]. The analysis of RR variability provides 3 parameters: 1) spectral power, between 0.01 and 1 Hz (total spectral power); 2) low frequency power (LF) which falls between 0.04 and 0.15 Hz and 3) high frequency power (HF) which is between 0.15 and 0.40 Hz. LF is an expression of sympathetic activity, HF reflects vagus nerve activity and the LF/HF ratio provides an indication of the sympathetic-vagal equilibrium.

Beta-blocking drugs have become widely used for the prevention of myocardial ischemia [14]. It is known that these drugs enhance vagal activity, and this may be one reason for their effectiveness [12]. In patients with chronic heart failure there is a loss of RR variability and it is remarkable to note that treatment with atenolol causes a normalization of the sympathetic-vagal equilibrium which goes hand in hand with clinical improvement. This observation, which was recently published in the American Heart Journal [13], gives an idea of the importance of the Holter test for the assessment of sympathetic-vagal equilibrium in high risk patients who need to undergo surgery.

The exercise induced tolerance test has maintained its role in the preoperative evaluation of the surgical patient at risk for coronary artery disease. Since intra- and postoperative myocardial ischemia is often caused by tachycardia, to the point that Mangano [15] concluded that at least half of the perioperative ischemic events are caused by tachycardia, it follows that a test which suggests ischemia under conditions of tachycardia is of fundamental importance. A positive exercise tolerance test should trigger the adoption of a series of measures for prevention and surveillance of myocardial ischemia as described elsewhere in this volume [16].

Unfortunately, the sensitivity and specificity of the exercise tolerance test are not very high (61 and 76% respectively) but better results can be obtained by combining the ECG assessment with the clinical behaviour of the patient during the test. The Duke Treadmill Score (DTS) has been proposed and is calculated using the following formula: DTS = exercise time – (5 X ST segment depression) – (4 X angina level) where time is expressed in minutes, ST depression in mm and angina level equals 0 when absent, 1 if it does not limit exercise and 2 if it limits exercise. The DTS may vary from – 25 to + 15. A score of > 5 is generally found in low risk patients, from + 4 to – 10 in intermediate risk patients, and a score ≤ 11 is associated with a high risk of coronary artery disease. The latter group of patients usually have to interrupt the test due to hypotension, ST aberrations > 3 mm, chest pain or malignant ventricular arrhythmias.

Show et al. recently tested the DTS on 2758 symptomatic patients [17] with good results. The DTS was judged useful in establishing the diagnosis and prognosis of patients with suspected coronary artery disease.

Therefore, the correct use of the exercise induced tolerance test is important to identify those patients in whom the prevention and early diagnosis of myocardial ischemia in the intraoperative and postoperative periods are of extreme importance. Manganol [18] showed that the incidence of myocardial ischemia in patients with pathological stress tolerance tests undergoing vascular surgery was 37% vs. 1.5% in patients with normal tests.

We can conclude that the ECG in its various forms (resting ECG, exercise tolerance test, Holter) retains a crucial role in the preoperative evaluation of patients with risk factors for coronary artery disease and permits accurate identification of patients who are at risk for ischemic events.

In the course of the above discussion we mentioned the importance of the early diagnosis and treatment of intra- and postoperative myocardial ischemia. The ECG plays a fundamental role in this regard. Beyond demonstrating arrhythmias which are often an expression of ischemia the ECG allows analysis of the ST segment which is important for the diagnosis of myocardial ischemia. Studies have shown that the sensitivity of simple visual ST segment analysis for the diagnosis of ischemia is very low and ranges from 0 to 45% [19, 20]. Computerized monitoring of ST depression undoubtedly improves both sensitivity and specificity but is still not ideal. This method provides an average sensitivity of 74% (range 60 to 78%) and specificity of 73% (range 69 to 80%) [21, 22].

This signifies that, compared to the Holter ECG, the modern techniques used for cardiac monitoring in the operating room and in the ICU fail to identify myocardial ischemia in 26% of cases and show modifications which are not due to ischemia in 27%. Thus, the false positive and false negative rates are unacceptably high in spite of the technological innovations of recent years.

What are the reasons for these poor results?

The main reason is related to which leads are employed. A single lead is undoubtedly insufficient, but the combined use of D2 and V5 substantially improves sensitivity. According to London et al. [23] the simultaneous use of these 2 leads provides a sensitivity of 80% (similar to the average 74% sensitivity obtained using other leads), and in order to reach a satisfactory sensitivity level (96%) it is necessary to add V4. But, how many operating room monitors allow the simultaneous reading of 3 leads?

The second cause lies in the types of software which the manufacturers of monitors employ. Leung [21] recently compared the performance of 3 different monitors and found that the Marquette, Hewlett Packard, and Datex models provided sensitivity levels of 75, 78 and 60% respectively and specificities of 89, 71 and 69%.

The third cause is the type of filter employed. The American Heart Association recommends the use of a 0.05 to 100 Hz bandwidth for ECG monitoring. Sometimes, the low cut-off is set at 0.5 Hz in order to reduce the isoelectric oscillations caused by mechanical ventilation or imperfect attachment of electrodes. This type of filter causes distortion of the ST segment which leads to interpretation errors as shown by Slogov et al. [24].

Tachycardia is the fourth cause. An increased heart rate can cause a depression of the J point of more than 1 mm and an ST segment depression which the system interprets as ischemia. This can simply be the consequence of repolarization phase modifications which accompany the tachycardia [25].

The fifth possible cause is the coexistence of conduction anomalies such as left bundle branch block or the Wolf-Parkinson-White Syndrome which can render ST segment interpretation impossible. Left ventricular hypertrophy is another condition which can cause important problems. In this case an ST segment depression of 1 mm may not be a true expression of ischemia and one may be tempted to raise the threshold to 1.5 mm as suggested for the exercise tolerance test. Since this would cause a reduction in sensitivity, we feel that, even in patients with left ventricular hypertrophy, it is better to maintain the 1 mm threshold for ischemia even though this may reduce specificity.

An improvement in the performance of presently available monitors seems to have been achieved with the new EASI Monitoring System produced by The Hewlett Packard Company. This monitor employs 4 chest electrodes plus a grounding electrode attached to the thigh. The electrodes are applied as shown in Figure 1 and permit the simultaneous visualization of 12 leads as in the traditional ECG with the advantage of requiring only 5 electrodes instead of 10. Its advantages over traditional systems are evident: by monitoring 12 leads, the early diagnosis of ischemia as well as the recognition of complex arrhythmias are facilitated. Compared to the classic ECG, the EASI System is superior for continuous monitoring since the traditional ECG requires a greater number of electrodes and wires which can be cumbersome and cause interference and artefacts.

The EASI System offers a better signal to noise ratio, is appreciated by patients and operating room personnel because it has fewer electrodes and having fewer channels makes it easier to memorize the monitoring system. While a traditional 12 lead ECG requires 8 channels, the EASI system has only 3.

Another advanced system produced by Hewlett Packard is the MIDA system (Myocardial Ischemia Dynamic Analysis). This system uses 8 electrodes (Frank type) to allow the continuous online analysis of 12 leads with advanced features such as the elaboration of trends in many parameters such as QRS, ST, QT, R-R

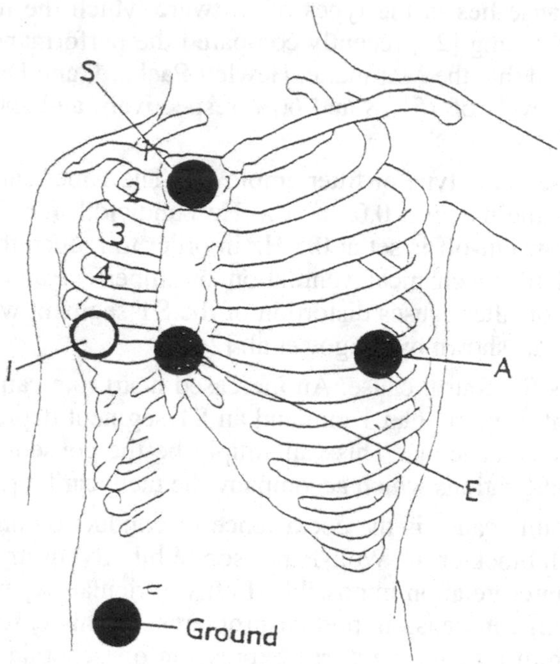

Fig. 1. Electrode placement for the "EASI monitoring system", which allows the 12 lead ECG continuous monitoring

interval, etc. The system also allows the operator to superimpose the present QRS-T complex and the baseline one in different colors so as to directly compare the curves over time.

From this discussion it should be evident that the ECG remains essential for the early diagnosis of ischemic events and that modern technology allows it to be used to its maximum by obtaining more continuous information than in the past.

We can state that the ECG signal elaborated by the current technologically advanced systems is the only truly useful instrument for the continuous monitoring of patients at risk for myocardial ischemia and/or arrhythmias in the perioperative period. Other methods such as TEE will never be able to be extended to large numbers of patients and therefore retain a marginal role (cardiac surgery patients, patients with bundle branch blocks, left ventricular hypertrophy and WPW syndrome where analysis of the ST segment and T waves is not reliable, and patients whose ECG leaves room for doubt). The percutaneous and transesophageal echocardiograms are very important diagnostic tests for ischemic heart disease but cannot be used for continuous monitoring in the perioperative period.

References

1. Garber MA, Solomon NA (1999) Cost effectiveness of alternative test strategies for the diagnosis of coronary artery disease. Ann Int Med 130:719-728
2. Palda VA, Detsky AS (1997) Perioperative assessment and management of risk from coronary artery disease. Ann Int Med 127:313-328
3. Daviglus ML, Liao Y, Greenland PG et al (1999) Association of nonspecific minor ST-T abnormalities with cardiovascular mortality. JAMA 281:530-536
4. Goldstein RE, Holmbar ES (1999) Prognostic indicators for coronary artery disease. Ready for the bedside? JAMA 281:565-566
5. Kemp HG, Eliott WC, Gorlin R (1967) The anginal syndrome with normal coronary arteriography. Trans Ass Am Physicians 80:50-70
6. Likoff W, Segal B, Kasparian H (1967) Paradox of normal selective coronary arteriograms in patients considered to have unmistakable coronary heart disease. N Eng J Med 276:1063-1066
7. Kemp HG (1973) Left ventricular function in patients with the anginal syndrome and normal coronary arteriograms. Am J Cardiol 32:375-376
8. Cannon RO, Boloban RS (2000) Chest pain in woman with normal coronary angiograms. N Eng J Med 342:885-886
9. Mehta RH, Eagle KA (2000) Missed diagnosis of acute coronary syndromes in the emergency rooms - Continuing challenges. N Eng J Med 342:1207-1209
10. Eisenberg M, Londo M, Leung J et al (1992) Monitoring for myocardial ischemia during noncardiac surgery: a technology assessment of transesophageal echocardiography and 12-lead electocardiography. JAMA 268:210-216
11. Van Boven AJ, Jukema JW, Crijns JGM et al (1995) Heart rate variability profiles in symptomatic coronary artery disease and preserved left ventricular function: relation to ventricular tachycardia and transient myocardial ischemia. Am Heart J 130:1020-1025
12. Cook JR, Bigger JT, Kleiger RE et al (1991) Effect of atenolol and diltiazem on heart period variability in normal persons. J Am Coll Cardiol 17:480-484
13. Jiunn Lee Lin, Hsiao Lung Chan, Chao Chen Du et al (1999) Long term Betablocker therapy improves automic nervous regulation in advanced congestive heart failure: a longitudinal heart rate variability study. Am Heart J 137:658-665
14. Raby KF, Brull SJ, Timimi F et al (1999) The effect of heart rate control in myocardial ischemia among high risk patients after vascular surgery. Anesth Analg 88:477-482
15. Mangano DT, SPI Research Group (1995) Preoperative assessment of the patient with cardiac disease. Curr Opin Cardiol 10:530-542
16. Mangano DT (1999) Assessment of the patient with cardiac disease. An anesthesiologic paradigm. Anesthesiology 91:1521-1526
17. Shaw LJ, Peterson ED, Shaw LK et al (1998) Use of prognostic treadmill score in identifying diagnostic coronary disease subgroups. Circulation 98:1622-1630
18. Mangano DT, Goldman L (1995) Preoperative assessment of patients with known or suspected coronary disease. N Eng J Med 333:1750-1756
19. Mangano DT, Hollenberg M, Fegert G et al (1991) Perioperative myocardial ischemia in patients undergoing noncardiac surgery: I. Incidence and severity during the 4 day perioperative period. The Study of Perioperative Ischemia (SPI) Research Group. J Am Coll Cardiol 17: 843-850
20. Mangano DT, Wong MG, London MJ et al (1991) Perioperative myocardial ischemia in patients undergoing noncardiac surgery: II. Incidence and severity during the 1st week after surgery. The Study of Perioperative Ischemia (SPI) Research Group. J Am Coll Cardiol 17: 851-857
21. Leung JM, Voskanian A, Bellows WH et al (1998) Automated electrocardiograph ST segment trending monitors: accuracy in detecting myocardial ischemia. Anesth Analg 87:4-10

22. Ellis JE, Shah MN, Briller JE et al (1992) A comparison of methods for the detection of myocardial ischemia detected during noncardiac surgery: Automated ST segment analysis system, electrocardiography and TEE. Anesth Analg 75:764-772
23. London MJ, Hollemberg M, Wong MG et al (1988) Intraoperative myocardial ischemia: localization by continuous 12 lead electrocardiography. Anesthesiology 69:232-241
24. Slogov S, Keats AS, David Y, Igo SR (1990) Incidence of perioperative myocardial ischemia detected by different electrocardiographic systems. Anesthesiology 73:1074-1081
25. Fleischer LA (2000) Real time intraoperative monitoring of myocardial ischemia in noncardiac surgery. Anesthesiology 92:1193-1288

Myocardial Contractility. Mechanism - Diagnosis - Therapy. Focus in General Anesthesia - Linked Problems

R. MUCHADA

Myocardial contractility is a cyclic phenomenon regulated by individual autonomous mechanisms. In each cycle, two defined phases, may be distinguished.

1. The systolic phase corresponding to the setting in tension of the myocardial fibers and their secondary stretch. This phase has as consequence the expulsion of a part of the blood volume contained in the ventricular cavities, denominated stroke volume (SV).
2. The diastolic phase, during which a progressive relaxation of the myocardial fibers takes place, allowing the filling, also progressive, of the ventricular cavities.

In the contraction phase as in the relaxation phase, the mechanical phenomena are manifested by precisely identifiable periods. During the systolic phase the isovolumetric contraction period is recognized (setting in tension of the fibres, without reduction in their length) and ejection period (expulsion of the SV, due to a rapid reduction of the length of the fibers). The diastolic phase is a proven period of isovolumetric relaxation, followed by the filling period, conditioned for the passive entry of blood in the ventricular cavities, completed by the secondary filling, made by the atrial contraction.

All these sequential mechanical modifications lead to three types of variations: 1) volume; 2) pressure; 3) timing. The appreciation and the measure of each either individually or together contribute to the evaluation of heart contractility and its organic or functional alterations.

All these modifications are the mechanical manifestation of biological phenomena that regulate myocardial contractility. The mechanisms of the myocardial contractile cycle can be described in the following way. The structure of the heart muscle allows easy inter-fibrillar communication, facilitating the ionic passage from one point to another of the muscular mass. During systole everything begins with the genesis of an action potential, generated in the sinus node, and driven by the specific fibers of the Purkinje's net. This action potential has some particular characteristics of its morphology and in its duration, which play an essential role in the activation of the transmembrane channels. In cardiac muscle, the action potential causes the opening of two types of channels: 1) the fast sodium channels; 2) another entire population of so-called slow calcium channels. This second population of channels differs from the fast sodium channels in being slower to open; but more important, they remain open for several tenths of a second. During this time, a large quantity of both calcium and sodium ions flows through these channels to the interior of the cardiac muscle fiber, and this maintains a prolonged period of depolarization, causing the plateau in the action potential. Furthermore, the calcium ions that enter the muscle during this action potential play an important role in helping to excite the muscle contractile process.

Immediately after the onset of the action potential, the permeability of the cardiac muscle membrane for potassium decreases about fivefold. This decreased potassium permeability may be caused by the excess calcium influx through the calcium channels just noted. Regardless of the cause, the decreased potassium permeability greatly decreases the outflow of potassium ions during the action potential plateau, and thereby prevents early return of the potential to its sting level. When the slow calcium-sodium channels do close, at the end of 200-300 ms and the influx of calcium and sodium ions ceases, the membrane permeability for potassium increases rapidly. This rapid loss of potassium from the fiber returns the membrane potential to its resting level, thus ending the action potential.

Following the action potential a phenomena called "excitation-contraction coupling" is produced. This is the mechanism by which the action potential causes the myofibrils of muscle to contract. When an action potential passes over the cardiac muscle membrane, it also spreads to the interior of the cardiac muscle fiber along the membranes of the transverse (T) tubules. The T tubule action potentials in turn act on the membranes of the longitudinal sarcoplasmic tubules to cause instantaneous release of calcium ions into the muscle sarcoplasm from the sarcoplasmic reticulum (SR). In another few thousandths of a second, these calcium ions diffuse into the myofibrils and catalyze the chemical reactions that promote sliding of the actin and myosin filaments along one another; this in turn produces the muscle contraction.

However, there is a second effect. In addition to the calcium ions released into the sarcoplasm from the cisternae of the SR, a large quantity of extra calcium ions diffuses into the sarcoplasm from the T tubules themselves at the time of the action potential. Indeed, without this extra calcium from the T tubules, the strength of cardiac muscle contraction would be considerably reduced because the SR of cardiac muscle is less well developed than that of skeletal muscle and does not store enough calcium to provide full contraction.

On the other hand, the T tubules of cardiac muscle have a diameter 5 times as great as that of the skeletal muscle tubules, which means a volume 25 times as great. Also, inside the T tubules is a large quantity of mucopolysaccharides that are electronegatively charged and bind an abundant store of even more calcium ions, keeping them always available for diffusion to the interior of the cardiac muscle fiber when the T tubule action potential occurs.

The strength of contraction of cardiac muscle depends to a great extent on the concentration of calcium ions in the extracellular fluids. The reason for this is that the ends of the T tubules open directly to the outside of the cardiac muscle fibers, allowing the same extracellular fluid that is in the cardiac muscle interstitium to percolate through the T tubules as well. Consequently, the quantity of calcium ions in the T tubule system, i.e., the availability of calcium ions to cause cardiac muscle contraction, depends to a great extent on the extracellular fluid calcium ion concentration [1].

The activation of slow sodium-calcium channels is determined by cAMP via phosphorylation regulated for the B 1 receptors by adenyl cyclase – ATP way. Relaxation is mediated predominantly by the uptake of calcium into the SR by the SR calcium ATPase pump (SERCA2). Phospholamban and its state of phosphorylation regulate the activity of SERCA2. Stimulation of the β-adrenergic receptor cascade leads to phosphorylation of phospholamban [2] and subsequent relief of the inhibition of SERCA2. Therefore, the phospholamban/SERCA2 interaction controls the calcium content of the SR and ultimately cardiac contractility.

At the end of the plateau of the cardiac action potential, the influx of calcium ions to the interior of the muscle fiber is suddenly cut off. The cAMP is inactivated to AMP via phosphodiesterase III [3]. The calcium ions in the sarcoplasm are rapidly pumped back into both the SR and the T tubules. As a result, the contraction ceases until a new action potential occurs [4, 5].

Diagnostic methods

The investigation of the biocellular stages of myocardial contraction is outside the scope of the anaesthetist, in the pre-anesthetic period, during general anesthesia, or in the follow-up post-anesthetic period. However, basic knowledge of these mechanisms can aid therapeutic selection, once the clinical diagnosis has been made.

During general anesthesia, the anesthetist can be confronted with two different situations: 1) a patient without myocardial pathology but presenting elements of decreased heart contractility; the recognition of this situation could be made using information from standard monitoring and from clinical evaluation of the situation; frequently it is not diagnosed; the patient will suffer the consequences of the missed Diagnosis; other times the diagnosis is made belatedly, due to insufficient information of the basic monitoring or erroneous interpretation of the clinical facts, leading to late detection, only when the compensatory stages have been bypassed and the patient is in a poor condition; 2) a patient with a contractility failure preceding the general anesthesia which is aggravated by the anesthetic act. In this case the delay in the diagnosis and treatment could be fatal or allow only a slow and progressive recovery, with risks of functional or organic sequelae; in both situations the fundamental problem is one of diagnosis of the altered contractility, to allow therapeutic selection, based on the fundamental knowledge of the mechanisms that regulate the contractility.

During the general anesthesia, most of the symptoms are hidden behind the action of the used products, the controlled ventilation, and by the difficulty in access for a clinical evaluation. For these reasons the monitoring data allowing the appreciation of the quality of the myocardial contractility are fundamentals.

Systolic period

Historically, the invasive methods provided interesting information, even if the practical difficulties reserved their use for a minority of patients. They evaluated the contractility by the measurement of the derived intraventricular pressure in relation to the necessary time to arrive at the maximum pressure, Dp/Dt, and (Dp/Dt)/Pt max (where Pt is the corresponding total pressure).

It is necessary to point out that these indexes are influenced by the pre- and the after-load conditions, reasons why their interpretation was difficult if these two conditions did not remain stable. Other indexes involving tele-systolic pressure/tele systolic volume ratio (PTS/VTS) were proposed to allow an evaluation of contractility independent of the load conditions [6].

However, the progressive introduction of ultrasound methods has allowed elimination of the risks imposed by the invasive methods, facilitating the studies, and enlarging the fields of application. The frequent use of echocardio graphic methods, mainly the transesophageal echocardiography (TEE), has contributed to real progress in the evaluation of the contractile function of the left ventricle [7]. The possibility of detecting morphological changes of the ventricle cavities, the synergy of the contraction, the reduction fraction, and the ejection fraction have made this the method of choice for the diagnosis of per myocardial contractility alterations during anesthesia.

However, there are some practice difficulties for the widespread application during general anesthesia. It is fundamentally a diagnostic method, not allowing the monitoring for long periods, as is necessary in certain long-duration general anesthesia with sudden changes, determined by the patient's individual reaction or surgical interference. The cost of TEE equipment is relatively high; the complexity of obtaining the signals and their interpretation needs a precise technique, based on specific method and experience, acquired in the clinical field; finally the introduction of some hypothetical elements and the subjective interpretation mean, even today, that this technique is reserved for a limited number of patients and used by a select body of professionals, trained in such a method.

Undoubtedly in the future, the miniaturization of the equipment, the improvement of the software, and the automation of the reconstruction of the signals will lead to a much more-wide application and allow objective interpretation of the obtained data.

While we wait the arrival of this new generation of systems, what do we have nowadays for the evaluation of myocardial contractility during anesthesia?

The data of standard monitoring (heart rate, ECG, arterial pressure, and central venous pressure) do not contribute any direct information on contractility. Swans Ganz's catheter and the thermodilution measurements also do not yield objective and direct data relative to contractility.

The systolic time intervals (STI) can partially solve the problem, since all the obtained information refers to the left ventricle and only to the systolic phase. Although the inconveniences of the methodology have been largely overcome by the technique proposed by our team [8], it is necessary to recognize that the brevity of the times on which the STI are measured makes extreme precision necessary. This precision can be obtained only when all the constants of time of the devices implied in the measure are known and integrated in the monitoring system.

The STI has the advantage of being easily and objectively measured, with a non-invasive technique, with data obtained, practically, in real time. The follow-up over long periods is possible. When they are integrated into a hemodynamic profile, they facilitate choice of therapy, the observation of the patient contractility modification status, the adjustment of the used product doses, and reconsideration of the initial treatment decision.

Two main component integrate the STI, the pre-ejection period (PEPi) and the left ventricle ejection time (LVETi). The first is, without a doubt, the more interesting for left ventricle contractility evaluation. The PEPi represents the time necessary to achieve the left intraventricular pressure at a level sufficient to open the aortic valve. It is therefore a parameter generated in the isovolumetric period of the contraction. Its duration is influenced by: 1) the contractility; 2) the diastolic arterial pressure (DAP); 3) the pre-load. Of these three parameters the second and the third can be evaluated with a simple hemodynamic monitoring system. When the pre-load is supposed correct and when the DAP remains stable, any change in the PEPi implies a modification of the contractility. Its augmentation indicates a need for a decrease of the contractility. Its reduction indicates a need for an improvement of the contractility.

But once again the anesthetist needs to integrate these data in as complete as possible a hemodynamic profile, to interpret the variations correctly. This includes ultrasound Doppler monitoring and other parameters that have been presented as useful to evaluate myocardial contractility.

The maximum peak aortic blood acceleration and its variations have been and are still used by some authors [9], as an index of the contractility status. However, it is necessary to remember that this parameter is measured once the aortic valve has been opened by the intraventricular pressure. As a consequence, its modifications do not only depend on the contraction of the left ventricle and the pre-load, but also on the after-load, the aortic compliance, the μ factor (blood viscosity), the mean intra-thoracic pressure, the vascular impedance, etc. Therefore, its variations depend on many factors and are much more complex to interpret than the PEPi variations.

However, it is necessary to recognize that the PEPi and sequential and continuous measurements of the peak of aortic blood acceleration, integrated in a hemodynamic profile, could have real interest for the identification of syndromes with contractility alteration during the systolic phase.

How can the anaesthetist recognize and diagnose a relaxation alteration in the diastolic period? The fundamental resource is at present TEE. All the other data from standard monitoring or other ultrasound information are only orientation indexes, which should be integrated in a clinical context. The tachycardia, the hyperkinetic syndromes, the PEPi reduction with increase of the maximum acceleration and without suspicion of hypovolemia are elements that could be taken into account, but are not absolute indicative measures of diastolic relaxation problems.

Interest in diagnosing altered myocardial contractility during the general anesthesia

All the narcotics used for the induction or the maintenance of general anesthesia cause a contractility myocardial depression.The effects of halogenated anesthetics on the myocardium have been studied extensively in vivo and in vitro in various animal species. During recent years, considerable knowledge has been obtained by new investigative methodologies, including molecular and cellular biology and animal models of disease. Important interactions of halogenated anesthetics with pharmacological agents on the myocardium have also been recently emphasized [10, 11], leading to a better knowledge of their effects on signal transduction.

Hanouz et al. [12] made an important contribution to our knowledge of the myocardial effects of halogenated anesthetics, using isolated atrial trabeculae fibers in isometric conditions, allowing comparison of the inotropic effects of the four main halogenated anesthetics (halothane, isoflurane, sevoflurane, and desflurane).

This study provides important information on the *negative inotropic* effect of halogenated anesthetics (halothane > sevoflurane, isoflurane > desflurane), confirming the previous results obtained in various animal species. These results also suggest that species differences in the myocardial effects are less important for halogenated anesthetics than for intravenous anesthetics.

Investigating desflurane action it was found that it may release intra-myocardial catecholamine stores in human myocardium. This effect explains why desflurane induces a *less-pronounced* negative inotropic effect compared with other halogenated anesthetics and probably contributes to the preserved hemodynamic conditions. However, this effect deserves further study to elucidate the origin of these catecholamines (nerve endings of extracardiac neurons, intrinsic cardiac neurons, non-neuronal adrenergic cardiac cells) and, overall, the beneficial or deleterious consequences of this release in healthy and diseased myocardium. Indeed, intra-myocardial catecholamines play a role in the maintenance of cardiac function and may interfere with ischemic preconditioning. The diastolic period is affected principally by halothane (negative lusiotropic action).

Another study [13] performed in animals leads to nearly the same conclusions concerning the decreased contractility effects of the volatile anesthetics, even if the myocardial contractility failure can be dissimulated by a decreased afterload in the whole organism.

The effect of intravenous anesthetics the contractility in vitro of human myocardium fibers has been described [14]. Propofol, thiopental, midazolam, etomidate, and ketamine induce a dose-dependent myocardial decreased contractility. With the current clinical doses this action is very weak for midazolam, etomidate, and propofol, and stronger for thiopental and ketamine. Even the morphinomimetic drugs, alone or associated with some other narcotic products, may have a depressive myocardial contractility action [15-17].

The explanation of this depressant action of practically all the inhaled and intravenous anesthetics is not yet very clear. It could be explained by interference with the myocardial endoplasmic reticule and its ionic reception/liberation, affecting myocardial contractility. This interference could be the result of a decrease of circulating endogenous cathecholamines, or of a decrease of the myocardial B1 receptor sensitivity to the actions of the cathecholamines, or of a functional and momentary reduction of the number of available receptors [18].

Treatment of decreased myocardial contractility

Knowing the depressive actions of general anesthesia on myocardial contractility and using the diagnostic and clinical evaluation and the data of an appropriate monitoring system, the anesthetist will be able to plan and to execute a therapeutic action, to quickly correct the anomaly.

The medications to be used should respond, in general, to the following premises: 1) introduced in an intravenous way; 2) administration in bolus and/or in continuous perfusion; 3) not aggressive for the peripheral veins; 4) immediate action; 5) short half-life (less than 10 min); 6) quick reversible action, spontaneously or with specific antidotes.

Considering these imperatives, the products are few that the anesthetist has at his disposal to treat altered contractility. From the pathophysiological point of view, we should consider two possibilities: 1) treatment of the decreased contractility; 2) treatment of an excess of the same one, leading to a hyperkinetic syndrome with dysfunction in the diastolic phase. A third eventuality could be considered that is represented by an alteration of the coronary perfusion, leading to a flaw of the contractility. The coronary flow can be functionally altered, during general anesthesia by an excessive decrease of the diastolic period (noxious tachycardia), a fall of the DAP (inferior limits tolerated 40 mmHg), with an alteration of the relationship DAP/HR, or even a diastolic "tetanization" of the myocardium (negative lusiotropic effect) committing the diastolic ventricular function.

In the first case, keeping in mind the depressive mechanisms of the general anesthetics, the common specific way is the use of beta-stimulant products. The product of choice, is, in our experience, Dobutamina. Used in perfusion in a specific venous way, the dose is individually variable. The administration of a 4 μg/kg per min can, in most cases, help to recover a diminished contractility, under general anesthesia. But an appropriate guide is to adapt the dose to bring the PEPi near to their normal value (135 ± 5 ms), without causing a tachycardia superior to 90 beats/min but producing a sensitive increase of the SV.

Another therapeutic option is the use of inhibitors of the phosphodiesterase III, which exercise a positive inotropic action due to the increase of cAMP, independent from the $beta_1$-receptors. However the vasodilator actions of these products (amrinona, enoximone can produce the desired result [19, 20]. In the second case, beta-blockers can be useful, mainly esmolol, for its specific pharmacodynamic characteristic [21, 22]. In the third case a vasoconstrictor-type alpha 1 can correct the alteration in the event of a decrease of DAP below 40 mmHg. To increase the diastolic time, reducing the heart rate, the esmolol is useful to re-establish a DAP/HR superior at 0.7.

Conclusion

At present everybody knows that general anesthetics have a potentially depressive action on myocardial contractility. Although the diagnosis of this alteration during anesthesia is imperfect, available methods allow us a better understanding and identification of the question. Myocardial contractility is one component of cardiovascular function that assures cellular metabolism and even the individual's life. Its alterations should be recognized and quickly treated to avoid the cellular metabolic problems with functional or organic consequences. To achieve these objectives, progress in technical monitoring is necessary and a change of anesthetic attitude, in the pathophysiological analysis of these problems, to open up and bring into routine application new therapeutic options.

References

1. Morgan IP (1991) Abnormal intracellular modulation of calcium as a major cause of cardiac contractile dysfunction. N Engl J Med 325:625-632
2. Koss KL, Kranias EG (1996) Phospholamban: a prominent regulator of myocardial contractility. Circ Res 79:1059-1063
3. Vittone L, Grassi A, Chiappe L et al (1981) Relaxing effect of pharmacological intervention increasing CAMP in the rat heart. Am J Physiol 240:H441-447
4. Brutsaert DL, Sys SU (1989) Relaxation and diastole of the heart. Physiol Rev 69:1228-1315
5. Chemla D, Lecarpentier Y, Martin JL et al (1986) Relationship between inotropy and relaxation in rat myocardium. Am J Physiol 250:H1008-1016
6. Merillon JP, Motté G, Lecarpantier Y et al (1977) Le rapport pression-volume télèsystolique ventriculaire gauche. Arch Mal Cœur 10:1013-1020
7. Shanewise JS, Cheung AT, Aronson S et al (1999) ASE/SCA guidelines for performing a comprehensive intraoperative multiplane transesophageal echocardiography examination: recommendation of the american society of Echocardiography and Society of Cardiovascular Task Force for Certification in Perioperative Transesophageal Echocardiography. Anesth Analg 89:870-884
8. Tournadre JP, Muchada R, Lansiaux S et al (1999) Measurement of systolic time intervals using a transeosphageal pulsed echo Doppler. Br J Anaesth 83:630-636
9. Stein PD, Sabbah HN (1976) Ventricular performance measured during ejection. Studies in patients of the rate of change of ventricular power. Am Heart 91:599-604
10. Hanouz JL, Vivien B, Gueugniaud PY et al (1998) Comparison of the effects of sevoflurane, isoflurane, and halothane on rat myocardium. Br J Anaesth 80:621-627
11. Gueugniaud PY, Hanouz JL, Vivien B et al (1997) Effects of desflurane in rat myocardium. Comparison with isoflurane and halothane. Anesthesiolgy 87:599-609
12. Hanouz JL, Massetti M, Guesne G et al (2000) In vitro, effect of desflurane, sevoflurane, isoflurane and halothane in isoleted human right atria. Anesthesiology 92:116-124
13. Hettrick DA, Pagel PS, Wariter C (1996) Desflurane, sevoflurane and isoflurane impair canine left ventricular-arterial coupling and mechanical efficiency. Anesthesiology 85:403-413
14. Gelissen HPMM, Epema AH, Henning RH et al (1996) Inotropic effects of propofol, thiopental, midazolam, etomidate, and ketamine on isolated human atrial muscle. Anesthesiology 84:397-403
15. Wong KC, Martin WE, Hornbein TF et al (1973) The cardiovascular effects of morphine sulfate with oxygen and without nitrous oxide in man. Anesthesiology 38:542-549
16. Kazmaier S, Hanekop G-G, Buhre W et al (2000) Myocardial consquences of remifentanil in patients with coronary artery disease. Br J Anaesth 578-583
17. Camu F, Royston D (1999) Inpatient experience with remifentanil. Anesth Analg 89:S15-21
18. Rusy BF, Kornai H (1987) Anesthetic depression of myocardial contractility: a review of possible mechanisms. Anesthesiology 67:745-766
19. Mancini D, Lejemtel T, Sonnenblick E (1985) Intravenus use of amrinone for the treatment of the failing heart. Am J Cardiol 56:8B-15B
20. Pagel PS, Hettrick DA, Warliter DC (1993) Amrinone enhances myocardial contractility and improves left ventricule diastolic function in conscious and anesthethetized chronically instrumented dogs. Anesthesiology 79:753-765
21. Nagatsu M, Spinale FG, Koide M et al (2000) Bradycardia and the role of B-blockade in the amelioration of left ventricular dysfunction. Circulation 101:653-659
22. Bristow MR (2000) B adrenergic receptor blockade in chronic heart failure. Circulation 101: 558-559

Hypocynetic and Hypercynetic Arrhythmias: Diagnosis, Management, Prevention

A.S. Montenero, D. Mangiameli, P. Franciosa

Arrhythmias arise through three potential mechanisms: 1) disorders of impulse formation, 2) disorders of impulse conduction, and 3) mixed disorders.

Disorders of impulse formation

Sinus node dysfunction or "sick sinus syndrome" includes various cardiac arrhythmias that have been classified in many ways. Sinoatrial disturbances associated with sinus node dysfunction include symptomatic sinus bradycardia, sinus arrest, sinoatrial block, and paroxysmal supraventricular tachycardia alternating with periods of bradycardia or even asystole. The definition of bradycardia varies from institution to institution, but it generally includes a rate less than 40-50 beats/min.

In sinus node dysfunction, symptoms should be correlated with the specific arrhythmia. However, many patients who have episodes of both tachycardia and bradycardia are often asymptomatic, while others are so symptomatic to require medication to treat the episodes of tachycardia. Meanwhile, the treatment of tachycardia exacerbates the tendency toward bradycardia. In most of these patients permanent pacing should be considered as treatment, either alone or in combination with antiarrhythmic drugs.

Disorders of impulse conduction

AV block is defined as an impairment of conduction from the atrium to and within the specialized conducting tissue of the ventricular septum, resulting in a complex variety of clinical and electrocardiographic (ECG) findings. AV block is traditionally classified into first-degree, second-degree, or third-degree (or complete heart block). It can be defined anatomically as occurring at a supra-Hisian, intra-Hisian, or infra-Hisian location. More specifically, if the patient has a QRS complex, there is a greater probability that the conduction disturbance is infra-Hisian.

Patients with abnormal AV conduction may be asymptomatic or may experience severe symptoms related to profound bradycardia or ventricular arrhythmias. Indications for permanent pacing in acquired AV block are listed in Table 1.

Table 1.

Necessary	Probably necessary	Probably not necessary
Symptomatic complete AV block intermittent or permanent	Asymptomatic complete AV block at any sites, permanent or intermittent	First-degree AV block
Second-degree AV block of any type associated with symptoms due to bradycardia	Asymptomatic Mobitz II, second-degree AV block	Asymptomatic Mobitz I, second-degree AV block
	Congenital complete AV block	

Indications for permanent pacing after myocardial infarction (MI) in patients experiencing AV block are related in large measure to the presence of intraventricular conduction defects. The requirement for temporary pacing in acute MI does not necessarily constitute an indication for permanent pacing, while the need for permanent pacing does not necessarily depend on the presence of symptoms. Indications for permanent pacing in post-MI AV block are listed in Table 2.

Table 2.

Necessary	Probably necessary	Probably not necessary
Mobitz II or complete AV block (symptomatic or asymptomatic)	New right bundle branch block with new left-axis deviation	First-degree AV block
Bilateral bundle-branch block	Left-anterior or left-posterior hemiblock alone	Asymptomatic Mobitz I AV block in inferior MI
Symptomatic bradyarrhythmias of any origin or mechanism	Transient bifascicular block	Asymptomatic or transient sinus or AV junctional (nodal) delay
	Tachycardia/bradycardia syndrome	Acquired new asymptomatic bradyarrhythmias
		Right bundle branch block

Trifascicular heart block causing symptoms is associated with a high mortality and a significant incidence of sudden death. Syncope or increased incidence of sudden death are uncommon in patients with bifascicular block. Thus, being unable to define the cause of syncope in the presence of bifascicular or trifascicular block, it appears reasonable to assume that the syncope may be due to transient complete AV block and therefore prophylactic permanent pacing is indicated. In symptomatic patients with syncope or near-syncope, an HV interval of 100 ms or greater is generally an accepted indication for permanent pacing. Indication for permanent pacing in bifascicular and trifascicular block are listed in Table 3.

Table 3.

Necessary	Probably necessary	Probably not necessary
Bifascicular block with intermittent complete AV block associated with symptomatic bradyarrhythmias	Bifascicular or trifascicular block with intermittent Mobitz II AV block without symptoms	Fascicular blocks without AV block or symptoms
Bifascicular block with intermittent Mobitz II AV block with symptoms attributable to the AV block	Bifascicular or trifascicular block with syncope thought to be due to bradyarrhythmias	Fascicular blocks with first degree AV block without symptoms

Mixed disorders

These include supraventricular and ventricular arrhythmias. The term "supraventricular arrhythmia" refers to several groups of abnormal rhythms ranging from permanent atrial fibrillation to paroxysmal sinus-tachycardia due to re-entry within the sinus node. Although supraventricular tachycardia can be broadly defined as any tachycardia requiring the atrium or the AV node, either in whole or in part, for its perpetuation, more-specific definitions will be provided for each of the common supraventricular arrhythmias. The atrial arrhythmias vary considerably in their rate and regularity, their clinical manifestations, and the setting in which they occur. These rhythms are abrupt in onset and termination, and are often seen in patients who do not have evidence of organic heart disease. In the majority of cases these arrhythmias are generally benign, but sometimes they can result in significant hemodynamic compromise. Some patients with Wolff-Parkinson-Withe (WPW) syndrome can be at risk of sudden death. Two major groups are included in the broad classification of supraventricular arrhythmias: the first includes all atrial and AV tachycardias, the second includes atrial flutter and atrial fibrillation.

Supraventricular tachycardia is defined electrocardiographically as a regular tachycardia of 140-240 beats/min during which the QRS is of normal duration unless bundle branch block or ventricular pre-excitation are present.

The term supraventricular tachycardia is generally used to describe any paroxysmal atrial or AV tachycardia that matches the above-mentioned ECG definition. When P waves are identifiable, the P wave morphology is often different from sinus P wave morphology, and the P wave may precede, coincide with, or follow the QRS complex. These does not include atrial flutter which, although a regular tachycardia, does not match these criteria.

Clinically supraventricular tachycardia is characterized by the sudden onset of a rapid, regular heart rate with termination that is equally abrupt. Symptoms depend on absence or presence of associated clinical problems. Usually palpitations greatly contribute to patient discomfort. Objectives of the evaluation of supraventricular tachycardia are first to confirm the presence of and determine the mechanism for an arrhythmia and whether or not this is related to any precipitating factors that might be important in treatment. Another objective is to determine the functional consequences of the arrhythmia as pre-syncope or syncope, fatigue, dyspnea, or chest pain. These aspects of the patient's clinical history will largely determine the extent and sequence of special diagnostic studies, including electrophysiological studies. Moreover, the frequency of arrhythmia is important in deciding the management; i.e., catheter ablation.

Clearly the most-important diagnostic test in the evaluation of these patients is an ECG recording during the tachycardia. For optimal rhythm analysis of ECGs, extreme care should be taken to record distinct atrial and ventricular activity with a 12-lead recording, and a long strip should be obtained.

Physiological maneuvers used in association with an ECG recording (i.e., carotid artery massage) increase vagal tone and influence the AV node by prolonging AV nodal conduction and refractoriness, thereby facilitating the recognition of P waves that were not previously apparent or stopping tachycardia. However, carotid artery massage has a all-or-none effect, either terminating or changing little or not at all, on supraventricular tachycardia due to an AV nodal re-entry or an accessory pathway.

Adenosine may be useful in differentiating an arrhythmia with 2:1 AV conduction from supraventricular tachycardia and sinus tachycardia. Most supraventricular tachycardias in which the AV node is a critical part of re-entrant circuit are terminated by an i.v. infusion of adenosine. Atrial flutter can be recognized because adenosine creates transient heart block and flutter becomes obvious. Adenosine may terminate supraventricular tachycardia, especially AV nodal re-entry tachycardia.

Identification of P waves during an episode of tachycardia with aberrant ventricular conduction is important to differentiate from ventricular tachycardia. When surface recordings, including special leads orientation, fail to provide clear records of P waves, esophageal recording should be considered. Bipolar electrodes can be placed in the esophagus so that they lie just behind the left atrium. If esophageal electrode recordings fail to help in the diagnosis of supraventricular tachycardia, the use of more-invasive ECG recording techniques will be necessary.

The electrophysiological evaluation (EFH) of supraventricular tachycardia involves recording electrograms from the right atrium, right ventricle, region of His bundle, and coronary sinus during programmed stimulation and during tachycardia. The goals of EFH are to determine the mechanism of the tachycardia, its site of origin, the tissues used to sustain the tachycardia, and the potential benefit of alternative therapeutic approaches, including antiarrhythmic drugs, antitachycardia pacing system, catheter ablation, and surgery. EFHs are indicated for patients who have significant symptoms associated with supraventricular tachycardia, including pre-syncope and syncope; patients with pre-excitation syndromes and those with AV nodal re-entry tachycardia, patients with refractory atrial ectopic tachycardia and atrial flutter.

Advances in the pharmacology of the arrhythmia drugs and refinements in catheter ablation techniques have considerably altered our ability to treat arrhythmias. Successful treatment of supraventricular arrhythmias requires that the physician be knowledgeable of the mechanism and cause of the arrhythmia, the natural history, and the various therapies available. Currently pharmacological therapy is no longer the first choice for treating supraventricular tachycardia, catheter ablation being the gold standard.

Treatment of supraventricular arrhythmias depends first on a careful diagnosis, which can be accomplished by recording standard ECG, 24-h Holter recording, or transtelephonic monitoring system. A careful search should be made for the other possible factors that may aggravate the arrhythmia. Electrolyte imbalance, acid-base disturbance, anemia, drug intoxication or other drug effect, diseases of the heart or lungs, or even central system abnormalities should be sought and corrected if possible.

The development of radiofrequency catheter ablation has greatly changed the field of the electrophysiològy and eliminated the potential risk of lifelong antiarrhythmic drug treatment thereby cutting expenses.

Acute supraventricular tachycardia with narrow QRS complex is a common arrhythmia, which usually causes symptoms even in normal patients. Vagal maneuvers can be attempted initially, if they fail the acute treatment should involve i.v. administration of adenosine or verapamil. Adenosine causes slowing and block in the AV node and the advantage is that the adenosine has a very short half-life and does not have the tendency to cause hypotension or negative inotropic effect. When a WPW syndrome is suspected, an i.v. administration of propaphenone or flecainide may be more efficacious, because these selectively prolong refractoriness in the accessory pathway.

Atrial flutter is an important yet relatively uncommon cardiac arrhythmia that is seen in pediatric practice but is, however, more common in adults. Atrial flutter is due to a single macrore-entrant circuit contained within the right atrium. To contain such a circuit within the atrium, an area of slowed conduction is necessary. This is classically in the isthmus between the coronary sinus orifice, the tricuspid annulus, and the inferior vena cava. Several subtypes of atrial flutter are recognized. Common or type I atrial flutter occurs when activation around the macrore-entrant circuit is cranio-caudal down the right atrial free wall traversing the isthmus of slowed conduction to complete the circuit by caudo-cranial activation of the inter-atrial septum. In type II or uncommon atrial flutter, activation is in the reverse direction, although this is usually a faster arrhythmia. The ECG shows regular atrial activity with a cycle length typically around 200 ms. The ventricular response may be regular or irregular. In the regular response there is a fixed mathematical relationship between the flutter waves and the resulting QRS complexes; 2:1 and 3:1 AV conduction is common. Sometimes there is a variable ventricular response rate. Exceptionally, there may be 1:1 AV conduction; in this circumstance very rapid ventricular rates are possible, with concomitant hemodynamic collapse and a potential threat to life. Atrial flutter is often a primary arrhythmia with no evidence of associated cardiovascular disease. As such the prognosis is good, although with repeated events, perhaps through deleterious atrial electrical and mechanical remodelling, atrial fibrillation may develop.

The large macrore-entrant circuit is remarkably resilient, so any interventions that interrupt the circuit must dramatically alter conduction and/or refractoriness. To terminate the arrhythmia, the class IC drugs propafenone and flecainide are probably best. They may operate by further slowing of conduction in the isthmus area, perhaps even to the point of creating a block. In the initial stages of loading with these agents, there is a risk of slowing the atrial flutter rate and, paradoxically, increasing the ventricular response through a change of AV conduction ratio. A recent development is the introduction of ibutilide. Given i.v., this agent offers a higher drug reversion rate than any other; its drawback is a risk of torsades de pointes although when used in hospital, this is unlikely to be fatal. A new therapeutic approach is RF ablation that offers at present primary success rates of more than 85%.

Patients who have an accessory pathway (AP) of AV conduction may develop circus movement tachycardia, otherwise known as atrioventricular re-entrant tachycardia (AVRT). Orthodromic AVRT is the most-common form. It occurs as a result of antegrade conduction through the normal AV conduction system and retrograde conduction to the atria via the AP. Less commonly, conduction occurs in the opposite direction resulting in antidromic AVRT. Tachycardia may also involve multiple APs, which may provide both antegrade and retrograde conduction and may alternate antegradely or retrogradely.

The normal atrioventricular annulus is composed exclusively of electrically inert fibrous tissue, with the AV node/His bundle acting as the sole route of electrical conduction between the atria and ventricles. Accessory AV pathways represent the developmental abnormalities of the AV ring and consist histologically of small fibers resembling normal myocardium, which can act as pathway of conduction. Pathways occur anywhere along the AV ring and are described as being 'left-sided, right-sided, or septal', and 'anterior, posterior, or lateral (or free wall)' in location. Left free wall pathways are the most frequent, followed by posteroseptal pathways. Right-sided APs are frequently subendocardial, while left-sided pathways commonly pass obliquely on the epicardial aspect of the annulus fibrosus in close proximity to the coronary sinus and great cardiac vein. The incidence of APs in the general population is 0.1-0.3% and is 3.4% in first-degree relatives of patients with pre-excitation. The incidence of APs is twice as frequent in males as in females.

When accessory pathways conduct antegradely, the QRS complex during sinus rhythm is the result of fusion between conduction over the AP and the normal AV conduction system. Such APs are termed 'manifest' and result in classic ECG appearances of the WPW syndrome (PR < 0.12 s, delta wave and a widened QRS). In certain patients with antegradely conducting APs, pre-excitation may not be obvious on the ECG. These 'latent' APs occur when ventricular activation through the normal AV conduction system predominates, as when the AP is located relatively far from the sinus node or when conduction through the AP is relatively slow. In some cases, APs are not capable of antegrade conduction and AP is said to be 'concealed' since pre-excitation is not present on the ECG. The majority of APs, like normal myocardium, display non-decremental electrophysiological properties, with no slowing of conduction in response to incremental rates of stimulation. APs usually have conduction velocities that are significantly faster than those of the normal AV conduction tissue. The prerequisites for the initiation of a re-entrant arrhythmia are an area of unidirectional conduction block and an area of slow conduction. Perpetuation of such a re-entrant circuit requires that the refractory period of any part of part of the circuit must be shorter than the tachycardia cycle length.

Since the normal AV conduction system is an integral part of the tachycardia circuit in AVRT (except in the unusual circumstance of pre-excited tachycardia using APs as both limbs of the circuit), AV nodal block will result in termination of tachycardia. This may be achieved by physiological maneuvers that increase vagal tone, such as the Valsalva maneuvers or carotid massage. AV block may also be achieved with use of pharmacological agents such as adenosine, calcium channel blockers, and beta-blockers. Both adenosine and verapamil may decrease the ERP of APs and thus may increase the ventricular rate during pre-excited AF. Termination of AVRT may also be achieved by influencing AP conduction characteristics with the use of antiarrhythmic such as class IA (disopyramide and procainamide) and class IC (propafenone and flecainide) drugs. However, termination is not as reliable with these agents as with adenosine. Rapid AF in patients with pre-excitation should be managed with DC cardioversion if the patient is compromised.

Catheter-based techniques can now permanently abolish the substrate for AVRT, with long-term success and low complication rates. Long-term drug therapy is generally not recommended for their pro-arrhythmic effects.

Ventricular arrhythmias occur in a wide variety of patients, ranging from the asymptomatic with an occasional premature ventricular complex (PVC) to the patient with malignant ventricular tachycardia associated with poor left ventricular function. This variability among patients makes the treatment of ventricular arrhythmia challenging and, at times, frustrating. The physician must decide whether a patient's rhythm disturbance warrants treatment on the basis of the degree of symptoms and the relative risk the patient has of experiencing significant complications, including sudden death. Whenever the patient need treatment, it should be carefully determined, since all antiarrhythmic drugs can worsen ventricular arrhythmia and facilitate ventricular tachycardia and sudden death.

The most-common mechanism of formation of ventricular arrhythmia is re-entry and the most-common source of re-entrant PVCs is found in the setting of myocardial ischemia. In an ischemic myocardium, the impulse encounters myocardial fibers that are functionally dissociated with regard to their conductive characteristics. This allows slow conduction of an impulse to occur with the ability to excite myocardium that is no longer refractory and to initiate a re-entrant arrhythmia.

Abnormal automaticity may be considered to explain other forms of idiopathic ventricular arrhythmia that usually arise from the right ventricular outflow tract. Ventricular tachycardia (VT) is a difficult clinical problem for the physician. The evaluation and treatment of such rhythm disturbances are complicated by the fact that it often occurs in life-threatening situations that dictate rapid diagnosis and therapy.

VT is due to abnormal impulses originating from areas of specialized conduction system or ventricular myocardium that are distal to the bundle of His. It is defined as three or more consecutive ectopic complexes with a rate of 100-250 beats/min. The ability of patients to tolerate an episode of VT generally depends on the rate of the tachycardia and the state of the patient's cardiovascular system. It is critically important, yet often difficult, to differentiate supraventricular tachycardia with aberrance from VT. On the ECG these arrhythmias have similar rates (100-250 beats/min), but commonly VT has AV dissociation, superior QRS axis, QRS with exceeding 140 ms, monophasic or biphasic right bundle branch block-shaped QRS complex in V1, and complexes with QR or QS in V6 with a left bundle-branch morphology. Recording atrial activity with a bipolar recording lead placed in the esophagus can often identify AV dissociation that was not apparent on the surface ECG.

With the advent of programmed stimulation, it has become possible to induce and terminate tachycardia by pacing techniques. Such techniques have improved our understanding of VT and have made the approach to therapy more rational. Therefore, EFH should be performed in patients who have serious, life-threatening ventricular arrhythmia because this form of evaluation provides an objective basis for the rational choice of therapy that may include drugs, pacing, catheter ablation, or an AICD.

Treatment of VT is a challenging problem and depends on many variables including the clinical setting in which VT arises, the left ventricular function, and associated cardiovascular and non-cardiovascular diseases.

Post-MI VT represent the more-difficult arrhythmia to be treated and left ventricular function is the most-important factor to be analyzed before starting any therapy. Today all patients with an EF < 25% should be referred to an AICD implantation; catheter ablation might be considered for patients with good ventricular function and single inducible monomorphic VT.

A novel approach to the diagnosis and treatment of atrial fibrillation

Atrial fibrillation (AF) is the most-common arrhythmia in clinical practice and exacts a huge social and economic cost; the medical community have been engaged in an intensive search for more effective means of treating AF.

The mortality risk in patients with AF has been reported to be twice as high as that in controls, and stroke is the most-important cause of death, occurring in up to 30% of patients aged 80-89 years and in up of 15% patients aged 50-59 years. Even in the absence of clinically apparent stroke, patients with AF, including those with lone AF, have a high incidence of silent cerebral infarction on computed tomographic scanning of the brain.

Therefore, valuable results have emerged that relate not only to an effective non-pharmacological treatment of AF, but also to an understanding of the main pathophysiological mechanism involved in the initiation and persistence of the arrhythmia.

The natural history

It should be noted that, even today, we do not know much about the evolution of the disease over time, and in particular its natural history in the different subgroups of patients. In fact the etiology of AF is various, sometimes patients have a definite non-cardiac etiology, as those with hormonal disease, sometimes they have a clear structural heart disease such as valvular disease, coronary artery disease, hypertension etc. In a few patients no structural heart disease can be detected, therefore their AF has been called “lone AF”.

Moreover, from the clinical standpoint the most widely accepted time-course classification is the so-called 3 P classification, recently proposed by Gallagher and Camm. AF can be defined as paroxysmal when terminated spontaneously, persistent when requiring pharmacological or electrical cardioversion to be terminated and permanent when all attempts to terminate fail.

Thus, because the mechanism of initiation and maintenance of AF is still controversial, it is likely that treatment should vary between subgroups of patients, but this has never been investigated comparatively and prospectively.

Electrophysiology of AF

Growing evidence suggests that the electrophysiological mechanisms that initiate and maintain AF may be multiple and are associated with different types of AF. During AF several different patterns of atrial activation may be detectable in the same patient, resulting from the simultaneous migratory re-entrant wavelets in both atria.

AF develops on an electrically unstable atrial substrate that is characterized by regional conduction delay and an increased dispersion of refractoriness that is triggered by early premature atrial beats. Moreover, anatomical and electrical studies have found specific regions, such as part of the low right atrium and the Koch triangle, that have different areas of conduction velocity.

Previous studies by Moe and Allessie have provided the experimental evidence that AF is based on multiple wandering wavelets that re-enter themselves or each other (multiple wavelets re-entry). These wavelets change continuously in number and directions whatever initiating mechanism is involved.

High-density mapping studies of the electrical excitation of the atria, performed during surgery in humans, showed a variable spectrum of atrial activation due to the complexity of the arcs of conduction block and areas of slow conduction. The direction, size, and shape of each wavelet evolve with time, determined by the complex interaction of activation wavefronts with spatially and temporally varying tissue excitability and refractoriness. It has been hypothesized that sustained AF can be determined by the magnitude of the tissue wavelength, defined as the product of refractoriness and conduction velocity. The atrium is activated at a very high rate, and local atrial activation varies continuously in cycle length and morphology.

A relationship between local atrial activation during AF and atrial refractoriness has been demonstrated previously, assuming that the shortest FF interval reflects local refractoriness because cardiac cells can be re-excited soon after the refractory period (leading circle re-entry). However, variation of cycle length during AF might be also caused by the fact that after recovery of the excitability the fibers are re-entered after a slight delay by one of the wandering wavelets. This might result in a small gap of excitability because the atrial fibers are not activated at their maximal rate (random re-entry).

While supportive evidence for the multiple wavelet theory has indeed accumulated, other experimental and potential arrhythmogenic mechanisms could underlie AF subsets. Recently we have reported the results of catheter mapping of the right atrium activation during induced AF.

The trabeculated right atrium and the atrial roof

We observed a remarkably stereotypical pattern of endocardial activation along the trabeculated right atrium and the roof characterized by discrete atrial electrograms, separated by an isoelectric baseline, with a continuous change in the activation sequence between clockwise and counter-clockwise fashion. Each sequence lasted a mean of 7 ± 5 cycles and a longer interval or pause preceded every single change of sequence. This characteristic sequence of events, defined by our group as "washing-machine phenomenon", allows us to speculate that this predominantly organized pattern of activation on the trabeculated right atrium might be explained by the anisotropic conduction properties and the anatomical barriers, such as the crista terminalis and the Eustachian ridge. The trabeculated right atrium (the old atrium) and the smooth right atrium (the new atrium) have different embryological origins and tissue-specific anisotropic conduction properties that, in canine myocardium, resulted in a predominant impulse propagation in a craniocaudal direction in the trabeculated right atrium, and a relatively poor transverse coupling along the crista terminalis.

A similar pattern of organized AF was reported in the studies of Lesh and Gaita that allows us to assume also in humans that anatomical barriers may favor "streaming" of excitation along the trabeculated right atrium. The degree of transverse coupling along the crista terminalis may reduce invasion of multiple wavelets coming from the septum and posterior wall, whereas clockwise or counter-clockwise rotation might be explained with variable line of functional block along the right atrial free wall.

The anterior septum

In most patients, simultaneous recordings from the anterior and medial area of the atrial septum showed more-fractionated electrograms making the pattern of AF fairly disorganized. The reduced organization of AF in this area may be related to the presence of multiple simultaneous inputs from left atrium, via Bachmann's bundle, and posterior-inferior septum.

The posterior-inferior septum and the coronary sinus

The atrial activation in the inferior septum was rather disorganized and neither synchronized to the activation sequence of the trabeculated right atrium nor to the anterior septum, and as in the anterior septum showed fractionated electrograms and variability of the isoelectric baseline. Finally, a variable degree of organization was shown into the coronary sinus, indicating that coronary sinus activation during AF is largely affected by the proximity of the Eustachian ridge, the isthmus, and the mitral valve annulus, as previously demonstrated by Lesh.

The left atrium

Jais et al. sequentially mapped different atrial regions in AF while evaluating patients for radiofrequency ablation. They noted that early activation during AF occurred in the vicinity of the pulmonary veins, although such recordings were also seen in the coronary sinus ostium or crista terminalis in a few patients.

The focal AF

Several studies have demonstrated that arrhythmogenic foci play a significant role in AF. In contrast to the common concept of the existence of simultaneous multiple re-entrant wavelets, there is a growing evidence that AF may be initiated by very fast and irregular focal atrial tachycardia. Depending on the focus rate, the ECG tracings document AF as well as monomorphic and irregular atrial tachycardia and extrasystoles of the same morphology. Mapping performed during different types of atrial arrhythmia showed that they were due to the same focus firing irregularly. Long cycle lengths were responsible for the surface ECG morphology of organized monomorphic tachycardia or "focal flutter", whereas at short cycle lengths an ECG pattern of AF was observed.

Atrial premature beats that initiate these so-called focal forms of AF have been identified in the pulmonary veins in 60-94% of patients. They trigger AF with bursts of rapid discharges and respond to local RF catheter ablation. The mechanism (abnormal automaticity versus microre-entry versus triggered activity) is unknown. The pulmonary vein foci exhibited unique characteristics, including deep venous origin unpredictable firing and complex delayed conduction to the left atrium with ectopic beats confined to the vein. This complex electrophysiological behavior matches the complex anatomical features of venous muscular bands; however these foci may represent all the arrhythmia substrate or have a role only in the initiation of AF.

Non-pharmacological therapies

Pacing to prevent AF: single-site permanent atrial pacing

This type of pacing (AAI or AAIR modes) has long been considered as antiarrhythmic in patients with paroxysmal AF. In recent years, three randomized, prospective studies have provided results that sometimes are conflicting. According to Andersen (the Danish study), patients with sick sinus syndrome dependent-AF, followed for 5.5 years, showed a significantly lower incidence of AF episodes and better survival when submitted to atrial pacing. In contrast, Lamas in the PASE study, followed 407 patients paced randomly with VVI or DDD mode and found that there was no significant mode-related difference in the incidence of AF in the overall group, and only a trend of significance favoring the subgroup of patients with sick sinus syndrome who were paced with a DDD mode. Recently the Canadian Trial of Physiologic Pacing (CTOPP) showed statistically non-significant evidence for physiological pacing reducing stroke or cardiovascular mortality when compared to ventricular pacing (physiological pacing reduced the rate of AF episodes to 2.87% vs. 3.75% for VVI mode). Therefore, these studies support the evidence that single atrial pacing may help to reduce the episodes of AF in patients with sick sinus syndrome, but not in patients with no other indications for pacing.

Pacing to prevent AF: multi-site permanent atrial pacing

Rationale for biatrial pacing and also for dual-site right atrial pacing resulted from the fundamental premise that intraatrial and interatrial delays are important to initiate and maintain AF. Both acute and long-term studies have been recently performed. The acute studies showed that biatrial pacing and dual-site atrial pacing can reduce the inducibility of AF, but some points need to be addressed. Questions may arise from protocol used to induce AF and type of patients studied. Number of extra stimuli may influence the sensitivity of the studies, as well as the lack of the left atrium evaluation and the different population of patients enrolled. Apart from the above, it is unknown whether acute studies are relevant to patients with spontaneous AF or whether they can predict responders and non-responders to long-term biatrial pacing.

With regards to long-term studies, permanent biatrial pacing and dual-site right atrial pacing have been applied to an increasing number of patients. The SYNBIACE study, the first prospective, randomized, crossover biatrial pacing study showed a trend towards a reduction in the incidence of atrial arrhythmias during biatrial pacing compared to DDD mode at 70 and 40 beats/min, without a clear real benefit. The DAPPAF study (Dual Atrial Pacing For Prevention of AF) compares the efficacy of dual-site, single-site, and support pacing modes for prevention of AF in patients with history of paroxysmal AF and a bradyarrhythmic indication for pacing. The primary endpoint of this study is to compare the time to first recurrence of clinically significant symptomatic AF with ECG verification and quality of life among the three treatment modes. The enrolment phase of this study has been completed and the patients are presently being followed, but the results are not yet available. However, other small non-randomized studies showed more than 50% success rate without drugs in patients with paroxysmal AF in term of prolonged time of AF recurrence and reduced time in AF. All studies mentioned above have demonstrated in a large number of patients that multi-site atrial pacing is, to date, one of the best methods for efficient prevention of AF over a long-term period. Moreover, unselected patients are comparable to patients selected with interatrial conduction disorders; therefore patients with atrial arrhythmias can have altered atrial substrates, which is probably at least in part corrected with the pacing. At this time, the respective efficacy of biatrial resynchronization and dual-site atrial pacing on AF prevention has not been compared. However, dual-site atrial pacing is technically simpler with a shorter procedure time, with stable pacing threshold and lead position. Thus, although the above results are encouraging, they should not be taken to prove the merit of the technique beyond all doubt, since most are based on studies not properly randomized.

The surgical treatment

Three different surgical approaches have been developed: the left atrial isolation, the corridor procedure, and the Maze operation. The former two methods have been abandoned because of poor results, high morbidity, or other disadvantages. Cox in 1987 introduced the Maze operation that creates a "maze" of the electrical propagation routes involving the atria in an attempt to make AF non-sustained. After three enhancements of the technique, the rate of sinus rhythm maintenance was reported to be 85%, but with the disadvantages of the extracorporeal circulation, the open thoracotomy, and the problems of atrial transport function during follow-up. Recently radiofrequency energy has been used to shorten the procedure time, but although these procedures showed a very high success rate, they cannot be applied to a wide population since only a limited number of AF patients should undergo cardiac surgery for other reasons.

The ablative treatment

Target sites for successful tachyarrhythmia ablation can be characterized as being either discrete anatomical findings critical to maintaining the arrhythmia, or electrophysiological markers that bode well for the procedure even though the electrophysiological-anatomical correlations may be incompletely understood. At present, techniques being studied for ablation of AF address neither known critical anatomical elements nor well-defined electrophysiological markers. Thus, catheter-based cure of AF must be considered highly investigational.

Nevertheless, because the clinical need for better therapy of AF is so great, there are a number of ongoing-efforts to develop devices and techniques for atrial ablation in order to restore sinus rhythm and atrial mechanical contraction. Do we need a cure for AF? Certainly yes, so our ability to intervene in patients with AF has just begun to allow us to develop more-detailed descriptions of mechanism. AF as such may come to be recognized as the common surface manifestation of multiple potential mechanisms. In the setting of AF this will be particularly important, since if one considers the current "gold standard" for curative intervention to be the extensive lesions produced during the Cox surgical maze operation, then recognition of AF mechanisms that require a less-extensive lesion set would be highly desirable. Recently, "focal trigger" in the pulmonary veins was described as the initiating event in many cases of AF, therefore we should consider that AF actually has two substrates or mechanisms: that for perpetuation of multiple re-entrant wavelets and that for the initiation of AF.

The hypothesis of Moe that during AF there are multiple wandering re-entrant wavelets, even if they are not truly wandering, combined with the concept that there must be an adequate spatial extent of contiguous electrically active tissue for wavelets to perpetuate, allows us to understand how compartmentalization of the atrial wall by using linear radiofrequency lesions may block the electrical conduction and prevent AF by depriving the wavelets of sufficient spatial extent through which to propagate. Therefore, creating long linear lesions can be though of as a means to disrupt the substrate for AF maintenance or perpetuation. Preliminary reports from different groups resulted in a variable degree of success rate that is mainly dependent upon the ablation technique, the type of catheters, and the patient population. In order to prevent gaps in the lesions and to reduce the risk of thrombus formation, a recent advance is the use of multi-electrode catheters that can be placed against the atrial wall to allow creation of a long linear lesion. However, linear lesions performed only in the right atrium are rarely as effective as curative therapy; therefore this technique should be considered as palliative when used alone or as part of a combined therapeutic approach when associated with drugs. On the other hand, to add lesions in the left atrium may result in an increased rate of complications, even if it may improve the success rate.

Interestingly, pre-dating the multiple wavelet concept was the hypothesis by Sherf that AF may result from a single focus firing at a rate so that the remainder of the atrium cannot follow synchronously. The important work of Haissaguerre et al. supports this notion of focal triggers, and their careful mapping studies has shown that many patients indeed have "focal AF".

The patients in whom this mechanism is easiest to demonstrate are younger, non-organic heart disease, and have frequent atrial premature beats, and runs of atrial tachycardia with a relatively constant P wave morphology, in addition to AF which may appear to degenerate from a burst of atrial tachycardia. What is particularly remarkable is the relative constancy of anatomical sites of origin for these focal triggers in one of the pulmonary veins. Because these tachycardias have a focal mechanism, they can be abolished using standard radiofrequency ablation electrode catheters; nonetheless the recurrence rate is very high and most patients require multiple procedures. Thus, while the pulmonary veins appear to be a crucial source of triggers initiating AF, and mapping and ablation of these triggers are curative in most patients with paroxysmal and persistent forms of AF, there are a significant number of potential limitations to completely cure AF with the available standard mapping and ablation technique. Limitations such as the complex three-dimensional branching structure of pulmonary veins, no consistent method of trigger induction, unpredictability of spontaneous firing, multiple pulmonary veins foci, etc. may limit the efficacy of the procedure; therefore an anatomically guided ablative approach has been recently developed in order to isolate the pulmonary vein orifices. The ongoing clinical trials will provide substantial data to understand whether this technique will make ablation of AF a true curative procedure. Many technical and scientific problems need to be addressed if we want to "cure" AF with an efficient and effective procedure, maybe targeting either the initiating or the maintaining mechanism.

Suggested readings

Adam M, Casnadi Z, Tondo C et al (1999) A novel microcatheter approach to the ablation of atrial fibrillation: safety and feasibility in 43 patients. For the REVELATION European Atrial Fibrillation Group. Eur Heart J, p 235

Adam M, Fischetti D, Pelargonio G et al (1999) Microcatheter ablation technique in paroxysmal atrial fibrillation: results of clinical follow up min pilot study. S J Am Coll Cardiol 33[Suppl]:A1203

Adam M, Montenero AS, Fischetti D et al (1999) A typical pattern of activation in the right atrium during paroxysmal atrial fibrillation: the washing-machine phenomenon. Cardiologia 44:63-68

Aktar M, Avitall B, Jazayeri M et al (1992) Role of implantable cardioverter defibrillator therapy in the management of high risk patients. Circulation 85[Suppl 1]:131-139

Alessie MA, Lammers WJEP, Bonke FIM et al (1985) Experimental evaluation of Moe's multiple wavelet hypothesis of atrial fibrillation. In: Zipes DP, Jalife J (eds) Cardiac arrhythmias. Grune and Stratton, New York, pp 265-276

Alessie MA, Rensma PL, Lammers WJEP et al (1989) The role of refractoriness conduction velocity and wavelength in initiation of atrial fibrillation in normal conscious dogs. In Attuel P, Coumel P, Janse MJ (ed) The atrium in health and disease. Futura Publishing, Mount Kisco, pp 27-41

Alessie MA, Kirkof GJ, Konings KT (1996) Unraveling the electrical mysteries of atrial fibrillation. Eur Heart J 17[Suppl C]:2-9

Anderson HR, Nielsen JC, Thomsen PE et al (1997) Long term follow up of patients from a randomized trial of atrial versus ventricular pacing for sick-sinus syndrome. Lancet 350:1210-1216

Becker AE (1996) Atrial anatomy: relationship to atrial flutter. In: Waldo AL, Touboul P (eds) Atrial flutter: advances in mechanism and management: Futura Publishing, Armonk, New York, pp 13-19

Bialy D, Lehmann MH, Schumacher DN et al (1992) Hospitalization for arrhythmias in the United States: importance of atrial fibrillation (abstract). J Am Coll Cardiol 19:41A

Bigger JT (1997) Prophylactic use of implantable cardiac defibrillators in patients at high risk for ventricular arrhythmias after coronary artery bypass graft surgery. N Engl J Med 337:1569-1575

Buxton AE, Fisher JD, Josephson ME et al (1993) Prevention of sudden death in patients with coronary artery disease: the Multicenter Unsustained Tachycardia Trial (MUSTT). Prog Cardiovasc Dis 36:215-216

Buxton AE, Waxman HL, Marchlinski FE et al (1984) Atrial conduction: effects of extrastimuli with and without atrial dysrhythmias. Am J Cardiol 54:755-761

Cairns JA, Connolly SJ, Roberts et al (1997) Randomised trial of outcome after myocardial infarction in patients with frequent or repetitive ventricular premature depolarizations: CAMIAT. Lancet 349:675-682

Camm AJ, Echt D, Pratt C et al (1997) Dofetilide in patients with left ventricular dysfunction and either heart failure or acute myocardial infarction: rationale, design, and patients characteristics of the DIAMOND studies. Clin Cardiol 20:704-710

Connolly SJ, Gent M, Roberts RS et al (1993) Canadian Implantable Defibrillator Study (CIDS): study design and organization. Am J Cardiol 72:103F-108F

Cosio FG, Goicolea A, Lopez-Gil M et al (1993) Catheter ablation of atrial flutter circuits. PACE 16:637-642

Cosio FG, Palacios J, Vidal JM et al (1984) Electrophysiologic studies in atrial fibrillation: slow conduction of premature impulses: a possible manifestation of the back-ground for reentry. Am J Cardiol 51:122-130

Cox JL, Boineau JP, Schuessler RB et al (1995) Modification of the Maze procedure for atrial flutter and fibrillation. Rationale and surgical results. J Thorac Cardiovasc Surg 100:473-484

Cox JL, Canavan TE, Schuessler RB et al (1991) The surgical treatment of atrial fibrillation. II. Intraoperative electrophysiological mapping and description of the electrophysiological basis of atrial flutter and atrial fibrillation. J Thorac Cardiovasc Surg 101:406-426

Default P, Saksena S, Prakash A et al (1998) Long-term outcome of patients with drug-refractory atrial flutter and fibrillation after single and dual-site atrial pacing for arrhythmia prevention. J Am Coll Cardiol 32:1900-1908

Fitts SM, Hill MRS, Mehra R et al (1998) Design and implementation of the Dual-site Atrial Pacing to Prevent Atrial Fibrillation (DAPPAF) Clinical Trial. J Interv Cardiac Elect 2:138-144

Gaita F, Riccardi R, Calò L et al (1998) Atrial mapping and radiofrequency catheter ablation in patients with idiopathic atrial fibrillation: electrophysiological findings and ablation results. Circulation 97:2136-2145

Gallagher JJ, Camm AJ (1998) Classification of atrial fibrillation. Am J Cardiol 82:18N-28N

Garg A, Finneran W, Mollerus M et al (1999) Right atrial compartmentalization using radiofrequency catheter ablation for management of patients with refractory atrial fibrillation. J Cardiovasc Electrophysiol 10:763-771

Haïssaguerre M, Jaïs P, Shah DC et al (1998) Spontaneous initiation of atrial fibrillation by ectopic beats originating in the pulmonary veins. N Engl J Med 339:659-666

Jaïs P, Haïssaguerre M, Shah DC et al (1997) A focal source of atrial fibrillation treated by discrete radiofrequency ablation. Circulation 95:572-576

Julian DG, Camm AJ, Frangin G et al (1997) Randomised trial of the effect of amiodarone on mortality in patients with left ventricular disfunction after recent myocardial infarction: EMIAT. Lancet 349:667-674

Konings KTS, Kirchof CJHJ, Smeets JRLM et al (1994) High density mapping of electrically induced atrial fibrillation in man. Circulation 89:1665-1680

Kuck K-H. Cardiac Arrhythmia Study Hamburg (CASH), ACC newsonline

Lamas GA, Orav EJ, Stambler BS et al (1998) Quality of life and clinical outcomes in elderly patients treated with ventricular pacing as compared with dual-chamber pacing. N Engl J Med 338:1097-1104

Lammers WJEP, Alessie MA, Rensma PL et al (1986) The use of fibrillation cycle length to determine spatial dispersion in electrophysiological properties and to characterize the underlying mechanism of fibrillation. New Trends Arrhythmias 2:109-112

Lau CP, Tse HF, Yu CM et al (1999) Dual-site right atrial pacing in paroxysmal atrial fibrillation without bradycardia (NIPP-AF study). PACE 22:804

Lesh MD, Guerra PJ, Roithinger FX et al (2000) Novel catheter technology for ablative cure of atrial fibrillation. J Interv Cardiac Electrophysiol 4:127-139

Mabo P, Daubert JC, Bohour A (1999) Biatrial synchronous pacing for atrial arrhythmia prevention. The SYMBIACE study. PACE 22:755

Mcanulty J, Halperin B, Knon J et al (1997) A comparison of antiarrhythmic drug therapy with implantable defibrillators in patients resuscitated from near fatal ventricular arrhythmias. N Engl J Med 337:1576-1583

Moe GK (1962) On the multiple wavelets hypotesis of atrial fibrillation. Arch Int Pharmacodyn Ther 140:183-188

Montenero AS, Adam M, Franciosa P et al (2000) The linear ablation of atrial fibrillation in the right atrium: can the isthmus ablation improve its efficacy? J Am Coll Cardiol (in press)

Moss AJ, Hall WJ, Cannom DS et al (1996) Improved survival with an implant defibrillator in patients with coronary disease at high risk for ventricular arrhythmia. N Engl J Med 335:1933-1940

Pakash A, Saksena S, Hill M et al (1997) Acute effects of dual-site right atrial pacing in patients with spontaneous and inducible atrial flutter and fibrillation. J Am Coll Cardiol 29:1007-1014

Papageorgiou P, Anselme F, Kirchof CJ et al (1997) Coronary sinus pacing prevents induction of atrial fibrillation. Circulation 96:2292-2296

Papageorgiou P, Monahan K, Boyle NG et al (1996) Site-dependent intraatrial conduction delay: relationship to initiation of atrial fibrillation. Circulation 94:384-389

Pappone C, Lamberti F, Rillo M et al (1998) Catheter ablation of atrial fibrillation using a no-fluoroscopic system. J Am Coll Cardiol 31[2 Suppl A]:202A
Petersen P, Madesn EB, Brun B et al (1987) Silent cerebral infarction in chronic atrial fibrillation. Stroke 18:1098-1100
Prakash A, Default P, Krol RB et al (1998) Regional right and left atrial activation patterns during single and dual-site atrial pacing in patients with atrial fibrillation. Am J Cardiol 15:1197-1204
Ramdat Misier AR, Opthof T, Van Hemel NM et al (1992) Increased dispersion of refractoriness in patients with idiopathic paroxysmal atrial fibrillation. J Am Coll Cardiol 19:1531-1535
Roithinger FX, Sippens Groenewegen A, Karch MR et al (1998) Organized activation during atrial fibrillation in man: endocardial and electrocardiographic manifestations. J Cardiovasc Electrophysiol 9:451-456
Saffitz JE, Kanther HL, Green KG et al (1994) Tissue-specific determinants of anisotropic conduction velocity in canine atrial and ventricular myocardium. Circ Res 74:1065-1070
Sherf D (1947) Studies on auricular tachycardia caused by aconitine administration. Proc Exp Biol Med 64:230-233
Skanes AC, Krahn AD, Yee R et al (1999) Physiologic pacing reduces progression to chronic atrial fibrillation. PACE 22:728
Whaten MS, Klein GJ, Yee R (1993) Classification and terminology of supraventricular tachycardia. Diagnosis and management of atrial tachycardias. Cardiol Clin 11:109-120
Wolff PA, Dawber TR, Thomas HE jr et al (1978) Epidemiologic assessment of chronic atrial fibrillation and risk of stroke: The Framingham study. Neurology 28:973-977
Wolff PA, Mitchell JB, Baker CS et al (1995) Mortality and hospital cost associated with atrial fibrillation (abstract). Circulation 92:I-140
Yu WC, Chen SA, Tai CT et al (1997) Effects of different atrial pacing modes on atrial electrophysiology: implicating the mechanism of biatrial pacing in prevention of atrial fibrillation. Circulation 96:2992-2996

Clinical Applications of the Transpulmonary Thermodilution Technique

G. Della Rocca, M.G. Costa, P. Pietropaoli

In recent reviews of outcome, there is considerable evidence that mortality from high-risk surgery is often close to 10%, depending on case selection and operator experience. The inclusion of emergency work will often increase this figure to 20% [1, 2]. Whilst there is still no single definitive test to decide what is a high-risk case, it is possible to produce subgroups of patients who may be expected to do poorly. Tissue hypoperfusion during surgery has been shown to be a portent of poor outcome. Whatever the cause of this problem, be it poor cardiovascular performance or reduced intravascular volume, the link between alterations in microvascular flow and the onset of multiple organ dysfunction (MODS) is strong. In order to optimize fluid therapy it is necessary to have an appropriate method for measuring absolute values of flow or preload. Actually the current clinical standard of practice used to evaluate cardiac preload and to guide fluid administration during anesthesia includes monitoring of central venous pressure (CVP), invasive arterial pressure (AP) and, in selected high-risk patients, invasive cardiac output (CO), pulmonary artery pressure (mPA) and pulmonary artery occlusion pressure (PAOP) monitoring with pulmonary artery catheter (PAC) [3]. However, pressures can only serve as indirect indicators of filling volumes. They are as well influenced by intrinsic factors like cardiovascular compliance and patterns of myocardial relaxation as by extrinsic factors like positioning of the patients and, specifically in ventilated patients, changes in intrathoracic pressure. This might influence accuracy regarding cardiac preload estimation in specific clinical situations. Moreover, there is still controversy concerning indications and negative side effects attributed to this method [4, 5].

Recently, a new monitor with which CO (COart) may also be measured by transpulmonary artery thermodilution indicator technique (TPID) with the injection done through a central venous line and the change in temperature sensed in a thermistor that is embedded in an arterial (femoral or axillary) catheter became available (PiCCO System, Pulsion Medical System, Munich, Germany) [6]. This "less-invasive" device based on the pulse contour analysis measures continuous cardiac output (PCCO) and with the TPID technique volumetric cardiac preload index such as Intra Thoracic Blood Volume (ITBV), Global End Diastolic Volume (GEDV) and "lung edema" Extra Vascular Lung Water (EVLWI). ITBV has been shown to have higher correlation with stroke index (SI) and cardiac index (CI) when compared to conventional filling pressures (CVP, PAOP) in critically ill patients and during major surgery, confirming its validity as a bedside volumetric preload index (Table 1) [7-11].

Table 1. ITBVI and GEDVI validation as cardiac preload index by comparison with CI, SVI, SI and EDAI

Authors	Year	Ref		pat	Data analyzed	r
Lichtwarck-Aschoff M. et al.	1996	10	Dobutamine hypovol. test	10 piglets	ITBVI/CI	0.78
Preisman S. et al.	1997	13	Graded hemorrhage	8 dogs	ITBV/CI ITBVI/SVI	0.91 0.91
Hinder F. et al.	1998	27	Cardiac surg + ICU	15	ΔITBVI/ΔEDAI	0.87
Godje O. et al.	1998	7	Cardiac ICU	30	ΔITBVI/ΔSVIart ΔITBVI/ΔCIart ΔGEDVI/ΔSVIart ΔGEDVI/ΔCIart	0.76 0.83 0.82 0.87
Borelli M. et al.	1998	11	ICU	9	ΔITBVI/ΔCI ΔGEDVI/ΔCI	0.672* 0.562*
Sakka S.G. et al.	1999	8	ICU	57	ITBVI/SI (first data) ITBVI/SI (second data)	0.66 0.67
Buhre W. et al.	2000	29	Neurosurgery	10	ITBV/SVI	0.78

* = r^2; ITBVI = intra thoracic blood volume index; GEDVI = global end diastolic volume index; CI = cardiac index; SVI = stroke volume index; SI = stoke index; EDAI = end diastolic area index; CIart = transpulmonary cardiac index recorded in femoral artery

Besides these parameters the PiCCO System continuously computes stroke volume variation (SVV), which is induced by changes in intrathoracic pressure due to mechanical ventilation. Hence, this parameter represents an online application based on the same principle as the systolic pressure variation (SPV) and its Δdown component, which has earlier been described as a highly sensitive preload parameter [12, 13].

Cardiac output monitoring

Major hemodynamic changes may occur during anesthesia for major surgical procedures or in critically ill patients, making the invasive monitoring of hemodynamic data, including continuous cardiac output (CO), desirable [14]. Methods for continuous or semicontinuous cardiac output monitoring with transesophageal echocardiography and electrical bio-impedance have been developed and investigated during anesthesia [15]. Actually, two techniques are available for the measurement of continuous cardiac output in clinical practice. The first is the continuous thermodilution technique with the application of small quantities of heat using a modified pulmonary artery catheter (PAC), described in detail elsewhere [16-18]. The second is the beat-to-beat measurement of continuous cardiac output from the arterial pulse contour analysis suggested as a reliable method in clinical practice [19-21]. The PiCCO System with a transpulmonary indicator dilution (TPID) technique, in which a thermistor-tipped catheter is placed in the femoral artery, enables the measurement of cardiac output by aortic thermodilution (COart) and computes CO continuously by an improved arterial pulse contour analysis (PCCO) without the need of an invasive PAC. Buhre et al. [20] and Gödje et al. [21] comparing continuous cardiac output obtained by pulse contour analysis with intermittent cardiac output obtained by arterial (COart) and pulmonary artery thermodilution (COpa) showed a correlation with a high accuracy and precision during and after coronary artery bypass grafting. Rodig et al. in a recent study compared two methods of continuous CO measurement, the pulse contour analysis and a continuous thermodilution technique (Opti-Q SvO_2/CCO, Abbott Critical Care System, Mountain View, CA, USA), with conventional intermittent thermodilution measurement in cardiac surgical patients [19]. The authors concluded that assessment of CO by pulse contour analysis and by thermodilution technique provided comparable measurements during coronary artery by-pass surgery. Several studies on critically ill patients reported excellent correlation and small variation in the agreement between COpa and CCO [16-18]. Bottiger in a recent study evaluated the CCO measurement as an alternative to COpa monitoring in intensive care in patients after cardiac surgery [16]. A good correlation between CCO and COpa and acceptable levels of accuracy and precision were generally found.

In a previous study of 22 patients undergoing double lung transplantation (DLT) and of 28 patients undergoing orthotopic liver transplantation (OLT) measurements of cardiac output by aortic thermodilution (COart) with an injection volume of at least 15 mL of cooled saline was shown to be as accurate as when measured by pulmonary artery thermodilution (COpa) (DLT $r = 0.90$, OLT $r = 0.93$). Good correlation and accuracy was also observed for continuous cardiac output obtained from PiCCO (PCCO) and PAC (Intellicath for CCO/SvO_2, Baxter Healthcare Corporation, Irvine, CA) (DLT $r = 0.84$, OLT $r = 0.84$) [22]. Currently available data indicate that transpulmonary cardiac output can be measured reliably and it is at least as accurate as pulmonary artery cardiac output in the clinical applications. The COart can be more accurate and less influenced by respiratory changes also.

Volumetric monitoring

Whilst for many years there was an acceptance that pressure could be used as an indirect measurement of the degree of circulatory volume, and hence flow, in the group of high-risk patients for whom this therapy may be critical, this link is tenuous and may be impossible to predict. If the accepted aim of fluid therapy is to optimize tissue perfusion, a direct tool for the measurement of flow is needed [1, 2]. Whilst the evidence is increasing as to the need for optimal flow prior to surgery, there remains doubt as to the best method for the measurement of this parameter. Despite the current controversy concerning its use, it may be that a PAC equipped with continuous cardiac output technology remains the historical closest to the aim and the better known device in the intensive care team [5]. At the present time the PiCCO System is able to evaluate the CO, the PCCO, the Global End-Diastolic Volume (GEDV) and to estimate the Intrathoracic Blood Volume (ITBV) and the Extra Vascular Lung Water (EVLW) with the TPID technique using single indicator dilution technique [23-26]. Direct assessment of intravascular volume status is a useful tool in anesthesia and, with this new device, nowadays we can monitor volumes during high-risk surgery and in critically ill patients.

When compared to CVP and PAOP, ITBV and GEDV may directly reflect cardiac preload in many experimental and clinical studies [7, 8]. ITBV is considered as an indicator of cardiac preload that is less influenced by changes in intrathoracic pressures and myocardial compliance. Gödje et al. [7] compared conventional parameters CVP and PAOP with ITBV and GEDV in thirty patients after coronary artery by-pass grafting (CABG). The linear regression analysis was computed between changes of preload dependent left ventricular stroke volume index (SVI) and cardiac index (CI) and the corresponding, presumably preload indicating parameters CVP, PAOP, ITBV and GEDV. No correlation was found between CVP versus SVI ($r = -0.09$) or CI ($r = 0.00$), and PAOP versus SVI ($r = -0.02$) or CI ($r = -0.01$). ITBVI correlated well with SVI and CI; coefficients were 0.76 and 0.83, respectively. Correlation coefficients of GEDVI versus SVI/CI were 0.82 and 0.87. This study confirmed the ITBV and GEDV as better cardiac preload index when compared with conventional CVP and PAOP in cardiac surgical patients. Sakka et al. [8] in a recent study compared each preload variable in the early phase of hemodynamic stabilization in 57 critically ill patients with sepsis or septic shock, confirming the controlled study of Lichtwarck-Aschoff et al. [10] and Gödje et al. [7] which demonstrated that ITBV is a more reliable indicator of preload than the cardiac filling pressures. Hinder et al. showed a high correlation between changes in ITBVI and end-diastolic area index (EDAI) performed with transesophageal echocardiography (TEE) during anesthesia and perioperative ICU stay in patients undergoing cardiac surgery [27].

Recent experimental and clinical data demonstrate that a single arterial thermodilution-derived ITBV (ITBV*) correlates well with the respective values measured by the double indicator technique [25, 26, 28]. Neumann, in an experimental model of lung injury performed with 13 mechanically ventilated pigs, showed that single thermodilution ITBV* and EVLW* compared to the same data obtained with the double indicator technique were reasonably accurate

[26]. Buhre et al. [29], comparing the double indicator ITBV versus the derived single indicator ITBV* in 10 patients undergoing anesthesia for neurosurgical procedures, observed that during surgery in supine and sitting position the relative changes in ITBV* values were similar to those assessed by double indicator dilution. The authors confirmed that the assessment of changes in ITBV* by single thermodilution is valid enough for clinical purposes and relatively less expensive when compared with the double indicator technique. Sakka et al. in a recent study compared the simpler approach using single arterial thermodilution derived measurements of ITBV and EVLW with the double-indicator technique. Structural regression analysis of the first two thermodilution measurements in a derivation population of 57 critically ill patients revealed ITBV = (1.25·GEDV) – 28.4 mL. This equation was then applied by the authors to all first measurements in a validation population of 209 critically ill patients and single-thermodilution ITBV ($ITBV_{ST}$) and EVLW ($EVLW_{ST}$) were calculated and compared to thermo-dye dilution derived values ($ITBV_{TD}$, $EVLW_{TD}$). Linear regression analysis yielded a strong correlation for $ITBV_{ST}$ ($r = 0.97$, $p < 0.0001$; bias 7.6 mL/m^2, SD 57.4 mL/m^2), and $EVLWI_{TS}$ ($r = 0.96$, $p < 0.0001$; bias –0.2 mL/kg, SD 1.4 mL/kg) confirming single thermodilution accuracy [28].

Several clinical applications of the TPID are reported in literature. Many authors described their experience with the PiCCO System particularly in high-risk patients during anesthesia for coronary artery by-pass surgery [6, 7]. Others studied the PiCCO System in particular surgery like neurosurgery, laparoscopic procedures and major abdominal surgery performed with blended anesthesia [29-32]. In a previous report we described the usefulness of volumetric monitoring during anesthesia and postoperative care in patients undergoing double lung transplantation for cystic fibrosis [33]. In the critically ill patients, affected by sepsis, ARDS, pump failure, etc., the volumetric monitoring showed to be more accurate in terms of CI, preload and "lung edema" monitoring when compared to PAC or TEE [8, 23, 28, 34, 35]. Its bedside, real time, repeatability procedures, without necessity to place an invasive PAC, and its independence from hand operation and mechanical ventilation, give to this monitor a useful clinical application.

CVP-a-line vs hemodynamic-volumetric intraoperative management

Conventional CVP and AP monitoring represents the standard monitoring during anesthesia for major surgery. The PiCCO System gives us the possibility to obtain many more parameters, not only hemodynamics but also volumetrics, with the same invasiveness, with the chance to optimize intravascular blood volume during anesthesia and in critically ill patients. In particular anesthesia for major surgery performed with a blended technique, with epidural analgesia, is extremely useful to reduce perioperative stress and to obtain a successful pain relief in the postop period. This technique presents intraoperative side effects such as vasoplegia related to the local anesthetics, with or without opioids, given through the epidural route.

We studied 61 patients scheduled for general abdominal surgery randomized in two groups according to the monitoring applied. Combined anesthesia (epidural + general anesthesia) was used in both groups. During surgical procedure volume replacement and vasoactive and inotropic drug support in the PiCCO group were managed using an algorithm based on ITBV monitoring (Fig. 1). In the PiCCO group the GEDVI, the ITBVI and the CI were significantly increased at the end of surgery versus the baseline after anesthesia induction. mAP was significantly increased either in the PiCCO or Control group at the end of surgery. CVP didn't change during the study in both groups. The perioperative management based on volumetric algorithm (Fig. 1) in the PiCCO group resulted in the reduction of vasoactive drug administration probably as a result of fluid balance based on GEDVI or ITBVI and the consequence was blood volume optimization. Diuresis was preserved in the PiCCO group without administration of diuretics. In the Control group the management based on conventional mAP, HR and CVP was not able to optimize volume replacement. As a result, vasoactive drugs were necessary to maintain hemodynamic stability. No difference in total volume loading performed with the two different algorithms was observed between groups, even if the administration per hours was different. An additional sign that volume replacement was insufficient in the Control group was the consumption of diuretics, higher in this group, to maintain urine output (1 mL/kg/h). In the PiCCO group, EVLWI increased slightly during the surgery; however, it decreased at the end of surgery with a subsequent significant increase in PaO_2/FiO_2.

Conclusion

Actually the PiCCO System finds a clinical application in the following fields:

1. *medical* - to optimize preload and cardiac function in patients with cardiac impairment (PCCO, SV, dPmx, EVLWI);
2. *surgical* - in high-risk patients undergoing major surgery, and in every major surgical procedure with the only limitation related to vascular surgery (apart from the axillary approach). Intraoperative management based on volumetric algorithm is able to optimize fluids and drugs administration (PCCO, ITBVI, EVLWI, SVV);
3. *intensive care unit* - in septic, cardiac, trauma and respiratory critically ill patients, this monitor allows us to obtain more data to optimize fluids, drugs and ventilatory setting which could reduce ventilatory days and intensive care lengths of stay (PCCO, ITBVI, EVLWI, SVV).

The possibility to obtain hemodynamic (CO) and volumetric values (GEDVI, ITBVI, EVLWI) with the same invasiveness (a central venous line and an arteri-

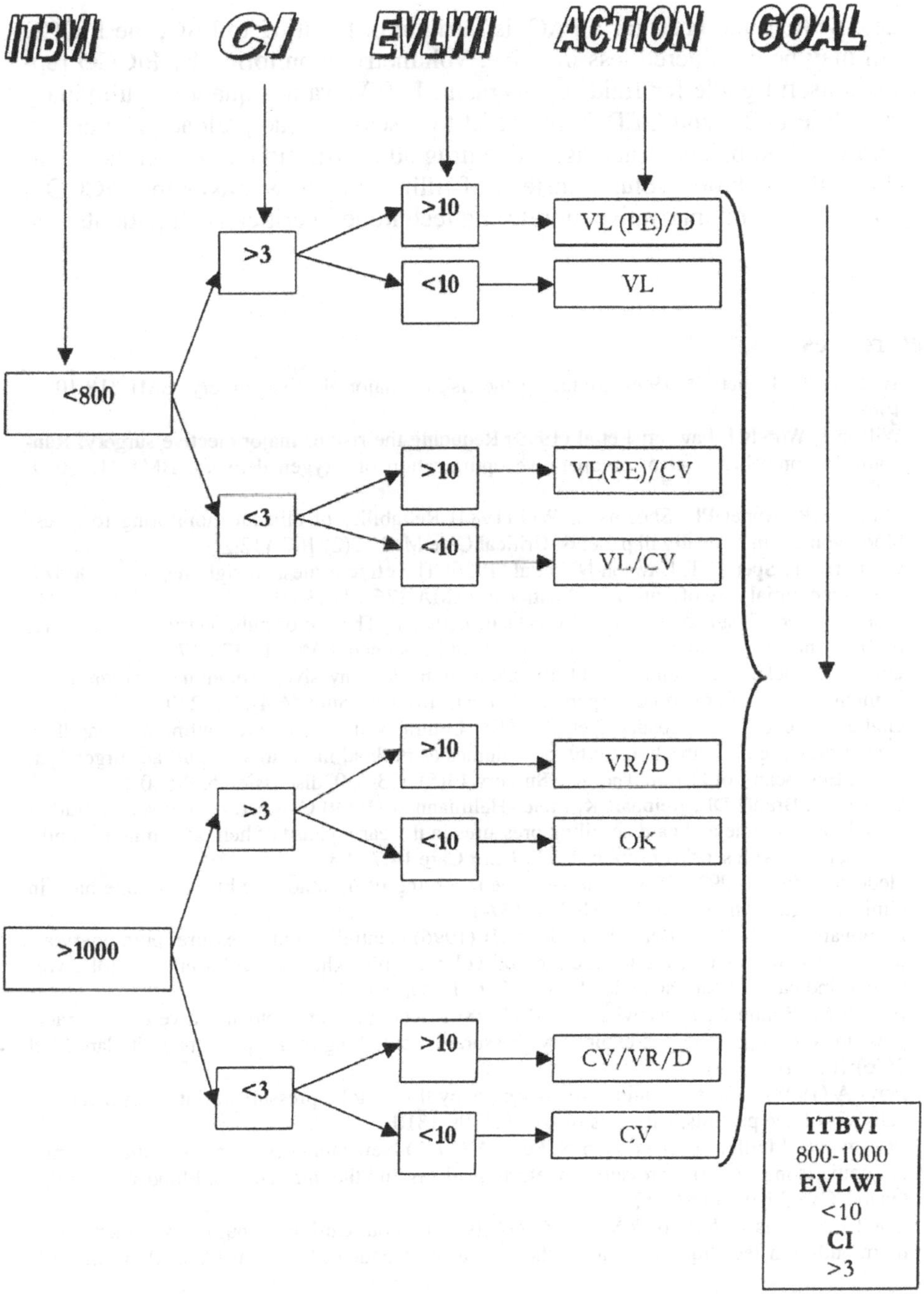

Fig. 1. Algorithm for hemodynamic-volumetric management in the PiCCO group
VL = volume loading (PE) plasma exp; D = diuretic drugs; VR = volume restriction; CV = cardiovascular drugs; ITBVI = intra-thoracic blood volume index; EVLWI = extra-vascular lung water index; CI = cardiac index

al line), without the need for a PAC, is intriguing. Relating to PAC, the PiCCO system may be considered less invasive. Volumetric monitoring by PiCCO represents a useful guide for fluid replacement: EVLW values quantify pulmonary edema while ITBV and GEDV are useful to assess cardiac preload. The ability to optimize fluid balance and vasoactive drug administration based on the quantified circulating blood volume instead of filling pressures makes the PiCCO a very interesting and innovative monitoring technique in critically ill patients.

References

1. Treasure T, Bennett D (1999) Reducing the risk of major elective surgery. BMJ 318:1087-1088
2. Wilson J, Woods I, Fawcett J et al (1999) Reducing the risk of major elective surgery: Randomized controlled trial of preoperative optimization of oxygen delivery. BMJ 318:1099-1103
3. Shippy CR, Appel PL, Shoemaker WC (1984) Reliability of clinical monitoring to assess blood volume in critically ill patients. Critical Care Med 12(2):107-112
4. Connors AF, Speroff T, Dawson NV et al (1996) The effectiveness of right heart catheterization in the initial care of critically ill patients. JAMA 276:889-897
5. Soni N (1996) Swan song for the Swan-Ganz catheter? The use of pulmonary artery catheter probably needs re-evaluation-but they should not be banned. BMJ 313:173-174
6. Godje O, Hoeke K, Lamm P et al (1998) Continuous, less invasive, hemodynamic monitoring in intensive care after cardiac surgery. J Thorac Cardiovasc Surg 46(4):242-249
7. Gödje O, Peyerl M, Seebauer T et al (1998) Central venous pressure, pulmonary capillary wedge pressure and intrathoracic blood volumes as preload indicators in cardiac surgery patients. European J of Cardio-Thoracic Surgery 13(5):533-539; discussion 539-540
8. Sakka SG, Bredle DL, Reinhart K, Meier-Hellmann A (1999) Comparison between intrathoracic blood volume and cardiac filling pressures in the early phase of hemodynamic instability of patients with sepsis or septic shock. J Crit Care 14:78-83
9. Hedenstierna G (1992) What value does the recording of intrathoracic blood volume have in clinical practice? Intensive Care Med 18:137-138
10. Lichtwarck-Aschoff M, Beale R, Pfeiffer UJ (1996) Central venous pressure, pulmonary artery occlusion pressure, intrathoracic blood volume, and right ventricular end-diastolic volume as indicator of cardiac preload. J Crit Care 11(4):180-188
11. Borelli M, Benini A, Denkewitz T et al (1998) Effects of continuous negative extrathoracic pressure versus positive end-expiratory pressure in acute lung injury patients. Crit Care Med 26(6):1025-1031
12. Perel A (1998) Assessing fluid responsiveness by the systolic pressure variation in mechanically ventilated patients. Anesthesiology 89:1309-1310
13. Preisman S, Pfeiffer U, Lieberman N, Perel A (1997) New monitors of intravascular volume: A comparison of arterial pressure waveform analysis and the intrathoracic blood volume. Intensive Care Med 23:651-657
14. Boldt J, Menges T, Wollbruck M et al (1994) Is continuous cardiac output measurement using thermodilution technique reliable in the critically ill patients? Critical Care Med 22:1913-1918
15. Stelzer H, Blazek G, Gabriel A et al (1991) Two-dimensional transesophageal echocardiography in early diagnosis and treatment of hemodynamic disturbances during liver transplantation. Transplantation Proceedings 23:1957-1958
16. Bottiger BW, Soder M, Rauch H et al (1996) Semi-continuous versus injectate cardiac output measurement in intensive care patients after cardiac surgery. Intensive Care Med 22:312-318

17. Greim CA, Roewer N, Thiel H, Laux Gand Schulte J (1997) Continuous cardiac output during adult liver transplantation: Thermal filament technique versus bolus thermodilution. Anesth Analg 85:483-488
18. Bottiger BW, Sinner B, Motsch J et al (1997) Continuous versus intermittent thermodilution cardiac output measurement during orthotopic liver transplantation. Anaesthesia 52:207-214
19. Rodig G, Prasser C, Keyl C et al (1999) Continuous cardiac output measurement: Pulse contour analysis vs thermodilution technique in cardiac surgical patients. Br J Anaesth 82: 525-530
20. Buhre W, Weyland A, Kazmaier S et al (1999) Comparison of cardiac output assessed by pulse-contour analysis and thermodilution in patients undergoing minimally invasive direct coronary artery bypass grafting. J Cardiothorac Vasc Anesth 13:437-440
21. Gödje O, Hoeke K, Lichtwarck-Aschoff M et al (1999) Continuous cardiac output by femoral arterial thermodilution calibrated pulse contour analysis: Comparison with pulmonary arterial thermodilution. Critical Care Med 27:2407-2412
22. Della Rocca G, Costa MG, Pompei L et al (2000) Pulse contour analysis vs thermodilution technique during lung and liver transplantation. Eur J Anesthesiology 17[Suppl 19]:A75
23. Sakka SG, Reinhart K, Meier-Helmann A (1999) Comparison of pulmonary artery and arterial thermodilution cardiac output in critically ill patients. Intensive Care Med 25:843-846
24. Godje O, Thiel C, Lamm P et al (1999) Less invasive, continuous hemodynamic monitoring during minimally invasive coronary surgery. Ann Thorac Surg 68:1532-1536
25. Buhre W, Bendyk K, Weyland A et al (1998) Assessment of intrathoracic blood volume. Thermo-dye dilution technique vs single thermodilution technique. Anaesthesist 47:51-53
26. Neumann P (1999) Extravascular lung water and intrathoracic blood volume: Double versus single indicator dilution technique. Intensive Care Med 25:216 219
27. Hinder F, Poelaert JI, Schmidt C et al (1998) Assessment of cardiovascular volume status by transoesophageal echocardiography and dye dilution during cardiac surgery. Eur J Anaesthesiology 15:633 640
28. Sakka SG, Rühl CC, Pfeiffer UJ et al (2000) Assessment of cardiac preload and extravascular lung water by single transpulmonary thermodilution. Intens Care Med 26:180-187
29. Buhre W, Weyland A, Bhure K et al (2000) Effects of the sitting position on the distribution of the blood volume in patients undergoing neurosurgical procedures. Br J Anaesth 84(3): 354-357
30. Hachenberg T, Holst D, Ebel C et al (1997) Effect of thoracic epidural anaesthesia on ventilation-perfusion distribution and intrathoracic blood volume before and after induction of general anaesthesia. Acta Anaesthesiol Scand 41:1142-1148
31. Hachenberg T, Ebel C, Czorny M et al (1998) Intrathoracic and pulmonary blood volume during CO_2-pneumoperitoneum in humans. Acta Anaesthesiol Scand 42:794-798
32. Della Rocca G, Costa MG, Pietropaoli P (2000) Conventional CVP/A line vs volumetric hemodynamic monitoring. J Anasth Intensiv 3:S21-S24
33. Della Rocca G, Costa MG, Coccia C et al (2000) Double lung transplantation in cystic fibrosis patients: Perioperative hemodynamic-volumetric monitoring. Transplantation Proceeding 32:104-108
34. Bindles AJGH, van der Hoeven JG, Meinders AE (1999) Pulmonary artery wedge pressure and extravascular lung water in patients with acute cardiogenic pulmonary edema requiring mechanical ventilation. Am J Cardiol 84:1158-1163
35. Davey-Quinn A, Gedney JA, Whiteley SM, Bellamy MC (1999) Extravascular lung water and acute respiratory distress syndrome. Oxygenation and outcome. Anaesth Intens Care 27: 357-362

VENTILATION

Respiratory Function - Monitoring and Modalities at the Bedside

P. Pelosi, N. Bottino, P. Caironi

By the term "monitoring", we mean the possibility to have a continual and/or a repetitive measure of a physiologic parameter that allows us to timely carry out diagnostic and/or therapeutic measures. The monitoring of respiratory function avails itself of some tools, such as arterial blood gases [1], pulse oximetry [2] and capnometry [3], that have already fit into the daily clinical practice. Instead, the parameters of respiratory mechanics are rarely measured in Intensive Care. Really, some measurements of respiratory mechanics are often easy to obtain, in particular in sedated and curarized patients, also because of the availability of ventilators with more and more refined technical functions and accurate displays.

In this chapter we will describe some technical supports for the measurement, in curarized subjects, of pulmonary volumes and some parameters of respiratory mechanics (compliance and resistance, partitioned into chest wall and pulmonary components, intrinsic positive end-expiratory pressure – $PEEP_i$ –, Pressure Volume curve), that could be routinely applied at the bedside in Intensive Care.

Lung volumes

Functional Residual Capacity (FRC) is the gas volume that remains in the respiratory system at the end of a relaxed expiration, when there is a balance between elastic retraction forces of the lung and expansive ones of the chest wall. From a physiologic point of view, FRC is one of the most relevant lung volumes, since it represents the gas volume that balances itself with pulmonary capillary blood; in several clinical conditions it may be appreciably decreased (as in the Acute Respiratory Distress Syndrome - ARDS) or increased (as during pulmonary emphysema). The measuring of FRC may provide us with important information for the treatment of hyposemic patients [4]. The more frequently utilised techniques to measure FRC are pletismography and the methods that use inert gas elimination, such as nitrogen washing/washout and helium [5, 6] and SF6 [7] dilution technique. While pletismography is difficult to carry out in patients admitted to Intensive Care Units, the multiple inert gas elimination techniques are easier to do.

Now, we will briefly describe a simplified method for measuring of FRC, based on helium dilution, we use in our unit [8, 9]. This method is based on the re-respiration, in a closed system, of a determined volume of an oxygen – helium mixture, with a known concentration. The total amount of helium remains unchanged and it dilutes itself into the initial volume and into the patient's FRC, since helium is poorly diffusable across alveolar-capillary membrane and, in particular, is poorly soluble in the blood. Strictly speaking, an anaesthesia balloon previously filled with 1.5 l of oxygen – helium mixture (87% oxygen, 13% helium) is linked up to the proximal part of endotracheal tube and is inflated in the respiratory system 10-15 times, to allow the achievement of balance between balloon and alveolar helium concentrations. The helium concentration of collected gas volume is measured through the helium analyser and FRC is computed according to the following formula:

$$FRC = [Vi * (He)_i/(He)_f] - Vi \quad (1)$$

where V_i and $(He)_i$ respectively represent the volume of the mixture previously introduced in the balloon (1.5 l) and the initial helium concentration of this one (13%), and $(He)_f$ is the final helium concentration, measured with the helium analyser.

The main limitation of these techniques consists of the possibility of measuring only the portion of lung volume that takes part in ventilation. The obtained value doesn't care about pulmonary regions completely excluded from the ventilation, and it may be affected by the occurrence of poorly ventilated lung units: as a consequence, the measurement will be poorly reliable in patients with Chronic Obstructive Pulmonary Disease (COPD), in which one of the most important pathophysiological alterations is an abnormality and an extreme variability of ventilation-perfusion ratio. Instead, in patients with acute respiratory failure, in which the prevalent alterations seem to be an alveolar consolidation, atelectasis and pulmonary collapse (i.e. non ventilated pulmonary units), the FRC measurement with helium dilution technique is more accurate.

Clinical implications

The determination of Functional Residual Capacity – or End-Expiratory Lung Volume (EELV), when a positive end-expiratory pressure (PEEP) is applied – is useful not only for quantifying the ventilated lung volume. In fact, the changes in end-expiratory lung volumes may point out the occurrence of alveolar recruitment and derecruitment, as a consequence of the variations of applied ventilatory parameters or the addition of other therapeutic manoeuvres. It's necessary to remember that a change in end-expiratory lung volume (Δ EELV) will really correspond to an alveolar recruitment (a positive value of Δ EELV) or derecruitment (a negative value of Δ EELV) only if we consider end-expiratory lung volume at the same ventilatory conditions (i.e. the same PEEP level). To compare different value of EELV measured at different value of PEEP, and to point out the possible occurrence of alveolar recruitment, it's necessary to carry out a Pressure Volume curve at the lower PEEP level or at atmospheric pressure (see Fig. 1). Therefore, it's possible to obtain the expected value of Δ EELV that is characteristic for lung parenchyma and pressure level (PEEP) considered. If the measured Δ EELV is higher than the expected value, there will be a recruitment and the difference between the measured and the expected lung volume will be an estimate of the extent of alveolar recruitment. On the contrary, if the measured value is lower than the expected one, there will be a derecruitment.

As it is shown in Figure 1, different Pressure Volume curves, effected at different PEEP level, may be compared through the measurement of EELV: when

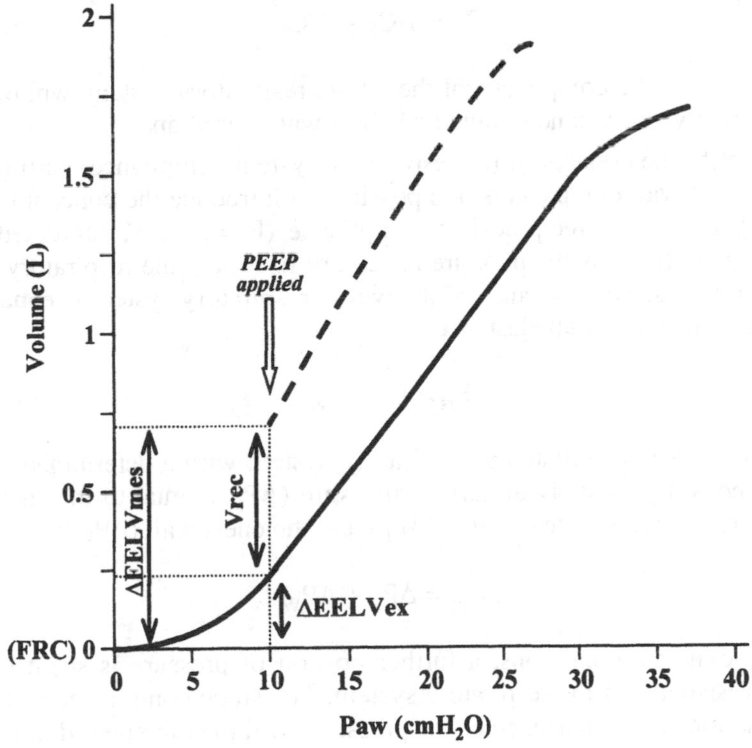

Fig. 1.

Pressure volume curve measured at FRC, 0 cm H_2O of PEEP (solid line), and at 10 cm H_2O of PEEP (dashed line). The curve measured at FRC allows us to estimate the increase of pulmonary volume expected at the end of expiration (Δ EELVex). From the difference between the increased volume measured (Δ EELVmes) and the expected one the recruited volume (Vrec) may be extracted. Δ EELVmes represents also the beginning point (on the volume axis) from which PV curve measured at 10 cm H_2O of PEEP has to be drawn; this last curve, in the presence of recruitment, will appear shifted on the top and on the left, compared to the PV curve measured at FRC

there has been an alveolar recruitment, the Pressure Volume curve at the correspondent PEEP level will appear shifted on the left and on the top.

Compliance

Compliance (C) defines a volume variation determined by a pressure variation ($C = \Delta V/\Delta P$, expressed in mL/cm H_2O), and it is graphically represented by the slope of the Pressure Volume curve. The compliance of the whole respiratory system depends on lung and chest wall compliance. From a physical point of view, the compliance corresponds to a capacity; therefore, the compliance of the respiratory system, that may be considered as the whole of lung and chest wall compliance (two capacities in succession), is equal to the sum of their reciprocals:

$$1/C_{rs} = 1/C_L + 1/C_W \quad (2)$$

where C_{rs} means the compliance of the whole respiratory system, while C_L and C_W respectively correspond to lung and chest wall compliance.

To simplify the concept of the respiratory system compliance, partitioned in lung and chest wall components, it's possible to introduce the concept of "elastance" (E), that is the reciprocal of compliance ($E = \Delta P/\Delta V$, expressed in cm H_2O/L); it is defined as the pressure necessary to inflate the respiratory system with a liter of gas. The elastance of the whole respiratory system is equal to the sum of lung and chest wall elastance:

$$E_{rs} = E_L + E_w \quad (3)$$

This means that to inflate the respiratory system with a determined gas volume it's necessary to apply an airway pressure (ΔP_{aw}) equal to the sum of the adequate pressure to inflate the lung (ΔP_L) and the chest wall (ΔP_W):

$$\Delta P_{aw} = \Delta P_L + \Delta P_W \quad (4)$$

During dynamic conditions, a further portion of pressure is spent to overcome the resistance of the respiratory system. The static compliance is different from "dynamic" compliance, since the pressure used to compute it doesn't comprise the pressure used to overcome the resistance of the respiratory system (due to airflow), but it comprises only the pressure necessary to expand the respiratory system with a gas volume (i.e. tidal volume).

The most utilised and simple method to apply at the bedside for measuring compliance and resistance of the respiratory system, with their components, is the rapid airway occlusion [9-12]. It's necessary to point out flow, tidal volume, airway pressure (P_{aw}) and esophageal pressure (P_{es}) values and/or tracks. Flow, volume and P_{aw} values are generally provided by ventilator displays (the most modern ventilator allows the visualisation of tracks). Alternatively, these variables may be recorded more proximally to the patient, through a pneumotagograph (that provides flow tracks, from which, through an integration, it is possible to obtain volume values) and a pressure transducer. Instead, to measure esophageal pressure (P_{es}) it is necessary to place into the esophagus (between the middle and the lower third) a balloon inflated with 0.5-1 ml of air, and connect it to a pressure transducer. P_{es} value measured in this way is indicative of mean pleural pressure, that in a positive pressure mechanically ventilated and paralysed patient is representative of the pressure spent expanding the chest wall component of the respiratory system (ΔP_W).

During a volume controlled ventilation, with a constant inspiratory flow inflation, while we are recording several tracks of the above mentioned variables, we have to occlude airway at the end of inspiration, through an end-inspiratory pause (pressing the end-inspiratory hold button of the ventilator). Airway occlusion has to be maintained until airway and esophageal pressure tracks decrease from a maximum value to an apparent plateau. Generally, a 4-5 seconds period is sufficient for this decrease, and during this brief lapse of time the pressure decrease caused by volume variation, because of gas exchange, may be considered negligible.

Figure 2 shows, respectively from the top to the bottom, flow, volume, airway pressure (P_{aw}) and esophageal pressure (P_{es}) tracks, during a respiratory cycle with volume controlled ventilation, in which a briefly end-inspiratory occlusion has been carried out. After the occlusion (the flow decreases to zero), in the airway pressure track an immediate decrease from P_{max} to the lower value of P_1 may be observed, with a following and slower decrease to a plateau value (P_2). Instead, in esophageal pressure track, there isn't the immediate decrease, and P_{es} directly and gradually decreases from the maximum value (P_{max}) to the plateau value (P_2). The plateau pressures (P_2) of P_{aw} and P_{es} represent the pressures due to the end-inspiratory elastic recoil of the whole respiratory system (in the P_{aw} track) and the chest wall (in the P_{es} track).

To compute the static compliance of the whole respiratory system (Cst,rs), it is sufficient to divide tidal volume (V_T) by the difference of pressure that tidal volume inflation has determined in airway pressure (ΔP_{aw}), as it is shown in the following formula:

$$Cst,rs = V_T/\Delta P_{aw} \tag{5}$$

where ΔP_{aw} is the difference between end-inspiratory (i.e., plateau pressure, P_2) and end-expiratory (i.e., 0 cm H_2O or the value of the PEEP applied) airway pressure. If intrinsic PEEP is present ($PEEP_i$), the value of ΔP_{aw} will be corrected by subtracting P_2 from the value of $PEEP_i$.

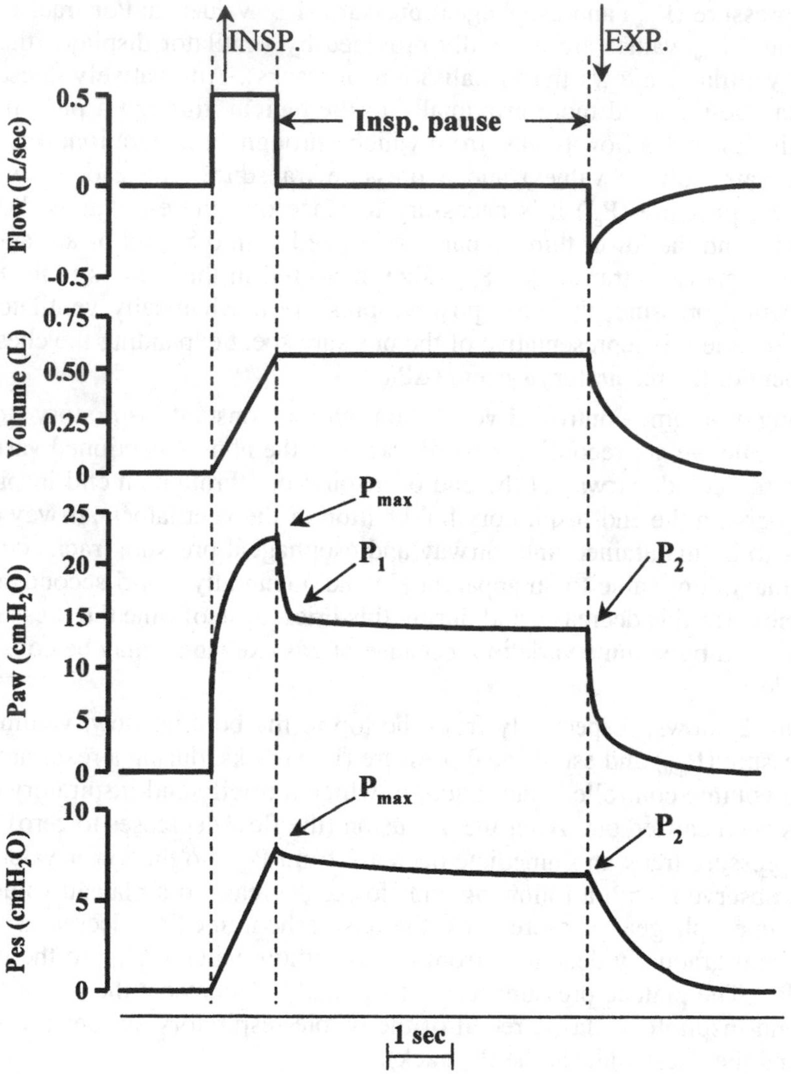

Fig. 2.

Respectively from the top to the bottom, flow, volume (extracted as integration of flow track), airway (P_{aw}) and esophageal pressure (P_{es}) tracks, after an end-inspiratory airway occlusion.
With an airway occlusion, the flow sharply decreases to zero. On P_{aw} track, airway pressure rapidly decreases from peak pressure (P_{max}) to a lower value (P_1), because of the resistance of the endotracheal tube and the tracheo-bronchial tree. Then, airway pressure slowly decreases from P_1 to plateau pressure (P_2), that indicates the pressure necessary to overcome viscoelastic resistance and the dishomogeneity of ventilation distribution due to time-constant inequalities in different tissues. After 4-5 seconds, the pressure decrease finishes to a balance (P_2, plateau pressure), that represents the elastic recoil of the respiratory system. On the P_{es} track, there is not a significant decrease immediately after airway occlusion (i.e., P_1 is not identifiable), but only a slow reduction from the peak (P_{max}) to a plateau (P_2) pressure, indicative of viscoelastic resistance that overcomes the chest wall

In the same way, since plateau pressure (P_2) of P_{es} represents, in a sedated and curarized patient, the pressure produced only by chest wall elastic recoil, the static compliance of the chest wall (Cst,w) may be computed according to the following formula:

$$Cst,w = V_T/\Delta P_{es} \quad (6)$$

where ΔP_{es} is the difference between end-inspiratory (P_2) and end-expiratory esophageal pressure.

The pressure produced by the elastic recoil of the lung component (ΔP_L or transpulmonary pressure) is equal, as it may be deducted from the equation 4, to the difference between ΔP_{aw} and ΔP_{es}. Therefore, lung static compliance may be computed as:

$$Cst,l = V_T/\Delta P_L = V_T/(\Delta P_{aw} - \Delta P_{es}) \quad (7)$$

Clinical implications

The measurement of respiratory mechanics partitioned in the chest wall and lung components presents important clinical implications in the ventilatory treatment of patients with acute respiratory failure (Acute Lung Injury or Acute Respiratory Distress Syndrome - ALI or ARDS). Now it is evident that, in ARDS of different etiologies, similar alterations in mechanical properties of the whole respiratory system may be due to a different alteration of chest wall and lung compliance [13, 14]. In ARDS of pulmonary origin, lung compliance is decreased, while chest wall compliance is near normal. Instead, ARDS of extrapulmonary origin is characterised by a pronounced decreased of chest wall compliance, in respect of a relatively normal lung compliance. In accordance with a prevalent alteration in lung or chest wall compliance, the same pressure applied to the airway will correspond to a different value of transpulmonary pressures (ΔP_L), which is the effective pressure that takes effect on the lung parenchyma. We have to expect, differently for ARDS of pulmonary and extrapulmonary origin, different effects from the application of PEEP or a recruitment manoeuvre [15]. In ARDS of extrapulmonary origin, there will be a greater recruitment, lung parenchyma will be more easily kept open, and there will be a smaller risk for barotrauma (smaller transpulmonary pressure), while the risk of haemodynamic alteration will be greater (high pleural pressures, due to the greater stiffness of chest wall). On the contrary, in ARDS of pulmonary origin, there will be a greater risk of lung overstretching, with a greater risk of barotrauma (high transpulmonary pressures), and a smaller potential for recruitment.

Resistance

A portion of the pressure provided by the ventilator is spent to overcome the resistance of the ventilatory circuit-patient system. Resistance is defined as the decrease of pressure due to the flow passage ($R = \Delta P/F$, expressed in cm H_2O/l/ sec).

From the same tracks (see Fig. 2) used for the compliance calculation, it is possible to extract the value of the total resistance of respiratory system, and it is possible to partition it in lung and chest wall components. In fact, while in static condition (with airway occlusion) the pressure recorded is only due to the elastic recoil of respiratory system (plateau pressure, P_2), in dynamic condition (immediately before airway occlusion) a greater value of pressure is recorded (peak pressure, P_{max}). The difference between the pressure pointed out in dynamic conditions (P_{max}) and that recorded without flow (P_2) just represents the portion of pressure due to resistance of the respiratory system. So, total resistance of respiratory system ("maximal" resistance - Rmax,rs) may be computed from P_{aw} track according to the following formula:

$$\text{Rmax,rs} = (P_{max}/P_2)/F_i \tag{8}$$

where F_i is the immediately previous inspiratory flow.

Moreover, analysing P_{aw} track, it is evident that, immediately after airway occlusion, there is a rapid decrease of pressure from the peak value to a lower value (P_1), followed by a slower decay to the plateau value. Therefore, in Rmax,rs value two different resistive components may be recognised:

– a resistive "ohmic" component of the respiratory system ("minimal" resistance - Rmin,rs), due to the resistance caused by endotracheal tube and by middle and great calibre airway, which is the cause of the P_{aw} decrease from peak pressure to P_1:

$$\text{Rmin,rs} = (P_{max} - P_1)/F_i \tag{9}$$

– An "additional" respiratory component (DR,rs), caused by stress relaxation (viscoelastic resistance) and/or by ventilation redistribution due to time-constant inequalities in different tissues of the respiratory system ("pendelluft" phenomenon). This "additional" component causes the following decrease of P_{aw} from P_1 to P_2:

$$\text{DR,rs} = (P_1 - P_2)/F_i = \text{Rmax,rs} - \text{Rmin,rs} \tag{10}$$

Instead, in the P_{es} track, there isn't a significant decrease of pressure immediately after airway occlusion (i.e., in the esophageal track a P_1 point is not identifiable). Therefore, Rmin essentially reflects airway "ohmic" resistance (lung component, i.e., Rmin,rs = Rmin,l), and the minimal "ohmic" component due to the chest wall (Rmin,w) may be considered negligible [11, 12]. As a consequence, the maximal resistance of chest wall (Rmax,w, which causes the decrease from P_{max} to P_2 in the esophageal pressure track) is entirely due to the viscoelastic properties of chest wall tissues:

$$Rmax,w = DR,w = (P_{max} - P_2)/F_i \tag{11}$$

where P_{max} and P_2 refer to the esophageal pressure track.

The lung "additional" resistance (DR,L) may be obtain according to the following subtraction:

$$DR,L = DR,rs - DR,w \tag{12}$$

DR,L and DR,w (i.e. Rmax,w) are due to stress relaxation and/or time-constant inequalities respectively of lung and chest wall tissues.

The lung maximal resistance (Rmax,L) is equal to:

$$Rmax,L = Rmin,L + DR,L \tag{13}$$

With the same flow, expiratory resistances are generally greater than inspiratory ones, also in a normal subject. The total expiratory resistance is difficult to measure, but it may be estimated, after the application of an end-inspiratory pause, from the airway pressure track according to the following formula:

$$R_{esp} = (P_2 - P_{esp})/F_{esp} \tag{14}$$

where P_{esp} represents the end-expiratory pressure (equal to zero or to the total PEEP value, including auto-PEEP), and F_{esp} is the expiratory flow peak.

Clinical implications

Airway resistance, in particular expiratory resistance, presents important consequences, also in a curarized patient, since it induces an increase of intrinsic PEEP and creates differences between mean airway and alveolar pressures. For simplicity, only inspiratory resistance is usually measured. It is important to remember that Rmax,rs, Rmax,L and Rmin,L values measured with the airway occlusion method represent the whole resistance between the point at which the pressure transducer takes place and the peripheral pulmonary units: therefore, they comprise the resistance of endotracheal tube and, eventually, the resistance due to a large part of the respiratory circuit. This "artificial" resistance is overcome by the ventilator during inspiration, but nevertheless it opposes patient deflation during expiration.

The measurement of respiratory resistance may be useful to evaluate the effectiveness of a broncodilator therapy [16]. However, the resistance is flow-dependent (it increases with a flow increase): so, to compare resistance values in different conditions we always have to apply the same inspiratory flow.

Pressure volume curve

The pressure volume curve (PV curve) represents the static relation between pressure and volume of the respiratory system. The main clinical application of the PV curve is in the understanding the mechanical properties and in driving the ventilatory treatment in ARDS patients. We will briefly describe several methods used to measure the PV curve, and then the morphology of PV curve and the information that we may extract from it in ARDS patients.

The simplest method to provide the PV curve is the "supersyringe" method [17, 18]. After having filled a supersyringe with a gas volume (1500-2000 ml) and being connected to the endotracheal tube, lung parenchyma are inflated with steps of 100 ml, a constant flow and with pauses of 1-2 seconds between steps. At the same time, pressure values reached at the end of each step are recorded. Then, the PV curve is drawn plotting pressure values with the respective volume values inflated. The main disadvantages of this technique are the necessity of using a supersyringe and the fact that we don't consider the continuous gas exchange and the variations of temperature and humidity of the gas inflated during the execution of the manoeuvre [19].

The second method is more complex, but it has the advantage of being able to be effected with any ventilators that are able to carry out end-inspiratory pauses. With constant minute volume and inspiratory flow, respiratory frequency is varied and the patient is ventilated with different tidal volumes (with an increase of the respiratory frequency the tidal volume decreases, and vice versa) [20]. An end-inspiratory pause is effected at each inflation: the PV curve is obtained by plotting the inspiratory plateau pressure values with the correspondent tidal volumes. With this technique the effects of continuous gas exchange are negligible and it's not necessary to disconnect the patient from the ventilator.

More recently, the continuous flow technique has been introduced [21]. After having inflated the patient through an automatic system that provides a low continuous flow, the resistive component of pressure due to the respiratory circuit and the airway are subtracted and a quasi-static PV curve of the respiratory system is constructed.

The pressure volume curve of ARDS patients generally presents a sygmoid shape, because of the presence of two inflection regions – lower and upper – (see Fig. 3). The initial slope of the curve is lower, meaning a worse compliance: it has been described that this start compliance is correlated to the extent of lung tissue that is normally aerated at atmospheric pressure, and, as a consequence, it may give an idea of the dimension of the non collapsed pulmonary regions [18]. The more central and more linear part of the curve presents a better compliance, while at higher pressures the slope decreases, suggesting that, at these pressure values, the prevalent phenomena are alveolar hyperinflation and overstretching.

Clinical implications

The shape of the pressure volume curve takes origin from regional differences in the mechanical properties of the ARDS lung. In the dependent lung regions atelectasis is more prevalent, since pulmonary units tend to collapse because of regional increase in pleural pressure and the weight of the overhanging lung tissue [22-24]. This phenomenon is still more emphasised at a volume equal to FRC, without any application of PEEP, when transalveolar pressure (defined as the difference between the inner alveolar pressure – P_{aw} – applied by the ventilator, and the alveolar external pressure – pleural pressure) is minimal. On the contrary, non dependent pulmonary units remain opened and relatively extensible, but they are subject to overstretching because of end-inspiratory peak pressures. These end-inspiratory pressures may provide transalveolar pressures sufficient to open the dependent alveolar units, that at the end of the following expiration will close, determining a continuous alveolar “opening and closing” movement within the respiratory cycle. To avoid this harmful alveolar collapse and reopening during every respiratory cycle, the target of mechanical ventilation in ARDS patient has to be opening and maintaining open the lung parenchyma [25], avoiding the end-expiratory collapse, and, at the same time, limiting inspiratory plateau pressure to avoid the overtstretching of the non dependent pulmonary units [26].

The PV curve seems to have more and more success for the guide of the ventilatory statement in ARDS patient. To assure an open lung at end expiration, some authors apply a PEEP level just above the pressure correspondent to the lower inflection zone of the PV curve [27, 28]. In fact, it has been suggested that the lower inflection zone may indicate the pressure at which occurs most of the potential for recruitment, and that the ratio between the slope of the PV curve after the lower inflection zone and the start compliance is useful to quantify the potential for recruitment (higher the ratio, higher the potential for recruitment) [18]. Moreover, to avoid alveolar overstretching we have to apply tidal volumes such that plateau pressure doesn’t exceed the upper inflection point: in this way, the whole respiratory cycle is set up within the “safety zone” of the PV curve of the respiratory system (see Fig. 3).

However, we have to be cautious in PV curve interpretation and in its use for the statement of the ventilatory pattern. In fact, it has been suggested that lower inflection zone indicates the beginning of alveolar recruitment, and it doesn’t indicate the pressures at which most of the recruitment has already been effected [29]. Moreover, inflection points may be lacking or be explained by inflection zones of the PV curve of the chest wall instead of the lung, leading to wrong in-

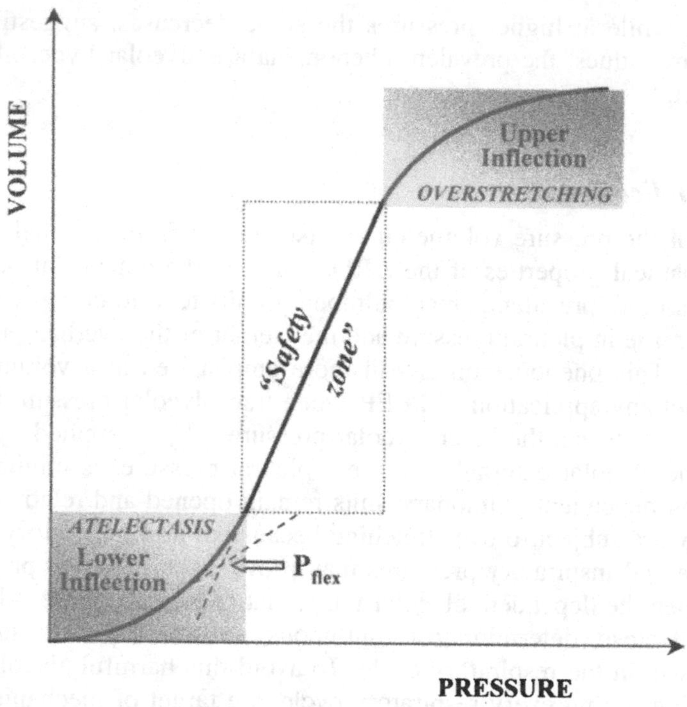

Fig. 3.

Pressure volume curve of the respiratory system of a patient affected by acute respiratory distress syndrome (ARDS). In the lower inflection zone the prevalent phenomena are the occurrence of atelectasis and alveolar derecruitment, while in the upper inflection zone alveolar overstretching prevails. Applying a PEEP level just above the lower inflection point (Pflex, the pressure correspondent to the intersection between the start compliance and the compliance of the linear portion of the PV curve) and limiting the inspiratory plateau pressure, the whole respiratory cycle is maintained within the "safety zone"

terpretations of the PV curve of the whole respiratory system [30, 31]. Moreover, it is necessary to stress that all the clinical information extracted from PV curve derives from the analysis of its inspiratory phase: it is useful to study alveolar recruitment, but it is not adequate to investigate expiratory phenomena, such as the application of PEEP [32].

In conclusion, further studies are necessary to mainly analyse the expiratory phase and the partitioning of the PV curve in lung and chest wall components. Therefore, it will be possible to better understand the physiological meanings of the information that may be extracted and the potential applications in the ventilatory treatment of ARDS patients.

References

1. Pilon CS, Leathley M, London R et al (1997) Practice guideline for arterial blood gas measurement in the intensive care unit decreases the numbers and increases appropriateness of test. Crit Care Med 25:1308-1313
2. Hess D, Kacmarek RM (1993) Techniques and devices for monitoring oxygenation. Respir Care 38:646-671
3. Bhavani-Shankar K, Moseley H, Kumar AY, Delph Y (1992) Capnometry and anaesthesia. Can J Anaesth 39:617-632
4. Hedenstierna G (1993) The recording of FRC - is it of importance and can it be made simple? Intensive Care Med 19:365-366
5. Fretschner R, Deusch H, Weitnauer A, Brunner JX (1993) A simple method to estimate functional residual capacity in mechanically ventilated patients. Intensive Care Med 19:372-376
6. Meneely GR, Ball COT, Kory RC et al (1960) A simplified closed circuit helium dilution method for the determination of the residual volume of the lungs. Amer J Med 29:824
7. Jonmarker C, Jansson L, Jonson B et al (1985) Measurement of functional residual capacity by sulfur hexafluoride washout. Anesthesiology 63:89-95
8. Damia G, Mascheroni D, Croci M, Tarenzi L (1988) Perioperative changes in functional residual capacity in morbidly obese patients. Br J Anaesth 60:574-578
9. Pelosi P, Cereda M, Foti G et al (1995) Alterations of lung and chest wall mechanics in patients with acute lung injury: effects of positive end-expiratory pressure. Am J Respir Crit Care Med 152:531-537
10. Dantzker DR, Brook LJ, Dehart P et al (1979) Ventilation-perfusion distributions in the ARDS. Am Rev Respir Dis 120:1039-1052
11. D'Angelo E, Robatto FM, Calderini E et al (1991) Pulmonary and chest wall mechanics in anesthetized and paralyzed humans. J Appl Physiol 70:2602-2610
12. Polese G, Rossi A, Appendini L et al (1991) Partitioning of respiratory mechanics in mechanically ventilated patients. J Appl Physiol 71:2425-2433
13. Pelosi P, Croci M, Chiumello D et al (1996) Direct or indirect lung injury differently affects respiratory mechanics during acute respiratory failure. Intensive Care Med 22:105
14. Gattinoni L, Pelosi P, Suter PM et al (1998) Acute respiratory distress syndrome due to pulmonary and extrapulmonary disease: different syndromes? Am J Respir Crit Care Med 158: 3-11
15. Pelosi P, Cadringher P, Bottino N et al (1999) Sigh in acute respiratory distress syndrome. Am J Respir Crit Care Med 159:872-880
16. Pesenti A, Pelosi P, Rossi N et al (1993) Respiratory mechanics and bronchodilator responsiveness in patients with the adult respiratory distress syndrome. Crit Care Med 21:78-83
17. Harf A, Lemaire F, Lorino H, Atlan G (1975) Etude de mécanique ventilatoire: application à la ventilation artificielle. Bull Eur Physiopathol Respir 11:709-729
18. Gattinoni L, Pesenti A, Avalli L et al (1987) Pressure-volume curve of total respiratory system in acute respiratory distress failure: computed tomographic scan study. Am Rev Respir Dis 136:730-736
19. Brochard L (1998) Respiratory pressure-volume curves. In: Tobin MJ (ed) Principles and practice of respiratory monitoring. McGraw-Hill Inc, New York, pp 597-616
20. Levy P, Similowski T, Corbeil C et al (1989) A method for studying the static volume-pressure curves of the respiratory system during mechanical ventilation. J Crit Care 4:83-89
21. Servillo G, Svantesson C, Beydon L et al (1997) Pressure-volume curves in the acute respiratory failure. Automated low flow inflation versus occlusion. Am J Respir Crit Care Med 155:1629-1636
22. Gattinoni L, Mascheroni D, Torresin A et al (1986) Morphological response to positive end-expiratory pressure in acute respiratory failure. Int Care Med 12:137-142
23. Gattinoni L, Pelosi P, Vitale G et al (1991) Body position changes redistribute lung computed tomographic density in patients with acute respiratory failure. Anesthesiology 74:15-23

24. Gattinoni L, Pelosi P, Crotti S, Valenza F (1995) Effect of positive end-expiratory pressure on tidal volume and recruitment in adult respiratory distress syndrome. Am J Respir Crit Care Med 151:1807-1814
25. Lachmann B (1992) Open up the lung and keep the lung open. Intensive Care Med 18: 319-321
26. Slutsky AS (1994) Consensus Conference on mechanical ventilation. Intensive Care Med Part I 20:64-79; Part II 20:150-162
27. Amato MB, Barbas CS, Medeiros DM et al (1998) Effect of a protective ventilation strategy on mortality in the acute respiratory distress syndrome. N Engl J Med 338:347-354
28. Ranieri VM, Suter PM, Tortorella C et al (1999) Effect of mechanical ventilation on inflammatory mediators in patients with acute respiratory distress syndrome: a randomized controlled trial. JAMA 282:54-61
29. Hickling KG (1998) The pressure-volume curve is greatly modified by recruitment. A mathematical model of ARDS lungs. Am J Respir Crit Care Med 158:194-202
30. Ranieri VM, Brienza N, Santostasi S et al (1997) Impairment of lung and chest wall mechanics in patients with acute respiratory distress syndrome: role of abdominal distension. Am J Respir Crit Care Med 156:1082-1091
31. Mergoni M, Martelli A, Volpi A et al (1997) Impact of positive end-expiratory pressure on chest wall and lung pressure volume curve in acute respiratory failure. Am J Respir Crit Care Med 156:846-854
32. Pelosi P, Gattinoni L (2000) Respiratory mechanics in ARDS: a siren for physicians? Intensive Care Med 26:653-656

Respiratory Physiology during Artificial Ventilation

G. HEDENSTIERNA

Subjects who undergo artificial ventilation show a different pattern of ventilation and lung blood flow distribution compared to what is seen during spontaneous breathing. These effects are secondary to an altered mechanical behaviour of the respiratory system. In addition, artificial ventilation is mostly undertaken in humans who are either anaesthetised or suffering from respiratory failure. Thus, most observations on the effects of artificial ventilation have been obtained in conditions that themselves may effect pulmonary function.

When analysing the effects of artificial ventilation, comparisons will be made with what must be considered the normal state, i.e. spontaneous breathing under resting conditions. This review will therefore begin with a short summery of pulmonary function in the healthy, spontaneously breathing subject. The focus will be on distributions of ventilation and blood flow and effects on gas exchange.

Spontaneous breathing

Ventilation

The air that is inspired will not be evenly distributed in the lung. During quiet breathing, most air goes to the lower, dependent regions, i.e. basal, diaphragmatic areas in the upright or sitting position, and to dorsal units in the supine position [1]. The lower, dependent lung will receive most of the air if the subject is in the lateral position. This is the combined effect of the curved pressure-volume relationship of the lung tissue (the "P-V curve") and the increasing pleural pressure down the lung. Thus, with increasing lung volume, more pressure is required to inflate the lung by a constant volume. In addition, the increasing pleural pressure in the gravitational direction causes transpulmonary pressure (Ptp) to decrease from top to bottom of the lung. In the upright position, apical lung regions are exposed to a higher Ptp than dependent, basal ones. Thus, upper and lower lung regions are positioned at different levels of the pressure-volume curve. During an inspiration, pleural pressure is lowered and causes lower lung regions to inflate more than upper ones, for a similar change in Ptp (it is assumed that pleural pressure changes uniformly in the pleural space). Thus, in the healthy subject, ventilation goes preferentially to the basal regions. The pleural pressure gradient is oriented in a vertical, gravitational direction, and that is why ventilation distribution changes with body position.

Airways become narrower during the expiration. If the expiration is deep enough, airways in dependent regions will eventually close. In young subjects closure may not occur until they have expired to residual volume. However, with increasing age, airway closure may occur above FRC [2]. The impediment of ventilation by the closure of airways seems to be the major explanation why arterial oxygenation decreases with age. Airway closure will play an even greater role in the supine position. This is because FRC is reduced, whereas airway closure is not affected by body position. Closure of airways may occur above FRC already at an age of 45-50 years, and in the 70-year-old subject airways may be continuously closed if closing capacity exceeds FRC plus the tidal volume.

Blood flow

Pulmonary artery pressure increases down the lung, an effect of the hydrostatic pressure that builds up on the way from top to bottom of the lung. This pressure increases by 1 cm H_2O per cm distance down the lung (or 0.74 mm Hg/cm vertical distance; blood has a density close to 1, or 1.04). There is thus less driving pressure to the top of the lung. Since the mean pulmonary artery pressure is approximately 12 mmHg at the level of the heart, it may approach zero in the apex of the lung in the upright position. No blood will then flow through the vessels. That part of the lung is called zone I, according to the nomenclature introduced by West [3] and associates. If arterial and capillary pressure exceeds alveolar pressure, as it will further down the lung because of the addition of hydrostatic pressure, a blood flow will be established. The perfusion pressure will be arterial minus alveolar pressures, as long as the latter pressure exceeds that of the pulmonary veins (zone II). This is different from the systemic circulation, where perfusion pressure is arterial minus venous pressure. Since pulmonary arterial pressure increases down the lung blood flow also increases down this zone. Further down the lung, both arterial and venous pressures exceed that in the alveoli, so that perfusion pressure is arterial minus venous pressure (zone III). Since both arterial and venous pressures increase to the same extent down this zone, hydrostatic pressure adding to both sides, perfusion pressure does not increase down the zone. Still, perfusion increases downwards, albeit it may be less than the increase in zone II. The explanation is that the increasing vascular pressure dilates the vessels down the lung, and by this means reduces the vascular resistance. Finally, blood flow decreases in the bottom of the lung. This zone IV is generally explained by an increasing interstitial pressure down the lung that compresses the extra-alveolar vessels. The vertical distribution of blood flow can thus be explained by the influence of gravitation on vascular, alveolar and interstitial pressures.

There is also an uneven distribution of blood flow in the non-gravitational plane [4]. This suggests that there are morphological and/or functional differences between lung vessels that, in addition to gravity, determine blood flow distribution.

Ventilation-perfusion match (VA/Q)

Since both ventilation and blood flow increase down the lung, they match each other fairly well from top to bottom of the lung. Ventilation is normally a little larger, by three-four times, than perfusion in upper regions and is smaller, by five-ten times, in the very bottom of the lung [3]. Non-gravitational inhomogeneity will also add to the VA/Q scatter. The result is a VA/Q match centred on a VA/Q ratio of one and with a range of ratios between 0.1 and 10 ("normal VA/Q").

Morphological and functional changes by anaesthesia and by ARDS

To understand the effects of artificial ventilation on pulmonary physiology we need also to know the impact of the conditions per se, that is the indications for applying ventilatory support. Thus, a short summary of the effects of anaesthesia and of acute respiratory failure and ARDS on morphology and function will be made here.

Anaesthesia

Anaesthesia in general lowers muscle tone, including the diaphragm and the intercostal muscles and this causes a decrease in FRC (for a review of pulmonary effects of anaesthesia, see [5]). The loss of muscle tone will also allow the transmission of the higher abdominal pressure and its higher vertical pressure gradient into the thoracic cavity. This contributes to the decrease in FRC but also to a greater regional difference in lung volume. Thus, upper, non-dependent alveoli may even expand during anaesthesia while at the same time the dimensions of the dependent alveoli are reduced. The decrease in volume promotes airway closure that occurs in lower lung regions. The fall in FRC with promotion of airway closure and the use of high oxygen fraction will also promote atelectasis formation in the most dependent lung regions. The atelectasis is thus a consequence of gas adsorption in small alveoli, possibly behind occluded airways. It is interesting to note that if muscle tone is preserved and FRC is not reduced, as with ketamine, no atelectasis is produced even when ventilating with 100% O_2. Also, if pure oxygen is avoided during induction and the subsequent anaesthesia no or very little of atelectasis is produced. The airway closure causes a ventilation/perfusion mismatch and the atelectasis true shunt. These two morphological and functional changes explain approximately three-fourths of the regularly occurring oxygenation impairment during anaesthesia.

The anaesthetic may also attenuate the hypoxic pulmonary vasoconstrictor response but it should be remembered that such attenuation would have no effect unless there is an underlying V_A/Q disturbance. Also, the frequently used anaesthetics will not impede HPV by more than 25% at clinical concentrations [6].

It is also well known that the compliance of the respiratory system is reduced during anaesthesia, and the resistance is increased [7]. A convincing explanation to these changes has not yet been offered, but they may be related to the decrease in lung volume with less ventilated parenchyma and reduced airway dimensions.

The anaesthetic may have cardio-depressant effects with decreases in cardiac output and vascular pressures [8]. Pulmonary blood flow may then be distributed more towards dependent regions and uppermost units may be poorly or not at all perfused (zone I). This exaggerates the VA/Q mismatch during anaesthesia by enhancing the shunt fraction and increasing the dead space.

Acute respiratory failure

Acute respiratory failure (ARF/ARDS) is characterised by pulmonary infiltrates [9], caused by extravasation of fluid, producing protein-rich pulmonary oedema that is later followed by fibrosis. The infiltrates can be seen on X-ray as densities. CT investigations have shown that most of the densities are in the dependent regions, indicating an influence of gravitational forces [10]. The densities have an attenuation of around 0 Hounsfield units (HU) which means that they do not contain air. They are qualitatively similar to the densities (atelectasis) seen during anaesthesia, but quantitatively much larger. Thus, in ARDS patients the amount of densities may account for up to 70-80% of the lung area on the CT compared to 4-8% in the lung of healthy, anaesthetised subjects. The apical regions are less compromised and the hilar and basal regions are more affected.

One of the hallmarks of ARF/ARDS is the reduction of lung compliance. The ARDS lung is usually referred to as a "stiff lung" due to the high pressures needed to inflate it. Interestingly, lung compliance is significantly correlated with the amount of normally inflated lung but not with the amount of poorly inflated or collapsed tissue [10]. The findings suggest that compliance is correlated to the air-containing part of the lung and not to the "amount of disease" (although the oedema accumulation expels air out of the lung, as mentioned above). These findings have brought forward the nickname "baby-lung" in ARDS.

In ARF/ARDS ventilation goes mainly to upper lung regions, a finding that may not be too surprising in view of the collapsed or consolidated dependent lung regions that are thus non-ventilated [10]. Perfusion, on the other hand, increases down the lung, in similar with the pattern in healthy lungs. However, two factors may modify the perfusion distribution to some extent. Firstly, the pulmonary hypertension that is a frequent finding in ARDS will raise blood flow in upper, non-dependent lung regions. Secondly, hypoxic pulmonary vasoconstriction and, possibly, mechanical compression of vessels will reduce blood flow in the atelectatic and consolidated, dependent regions. However, there will still be a large blood flow through the lower, non-ventilated lung units [11].

While lung compliance is correlated with the normally inflated part of the lung (see above), the gas exchange impairment is strongly related to the amount of disease, i.e. the non-inflated tissue mass. Thus, the impairment of arterial oxygenation and the venous admixture ("shunt") correlate with the quantity of non-inflated lung tissue [10]. This suggests that the shunt (VA/Q = 0; i.e. perfusion of the atelectatic and consolidated tissue) is the main cause of hypoxemia in ARDS. Most patients show in addition increased scatter of VA/Q ratios ("mismatch") with perfusion of low V_A/Q regions (VA/Q < 0.1) and ventilation of high VA/Q regions (VA/Q > 10) [12]. The former is reasonably explained by airway narrowing by oedema and redistribution of blood flow by hypoxic pulmonary vasoconstriction and the latter by regional over-ventilation in relation to blood flow.

Artificial ventilation

This review will focus on intermittent positive pressure ventilation that is dominating the field of artificial ventilation. A short historical review will be made first and a few comments on intermittent negative pressure ventilation will also be made.

Short historical review

There are different ways of delivering ventilation by artificial means. Vesalius reported already in 1543 that intermittent finger pressure on the chest of a frog caused air to be pushed out and in to the animal. Sauerbruch applied a continuous positive airway pressure (CPPV, V for ventilation) by a face mask in the begining of the early 1900s to inflate the lungs. It was later discovered that if the face mask was disconnected intermittently, the patient appeared to be much better oxygenated. The intermittent positive pressure ventilation (IPPV) was rediscovered! During the recurrent polio epidemics in the years 1930-1950, intermittent negative pressure ventilation (INPV) was developed and executed by means of tank respirators that enclosed the patient, save his or her head. By using a cuirass INPV could be applied around the chest only. The dominance of the tank ventilator ended when efficient positive pressure ventilators had been developed. The Engström respirator was one of the first to come out on the market in the early 1950s; this was a sturdy and reliable piston pump with an ingenious bag-in-bottle principle to deliver the tidal volume. Finally, the "electronic" ventilators with computer-controlled pneumatic systems succeeded the "mechanical" machines. The first machine that appeared on the market was the Siemens 900 around 1970. These engineering advancements founded the basis for the multitude of ventilator modes that have appeared during the last 20 years.

It may be worth mentioning that the whole patient can be enclosed in a tank (also his or her head) and be ventilated by varying the pressure in the tank: the barospirator by Thunberg. When pressure is increased, air is compressed and forced into the lungs until pressure is equilibrated between alveoli and room. Distribution of air in the lungs will depend solely on airway resistance, since there is no lung expansion. The principle was used for artificial ventilation in operation rooms with the surgical staff being exposed to the same pressure variation as the patient. It did not become widely accepted because the pressure variation caused discomfort, the eardrums flapping in and out.

Intermittent positive pressure ventilation

With intermittent positive pressure ventilation (IPPV), air or a gas mixture is pushed into the airway by raising the pressure at the airway opening to above that in the alveoli. This can be achieved by blowing mouth-to-mouth, by squeezing a rubber balloon and by means of a ventilator. The pressure has to overcome 1) the resistance to gas flow in the airways (airway resistance, Raw), 2) the resistance caused by the sliding of different lung tissues over each other (tissue resistance, Rtis), 3) the elastic recoil of the alveolar wall (lung elastance; its inverse expression, the compliance, is more commonly used, Clung), 4) the elastance of the chest wall (again, the inverse, chest wall compliance, Ccw, is more commonly used, and 5) the resistance in the chest wall (Rcw). It follows that there are many morphological and functional disturbances that can affect the pressure required to inflate the lungs with gas. It should also be remembered that, when comparing pressure during mechanical ventilation with that during spontaneous breathing, pressure at the same measurement point reflects different components of the respiratory system. Thus with spontaneous breathing, airway opening pressure (Pao) is obviously atmospheric unless continuous positive airway pressure (CPAP) or a negative pressure (whatever the reason would be) is applied. The driving pressure is Pao minus pleural pressure (Ppl). During a maximum inspiration Ppl may reach –25 to –30 cm H_2O. If the lungs of the same subject were to be inflated by positive pressure to vital capacity (or more correct, to total lung capacity), then a Pao of +40 cm H_2O would be required. The seemingly higher pressure than during spontaneous breathing is because the pressure to overcome elastic and resistive forces in the chest wall is visible during mechanical ventilation but not during spontaneous breathing. Ppl during spontaneous breathing overcomes the elastic and resistive forces in the lung, as said above, whereas during positive pressure ventilation it overcomes these forces in the chest wall. To allow a comparison between spontaneous breathing and positive pressure ventilation, the transpulmonary pressure (Ptp = Pao – Ppl) must be compared and the comparison is limited to the lung. Chest wall mechanics are impossible to measure during spontaneous breathing under clinical conditions, but require trained volunteers.

The volume inflated for a given Ptp should be the same during spontaneous breathing and mechanical, positive pressure ventilation. Also, gas distribution should be the same. Thus, the differences in tidal volume and in gas distribution that are common when comparing the two modes of ventilation must be explained by other, coexisting factors. Anaesthesia, muscle relaxation and probably heavy sedation lower FRC. Airways become narrower and the resistance to gas flow increases, more so in dependent lung regions. The fall in FRC also promotes airway closure This will alter the distribution of gas towards upper regions. Reduced alveolar size shortens the time to collapse by adsorption of gas, atelectasis being another mechanism behind altered distribution of gas [5]. Moreover, the reduced number of alveoli accessible for ventilation will lower Clung and decrease tidal volume for a given Ptp. To this may be added possible decreases in surfactant release or function by the anaesthetic [13] and effects on pulmonary vascular tone with concomitant changes in pulmonary blood volume [14]. These changes may add to the other ones in reducing Clung. All these factors will also apply in various conditions of acute respiratory failure.

Positive pressure ventilation has a more clear effect on circulation, compared to spontaneous breathing, than it has on ventilation. Thus, the higher intrathoracic pressure impedes venous return and lowers cardiac output. The pressure increase may also cause a, or increase an existing, zone I (where alveolar pressure exceeds capillary pressure) with elimination of blood flow in uppermost lung regions [15] (not completely, there is a tiny, persisting perfusion of so-called alveolar corner vessels) [16]. This causes an increase in alveolar dead space and reduces the part of the tidal volume that can be used for gas exchange. To compensate for this "loss", minute ventilation must be increased, and this has to be accomplished by raising airway pressure, followed by further increase in zone I! Zone IV (the bottom-most zone where perfusion is decreasing), on the other hand, is reduced. This is a consequence of the squeezing of blood flow down the lung towards the bottom. Since atelectasis and airway closure are located there, shunt and perfusion of "low VA/Q" regions increase by positive pressure ventilation unless the positive pressure opens up collapsed regions and widens narrow airways. This will be discussed in a following paragraph, on PEEP.

Positive pressure ventilation may also affect pulmonary vascular resistance (PVR), but the major mechanism is probably via any effect on lung volume. PVR is lung volume dependent, having a minimum around FRC. It increases when lung volume is increased, because of compression of alveolar capillaries. It increases when lung volume goes down below FRC, because of compression of extra-alveolar lung vessels [17].

The increase in intrathoracic pressure is accompanied by an increase in pulmonary vascular pressure. However, the increase is less than that in intrathoracic pressure. If anything, less leakage of plasma to the interstitial tissue should occur. The raised intrathoracic pressure impedes lymph flow in the lung and there are reports on dramatic increases in lymph flow when spontaneous breathing was resumed in animal experiments [18]. Impeded lymph flow may suggest fluid accumulation in the tissue, unless the net capillary leakage is reduced to the same extent.

Positive end-expiratory pressure (PEEP) is frequently used as a means of improving oxygenation of blood. It can be considered an extension of positive pressure ventilation. PEEP increases lung volume and may open up collapsed lung regions. Such recruitment should improve oxygenation. However, the additional increase in intrathoracic pressure impedes cardiac output further and forces lung blood flow even more down the lung [15]. This may result in an increased fractional perfusion of remaining atelectatic lung tissue, so that shunt even is increased [5]! PEEP appears to impede further the lymph drainage of the lung and to increase interstitial lung fluid ("lung water") [19], although contradictory results have been published.

PEEP may cause over-distension of alveoli and even damage, so-called volo/barotrauma [20]. It may be assumed to occur mainly in upper lung regions. This is because of the larger initial inflation of the upper lung regions, until dependent regions are reopened, if it at all occurs [21]. However, in ARDS, the damage seems to predominate in the lower lung regions [22]. This has been proposed to be due to "shear stress failure", i.e. the opening and closing of lung units with each tidal breath [23]. That cyclic collapse and reopening of dependent lung tissue occurs has recently been shown in animal experiments [24, 25]. If cyclic collapse is the mechanism of volo/barotrauma, PEEP should be advocated to prevent intermittent collapse of lung units.

Different modes of positive pressure ventilation have been tried in order to improve gas exchange in ARDS as well as in experimental studies. Only a few of these modes will be discussed here to illustrate the effects on ventilation distribution, gas exchange and lung integrity. The change in the inspiratory to expiratory (I:E) ratio from the conventional 1:2 to 2:1-4:1, so-called inverse ratio ventilation (IRV), was initially reported to improve oxygenation, sometimes dramatically [26, 27]. IRV is normally performed in the pressure-controlled mode, which results in an early rapid increase in airway pressure and inspiratory flow. This rapid flow increase was thought to open up closed airways and the long inspiratory phase to promote alveolar recruitment. Although these may be possible mechanisms, the major effect is more likely executed by an interrupted expiration due to the short expiratory time. This creates an intrinsic PEEP that keeps alveoli recruited. Comparisons with conventional mechanical ventilation (CMV) with an extrinsic PEEP of the same magnitude as that produced intrinsically by IRV have, however, shown no advantage for the IRV technique [28, 29]. It may be hypothesised that IRV would promote aeration of lung units with long time constants, due to the short expiratory time that is available, and that this would keep more collapsible units open to a higher degree than CMV. However, experimental data suggest the opposite. Thus, upper, already well-aerated lung regions become even more aerated with IRV and lower, dependent regions are less expanded in comparison with CMV with essentially the same mean airway pressure and extrinsic/intrinsic PEEP (20 and 17 cm H_2O in CMV and IRV, respectively) [30]. Lung blood flow distribution, assessed by the injection of radioactive microspheres, showed no consistent difference between the two ventilatory modes but shunt, assessed by multiple inert gas elimination technique, was much higher with IRV. This suggests that the major difference between the two modes is in the aeration and recruitment of alveoli and this was better with CMV.

Another aspect is whether to maintain some spontaneous ventilation even in severe lung damage. Airway pressure release ventilation (APRV) allows an essentially unrestricted spontaneous breathing from a pre-set positive airway pressure, with the addition of short releases of the airway pressure to a pre-set lower airway pressure, mimicking an expiration and subsequent inspiration [31]. Putensen and co-workers showed better oxygenation in experimental animals, and subsequently in human patients who where breathing spontaneously as little as 10% of their total ventilation in an APRV mode (also called BIPAP), compared to 100% mechanical ventilation [32, 33]. Preliminary experimental data from our group show a dose-dependent improvement in oxygenation with increasing fraction of spontaneous ventilation. Moreover, the animals that had been breathing spontaneously (between 50 and 100% of total ventilation) showed a reduction in the pulmonary artery pressure and increase in PaO_2 6 hours after induction of lung damage compared to earlier phases of lung damage. Pigs on continuous mechanical ventilation, on the other hand, showed no recovery during the study period. Although the data are preliminary, they suggest that spontaneous breathing may also promote lung healing as compared to CMV. Further research is required before making a definite conclusion.

Intermittent negative pressure ventilation

By lowering the pressure on the outside of the body, the chest wall is expanded, both the rib cage and the diaphragm – the latter by the expansion of the abdominal wall. The lung is expanded and air is sucked into the alveoli. This may appear more similar to spontaneous breathing than intermittent positive pressure ventilation and certainly is. However, it is a general misconception that INPV offers the advantage over IPPV of better preservation of cardiac output. It is based on the knowledge that the lowering of intra-thoracic pressure will increase the return of venous blood to the right ventricle. However, the tank respirator, with the application of sub-atmospheric, "negative" pressure around the whole body, will not suck blood into the thorax, since no increased pressure gradient between extra- and intra-thoracic vessels is produced. Obviously, it will be different with the cuirass ventilator.

Conclusions

It can thus be concluded that artificial ventilation has little effect on distribution of inspired air, provided that all other factors that may influence such distribution remain constant. This is seldom the case. The use of anaesthetics, sedatives and muscle relaxants, together with artificial ventilation, lower muscle tone and FRC and increase the vertical pleural pressure gradient. These changes will modify gas distribution and shift it towards upper, non-dependent lung regions. Positive pressure ventilation will also affect distribution of lung blood flow, forcing it down towards dependent lung regions. This will create a ventilation-perfusion mismatch, and even shunt.

References

1. Milic-Emili J, Henderson JAM, Dolovich MB et al (1966) Regional distribution of inspired gas in the lung. J Appl Physiol 21:749-759
2. Leblanc P, Ruff F, Milic Emili J (1970) Effects of age and body position on "airway closure" in man. J Appl Physiol 28:448-451
3. West JB (1977) Blood flow. In: West JB (ed) Regional differences in the lung. Academic Press, New York, pp 85-165
4. Glenny RW, Lamm WJ, Albert RK, Robertson HT (1991) Gravity is a minor determinant of pulmonary blood flow distribution. J Appl Physiol 71:620-629
5. Hedenstierna G (1998) Gas exchange pathophysiology during anesthesia. Anesthesiol Clin N Am 16:113-127
6. Marshall BE (1989) Effects of anesthetics on pulmonary gas exchange. In: Stanley TH, Sperry RJ (eds) Anesthesia and the lung. Kluwer Academic Press, London, pp 117-125
7. Don H (1977) The mechanical properties of the respiratory system during anesthesia. Int Anesthesiol Clin 15:113-136
8. Merin RG (1975) Effects of anesthetics on the heart. Surg Clin North Am 55:759-774
9. Ashbaugh DG, Bigelow DB, Petty TL, Levine BE (1967) Acute respiratory distress in adults. Lancet 2:319-323
10. Gattinoni L, Pesenti A, Bombino M et al (1988) Relationships between lung computed tomographic density, gas exchange, and PEEP in acute respiratory failure. Anesthesiology 69: 824-832
11. Schuster DP, Haller J (1990) Regional pulmonary blood flow during acute pulmonary edema: a PET study. J Appl Physiol 69:353-361
12. Mélot C (1994) Ventilation-perfusion relationships in acute respiratory failure. Thorax 49: 1251-1258
13. Wollmer P, Schairer W, Bos JAH et al (1990) Pulmonary clearance of ^{99m}Tc-DTPA during halothane anesthesia. Acta Anaesthesiol Scand 34:572-575

14. Hedenstierna G, Strandberg A, Brismar B et al (1985) Functional residual capacity, thoracoabdominal dimensions, and central blood volume during general anesthesia with muscle paralysis and mechanical ventilation. Anesthesiology 62:247-254
15. West JB, Dollery CT, Naimark A (1964) Distribution of blood flow in isolated lung: relation to vascular and alveolar pressures. J Appl Physiol 19:713-724
16. Hedenstierna G, White FC, Mazzone R, Wagner PD (1979) Redistribution of pulmonary blood flow in the dog with PEEP ventilation. J Appl Physiol 46:278-287
17. Harris P, Heath D (1986) The human pulmonary circulation. Churchill Livingstone, New York
18. Blomqvist H, Frostell C, Pieper R, Hedenstierna G (1990) Measurement of dynamic lung fluid balance in the mechanically ventilated dog. Theory and results. Acta Anaesthesiol Scand 34:370-376
19. Frostell C, Blomqvist H, Hedenstierna G et al (1987) Thoracic and abdominal lymph drainage in relation to mechanical ventilation and PEEP. Acta Anaesthesiol Scand 31: 405-412
20. Dreyfuss D, Saumon G (1993) Role of tidal volume, FRC, and end-inspiratory volume in the development of pulmonary edema following mechanical ventilation. Am Rev Respir Dis 148: 1194-1203
21. Gattinoni L, Pelosi P, Crotti S, Valenza F (1995) Effects of positive end-expiratory pressure on regional distribution of tidal volume and recruitment in adult respiratory distress syndrome. Am J Respir Crit Care Med 151:1807-1814
22. Gattinoni L, Bombino M, Pelosi P et al (1994) Lung structure and function in different stages of severe adult respiratory distress syndrome. JAMA 271:1772-1779
23. Muscedere JG, Mullen JB, Gan K, Slutsky AS (1994) Tidal ventilation at low airway pressures can augment lung injury. Am J Respir Crit Care Med 149:1327-1334
24. Neumann P, Berglund JE, Mondejar EF et al (1998) Dynamics of lung collapse and recruitment during prolonged breathing in porcine lung injury. J Appl Physiol 85:1533-1543
25. Neumann P, Berglund JE, Mondejar EF et al (1998) Effect of different pressure levels on the dynamics of lung collapse and recruitment in oleic acid-induced lung injury. Am J Resp Crit Care Med 158:1636-1643
26. Andersen JB (1989) Ventilatory strategy in catastrophic disease. Inversed ratio ventilation (IRV) and combined high frequency ventilation (CHFV). Acta Anaesthesiol Scand 33: 145-148
27. Tharratt RS, Allen RF, Albertson TE (1988) Pressure controlled inverse ventilation in severe adult respiratory failure. Chest 94:755-762
28. Lessard MR, Guerot E, Lorino H et al (1994) Effects of pressure controlled ventilation with different I:E ratios versus volume controlled ventilation on respiratory mechanics, gas exchange and hemodynamics in patients with adult respiratory distress syndrome. Anesthesiology 80:983-991
29. Chan K, Abraham E (1992) Effects of inverse ratio ventilation on cardiorespiratory parameters in severe respiratory failure. Chest 192:1556-1561
30. Neumann P, Berglund J, Andersson LG et al (2000) Effects of inverse ratio ventilation and positive end-expiratory pressure in oleic acid-induced lung injury. Am J Respir Crit Care Med 161:1537-1545
31. Downs JB, Stock MC (1987) Airway pressure ventilation. A new concept in ventilatory support. Crit Care Clin 15:49-61
32. Putensen C, Räsänen J, Lopez FA (1994) Ventilation-perfusion distributions during mechanical ventilation with superimposed spontaneous breathing in canine lung injury. Am J Resp Crit Care Med 150:101-108
33. Putensen C, Mutz NJ, Putensen-Himmer G, Zinserling J (1999) Spontaneous breathing during ventilatory support improves ventilation-perfusion distributions in patients with acute respiratory distress syndrome. Am J Respir Crit Care Med 159:1241-1248

Capnography: Basic Concepts

P.V. ROMERO

Carbon dioxide (CO_2)elimination is a specific task of the lung. While CO_2 production is basically a metabolic matter, the elimination of CO_2 is performed by the lung by integrating alveolar perfusion, and alveolar ventilation, and alveolar exchange functions. The way the lung performs CO_2 elimination is a reflection of the efficacy, regulation, and matching of alveolar ventilation and perfusion. Expiratory CO_2 signal (instantaneous CO_2 concentration, or CO_2 contents, or partial pressure in expiratory gas) or capnogram yield an important amount of information about the functional status of the gas exchange in the lung: the efficacy of lung in eliminating CO_2, and the functional status of alveolar gas exchange.

Classically three distinct phases have been identified in the capnogram versus time [$FECO_2(t)$], and in the capnogram versus volume [$FECO_2(v)$] curves [1]: Phase I has no CO_2 elimination, and roughly corresponds to the exhalation of the gas content of the anatomical dead space; phase II is a transition phase during which $FECO_2$ increases progressively, and phase III or "alveolar phase" is a plateau during which $FECO_2$ increases more or less linearly with expired volume, with a smooth slope in normal subjects and a steeper slope in patients with abnormalities of ventilatory distribution. The identification of these phases cannot be performed without a visual identification of those points that better define the transition between I-II and II-III phases.

For many years, lung physiologists have studied ways of interpreting expiratory CO_2 signal in order to obtain information about lung and alveolar function, and sometimes to analyze some of the different aspects of lung function in relation to the gas exchange function and sometimes to obtain a global index to identify pulmonary dysfunction. Historically, we can describe three periods, which are related to the development of CO_2 analyzers. In a first period, the CO_2 content of expiratory gas was done by chemical analysis or the response of the analyzers was so low, that CO_2 signal could not be analyzed at the time of the trial. In this period capnography was based on the assumptions underlying the ideal alveolar gas hypothesis, and alveolar sampling was performed by means of devices activated by the volume signal. In a second period, relatively fast analyzers (infrared chambers, mass spectrometry) were available for on-line measurement of CO_2 expiratory signal by sidestream sampling, with only small phase lags with the real time. Capnography versus time signals were obtained and used in order to obtain data about lung function in a more analytical way; the two-compartment lung model allowing to description of the classical phases of the capnogram. In a third period, the development of main stream analyzers allowed the capnographic signal to be obtained in real time, and by plotting it against expiratory volume volumetric capnography was born. Volumetric capnography allowed measurement of anatomical dead space, and assessment of parameters of alveolar inhomogeneity based on the assumption of sequential gas elimination [2, 3].

In this chapter we will first describe the most-important points in this evolution, as well as some usual parameters derived from the capnographic signal. New developments of capnography based on the use of parameters that are easily handled by computer will compose the second part of the chapter.

Basic model assumptions

As in practically all applied physiological measurements, prior model assumptions are imperative. This is because we need to have a physiological basis for signal parameters, and to interpret the results in the least- speculative way possible. On the other hand, a model allows implementation of advances in our knowledge, to define the limits of the application of a technique, and to correct the assumption if necessary.

The two serial compartments model

In the case of capnography the model generally used has been the so called two serial compartments model (Fig. 1). This model arises from the assumption that the lung, as exchanger, is composed of two compartments placed in series: anatomical dead space and alveolar compartment. Anatomical dead space is the volume of gas contained in conducting airways. As a general rule, VDanat is considered as the volume of gas that does not participate in the gas exchange, anatomically placed between alveoli and airways opening. The serial position of this volume in respecti to the gas exchange area makes it unavoidable during tidal breath. Part of tidal volume (VT) will be wasted in the renewal of this area and, therefore, will not participate in gas exchange. The amount of tidal volume that reaches the gas exchange area is called alveolar volume (VA). Unlike VDanat, VA does not reflect a real volume in a dimensional sense, but the fraction of VT that is used in the turnover and renewal of alveolar gas contents. This two-compartment model assumes that dead space is exclusively composed of serial or anatomical dead space. On this basis Bohr [4], in 1891, described the equation that allowed the first capnographic approach to the evaluation of gas exchange function of the lung. Bohr sampled the end expiratory gas and ana-

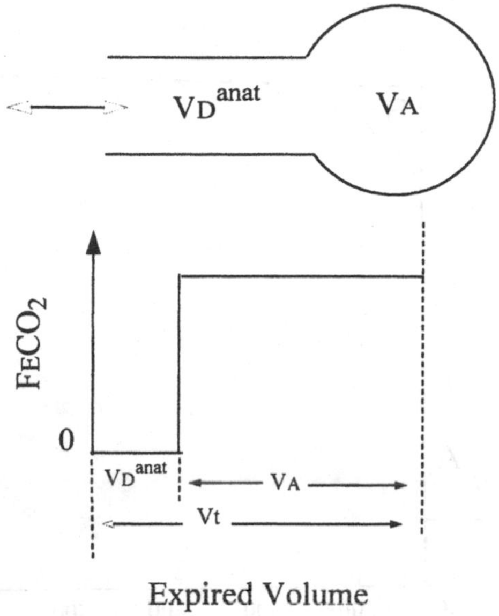

Fig. 1. The two-compartment basic model

lyzed it, as well as measured the average expiratory concentration of CO_2 and minute expiratory volume. He reasoned as follows: all CO_2 is, by definition, exhaled by the alveolar exchange area, and consequently we can write

$$VCO_2 = VT \cdot f \cdot FECO_2 = VA \cdot f \cdot FACO_2$$

or tidal CO_2 elimination of CO_2 is equal to alveolar CO_2 elimination (f is breathing frequency). As tidal volume can be divided into the alveolar and dead space components we can write:

$$VT \cdot FECO_2 = (VT\text{-}VD) \cdot FACO_2$$

and VD is easily calculated.

Later in the 1940s, when fast side stream expiratory gas analyzers were available, Fowler [5] described another method, based on a geometrical reconstruction of the expiratory capnogram (or nitrogenogram) in order to fit the two-compartment model. This method is known as the equal area method, and is described in Figure 2. Variations of this method are the measurement of dead space from an alternative alveolar value taken at mid-alveolar plateau [6], or the measurement of dead space using phase II inflection [7]. In all these methods dead space volume is estimated by the best fit of an idealized step response of gas washout to the observed expired waveform. In each method, there is an as-

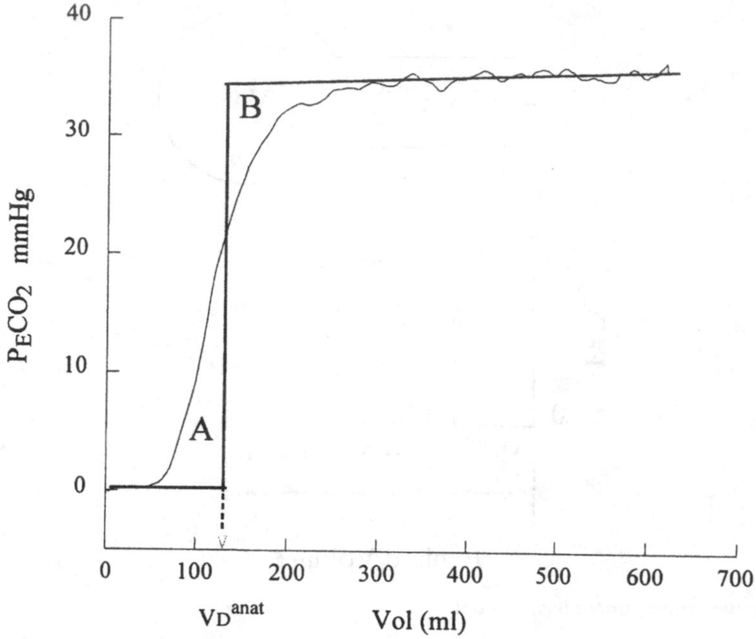

Fig. 2. Measurement of anatomical dead space by reconstruction of the two-compartment model: the Fowler's equal area method

sumption that the expired waveform is a mixture of dead space and alveolar gas. Computation of dead space involves allocation of a proper fraction of the breath to alveolar gas with the remainder assigned to dead space (Fig. 2). Expired gas to the right of the line, indicating dead space, is assigned to alveolar gas. Gas to the left is assigned to dead space. Shaded regions show deficient alveolar gas below the assumed alveolar value (*B*) or dead space with non-zero expired concentration (*A*). These regions must be balanced.

The three-compartment model

The simplest model that introduces ventilation/perfusion (V/Q) inequalities in the capnographic evaluation of lung exchange function is the three-compartment model. It consists of two parallel compartments, connected to a serial dead space (Fig. 3). However, this model requires an arterial concentration of CO_2. Alveolar parallel compartments are assumed to have their own ventilation and alveolar partial pressures of CO_2 that are either equal to the arterial PCO_2 or zero, for the alveolar compartment and the so called alveolar (or parallel) dead space, respectively. The main assumption underlying this model was proposed by Enghoff [8] in 1931, who suggested that, in ventilated alveoli, $pACO_2$ always

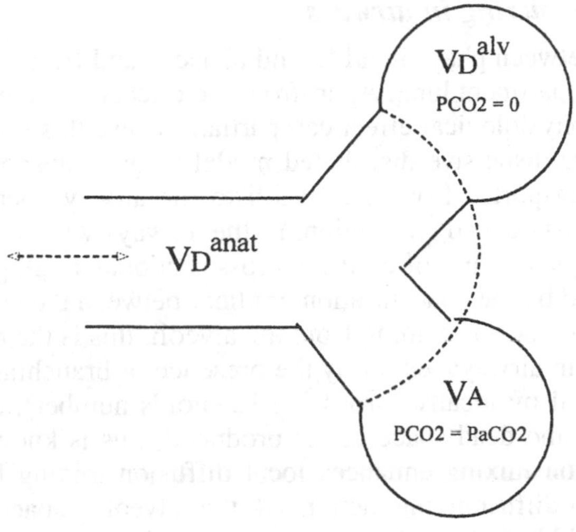

Fig. 3. Three-compartment model. VD^{alv} does not reflect on the capnogram, but it requires arterial PCO_2 measurement

matches $paCO_2$, whereas areas without perfusion have a $pACO_2$ equal to zero. By substituting alveolar CO_2 with arterial CO_2 in the Bohr equation a new value of dead space is obtained. This is widely accepted as physiological dead space (Vdphys):

$$Vdphys = (PaCO_2 - PECO_2) \cdot VT/PaCO_2$$

In the absence of alveolar dead space $pACO_2 = paCO_2$ and Bohr and Enghoff equations are identical. So, the main effect of alveolar dead space is to generate an alveolar-arterial gradient of CO_2. The all or none assumption introduced in this model has to be smoothed to interpret the evaluation of V/Q mismatching effects. Alveolar CO_2 partial pressure is a result of the V/Q regional relationship. Every given alveolar region, having a fixed V/Q, can be considered to be composed of two compartments, one composed of the ventilation fraction ideally matching perfusion in order to have $pACO_2 = paCO_2$. The rest of the alveolar ventilation is wasted ventilation, whose effect is to reduce $pACO_2$ from the ideal $paCO_2$ to its actual value. Alveolar ventilation is, therefore, the sum of all regional alveolar ventilatory fractions, whereas alveolar dead space ventilation is the sum of all the regional wasted ventilatory fractions.

The three-compartment model requires a measurement of arterial $paCO_2$, and therefore cannot be considered as a non-invasive technique. For this reason volumetric capnography developed on the basis of the two-compartment model in order to obtain information about pulmonary function.

Introducing gas mixing in airways

The transitions between phase I and II, and phase II and III are smoother than in the ideal two-compartment lung. Apart from the effects of the measurement system response, a physiological effect can partially cause this effect. It is thought to be a convective-dispersive distributed model of gas transport in the airways [2, 9]. CO_2 is transported from the alveoli to the airway opening by the flow stream, a mechanism called convection. In the airways where convection is low (peripheral airways, because of their big cross sectional area), gas molecule diffusion is enhanced by the concentration gradient between the gas inside the conducting airway and the gas coming from the alveoli; this is the diffusion mixing. At certain points in airways, either by the presence of branching or by turbulent streams (in general by locally surpassing Reynolds number), an active mixing between alveolar and dead space gas is produced; this is known as convection mixing. Convection mixing enhances local diffusion mixing by a mechanism called convection-diffusion interaction. If the alveolar space were perfectly mixed, there would be a discontinuity (i.e., a step change) between phases I and III. The asymmetrical branching pattern of airways with different effective lengths induces a temporal distribution of convection-diffusion interactions [10]. This can be modelled as a temporal compartment of mixing taking place in the anatomical dead space, during exhalation of alveolar gas, until a complete lavage of dead space contents is performed. The impulse response of this compartment is a decreasing function [11], that can be approached exponentially (but is not necessarily exponential), as observed in Figure 4. The convective-dispersive distributed model of gas transport in the airways explains the phase I to phase II smooth transition, but not completely phase II to phase III transition, nor the phase III slope, if we take into account local or regional differences in V/Q, and ventilation inhomogeneities.

Alveolar distribution and the sequential gas exhalation model

We now consider that, instead of a single alveolus, we have an infinite number, and that CO_2 elimination is continuously distributed through the lung. For a given alveolus or homogeneous alveolar region, CO_2 elimination depends on the local ventilation and the local CO_2 concentration. Local ventilation will depend on pulmonary mechanics, while $FACO_2$ depends on local V/Q matching. Alveolar ventilation and V/Q distribution (the globally called lung homogeneity) are responsible for the actual shape of capnogram as a function of volume (the capnogram as a function of time depends also on the pattern of the expiratory flow). The more homogeneous the lung, the more the capnographic shape matches the two-compartment model. With smooth but short transitions between phase I and II, and II and III, the more sharp the slope of phase II, and the more flat the slope of phase III. In contrast, as lung inhomogeneity increases, the phase II slope decreases, the transition between phase II and III, and to a lesser degree between phase I and II smooths, and the slope of phase III increas-

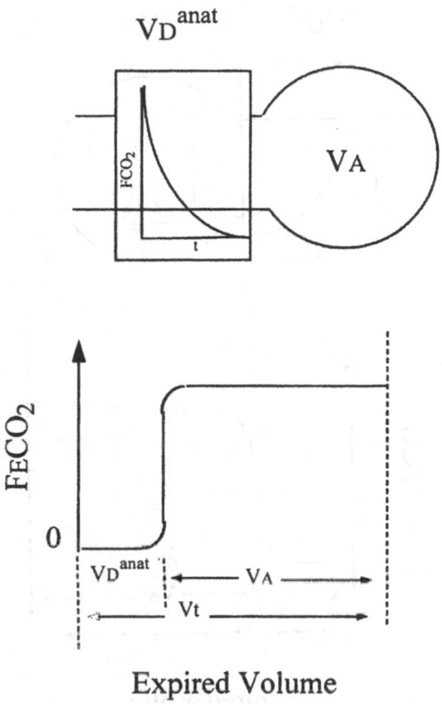

Fig. 4. The two-compartment model with an airway mixing function, involving the capnogram in Figure 1. Notice the smoothing of the transitions

es (Fig. 5). The sequential gas exhalation model establishes a temporal sequence of events during expiration. True alveolar dead space (i.e., without any alveolar mixing) is exhaled during phase I. Phase I to II transition and phase II correspond to the convection-diffusion in airways. Phase II to III transition and alveolar plateau reflect the interaction between alveolar inhomogeneity and airways mixing. The slope of phase III has been simulated as a convective process in which inhomogeneous lungs have not only different alveolar CO_2 concentrations at the end of inspiration, but also have a continuous distribution of time constants [2, 12].

The CO_2 elimination versus volume curve

An important issue for computer processing of the capnographic signal is the capnographic recording by avoiding the visual recognition of reference points on the curve. The measurement of many of the classical parameters of the temporal or volumetric capnography requires a visual identification of those points

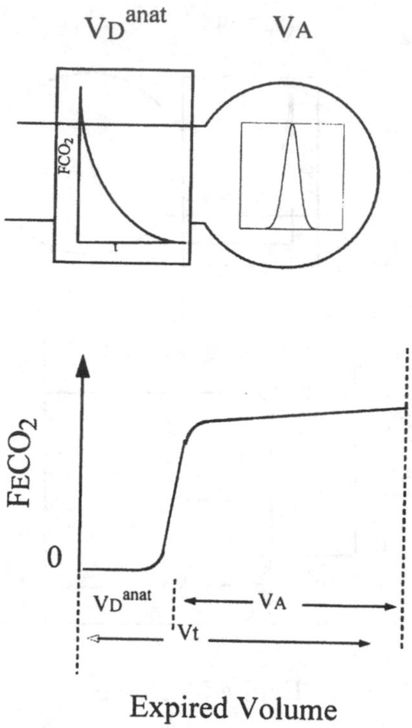

Fig. 5. The two-compartment model with an airway mixing function and a Gaussian distribution of alveolar ventilation, assuming a constant alveolar perfusion. Notice the generation of an alveolar slope

that better define the transition between I-II and II-III phases. Computerized procedures have been unsuccessful because of the smooth transitions between phases, especially in patients.

A new approach to the volumetric capnography is the use of the CO_2 elimination versus volume [VCO_2 (v)] curve instead of CO_2 concentration (or partial pressure) versus time or volume [13]. Model assumptions are essentially the same. In an ideal two-compartment model, the CO_2 elimination pattern would show two phases: a first phase with no CO_2 elimination and a second linear increase of VCO_2 with volume (Fig. 6). There would be a sharp transition between the two phases at the point where the anatomical dead space gives way to alveolar gas exhalation. The slope of the increasing branch of VCO_2 (v) curve is the alveolar pressure ($FACO_2$) at the end of the preceding inspiration, according to the equation

$$VCO_2 = VCO_2tot - FACO_2 \cdot (Vt\text{-}V) \quad [3]$$

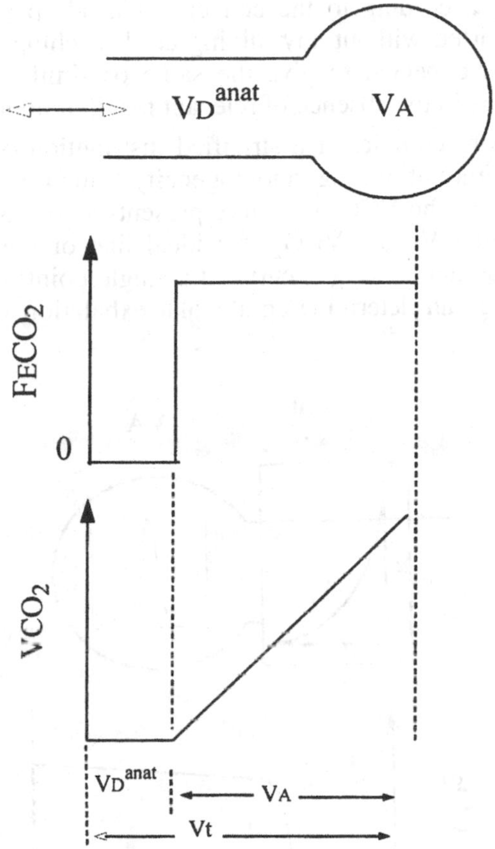

Fig. 6. The two-compartment basic model and the curve VCO_2 (v)

where VCO_2tot is the total amount of CO_2 eliminated in this breath and Vt is tidal volume.

If this simple model is used with the impulse response of the airways mixing, the transition between dead space and alveolar volume smooths, but the increasing lip of the VCO_2 exhalation versus volume is still linear, and will remain unmodified in the absence of alveolar inhomogeneity. Extrapolation of this line to $VCO_2 = 0$ gives the value of anatomical dead space (Langley's modified method) [14]. The computational definition for serial dead space volume (VD^{aw}) depends on the conceptual model. In both Fowler and Langley methods, the expired concentration-volume or elimination-volume curves with a linearized alveolar plateau are compared to the ideal step response. The line separating equal areas in the $FECO_2$ (v) curve or the linear extrapolation of the alveolar segment in the VCO_2 (v) curve try to reproduce the ideal conditions, and try to define VD^{aw} according to the concept of dead space as the region in which gas is transported without any mixing until reaching the alveolar space. Therefore, VD_{Lan} is expected to give the same or similar value as Fowler's method of equal areas in the absence of relevant parallel inhomogeneities.

The model is more complex if a stratified distribution of VCO_2 is considered. If a "normal" amount of lung inhomogeneity is incorporated into the model, the increasing lip of the VCO_2 (v) curve presents a concave upward bending (Fig. 7). For the same Vt and $\dot{V}CO_2$, the ideal line of the two-compartment model cross as the actual VCO_2 (v) curve at a single point. As far as this point can be identified, we can determine an alveolar exhalation volume (VAE) (be-

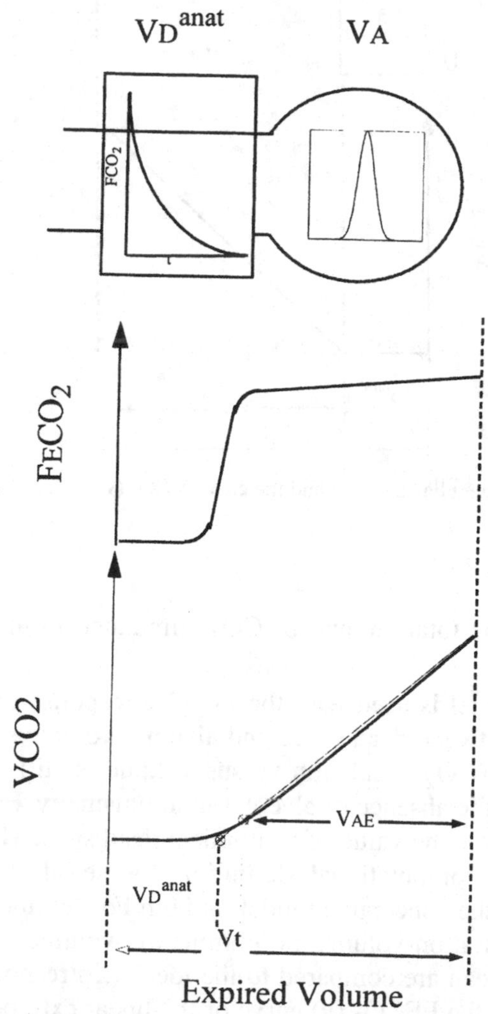

Fig. 7. Two-compartment sequential exhalation model: $FECO_2$ (v) and VCO_2 (v) curves

tween this point and the end expiratory point), an airways dead space by extrapolation, and an intermediate volume, proportional to the amount of inhomogeneity and airways mixing.

How to determine the crosspoint between the ideal and the real curve?

The linear part of the VCO_2 (v) curve at the end of expiration has a slope equal to the end tidal CO_2 concentration:

$$VCO_2 = VCO_2\ (tot) - FETCO_2 \cdot (Vt\text{-}V)$$

If we compare with equation 3, it is evident that the only difference between both lines is the slope. We can therefore establish the following identity

$$VCO_2\ (tot) - FACO_2 \cdot (Vt\text{-}V) = VCO_2\ (tot) - k \cdot FETCO_2 \cdot (Vt\text{-}V)$$

which shows that a single parameter (k) which allows us to determine the straight line that would define an ideal homogenous behavior

$$k = FACO_2/FETCO_2$$

is related to the physiological end tidal-arterial gradient, if we assume that in normal lungs $pACO_2 \simeq paCO_2$. From values obtained in the literature for normal CO_2 gradients, the value of k would be in the range of 0.94-0.95.

We can therefore determine VAE as the crossing point between the actual VCO_2 (v) curve and the straight line described by:

$$VCO_2 = VCO_2\ (tot) - k \cdot FETCO_2 \cdot (Vt\text{-}V)$$

the magnitude 1-k is called the dead space allowance (DSA) because it corresponds to the physiological or normal amount of pulmonary heterogeneity (plus airway mixing) that shifts the VCO_2 (v) curve from the ideal two-compartment behavior. Once we define the normal value of DSA (we can accept a value of 6%, or 0.06, to be as tolerant as possible), we can calculate the value of VAE in normal subjects and in patients. VAE is presented as a fraction of tidal volume: VAE/Vt. Also we can define an index of ventilatory efficiency (IVE) if we refer to VAE as a percentage of Vt-VDanat, so that the normal value would be 100%, and would decrease as pulmonary heterogeneity increases:

$$IVE = VAE/(Vt\text{-}VD^{anat})$$

The value of VAE/VT is the fraction of tidal volume that corresponds to alveolar volume with a level of heterogeneity lower than 6% (DSA = 0.06). The meaning of DSA is related to the divergence between the real lung and the ideal modelled lung behaviors. Even in the most-perfect normal lung, an ideal two-compartment behavior is unrealistic. A certain amount of parallel inhomogeneity is always present, and convection diffusion interactions in airways [15, 17] prevent an all or none pattern of CO_2 elimination at airway opening. Therefore a smooth bending is observed in the rising lip of the VCO_2 (v) curves in normal subjects. Accordingly, DSA is used to account globally for physiological factors implied in the real response of the system [9].

Measurement of VAE/VT

The principle of VAE determination is presented in Figure 8 on a curve from a normal subject. After a certain amount of gas has been exhaled, VCO_2 increases progressively to reach VCO_2tot at the end of expiration. The increase in VCO_2 is slightly non-linear because of alveolar heterogeneity. At the very end of expiration, it is assumed that gas is coming from alveolar air spaces, according to the simplifying hypothesis of sequential lung emptying. By assuming a given amount of non-linearity due to physiological alveolar inhomogeneity, we can determine a point in the VCO_2 (v) curve representing the hypothetical beginning of alveolar gas ejection. To perform this measurement we proceed as follows:

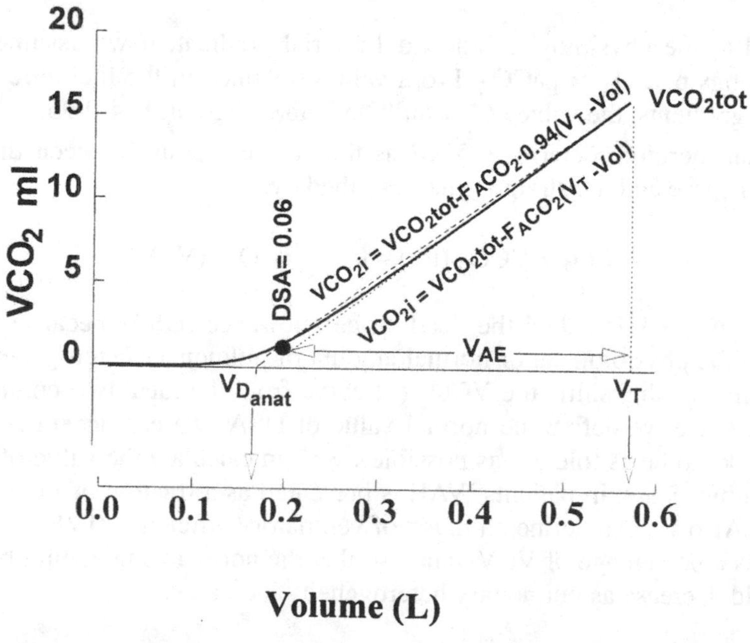

Fig. 8. Measurement of VAE and VD^{anat} from the VCO_2 (v) curve

first we select the final part of the curve (in the present case the last 50 points) to obtain $FETCO_2$, then we multiply $FETCO_2$ by 0.94 to obtain:

$$VCO_2 = VCO_2tot - 0.94 \cdot FACO_2 \cdot (Vt\text{-}V)$$

This line will cross the measured VCO_2 (v) curve somewhere between the end expiration and the knee of the curve. The volume between this crossing point and the end expiration is VAE.

Measurement of serial dead space by Langley's modified method

Linear regression was applied to the segment of the VCO_2 (v) curve corresponding to VAE. The regression line was extrapolated to obtain the volume at zero VCO_2. The volume expired from the beginning of expiration to this point would correspond to Langley's serial dead space (VD_{Lan}).

In our previous studies [9, 18], performed in intubated normals and patients, VAE/VT seemed to account well for the lung impairment, correlating with other indexes of ventilatory maldistribution, and presenting a lesser of tidal dependence volume than other capnographic parameters.

References

1. Fletcher R, Jonson B, Cumming G et al (1981) The concept of dead space with special reference to the single breath test for carbon dioxide. Br J Anaesth 53:77-88
2. Engel LA (1985) Intraregional gas mixing and distribution. In: Engel LA, Paiva M (eds) Gas mixing and distribution in the lung. Dekker, New York, pp 287-358
3. Nunn JF (1993) Applied respiratory physiology, 4th edn. Distribution of pulmonary ventilation and perfusion. Anatomical dead space. Butterworth Heinemann, Oxford, pp 172-175
4. Bohr C (1891) Über die Lungenathmung. Skand Arch Physiol 2:236
5. Fowler WS (1948) Lung function studies. II. The respiratory dead space. Am J Physiol 154: 405-416
6. Lacoste J (1972) Etude des echanges et de lèchangeur oulmonaire: les ductances partielles et globale. Bull Physiopath Resp 8:146-148
7. Fletcher R (1985) Dead space: invasive and non invasive. Br J Anaesth 57:245-249
8. Enghoff H (1931) Zur Frage des schlädlichen Raumes bei der Atmung. Skand Arch Physiol 63:15
9. Romero PV, Lucangelo U, Lopez-Aguilar J et al (1997) Physiologically based indices of volumetric capnography in patients receiving mechanical ventilation. Eur Respir J 10:1309-1315
10. Scherer PW, Shendalman LH, Greene NM (1972) Simultaneous diffusion and convection in single breath lung washout. Boll Math Biophys 34:393-412
11. Paiva M, Engel LA (1987) Theoretical studies on gas mixing and ventilation distribution in the lung. Physiol Rev 67:750-796
12. Paiva M, Van Muylem A, Ravez P et al (1984) Inspired volume dependence of the slope of alveolar plateau. Respir Physiol 56:309-325
13. Romero PV, Lopez-Aguilar J, Lucangelo U et al (1995) Alveolar ejection ratio elucidated from VCO_2 versus Vt curves (abstract). Intensive Care Med 21:45S

14. Langley F, Even O, Duroux P et al (1975) Ventilatory consequences of unilateral pulmonary occlusion. Les Colloques de l'Institut National de la Santé et de la Recherche Mèdicale (INSERM) 51:209-212
15. Nunn JF, Hill DW (1960) Respiratory dead space and arterial to end-tidal CO_2 tension difference in anesthetized man. J Appl Physiol 15:383-389
16. Meyer M, Mohr M, Schulz H et al (1990) Sloping alveolar plateaus of CO_2, O_2 and intravenously infused C2H2 and CHClF2 in the dog. Respir Physiol 81:137-152
17. Sidel GM, Lewis SM (1989) Distribution of ventilation. In: Chang HK, Paiva M (eds) Respiratory physiology: an analytical approach. Dekker, New York, pp 195-243
18. Blanch L, Lucangelo U, Lopez-Aguilar J et al (1999) Volumetric capnography in patients with acute lung injury: effects of positive end expiratory pressure. Eur Respir J 13:1048-1054

Capnography in Patients with Acute Respiratory Distress Syndrome

LL. BLANCH, U. LUCANGELO, P.V. ROMERO

Capnography is a technique that permits recognition of CO_2 concentration changes in the patient's airway during the respiratory cycle. The ability to measure a patient's inspired and expired CO_2 has existed for many years. In the past 10 years, this technology has evolved so that it is now available in many intensive care units.

To correctly analyze a capnogram, the following steps must be systematically evaluated. First, it is important to recognize whether or not there is exhaled CO_2. This is very important for early recognition of esophageal intubations. Second, the four phases of the waveform should be analyzed. The capnogram represents total CO_2 eliminated by the lungs, given that no gas exchange occurs in the airways. Expired gas contains CO_2 from three sequential compartments: phase I contains gas from apparatus and anatomical dead space, phase II represents increasing CO_2 concentration resulting from progressive emptying of alveoli, and phase III represents essentially alveolar gas. Phase III is often referred to as the plateau and its appearance is flat or with a small positive slope. The highest point is the end-tidal pCO_2. Therefore, the expiratory capnogram is a technique that provides qualitative information on the waveform patterns associated with mechanical ventilation and quantitative estimation of arterial pCO_2 from the end-tidal pCO_2, which is normally located immediately before the next inspiration. Additionally, the minimum pCO_2 as well as the calculation of the arterial minus end-tidal pCO_2 gradient should be performed. When all this information is analyzed, we can search for causes of hypo-or hypercapnia if present, such as inadequate alveolar ventilation, CO_2 rebreathing, or excessive CO_2 output. Changes in the morphology of the capnographic curve often indicate ventilatory maldistribution. In order to quantify these problems, several indexes based on the geometrical analysis of the curve have been developed, of these alveolar plateau slope is the most frequently used [1-4].

Physiological principles

When expiratory partial CO_2 pressure is plotted as a function of time [$p_ECO_2(t)$ curve], expiratory flow has to be taken into account, even in healthy subjects.

This constraint has lead to the use of volumetric capnography, i.e., the expiratory partial pressure of CO_2 as a function of volume or $p_ECO_2(V)$ curve, which seems more useful and clinically reliable than capnography as a function of time [5]. Nonetheless, alveolar slope indexes are highly dependent on the visual criterion used to define phase III [6]. Indeed, by-eye identification of significant points on the curve is still necessary. This makes computerized analysis of the curve more difficult, and limits the use of volumetric capnography in current clinical practise.

An improvement in volumetric capnography is represented by the use of the CO_2 elimination versus volume curve [$VCO_2(V)$ curve], which has been successfully used in the measurement of anatomical dead space by linear back extrapolation of the increase of VCO_2 with volume [5, 7]. A simple, physiologically based assumption allows identification of the fraction of tidal volume corresponding to the exhalation of alveolar gas (VAE). This process can be easily computerized, and could represent a substantial improvement in the automatization of the quantitative analysis of the curve. The quotient between V_{AE} and tidal volume (V_{AE}/V_T ratio), related to the ventilatory efficiency, would be a new concept in volumetric capnography (Fig. 1).

According to the simplified hypothesis of sequential gas emptying, early expiration contains gas from apparatus and VD_{aw}, and afterwards from the alveoli, with a clear transition between both phases in a homogeneous lung. In disease, a serial stratification occurs as the lung becomes inhomogeneous. Consequently, the transition between airways and alveolar phases becomes blurred or rather difficult to identify. According to this model, "pure" alveolar gas in this situation can only be collected at the end of expiration [8].

Even in a normal lung, complete homogeneity between lung units is unrealistic. Therefore, a level of tolerance should be allowed to account for the physiological inhomogeneity, as well as for the convection-diffusion interaction that occurred in the airways. This tolerance has been called in our previous studies "dead space allowance" (DSA), and modulates V_{AE} determination on the volumetric CO_2 elimination ($VCO_2(v)$) curve [5, 9].

According to the model of sequential gas emptying, V_{AE} represents the fraction of tidal volume that corresponds to alveolar volume with a level of heterogeneity lower than DSA. The level of DSA was based on a previous study where we assessed intra- and inter-individual variability and noise-to-signal ratio in normal intubated subjects receiving mechanical ventilation. A DSA of 5% had the best reproducibility and lower noise-to-signal ratio [9]. As expected, in normal subjects V_{AE} corresponds narrowly to the difference between expired tidal volume and VD_{aw} measured either by Fowler [10] or Langley [7] methods (personal observations). In disease, alveolar heterogeneity is more prominent and V_{AE} (measured at 5% DSA) is progressively lower, and parametrizes the progressive bending of the raising limb of the $VCO_2(v)$ curve. These phenomena are the consequence of the increased alveolar heterogeneity present during disease, irrespective of its origin (Fig. 1).

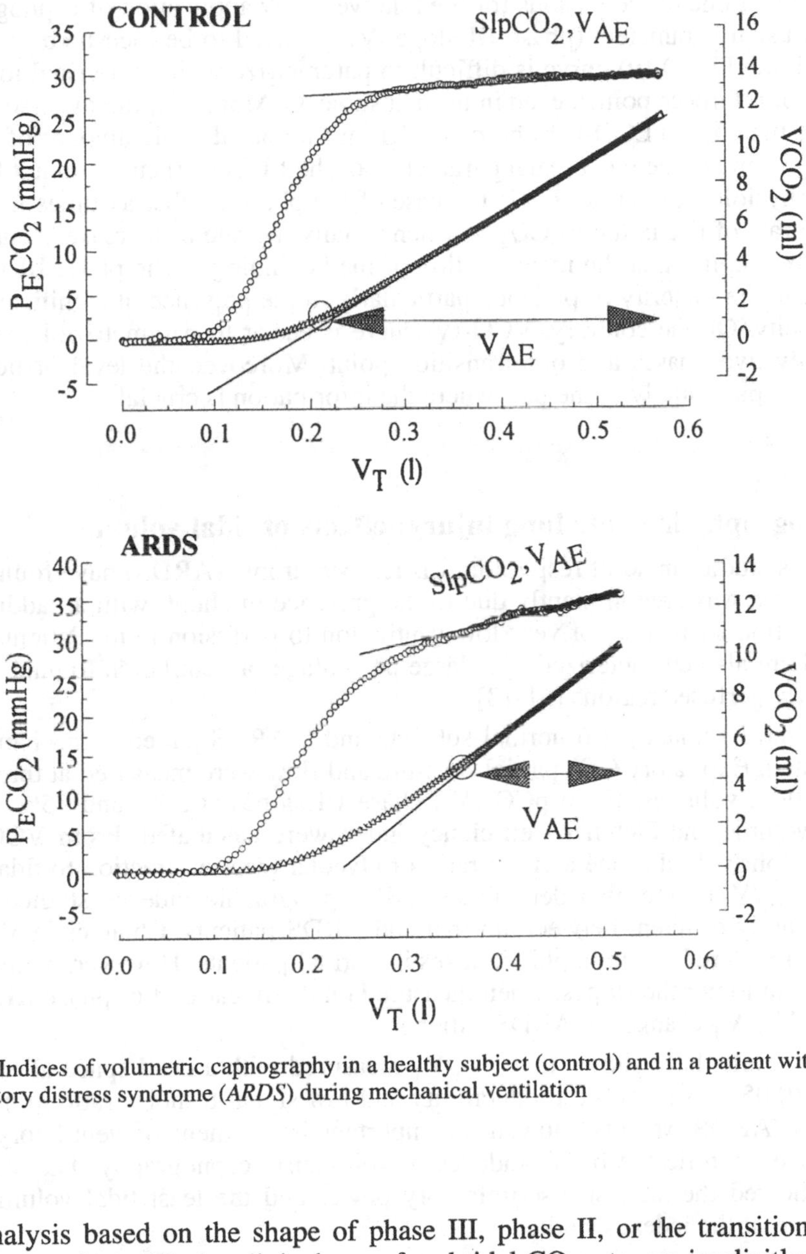

Fig. 1. Indices of volumetric capnography in a healthy subject (control) and in a patient with acute respiratory distress syndrome (*ARDS*) during mechanical ventilation

Analysis based on the shape of phase III, phase II, or the transition from phase II to phase III, the clinical use of end tidal CO_2, etc. are implicitly based on the model of serial compartments, and the simplified hypothesis of serial alveolar gas exhalation. In other studies, the so-called alveolar sampling is frequently based on the same model. Another point is related to our purpose of obtaining reliable and easily computerized parameters in order to increase the understanding and clinical use of capnography to monitor respiratory function. We believe that one of the reasons for the relatively low application of capnography is that usual parameters (phase III slope, VD_{aw}) need to be measured by hand. Indeed, the $FECO_2(v)$ curve is difficult to parametrize without a visual identification of reference points, even in normal subjects. Moreover, the most-sensitive part of the curve $FECO_2(v)$, the phase III, has a considerable amount of noise. Finally, some of the most-usual parameters of the $FECO_2(v)$ curve do not have a clear physiological basis; this is the case of the phase III that assumes linearity for the rate of rise in the $FECO_2(v)$ when usually the rate of increase is curvilinear. This implies that the identification of the beginning of the phase III is subjective in the majority of patients, particularly in the presence of significant heterogeneity. On the contrary, $VCO_2(v)$ curve is easier to parametrize because it has only two phases and one transition point. Moreover, the level of noise is very low, particularly in the part where the information is crucial.

Capnography in acute lung injury: effects of tidal volume

Previous studies in adult respiratory distress syndrome (ARDS) have found that hypoxemia was predominantly due to the presence of shunt, with an additional contribution by regions of very low ventilation to perfusion ratio. Patients with ARDS are also characterized by a large percentage of ventilation to unperfused or poorly perfused regions [11-13].

We have studied [5] 6 normal subjects and 5 ARDS patients, mechanically ventilated. Expiratory CO_2 partial pressure and flow were measured at three different tidal volumes. From $pCO_2(V)$, phase III slopes at 50% and 75% of expired volume and Fletcher's efficiency index were calculated. From $VCO_2(V)$ curve, Bohr's dead space and the ratio of alveolar ejection fraction to tidal volume (V_{AE}/V_T) were also determined. All capnographic indexes studied were significantly different between normal and ARDS patients. Changes in V_T significantly altered capnographic indexes in normal patients. However, neither the V_{AE}/V_T ratio nor the slopes, when measured on the linear part of phase III, were affected by V_T changes in ARDS patients.

Our results have shown that V_{AE}/V_T measured with a dead space allowance of 5% (0.05) has a good reproducibility and low signal-to-noise ratio in normal patients. ARDS patients showed an important impairment of ventilatory performance, as reflected by all indexes of volumetric capnography. The V_{AE}/V_T ratio showed the highest discriminatory power and the least tidal volume dependence of the indexes studied.

Volumetric capnography has been proposed as a better way to assess ventilatory maldistribution than the usual temporal capnography, because it is less sensitive to changes in expiratory time and expiratory flow [6, 14]. Recently, the $VCO_2(V)$ curve has been used to determine the anatomical dead space in both adults and children [5, 15]. This method assumes a linear increase of VCO_2 with volume during expiration.

Figure 1 shows that the $VCO_2(V)$ curve can be divided into three parts: a first flat section ($VCO_2 = 0$) corresponding to phase I on the $FCO_2(V)$ curve; a second transitional part, where VCO_2 begins to increase, which corresponds roughly to phase II, and finally a quasi-linear increase of VCO_2 with volume, related to the alveolar plateau or phase III on the expired capnogram.

The less heterogeneous the alveolar ventilatory distribution, the more linear the increase of VCO_2i with volume (and more rectangular the shape of the $FCO_2(V)$ curve). If we accept a fixed degree of physiological heterogeneity, a magnitude directly related to the alveolar plateau can be measured from the rising section of the curve. We have termed it alveolar ejection volume or V_{AE}, instead of alveolar plateau, because it includes part of phase II in the conventional capnographic [$FCO_2(V)$] curve (Fig. 1). The index V_{AE} has a similar physiological significance to that of the alveolar plateau in the sense that both define the fraction of V_T related to the ejection of alveolar gas. However, the difference between both indexes lies in the assumption of linearity of phase III on the expired capnogram. Physiologically the rate of rise of expired CO_2 as a function of expired volume is expected not to be linear, as a consequence of the sequential emptying of lung units with different time constants [16-18].

Alveolar sequential emptying is considered to define phase III in an expired capnogram [8, 19]. Most of the problems involved in an accurate and reproducible measurement of phase III are related to the identification of the breaking point from which expired air corresponds to alveolar air. Geometrical methods have proved to be sensitive enough for clinical applications [3, 6]. However, computerized calculation of these indices in real time is technically difficult, as they need either a visual identification of the phase II, phase III transition point, or a by-eye fitting of phase III. One of the possible advantages of a physiologically based volumetric approach is to avoid the visual identification of significant points in the curve in order to computerize some of the measurements, including the back extrapolation method for anatomical dead space measurement [6, 7].

Volumetric capnography has shown important distribution abnormalities in ARDS patients, with respect to anesthetized normal patients, during artificial ventilation. V_{AE}/V_T is a reproducible and sensitive index to assess ventilatory maldistribution, which easy to computerize and relatively insensitive to tidal volume changes in patients [5].

Capnography in acute lung injury: effects of positive end-expiratory pressure

Positive end-expiratory pressure (PEEP) is commonly applied to improve oxygenation in patients with ARDS. Several studies analyzed the effect of PEEP on respiratory system mechanics and found increases in additional resistance (DR) at high PEEP levels [20-22]. Recently, Pelosi et al. [23] demonstrated that the increased respiratory system resistance in acute lung injury (ALI) was caused by the reduction in lung volume. PEEP increased specific additional resistance (DR corrected for total end-expiratory lung volume) only for PEEP equal or higher than 10 cm H_2O. Accordingly, these authors suggested that PEEP may change the viscoelastic properties of the lung by overdistending previously aerated lung regions. These changes in ventilation distribution might probably alter the pattern of exhaled PCO_2.

The effects of PEEP on volumetric capnography and respiratory system mechanics were studied [24] in 17 mechanically ventilated patients with ALI (9 patients with moderate ALI – ALI group – and 8 patients with severe ALI – ARDS group) and in 8 normal anesthetized and paralyzed subjects (control group). We recorded tracheal pressure, airflow, and expired capnograms as a function of expired volume during mechanical ventilation in control mode and at different levels of PEEP (0, 5, 10, 15 cm H_2O). Using the airway occlusion technique during constant airflow inflation, we measured total respiratory system static compliance (Cst) and total respiratory system resistance (Rmax). Rmax includes airway resistance (Rmin) and additional resistance (DR). From expiratory CO_2 partial pressure and instantaneous CO_2 elimination curves we measured the alveolar ejection volume as a fraction of tidal volume (V_{AE}/V_T), the phase III slopes of expired CO_2 curves beyond V_{AE} ($SlpCO_2, V_{AE}$), and total physiological dead space (V_D/V_T,Bohr). We found that Crs were markedly decreased in ARDS patients ($p < 0.01$). At PEEP 0 cm H_2O, Rmax was increased in ALI and in ARDS (9 ± 51 cm H_2O/l per s and 11 ± 10.6 cm H_2O/l per s, respectively) compared with control patients (± 40.5 cm H_2O/l per s) ($p < 0.01$). No differences in Rmax, Rmin, and DR were observed between ALI and ARDS. Total physiological dead space and $SlpCO_2, V_{AE}$ were higher in ALI patients (0.52 ± 0.01 and 13.9 ± 0.7 mmHg/l, respectively) compared with control patients (0.46 ± 0.01 and 7.7 ± 0.4 mmHg/l, $p < 0.01$ respectively) and in ARDS patients (0.61 ± 0.02 and 24.9 ± 1.6 mmHg/l, $p < 0.01$, respectively) compared with ALI patients. V_{AE}/V_T decreased in the same fashion (0.6 ± 0.01 in control group, 0.43 ± 0.01 in ALI group, and 0.31 ± 0.01 in ARDS group, $p < 0.01$). Only at PEEP 15 cm H_2O did DR increase significantly in ALI and ARDS patients ($p < 0.05$). Nevertheless, PEEP had no effect on V_{AE}/V_T, $SlpCO_2, V_{AE}$, and V_D/V_T,Bohr in any group (Fig. 2). Significant correlation were found between capnographic indices (V_{AE}/V_T and $SlpCO_2, V_{AE}$) and lung injury score ($p < 0.01$), and with respiratory mechanics measurements ($p < 0.001$).

The results of the study of Blanch et al. [24] demonstrate that the severity of disease affects volumetric capnographic indices and the mechanical properties of the respiratory system. A relationship was established between alterations in respiratory system mechanics due to disease and volumetric capnographic indices. Increasing PEEP improved Cst in normal subjects and worsened DR in patients with respiratory failure, but did not affect volumetric capnographic indices.

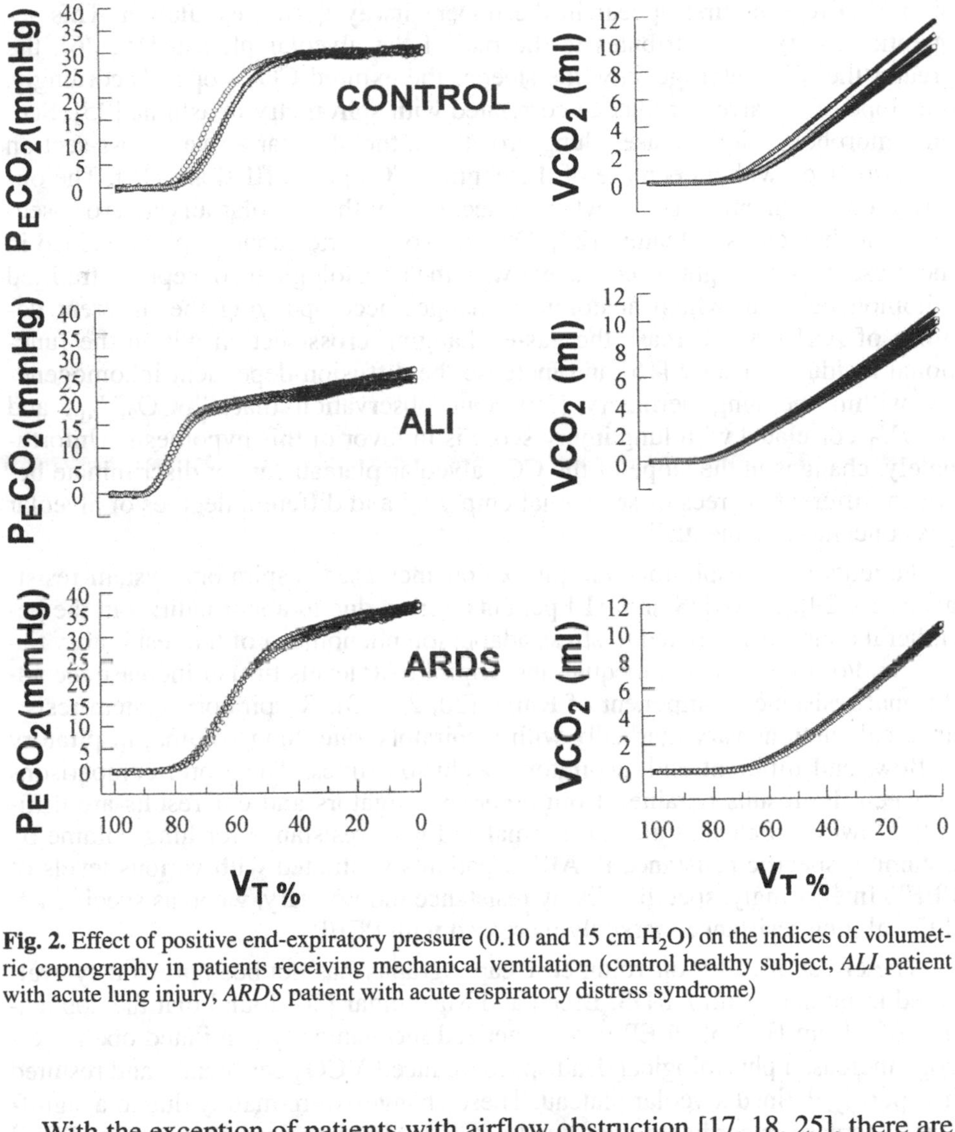

Fig. 2. Effect of positive end-expiratory pressure (0.10 and 15 cm H_2O) on the indices of volumetric capnography in patients receiving mechanical ventilation (control healthy subject, *ALI* patient with acute lung injury, *ARDS* patient with acute respiratory distress syndrome)

With the exception of patients with airflow obstruction [17, 18, 25], there are no data in the literature that evaluate the shape of the capnogram in patients with respiratory failure. In this investigation, we confirmed our preliminary data that capnographic shape is altered in ARDS and ALI patients [5]. Moreover, the application of PEEP, an intervention that increases lung volume and alters respiratory system mechanics, did not affect $SlpCO_2$, V_{AE}, and V_{AE}/V_T. Two physiological explanations could be considered to analyze these results.

First, the almost-rectangular shape of the expired capnogram depends on the homogeneity of the gas distribution and alveolar ventilation [15, 26, 27]. Lung heterogeneity creates regional differences in CO_2 concentration and gas from high V/Q regions first appear in the upper airway during exhalation. This sequential emptying contributes to the rise of the alveolar plateau [16, 26], the greater the V/Q heterogeneity, the steeper the expired CO_2 slope. Accordingly, the slope of the alveolar plateau correlated with spirometry in asthma [25]. Second, morphometric increases (lung growth) in the alveolar airway cross-section are associated with a decrease of the expired CO_2 phase III slope [15]. The opposite occurs in emphysema, where a decrease in the alveolar airway cross-section is a characteristic feature [28]. Data on volumetric capnography obtained in the present study might be consistent with the physiological concept of stratified inhomogeneity, in which anatomical changes accompanying the different degrees of ALI may decrease the gas-exchanging cross-section within the functional residual capacity [15] and increase the diffusion-dependent inhomogeneity within the lung periphery [26]. Our observation that $SlpCO_2$,V_{AE}, and V_{AE}/V_T correlated with lung injury score is in favor of this hypothesis. Unfortunately, changes in the slope of the CO_2 alveolar plateau cannot discriminate between different degrees of sequential emptying and different degrees of alveolar gas concentration inequality.

Patients with respiratory failure exhibit increased respiratory system resistance [20, 29]. In ARDS and ALI patients, this is due to abnormalities in the peripheral component related to stress adaptation phenomena of the respiratory tissues and/or time constant inequalities. High PEEP levels further increase the additional resistance component of Rmax [20, 22, 23]. Respiratory system resistance calculations vary markedly with respiratory rate, lung volume, inspiratory airflow, and different end-inspiratory occlusion times. Therefore, comparisons between the results obtained from other investigators and our results are difficult. However, Pelosi et al. [23] normalized lung resistance for lung volume by obtaining specific resistance in ARDS patients ventilated with various levels of PEEP. Interestingly, specific airway resistance did not vary, whereas specific additional lung resistance markedly increased with PEEP.

The effect of PEEP on volumetric capnography has not been previously evaluated in humans with ARDS. Breen and Mazumdar [30] found that the application of 11 cm H_2O of PEEP in anesthetized mechanically ventilated open chest dogs increased physiological dead space, reduced VCO_2 per breath, and resulted in a poorly defined alveolar plateau. These changes were mainly due to a significant decrease in cardiac output due to PEEP. Although cardiac effects of PEEP were not measured in the present investigation, V_D/V_T,Bohr did not change significantly with PEEP. Because V_D/V_T,Bohr is heavily influenced by variations in cardiac output, we can reasonably reject a hemodynamic effect of PEEP on our capnographic measurements. Recently, Smith and Fletcher [31] studied the effects of PEEP in a population of patients immediately after heart surgery and also found that PEEP appeared to have little effect on volumetric capnography.

Studies with computed tomographic scan revealed that PEEP overdistended previously inflated lung units [11], supporting the concept that high PEEP changes the viscoelastic properties of lung tissues [23]. Potential contributors to the viscoelastic behavior are contractile elements of the alveolar ducts and septa, parenchyma and airway smooth muscles, and the alveolar lining film [32]. All these elements are affected in patients with respiratory failure and are related to the decreased Cst and increased respiratory system resistance. Moreover, in contrast to other studies that found that amelioration of bronchospasm normalizes the slope of alveolar plateau [25], we were unable to show any modification in the studied capnographic indices at different PEEP levels in any group. These findings suggest that high PEEP in ARDS and ALI mostly increase stress relaxation and viscoelastic phenomena (increase in DR at PEEP 15 cm H_2O in the ALI and the ARDS groups). The observation that time constants did not change when different PEEP levels were applied is in favor of this theory. However, a limitation in this explanation is that capnography reflects global lung behavior. Therefore, if PEEP produced opposite regional effects on ventilation or in perfusion, the lack of changes in $V_{AE}V_T$ and $SlpCO_2,V_{AE}$ with PEEP cannot distinguish between viscoelastic behavior or pendelluft for the same increase in additional resistance. Finally, the results of Blanch et al. [24] are in agreement with the concept that the ARDS lung, independent of the location of the lung densities, is globally affected by the disease [12].

Only in normal subjects did Cst increase with PEEP. This observation coincides with earlier observations in anesthetized humans [33], suggesting that airway closure appears at the reduced functional residual capacity induced by anesthesia. This explanation is supported by computed tomography studies in anesthetized patients showing lung collapse in dependent lung zones, which completely re-expand after PEEP therapy [13]. The fact that volumetric capnographic indices remained within the normal range in normal subjects and were unaltered after PEEP therapy suggests that volumetric capnographic indices reflect primarily alterations in ventilated lung areas and lung collapse of dependent areas, although containing very low volume, do not affect these measurements (Fig. 2).

In conclusion, in mechanically ventilated patients: 1) the severity of the lung injury correlates with indices derived from volumetric capnography, such as $SlpCO_2,V_{AE}$ and V_{AE}/V_T; 2) individual changes in respiratory system mechanics are related to changes in volumetric capnography indices; 3) application of PEEP did not alter volumetric capnographic indices but significantly increased additional respiratory system resistance. These findings indicate that indices derived from volumetric capnography might be useful to assess the severity of the respiratory failure.

Capnography during weaning from mechanical ventilation

The decision to start a weaning trial in a critically ill patient often implies that patients have correct arterial blood gases. The fact that capnography could provide a non-invasive tool to assess alveolar ventilation and thereby $paCO_2$ induced some investigators to evaluate the utility of capnography during weaning periods [34]. However, these studies have yielded controversial results. Whereas some authors found that patients monitored with pulse oximetry and capnography required less blood gas sampling, others found that variations in $petCO_2$ did not correctly indicate changes in $paCO_2$ in patients with parenchymal lung disease, particularly patients with emphysema. To analyze this clinical problem, we evaluated the relationship between $paCO_2$ and $petCO_2$ before weaning and during a weaning trial, and to determine the ability of $petCO_2$ to identify clinically relevant episodes of hypercapnia. Interestingly, we found that monitoring of $petCO_2$ and pulse oximetry provided good assessment of hypercapnic episodes and of impairments in oxygenation, when present, during weaning from mechanical ventilation. Although in this study, capnography did not appear to provide 100% accuracy in detecting minor changes in $paCO_2$ and the high number of false positives may result in arterial blood sampling in patients who do not present with a failure of ventilation, continuous $petCO_2$ monitoring might obviate arterial blood sampling in half of the patients. Accordingly, while not entirely replacing invasive arterial determinations, capnography seems reliable for use as a non-invasive tool for assessing alveolar ventilation during weaning in general intensive care patients [35].

References

1. Hess D (1990) Capnometry and capnography: technical aspects, physiologic aspects, and clinical applications. Respir Care 35:557-576
2. Blanch Ll, Fernandez R, Benito S et al (1987). Effect of PEEP on the arterial minus end-tidal carbon dioxide gradient. Chest 92:451-454
3. Blanch Ll, Fernandez R, Artigas A (1991) The effect of autoPEEP on the $PaCO_2$-$PetCO_2$ gradient and expired CO_2 slope in critically ill patients during total ventilatory support. J Crit Care 6:202-210
4. Falk JL, Racko, EC, Harry Weil M (1988) End-tidal carbon dioxide concentration during cardiopulmonary resuscitation. N Engl J Med 318:607-611
5. Romero PV, Lucangelo U, Lopez-Aguilar J et al (1997) Physiologically based indices of volumetric capnography in patients receiving mechanical ventilation. Eur Respir J 10:1309-1315
6. Fletcher R, Jonson B, Cumming G, Brew J (1981) The concept of deadspace with special reference to the single breath test for carbon dioxide. Br J Anaesth 53:77-88
7. Langley F, Even P, Duroux P (1976) Ventilatory consequences of unilateral pulmonary artery occlusion. In: Distribution des echanges gaseaux pulmonaires. INSERM, Paris, France, pp 209-212
8. Piiper J, Scheid P (1987) Diffusion and convection in intrapulmonary gas mixing. In: Fishman AP, Farhi LE, Tenney SM, Geiger SR (eds) Handbook of physiology, Section 3. The respiratory system, vol IV. American Physiological Society, Bethesda, Maryland, pp 51-69
9. Romero PV, Lopez-Aguilar J, Lucangelo U, Blanch Ll (1995) Alveolar ejection ratio elucidated from VCO_2 versus VT curves. Intensive Care Med 21:S45
10. Fowler WS (1948) Lung function studies. II. The respiratory deadspace. Am J Physiol 154: 405-410
11. Gattinoni L, Pelosi P, Crotti S, Valenza F (1995) Effects of positive end-expiratory pressure on regional distribution of tidal volume and recruitment in adult respiratory distress syndrome. Am J Respir Crit Care Med 151:1807-1814

12. Tomashefski JF Jr (1990) Pulmonary pathology of the adult respiratory distress syndrome. Clin Chest Med 11:593-619
13. Pelosi P, Crotti S, Brazzi L, Gattinoni L (1996) Computed tomography in adult respiratory distress syndrome: what has it taught us? Eur Respir J 9:1055-1062
14. Fletcher R, Jonson B (1984) Deadspace and the single breath test for carbon dioxide during anaesthesia and artificial ventilation. Br J Anaesth 56:109-119
15. Ream RS, Screiner MS, Neff JD et al (1995) Volumetric capnography in children. Influence of growth oh the alveolar plateau slope. Anesthesiology 82:64-73
16. Meyer M, Mohr M, Schulz H, Piiper J (1990) Sloping alveolar plateaus od CO_2, O_2, and intravenously infused C_2H_2 and $CHClF_2$ in the dog. Respir Physiol 81:137-152
17. Blanch Ll, Fernandez R, Saura P et al (1994) Relationship between expired capnogram and respiratory system resistance in critically ill patients during total ventilatory support. Chest 105:219-223
18. Kars AH, Goorden G, Stijnen T et al (1995) Does phase 2 of the expiratory versus volume curve have diagnostic value in emphysema patients? Eur Respir J 8:86-92
19. DuBois AB, Fowler RC, Soffer A, Fenn WO (1952) Alveolar CO_2 measured by expiration into the rapid infrared gas analyzer. J Appl Physiol 4:526-534
20. Pesenti A, Pelosi P, Rossi N et al (1991) The effects of positive end-expiratory pressure on respiratory resistance in patients with the adult respiratory distress syndrome and in normal anesthetized subjects. Am Rev Respir Dis 144:101-107
21. Ranieri VM, Eissa NT, Corbeil C et al (1991) Effects of positive end-expiratory pressure on alveolar recruitment and gas exchange in patients with the adult respiratory distress syndrome. Am Rev Respir Dis 144:544-551
22. Eissa NT, Ranieri VM, Corbeil C et al (1992) Effects of PEEP on the mechanics of the respiratory system in ARDS patients. J Appl Physiol 73:1728-1735
23. Pelosi P, Cereda M, Foti G et al (1995) Alterations of lung and chest wall mechanics in patients with acute lung injury: effects of positive end-expiratory pressure. Am J Respir Crit Care Med 152:531-537
24. Blanch Ll, Lucangelo U, Lopez-Aguilar J (1999) Volumetric capnography in patients with acute lung injury: effects of positive end-expiratory pressure. Eur Respir J 13:1048-1054
25. You B, Peslin R, Duvivier C et al (1994) Expiratory capnography in asthma: evaluation of various shape indices. Eur Respir J 7:318-323
26. Engel LA (1985) Intraregional gas mixing and distribution. In: Engel LA, Paiva M (eds) Gas mixing and distribution in the lung. Marcel Dekker, New York, pp 287-358
27. Fowler WS (1948) Lung function studies. II. The respiratory dead space. Am J Physiol 154:405-416
28. Schwardt JD, Neufeld GR, Baumgardner JE, Scherer PW (1994) Noninvasive recovery of acinar anatomic information from CO_2 expirograms. Ann Biomed Eng 22:293-306
29. Wright PE, Bernard GR (1989) The role of airflow resistance in patients with the adult respiratory distress syndrome. Am Rev Respir Dis 139:1169-1174
30. Breen PH, Mazumdar B (1996) How does positive end-expiratory pressure decrease CO_2 elimination from the lung? Respir Physiol 103:233-242
31. Smith RPR, Fletcher R (2000) Positive end-expiratory pressure has little effect on carbon dioxide elimination after cardiac surgery. Anesth Analg 90:85-88
32. Hoppin FG, Stothert JC, Greaves IA et al (1986) Lung recoil: Elastic and rheological properties. In: Handbook of physiology. The respiratory system. Mechanics of breathing, part I, section 3, vol III. American Physiological Society, Bethesda, pp 195-215
33. D'Angelo E, Calderini E, Torri G et al (1989) Respiratory mechanics in anesthetized paralyzed humans: effects of flow, volume, and time. J Appl Physiol 67:2556-2564
34. Hess D, Schlottag A, Levin B et al (1991) An evaluation of the usefulness of end-tidal PCO_2 to aid weaning from mechanical ventilation following cardiac surgery. Respir Care 36:837-843
35. Saura P, Blanch Ll, Lucangelo U (1996) Utility of capnography to detect hypercapnic episodes during weaning from mechanical ventilation. Intensive Care Med 22:374-381

Volumetric Capnography in Anaesthesia

U. Lucangelo, Ll. Blanch, S. Vatua

In the last twenty years, capnography has become routinely used in monitoring in all operating rooms and in most critical care units to ensure patient's safety, as suggested by the Society of Critical Care Medicine [1-4]. However, only recently have technological developments resulted in the availability of capnography at the patient's bedside, to measure variations in carbon dioxide concentration (CO_2) and tidal volume simultaneously, during the respiratory cycle. This "combined" monitoring device (Novametrix CO_2SMO^+, Novametrix Medical System, Wallinford, CT, USA) that can measure at the same time the carbon dioxide partial pressure of expired gas ($PECO_2$) and the airflow, made it possible to plot CO_2 concentration against expired volume (achieved by the integration of flow signal), thus obtaining the "volumetric capnogram". This curve has been used successfully in the measurement of the anatomical dead space and in the detection of ventilatory disturbances [5, 6]. The purpose of this chapter is to illustrate the theoretical background and the clinical usefulness of monitoring volumetric capnography in the perioperative period. Moreover, the alveolar ejection volume tidal volume ratio (VAE/VT) will be analysed as a new capnographic index in the detection of lung function impairment before, during and after surgery [7, 8].

Theoretical considerations

The volumetric capnogram, unlike time capnography, plots carbon dioxide partial pressure ($PECO_2$) as a function of expired volume during a single breath [9]. The capnographic trace is typically divided into three phases: phase I, corresponds to the expiration of gas from the apparatus and anatomical dead space, where CO_2 is practically undetectable because of its low concentration in the atmospheric air; phase II is characterised by a very rapid rise in CO_2, corresponding to the mixture of alveolar gas with air in the conducting airway; phase III, also known as alveolar plateau, corresponds to the elimination of alveolar air [7] (Fig. 1).

With correct sampling techniques end-tidal PCO_2 ($PETCO_2$) is assumed to be equivalent to alveolar carbon dioxide tension ($PACO_2$) which at the same

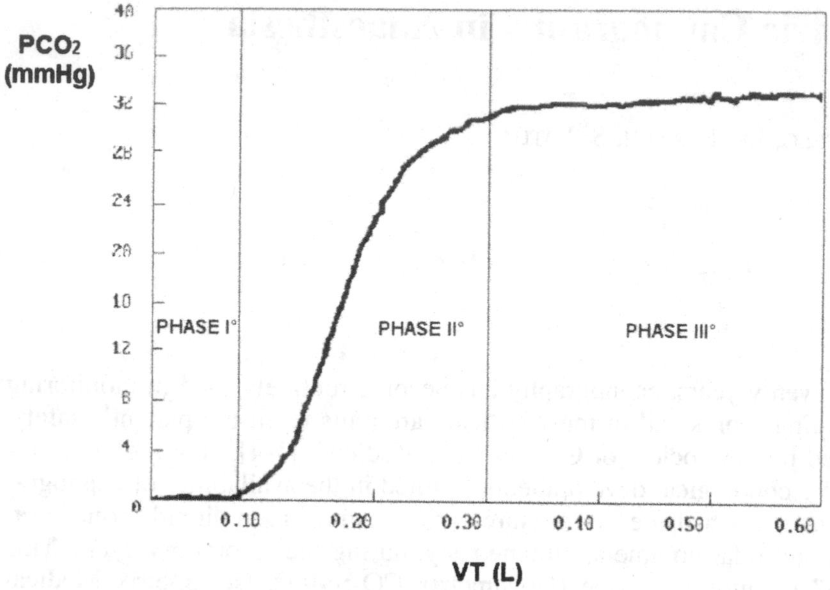

Fig. 1. The three phases of the volumetric capnogram

time reflects the arterial carbon dioxide concentration ($PaCO_2$). Under normal circumstances there is a difference of 2-5 mmHg between the arterial and alveolar CO_2 values (α-$ADCO_2$) but this can pathologically increase considerably with dead space [1, 9-11]. The normal volumetric capnogram has a rapid S-shaped upswing and an almost linear plateau indicating gas distribution and alveolar ventilation homogeneity. The slope of the alveolar plateau depends on the emptying patterns of the different alveoli with different ventilation/perfusion (V/Q) ratios. If all the alveoli had the same PCO_2 and V/Q ratios, the alveolar plateau would be perfectly horizontal. However, this "ideal" situation does not occur even in normal lungs because of the wide range of alveoli with different V/Q ratios. Therefore, the slope of phase III of the normal capnogram derives from a temporal mismatching between perfusion and ventilation (when perfusion is highest at the end of expiration ventilation is lowest) and from a spatial mismatching, because of the different emptying times between alveolar units, for instance alveoli with low V/Q ratios empty latter during expiration contributing to rising the slope of phase III [2]. All of these factors occur simultaneously. While changes in amplitude of the capnographic curve suggest haemodynamic impairments, changes in the morphology are the expression of V/Q disturbances.

In order to quantify these disturbances several indices based on geometrical analysis of the curve have been developed and among them the slope of phase III is one of the most frequently used [7].

Volumetric capnography also gives the opportunity to determine physiological dead space and its components with the equal area method. This method consists in tracing two lines: one is the back extrapolation of the phase III slope; the second is a vertical line passing through phase II, positioned so that the two areas "p and q" are equal [12]. If arterial CO_2 tension is measured during $PECO_2$ recording another horizontal line can be traced on the SBT-CO_2 trace delimiting the areas Y and Z that correspond to alveolar dead space and anatomical dead space respectively. The area under the curve, X, is the CO_2 volume that effectively participates to gas exchange. Physiologic dead space can be calculated from the sum of the Z and Y area[10-13]. From the SBT-CO_2 the carbon dioxide elimination (VCO_2) can also be calculated and corresponds to the sum of the areas X and p. This information can be easily obtained with a combined CO_2/flow sensor (Novametrix CO_2SMO^+, Novametrix Medical System, Wallinford, CT, USA). By plotting VCO_2 as a function of tidal volume the alveolar ejection volume fraction can be calculated.

Alveolar ejection volume ratio

As described in our previous study in acute lung injury (ALI), ARDS patients and healthy subjects, we defined the alveolar ejection volume fraction (VAE/VT). This index is based on the hypothesis of sequential gas emptying and corresponds to a fraction of tidal volume free from dead space contamination, assuming a fixed amount of dead space of 5%. By plotting VCO_2 as a function of expired volume (VCO_2/VT) we obtain the curve shown in Figure 3. The gradual VCO_2 increase cannot be linear because of the contamination from alveolar, anatomical and instrumental dead space. At the very end of expiration, exhaled gas comes only from the alveoli representing pure alveolar gas [7, 8]. VAE/VT seemed to account well for the amount of lung impairment, correlated well with other indexes of ventilatory maldistribution, and was less dependant on tidal volume. For this reason the aim of this pilot study was to evaluate the clinical usefulness of measuring VAE/VT during the perioperative period that is frequently characterised by ventilatory disturbances.

Pulmonary function in the perioperative period

The postoperative period, after abdominal or thoracic surgery, can be associated to important ventilation and gas exchange impairments [14-16]. The exact incidence of postoperative pulmonary complications is difficult to establish because of imprecision and heterogeneity of clinical studies, where frequency ranges between 4 and 80% [17]. One of the major causes of impaired gas exchange is the formation of atelectasis and shunt. The exact mechanism by which atelectasis develops, during and after anaesthesia, has not yet been completely established

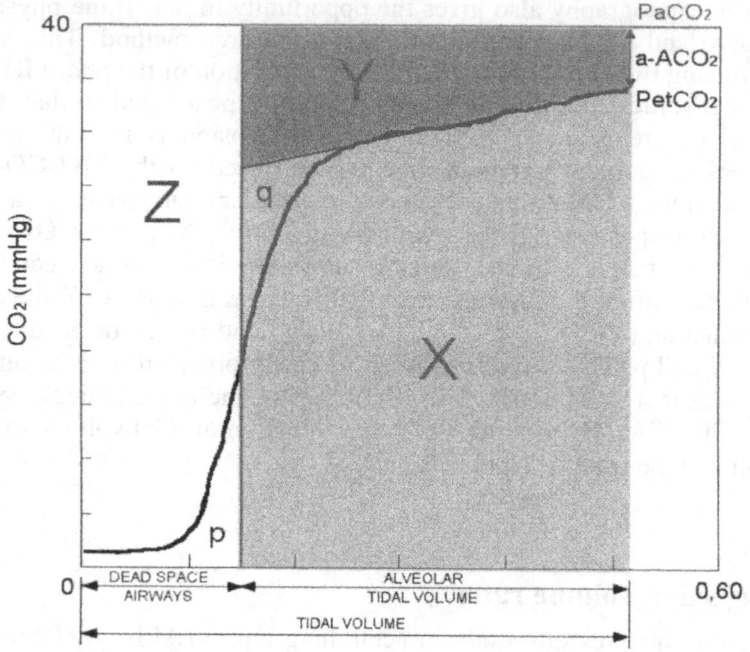

Fig. 2. Equal area method (for further explanation see text)

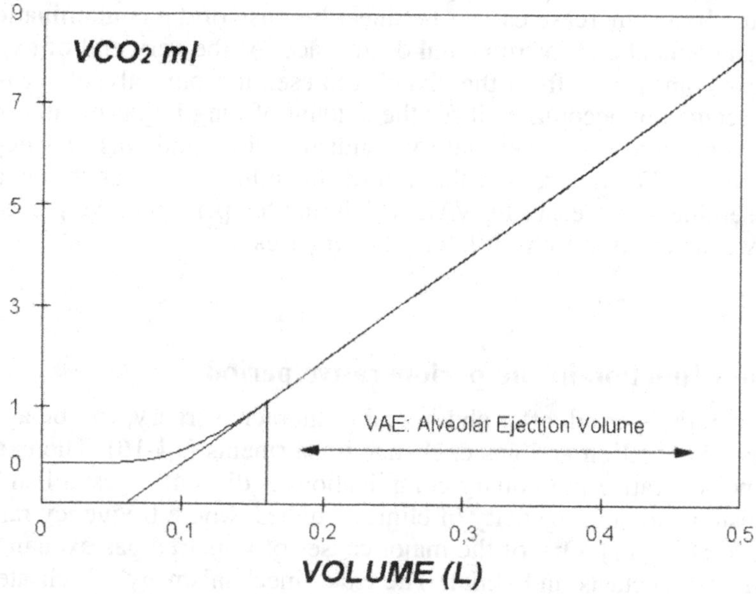

Fig. 3. VAE

[18]. Right after the induction of anaesthesia there is a reduction of functional residual capacity (FRC) that seems to be responsible for atelectasis formation. This depends not only on gas reabsorbtion, but also on compression of lung tissue by the cephad shift of the diaphragm. During the postoperative period, patients breathe more rapidly and with small tidal volumes, as they are unable to breathe more deeply because of the residual effects of anaesthesia, pain immobilisation, and reduced sensitivity to hypoxemia and hypercarbia. Their inspiratory capacity and their ability to cough effectively is reduced. All these factors may contribute to atelectasis formation and impaired gas exchange [15-19]. Immediately following upper abdominal surgery vital capacity (VC) is normally reduced approximately to 40% of preoperative values and remains depressed for at least 10-14 days. Information on when full recovery from upper abdominal surgery occurs is lacking because most studies end within 5 days after surgical operation, because of patient's discharge. Lower abdominal surgery is characterised by smaller changes in VC and FRC which normally return to preoperative values after 3 days [20].

The purpose of our study was to evaluate the behaviour of VAE/VT during the perioperative period in a group of 11 patients undergoing general surgery, and in 6 patients undergoing thoracic surgery involving lung exeresis. Volumetric capnography was obtained in spontaneously breathing awake patients before anaesthesia (*pre*), post intubation and mechanical ventilation (*intub*), at incision (*incis*), in the mid-operative time (*intraop*), and after spontaneous breathing recovery (*rec*) (Fig. 4). During thoracic surgery, volumetric capnography was obtained in spontaneously breathing awake patients before anaesthesia (*pre*), post intubation and mechanical ventilation (*int*), after lateral decubitus positioning (*lat*), after thorax opening (*open*), during steady ventilation of the dependent

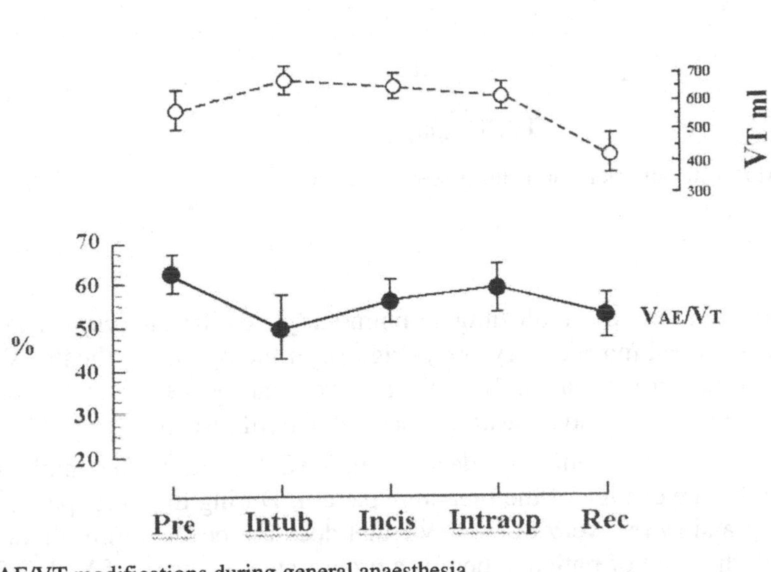

Fig. 4. VAE/VT modifications during general anaesthesia

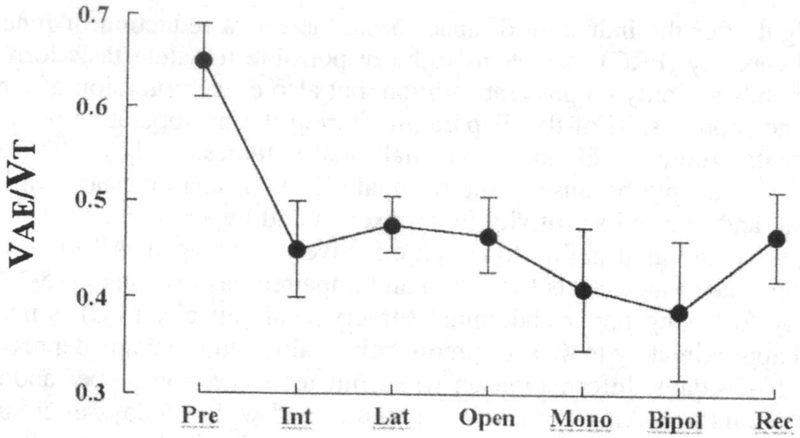

Fig. 5. VAE/VT modifications during thoracic surgery

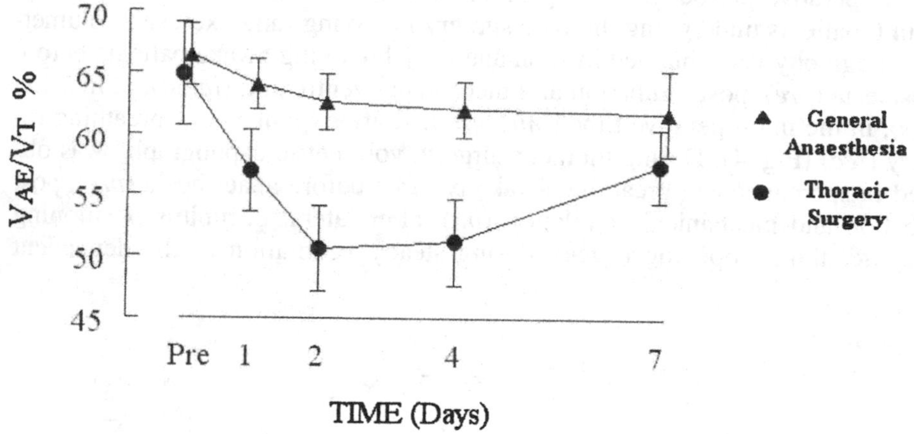

Fig. 6. VAE/VT modification during the postoperative period

lung (*mono*), after re-establishing bi-pulmonary ventilation (*bipol*), and after spontaneous breathing recovery (*rec*) (Fig. 5). In the operating theatre VAE/VT was measured during haemodynamic and ventilatory steady state condition. These variables were also measured twice a day until discharge (Fig. 6).

Results showed a significant decrease in VAE/VT right after intubation unexplained by the change of the breathing pattern. During the intraoperative period there is a slow recovery of VAE/VT that does not occur during thoracic surgery. In both group of patients there is a progressive recovery of VAE/VT without ever reaching preoperative values. These preliminary results suggest that VAE/VT is a useful non-invasive index of lung function recovery. However further clinical research is needed.

References

1. Hess D (1993) Capnography: technical aspects and clinical applications. In: Kakmarek RM, Hess D, Stoller JK (eds) Monitoring in respiratory care. Mosby, St Louis, pp 375-406
2. Hess D (1990) Capnometry and capnography: technical aspects, physiologic aspects, and clinical applications. Respiratory Care; Vol 35, 6:557-576
3. Bhavani-Shankar K, Moseley H, Kumar AY, Delph Y (1992) Capnometry and anaesthesia. Review article. Can J Anaesth 39(6):617-632
4. AARC Clinical Practice Guideline (1995) Capnography/capnometry during nechanical ventilation. Respir Care 40(12):1321-1324
5. Society of Critical Care Medicine: Task force on guidelines (1998) Recommendations for services and personnel for delivery of care in a critical care setting. Crit Care Med 16(8): 809-811
6. Breen PH (1996) The American Society of Anestesiologists, Inc. Respiratory concerns during anesthesia. An update
7. Romero PV, Lucangelo U, Lopcz Aguilar J et al (1997) Physiologically based indices of volumetric capnography in patients receiving mechanical ventilation. Eur Respir J 10:1309-1315
8. Blanch Ll, Lucangelo U, Lopez Aguilar J et al (1999) Volumetric capnography in patients with acute lung injury: effects of positive end-expiratory pressure. Eur Respir J 13:1048-1054
9. Ward KR, Yealy DM (1998) End – tidal carbon dioxide monitoring in emergency medicine, Part 1: Basic priciples. Acad Emerg Med 5:628-636
10. Bhavani-Shankar K, Kumar AY, Moseley HSL, Ahyee-Hallsworth R (1995) Terminology and the current limitations of time capnography: a brief review. J Clin Monit 11:175-182
11. Lucangelo U, Beltrame F, Antonaglia V et al (1996) Monitoraggio capnografico della funzione respiratoria durante ventilazione meccanica. Aspetti di fisiologia, clinici e di monitoraggio in anestesiologia. A cura di Giron GP, Gullo A. APICE, Trieste
12. Fowler WS (1948) Lung function studies. II. The respiratory dead space. American J Physiol 154:405-416
13. Graig DB (1981) Postoperative recovery of pulmonary function. Anesthesia and Analgesia 60;1:46-52
14. Rehder K (1979) Anesthesia and the respiratory system. Can Anaesth Soc J 26:451-462
15. Lindberg P, Gunnarsson L, Tokics L et al (1992) Atelectasis and lung function in the postoperative period. Acta Aaesthesiol Scand 36:546-553
16. Christensen EF, Schultz P, Jensen OV et al (1991) Acta Anaesthesiol Scand 35:97-104
17. Engberg G, Wilklund L (1988) Pulmonary complications after upper abdominal surgery: their prevention with intercostal blocks. Acta Anaesthesiol Scand 32:1-9
18. Hedenstierna XYZ, Tokics L, Strandberg A et al (1986) Correlation of gas exchange impairment to development of atelectasis during anaesthesia and muscle paralysis. Acta Anaesthesiol Scand 30:183-191
19. Strandberg A, Tokics L, Brismar B et al (1986) Atelectasis during anaesthesia and in the postoperative period. Acta Anaesthesiol Scand 30:154-158
20. Graig DB (1981) Postoperative recovery of pulmonary function. Anesthesia and Analgesia 60:46-52

Disturbances of Alveolar Capillary Permeability Pathomechanisms and Pharmaceutical Interactions

H. GERLACH

Formation of pulmonary edema is a major problem in critical care medicine, and initial diagnostics focus to distinguish between the two forms, so-called cardiogenic and non-cardiogenic lung edema. Whereas the first is predominantly based on increased hydrostatic filtration pressure and will not be discussed in the following chapter, the second is due to increased vascular permeability. The prototypic example of non-cardiogenic pulmonary edema is the acute lung injury (ALI) or, in its aggravated form, the acute respiratory distress syndrome (ARDS).

Normal water homeostasis in the lung is based on a balance among the so-called Starling forces: a vascular-to-extravascular hydrostatic pressure gradient, a similar but directionally opposite oncotic pressure gradient, and the "leakiness" or "permeability" of the alveolo-capillary endothelial membrane to protein [1, 2]. Despite this commonly accepted model, the diagnosis of non-cardiogenic pulmonary edema, and therefore of ARDS, is still usually made by inference: when pulmonary edema occurs in the setting of normal hydrostatic pressures (estimated either clinically or from the pulmonary artery wedge pressure), the pathogenesis is generally assumed to be non-cardiogenic. Conversely, if the wedge pressure is elevated, the primary mechanism for pulmonary edema is assumed to be due to increased pulmonary hydrostatic pressures, not increased vascular permeability. Importantly, patients with increased pulmonary hydrostatic pressures, regardless of other considerations, are usually excluded from clinical trials of new therapies for ARDS. Of course, there is no reason why vascular permeability and hydrostatic pressures cannot both be elevated simultaneously.

Conversely, pulmonary venous hypertension (and thus pulmonary capillary hypertension) can occur without increasing the wedge pressure per se. In addition, any change in pulmonary vascular permeability from lung injury must surely cover a wide spectrum of abnormality, and not simply be "normal" or "increased". For all these reasons, a strategy in which lung injury is determined only by inference and exclusion is unsatisfactory. To fully characterize the pathogenesis of pulmonary edema, the relative contribution of both hydrostatic pressures and permeability should be quantified. The importance of these issues has been recognized, and vascular permeability measurements should be important to the diagnosis and evaluation of acute lung injury. In the ATS/ESICM report [3], the Consensus Conference committee declared that "the difficulty in determining the incidence and outcome of ARDS is largely due to the heterogeneity and lack of definitions for the underlying disease processes [and] the lack of definition for ARDS...". In response, they recommended that acute lung injury be defined as "a syndrome of inflammation and increasing permeability that is associated with a constellation of clinical, radiological, and physiological abnormalities that cannot be explained by, but may coexist with, left atrial or pulmonary capillary hypertension", and that ARDS be defined simply as a more-severe form of acute lung injury. They recommended, however, that this distinction in severity should be based solely on differences in oxygenation [3]. This approach can be expected to be insensitive, underestimating pathophysiologically important mechanisms leading to functional abnormalities as a result of a breakdown in the pulmonary endothelial barrier, leading first to proteinaceous alveolar edema, and then, as a consequence, to altered respiratory system mechanics and hypoxemia.

In the following, basic cellular mechanisms regulating alveolar capillary permeability are presented; furthermore, both clinical as well as experimental strategies to quantify lung edema are discussed. The overall objective is to consider the role of the alveolar epithelial and endothelial barrier in the development and resolution of acute lung injury and ARDS.

Morphology and fluid balance

The alveolar capillaries in the lung are surrounded by an interstitial space, which is separated from the airspaces by the alveolar epithelial barrier. Under normal conditions, some fluid and a small amount of protein filters into the interstitium from the lung capillaries through small gap junctions in the endothelium [4]. The tight junctions between the cells of the normal alveolar epithelium are much tighter than the gap junctions between endothelial cells [5]. Thus, the alveolar epithelium offers substantial resistance to the passive movement of liquid and protein into the alveoli. Until approximately the mid 1980s, fluid movement across the alveolar barrier was thought to depend entirely on passive hydrostatic forces [6]. Hydrostatic pulmonary edema develops because of elevated pressure within the pulmonary microcirculation, usually because of left heart failure. In contrast, permeability pulmonary edema develops because of an increase in the permeability of the lung endothelial barrier leading to an abnormal extravascular accumulation of fluid. Both experimental and clinical work demonstrated that alveolar flooding in hydrostatic or increased permeability pulmonary edema occurred when the quantity of edema fluid in the lung interstitium exceeded the capacity of the interstitial space, resulting in bulk flow of the interstitial fluid into the air spaces of the lung [7]. Moreover, in both hydrostatic and increased permeability pulmonary edema, there is a rise in the net flux of fluid from the vascular to the interstitial space of the lung. Approximately 500 ml of edema fluid can collect in the interstitium of the lung before the pressure is high enough for edema fluid to break through the epithelium and flood the airspaces [4].

Pulmonary edema fluid contains both liquid and protein. Initial samples of pulmonary edema fluid from patients with cardiac failure have a protein concentration that generally ranges from 2 to 4 g/100 ml. In patients with increased permeability pulmonary edema, the edema fluid has a protein concentration between 4 and 6 g/100 ml [8]. The distinction between hydrostatic and increased permeability mechanisms for pulmonary edema formation can usually be made by analyzing the ratio of the protein concentration in pulmonary edema fluid to the protein concentration in plasma [4, 8]. If the ratio is less than 0.65, then the edema fluid is a transudate, diagnostic of hydrostatic forces causing the extravascular accumulation of edema fluid in the lung. If the ratio is greater than 0.75, the pulmonary edema fluid reflects an increase in permeability; if the ratio is between 0.65 and 0.75, then the type of pulmonary edema is indeterminate [9]. The cellular content of the edema fluid depends on associated conditions, such as hemorrhage or inflammation. There are always red blood cells, and usually a few monocytes and neutrophils in hydrostatic pulmonary edema; in most causes of increased permeability, the number of neutrophils is greater [10, 11].

The sites or locations of airspace flooding have never been established with certainty, although some studies suggest that in some cases alveolar edema may develop from the passage of interstitial fluid through distal extra-alveolar epithelial locations with retrograde filling of the alveoli [12]. However, some severe cases of ARDS, caused by low pH gastric aspiration, sepsis, or some types of necrotizing pneumonia, can cause direct injury to the alveolar epithelial barrier with denuding of the alveolar epithelial type I cells [13]. When this type of injury develops, direct translocation of interstitial edema fluid into the alveoli occurs.

In contrast to formation of pulmonary edema by translocation of water and protein into the interstitial and alveolar space, the other scale of fluid balance in the lung comprises mechanisms of fluid removal. Several experimental studies, most of which were performed by the group of Matthay et al. [14-16], demonstrated that removal of free alveolar water can not be accounted for by a simple hydrostatic force or oncotic mechanisms. Matthay's findings provided strong evidence to support the hypothesis that an active ion transport system was driving the reabsorption of excess alveolar fluid and that the mechanism depended at least in part on sodium transport. Concurrent work on alveolar epithelial type II cells in vitro demonstrated that these cells were capable of transporting sodium from the apical to the basal surface in cultured monolayers [17, 18]. Thus, these results from both in vivo and in vitro studies provided further evidence that removal of alveolar fluid across the epithelial barrier depended primarily on a sodium transport system. Hence, the process of alveolar fluid reabsorption requires an active process and does not depend on lung inflation or transpulmonary pressure. One of the important findings of the experimental studies has been that an intact alveolar epithelial barrier is required for net alveolar liquid clearance to take place. In other words, in order for the active ion transport system to work optimally, there needs to be a sufficiently tight alveolar epithelial barrier so that passive movement between the two spaces is minimal. The epithelial barrier under some pathological conditions can still remove some excess alveolar fluid, but the rate of clearance is usually slower. Our current understanding of the mechanisms regulating alveolar fluid reabsorption can be summarized as follows (Fig. 1).

The first step in the removal of excess alveolar fluid depends on sodium uptake by the apical surface of alveolar type II cells [19]. Once the sodium has entered the alveolar epithelial cell, it is then extruded into the lung interstitium by the Na^+,K^+-ATPase system along the basolateral surface of alveolar type II cells [20]. The active movement of sodium is followed by chloride through transcellular pathways that have not been identified. The water fraction appears to move through specific transcellular water channels [21]. In addition, more-recent studies have indicated that there are several specific water channels in the lung [22, 23].

In addition to aqueous liquid, a considerable quantity of protein needs to be removed from the alveoli in lung edema. Experimental studies have indicated that soluble protein is removed from the air spaces primarily by diffusion between alveolar epithelial cells [24]. Evidence for this conclusion is based in part on the clearance of molecules across the epithelium at a rate inversely related to

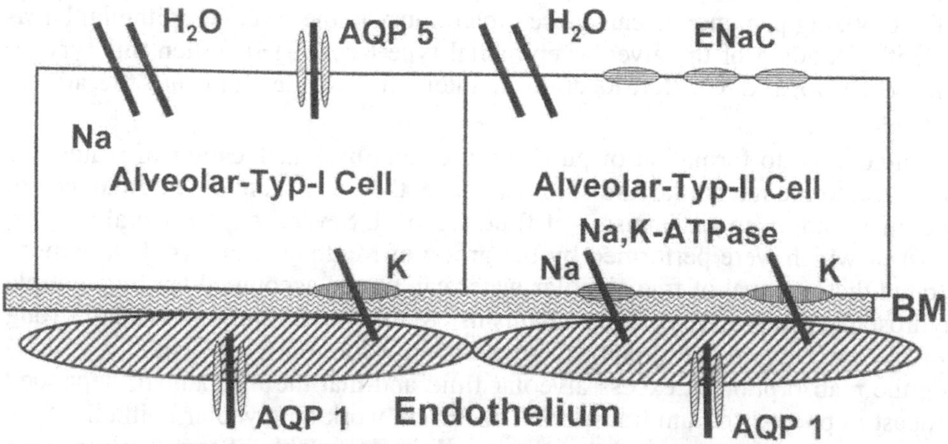

Fig. 1. Active water transport: removal of excess alveolar fluid depends on sodium uptake by the apical surface of alveolar type II cells (*right side*, *ENaC* epithelial sodium channel). Once the sodium has entered the alveolar epithelial cell, it is then extruded into the lung interstitium by the Na^+,K^+-ATPase system along the basolateral surface of alveolar type II cells. Additional water moves through specific transcellular water channels, called aquaporines (*AQP*). Several subtypes of aquaporines exist and are expressed on different cell types (*BM* basal membrane)

molecular size [25]. There is some endocytosis and transcytosis of protein by alveolar epithelial cells, although most in vivo studies indicate that this mechanism cannot account for the majority of alveolar protein clearance when large quantities have entered the airspaces [24, 25]. Mucociliary clearance is another minor pathway, as is protein degradation and macrophage engulfment, at least in the uninjured lung [24]. However, in the setting of lung injury, in which precipitation of protein occurs in the alveoli, the mechanism for removal of excess protein may include a more-important role for alveolar macrophage engulfment and protein degradation.

Pathomechanisms of disturbed alveolar permeability

Until recently, little work had been done on the role of the alveolar epithelial barrier in acute lung injury nor the mechanisms by which it is injured. The best morphological evidence for injury to the alveolar epithelial barrier derives from the ultrastructural studies of Bachofen and Weibel [13, 26] in the mid 1970s on patients who died with acute lung injury. These classic investigations established that there was evidence of both endothelial and epithelial injury in the first few days following acute lung injury, often with denuding of type I alveolar epithelial cells with vacuolization and evidence of injury to alveolar type II cells as well. In the subacute phase (day 5-10), there was still evidence of alveolar epithelial barrier injury in many patients, particularly those with sepsis, but there was also proliferation of alveolar epithelial type II cells in an apparent attempt to form a new epithelial barrier following the necrosis of type I cells.

Much early experimental work on the pathogenesis of acute lung injury focused on mechanisms of endothelial damage. It was possible to study the early phase of acute lung injury by using the isolated perfused lung preparation, in which net weight gain could be used as an index of endothelial damage. Furthermore, the injection of a vascular protein tracer could be used as a marker of pulmonary endothelial injury by measuring its escape from the circulation as well as its accumulation in the lung. Considerable work has been done on both neutrophil-dependent [27] and neutrophil-independent [28] mechanisms of acute lung endothelial injury using these models.

In clinical conditions in which there is injury to both lung endothelial and epithelial barriers, such as blood-borne sepsis, primary lung infection, and gastric aspiration, there is morphological and physiological evidence for injury to both the endothelial and epithelial barriers of the lung [8, 13]. It has been suggested that barotrauma in patients with acute lung injury may be primarily a function of the extent of lung injury and the damage to the alveolar epithelial barrier [29]. If there is a sufficient increase in lung interstitial edema from any cause, a rise in lung interstitial pressure alone will lead to alveolar flooding. The exact site for movement of edema fluid from the interstitium into the air spaces has not been identified clearly, although some evidence suggests that there may be flooding in terminal or respiratory bronchioles, where epithelial junctions might not be as tight as they are in the alveolar epithelial barrier [30]. In this model, pulmonary edema fluid would fill the alveoli in a retrograde fashion. After interstitial edema has flooded the air spaces of the lung and the increase in lung microvascular pressure has returned towards normal, the alveolar epithelial barrier rapidly regains its tight barrier properties, allowing reabsorption of excess alveolar fluid. Thus, when hydrostatic pulmonary edema results in alveolar flooding, it is associated with an increase in alveolar epithelial barrier permeability, probably from a transient opening of tight junctions in the distal pulmonary epithelium.

This concept of alveolar flooding from high-pressure pulmonary edema may also be relevant to some forms of increased permeability pulmonary edema, in which the acute lung injury may be primarily confined to the lung endothelial barrier. In these cases, there may be a rapid accumulation of protein-rich edema fluid in the lung interstitium, which then results in alveolar flooding if there is a sufficient increase in the total quantity of lung interstitial edema fluid, as in uncomplicated hydrostatic pulmonary edema. In this case, the injury may be confined primarily to the lung endothelium without any actual injury to the epithelial barrier. We have clinical evidence for this pattern of acute lung injury in some patients who rapidly reabsorb some of their protein-rich alveolar edema within a short time [8, 25]. This kind of acute lung injury, which may be more typical of transient lung endothelial injury, seems to be associated with blood product reactions, surgery involving cardiopulmonary bypass, and high-altitude or neurogenic pulmonary edema, in which there may be a combination of both increased pressure and increased permeability primarily affecting the lung endothelial barrier.

Some patients with acute lung injury, especially associated with sepsis, have persistent alveolar flooding and persistently poor arterial oxygenation. These patients characteristically have little evidence of reabsorption of alveolar edema, at least within 12-24 h of the development of acute lung injury [8]. After an initial phase of severe alveolar flooding with protein-rich edema fluid, some patients begin to reabsorb some excess alveolar fluid within 6-12 h [8, 25]. This phase of alveolar reabsorption is associated with a decrease in edema fluid on the chest radiograph and an improvement in arterial oxygenation. Experimentally, the same phenomena have been reported in different models. The clinical studies have supported the hypothesis that the ability to reabsorb some alveolar edema fluid in the first 12 h after the development of acute lung injury is a favorable prognostic finding, associated with a mortality of only 20%. In contrast, the inability to reabsorb alveolar edema fluid early in the course of acute lung injury is associated with a mortality of nearly 80% [8]. Thus, the function of the alveolar epithelial barrier early in the course of acute lung injury may be a useful prognostic index, perhaps because of the central importance of damage to the alveolar epithelial barrier in acute lung injury [31].

It is possible that inflammatory cells also contribute to the barrier injury in pneumonia, although it appears that neutrophils are primarily protective in this setting. Other investigators have provided evidence that oxygen radicals may be important mediators of injury under certain conditions, such as oxygen toxicity or noxious gases, including nitrogen dioxide [32, 33]. Neutrophils may play a role in injuring the epithelial barrier in certain types of acute lung injury, such as gastric aspiration [34] or even septicemia, although further work on this hypothesis is required.

Identification of increased pulmonary permeability

As with pulmonary edema, a number of techniques that are appropriate for clinical application have been developed to evaluate pulmonary vascular permeability. The most straightforward method is to simply sample and analyze alveolar edema fluid for its protein concentration. If the endothelial barrier is intact, the protein concentration in the fluid should be significantly less than that in plasma. The epithelial barrier is clearly breached in most patients with acute lung injury, as evidenced by the presence of alveolar edema, both radiographically and clinically. Hence, with injury, the concentration of protein in the edema fluid should approach that of plasma. Direct evidence for an increase in alveolar epithelial barrier permeability was derived from studies in which it was demonstrated that patients with acute lung injury had an initial alveolar edema protein concentration that was higher (75% or greater) than that of plasma [35]. Furthermore, experimental studies demonstrated that in the presence of acute lung injury there was flooding of the air spaces with protein-rich pulmonary edema fluid [7]. Thus, both morphological and physiological evidence suggests that the clinical syndrome of acute lung injury or ARDS includes flooding of the air spaces with protein-rich edema fluid and a loss of a primary protective function of the alveolar epithelial barrier. However, sampling errors, dilution with lavage fluid, or fluid resorption during edema resolution could all potentially affect the relationship between injury and the assessment of that injury by this simple technique.

The protein concentration of alveolar edema fluid can be determined from samples obtained [by direct aspiration from distal airways or via bronchoalveolar lavage (BAL)]. In directly obtained samples, the protein concentration in the fluid should be significantly less than that in plasma if the endothelial barrier is intact and continues to truly function as a semi-permeable membrane (edema-to-plasma protein ratio < 0.65). However, with injury, the concentration of protein in the edema fluid should approach that of plasma (ratio > 0.75). Patients with values between 0.65 and 0.75 are not readily classified. The technique for obtaining alveolar edema fluid by direct aspiration is straightforward, although not always successful. A suction catheter with a 14 to 18-gauge catheter attached is blindly advanced through an endotracheal tube until it reaches a "wedged" position. Fluid is collected with gentle suction into a standard suction trap, sometimes after several attempts, and sometimes only after patient repositioning. In some instances, all maneuvers are unsuccessful and no fluid at all is obtained.

While this method is safe, quick, non-invasive, and inexpensive, it can only be performed in intubated patients. Also, it underestimates injury at times, since proteins in the alveolar space that precipitate into hyaline membranes will not be represented in the fluid sample. Furthermore, as the edema resolves, the protein concentration in the remaining fluid will increase. Since edema may begin to resolve within hours of the onset of injury, the direct sampling method should lose specificity with time. In general, the measurements of protein concentration from directly sampled alveolar fluid can only be used to differentiate hydrostatic from permeability forms of pulmonary edema when the samples are obtained within several hours of the onset of injury.

Perhaps the most-common clinical method of determining whether or not the integrity of the capillary endothelial barrier has been compromised is to measure the time-dependent accumulation of an intravenously administered radioactively labelled protein tracer into lung tissue [36, 37]. Both albumin and transferrin (with approximately comparable molecular weights) have been used as protein tracers; technetium^{99m}, gallium^{68}, and indium^{113m} have been used as the radioactive labels. After the radioactive tracer is injected intravenously, activity within lung tissue is detected and recorded for minutes to hours with one of several kinds of external radiation detection devices: probes, gamma cameras, or positron emission tomography (PET) cameras have all been used successfully. Since these devices cannot distinguish whether activity within the lung tissue originates from the blood or extravascular space, similar time-activity data must be simultaneously obtained from the blood, either by measuring activity within the cardiac blood pool of the right or left ventricle with the same external detection system, or by measuring the protein activity in separately obtained blood samples [37]. The blood volume within the lung tissue region-of-interest must also be determined, either by using a single protein tracer and assuming that all the protein activity at the beginning of the data collection period is intravascular (in which case one must also assume that intravascular volume does not change during the data collection period), or by using a second tracer which can be assumed to remain intravascular (usually radioactively labelled red blood cells). The latter option is theoretically attractive since changes in intravascular volume during the data collection period can also be monitored (usually about 1-2 h) [37]. However, there is little reason to believe that intravascular volume in fact changes in a unidirectional manner during this brief period of time in clinically stable subjects. Furthermore, it was shown that such measurements are a sensitive and probably accurate, even though non-specific, marker of injury, and do correlate well with morphological indices of injury. Other techniques based on indicator-dilution methods or on the pulmonary uptake of an inhaled radiolabelled aerosol, are unlikely to be used extensively because of either complexity or technical artifacts that interfere with data interpretation.

For clinical use, the radiographic identification and quantification of lung edema still is the first-choice tool. The clinical and radiological manifestations of acute pulmonary edema are generally well established. However, pulmonary edema may also demonstrate unusual findings. Gluecker et al. [38] recently divided pulmonary edema into four main categories on the basis of pathophysiology [38]: 1) increased hydrostatic pressure edema, 2) permeability edema with diffuse alveolar damage (DAD), 3) permeability edema without DAD, and 4) mixed edema due to simultaneous increased hydrostatic pressure and permeability changes. Pulmonary edema was categorized according to a classification scheme. Atypical pulmonary edema was defined as lung edema with an unusual radiological appearance but with clinical findings that were usually associated with well-known causes of pulmonary edema. Unusual forms of pulmonary edema were defined as lung edema from unusual causes (i.e., rare diseases or rare manifestations of common diseases).

In patients with increased hydrostatic pressure edema, two pathophysiological and radiological phases are recognized in the development of pressure edema: interstitial edema and alveolar flooding or edema. These phases are virtually identical for left-sided heart failure and fluid overload, the two most frequently observed causes of pressure edema in intensive care and emergency patients. The intensity and duration of both phases are clearly related to the degree of increased pressure, which is determined by the hydrostatic-oncotic pressure ratio. Interstitial edema occurs with an increase of 15-25 mmHg in mean transmural arterial pressure and results in the early loss of definition of subsegmental and segmental vessels, mild enlargement of the peribronchovascular spaces, the appearance of Kerley lines, and subpleural effusions. If the quantity of extravascular fluid continues to increase, the edema will migrate centrally, with progressive blurring of vessels, first at the lobar level and later at the level of the hilum. At this point, lung radiolucency decreases markedly, making identification of small peripheral vessels difficult. Peribronchial cuffing becomes apparent, particularly at the perihilar areas. With increases in transmural pressure greater than 25 mmHg, fluid drainage from the extravascular compartment is at maximum capacity and the second phase (alveolar flooding) commences, leading to a sudden extension of edema into the alveolar spaces. Some investigators have observed that, with such pressure increases, the onset of alveolar edema may also be associated with direct pressure-induced damage to the alveolar epithelium [39].

ARDS occurs without an increase in pulmonary capillary pressure and represents the most-severe form of permeability edema associated with diffuse alveolar damage (DAD). DAD may be the direct result of a local precipitating factor or may occur secondary to some systemic condition. Primary or direct injuries to the alveolar and vascular endothelium of the lung usually result from the exposure of these cells to chemical agents, infectious pathogens, gastric fluid, or toxic gas, which destroy or severely damage the cells. Secondary damage is due to a systemic biochemical cascade creating oxidating agents, inflammatory mediators, and enzymes, which also harm these endothelial cells during sepsis, pancreatitis, severe trauma, or blood transfusion. ARDS encompasses three often overlapping stages. The first (exudative) stage is characterized by interstitial edema with a high protein content that rapidly fills the alveolar spaces and is associated with hemorrhage and ensuing hyaline membrane formation. The rapid extension of edema into the alveolar spaces probably explains why findings that are typically seen in interstitial edema (e.g., Kerley lines) are not prominent in ARDS. The second (proliferative) stage manifests as organization of the fibrinous exudate. Following this organization, one observes the regeneration of the alveolar lining and thickening of the alveolar septa. The third (fibrotic) stage is characterized by varying degrees of scarring and formation of subpleural and intrapulmonary cysts.

The early exudative stage demonstrates few radiological findings. Initially, interstitial edema is observed, followed rapidly by perihilar areas of increased opacity. The progression from interstitial edema to the filling of alveolar spaces corresponds to the appearance of widespread alveolar consolidation on air bronchograms. Compared with hydrostatic edema, the alveolar edema in ARDS usually has a more-peripheral or cortical distribution. Radiological signs that are typically seen in cardiogenic edema (e.g., cardiomegaly, apical vascular redistribution, Kerley lines) are absent. Despite the presence of diffuse, homogeneous DAD, ARDS usually displays a gravitational gradient that is easily visualized by computed tomography (CT) and can be modified by changing the patient's position [40]. This suggests that atelectasis is also an important factor in the inhomogeneous regional distribution of ARDS. Furthermore, this gravitational pattern can help exclude concomitant infectious processes because such dependent atelectasis is more common in patients with early ARDS without pneumonia [41].

With progression of the disease into the proliferative stage, an inhomogeneous pattern of ground-glass areas of increased opacity is seen, along with early modifications due to fibrosis. During the fibrotic stage, subpleural and intrapulmonary cystic lesions may be observed and may be the direct cause of pneumothoraces. Recurrent exudative episodes can still occur in the proliferative and fibrotic stages of ARDS, resulting in mixed radiological findings that demonstrate parts of all three stages simultaneously. Atypical ARDS, which is characterized by a predominance of anterior airspace consolidations in supine patients, was observed in about 5% of patients who underwent CT during the exudative stage. The pathophysiological explanation for this finding remains unclear, but may involve regional differences in mechanically assisted ventilation pressures.

The absence of cellular damage in DAD is often not provided pathologically but may be inferred from the clinical and radiological course of the disease, because rapid regression is often observed, with ventilatory improvements occurring within a short period of time. Although some degree of DAD may occur, damage remains minor and usually only partially affects patient outcome [38]. Examples for this form of pulmonary edema are: heroin-induced lung edema, pulmonary edema after therapeutic administration of cytokines in cancer patients, and high-altitude pulmonary edema.

The mixed edema due to simultaneous increased hydrostatic pressure and permeability changes is seen in neurogenic pulmonary edema in up to 50% of patients who have suffered a severe brain insult such as trauma, subarachnoid hemorrhage, stroke, or status epilepticus [42]. Differentiation of neurogenic pulmonary edema from simple fluid overload or postextubation edema may be difficult if not impossible in trauma patients or immediately following surgery. Its cause remains controversial, but probably involves a combination of factors associated with hydrostatic edema and factors associated with permeability edema without DAD. The cellular mechanisms that cause capillary leakage are also not well understood. Modifications in neurovegetative pathways are probably the cause of sudden, significant increases in microvascular pressure in the lungs, particularly in the pulmonary venules. This leads to reduced venous outflow, which in turn causes pulmonary capillary and arterial hypertension. In addition, there are probably direct effects of various mediators that cause leakage of vascular endothelial cells and cell junctions. Conventional chest radiography demonstrates the presence of bilateral, rather homogeneous airspace consolidations, which predominate at the apices in about 50% of cases.

Hemodynamic parameters can be used for identification and characterization of pulmonary edema. Pulmonary artery catheters are frequently used to assess hydrostatic pressure in intensive care patients. Pulmonary capillary wedge pressure has been shown to reflect left atrial pressure and correlates well with the radiological features of congestive heart failure and pulmonary venous hypertension. However, in acute heart failure, a time lag is often observed between the increased pulmonary capillary wedge pressure and the radiological manifestation of pulmonary edema due to the relatively slow movement of water through the widened capillary endothelial cell junctions [43]. Similarly, as pulmonary edema resolves, the radiological findings will persist with decreasing or even normal pulmonary capillary wedge pressure.

A wide variety of other techniques have also been evaluated for the purpose of measuring the accumulation of excess extravascular lung water (EVLW), including indicator-dilution methods, X-ray CT, nuclear magnetic resonance imaging, and PET, among others. With the exception of the indicator-dilution approach, however, none of these have much chance of wide clinical implementation, because of problems with accuracy, cost, or complexity. At present, the most clinically appropriate method to quantify EVLW in patients with acute lung injury is by indicator-dilution methods. The theoretical foundation for these techniques is quite consistent, despite differences in indicators, technology, or methods of analysis. In general, temperature-time or concentration-time data are first generated in the course of determining EVLW [44]. These data are then analyzed by so-called mean transit time or slope-volume approaches. The former strategy is based on a rationale similar to that used to measure cardiac output by the familiar "thermodilution" method. While the theory underlying these measurements is well understood [44], commercially available equipment may have seriously biased the interpretation of performance in experimental and clinical settings. A number of studies have suggested that EVLW measurements could be used to help plan respiratory, diuretic, fluid, or other intensive care therapy. However, measurements of vascular permeability, including EVLW, have never been incorporated into any clinical trial of therapy for pulmonary edema. Finally, the cost-benefit ratio of using such measurements in patients remains to be determined.

Pharmacological interactions in alveolar permeability

Although the increased pulmonary alveolar permeability is mostly induced by the disease itself, there are many pharmacological interactions that are able to aggravate or ameliorate pulmonary edema. For instance, upregulation of cyclooxygenase is an important event in the generation of thromboxane (TxA_2) during acute inflammatory states leading to severe respiratory distress. TxA_2 has been incriminated as an important mediator of the pulmonary microvascular dysfunction that characterizes tissue ischemia and reperfusion injury [45]. In these conditions, as well as others, TxA_2 has been shown to cause vasoconstriction and enhanced microvascular permeability. Cyclooxygenase catalyzes the incorporation of molecular oxygen into arachidonic acid; subsequent peroxidation yields prostaglandin H_2 (PGH_2), the precursor for the synthesis of TxA_2 and PGE_2, PGI_2, and $PGF_{2\alpha}$. In general, each of these cyclooxygenase products is released by the lung in response to a particular inflammatory stimulus, albeit in varying amounts [46].

Despite their common origin, the physiological effects of these substances on the pulmonary microvasculature are diverse. For example, TxA_2 and $PGF_{2\alpha}$ are constrictors of the pulmonary vasculature in rats, whereas PGI_2 is a potent vasodilator [47]. Furthermore, TxA_2 profoundly increases microvascular permeability, whereas the other agents have little, if any, effect by themselves [48]. Several investigators have reported that PGE_2 and PGI_2 might enhance the effects of histamine, bradykinin, and interleukin-1 on microvascular permeability [49, 50]. This observation, as well as the frequency with which PGE_2 and other prostaglandins are released with TxA_2 during acute inflammatory states, led investigators to postulate that PGE_2, PGI_2, and $PGF_{2\alpha}$ potentiate the proinflammatory effects of TxA_2 on the pulmonary microvasculature. Recently, Wright et al. [51] confirmed in an experimental study that several prostaglandins, which are also used clinically, increase the effects of TxA_2-receptor activation on pulmonary microvascular permeability. In contrast, inhibitors of cyclooxygenase, e.g., indomethacin, were demonstrated to exert a beneficial effect in this model

[51]. So far, however, clinical trials have not been able to evaluate this pharmacological approach as a useful way to treat pulmonary edema.

Polymorphonuclear leukocytes become primed by inflammatory agents released at sites of injury or circulating in the vasculature [52]. On attachment to vascular endothelial cells and/or after emigration into the underlying tissue, polymorphonuclear leukocytes become activated, resulting in the release of highly toxic reactive oxygen species such as hydrogen peroxide (H_2O_2) and cytoplasmic granules. H_2O_2 generated extracellularly can freely enter the endothelial cell where it has been shown to target and affect various cellular components [53]. These cellular changes ultimately result in an increase in the passage of protein and water across the vascular endothelium, leading to edema, abnormalities in gas exchange, and finally pulmonary insufficiency or ARDS [54]. However, the effect of H_2O_2, or any other oxidant, on transvascular protein clearance under nonisogravimetric conditions, where both the diffusive and convective clearances of protein can be affected, has not been evaluated in an intact vasculature.

Previous studies have demonstrated the permeability decreasing activity of cAMP-enhancing agents using a variety of inflammatory agents, diseases, and syndromes [55]. However, the ability of cAMP-enhancing agents to prevent a H_2O_2 or any oxidant-induced increase in transvascular protein clearance in an intact vasculature has not been evaluated. Drug therapy to increase intracellular levels of cAMP can take on many forms, such as stimulation of the β_2-adrenergic receptor by isoproterenol, stimulation of adenylate cyclase by forskolin, the use of a cell-permeable analogue such as 8-bromo-cAMP, or inhibition of phosphodiesterases that metabolize cAMP to 5′-AMP. Recent developments in the literature would suggest that H_2O_2 and/or its metabolite, the hydroxyl radical ($^{\cdot}OH$), may adversely affect β_2-adrenergic receptors. Thus the use of agonists that stimulate β_2-adrenergic receptors may not be as effective as, for example, drugs that inhibit cAMP metabolism in preventing an oxidant-induced increase in transvascular protein clearance.

Waypa et al. [56] performed a study to determine whether H_2O_2 increases the diffusive and convective clearances of albumin across an intact vasculature under nonisogravimetric conditions. They also determined the efficacy of post-treatment with cAMP-enhancing agents that function to either stimulate production or inhibit metabolism of cAMP on prevention of the increased transvascular albumin clearance induced by H_2O_2. It was found that H_2O_2 increased the convective and diffusive clearances of albumin across an intact pulmonary vasculature. Furthermore, inhibition of cAMP metabolism by a phosphodiesterase inhibitor more effectively attenuated the H_2O_2-induced increases in convective albumin clearance and lung weight compared with stimulation of cAMP production by isoproterenol [56].

Studies in the fetal lung have indicated that elevated plasma levels of epinephrine may be important in hastening reabsorption of fetal lung fluid at the time of birth [57]. Exogenous administration of β-adrenergic agonists, either intravenously or directly into the distal air spaces, markedly increased alveolar liquid clearance in several species [15] and most recently in the human lung [58]. Matthay [59] extended these observations to study the possible effect of catecholamines under pathological conditions, examining the effects of both endogenous as well as exogenously administered catecholamines.

Pathological conditions which were associated with a marked increase in circulating catecholamine levels might be associated with an acceleration in alveolar fluid clearance. To test this possibility, septic shock and metabolic acidosis was induced with a bolus dose of intravenous *P. Mesa* in anesthetized, ventilated rats [59]. As expected, there were markedly elevated levels of epinephrine detectable in the circulating plasma. To further confirm that accelerated alveolar fluid clearance might be due to the increased circulating levels of epinephrine, similar studies were performed in rabbits. These experimental studies may have major implications for the potential role of circulating catecholamines under some pathological conditions [59]. Elevated levels of circulating catecholamines may help to protect against flooding, providing that the epithelial barrier is sufficiently intact, particularly in patients with shock from sepsis, hypovolemia, trauma, or cardiac failure. Further studies are needed to define in more detail the clinical conditions under which this mechanism may function, and to determine if alveolar fluid clearance in acute lung injury can be accelerated with β-adrenergic agonists. These agents might also be beneficial because they have been shown to increase surfactant secretion from alveolar type II cells and to decrease endothelial injury in some experimental models [60]. Furthermore, they might be useful in reversing some of the increase in airway resistance that has been reported in some patients with acute lung injury [61]. Finally, their mild vasodilating properties might reduce lung microvascular pressures, thus reducing the accumulation of pulmonary edema fluid in the lung.

Additional pharmacological approaches were tested to reduce pulmonary edema: the effects of volatile anesthetics on ischemia/reperfusion (IR)-induced lung injury are not clear. Previous studies have shown that these agents could protect against IR-induced injury of the heart, the brain, and the liver [62]. It was shown that isoflurane could attenuate IR-induced injury in rabbit lung. Volatile anesthetics could significantly inhibit the release of tumor necrosis factor-α (TNF-α) in vitro [63]. These studies suggest that volatile anesthetics may protect against IR-induced lung injury by inhibiting the release of TNF-α. Liu et al. [64] investigated whether administration of volatile anesthetics (isoflurane and sevoflurane) before ischemia could inhibit the release of TNF-α and protect the lung against IR-induced injury in an isolated rat lung model. They found that these two volatile anesthetics administered before ischemia indeed attenuated IR-induced injury in isolated rat lungs, measured by lung weight, coefficient of filtration, increase of lactate dehydrogenase activity, and TNF-α as well as nitric oxide metabolites in the perfusate [64].

Platelet-activating factor (PAF) is a proinflammatory lipid mediator that is thought to contribute to a variety of inflammatory lung diseases, such as asthma or ARDS. In addition, PAF has been shown to contribute to pulmonary injury from extrapulmonary lesions, such as intestinal IR [65]. Direct administration of PAF causes pulmonary edema, mucus secretion, and reduced ciliary beat frequency. The mechanisms of the PAF-induced alterations in lung functions are only partly understood. TxA_2 derived from cyclooxygenase-1, and to a lesser extent also leukotrienes, are responsible for the PAF-induced bronchoconstriction and vasoconstriction. The mechanisms of the PAF-induced edema formation, however, are largely unknown. PAF has been shown to play an important role in many models of pulmonary edema such as those induced by lipopolysaccharides (LPS), interleukin-2 (IL-2), or pulmonary as well as intestinal IR [65]. The few drugs that have been identified to ameliorate PAF-induced alterations in pulmonary vascular permeability are steroids, cAMP-raising agents, vitamin D_3, and copolymer of polyinosinic and polycytidylic acids (polyIC). Two other agents, i.e., heparin sulfate and dextrane sulfate probably act by direct binding of PAF. Thus, any new agent that prevents PAF-induced edema is of both mechanistic and clinical interest.

Quinolines such as quinine, quinidine, or chloroquine are best known as antimalaria drugs or antiarrhythmics. Beyond this, a number of investigations support the hypothesis that quinolines possess anti-inflammatory properties. For instance, hydroxychloroquine was studied as an antiasthma drug in humans with promising results [66]. Falk et al. [67] investigated the antiphlogistic properties of quinolines in order to gain more insight into the mechanism of PAF-induced edema formation, and found that pretreatment with quinine in vivo prevented not only PAF-, but also endotoxin-induced edema formation. In addition, in vivo quinine prevented the endotoxin-induced release of TNF-α. Furthermore, in perfused lungs quinine reduced the PAF-induced increases in airway and vascular resistance, as well as TxA_2 release. These findings demonstrate the following anti-inflammatory properties of quinolines: reduction of TxA_2 and TNF formation; reduction of PAF-induced vasoconstriction and bronchoconstriction; and attenuation of PAF- and LPS-induced edema formation. Hence, the PAF- induced edema consists of two separate mechanisms, one dependent on an unknown cyclooxygenase metabolite, the other one sensitive to quinolines. Therefore, future clinical studies using this type of drug definitely merit further attention.

There are many additional studies with different approaches – too many to go into detail. One common conclusion of all these trials is that the pharmacological approach to increased pulmonary alveolar permeability seems to be possible but needs a lot of work in the future, both clinical and experimental.

Conclusion

Both in vivo and in vitro studies have established the critical role of the alveolar epithelial and endothelial barrier in formation and resolution of pulmonary edema. Several processes are involved, including active cellular transport mechanisms, which are responsible for the physiological clearance of liquids, proteins, and cells. Pathogenesis of increased alveolar permeability is various, and simply quantifying the amount of pulmonary edema does not distinguish whether the etiology represents a hydrostatic form of pulmonary edema or one due to lung injury per se (with its associated increase in vascular permeability). Accordingly, a quantitative measure of pulmonary edema, while a desirable component of a lung injury evaluation, cannot by itself be sufficient. New knowledge regarding the role of the alveolar epithelial barrier in regulating lung fluid balance (sodium and water transport) under normal and pathological conditions has made it possible to appreciate the critical role of the alveolar barrier in patients with acute lung injury, and the function of the barrier appears to be a major prognostic factor in clinical acute lung injury. Recent studies have provided some new insights into neutrophil-dependent and neutrophil-independent mechanisms responsible for alveolar barrier injury. There are promising future directions for therapeutic interventions directed specifically at the alveolar barrier. β-adrenergic agonists might be of value in some patients because of their potential to accelerate alveolar fluid clearance and increase surfactant production. Furthermore, in the future, prevention or treatment of nosocomial bacterial pneumonia would serve both to protect the alveolar epithelial barrier and also to provide a much needed additional treatment for pulmonary infections in ARDS. Finally, recent work on mechanisms of alveolar epithelial repair after lung injury has provided new insights into its recovery.

References

1. Staub NC (1978) The forces regulating fluid filtration in the lung. Microvasc Res 15:45-55
2. Staub N (1974) Pulmonary edema. Physiol Rev 54:678-721
3. Bernard GR, Artigas A, Grigham KL et al (1994) The American-European Consensus conference on ARDS: definitions, mechanisms, relevant outcomes, and clinical trial coordination. Am J Respir Crit Care Med 149:818-824
4. Matthay MA (1985) Pathophysiology of pulmonary edema. Clin Chest Med 6:301-314
5. Schneeberger-Keeley EE, Karnowsky MJ (1971) The influence of intravascular fluid volume on the permeability of the newborn and adult mouse lungs to ultrastructural protein tracers. J Cell Biol 49:319-327
6. Taylor AE, Guyton AC, Bishop VS (1965) Permeability of the alveolar membrane to solutes. Circ Res 16:353-362
7. Vreim CF, Snashall PD, Demling RH (1976) Lung lymph and free interstitial fluid protein composition in sheep with edema. J Appl Physiol 230:1650-1653
8. Matthay MA, Wiener-Kronish JP (1990) Intact epithelial barrier function is critical for the resolution of alveolar edema in humans. Am Rev Respir Dis 142:1250-1257
9. Matthay MA, Eschenbacher WL, Goetzl EJ (1984) Elevated concentrations of leukotriene D4 in pulmonary edema fluid of patients with the adult respiratory distress syndrome. J Clin Immunol 4:479-483
10. Ratnoff WD, Matthay MA, Wong MYS (1988) Sulfidopeptide-leukotriene peptidases in pulmonary edema fluid from patients with the adult respiratory distress syndrome. J Clin Immunol 8:250-258

11. Cohen AB, Stevens MD, Miller EJ (1993) Neutrophil-activating peptide-2 in patients with pulmonary edema from congestive heart failure or ARDS. Am J Physiol 264:L490-L495
12. Gee MH, Williams DO (1979) Effect of lung inflation on perivascular cell fluid volume in isolated dog lung lobes. Microvasc Res 19:209-216
13. Bachofen H, Weibel ER (1977) Alterations of the gas exchange apparatus in adult respiratory insufficiency associated with septicemia. Am Rev Respir Dis 116:589-615
14. Matthay MA, Berthiaume Y, Staub NC (1985) Long-term clearance of liquid and protein from the lungs of unanesthetized sheep. J Appl Physiol 59:928-934
15. Berthiaume Y, Broaddus VC, Gropper MA et al (1988) Alveolar liquid and protein clearance from normal dog lungs. J Appl Physiol 65:585-593
16. Matthay MA (1985) Resolution on pulmonary edema: mechanisms of liquid, protein, and cellular clearance from the lung. Clin Chest Med 6:521-545
17. Mason RJ, William MC, Widdicombe JH (1982) Transepithelial transport by pulmonary alveolar type II cells in primary culture. Proc Natl Acad Sci U S A 79:6033-6037
18. Goodman BE, Fleischer RS, Crandall ED (1983) Evidence for active sodium transport by cultured monolayers of pulmonary alveolar epithelial cells. Am J Physiol 245:C79-C83
19. Matalon S (1991) Mechanisms and regulation of ion transport in adult mammalian alveolar type II pneumocytes. Am J Physiol 261:C1-C12
20. Saumon G, Basset G (1993) Electrolyte and fluid transport across the mature alveolar epithelium. J Appl Physiol 74:1-15
21. Verkman AS (1992) Water channels in cell membranes. Annu Rev Physiol 54:97-108
22. Folkesson HG, Matthay MA, Hasegawa H (1994) Transcellular water transport in lung alveolar epithelium through mercurial-sensitive water channels. Proc Natl Acad Sci U S A 91:4970-4974
23. Hasegawa H, Ma T, Skach W (1994) Molecular cloning of a mercurial-insensitive water channel expressed in selected water transporting epithelia. J Biol Chem 269:5497-5500
24. Berthiaume Y, Albertine KH, Grady M (1989) Protein clearance from the air spaces and lungs of unanesthestized sheep over 144 h. J Appl Physiol 67:1887-1897
25. Hastings RH, Grady M, Sakuma T, Matthay MA (1992) Clearance of different-sized proteins from the alveolar space in humans and rabbits. J Appl Physiol 73:1310-1316
26. Bachofen M, Weibel ER (1982) Structural alterations of lung parenchyma in the adult respiratory distress syndrome. Clin Chest Med 3:35-56
27. Wortel CH, Doerschut CM (1993) Neutrophil and neutrophil-endothelial cell adhesion in adult respiratory distress syndrome. New Horiz 1:631-637
28. Ognibene FC, Martin SE, Parker MM (1986) Adult respiratory distress syndrome in patients with severe neutropenia. N Engl J Med 315:547-551
29. Schnapp LM, Chin DP, Szaflarski N, Matthay MA (1995) Frequency and importance of barotrauma in 100 patients with acute lung injury. Crit Care Med 23:272-278
30. Conhaim RL (1989) Airway level at which edema liquid enters the airspace of isolated dog lungs. J Appl Physiol 67:2234-2242
31. Matthay MA, Folkesson G, Campagna A, Kheradmand F (1993) Alveolar epithelial barrier and acute lung injury. New Horiz 1:613-622
32. Bauer ML, Beckman JS, Bridges RJ (1992) Peroxynitrite inhibits sodium uptake in rat colonic membrane vesicles. Biochim Biophys Acta 1104:87-94
33. Kim KJ, Suh DJ (1993) Asymmetric effects of H_2O_2 on alveolar epithelial barrier properties. Am J Physiol 264:L308-L315
34. Folkesson HG, Matthay MA, Hébert C, Broaddus VC (1995) Acid aspiration-induced lung injury in rabbits is mediated by interleukin-8-dependent mechanism. J Clin Invest 96:107-116
35. Fein A, Grossmann RF, Jones JG (1979) The value of edema fluid protein measurement in patients with pulmonary edema. Am J Med 67:32-39
36. Roselli RJ, Riddle WR (1989) Analysis of non-invasive macromolecular transport measurements in the lung. J Appl Physiol 67:2343-2350
37. Schuster DP (1995) What is acute lung injury? What is ARDS? Chest 107:1721-1726

38. Gluecker T, Capasso P, Schnyder P et al (1999) Clinical and radiologic features of pulmonary edema. Radiographics 19:1507-1531
39. Bachofen H, Schurch S, Weibel ER (1993) Experimental hydrostatic pulmonary edema in rabbit lungs: barrier lesions. Am Rev Respir Dis 147:997-1004
40. Gattinoni L, Pelosi P, Vitale G et al (1991) Body position changes redistribute lung computed-tomographic density in patients with acute respiratory failure. Anesthesiology 74:15-23
41. Winer-Muram HT, Steiner RM, Gurney JW (1998) Ventilator-associated pneumonia in patients with adult respiratory distress syndrome: CT evaluation. Radiology 208:193-199
42. Ell Sr (1991) Neurogenic pulmonary edema. A review of the literature and a perspective. Invest Radiol 26:499-506
43. Fleischner FG (1967) The butterfly pattern of acute pulmonary edema. Am J Cardiol 20: 39-46
44. Effros RM (1985) Lung water measurements with the mean transit time approach. J Appl Physiol 59:673-683
45. Turnage RH, LaNoue JL, Kadesky KM et al (1997) Thromboxane A_2 mediates increased pulmonary microvascular permeability after intestinal reperfusion. J Appl Physiol 82:592-598
46. Demling RH, Smith M, Gunther R et al (1981) Pulmonary injury and prostaglandin production during endotoxemia in conscious sheep. Am J Physiol Heart Circ Physiol 240:H348-H353
47. Barnard, JW, Ward RA, Adkins WK, Taylor AE (1992) Characterization of thromboxane and prostacyclin effects on pulmonary circulation. J Appl Physiol 72:1845-1853
48. Misselwitz B, Brautigam M (1996) A comparative study of the effects of iloprost and PGE_1 on pulmonary arterial pressure and edema formation in the isolated perfused rat lung model. Prostaglandins 51:179-190
49. Williams TJ (1979) Prostaglandin E_2, prostaglandin I_2 and the vascular changes of inflammation. Br J Pharmacol 65:517-524
50. Williams TJ, Jose PJ, Wedmore CV et al (1983) Mechanisms underlying inflammatory edema: the importance of synergism between prostaglandins, leukotrienes and complement-derived peptides. Adv Prostaglandin Thromboxane Leukot Res 11:33-37
51. Wright JK, Kim LT, Rogers TE, Turnage RH (2000) Prostaglandins potentiate U-46619-induced pulmonary microvascular dysfunction. J Appl Physiol 88:1167-1174
52. Ward PA, Till GO, Kunkel R, Beauchamp C (1983) Evidence for role of hydroxyl radical in complement and neutrophil-dependent tissue injury. J Clin Invest 72:789-801
53. Hyslop PA, Hinshaw DB, Halsey WA Jr et al (1988) Mechanisms of oxidant-mediated cell injury. J Biol Chem 263:1665-1675
54. Chollet-Martin S, Montravers P, Gibert C et al (1992) Subpopulation of hyperresponsive polymorphonuclear neutrophils in patients with adult respiratory distress syndrome. Am Rev Respir Dis 145:990-996
55. Minnear FL, DeMichele MAA, Leonhardt S et al (1993) Isoproterenol antagonizes endothelial permeability induced by thrombin and thrombin receptor peptide. J Appl Physiol 75: 1171-1179
56. Waypa GB, Morton CA, Vincent PA et al (2000) Oxidant-increased endothelial permeability: prevention with phosphodiesterase inhibition vs. cAMP production. J Appl Physiol 88:835-842
57. Olver RE, Ramsden CA, Strang LB, Walters V (1986) The role of amiloride-blockable sodium transport in the adrenaline-induced lung liquid absorption in the fetal lamb. J Physiol 376:321-340
58. Sakuma T, Okaniwa G, Nakada T (1994) Alveolar fluid clearance in the resected human lung. Am J Respir Crit Care Med 150:305-310
59. Matthay MA (1994) The function of the alveolar epithelial barrier under pathological conditions. Chest 105:67S-74S
60. Minnear FL, Johnson A, Malik AB (1986) Adrenergic modulation of pulmonary transvascular fluid and protein exchange. J Appl Physiol 60:266-274
61. Bell RC, Coalson J, Smith JD, Johanson WG (1983) Multiple organ failure and infection in adult respiratory distress syndrome. Ann Intern Med 99:293-298

62. Patel P, Drummond J, Cole D et al (1998) Isoflurane and pentobarbital reduce the frequency of transient ischemic depolarizations during focal ischemia in rats. Anesth Analg 86:773-780
63. Mitsuhata H, Shimizu R, Yokoyama M (1995) Suppressive effects of volatile anesthetics on cytokine release in human peripheral blood mononuclear cells. Int J Immunopharmacol 17: 529-534
64. Liu R, Ishibe Y, Ueda M (2000) Isoflurane-sevoflurane administration before ischemia attenuates ischemia-reperfusion-induced injury in isolated rat lungs. Anesthesiology 92:833-840
65. Chung KF (1992) Platelet-activating factor in inflammation and pulmonary disorders. Clin Sci 83:127-138
66. Charous B, Halpern B, Steven G (1998) Hydroxychloroquine improves airflow and lower circulating IgE levels in subjects with moderate symptomatic asthma. J Allergy Clin Immunol 102:198-203
67. Falk S, Göggel R, Heydasch U et al (1999) Quinolines attenuate PAF-induced pulmonary pressor responses and edema formation. Am J Respir Crit Care Med 160:1734-1742

Local and Systemic Effects of Hypercapnia

G. SERVILLO, E. DE ROBERTIS, M. COPPOLA, R. TUFANO

In intensive care acute hypercapnia is mainly encountered in acute respiratory failure, in cardiorespiratory arrest, and during mechanical ventilation. In the latter circumstance, it can be non-intentional (ventilator malfunction, extreme derangement of lung mechanics) or intentional (permissive hypercapnia).

In acute respiratory failure, the most-severe hypercapnia is observed in suddenasphyctic asthma, often characterized by an initial $paCO_2$ above 100 mmHg and an arterial pH close to 7.0 [1, 2]. If treatment is promptly established, resolution of airway obstruction is generally fast, with normocapnia usually regained in hours. In such conditions the transient severe respiratory acidosis is well tolerated and survival common. In cardiorespiratory arrest, it is impossible to evaluate the tolerance to hypercapnia because of the associated anoxia.

Permissive hypercapnia, or controlled mechanical hypoventilation, is a strategy for the management of patients requiring mechanical ventilation, in which priority is given to the prevention or limitation of severe pulmonary hyperinflation over the maintenance of normal alveolar ventilation.

Few studies of the clinical application of permissive hypercapnia are available. Permissive hypercapnia was first described in 1984 in patients ventilated for asthma [3]. In these patients a reduction of complications induced by mechanical ventilation and a decrease in mortality were observed. Such results have been subsequently confirmed. Today the use of hypercapnic hypoventilation during asthma is well accepted. In 1990 a retrospective non-controlled study of ventilated patients with acute respiratory distress syndrome showed that in patients ventilated with a peak pressure of 40 cm H_2O, a mild hypercapnia (40-70 mmHg) was well tolerated; in some cases it was higher than 100 mmHg and reached 140 mmHg [4]. The mortality, calculated by three different prognostic indexes, was less than expected. Other prospective studies, although not randomized have confirmed these interesting results on mortality. More recently a few randomized studies have been published on the effects of a protective ventilatory strategy based on reduced tidal volumes. However, their conclusions are not univocal and are difficult to interpret.

But what are the effects of hypercapnia? The most-important effects of hypercapnia on the function of any organ result from a complex interplay between local effects of CO_2 on proton concentration and effects mediated by the activation of the sympathoadrenergic system [5, 6]; the latter are subject to important interspecies variation, and are heavily influenced by anesthesia. However, the bulk of investigation in this field has been performed on isolated preparations and anesthetized animals, with relatively few studies performed in humans. Therefore, extrapolation of most experimental results to the clinical situation must be done with extreme caution. Acute hypercapnia has a myriad of effects, affecting almost any physiological function. In the following, we shall focus on effects of potential significance to the intensivist.

Effects of hypercapnia on the cell

Because of the free diffusibility of CO_2 across cell membranes, a sudden increase in extracellular pCO_2 will decrease the intracellular pH (pHi). Due to the abundance of carbonic anhydrase in the cytosol, intracellular acidosis occurs rapidly [7]. The latter is responsible for most of the effects of hypercapnia. However, several immediate or late compensatory mechanisms are able to partly compensate for the variations in pHi in the presence of severe hypercapnia. In fact, a reduction of pHi (6.9-7.2) does not modify the energetic cellular state. A severe acidosis may have a protective effect on the hypoxic cell. Finally, acidosis inhibits the activity of contractile elements and deregulates the electric properties of excitable cells.

Effects of hypercapnia on the cardiocirculatory system

Hypercapnia induces an acute deterioration of ventricular performance. The myocardial response to acute respiratory acidosis is mainly characterized by an impairment in contractility that is entirely reversible [8]. The principal mechanism responsible for the fall in cardiac contractile force is explained by a rapid diffusion of CO_2 into cells with consequent intracellular acidosis, which interferes with myofilament responsiveness to calcium [9].

CO_2 is a potent coronary vasodilator, and hypercapnia produces a substantial increase in coronary flow, together with a rise in coronary sinus pO_2 [10], independent of myocardial oxygen consumption [11]. Response to CO_2 is likely to be different in the presence of heart failure or diminished coronary reserve.

The hemodynamic response to hypercapnia is characterized by an increase in cardiac output, heart rate, and stroke volume, and a decrease in systemic vascular resistance [12, 13]. This response represents the balance between the depressant effects of CO_2 on mechanical performance and its indirect effects on peripheral chemoreceptors and vasomotor centers, which improve both sympathetic nervous activity and catecholamine secretion. On the other hand, hypercapnia may adversely affect right ventricular performance in patients with previously impaired right ventricular systolic function. Respiratory acidosis induces pulmonary arteriolar vasoconstriction, thus leading to pulmonary hypertension and an increase of both end-diastolic and end-systolic right ventricular volumes [14]. The hypercapnia produces arrhythmogenic effects, especially ventricular ones, that require further investigation.

Effects of hypercapnia on oxygen delivery

Increased pCO_2 produces a rightward shift of the oxygen dissociation curve, promoting the release of oxygen to the tissues. This effect is related to two mechanisms: the increase in H^+, as CO_2 is hydrated in carbonic acid, and the formation of carbamino compounds from the reaction between CO_2 and n-terminal amino acids of the hemoglobin chains.

The decreased affinity of hemoglobin for oxygen may compromise the O_2 loading in alveolar capillaries, an effect of minimal significance when pO_2 is in the normal range, but dramatic in the presence of pulmonary disease and hypoxemia [15].

Effects of hypercapnia on the central nervous system

Hypercapnia acts on the central nervous system by reducing intracellular and extracellular pH; the effects on the oxygen consumption of the brain are controversial even if the available studies suggest that the oxygen demand of the brain does not change or even decreases under hypercapnic conditions [16-18].

In normal subjects hypercapnia increases the cerebral blood flow [19, 20]; this effect is partly mediated by the concomitant arterial hypertension, which increases cerebral perfusion pressure, and in part by cerebral vasodilatation, which reduces cerebral vascular resistance.

Hypercapnia reversibly increases intracranial pressure because of the enlargement of cerebral blood volume secondary to the diminished vascular tone in the face of maintained or raised vascular pressure [21, 22].

Theoretically the CO_2 has anesthetic properties on the basis of its lipid solubility, but anesthesia by CO_2 alone requires a much higher partial pressure (> 200 mmHg) [23]; in addition to being an anesthetic, CO_2 also has stimulant properties on the central nervous system, the best-known being the stimulation of respiratory drive, which becomes maximal for pCO_2 in the range of 100-150 mmHg [5].

Other effects of hypercapnia

Acute hypercapnia reduces the contractility and the endurance of skeletal muscle, in particular that of diaphragm [24, 25]; it would be interesting to know how fast the respiratory muscles recover their strength and endurance upon return to normocapnia after hypercapnic exposure of a few hours or a few days, to understand whether weaning from the ventilator will be difficult.

Normoxemic hypercapnia increases the secretion of epinephrine, norepinephrine, adrenocorticotropic hormone, cortisol, aldosterone and antidiuretic hormone [5, 6, 26, 27].

The inhalation of up to 10% CO_2 has no effect on airway resistance but probably reduces the expiratory flow because it causes laryngeal narrowing [28].

Hypercapnia has been shown experimentally to increase sodium and chloride absorption in the gut [29], but whether it increases the risk of acute gastrointestinal bleeding by stimulating gastric secretion of H^+ remains to be established.

The high level of CO_2 in the portal venous blood increases portal resistance and reduces portal flow, whereas slight changes in the opposite direction are noted in the hepatic arterial circulation, with an overall reduction of total hepatic blood flow [30].

Studies on dogs have shown that mild acute normoxic elevations of $paCO_2$ (< 70 mmHg) led to either a moderate fall [31] or a moderate increase of renal vascular resistance, with relatively little impact on renal blood flow and glomerular filtration rate. More-severe acute respiratory acidosis ($paCO_2$ > 100 mmHg) results in more-pronounced renal vasoconstriction with a concomitant fall of renal blood flow, glomerular filtration rate, and possibly urine output [31].

Conclusions

All the recent studies seem to suggest that normocapnia is no longer an endpoint and that hypercapnia is not so detrimental. For instance, some authors are also proposing instead of a permissive hypercapnia a therapeutic hypercapnia [32, 33]. However, effects of changes in $paCO_2$ and pH on organ function, particularly in critically ill patients, are still not clear and more studies and clinical trials are needed.

References

1. Wasserfallen JB, Schaller MD, Feihl F, Perret CH (1990) Sudden asphyxic asthma: a distinct entity? Am Rev Respir Dis 142:108-111
2. Molfino NA, Nannini LJ, Martelli AN, Slutsky AS (1991) Respiratory arrest in near-fatal asthma. N Engl J Med 324:285-288
3. Darioli R, Perret C (1984) Mechanical controlled hypoventilation in status asthmaticus. Am Rev Respir Dis 129:385-387
4. Hickling KG, Henderson SJ, Jackson R (1990) Low mortality associated with low volume pressure limited ventilation with permissive hypercapnia in severe adult respiratory distress syndrome. Intensive Care Med 16:372-377
5. Nunn JF (1987) Applied respiratory physiology. The effects of changes in carbon dioxide tension, 3rd edn. Butterworth, London, pp 460-470
6. Brofman JD, Leff AR, Munoz NM et al (1990) Sympathetic secretory response to hypercapnic acidosis in swine. J Appl Physiol 69:710-717
7. Thomas RC (1984) Experimental displacement of intracellular pH and the mechanism of its subsequent recovery. J Physiol (Lond) 354:3-22
8. Tang WC, Weil MH, Gazmuri RJ et al (1991) Reversible impairment of myocardial contractility due to hypercarbic acidosis in the isolated perfused rat heart. Crit Care Med 19:218-224
9. Orchard C, Kentish J (1990) Effects of changes of pH on the contractile function of cardiac muscle. Am J Physiol 258:C967-C981
10. Case RB, Greenberg H, Moskowitz R (1975) Alterations in coronary sinus PO_2 and O_2 saturation resulting from PCO_2 changes. Cardiovasc Res 9:167-177
11. Wexels JC, Myhre ES (1987) Hypocapnia and hypercapnia in the dog: effects on myocardial blood-flow and haemodynamics during beta- and combined alpha- and beta-adrenoceptor blockade. Clin Physiol 7:21-33
12. Blackburn JP, Conway CM, Leigh JM et al (1972) $PaCO_2$ and the pre-ejection period: the $PaCO_2$/inotropy response curve. Anesthesiology 37:268-276
13. Prys-Roberts C, Kelman GR, Greenbaum R, Robinson RH (1967) Circulatory influences of artificial ventilation during nitrous oxide anaesthesia in man. II. Results: the relative influence of mean intrathoracic pressure and arterial carbon dioxide tension. Br J Anaesth 39:533-548
14. Viitanen A, Salmenperä M, Heinonen J (1990) Right ventricular response to hypercarbia after cardiac surgery. Anesthesiology 73:393-400
15. McLellan TM (1991) The influence of a respiratory acidosis on the exercise blood lactate response. Eur J Appl Physiol 63:6-11
16. Siesjö BK (1980) Cerebral metabolic rate in hypercarbia – a controversy. Anesthesiology 52:461-465
17. Berntman L, Dahlgren N, Siesjö BK (1979) Cerebral blood flow and oxygen consumption in the rat brain during extreme hypercarbia. Anesthesiology 50:299-305
18. Prough DS, Rogers AT, Stump DA et al (1990) Hypercarbia depresses cerebral oxygen consumption during cardiopulmonary bypass. Stroke 21:1162-1166
19. Edvinsson L, McKenzie ET, McCulloch J (1993) Cerebral blood flow and metabolism. Changes in arterial gas tensions. Raven, New York, pp 524-552
20. Miller JD (1987) Cerebral blood flow variations with perfusion pressure and metabolism. In: Wood JH (ed) Cerebral blood flow. Physiologic and clinical aspects. McGraw-Hill, New York, pp 119-130
21. Lanier WL, Weglinski MR (1991) Intracranial pressure. In: Cucchiara RF, Michenfelder JD (eds) Clinical neuroanesthesia. Churchill Livingstone, New York, pp 77-110
22. Miller JD, Sullivan HG (1979) Severe intracranial hypertension. In: Trubuhovich RV (ed) Management of acute intracranial disaster. Little Brown, Boston, pp 19-35
23. Eisele JH, Eger EI, Muallem M (1967) Narcotic properties of carbon dioxide in the dog. Anesthesiology 28:856-865
24. Juan G, Calverley P, Talamo C et al (1984) Effect of carbon dioxide on diaphragmatic function in human beings. N Engl J Med 310:874-879

25. Gomes Vianna L, Koulouris N, Lanigan C, Moxham J (1990) Effect of acute hypercapnia on limb muscle contractility in humans. J Appl Physiol 69:1486-1493
26. Chen HG, Wood CE (1993) The adrenocorticotropic hormone and arginine vaspressin responses to hypercapnia in fetal and maternal sheep. Am J Physiol 264:R324-330
27. Raff H, Roarty TP (1988) Renin, ACTH and aldosterone during acute hypercapnia and hypoxia in conscious rats. Am J Physiol 254:R431-R435
28. Butler J, Caro CG, Alcala R, DuBois AB (1960) Physiological factors affecting airway resistance in normal subjects and in patients with obstructive respiratory disease. J Clin Invest 39:584-591
29. Charney AN, Feldman GM (1984) Systemic acid-base disorders and intestinal electrolyte transport. Am J Physiol 247:G1-G12
30. Gelman S, Ernst EA (1977) Role of pH, PCO_2, and O_2 content of portal blood in hepatic circulatory autoregulation. Am J Physiol 233:E255-E262
31. Bersentes TJ, Simmons DH (1967) Effects of acute acidosis on renal hemodynamics. Am J Physiol 212:633-640
32. Laffey JG, Kavanagh BP (1999) Carbon dioxide and critically ill – too little of a good thing? Lancet 354:1283-1286
33. Laffey JG, Engelberts D, Kavanagh BP (2000) Buffering hypercapnic acidosis worsens acute lung injury. Am J Respir Crit Care Med 161:141-146

Monitoring Respiratory Mechanics by Forced Oscillation in Ventilated Patients

R. FARRÉ

The forced oscillation technique (FOT) is a non-invasive procedure particularly useful for assessing respiratory mechanics during ventilation since application of the method does not require patient co-operation and does not interfere with the normal or artificial ventilation cycle [1, 2]. The technique is based on the application of a small pressure oscillation to the respiratory system and on computing patient mechanics from the pressure and flow signals recorded at the airway opening. In conventional FOT measurements the oscillation pressure is applied at a frequency greater than the ventilation rate of the patient. The basic assumption of FOT is that the pressure component generated by the patient's breathing muscles at the forced oscillation frequency is negligible. Accordingly, respiratory mechanics may be assessed by simply measuring pressure and flow at the airway opening regardless of the fact that the patient is breathing spontaneously or with ventilatory support.

The FOT is, therefore, applicable to monitoring respiratory mechanics in patients subjected to artificial ventilation [3-5]. Indeed, in contrast to the conventional occlusion techniques, FOT does not require patient paralysis or interfering with the ventilator pattern to perform particular manoeuvres. Consequently, FOT is also applicable during non-invasive ventilatory support and during the process of weaning [6]. As a result of the methodological advances in the last years, FOT may be easily applied for monitoring the respiratory mechanics of the patient in the clinical setting of mechanical ventilation.

Forced oscillation set-up

Figure 1 is a diagram of the setup to apply FOT during artificial ventilation through a conventional interface (endotracheal tube or mask). Although this figure shows a ventilator with inspiratory and expiratory lines, which is the most usual type in invasive ventilation, FOT may also be applied when using a kind of ventilator that includes only one tubing and an exhalation port. The only change in the conventional ventilation setup required by FOT is the connection of a forced oscillation generator between the ventilator and the patient (Fig. 1).

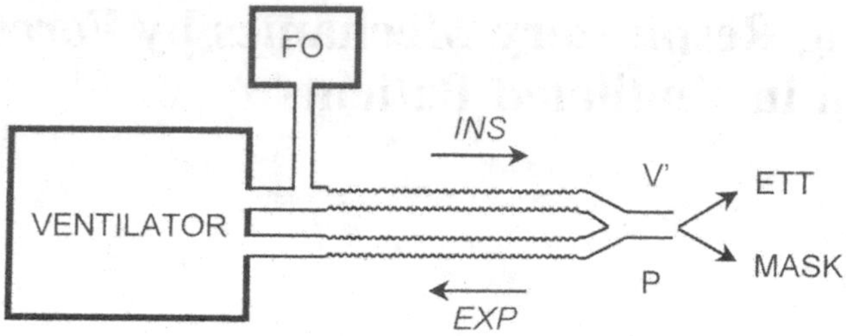

Fig. 1. Diagram of the conventional setting to monitor respiratory mechanics by the forced oscillation technique during mechanical ventilation. FO: forced oscillation generator; INS: inspiration; EXP: expiration; ETT: endotracheal tube; P, V′: pressure and flow recorded at the airway opening, respectively

This FOT generator is an oscillating pump capable of superimposing a low-pressure oscillation (typically 2 cm H_2O peak-to-peak) onto the pressure wave generated by the mechanical ventilator. As the oscillation pressure is applied during the normal cycling of the ventilator, the ventilation mode is not modified by FOT measurements.

The FOT generator should be able to withstand the inspiratory high pressure at the airway opening. This may be achieved by enclosing the rear part of a loudspeaker in a small chamber [3], by servocontrolling a loudspeaker [7] or by using a device that simultaneously generates the pressure applied to the patient and the oscillation pressure [8]. Pressure and flow are measured at the airway opening by means of a pressure transducer and a pneumotachograph plus a differential pressure transducer, respectively. These signals are analogically low-pass filtered, sampled and analysed in a microcomputer. To accurately measure pressure and flow, the frequency response of the transducers and of the pneumotachograph [9] and its common-mode rejection ratio should be calibrated and adequately compensated [10, 11]. To avoid artefacts due to the non-linear resistance of the endotracheal tube, pressure may be recorded at the trachea with a special tube [12] or by a catheter [4]. Another possibility to overcome the tube non-linearity is to digitally compensate for the influence of the tube by means of a calibration procedure [3]. Application of FOT through a mask is particularly sensitive to air leaks owing to inadequate mask fitting [6, 13, 14].

Figure 2 shows an cxample of the pressure and flow signals recorded at the airway opening when a sinusoidal forced oscillation at a frequency of 5 Hz was applied through a face mask during non-invasive pressure-support ventilation (Servo 300, Siemens) in a patient with a severe chronic obstructive pulmonary disease (COPD). The figure illustrates that the low amplitude oscillation pressure and the induced oscillatory flow were superimposed onto the ventilator waveforms. Figure 2 also illustrates that the application of FOT does not interfere with the normal ventilation cycle.

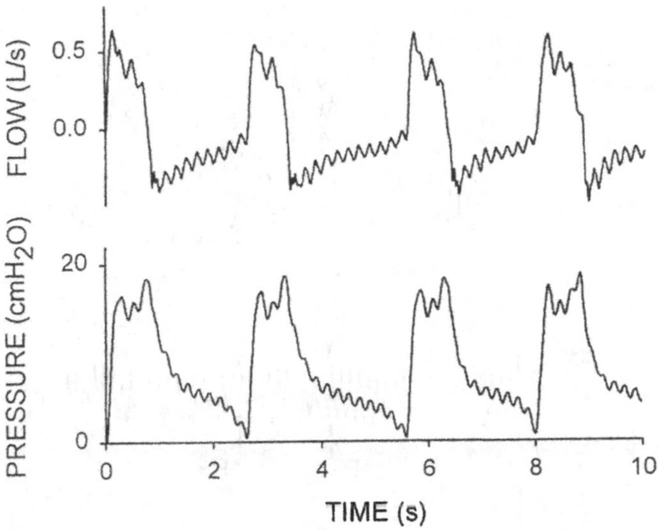

Fig. 2. Flow and pressure signals recorded at the mask during a forced oscillation measurement at 5 Hz carried out during non-invasive pressure-support ventilation in a patient with a chronic obstructive pulmonary disease

Oscillatory impedance, resistance and reactance

Assessment of respiratory system mechanics by FOT requires the processing of the pressure and flow signals recorded at the airway opening (Fig. 2). As shown by the example in Figure 3, the recorded signals provide direct and intuitive information about the magnitude of the mechanical load of the patient's respiratory system. This figure shows the flow and pressure signals recorded at the nasal mask in a patient with the obstructive sleep apnea/hypopnea syndrome subjected to a continuous positive airway pressure (CPAP) during sleep. As indicated by the abnormal inspiratory flow contour the value of CPAP applied was not able to avoid inspiratory flow limitation. The 5 Hz oscillatory flow exhibited an amplitude that greatly changed along the breathing cycle, being smaller during inspiration ($\Delta V'_1$) than during expiration ($\Delta V'_2$). This change in oscillatory flow amplitude contrasts with the fact that the oscillatory pressure applied was slightly higher during inspiration (ΔP_1) than during expiration (ΔP_2). The quotient between the amplitude of oscillatory pressure (ΔP) and the amplitude of oscillatory flow ($\Delta V'$) is defined as the amplitude of oscillatory impedance ($|Z_{rs}| = \Delta P/\Delta V'$) and is an index to quantify the total mechanical load of the patient's respiratory system at the oscillation frequency. Indeed, the higher $|Z_{rs}|$, the greater the pressure amplitude (ΔP) required to induce a given flow ($\Delta V'$). In the example of Figure 3, the amplitude of impedance computed along the breathing cycle is shown in the bottom panel. $|Z_{rs}|$ shows high values due to upper airway

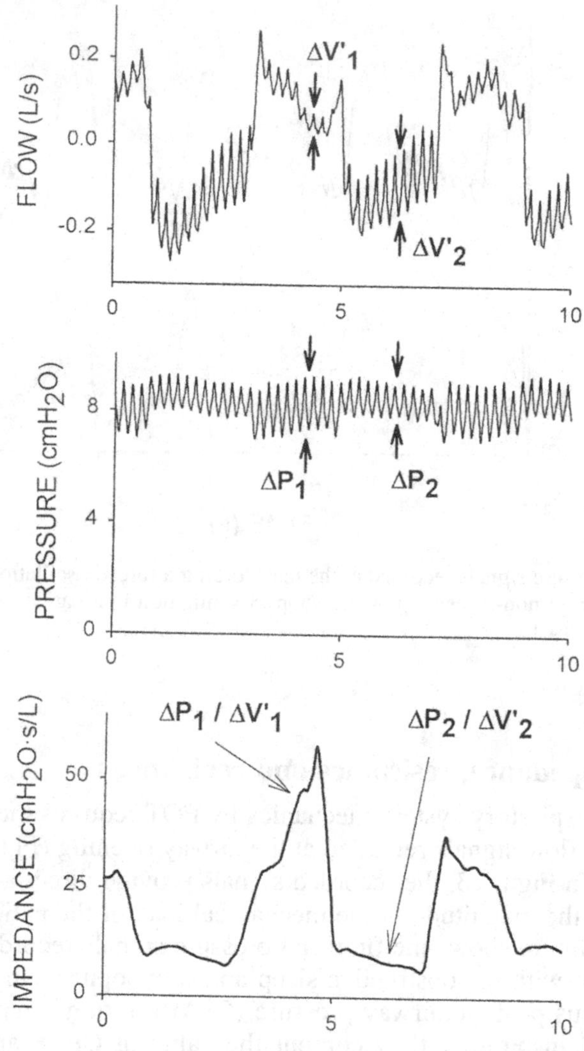

Fig. 3. Flow (positive during inspiration) and pressure signals recorded at the mask and amplitude of respiratory impedance computed in a patient with the obstructive sleep apnea/hypopnea syndrome. FOT was applied at 5 Hz during sleep when the patient was subjected to suboptimal CPAP. ΔP_1 and ΔP_2 are the amplitudes of oscillation pressure at two instants during inspiration and expiration, respectively. $\Delta V'_1$ and $\Delta V'_2$ are the amplitudes of the corresponding oscillatory flow. Impedance amplitude is computed as the ratio between the amplitudes of oscillatory pressure and flow along the breathing cycle

obstruction during inspirations and low impedance values during normal expirations. A more detailed analysis of these oscillatory pressure and flow signals would show that the pressure and flow FOT components did not oscillate in phase and that the relative phase angle (ϕ_{rs}) also showed a phasic pattern. The pair of values $|Z_{rs}|$ and ϕ_{rs} completely characterises the mechanical properties of the respiratory system at the frequency of oscillation. The value of ϕ_{rs} depends on the balance between the different kinds of mechanical properties (resistive, elastic, inertial) determining the mechanics of the respiratory system.

Although $|Z_{rs}|$, and to a lesser extent ϕ_{rs}, are very intuitive indices of the mechanical load of the patient, the oscillatory impedance may also be characterised by an equivalent representation in terms of the oscillatory pressure component in phase with flow and in terms of the oscillatory pressure component in phase with volume. This representation consists of computing the effective resistance (R_{rs}; $R_{rs} = |Z_{rs}| \cdot \cos(\phi_{rs})$) and reactance ($X_{rs}$; $X_{rs} = |Z_{rs}| \cdot \sin(\phi_{rs})$) of the respiratory system. The characterisation of oscillatory impedance by the pair of values $|Z_{rs}|$ and ϕ_{rs} or by the pair R_{rs} and X_{rs} is equivalent: $|Z_{rs}| = (R_{rs}^2 + X_{rs}^2)^{1/2}$ and $\phi_{rs} = \tan^{-1}(X_{rs}/R_{rs})$. The representation of oscillatory mechanics in terms of R_{rs} and X_{rs} is particularly useful when the respiratory system is interpreted with a mechanistic model. For instance, if the respiratory system is modelled by a resistance (R), an inertance (I) and an elastance (E), it can be shown [1] that $R_{rs} = R$ and that $X_{rs} = 2\pi \cdot f \cdot I - E/(2\pi \cdot f)$. Therefore, when applied to a simple R-I-E model, the FOT results in a R_{rs} which does not depend on frequency and in a frequency dependent X_{rs}. The reactance component associated with E is negative and inversely increases with frequency. By contrast, the reactance component associated with I is positive and increases linearly with frequency. Consequently, reactance is mainly determined by elastance E at low frequencies and by inertance I at high frequencies.

Monitoring respiratory mechanics in ventilated patients

The FOT provides a time resolution high enough to track the changes of respiratory mechanics along the breathing cycle [15-17]. Figure 4 shows the data obtained in a patient with severe COPD subjected to non-invasive ventilation with CPAP through a face mask at the resolution phase of an exacerbation of the disease. The figure shows the flow signal after applying a low-pass filter to eliminate the 5 Hz oscillatory component during the FOT measurement. Patient impedance exhibited a marked phasic pattern with the breathing cycle: impedance amplitude was considerably high during expiration. This increase in expiratory impedance was attributed to the expiratory flow limitation phenomena characterising severe COPD [3]. A more detailed analysis of the impedance changes in terms of its resistance (R_{rs}) and reactance (X_{rs}) components (Fig. 4) showed a periodic R_{rs} pattern with higher values during expiration than inspiration. Moreover, X_{rs} exhibited very negative values during expiration and was almost nil

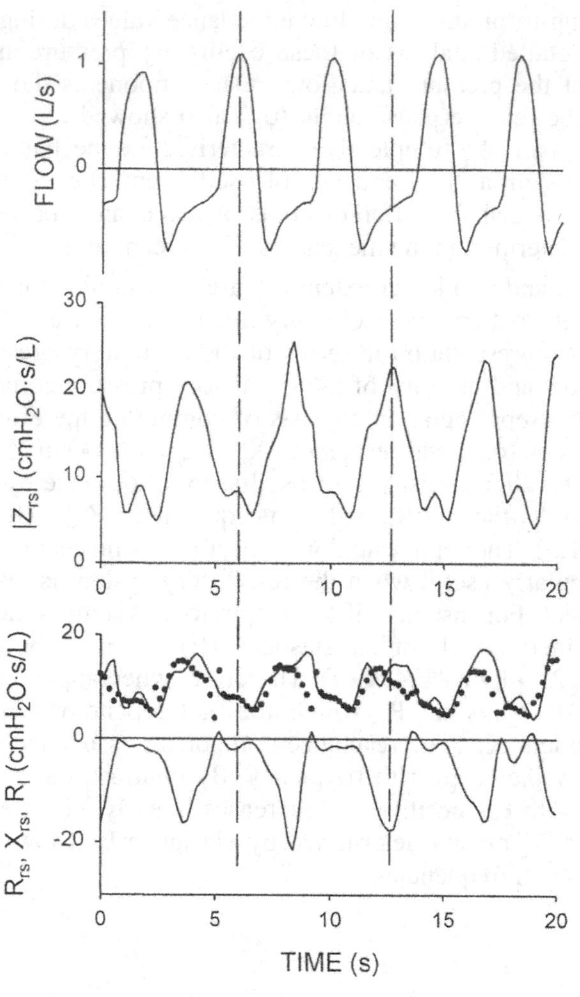

Fig. 4. FOT results obtained during non-invasive CPAP application in a patient with severe COPD. *Top*: The 5 Hz oscillatory component in the flow signal (positive during inspiration) shown in the figure was eliminated by digital filtering. *Center*: Patient impedance ($|Z_{rs}|$) was markedly increased during expiration. *Bottom*: R_{rs} and X_{rs} showed the same phasic pattern as $|Z_{rs}|$. Lung resistance (R_l) simultaneously computed by means of an oesophageal balloon is also shown (•)

during inspiration. This marked decrease in reactance has been interpreted in terms of the bronchial wall movement during expiratory flow limitation [3, 18, 19]. As illustrated in the figure, the values of R_{rs} measured by FOT were well correlated with lung resistance computed by means of the conventional oesophageal balloon technique [17]. It is worth noting that R_{rs} and X_{rs} were monitored in a non-invasive way from only recording pressure and flow at the airway opening.

Besides performing a detailed tracking of respiratory mechanics during the breathing cycle (Fig. 4), the FOT may be also applied to obtain a mean index of respiratory resistance and reactance over the whole breathing cycle in order to assess the degree and evolution of a patient's respiratory mechanics [20, 21]. Figure 5 shows an illustrative example corresponding to a patient with severe COPD. In this figure both R_{rs} and X_{rs} correspond to the mean values over the whole breathing cycle. When the patient was in sitting position in the base line (CPAP = 0), R_{rs} and X_{rs} were higher and more negative, respectively, than the normal values corresponding to a healthy subject. The degree of respiratory obstruction is also reflected by the relatively high oesophageal pressure swings (about 15 cm H_2O • s/L) simultaneously recorded in the patient. When the patient changed to supine at the same CPAP = 0, R_{rs} increased by about 50% and X_{rs} was about 100% more negative, indicating a marked increase in the mechanical load of the patient. This increase in the respiratory mechanics indices, which could be attributed to enhanced expiratory flow limitation in supine, is also reflected by the fact that the amplitude of oesophageal pressure swings increased by about 100%. When the supine patient was subjected to a CPAP value of 12 cm H_2O, respiratory impedance (and oesophageal pressure effort) consid-

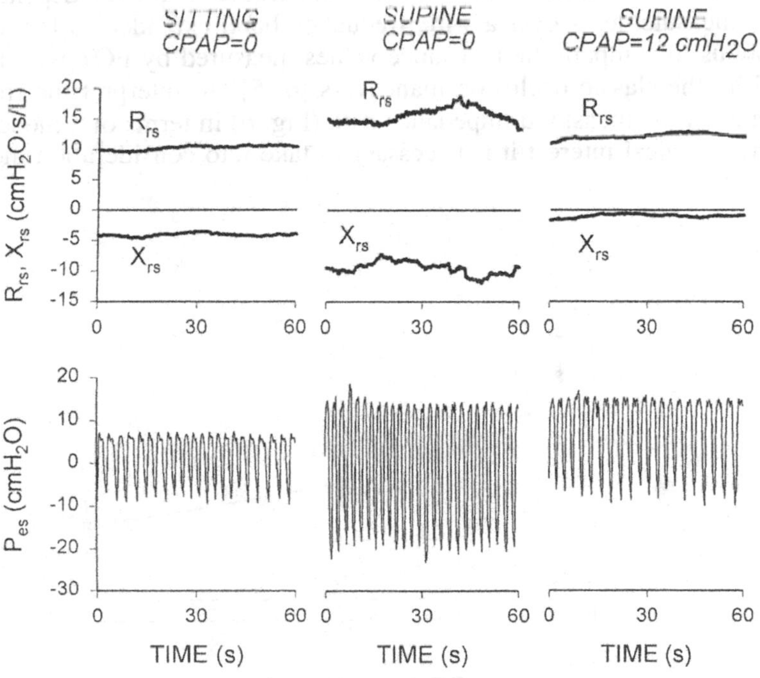

Fig. 5. Respiratory resistance (R_{rs}) and reactance (X_{rs}) measured by FOT (5 Hz) in a COPD patient at CPAP = 0 in sitting (left) and in supine (center) and in supine at CPAP = 12 cm H_2O (right). Inspiratory effort is illustrated by the swings of the oesophageal pressure simultaneously recorded in the patient (P_{es}, bottom)

erably improved (Fig. 5). This simple example suggests how FOT may be a simple and non-invasive tool for assessing respiratory mechanics and for providing information to optimise the artificial ventilatory support.

The two previous examples in Figures 4 and 5 correspond to the most simplified version of the FOT consisting of applying a sinusoidal oscillation. However, FOT may also be used to simultaneously explore R_{rs} and X_{rs} at several frequencies. To this end, the sinusoidal oscillation is replaced by a more complex signal containing all the frequencies to be assessed. However, the reliability of the measured impedance values can be reduced because the signal-to-noise ratio at each frequency component is decreased when compared with sinusoidal oscillation. This reduction in the signal-to-noise ratio is due to the fact that the peak-to-peak amplitude of the FOT signal should be kept within a range (± 1 cm H_2O • s/L) so as to ensure linearity. Figure 6 corresponds to a particular application of multifrequency FOT measurements in mechanically ventilated and paralysed patients from the typical values of breathing frequencies (about 0.25 Hz) to higher frequencies. This figure illustrates that intubated and mechanically ventilated patients due to an exacerbation of COPD [4] show resistance values much higher than intubated and mechanically ventilated patients with a healthy respiratory system [22]. Moreover, Figure 6 also indicates that, in contrast to healthy subjects, the COPD patients exhibited a considerable frequency dependence of R_{rs}. FOT measurements over a wide frequency band extended to low frequencies allow us to compare the resistance values measured by FOT with the ones obtained by the classic occlusion maneuvers [4, 5]. To interpret the frequency dependence of the measured impedance data (Fig. 6) in terms of a model with a patho-physiological interest it is necessary to take into consideration the differ-

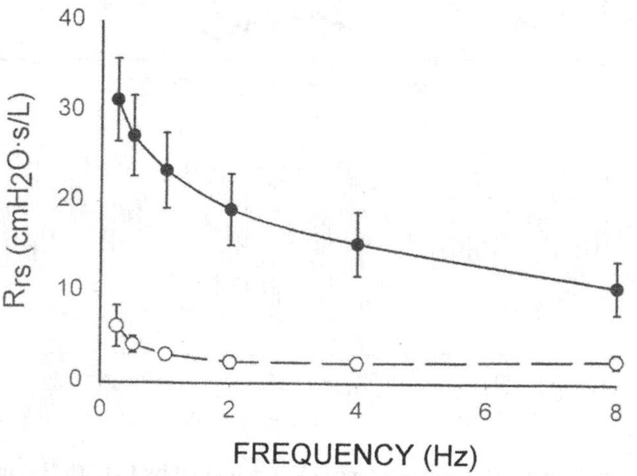

Fig. 6. Respiratory resistance (R_{rs}) between 0.25 and 8 Hz measured by FOT in intubated and paralyzed COPD patients (•) and healthy subjets (∘). FOT measurements were carried out at an expiratory pause during mechanical ventilation. Data are mean ± SD

ent mechanisms that determine the behaviour of the respiratory system: serial and/or parallel inhomogeneities [23] and viscoelasticity of respiratory tissues [3, 4]. As the influence of these mechanisms varies with frequency, the frequency band explored may be modified depending on the patho-physiological aim of the measurement. Accordingly, low frequencies are most suitable for studying tissue properties while high frequency measurements provide more sensitive data of the airway characteristics.

In conclusion, FOT allows an easy assessment of respiratory mechanics during non-invasive and invasive mechanical ventilation both in spontaneously breathing and in paralysed patients. The time and frequency dependence of respiratory impedance reflect the interaction of the elastic, resistive and inertial properties of the whole respiratory system and may be interpreted in terms of models with a patho-physiological interest. The FOT may be a useful tool for monitoring the status and evolution of respiratory mechanics in the ventilated patient and could be helpful in optimising the ventilator settings and the weaning process.

References

1. Navajas D, Farré R (1999) Oscillation mechanics. In: Milic-Emil J (ed) Respiratory mechanics. European Respiratory Monograph, vol 4, Monograph 12:112-140
2. Van de Woestijne K (1993) The forced oscillation technique in intubated, mechanically-ventilated patients (ed). Eur Respir J 6:767-769
3. Peslin R, Felicio-da SJ, Duvivier C, Chabot F (1993) Respiratory mechanics studied by forced oscillations during artificial ventilation. Eur Respir J 6:772-784
4. Farré R, Ferrer M, Rotger M et al (1998) Respiratory mechanics in ventilated COPD patients: forced oscillation versus occlusion techniques. Eur Respir J 12:170-176
5. Beydon L, Malassiné P, Lorino AM et al (1996) Respiratory resistance by end-inspiratory occlusion and forced oscillations in intubated patients. J Appl Physiol 80:1105-1111
6. Farré R, Gavela E, Rotger M et al (2000) Noninvasive assessment of respiratory resistance in severe chronic respiratory patients with nasal CPAP. Eur Respir J 15:314-319
7. Farré R, Ferrer M, Rotger M, Navajas D (1995) Servocontrolled generator to measure respiratory impedance from 0.25 to 26 Hz in ventilated patients at different PEEP levels. Eur Respir J 8:1222-1227
8. Farré R, Rotger M, Montserrat JM, Navajas D (1997) A system to generate simultaneous forced oscillation and continuous positive airway pressure. Eur Respir J 10:1349-1353
9. Delavault E, Saumon G, Georges R (1980) Identification of transducer defect in respiratory impedance measurements by forced random noise. Correction of experimental data. Resp Physiol 40:107-117
10. Peslin R, Jardin P, Duvivier C, Begin P (1984) In-phase rejection requirements for measuring respiratory input impedance. J Appl Physiol 56:804-809
11. Farré R, Navajas D, Peslin R et al (1989) A correction procedure for the asymmetry of differential pressure transducers in respiratory impedance measurements. IEEE Trans Biomed Eng 36:1137-1140
12. Navajas D, Farré R, Rotger M, Canet J (1989) Recording pressure at the distal end of the endotracheal tube to measure respiratory impedance. Eur Respir J 2:178-184
13. Farré R, Peslin R, Rotger M, Navajas D (1997) Inspiratory dynamic obstruction detected by forced oscillation during CPAP. Am J Respir Crit Care Med 155:952-956

14. Badia JR, Farré R, Kimoff J et al (1999) Clinical application of the forced oscillation technique for CPAP titration in the sleep apnea/hypopnea syndrome. Am J Respir Crit Care Med 160:1550-1554
15. Cauberghs M, Van-de-Woestijne K (1992) Changes of respiratory input impedance during breathing in humans. J Appl Physiol 73:2355-2362
16. Peslin R, Ying Y, Gallina C, Duvivier C (1992) Within-breath variations of forced oscillation resistance in healthy subjects. Eur Respir J 5:86-92
17. Farré R, Peslin R, Rotger M et al (1999) Forced oscillation total respiratory resistance and spontaneous breathing lung resistance in COPD patients. Eur Respir J 14:172-178
18. Vassiliou M, Peslin R, Saunier C, Duvivier C (1996) Expiratory flow limitation during mechanical ventilation detected by forced oscillation method. Eur Respir J 9:779-786
19. Peslin R, Farré R, Rotger M, Navajas D (1996) Effect of expiratory flow limitation on respiratory mechanical impedance: a model study. J Appl Physiol 81:2399-2406
20. Ducharme FM, Davis GM (1997) Measurement of respiratory resistance in the emergency department: feasibility in young children with acute asthma. Chest 111:1519-1525
21. Ducharme FM, Davis GM (1998) Respiratory resistance in the emergency department: a reproducible and responsive measure of asthma severity. Chest 113:1566-1572
22. Navajas D, Farré R, Canet J et al (1990) Respiratory input impedance in anesthetized paralyzed patients. J Appl Physiol 69:1372-1379
23. Similowski T, Bates JHT (1991) Two-compartment modelling of respiratory system mechanics: gas redistribution or tissue rheology. Eur Respir J 4:353-358

Optimizing Patient Interface with Ventilation

A. JUBRAN

The primary goal of mechanical ventilation is to rest a patient's respiratory muscles. Unfortunately, many physicians assume that the mere act of connecting a patient to a ventilator will rest his muscles. In fact, with inappropriate settings the patient's work of breathing may be greater than if he was taken off the ventilator.

The importance of providing sufficient respiratory muscle rest is highlighted in a study in healthy subjects in which twitch transdiaphragmatic pressure was measured by stimulating their phrenic nerves [1]. Diaphragmatic fatigue was then induced by having them breathe through a resistor to the limits of tolerance. This caused a decrease in their twitch pressures, and importantly, the reduction in twitch pressure was still evident after 24 h. Thus, if, as we suspect is likely, patients develop respiratory muscle fatigue, they are going to require a considerable period of rest to recover. If a muscle receives too much rest, it may develop atrophy. A marked decrease in contractility was noted in three baboons after 11 days of controlled mechanical ventilation [2].

Assisted modes of ventilation

The most-common assisted modes are assist-control ventilation, intermittent mandatory ventilation, and pressure support ventilation. Which of these methods of mechanical ventilation is best designed to achieve the desirable amount of rest? Surprisingly, we have relatively little information on these major clinical questions.

In the assist-control mode, the ventilator delivers a breath either when triggered by the patient's inspiratory effort, or independently if such an effort does not occur within a preselected period of time. The pressure required to achieve the set tidal volume may be provided solely by the machine or in part by the patient. The amount of active work performed by the patient during assist-control ventilation is dependent on trigger sensitivity and inspiratory flow settings. Even when these settings are selected appropriately, patients perform about one-third of the work performed by the ventilator during passive ventilation [3].

With intermittent mandatory ventilation, the patient receives positive pressure breaths from the ventilator at a preset volume and rate, but the patient can also breathe spontaneously between the mandatory breaths. When this mode was first introduced, it was thought to represent a significant advance as it combines some assisted breaths from the ventilator (which should rest the muscles) and it also allows the patient to breathe spontaneously (and so prevent atrophy). However, patients have difficulty in adapting to the intermittent aspect of ventilator assistance, and studies have indicated that inspiratory efforts were similar in the assisted and spontaneous breaths [4]. The reason for this is that with intermittent unloading, the patient's respiratory centers do not know if they are responsible for generating the next breath or if they will receive assistance from the ventilator. Once the respiratory centers begin to fire, they can not be switched off, and the amount of patient work is not different from the spontaneous breaths.

Pressure support ventilation differs from assist control ventilation and intermittent mandatory ventilation in that the physician sets a level of pressure to augment every effort. The patient can alter respiratory frequency, inspiratory time, and tidal volume. There is no flow setting with pressure support, although the initial peak flow rate determines the speed of pressurization and the initial pressure ramp profile. Pressure support is very effective in decreasing the work of breathing, although the degree of inspiratory muscle unloading is variable among patients.

In a study comparing patient effort during assisted modes of ventilation, Leung et al. [5] observed a decrease in pressure-time product as the level of support was increased with intermittent mandatory ventilation and pressure support ventilation. The rate of change in pressure-time product did not differ between the two modes over the entire span of assistance. However, from 0 to 60% of assistance, the decrease in the pressure-time product was significantly greater for pressure support, whereas between 60 and 100% of support, the decrease in pressure-time product is greater with intermittent mandatory ventilation.

The dissimilar pattern of pressure support and intermittent mandatory ventilation can be explained by different effects of these modes on the two elements of pressure-time product/min, namely pressure-time product/breath and frequency. Pressure-time product/breath decreased linearly as intermittent mandatory ventilation was increased, whereas it reached a plateau when pressure support ventilation was increased from 0 to 60%. The dissimilar pattern in pressure-time product is likely due to the need for continued patient effort to ensure flow delivery during pressure support, whereas with intermittent mandatory ventilation, the mandatory breaths deliver a preset tidal volume even when patient effort is minimal or absent. As the level of pressure support ventilation was increased, respiratory frequency decreased linearly. For intermittent mandatory ventilation, there is very little fall in frequency until 80% of maximum support is attained, at which point frequency decreases abruptly. The abrupt decrease in frequency at 80% may have arisen because the mandatory breaths achieved sufficient alveolar ventilation, and the patient did not need to add intervening spontaneous breaths to achieve overall ventilation.

It is extremely common to combine pressure support ventilation with intermittent mandatory ventilation. When pressure support ventilation of 10 cm H_2O was added to a given level of intermittent mandatory ventilation, a marked decrease in inspiratory pressure-time product during the mandatory breaths and a decrease in respiratory drive (dP/dt) during the intervening breaths was observed [5]. These two changes were significantly correlated with each other (r = 0.67). In other words, the addition of pressure support to intermittent mandatory ventilation caused a reduction in respiratory drive during the intervening breaths, which facilitated greater respiratory muscle unloading during the mandatory breaths.

The degree of ventilatory unloading by the ventilator depends on the synchronization between the ventilator-delivered gas flow and the patient's ventilatory demand. Factors that determine patient-ventilator interaction are listed in Table 1. Problems during mechanical ventilation can arise at the time of triggering and with delivery of flow during the inflation phase. Significant problems can also arise at the switchover between mechanical inflation and expiration.

Table 1. Patient-ventilator synchronization

Inspiration
– Triggering
– Flow demand
Expiration
– Inspiration-expiration switchover
– Circuit impedance

Triggering

The actual change in airway pressure with ventilator triggering can be divided into two phases [6]. The trigger phase refers to the time between the onset of patient effort and the onset of flow delivery. The post-trigger phase refers to the time from the onset of flow to the maximum decrease in airway pressure.

Factors that influence the efficacy of triggering attempts include the responsiveness of the machine, patient's inspiratory drive, inspiratory muscle strength, elastic recoil, persistence of expiratory muscle activity, and the time constant (Table 2).

Ventilator responsiveness has significantly improved with the latest generation of ventilators, which exhibit a shorter delay between the onset of the decrease in pressure and the onset of flow delivery. Also, the decrease in pressure necessary for triggering is much less. Responsiveness is even better for flow-

Table 2. Triggering modifying factors

– Responsive machine
– Inspiratory drive
– Inspiratory muscle strength
– Elastic recoil
– Expiratory muscle persistence
– Time constant

triggering than for pressure triggering. However, improvements in machine responsiveness do not necessarily translate into improvements in clinical outcome. In patients during acute respiratory failure, triggering effort was decreased by flow triggering, but the overall effect was rather small, and, in particular, post-triggering effort was similar to that with pressure triggering [7].

In an assisted mode, the patient is dependent on adequate respiratory drive to generate inspiratory efforts that can trigger the ventilator. In ventilator-dependent patients, the magnitude of the patient's respiratory drive, quantified as dP/dt, was a major determinant of the inspiratory work performed after triggering [5]. That is, once the patient has triggered the machine, he does not switch off his respiratory motor output, and the amount of drive at the onset of the triggered breath determines how much, or how little, rest the ventilator is capable of achieving. Likewise, Alberti et al. [8] found that $P_{0.1}$, another measure of respiratory drive at the onset of triggering, was closely related to work breathing in ten patients receiving pressure support.

Patient's respiratory effort, quantitated as pressure-time product, increases as the level of pressure support is decreased from an optimal level of 100%. The pressure-time product, however, during the trigger phase remained constant [5]. This constancy of pressure-time product during triggering probably resulted from different factors becoming operational at different levels of support. At a low level of support, dP/dt is high but triggering time is short, resulting in a large change in pleural pressure over a short time. At a high level of pressure support, drive is low but triggering time is prolonged, resulting in a small change in pleural pressure over a longer period of time.

Failed attempts at triggering occur more frequently than are generally recognized and result in marked dysynchrony between a patient's inspiratory neuronal activity and the action of the machine. Non-triggering efforts constitute as much as 30% of total inspiratory attempts depending on the ventilator mode and the patient's respiratory mechanics. With partial modes of assistance, namely pressure support and intermittent mandatory ventilation, non-triggering progressively increased as the level of ventilatory assistance was increased.

In 11 ventilator-dependent patients, Leung et al. [5] reported that at each ventilator setting, patient effort during non-triggering efforts is higher than that during the triggering phase that opened the inspiratory valve. Also, the breaths preceding the non-triggering efforts have a shorter expiratory time and total respiratory time, and higher tidal volume and dynamic intrinsic positive end expiratory pressure ($PEEP_i$) than did the breaths preceding triggering efforts. These observations indicate that ineffective triggering did not result from a decrease in the magnitude of inspiratory effort, but rather from inspiratory efforts that were premature and insufficient to overcome the elevated elastic recoil pressure associated with dynamic hyperinflation.

Inspiratory flow settings

Many ventilator-supported patients have increased respiratory motor output. If the inspiratory flow setting is insufficient to meet a patient's ventilatory demands, work of breathing will increase [9]. While respiratory discomfort results from an excessive as well as an inadequate flow setting, discomfort is 7 times greater when flow is set at 30% or less of a healthy subject's preferred level than when it is set at 300% above the preferred level [10]. When adjusting the flow rate and triggering sensitivity, it is helpful to examine the contour of the airway pressure waveform. Ideally the waveform should show a smooth rise and convex appearance during inspiration.

Studies in healthy subjects and intubated patients demonstrate that increasing the inspiratory flow rate causes an increase in patient's respiratory frequency and respiratory drive [11, 12]. This flow-associated alteration in frequency has been shown to be independent of breathing route, inspired gas temperature, and delivered tidal volume, and persists after anesthesia of the airway. A change in inspired tidal volume has also been shown to be associated with a change in frequency during wakefulness and sleep under both isocapnic and hypocapnic conditions [13].

When studying the effects of a change in a ventilator's flow or tidal volume, it is important to control for the ventilator inspiratory time. When tidal volume is increased and inspiratory flow is kept constant, ventilator inspiratory time must increase; when inspiratory flow is increased and tidal volume is kept constant, ventilator inspiratory time must decrease. To address this issue, Laghi et al. [14] employed four protocols in healthy volunteers receiving assist-control ventilation. When tidal volume was fixed and flow was delivered at 30, 60, and 90 l/min, frequency increased as a function of the increase in flow and the decrease in ventilator inspiratory time. When flow was held constant and tidal volume was changed from 0.5 to 1.5 l, frequency increased as a function of the decrease in tidal volume and ventilator inspiratory time. When flow was increased from 60 to 90 l/min and ventilator inspiratory time was held constant, frequency did not change. When flow and tidal volume were held constant and ventilator inspiratory time was varied by applying inspiratory pauses, frequency decreased as a function of the increase in ventilator inspiratory time. These observations demonstrate that the imposed ventilator inspiratory time during mechanical ventilation can determine frequency independently of delivered inspiratory flow and volume.

Inspiration-expiration switchover

The switch from inspiration to expiration during spontaneous breathing occurs abruptly. Attempting to synchronize the end of inspiratory assistance from the ventilator with the end of patient's neural inspiratory time is difficult and the extent to which they coincide varies with the mode of ventilation.

During pressure support ventilation, the termination of machine assistance is based on a decrease in the inspiratory flow rate to a preset level, such as 25% of the peak inspiratory flow value. Patients who have a prolonged time constant require more time for flow to reach this threshold. Accordingly, the expiratory neurons will become impatient and start to fire, causing contraction of the expiratory muscles during inflation. Of 12 patients with chronic obstructive pulmonary disease receiving pressure support of 20 cm H_2O, 5 recruited their expiratory muscles during the inflation phase of the ventilator [15, 16]. The patients displaying this phenomenon had an average time constant of 0.54 s compared with an average time constant of 0.38 s in the patients who did not display expiratory muscle recruitment during the inflation phase.

Expiratory muscle activity

Activation of the expiratory muscles during mechanical inflation can also interfere with a patient's ability to trigger the next breath. In a detailed investigation of the importance of the timing and magnitude of expiratory muscle activity in causing patient-ventilator asynchrony, Parthasarathy et al. [16] induced airflow limitation using a Starling resistor in healthy volunteers. The degree of synchronization between the onset of a patient's expiratory muscle activity and the point that machine inflation ended was expressed in terms of phase angle. If the start of the eletromyogram (EMG) and the end of mechanical inflation coincide, phase angle is zero. If EMG activity commenced after the end of mechanical inflation, the phase angle will have a positive value; and if expiratory muscle activity started before the end of mechanical inflation, the phase angle will have negative units.

In the presence of airflow limitation and at a pressure support of 10 and 20 cm H_2O, the subject had repeated episodes of non-triggering. The phase angle of non-triggering attempts was significantly more negative than for triggering attempts. This means that in the case of non-triggering attempts, the expiratory muscles were active for a longer period before the switching off of mechanical inflation. In other words, the continuation of mechanical inflation into neural expiration caused shortening of the time available for unopposed expiratory flow; this will cause the elastic recoil to be higher at the point of the next triggering attempt and increase the likelihood that triggering will fail.

In conclusion, synchronization of the activity of the different respiratory muscle groups with the cycling of the ventilator is quite complex. Problems can arise at the onset of mechanical inflation – during triggering – and also at the termination of mechanical inflation – at the point of switchover from inspiration to expiration. Synchronization of the neuromuscular activity with the cycling of the machine is a key factor in achieving a desirable level of respiratory muscle rest. Our current methods for detecting these problems are extremely crude and in need of considerable refinement.

References

1. Laghi F, D'Alfonso N, Tobin MJ (1995) Pattern of recovery from diaphragmatic fatigue over 24 hours. J Appl Physiol 79:539-546
2. Anzueto A, Peters JI, Tobin MJ et al (1997) Effects of prolonged controlled mechanical ventilation on diaphragmatic function in healthy adult baboons (see comments). Crit Care Med 25:1187-1190
3. Marini JJ, Capps JS, Culver BH (1985) The inspiratory work of breathing during assisted mechanical ventilation. Chest 87:612-618
4. Imsand C, Feihl F, Perret C et al (1994) Regulation of inspiratory neuromuscular output during synchronized mechanical ventilation. Anesthesiology 80:13-22
5. Leung P, Jubran A, Tobin MJ (1997) Comparison of assisted ventilator modes on triggering, patient effort, and dyspnea. Am J Crit Care Med 155:1940-1948
6. Sassoon CSH, Gruer SE (1995) Characteristic of the ventilator pressure- and flow-trigger variables. Intensive Care Med 21:159-168
7. Aslanian P, El Atrous S, Isabey D et al (1998) Effects of flow triggering on breathing effort during partial ventilatory support. Am J Respir Crit Care Med 157:135-143
8. Alberti A, Gallo F, Fongaro A et al (1995) $P_{0.1}$ is a useful parameter in setting the level of pressure support ventilation. Intensive Care Med 21:547-553
9. Tobin MJ, Laghi F, Jubran A (1998) Respiratory muscle dysfunction in mechanically ventilated patients. Mol Cell Biochem 179:87-98
10. Manning HL, Molinary EJ, Leiter JC (1995) Effect of inspiratory flow rate on respiratory sensation and pattern of breathing. Am J Respir Crit Care Med 151:751-757
11. Puddy A, Younes M (1992) Effect of inspiratory flow rate on respiratory output in normal subjects. Am Rev Respir Dis 146:787-789
12. Corne S, Gillespie D, Roberts D et al (1997) Effect of inspiratory flow rate on respiratory rate in intubated ventilated patients. Am J Respir Crit Care Med 156:304-308
13. Tobert DG, Simon PM, Stroetz RW et al (1997) The determinants of respiratory rate during mechanical ventilation. Am J Respir Crit Care Med 155:485-492
14. Laghi F, Karamchandani K, Tobin MJ (1999) Influence of ventilator settings in determining respiratory frequency during mechanical ventilation. Am J Respir Crit Care Med 160:1766-1770
15. Jubran A, Van de Graaff WB, Tobin MJ (1995) Variability of patient-ventilator interaction with pressure-support ventilation in patients with COPD. Am J Respir Crit Care Med 152:129-136
16. Parthasarathy S, Jubran A, Tobin MJ (1998) Cycling of inspiratory and expiratory muscle groups with the ventilator in airflow limitation. Am J Respir Crit Care Med 158:1471-1478

Prevention of Acute Respiratory Failure by Optimal Ventilator Settings: The Open Lung Concept

D. SCHREITER, L. SCHEIBNER, S. KATSCHER, C. JOSTEN

The introduction of artificial ventilation into clinical practice opened up completely new horizons in the fields of anaesthesia and intensive care medicine; however this very ventilation, which is supposed to take over the respiratory function, is being blamed for acute respiratory failure. High peak pressures and tidal volumes are regarded as the main causes of such ventilation-induced lung damage [1-3]. Clinically this can lead to a surfactant damage and a tendency for the lungs to collapse [4].

Animal studies showed that even in conventionally ventilated lungs that were healthy at the outset, there was an increase in the release of TNF and chemokines [5, 6]; in addition, granulocytes started to migrate into the lung [7]. This means that mechanical ventilation can, itself, trigger an inflammatory reaction [8, 9]. Any secondary damage will depend on how damaged the lungs were in the first place. When a lung is unevenly damaged, as in cases of severe contusion, and is being ventilated at "normal" pressures, intermittent overstretching, which mainly tends to affect healthy alveoli, stimulates the ion channels and this, in turn, triggers mediator release [10]. The result is a reinforcement of the SIRS.

Artificial ventilation can thus induce the very disorder that it was meant to treat. Are there any ventilation strategies that will protect the lungs and minimize secondary lung damage of this type (Table 1)?

The application of a constant tidal volume is guaranteed by the conventional volume-controlled ventilation. In a damaged lung, the maintenance of a constant volume leads to high respiratory pressures causing a further increase of the morphological lung damage [2]. It is generally agreed that the way to avoid this vicious circle is to ventilate under constant pressure keeping the tidal volume as low as possible based on a high PEEP. Shear forces and overstretching need to be kept as low as possible. The resulting hypoventilation and consecutive hypercapnia along with their side-effects are tolerated [11-15].

After damage to the surfactant system, the full impact of the forces at the gas/water boundary is brought to bear upon affected portions of the lung. The reciprocal relationship between pressure and alveolar-radius according to the law of Laplace represents the physical basis of the "Open Lung concept" [16,

Table 1. Overview of ventilatory strategies

	Conventional	Consensus	Open-lung-concept
		Amato MBP et al. (1995) Am J Resp Crit Care Med 152, 1835 [11]	Lachmann B (1992) Intensive Care Med 18, 319 [17] Schreiter D et al. (1999) of Langenbeck Arch, 909 [18]
Goal of therapy	Normoventilation	Lung protection	Lung protection
Flow	Constant flow	Decelerated flow	Decelerated flow
Ventilation mode	VC	PC(-IRV)	(HF-)PC-IRV
Respiratory frequency	Physiological frequency	Physiological frequency	60-100/min
Tidal volume	12 ml/kg body weight	< 6 ml/kg body weight	< 6 ml/kg body weight
Peak pressures	Consecutive in constant volumes	< 40 mbar	< 40 mbar temporary recruitment 50-65(-80) mbar
PEEP	2-5 mbar	10-16 mbar (2 mbar > p_{flex})	Total PEEP 16-22 mbar set-PEEP 8-10 mbar + intrinsic PEEP
Aimed PO_2	= 60 mmHg	= 60 mmHg	= 100 mmHg
Aimed PCO_2	Normocapnia	= 80 mmHg permissive hypercapnia	= 35 mmHg

17]. Using this concept developed by Lachmann the atelectatic portions of the lung are opened up by a temporarily high peak pressure and kept open by a sufficiently high PEEP until the regeneration of the surfactant system. The application in the pressure-controlled mode with decelerated flow is inevitable [16, 17]. As a result of the successful recruiting and the improvement of lung compliance, oxygenation will increase rapidly and the PCO_2 will be normal [16-18]. Whether there is a reduction of shear forces and a release of mediators, or whether an additional inflammatory reaction is induced by the volutrauma of the nonaffected alveoli during the initial opening procedure, are the focus of our current experimental and clinical studies.

Prevention of respiratory failure in patients with healthy lungs during artificial ventilation

Anaesthesia, relaxation, intubation and supine position reduce the FRC by more than one litre, due to the decrease in chest diameter together with the cranial diaphragm shift [19, 20]. If the FRC is reduced to below a critical level, minor airways will be more likely to collapse and there will be a greater risk of atelectases in dependent portions of the lung with resulting ventilation-perfusion imbalance. It had been shown that dorsobasal atelectases occur in approximately 90% of anaesthetised patients, i.e. in patients with initially sound pulmonary function [21, 22].

The mandatory ventilation of the sound lung during general-anaesthesia or postoperative artificial ventilation is to ensure a constant tidal volume using a ventilation mode with constant flow and time trigger. The disturbance of ventilation developing even in the sound lung together with the formation of compartments of different time-constants could result in overstretching of compartments with normal time-constant and a decrease in aeration of compartments with long time-constant. Besides the ventilation-perfusion imbalance with resulting disturbance of oxygenation, increasing peak pressures (particularly in the areas with low resistance and low compliance) and overstretching of the compartments with short time constant occur. The uneven ventilation leads to intrapulmonary shear forces and further traumatization of the parenchyma by a baro- and volutrauma of the lung. Studies have shown that artificial ventilatory modes with high tidal volumes and high peak pressures cause a decrease in surfactant, leading to an increased tendency of the lung to collapse [4].

In pig studies we have shown dorsobasal atelectases by computer tomography 120 minutes after general anaesthesia depending on the height of PEEP. At a PEEP of 2 mbar there were ventilation disturbances in all animals, and at a PEEP of 5 mbar in over 50% of the animals. To recruit the atelectatic portions of the lung using the "Open Lung Concept" a peak pressure of 37 (30-55) mbar was necessary in the group with low PEEP (Fig. 1). In animals ventilated at a PEEP of 5 mbar we had to use a peak pressure of 33 (30-55) mbar. The opening pressures were defined by morphological signs in the CT and by functional data

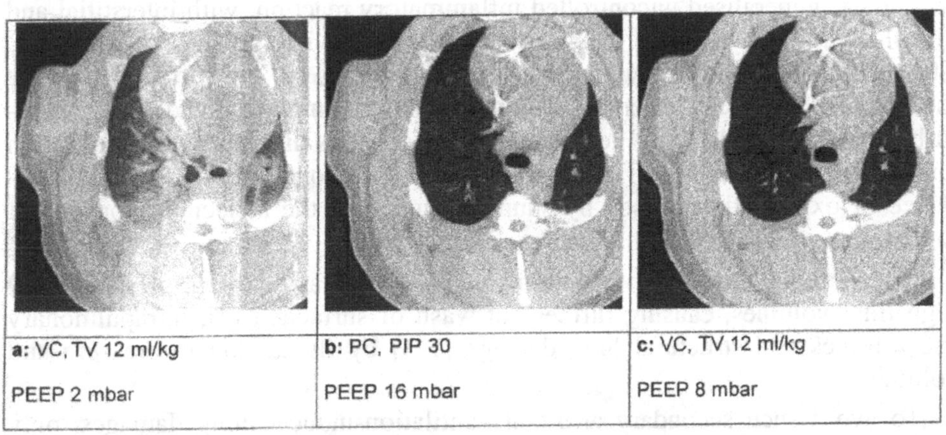

Fig. 1. a: Dorsobasal atelectases after 120′ endotracheal anaesthesia (pig); b: recruiting with temporary application of 30 mbar; c: securing the result by a PEEP of 8 mbar

from the online blood-gas analysis. After successful recruitment we needed lower pressure amplitudes at a PEEP of 8 mbar to reach the same tidal volumes as before. In another group ventilated at a PEEP of 8 mbar from the very beginning, no atelectases were found after the same time period.

The PEEP needs to be kept high enough to stabilise the alveoli and raise FRC. This should be regarded as the key factor in the prevention of ventilation induced lung damage. PEEP must be no lower than 5 mbar during intubation anaesthesia. If a patient with initially sound lungs has to be ventilated over a lengthy period this should be carried out usually in pressure-controlled mode based on a PEEP of no less than 8 mbar. The lung has to be open, or to have been opened up, for this to be done. The pathophysiological mechanisms that give rise to atelectases under anaesthesia and during ventilation are not the only cases of ventilation problems; these can also be exacerbated by surgical suction or compression caused either by diaphragm displacement or by intra-horacic procedures. Peak pressures of up to 40 mbar to achieve intermittent recruitment and a PEEP held at no lower than 8 mbar will deliver a physiological ventilation-perfusion ratio with the best oxygenation, will improve compliance, minimize the pressure amplitudes and prevent secondary lung damage by reduction of shear forces and release of cytokines. The "Open Lung Concept" should be regarded as prophylaxis, with an additional effective action in preventing ventilation-induced lung damage.

Therapy and avoidance of secondary damages in acute lung injury by adequate artificial ventilation strategies

The pathomorphological substrate of acute respiratory failure or ARDS represents direct primary parenchymal damage caused by trauma or infection and a secondary, generalised uncontrolled inflammatory reaction, with interstitial and alveolar capillary oedema, leading to interference with the surfactant system. The resultant increased liquid storage and the increase of the surface tension at the alveolar interfaces leads to a decrease of lung compliance and a severe disturbance of gas exchange. There is an inhomogeneous distribution of ventilation and perfusion in the lung. The most important functional problem is the disturbance of oxygenation caused by shunt perfusion of the atelectatic portions of the lung.

Conventional artificial ventilation leads to increasing peak pressures and high tidal volumes, causing further out wash of surfactant [4], intrapulmonary shear forces and structural lung damage [1-3] by fluctuation in pressure and volume.

To avoid such secondary artificial ventilation-induced lung damages, only low tidal volumes should be applied on a PEEP higher than the low flexion point. As a side-effect, permissive hypercapnia is to be tolerated.

If it is possible to recruit atelectatic lung sections by temporary crossing of a certain opening pressure, the pressure-volume ratio is transferred into a region where lower pressures are necessary to ventilate higher volumes. The oxygenation area will be much larger.

In our own studies pigs were ventilated with the "New Approach" (Amato) [11] and the "Open Lung Concept" after setting an experimental lung contusion under standardized conditions [16-18]. In the "Open Lung" group we reached a significantly faster and higher increase of the Horowitz-Quotient (Fig. 2a) and compliance (Fig. 2b). Average peak pressure necessary, defined by morphological (CT) and PO_2, data was 60 (50-80) mbar.

In both groups, a PEEP needed for alveolar stabilization of approximately 16 mbar was found. Whereas this expiratory minimum pressure in the Amato group was applied by a static set-PEEP, we used regional dynamic PEEP in the "Open Lung" group. This intrinsic PEEP is produced by means of a pressure-controlled inverse ratio ventilation at high frequency leading to a very short expiration period, so that the affected areas of the lung (short time constant) are unable to empty themselves completely. An external PEEP of 8-10 mbar was necessary to stabilise the healthy alveoli (short time constant).

Besides lower oxygenation due to slower recruiting, hypercapnia was the most limiting factor in the "New Approach" group ventilated at normal frequencies (20-25) and static PEEP. PCO_2 levels up to 80 mmHg were tolerated. Animals of this group needed higher dosages of sedation and higher pressure amplitudes than those of the Lachmann group. The overall better results in the "Open lung" animals were based on better recruitment and on the advantages of the intrinsic PEEP. The high respiratory frequencies in this group allowed a frequency-controlled balance (40-100/min) between hyperventilation and deadspace-ventilation into an easy respiratory alkalosis. It had to be accepted no permissive hypercapnia (Fig. 2c). Figures 2 and 3 show functional and morphological results of 24 hours' artificial respiration therapy (consensus and "Open Lung Concept") after experimental lung-contusion in pigs.

In a clinical study in polytraumatised patients with severe chest injury we achieved similar good results.

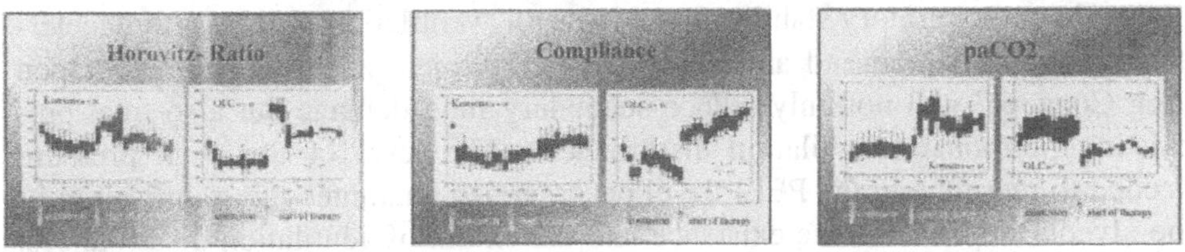

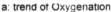

a: trend of Oxygenation b: trend of Compliance c: trend of pa_{CO2}

Fig. 2. Functional results of 24 hours' artificial respiration therapy (consensus and "open lung concept") after experimental lung-contusion in pigs

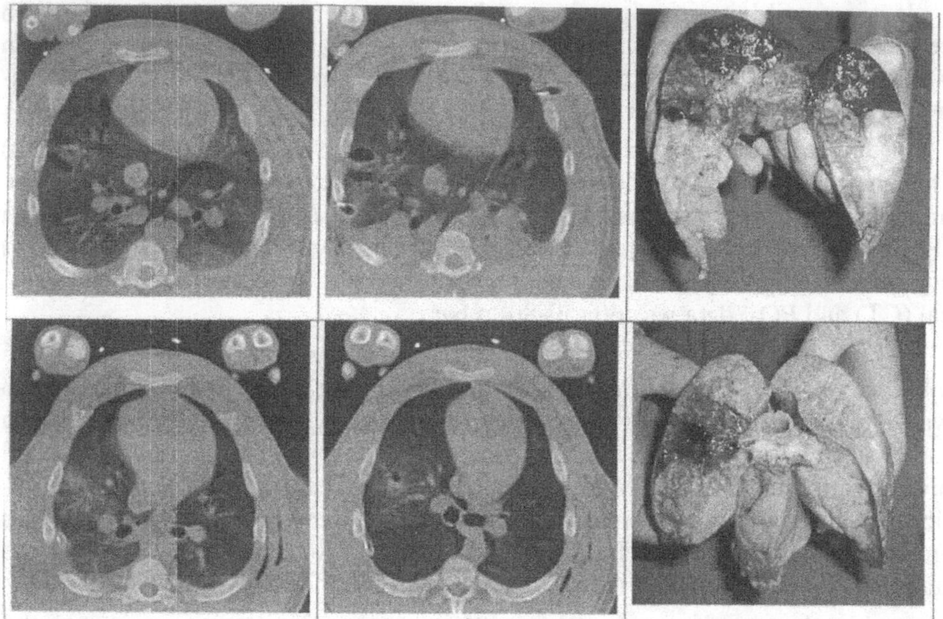

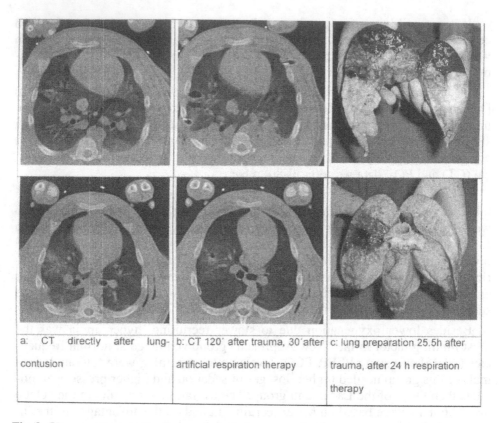

a: CT directly after lung-contusion	b: CT 120´ after trauma, 30´after artificial respiration therapy	c: lung preparation 25.5h after trauma, after 24 h respiration therapy

Fig. 3. (Upper row): example of a morphological course under "consensus ventilation"; (low row): example of a morphological course under "open lung concept"

Conclusion

Secondary lung damages caused by mechanical artificial ventilation can occur in patients with normal pulmonary function at the outset, and are even more deleterious in patients with pre-existing pulmonary insufficiency.

Sufficient expiratory stabilisation of alveoli, ventilation modes with decelerated flow application and an intermittent recruitment according to the "Open lung Concept" will not only reduce secondary lung damage but also treat pre-existing pulmonary ventilation disturbances. The level of the peak pressure needed to recruit, and the PEEP level necessary to guarantee the stabilisation of the alveoli, depends on the existence and the extent of ventilation disturbances. To define those levels exactly, online blood gas analysis is used preferably combined with morphological signs of chest CT. But based on present experimental and clinical experiences it should be possible to carry out the "Open Lung" procedure controlled by intermittent blood gas analysis. Because of verifiable and reproducible successes shown above, this causal artificial ventilation concept is becoming more widely used in anaesthesia and intensive-care-medicine.

References

1. Dreyfuss D, Saumon G (1992) Barotrauma is volutrauma, but which volume is the one responsible? Intensive Care Med 18:139
2. Dreyfuss D, Saumon G (1993) Role of tidal volume, FRC and end-inspiratory volume in the development of pulmonary edema following mechanical ventilation. Am Rev Respir Dis 148:1194-1203
3. Dreyfuss D, Saumon G (1998) Ventilator-induced lung injury. Am J Respir Crit Care Med 157:294-323
4. Houmes RJ, Bos JAH, Lachmann B (1994) Effects of different ventilator settings on lung mechanics: with special reference to the surfactant system. Appl Cardiopulm Pathophysiol 5:117-127
5. von Betmann AN, Brasch F, Müller K et al (1996) Prolonged hyperventilation is required for release of tumor necrosis factor but not IL-6. Appl Cardiopulm Pathol 6:171
6. von Betmann AN, Brasch F, Nüsing R et al (1998) Hyperventilation induces release of cytokines from perfused mouse lung. Am J Respir Crit Care Med 157:263
7. Sugiura M, McCulloch PR, Wren S et al (1994) Ventilator pattern influences neutrophil influx and activation in atelectasis-prone rabbit lung. J Appl Physiol 77:1355
8. Chiumello D, Pristine G, Slutsky AS (1999) Mechanical ventilation affects local and systemic cytokines in an animal model of acute respiratory distress syndrome. Am J Respir Crit Care Med 160:109
9. Verbrugge SJC, Uhlig S, Neggers SCMM et al (1999) Different ventilation strategies affect lung function but do not increase tumor necrosis factor-alpha and prostacyclin production in lavaged rat lungs in vivo. Anesthesiology 51:1834
10. Uhlig S (2000) Beatmungsinduzierte Lungenschäden - Gibt es sie? Journal für Anästhesie und Intensivbehandlung I;2000:208
11. Amato MBP, Barbas CSV, Medeiros DM et al (1995) Beneficial effects of the "Open lung approach" with low distending pressures in acute respiratory distress syndrome. Am J Respir Crit Care Med 152:1835-1846
12. Gattinoni L, Pelosi P, Vitale G et al (1991) Body position changes redistribute lung computed-tomographic density in patients with acute respiratory failure. Anesthesiology 74:15
13. Hickling KG, Henderson S, Jackson R (1990) Low mortality associated with low volume pressure limited ventilation with permissive hypercapnia in severe adult respiratory distress syndrome. Intens Care Med 16:372
14. Hickling KG, Walsh J, Henderson S, Jackson R (1994) Low mortality rate in adult respiratory distress syndrome using low-volume, pressure-limited ventilation with permissive hypercapnia: a prospective study. Crit Care Med 22:1568
15. Slutsky AS (1994) Consensus conference on mechanical ventilation - January 28-30, 1993 at Northbrook, Illinois, USA. Intensive Care Med 20:64-79
16. Böhm S, Lachmann B (1996) Pressure-control ventilation - Putting a mode into perspective. Int J Intensive Care. Spring
17. Lachmann B (1992) Open up the lung and keep the lung open. Intensive Care Med 18: 319-321
18. Schreiter D, Abitzsch D, Scheibner L et al (1999) Das Open Lung Concept - Ein neues Beatmungsregime beim schweren Thoraxtrauma. Deutsche Gesellschaft für Chirurgie, Kongressband, pp 909-912

19. Bein Th, Reber A (1999) Atelektasen während Anästhesie und Intensivbehandlung - Entstehungsmechanismen und Therapiemöglichkeiten. Anästesiol Intensivmed 6(40):477-486
20. Hedenstierna G, Strandberg Å, Brismar B et al (1985) Functional residual capacity, thoracoabdominal dimensions and central blood volume during general anesthesia with muscle paralysis and mechanical ventilation. Anesthesiology 62:247-254
21. Reber A, Engberg G, Sporre B et al (1996) Volumetric analysis of aeration in the lungs during general anaesthesia. Br J Anaesth 76:760-766
22. Rothen HU, Sporre B, Engberg G et al (1995) Prevention of atelectasis during general anaesthesia. Lancet 345:1387-1391

Prevention of Acute Respiratory Failure by Early Surfactant Application

J.J. HAITSMA, B. LACHMANN

An alveolus is the minimal functional entity of the lung; its physiology and subsequent behavior allow normal gas exchange and thus help sustain life. Disturbance of this 'normal' alveolar physiology leads to diminished gas exchange and subsequent impairment of lung function. A 'healthy' alveolus has the ability to lower its surface tension at the air liquid interface, parallel with a reduction in alveolar radius, keeping the pressure required to keep the alveolus open stable, even at a smaller radius, and thus keeping the alveolus constant. This phenomenon of the lung was first described by von Neergaard in 1929 [1]. However, the law describing this correlation was discovered by Pierre-Simon, marquis de Laplace (1749-1827), a French astronomer and mathematician. He formulated the law (nowadays referred to as the law of Laplace): $p = 2\gamma/r$, in which p is the pressure inside a bubble, γ is the surface tension at the air liquid interface of the bubble, and r the radius of a bubble. This law transferred to an alveolus means that p is the pressure inside an alveolus that keeps the alveolus stable, γ is the surface tension at the air liquid interface, and r the radius of the alveolus.

The ability of an alveolus to dynamically lower its surface tension in response to changes in alveolar radius is dependent on pulmonary surfactant (SURFace ACTive AgeNT). When this surfactant system is inactivated by proteins, as observed in many diseases [2], this disturbs the delicate balance that exists across an alveolus, resulting in a net flow of fluids into the alveolus, increasing surface tension resulting in end-expiratory alveolar collapse and further surfactant inactivation. This chain of events can spread across the lung due to further alveolar flooding, and subsequently leads to further surfactant inactivation by plasma proteins [3]. The collapse of alveoli at the end of expiration also dramatically increases traction forces on neighboring alveoli, resulting in so-called shear forces, which damage the integrity of the alveolar capillary membrane, increasing intercellular gaps, resulting in the loss of surfactant into the blood stream, cytokine release, and finally alveolar flooding. Thus, a vicious cycle of self-perpetuating lung injury is created that leads to acute respiratory failure.

Acute respiratory failure

Acute respiratory failure (ARF) has a mortality rate above 40% [4]. In spite of increased knowledge of the disease and technological advances in respiratory support, mortality has not decreased during the last 20 years. ARF patients often require a prolonged stay in the ICU. According to a recent study on costs and length of stay in acute respiratory distress syndrome (ARDS) patients, non-survivors had a mean stay in the ICU of 23 days and a cost of US$ 43,000, compared with a 30-day admission period for survivors and a mean cost of US$ 50,000 [5].

In ARF the deficiency of (active) surfactant leads to the progressive deterioration of lung function. If one can reverse the surfactant deficiency one can expect also to improve lung function, and ultimately this may reduce the mortality rate in ARF patients. Therefore, it would be logical to supplement the ARF lung with exogenous surfactant.

Exogenous surfactant therapy

Exogenous surfactant therapy has been used since 1980 with great success and with minimal side-effects in more than 400,000 premature infants suffering from respiratory distress syndrome (RDS). However, only limited clinical data are available on exogenous surfactant therapy in adult patients. Our group was the first to show that exogenous surfactant instillation dramatically improved gas exchange in a patient suffering from ARDS [6].

In a randomized controlled study, Gregory et al. [7] demonstrated that maximum improvement of oxygenation, minimum ventilatory requirements, and the lowest mortality rate were obtained in ARDS patients by using exogenous natural surfactant at sufficiently high doses (400-800 mg/kg). Similarly, in a group of ten patients with established severe ARDS and sepsis, Walmrath et al. [8] showed that bronchoscopic application of a natural surfactant resulted in an *"immediate, impressive, and highly significant improvement of arterial oxygenation in all patients, due to a marked reduction of shunt flow"*.

Thus, these first preliminary clinical data suggest that exogenous surfactant improves lung function, reduces mortality, and decreases ventilator requirements in ARDS patients.

However, adult patients require higher dosages of surfactant to overcome the surfactant inhibitors present in ARF lungs. Furthermore, due to accumulation of proteins over time in ARF, the dosage of surfactant needs to be higher in comparison with the dosage needed for the treatment of RDS to compensate for the dose-dependent inhibitory effect of proteins on surfactant [3]. Therefore, it would be wise to start with surfactant therapy as soon as possible.

Early treatment with surfactant

Our group showed that respiratory failure induced by aspiration of hydrochloric acid could be prevented when exogenous surfactant was given before deterioration of lung function (i.e., within 10 min of acid aspiration), whereas after the development of respiratory failure, exogenous surfactant served only to prevent further decline of lung function but did not restore gas exchange [9]. When treatment starts at a later stage of lung injury, the amount of inhibitory proteins that have accumulated in the lung require larger amounts of surfactant, or several consecutive administrations, to improve lung function.

If surfactant can prevent aspiration-induced lung injury, we speculated that treatment with surfactant could diminish the lung injury observed by ventilation-induced lung injury (VILI). Therefore, using a standard model of VILI, we investigated whether administration of exogenous surfactant has any beneficial effects. In the animals ventilated with high peak inspiratory volumes and low levels of positive end-epiratory pressure (inducing VILI), we demonstrated that surfactant prevented impairment of oxygenation and deterioration of lung mechanics, and reduced the permeability to Evans blue [10]. Because preventive treatment with surfactant helps to reduce lung injury, could treatment with exogenous surfactant therefore be used to prevent ARF?

Prevention of ARF by surfactant therapy

Although to date no clinical studies have investigated whether surfactant can help prevent ARF, observations in animal models [7, 10, 11] warrant further investigation to establish whether ARF can be prevented by surfactant application.

1. Exogenous surfactant beneficially influences the alveolar defense against bacteria, thus reducing the susceptibility of the lung for ventilator-associated pneumonia [11].
2. Surfactant application has been shown to dramatically improve lung function, facilitating the weaning process and thus shortening the stay in the ICU [7].
3. Mechanical ventilation itself can augment lung injury, thus protection of lungs already ‘at risk’ could diminish their susceptibility to lung injury, shortening the stay in the ICU [10].
4. Preventive application of surfactant requires lower amounts of surfactant and could help reduce overall costs by shortening the ICU stay.

Future considerations

Exogenous surfactant instillation offers an additional therapeutic tool in the treatment of ARF patients, especially when treatment is started as early as possible to prevent further deterioration of lung function and increased alveolar protein load. Early treatment could help reduce the stay in the ICU of ARF patients and thus reduce overall costs. However, before surfactant becomes a routine therapy for ARF, the randomized clinical trials that are currently taking place have to confirm all the benefits expected from exogenous surfactant instillation.

References

1. von Neergaard K (1929) Neue Auffassungen über einen Grundbegriff der Atemmechanik; Die Retraktionskraft der Lunge, abhangig von der Oberflachenspannung in den Alveolen. Z Ges Exp Med 66:373-394
2. Gommers D, Lachmann B (1993) Surfactant therapy: does it have a role in adults? Clin Intensive Care 4:284-295
3. Lachmann B, Eijking EP, So KL, Gommers D (1994) In vivo evaluation of the inhibitory capacity of human plasma on exogenous surfactant function. Intensive Care Med 20:6-11
4. Luhr OR, Antonsen K, Karlsson M et al (1999) Incidence and mortality after acute respiratory failure and acute respiratory distress syndrome in Sweden, Denmark, and Iceland. The ARF Study Group. Am J Respir Crit Care Med 159:1849-1861
5. Valta P, Uusaro A, Nunes S et al (1999) Acute respiratory distress syndrome: frequency, clinical course, and costs of care. Crit Care Med 27:2367-2374
6. Lachmann B (1987) The role of pulmonary surfactant in the pathogenesis and therapy of ARDS. In: Vincent JL (ed) Update in intensive care and emergency medicine. Springer Verlag, Berlin Heidelberg New York, pp 123-134
7. Gregory TJ, Steinberg KP, Spragg R et al (1997) Bovine surfactant therapy for patients with acute respiratory distress syndrome. Am J Respir Crit Care Med 155:1309-1315
8. Walmrath D, Gunther A, Ghofrani HA et al (1996) Bronchoscopic surfactant administration in patients with severe adult respiratory distress syndrome and sepsis. Am J Respir Crit Care Med 154:57-62
9. Eijking EP, Gommers D, So KL et al (1993) Surfactant treatment of respiratory failure induced by hydrochloric acid aspiration in rats. Anesthesiology 78:1145-1151
10. Verbrugge SJ, Vazquez de Anda G, Gommers D et al (1998) Exogenous surfactant preserves lung function and reduces alveolar Evans blue dye influx in a rat model of ventilation-induced lung injury. Anesthesiology 89:467-474
11. Lachmann B, Gommers D (1993) Is it rational to treat pneumonia with exogenous surfactant? Eur Respir J 6:1427-1428

Optimization of Oxygenation During One-Lung Ventilation

G. DELLA ROCCA, M. PASSARIELLO, P. PIETROPAOLI

Pulmonary surgery is not an absolute indication for one-lung ventilation (OLV), nevertheless many surgeons are used to operating with the lung collapsed, which minimizes lung trauma from retractors, helps to visualize pulmonary anatomy and facilitates surgical manipulation. The recent improvement of endoscopic techniques and the expansion of surgical and diagnostic procedures performed through video-assisted thoracoscopy (VAT) have led to an increase of the indications and employment of one-lung ventilation. VAT requires a well collapsed lung and may thus be included in the absolute indications for OLV (Table 1).

Table 1. Indications for one lung ventilation

Absolute	Relative
Massive hemorrhage	Pneumonectomy
Infections	Lobectomy
Lung lavage	Aortic thoracic aneurysm
Bronchpleural fistula	Surgery of esophagus
Thoracoscopy	

Physiology of one-lung ventilation

In the awake person a good match between ventilation and perfusion in the lungs provides a normal oxygenation, a low intrapulmonary shunt (Qs/Qt ratio < 10%) and a low alveolar-arterial difference in oxygen tension ($PA\text{-}aO_2 < 10$-15 mmHg).

General anesthesia with muscle paralysis and mechanical ventilation causes some changes in the respiratory function (reduction of Functional Residual Capacity-FRC) which is associated with an increase in intrapulmonary shunt. The employment of inspired oxygen fractions higher than 21% avoids hypoxemia during anesthesia.

During one-lung ventilation (OLV) the non dependent lung is collapsed and the dependent lung is mechanically ventilated. OLV creates thus a mandatory right-to-left transpulmonary shunt through the non-ventilated lung which results in a decreased PaO_2 for the same FiO_2 and hemodynamic and metabolic status compared to two-lung ventilation (TLV). Fortunately, however, both passive mechanical and active vasoconstrictor mechanisms prevent the PaO_2 from decreasing as much as might be expected. The passive mechanisms which are responsible for a reduction of blood flow to the nondependent lung are gravity and surgical manipulation and ligation of pulmonary vessels. However, the most significant reduction of blood flow to the nondependent lung is caused by an active vasoconstrictor mechanism, the *hypoxic pulmonary vasoconstriction* (HPV). HPV causes an increase of pulmonary vascular resistance (PVR) in the atelectatic portions of the lung (i.e. the nondependent lung during OLV) diverting blood flow to normoxic or hyperoxic ventilated lung. HPV thus minimizes the amount of Qs/Qt flow that occurs through the hypoxic non ventilated lung. Numerous clinical studies have found that intrapulmonary shunt during OLV is usually not greater than 20-25% of cardiac output as opposed to the 35-45% that may be expected in the absence of HPV [1]. The choice of the anesthetic technique for OLV must take into consideration the effects of drugs on oxygenation and therefore on HPV. HPV can raise PaO_2 from potentially dangerous levels to higher and safer ones; on the contrary, inhibition of HPV may cause or contribute to hypoxemia during anesthesia. Many drugs can inhibit HPV, including anesthetics. In several experimental studies halogenated anesthetics were found to inhibit HPV in a dose-related manner, whereas intravenous anesthetics do not. However most recent studies concluded that employment of doses up to 1 MAC of halogenated anesthetics can safely be used during OLV without inhibiting HPV and decreasing PaO_2 any more than does intravenous anesthesia [2-6]. Thus, overall the potent inhaled anesthetics are the drugs of choice during thoracic surgery; in the presence of cardiovascular instability or poor oxygenation, when depression of HPV has to be avoided a balanced technique may be chosen.

Thoracic epidural analgesia is frequently used intraoperatively in addition to general anesthesia and for postoperative pain relief. Although the optimal anesthetic technique for pulmonary surgery has not yet been defined [7, 8], thoracic epidural analgesia with local anesthetics and opioids combined with general anesthesia has become very popular worldwide. In particular postoperative pain management with epidural analgesia has been proven to improve postoperative mortality and morbidity and positively affect pulmonary function. Patients receiving postoperative epidural analgesia have demonstrated decreased incidences of postoperative pneumonia, respiratory failure and atelectasis [9]. The greatest benefit from epidural techniques has been shown in patients at high risk for pulmonary morbidity, that underwent intraoperative epidural anesthesia and continued epidural analgesia after surgery. However, thoracic epidural analgesia also influences HPV: on one side epidural analgesia allows reduction of intraoperative concentrations of inhaled and intravenous anesthetics, but on the other side induces, through vasoplegia, a reduction of PVR, an increase of pulmonary blood flow to the nondependent lung and of intrapulmonary shunt [10].

Vasodilators, such as nitroglycerin or sodium nitroprusside also can inhibit HPV, as opposed to vasoconstrictors such as epinephrine, norepinephrine, phenylephrine, ephedrine and, more recently, almitrine that enhance HPV.

Conventional management of OLV

The aim of intraoperative management during OLV is the prevention of hypoxemia while providing good surgical exposure. Proper management of OLV consists of the following steps (Table 2):

Table 2. Conventional interventions to maintain oxygenation during one lung ventilation

High FiO_2 (up to 1)
Tidal volume = 10 ml/kg
Respiratory rate 10-16 ($PaCO_2$ = 35-40 mmHg)
CPAP to non-dependent lung
PEEP to dependent lung
Intermittent two lung ventilation (FiO_2 = 1)

Proper airway management. The first step in prevention of hypoxemia during OLV is a proper management of the airway. Repeated suctioning, a careful observation of alteration of airway pressures and a correct position of the double-lumen tube (DLT) are fundamental during OLV for maintenance of oxygenation. When using a right-sided DLT, adequate ventilation to the right upper lobe should always be confirmed with the help of fiberoptic bronchoscopy. When using a left-sided DLT for right thoracotomy, where the patient is dependent on the left lung, the tip of the left-sided tube may block the left upper lobe bronchus. Thus, if hypoxemia occurs during a right thoracotomy with a left-sided DLT, the correct position of the tube should be reconfirmed with fiberoptic bronchoscopy.

High FiO_2. Although the theoretical possibility of absorption atelectasis and O_2 toxicity exists, the benefits of ventilating the dependent lung with high FiO_2 (up to 100%) far exceed risks. A high FiO_2 will cause pulmonary vasodilation and promote blood flow distribution to the dependent lung. Nitrous oxide can be safely used during OLV with continuous monitoring of pulse oxymetry if $FiO_2 = 1$.

Tidal Volume = 10 ml/kg. A tidal volume less than 10 ml/kg can promote atelectasis in the dependent lung. A tidal volume greater than 10 ml/kg can increase airway pressure and PVR, thereby decreasing blood flow to the dependent lung.

Respiratory rate should be set to maintain a $PaCO_2$ = 35-40 mmHg. OLV usually requires a 20-30% increase of the respiratory rate used for TLV because of the 20% reduction of tidal volume. Hypocapnia should be avoided because it can inhibit HPV in the nondependent lung and because the airway pressure increase associated with hyperventilation causes a rise of PVR in the dependent lung and an unfavorable blood flow distribution. In selected patients (COPD, lung volume reduction surgery, lung transplantation) permissive hypercapnia is preferable to reduce the risk of barotrauma.

CPAP to nondependent lung. Positive airway pressure can be applied selectively to the non ventilated lung, causing a continuous distension by O_2 and patency of the operative lung airways. The beneficial effect of CPAP is not secondary to the positive pressure effect, potentially causing blood flow diversion to the dependent perfused lung, but from distending the alveoli with oxygen: some O_2 uptake is so allowed by the blood flow directed to the nondependent lung, resulting in an improvement of Va/Qc mismatch and an increase of PaO_2. Low levels of CPAP (5-10 cm H_2O) are usually able to correct severe hypoxemia [11] without hemodynamic implications although surgical exposure may be compromised.

PEEP to dependent lung. During OLV the dependent lung has a reduced FRC and is at risk of atelectasis; several attempts have been made to improve PaO_2 by treating the ventilated dependent lung with PEEP, in order to increase FRC and prevent airway closure at end expiration and improve Va/Qt relationship in the dependent lung. However application of PEEP can increase PVR in the dependent lung and shunt blood up to the non ventilated nondependent lung, causing no improvement in oxygenation. No PEEP should, thus, be used routinely to avoid unnecessarily increasing of PVR in the dependent lung [11-13].

Intermittent TLV. Periodic ventilation of nondependent lung causes some O_2 to remain in the non ventilated lung, allowing O_2 uptake by the blood flow directed to the operative lung. The major implication is obviously the suboptimal surgical exposure related to the periodical insufflation of the operative lung.

Non-conventional management of OLV

Although several tools are in the anesthesiologist's hand to maintain oxygenation during OLV, hypoxemia may still occur. Despite careful airway management hypoxemia (PaO_2/FiO_2 < 100) may still occur and a PaO_2 < 60 mmHg may be life-threatening. Thus, several additional interventions have been investigated in order to prevent hypoxemia during OLV (Table 3).

Table 3. Non conventional treatment of hypoxemia during OLV

High frequency jet ventilation to non-dependent lung
Inhaled nitric oxide to dependent lung
Inhaled nitric oxide to dependent lung + almitrine i.v.
Inhaled nitric oxide to dependent lung + vasoconstrictors (phenylephrine, norepinephrine)
Inhaled nitric oxide + inhaled aerosolized prostacyclin to dependent lung

High frequency jet-ventilation (HFJV) [14-19] has been employed in order to allow O_2 uptake and CO_2 removal in the nondependent lung with minimal surgical interference and with improvement of hypoxemia (RR = 150-200 breaths/min, Ve = 10-15 l/min).

Several interventions have been investigated in order to perform a pharmacologic *modulation of pulmonary circulation* with the aim of optimizing the capability of the dependent lung to accept blood flow through the administration of inhaled vasodilators and enhancing HPV and diversion of blood flow from the nondependent lung through the infusion of pulmonary vasoconstrictors.

Inhaled nitric oxide (iNO) is a potent pulmonary vasodilator which selectively dilates vessels in the well ventilated alveoli [20, 21]. Endogenous NO is produced in the endothelium from the L-arginine metabolic pathway that requires the enzyme NO-synthase, and diffuses into the adjacent vascular smooth muscle to cause relaxation and vasodilation. Clinically used vasodilators such as nitroprusside and nitroglycerin also exert their effects by releasing NO intracellularly, but worsen gas exchange because vasodilation occurs also in non ventilated alveoli, thus increasing intrapulmonary shunt. Inhaled NO, instead, promotes vasodilation only in well ventilated alveoli, and because of its rapid inactivation by hemoglobin it does not have effect on adjacent alveoli or on the systemic circulation. INO has been shown to improve oxygenation in ARDS patients by reducing intrapulmonary shunt and improving Va/Qc [22-26]. Several investigators [20, 27, 28] administered iNO during OLV in order to promote vasodilation in the dependent ventilated lung and enhance the dependent lung capability to accept blood flow; results are, however, controversial. Most investigators did not obtain improvements in oxygenation, while Moutafis [27] showed that iNO alone was not able to influence PaO_2 during OLV, but could improve oxygenation if combined with the infusion of almitrine, a vasoconstrictor that enhances HPV. Probably other vasoconstrictors, such as norepinephrine and phenylephrine may be used in the place of almitrine which is not available any more. The synergistic vasodilator effect of iNO and inhaled aerosolized prostacyclin (IAP) has been employed in various clinical conditions, included ARDS [29], pulmonary hypertension [30-32] and lung transplantation [33]. INO in addition to IAP seems to be effective in reducing pulmonary artery pressure and be able to improve oxygenation by reducing intrapulmonary Va/Qc mismatch [29].

Conclusions

Optimization of oxygenation during OLV is a complicated and debated issue: on one side anesthesia for thoracic surgery frequently determines a worsening of oxygenation by the employment of one-lung ventilation itself, the administration of general anesthetics, either inhaled or intravenous, and of epidural analgesia that alter HPV, on the other hand many interventions are still under investigation with the aim of restoring normal HPV and providing adequate tissue oxygenation during pulmonary surgery. Current studies about the employment of selective inhaled pulmonary vasodilators and intravenous vasoconstrictors have led to promising results and need further investigations.

References

1. Benumof JL (1985) One-lung ventilation and hypoxic pulmonary vasoconstriction: Implications for anesthetic management. Anesth Analg 64:821-833
2. Fujita Y, Yamasaki T, Takaori M, Sekioka K (1993) Sevoflurane anaesthesia for one-lung ventilation with PEEP to the dependent lung in sheep: Effects on right ventricular function and oxygenation. Can J Anaesth 40:1195-1200
3. Benumof JL, Augustine SD, Gibbons JA (1987) Halothane and isoflurane only slightly impair arterial oxygenation during one-lung ventilation in patients undergoing thoracotomy. Anesthesiology 67:910
4. Steegers PA, Backx PJ (1990) Propofol and alfentanil anesthesia during one-lung ventilation. J Cardiothorac Anesth 4:194-199
5. Carli F, Stribley GC, Clark MM (1983) Etomidate infusion in thoracic anaesthesia. Anaesthesia 38:784-788
6. Abe K, Mashimo T, Yoshiya I (1998) Arterial oxygenation and shunt fraction during one-lung ventilation: A comparison of isoflurane and sevoflurane. Anesth Analg 86:1266-1270
7. Temeck BK, Schafer PW, Park WY, Harmon JW (1989) Epidural anesthesia in patients undergoing thoracic surgery. Arch Surg 124:415-418
8. Tenling A, Joachimsson PO, Tyden H et al (1999) Thoracic epidural anesthesia as an adjunct to general anesthesia for cardiac surgery: Effects on ventilation-perfusion relationships. J Cardiothorac Vasc Anesth 13:258-264
9. Yeager MP, Glass DD, Neff RK, Brinck-Johnson T (1987) Epidural anesthesia and analgesia in high-risk surgical patients. Anesthesiology 66:729-736
10. Stephen GW, Lees MM, Scott DB (1969) Cardiovascular effects of epidural block combined with general anesthesia. Br J Anaesth 41:933-938
11. Cohen E, Eisenkraft JB, Thys DM et al (1988) Oxygenation and hemodynamic changes during one-lung ventilation: Effects of CPAP10, PEEP10, and CPAP10/PEEP10. J Cardiothorac Anesth 2:34-40
12. Aalto-Setala M, Heinonen J, Salorinne Y (1975) Cardiorespiratory function during thoracic anaesthesia: A comparison of two-lung ventilation and one-lung ventilation with and without PEEP5. Acta Anaesthesiol Scand 19:287-295
13. Slinger PD, Hickey DR (1998) The interaction between applied PEEP and auto-PEEP during one-lung ventilation. J Cardiothorac Vasc Anesth 12:133-136
14. El-Baz N, Jensik R, Faber LP, Faro RS (1982) One-lung high-frequency ventilation for tracheoplasty and bronchoplasty: A new technique. Ann Thorac Surg 34:564-571
15. Jenkins J, Cameron EW, Milne AC, Hunter RM (1987) One lung anaesthesia. Cardiovascular and respiratory function compared during conventional ventilation and high frequency jet ventilation. Anaesthesia 42:938-943

16. Nakatsuka M (1995) 1988: Unilateral high-frequency jet ventilation during one-lung ventilation for thoracotomy. Updated in 1995. Ann Thorac Surg 59:1610
17. Pavlik M, Ctvrteckova D, Zvonicek et al (1999) The improvement of arterial oxygenation during one-lung ventilation-effect of different CPAP levels. Acta Chir Hung 38:103-105
18. Maroof M, Khan RM, Bhatti TH (1995) CPAP with air and oxygen to non-ventilated lung improves oxygenation during one lung anaesthesia. JPMA J Pak Med Assoc 45:43-44
19. El-Baz N, El-Ganzouri A, Gottschalk W, Jensik R (1981) One-lung high-frequency pressure ventilation for sleeve pneumonectomy: An alternative technique. Anesth Analg 60:683-686
20. Rich GF, Murphy GD, Roos CM, Johns RA (1993) Inhaled nitric oxide. Selective pulmonary vasodilation in cardiac surgical patients. Anesthesiology 78:1028-1035
21. Rich GF, Lowson SM, Johns RA et al (1994) Inhaled nitric oxide selectively decreases pulmonary vascular resistance without impairing oxygenation during one-lung ventilation in patients undergoing cardiac surgery. Anesthesiology 80:57-62
22. Dellinger RP, Zimmerman JL, Taylor RW et al (1998) Effects of inhaled nitric oxide in patients with acute respiratory distress syndrome: Results of a randomized phase II trial. Inhaled Nitric Oxide in ARDS Study Group [see comments]. Crit Care Med 26:15-23
23. Rossaint R, Falke KJ, Lopez F et al (1993) Inhaled nitric oxide for the adult respiratory distress syndrome. N Engl J Med 328:399-405
24. Krafft P, Fridrich P, Fitzgerald RD et al (1996) Effectiveness of nitric oxide inhalation in septic ARDS. Chest 109:486-493
25. Michael JR, Barton RG, Saffle JR et al (1998) Inhaled nitric oxide versus conventional therapy: Effect on oxygenation in ARDS [see comments]. Am J Respir Crit Care Med 157:1372-1380
26. Rossaint R, Gerlach H, Schmidt-Ruhnke H et al (1995) Efficacy of inhaled nitric oxide in patients with severe ARDS. Chest 107:1107-1115
27. Moutafis M, Liu N, Dalibon N et al (1997) The effects of inhaled nitric oxide and its combination with intravenous almitrine on PaO_2 during one-lung ventilation in patients undergoing thoracoscopic procedures. Anesth Analg 85:1130-1135
28. Wilson WC, Kapelanski DP, Benumof JL et al (1997) Inhaled nitric oxide (40 ppm) during one-lung ventilation, in the lateral decubitus position, does not decrease pulmonary vascular resistance or improve oxygenation in normal patients [see comments]. J Cardiothorac Vasc Anesth 11:172-176
29. Van Heerden PV, Blythe D, Webb SA (1996) Inhaled aerosolized prostacyclin and nitric oxide as selective pulmonary vasodilators in ARDS-a pilot study. Anaesth Intensive Care 24: 564-568
30. Haraldsson A, Kieler-Jensen N, Ricksten SE (1996) Inhaled prostacyclin for treatment of pulmonary hypertension after cardiac surgery or heart transplantation: A pharmacodynamic study. J Cardiothorac Vasc Anesth 10:864-868
31. Mikhail G, Gibbs J, Richardson M et al (1997) An evaluation of nebulized prostacyclin in patients with primary and secondary pulmonary hypertension [see comments]. Eur Heart J 18: 1499-1504
32. Olschewski H, Walmrath D, Schermuly R et al (1996) Aerosolized prostacyclin and iloprost in severe pulmonary hypertension. Ann Intern Med 124:820-824
33. Della Rocca G, Coccia C, Pugliese F (2000) Hemodynamic and oxygenation changes of combined therapy with inhaled nitric oxide and inhaled aerosolized prostacyclin. J Cardiothorac Vasc Anesth (in press)

Management of Lung Separation: The Difficult Airway

E. COHEN

The increasing popularity of video-assisted thoracoscopy (VAT) can be attributed to the fact that a considerable number of procedures, diagnostic or therapeutic, can be performed with VAT. Unlike the conventional thoracoscopy, during VAT the lung should be well collapsed to allow the surgeon an optimal view of the surgical field and to palpate the lesion in the lung parenchyma. When the separation of the lung is strictly indicated, use of "difficult tubes", such as double-lumen tube (DLT) or Univent tube, cannot be avoided despite the presence of a difficult airway. This review will discuss the alternative devices to assist in lung separation in a patient with a difficult airway and is adopted from Cohen and Benumof [1].

Indications for one lung ventilation: what has changed?

The indications for one-lung ventilation (OLV) are classified either as absolute or as relative. The absolute indications include life-threatening complications, such as massive bleeding, and abscess formation, where the non-diseased contralateral lung, must be protected from contamination from the diseased lung. Broncho-pleural and giant unilateral bullae may rupture under positive pressure and ventilatory exclusion is mandatory. Finally, during bronchopulmonary lavage for alveolar proteinosis or cystic fibrosis, prevention of the contralateral lung drowning is absolutely necessary. Recently, the popularity of VAT [2] has increased because a considerable number of procedures, such as lung biopsy, plural exploration and biopsy, random wedge resections, resection of a solitary lung lesion, talc insufflation, or pleuroabrasion, can be performed with VAT. In most circumstances these procedures are performed under general anesthesia. A well-collapsed lung is essential to allow the surgeon proper visualization of the operative field, and to permit adequate resection. In the past, when faced with a difficult intubation and a single-lumen tube (SLT) with intermittent ventilation, compressing the lung with lap pads and a low tidal volume were used. Only on rare occasions was there the need for an absolute lung separation in a patient with a difficult airway. During the last few years VAT was introduced to clinical practice. Unlike conventional thoracoscopy, VAT allow for an extensive variety of diagnostic and therapeutic procedures. The improvements in video endoscopic surgical equipment and a growing enthusiasm for minimally invasive surgical approaches brought VAT to the practice of surgery for diagnostic and therapeutic procedures. In most cases general anesthesia with one lung ventilation is required. Because of its common use today, VAT significantly increases the number of cases that require lung separation and the number of patients who also have a difficult airway.

Methods of lung separation in the patient with a difficult airway

An airway may be termed difficult when conventional laryngoscopy reveals a grade III view (just epiglottis) or a grade IV view (just soft palate). Furthermore, depending on the type and the length of surgery and the degree of fluid shift during surgery, an airway that initially was not classified as difficult may become difficult secondary to facial edema, the presence of secretions and laryngeal trauma from the initial intubation. A logical approach to lung separation is described in Figure 1. When the separation of the lung is strictly indicated, use of tubes that are difficult to insert, such as DLT or a Univent tube [3], cannot be avoided despite the presence of a difficult airway. If the patient has a recognized difficult airway awake, intubation with fiberoptic bronchoscopy (FOB) can be attempted using DLT/Univent/or a SLT [4]. The same approach may be use for the patient with an unrecognized difficult airway and failure to intubate with conventional laryngoscopy. When using a DLT over a fiberoptic bronchoscope (FB), one should bear in mind that it is a bulky tube with a large external diameter, and because of the length of the DLT, only a limited part of the FB is available for manipulation. In addition, the mismatch between the flexibility of the FOB and the rigidity of the DLT make it harder to pass over the FOB [5]. The Univent tube has the same bulky external diameter and is also often hard to pass through the vocal cords, particularly in an awake patient. In some cases advancing the bronchial blocker of the Univent tube can serve to facilitate the passage through the larynx. Following a successful intubation with a DLT or a Univent tube, OLV can be immediately established [6, 7]. If these difficult tubes are not able to be inserted over a FOB, than a SLT should be use to establish an airway.

SLT can be successfully placed

If failure to provide a lung separation could result in a life-threatening situation, there are two possibilities to provide a OLV when a SLT is in place. First, depending on the indication for lung isolation, a tube exchanger can be used to switch to a DLT or a Univent tube. The second possibility is to direct a bronchial blocker (BB) through the SLT into the selected mainstem bronchus. These two methods, however, offer a limited protection or inadequate seal in

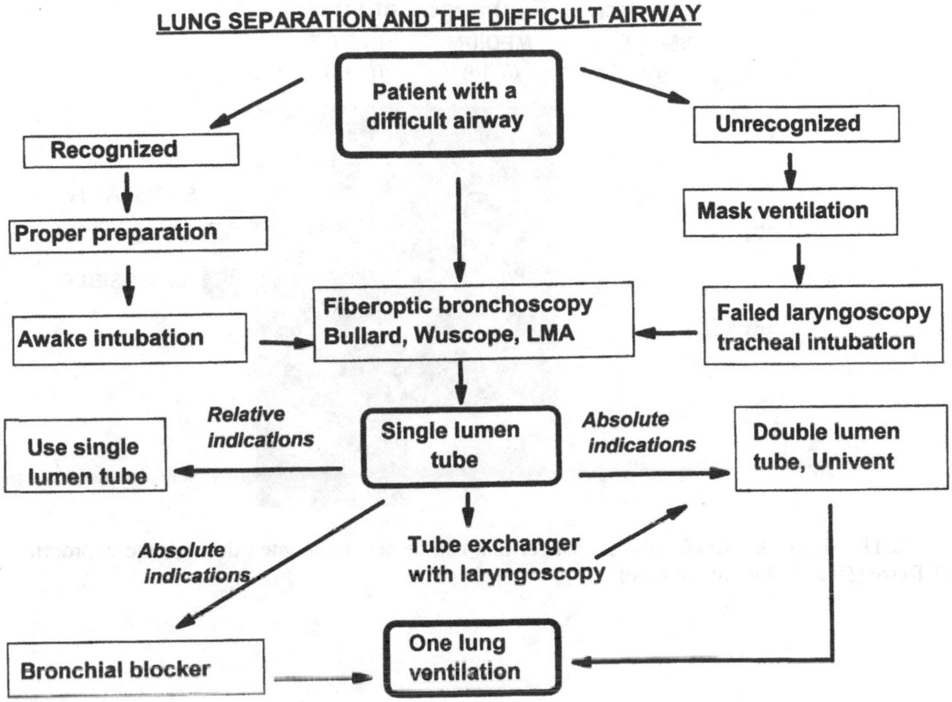

Fig. 1. Approach to lung separation in the difficult airways (*LMA*. Fastrach, laryngeal mask airways)

cases such a lung lavage, pulmonary abscess, or hemoptysis. For these procedures, DLT is without a doubt the tube of choice.

The use of a tube exchanger

Several tube exchanger are available (Cook Critical Care, Bloomington, Iowa, USA). All of these airway guides are commercially made, are depth marked in centimeters, are available in a wide range of outer diameters, and are easily adapted for either oxygen insulation or jet ventilation. The airway guide may be used for inserting a SLT, changing a SLT to one of the difficult tubes, or simply inserting a difficult tube. Critical details to bear in mind to maximize benefit and minimize risk of airway guides are as follows. *First*, the size of the airway guide and the size of the difficult tube must be determined and should be tested in vitro before the use of the airway guide. The diagram in Figure 2 shows the size of the Cook tube exchanger that can be accommodated through the appropriate DLT size. *Second*, the airway guide should never be inserted against a resistance, the clinician must always be cognizant of the depth of insertion. Two re-

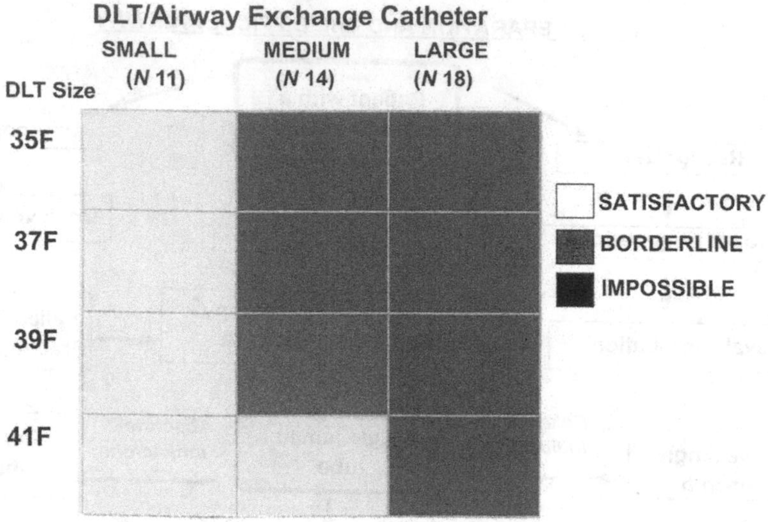

Fig. 2. The size of the Cook tube exchanger that can be accommodated through the appropriate DLT size (*DLT* double-lumen tube)

ported perforations of the tracheobronchial tree have occurred [8, 9]. *Third*, a jet ventilator should be immediately available in case the new tube does not follow the airway guide into the trachea, and the jet ventilator should be preset at 25 p.s.i by the use of an additional in-line regulator [10]. *Finally*, when passing any tube over an airway guide, a laryngoscope should be used, to facilitate passage of the tube over the airway guide past supraglottic tissues.

The Univent tube

The Univent tube (Univent, Fuji Systems, Tokyo, Japan) is a novel new means of achieving bronchial blockade. The BB technique has been modified so that the BB is passed along a single-lumen endobronchial tube. The BB is housed in a small anterior lumen containing a thin (2 mm internal diameter) tube with a distal balloon (blocker tube). The blocker tube can be advanced beyond the tip of the tracheal tube into a mainstem bronchus to serve as a blocker (Fig. 3). Prior to intubation, the blocker cuff is deflated and the blocker is completely retracted into the small lumen. Intubation is carried out as a routine with SLT. The tracheal tube is than rotated to the side to be occluded, and under direct visualization with a FOB, the blocker is manipulated into the desired mainstem bronchus. To achieve lung separation the blocker cuff is inflated, under direct vision to seal the bronchial lumen (6-7 ml of air). The Univent tube has the advantage of using a SLT instead of a DLT, and there is no need to change over at the end of the procedure if postoperative ventilatory support is required. It is al-

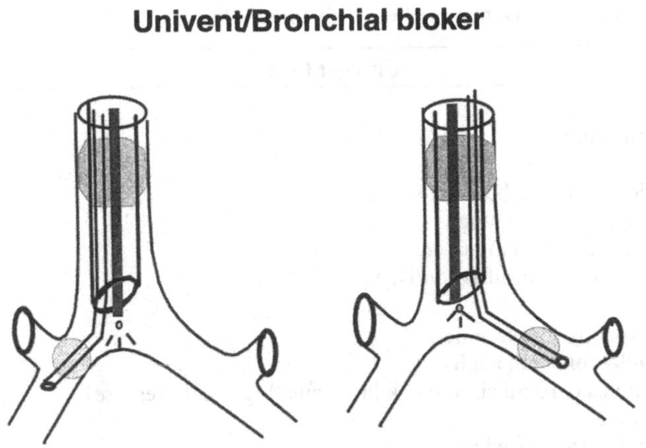

Fig. 3. Positioning of the Univent tube in the right and left main bronchus

so possible to suction through the blocker lumen or to apply continuous positive airway pressure to improve oxygenation in case of hypoxia. The disadvantages of the tube are: the enteral diameter is relatively large, the blocker can dislocate during surgical manipulation, and satisfactory bronchial seal and lung separation are sometimes hard to achieve. Finally, the relatively small diameter of the blocker lumen makes it more difficult to remove secretion (Table 1).

The use of a BB

An independently passed BB may be used in conjunction with a SLT to obtain lung isolation or OLV, thereby avoiding the use of a difficult tube in a patient with a difficult airway. The most commonly used independent BB is a Fogarty embolectomy catheter, which has occlusion balloons that range in size from 3 to 6 ml [11]. In brief, the technique sequentially consists of passing a FOB through a bronchoscopy elbow down a SLT, visualizing the carina, passing the Fogarty BB into the appropriate mainstem bronchus, and withdrawing the FOB. As with airway guides, the anticipated materials (FOB, Fogarty catheter, and SLT) must be tested in advance, in vitro, for compatibility of fit and ability to maintain continuous ventilation during placement. Also, the Fogarty occlusion catheter comes with a wire stylet in place and the wire stylet must be curved at the distal end into a hockey stick shape before passage through the bronchoscopy elbow and down the SLT.

Several limitations to the use of BB are: the difficulty to direct the BB into the desired bronchus even with the help of FB and the inability to effectively suction the airways distal to the blockers. Finally, during the surgical manipulation the BB may inadvertently slips into the trachea causing a life-threatening

Table 1. Advantages and disadvantages of the Univent tube/blocker

Univent tube
Advantages
– it is a single-lumen tube
– reintubation is unnecessary
– can block whole lung or a lobe/segment
– can be used for right and left lung
– blockers tubes contain a 2-mm lumen suction/CPAP/oxygen insufflation/HFV
Disadvantages
– requires bronchoscopy for placement
– too large and bulky for small adults
– blocker cuff requires 6-10 ml air to block bronchus (high cuff pressure)
– relatively expensive
– not ideal for right-sided procedures
– blocker may dislocate
– slow lung collapse by absorption
– *not recommended for absolute indication*

(*CPAP* continuous positive airway pressure, *HFV* high frequency ventilation)

airway obstruction. Attempts to overcome these problems were made by developing a snare-guided bronchial blocker (Cook, Bloomington, Ind., USA). The FB is passed through the loop and guided into the desired bronchus, then the BB is slid over the FB into the selected bronchus. Bronchoscopic visualization confirms blocker placement and occlusion. The string may than be removed and a 1.8-mm lumen may be used as a suction port or for oxygen insufflation. The disadvantage of this device is the high cost and the inability to reinsert the string once it has been pulled out, losing the ability to redirect the BB if necessary. Finally, the external diameter is somewhat larger and requires a large-size SLT (at least 8.0 mm) to be able to accommodate the BB.

The SLT was not successfully placed with FOB

If one cannot place a SLT with the aid of a FOB, and the patient's condition is stable, the clinician may use some alternative devices to assist in placement of the SLT. There are several commercially available laryngoscopes that can facilitate endobronchial intubation. (It is beyond the purpose of this manuscript to provide a detailed description of these devices). The two best-known are the Bullard laryngoscope (Circon, ACMI, Stamford, Conn., USA) [12, 13] and the Wu laryngoscope (Achi, Dublin, Calif., USA) [14, 15]. The Bullard laryngoscope is an anatomically shaped, rigid instrument that uses a fiberoptic bundle to obtain an indirect view of the larynx. Thus, the oral, pharyngeal, and tracheal axes do not have to be aligned to view the larynx. The Wu laryngoscope uses a similar concept but consists of a rigid blade portion and a separate flexible fiberoptic portion [16]. Clinician preference and experience play a major role in the degree of successful intubation. Successful use of these devices requires a relatively lengthy learning curve, and the time to first practice the use of these scopes is not when faced with a difficult airway. The LMA Fastrach (Laryngeal Airway Mask, Gensia, San Diego, Calif., USA) a new version of the conventional LMA, is commercially available and is a reasonable alternative. First, it allows ventilation of the patient during the airway manipulation and second, this new form of the LMA permits an insertion of a large-diameter SLT (8.0 mm). For a successful intubation using this device, experience plays an important role. In addition, unlike the conventional LMA, only a special SLT provided by the manufacturer as part of the LMA Fastrach package may be used. Finally, the conventional LMA can always be used for fiberoptic intubation through the LMA lumen [17, 18]. In rare cases, when none of these methods results in a successful endotracheal intubation, the plan to perform the procedure should be reevaluated. If a "cannot ventilate cannot intubate" situation develops, a Combitube (Kendall Sheridan Catheter, Argyl, N.Y., USA) can be inserted to allow ventilation [19].

Conclusion of the procedure

Depending on the extent and the length of the procedure, and the degree of fluid shift, an airway, initially not classified as difficult, may become difficult secondary to facial edema, secretion, and laryngeal trauma from the initial intubation. In these cases, when planning to provide lung separation, the postoperative period should be considered and the appropriate tube should be placed. Many procedures not considered to be absolute indications for lung separation, are lengthy and complex. For example, complex lung resection with or without chest wall resection, thoraco-abdominal esophagogastrectomy, thoracic aortic aneurysm resection with or without total circulatory arrest, or an extensive vertebral tumour resection, may result in facial edema, secretion, and hemoptysis that will require postoperative ventilatory support. Other indications for postoperative ventilatory support are marginal respiratory reserve, unexpected blood loss, or fluid shift, hypothermia, and inadequate reversal of muscle paralysis.

If a Univent tube was used to provide OLV, the BB may be fully retracted and the Univent tube can serve as a SLT. If an independent BB was used, then the BB is removed to leave the SLT in place (Fig. 4). The problem arises when a DLT was inserted for OLV. With a difficult airway and facial edema, DLT may be left in place. If the decision to leave the DLT in place is made, it is important to bear in mind that the ICU staff is generally less experienced in managing a DLT, which may easily dislocate. If the DLT is left in the endobronchial position, then the patient should be paralyzed to avoid malposition of the DLT. Another possibility is to withdrawn the DLT to the 19 to 20-cm mark, so that the

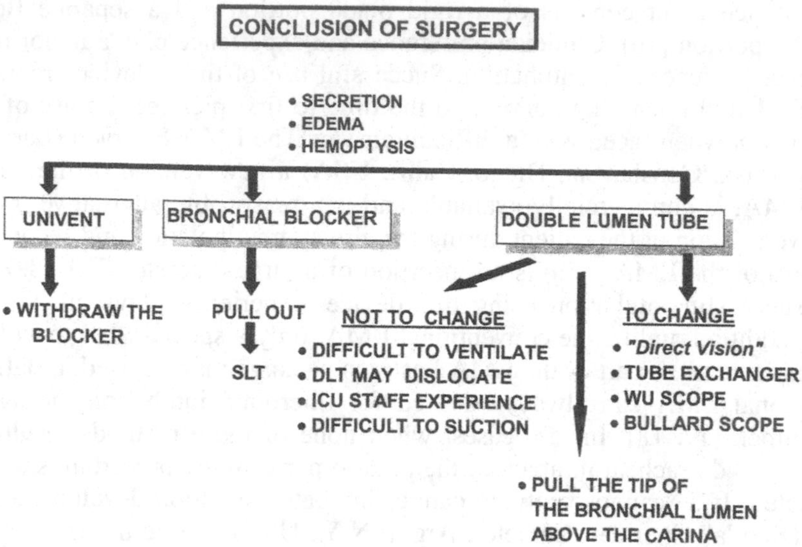

Fig. 4. The conclusion of surgery: a reasonable approach for the conclusion of the procedure (*SLT* single-lumen tube, *ICU* intensive care unit)

endobronchial lumen is supracarinal, and ventilate both lungs through both lumens. In addition, it is more difficult to suction thorough the DLT lumen and a longer suction catheter is needed to reach the tip of the endobronchial lumen. Extubation directly from the DLT should be considered following diuresis and steroid therapy to allow reduction of the facial edema. If the decision to change the DLT to SLT is made, it should not be accomplished blindly. A tube exchanger should invariably be used to conserve access to the airways, as discussed above. The exchange of the tubes may be performed under direct vision using a Bullard or the Wu scope. With these scopes the tube exchanger or a stylet can be placed under vision through the vocal cords alongside the existing tube to allow passing a SLT over.

In summary, the clinician should be able to master different methods of lung separation and make him-herself familiar with the available devices to provide OLV and optimal, safe management of the patient. In addition, one should plan in advance for the postoperative period when choosing the methods of lung separation. Finally, in these cases, a close dialogue with the surgical team is of vital importance.

References

1. Cohen E, Benumof J (1999) Lung separation in the patient with a difficult airway. Curr Opin Anesthesiol 12:29-35
2. Rau B, Huneerbein M, Below C et al (1998) Video-assisted thoracic surgery. Staging and management of thoracic tumors. Surg Endosc 12:133-136
3. Benumof J (1998) Difficult tubes and difficult airways. J Cardiothorac Vasc Anesth 12: 131-132
4. Taylor PA, Towey RM (1972) The broncho-fiberscope as an aid to endotracheal intubation. Br J Anaesth 44:611-612
5. Ransom ES, Carter SL, Mund GD (1995) Univent tube: a useful device in patients with difficult airways. J Cardiothoracic Vasc Anesth 9:725-727
6. Patane PS, Shell BA, Mahla ME (1990) Awake fiberoptic endobronchial intubation. J Cardiothorac Anesth 4:229-231
7. Baraka A (1996) The Univent tube can facilitate difficult intubation in a patient undergoing thoracoscopy. J Cardiothorac Vasc Anesth 10:693-694
8. Hagihira S, Takshina M, Mori T et al (1998) One lung ventilation patients with difficult airways. J Cardiothorac Anesth 12:186-188
9. DeLima L, Bishop M (1991) Lung laceration after tracheal extubation over a plastic tube changer. Anesth Analg 73:350-351
10. Seitz PA, Gravenstein N (1989) Endobronchial rupture from endotracheal reintubation with an endotracheal tube guide. J Clin Anesth 1:214-217
11. Benumof JL, Gaughan SD (1992) Concerns regarding barotrauma during jet ventilation. Anesthesiology 76:1072-1073
12. Ginsberg RJ (1981) New technique for one-lung anesthesia using an endobronchial blocker. J Thorac Cardiovasc Surg 8:542-546
13. Baraka A, Muallem M, Sibai AN (1991) Facilitation of difficult tracheal intubation by the fiberoptic bullard laryngoscope. Middle East J Anesthesiol 11:73-77
14. Watts AD, Gelb AW, Rach DB et al (1997) Comparison of Bullard and Macintosh laryngoscopes for endobronchial intubation of patients with a partial cervical spine injury. Anesthesiology 87:1335-1342
15. Wu T, Chou H (1994) A new laryngoscope: the combination intubating device. Anesthesiology 81:1085
16. O'Neill D, Capan L, Sheth R (1998) Flexiguide intubation guide to facilitate airway management with WuScope system. Anesthesiology 89:454
17. Joshi S, Sciacca R, Young W et al (1998) A prospective evaluation of clinical tests for placement of laryngeal mask airways. Anesthesiology 89:114-116
18. Verghese C, Berlet J, Kapila A et al (1998) Clinical assessment of the single use laryngeal mask airway – the LMA Unique. Br J Anaesth 80:677-679
19. Bishop M, Kharasch E (1998) Is combitube a useful emergency airway device for anesthesiologists? Anesth Analg 86:1141-1142

Use of Alternative Techniques in a Difficult Tracheal Intubation

F. AGRÒ, R. CATALDO, G. BARZOI

Difficulty in managing the airways is the single most-important cause of major anesthesia-related morbidity and mortality [1]. In clinical practice, difficult intubation often corresponds to a difficult laryngoscopy, defined as failure to visualize the larynx after neck flexion and external cricoid pressure [2]. It occurs in 1.5 to 8.5% of general anesthetics [3].

In 91.9% of difficult intubations, the clinician can visualize at laryngoscopy only the epiglottis [4]. Cormack and Lehane [5] defined this kind of view as a grade 3. The gold standard for airway management is the tracheal intubation, there are, however, situations in which tracheal intubation cannot be performed because of difficulties with direct laryngoscopy. A good anesthetic examination may allow anticipation of 98% of difficult intubations [2]; in these cases it is possible to perform fiberoptic techniques (fiberoptic scope, Bullard laryngoscopy, etc.), which may be helpful to solve the problem.

Greater problems occur when the difficult tracheal intubation cannot be predicted (1-3.5%) [3] or in an emergency, when a fiberoptic scope may be not available and/or the medical team cannot use it properly, or when a lot of blood and secretions do not allow a good view.

In order to minimize the possibilities of failure, it is important that the anesthesiologist has a wide range of solutions to deal successfully with unpredicted or predicted difficult intubations. The use of alternative devices of low cost, easily available and transportable, which require simple materials and permit immediate intervention in in- and out- patient emergency cases, increase the possibility of success.

Trachlight and direct laryngoscopy

The gum elastic bougie (GEB), or Eschmann tracheal tube introducer, is commonly used in anesthetic practice in cases of difficult airways. It is the favored aid used in the United Kingdom and several authors recommend using the GEB whenever a good view of the glottis cannot be immediately obtained [6-9].

Several anesthesiologists have tested the efficacy of the GEB in association with direct laryngoscopy and some consider the success rate of intubation with the GEB is higher than with the stylet, whenever a difficult airway is encountered [10-15].

Although tracheal intubation with GEB may be helped by clicks, hold up sign, and capnography [8, 12], it may be considered a blind technique whose success rate depends on the clinician's skill, ability, and experience.

In 1957, Macintosh [16] described a lighted stylet as an aid to intubation, and the device was claimed to combine the best features of a rigid metal and a gum elastic introducer. Since 1957 many authors have published studies [17-21] on possible advantages and uses of the lighted stylet and technical progress has created more-sophisticated and easier to use devices. The transillumination is based on the principle that a source of light brought into the trachea results in clearly visible and defined transcutaneous illumination, while no illumination can be observed with the light source in the esophagus [22]. A lightwand uses the principle of transillumination of the soft tissues of the anterior neck to guide the tip of the endotracheal tube (ET) into the trachea. It also takes advantage of the anterior (superficial) location of the trachea relative to the esophagus.

The Trachlight is the latest lighted stylet [23], it consists of three parts: a reusable handle, a flexible wand, and a stiff, retractable stylet. The light emitted by the Trachlight is extremely bright, with minimal heat production. After 30 s of illumination, the lightbulb blinks to minimize heat production and avoid extended intubations. The Trachlight is prepared with the lighted stylet passing into the tracheal tube (TL-ETT), so that the mark 19 of the stylet corresponded to 19 cm of the tube. Then it is bent like a hockey stick and inserted with the dominant hand. An unclear and ill-defined transillumination means that the tip of the TL-ETT is in the hypopharynx or at the beginning of the esophagus.

If the tip of the TL-ETT is in the rear of the tongue (in the glosso-epiglottic fold), intubation is impossible. This situation may commonly occur when the Trachlight is used alone.

Hung et al. [23] described a combined use of Trachlight (TL) and direct laryngoscopy (DL) (use of TL in case of unsuccessful intubation with DL and use of DL in case of unsuccessful intubation with TL). Biehl threaded a particular lighted stylet (Tube Stat) through the Murphy's hole of the ET [24].

We are performing a study to evaluate a combined technique of DL and lighted stylet to manage difficult airways. We have enrolled 188 patients to date, scheduled for elective surgery requiring tracheal intubation. After performing a DL, we simulate a Cormack grade 3. A lighted stylet (Trachlight) is bent as a hockey stick and an ET is mounted on it. While laryngoscopy is performed, the Trachlight is placed and tracheal intubation is attempted only when the neck transillumination is correct. In 138 patients (73.4%), tracheal intubation was obtained at the first attempt; in 34 patients (18.1%) tracheal intubation was performed at the second attempt; in 16 patients (8.5%) tracheal intubation was successful at the third attempt. At present all patients have been intubated with the combined technique without complications. The esophagus was never intubated because the intubation was never attempted without seeing a clear and well-defined glow.

In our opinion the lighted stylet using the property of the transillumination of the neck may be a good solution to guide the ET into the trachea in cases of difficult laryngoscopy.

The GEB is commonly used in the United Kingdom. In other countries, it is not always available and some clinicians are not able to use it. With the combined technique, we obtained a success rate of 91.5% at the second attempt. However, this rate is lower than that of the GEB [17], and is higher than that of the rigid stylet [17]. At the third attempt (within 45 s), we obtained a success rate of 100%.

The DL+TL technique enables intubation to be accomplished without the need for feeling clicks and hold up. Moreover, it reduces the risk of esophageal intubation and it may be useful in the emergency room or in all cases of unanticipated difficult intubations, as well as in outpatients' emergency, since it does not require any particular equipment.

In conclusion, the combined technique (DL+TL) may be a valid alternative in managing unanticipated difficult intubations whenever the fiberscope is not readily available or its use is technically impossible (blood and/or a lot of secretions, emergency) or the GEB is not a feasible choice (unskilled clinician, device not available).

Cuffed oropharyngeal airway as an aid for tracheal intubation

The laryngeal mask airway (LMA) has been used as a guide for blind intubation or with the aid of a lightwand [25]. This technique has varied success (19-93%), which depends on experience and the use of an adequate-size LMA that offers correct alignment with the laryngeal inlet. Fiberoptic-guided intubation via the LMA has a higher success rate (96%), but the equipment is not always available. The Trachlight may also be used to facilitate tracheal intubation with a semi-blind technique via LMA or LMA Fastrach [26]. In our department we have studied a new technique using the cuffed oropharyngeal airway (COPA) and a lightwand as an aid for tracheal intubation. The COPA was first described by Greenberg et al. [27, 28], as an airway for the spontaneously breathing patient during anesthesia. The device is a modified Guedel airway with an inflatable distal cuff and a proximal 15-mm connector for the breathing circuit. The cuff is inflated through a one-way valve and a pilot balloon that emerges from the COPA tube at the flange. The flange at the proximal end is fitted with two posts for a securing strap, which is used to stabilize the device at the mouth against the upper teeth or gums. The COPA is available in four sizes: 8, 9, 10, and 11 (the distance between the flange and the distal tip measured in millimeters). It is inserted as a Guedel, with a rotating movement. When inflated, the cuff is broad and flattened posteriorly, with a pointed shape more anteriorly. The COPA lies just above the vocal cords, allowing ventilation during intubation with the fiberscope.

We verified the usefulness of the COPA as a device to guide a tracheal tube using a semiblind technique with a lightwand (Agrò et al. submitted for publication). Ten anesthetized patients undergoing elective surgery were analyzed. We selected and positioned a correct size of COPA for each patient. A lightwand (Trachlight) was then inserted into the COPA to confirm correct placement of this device. The lightwand was then removed and the first portion of a Patil's tube exchanger (TE) was inserted and connected by a 15-mm connector with the breathing circuit, and its position was confirmed by end-tidal CO_2 values during ventilation. Patients were then paralyzed and ventilation through the first portion of the TE reconfirmed. The COPA was removed, and the second portion of TE was connected and used as a guide for a tracheal intubation. This combined technique had a success rate of 6 of 10 patients and could be used for airway management if a fiberscope or other device such as a Combitube, LMA, or LMA Fastrach was not available.

Adequate sedation of the patient is necessary to prevent the physiological responses induced during this procedure. It is important not to precipitate laryngeal spasm, vocal cord closure, or laryngeal movement. In all patients hemodynamic parameters remained stable. Hence, this technique may be suitable for patients with pre-existing hypertension, cardiovascular disease, or head injuries.

The COPA is a useful device that also allows patient ventilation with a self-inflating bag. We suggest that it has a potential role in first aid, because it is easy to position. Moreover, it does not require the use of mioresolution. The semiblind tracheal intubation technique using a COPA (with previous Trachlight test) and TE or other device, such as a GEB, may be a satisfactory alternative when an anesthetist is not able to secure the airway with direct laryngoscopy or when other devices such as fiberoptic intubating laryngoscope [30] or the Aintree intubation catheter [29] are not available.

It is most important to choose the correct size of COPA to permit alignment with the laryngeal inlet. The COPA cuff was designed so that, when inflated, it displaces the base of the tongue, forming an airtight seal with the pharynx and elevating the epiglottis from the posterior pharyngeal wall, and providing a clear airway. The patient may be ventilated, but intubation is not possible if the COPA is not precisely aligned with the laryngeal inlet. We think that this alignment is related to the COPA length, as well as to the cuff volume. The results of this study seem to suggest that it is a simple, atraumatic technique, which requires only a short period of training.

The dental mirror technique

The "dental mirror technique" is a new method, which may be used in all these cases; it was first described by Patil et al. [31] as an aid to tracheal intubation in a 2.5-month-old full-term infant, instead of DL. Recently, Gabhash [32] described the technique as an aid to see the tube between the vocal cords and to determine quickly the probable presence of the tube in the esophagus.

Esophageal intubation occurs in 5% of children and 6% of adults. "Dental mirror" allows a reduction in morbidity due to undetected tracheal tube misplacement (27% of predicted difficult intubations) [33].

Good manual dexterity is necessary to use this device in every unpredicted difficult airway situation and in respiratory emergencies, where orotracheal intubation is imperative. This ability may be first acquired with manikins and/or cadavers, and then in patients (ASA 1-2, Cormack-Lehane grade 1-2) undergoing elective surgery.

A mirror, like the ones for indirect laryngoscopy, previously warmed to avoid dimming, is placed with the dominant hand in the oropharynx in front of the uvula, with a downward angle of inclination of 40-50°. In this way the anesthesiologist can see the larynx and the vocal cords.

In the mirror image, the anterior commissure of the larynx is visible on the upper part of the mirror. In order to keep the mirror steady, the handle is held by the thumb of the hand performing the laryngoscopy against the oropharynx. The anesthesiologist uses a two-part intubation catheter (TE., 18 F Ø and 63 cm long, produced by Cook), which is formed by an intubation part and an extension part. Thanks to the mirror image of the vocal cords, the intubation part of the catheter is placed in front of the mirror, with the stylet curved so that it coincided with the curve of the laryngoscope blade. The anesthesiologist advances the catheter into the trachea while an assistant removes the stylet. The intubation catheter is then connected by a 15-mm adapter to an anesthesia circuit, so its position is confirmed by ventilation. Finally, the extension part is connected to the intubation part and an ET (7.5 mm Ø in female and 8 mm Ø in males) is threaded over the TE and the latter is then removed.

When properly learned, the technique allows us to approach: 1) cases of unpredicted difficult orotracheal intubation (Cormack-Lehane grade 2-3); 2) cases of suspected cervical fracture (when it is not possible to align mouth-pharynx-larynx axis), if a fiberoptic scope is not available; 3) cases where the view of "aditus ad laringem" is not possible for anatomical reasons (high and anterior glottis).

We have studied ten patients, three males and seven females, simulating a Cormack-Lehane grade 3, during DL [34]. The preliminary findings indicate that the technique is easy to use, reliable, cheap, with a short learning curve, and readily available. It is not possible to use it in patients with Cormack-Lehane grade 4 and an interincisor gap < 2 cm, because DL cannot be performed, as well as when there is a dimming of the mirror or the presence of blood and secretions. Furthermore, the clinician's skill is fundamental for performing this technique.

Magnetic intubation

A potential aid in airway management, especially in emergencies, is represented by the use of magnetic orotracheal intubation. This technique was described by Patil et al. [35] in a study carried out on 40 selected elective surgery patients. It has shown great potential as a possible alternative technique to simple DL. In order to successfully apply this technique in difficult intubations, it is important to have acquired experience and skill during theoretical and practical training, first on manikins, then in selected cases (ASA I/II), without predictive indexes for difficult tracheal intubation (Mallampati grade I/II). This technique may be very useful in unpredicted difficult intubations due to anatomical alterations (high and anterior glottis), or in the presence of blood, edema, and/or secretions.

After placing the patient in the sniffing position, the anesthesiologist performs a DL. An assistant places a cobalt magnet (approximately 2 cm x 2 cm x 1cm, 6 oz in weight) in the midline over the thyroid cartilage; the thyroid surface of the magnet is concave to fit the physiological anatomical convexity in the neck.

The anesthesiologist uses a two-part translucent 18-Fr intubation catheter (produced by Cook) reinforced by a metallic stylet. The intubation part of this catheter, 30 cm long, is inserted blindly behind the epiglottis in order to allow the magnet to pull the stylet and the catheter close to the glottic opening. When the anesthesiologist feels the magnetic attraction, (i.e., the catheter with the stylet is maintained in the midline by the magnet), the catheter is threaded over the stylet into the trachea and the stylet is removed. The intubation catheter is then connected by a 15-mm adapter to an anesthesia circuit, to confirm its position by the auscultation of the chest and by measuring the end-tidal CO_2. The adapter is removed, the first catheter extended with an extension part (30 cm long), and used as a guide to insert the ET (7.5 mm Ø in females and 8 mm Ø in males) into the trachea. The proper position of the ET is confirmed by auscultation of the chest and capnography. Magnetic intubation seems to be a safe, reliable technique, with a wide range of applications and a low cost [36]. This technique uses a device that is readily available and easily portable, so that it may also be used outside of the hospital (ambulance, helicopter). Finally, it is a fast and simple procedure, which requires a short training.

It is important to remember that the presence of a pacemaker (either in the patient or in the clinician) is an absolute contraindication for the use of this technique. Other limiting factors include Cormack-Lehane grade 4 and an inter-incisor gap < 2 cm, because DL cannot be performed.

Conclusion

When a difficult intubation is anticipated, it is necessary to have equipment immediately available and intubation is preferably achieved with the patient consciuos and with a fiberscope. Alternative devices may be used when a difficult intubation is not anticipated, especially in an emergency or for outpatients.

References

1. Benumof JL (1991) Management of the difficult adult airways. With special emphasis on awake tracheal intubation. Anesthesiology 75:1087-1110
2. Latto IP (1997) Difficult intubation. In: Latto IP, Vaughan RS (eds) Difficulties in tracheal intubation. Saunders, Philadelphia
3. Crosby ET, Cooper RM, Douglas MJ et al (1998) The unanticipated difficult airways with recommendations for management. Can J Anaesth 45:757-776
4. Koay CK (1998) Difficult tracheal intubation-analysis and management in 37 cases. Singapore Med J 39:112-114
5. Cormack RS, Lehane J (1984) Difficult tracheal intubation in obstetrics. Anaesthesia 39: 1105-1111
6. Sofferman RA, Johnson DL, Spencer RF (1997) Lost airways during anesthesia induction: alternatives for management. Laryngoscope 107:1476-1482
7. Nocera A (1996) A flexible solution for emergency intubation difficulties. Ann Emerg Med 27:665-667
8. Williamson JA (1993) The Australian incident monitoring study. Difficult intubation: an analysis of 2000 incident reports. Anaesth Intensive Care 21:602-607
9. Nolan JP, Wilson ME (1993) Orotracheal intubation in patients with potential cervical spine injuries. An indication for the gum elastic bougie. Anaesthesia 48:630-633
10. Nolan JP, Wilson ME (1992) An evaluation of the gum elastic bougie. Intubation times and incidence of sore throat. Anaesthesia 47:878-881
11. Dogra S, Falconer R, Latto IP (1990) Successful difficult intubation. Tracheal tube placement over a gum-elastic bougie. Anaesthesia 45:774-776
12. Kidd JF, Dyson A, Latto IP (1988) Successful difficult intubation. Use of the gum elastic bougie. Anaesthesia 43:822
13. Gataure PS, Vaughan RS, Latto IP (1996) Simulated difficult intubation. Comparison of the gum elastic bougie and the stylet. Anaesthesia 51:935-938
14. Mackersie AM (1997) Comparison of the gum elastic bougie and the stylet. Anaesthesia 52:396
15. Benumof JL (1997) Comparison of the gum elastic bougie and the stylet. Anaesthesia 52: 385-386
16. Macintosh RR (1957) Illuminated introducer for endotracheal tubes. Anaesthesia 12:223
17. Yamamura H (1959) Device for blind nasal intubation. Anesthesiology 20:221
18. Ducrow M (1978) Throwing light on blind intubation. Anaesthesia 33:827-829
19. Vollmer TP, Stewart RD, Paris PM et al (1985) Use of a lighted stylet for guided orotracheal intubation in the prehospital setting. Ann Emerg Med 14:324-328
20. Ellis DG, Stewart RD, Kaplan RM et al (1986) Success rate of blind orotracheal intubation using a transillumination technique with lighted stylet. Ann Emerg Med 15:138-142
21. Ellis DG, Jakymec A, Kaplan RM et al (1986) Guided orotracheal intubation in the operating room using a lighted stylet: a comparison with direct laryngoscopy technique. Anesthesiology 64:823
22. Lipp M, De Rossi L, Daublander M, Thierbach A (1996) The transillumination technique. An alternative to conventional intubation? Anaesthesist 45:923-930

23. Hung OR, Pytka S, Morris I et al (1995) Clinical trial of a new lightwand device (Trachlight) to intubate the trachea. Anesthesiology 83:509-514
24. Biehl JW, Bourke DL (1997) Use of the lighted stylet to aid direct laryngoscopy. Anesthesiology 86:1012
25. Agrò F, Brimacombe J, Carassiti M et al (1998) Lighted stylet as an aid to blind tracheal intubation via the LMA. J Clin Anesth 10:263-264
26. Agrò F, Brimacombe J, Carassiti M et al (1998) Use of a lighted stylet for intubation via laryngeal mask airway. Can J Anaesth 45:556-560
27. Greenberg RS, Toung T (1992) The cuffed oropharyngeal airway – a pilot study. Anaesthesiology 77:A558
28. Greenberg RS, Brimacombe J, Berry A et al (1998) A randomized controlled trial comparing the cuffed oropharyngeal airway and the laryngeal mask airway in spontaneously breathing anaesthetized adults. Anaesthesiology 88:970-977
29. Greenberg RS (1999) Cuffed oropharyngeal airway (COPA) as an adjunct to fibreoptic tracheal intubation. Br J Anaesth 82:395-398
30. Hawkins M, O'Sullivan E, Charters P (1998) Fibreoptic intubation using the cuffed oropharyngeal airway and Aintree intubation catheter. Anaesthesia 53:891-894
31. Patil VU, Sopchak AM, Thomas PS (1993) Use of a dental mirror as an aid to tracheal intubation in an infant. Anaesthesiology 78:619-620
32. Gabash MB (1997) Use of the mirror of indirect laryngoscopy for detection of esophageal intubation. Acta Anaesthesiol Scand 41:950
33. Morray JP (1993) A comparison of paediatric and adult anaesthesia closed malpractice claims. Anesthesiology 78:461
34. Agrò F, Cataldo R, Antonelli S et al (1999) Tracheal intubation with the aid of a "dental mirror". Resuscitation 42:247-250
35. Patil V, Buckingham T, Willoughby P et al (1994) Magnetic orotracheal intubation: a new technique. Anesth Analg 78:749-752
36. Agrò F, Cataldo R, Mattei A et al (1999) Tracheal intubation with the aid of a magnet. Resuscitation 42:73-75

Outcome of Patients Treated with Non-Invasive Ventilation in Intensive Care Unit

G. CONTI, I. MONTEFERRANTE, R. MAVIGLIA

Mechanical ventilation by endotracheal tube (ETT) is an accepted, lifesaving procedure for patients with acute respiratory failure, after the failure of conventional therapy with oxygen and drugs. However, the presense of an ETT affects the defence mechanisms against airway infection, increasing the risk of complications such as pneumonia and sinusitis. Moreover, endotracheal intubation is an invasive procedure that causes complications and morbidity, and can worsen the condition of the critically ill patients. Sedation or anesthesia may be needed, with further potential adverse effects. For example, endotracheal intubation can damage the airway mucosa causing ulceration, inflammation or edema, submucosal hemorrhage, and may result in life-threatening complications such as airway stenosis [1, 2].

Non-invasive ventilation (NIV) with nasal or face masks is a valuable approach, because it can reduce patient discomfort, complications, and damage caused by the ETT. NIV can also be used early in the treatment of the exacerbation, and allows the maintenance of speech and swallowing reflexes, with psychological advantages and the preservation of airway defense mechanisms.

NIV in patients with exacerbations of chronic obstructive pulmonary disease

The main mechanism causing respiratory failure in patients with obstructive lung disease is dynamic hyperinflation, which occurs with increased airway resistance, preventing complete expiration before the onset of the next inspiratory effort. Dynamic hyperinflation alters diaphragm shape, reducing its strength and endurance. A small further increase in airflow resistance (from increased airway secretions or bronchospasm) or an increase in ventilatory demand (from fever or infection) can cause respiratory muscle fatigue, producing rapid shallow breathing with wasted ventilation, hypercapnia, and respiratory acidosis. The work of breathing has to increase to overcome the threshold load at the start of inspiration represented by auto-positive endexpiratory pressure (PEEP), and also to increase the tidal volume when airway resistance is severely increased.

NIV can be used to overcome the cause of the increase in work of breathing: the combination of PEEP and positive pressure ventilation or pressure support ventilation can offset the auto-PEEP level (thus eliminating this inspiratory additional load) and reduce the work that the inspiratory muscles must perform to produce the tidal volume. When appropiate levels of inspiratory pressure are administered, tidal volume increases and respiratory rate decreases. Under these conditions NIV can rapidly reduce $paCO_2$, and restore normal values of pH [3]. Brochard et al. [3] showed that NIV can reduce diaphragmatic electromyographic activity.

It is important to realize when treating such patients that the level of external PEEP must never exceed the amount of auto-PEEP, to avoid an iatrogenic increase of hyperinflation. When values of external PEEP equivalent to 80% of the auto-PEEP are administered with face-mask ventilation, no change of end-expiratory volume occurs [4].

Methods of applications

NIV can be administered to chronic obstructive pulmonary disease (COPD) patients both with nasal and full-face masks. A nasal mask is usually well-tolerated as it causes less claustrophobia and discomfort, and it allows eating, drinking, and expectorating; however, it offers fewer advantages in patients with severe acute respiratory failure who normally breathe through the mouth and are less co-operative.

A full-face mask increases dead-space (this can be partially solved with specific space-reducers), is less well-tolerated but has fewer airleaks, and should be used in patients affected by severe decompensation, or when the nasal mask has failed.

Masks are usually fixed to the patient with elastic headbands, to obtain a close and continuous fit on the skin surface: this is crucial to avoid airleaks and problems with trigger function, but can cause skin necrosis. In our experience skin necrosis occurs in 15% of COPD patients treated with NIV for more than 72 h; however, after discontinuation of NIV, the skin lesions heal rapidly, usually in 7-10 days.

These lesions can be reduced by placing adhesive dressings on points of major pressure (usually the bridge of the nose) to increase the surface for pressure dissipation and reduce the depth of skin necrosis. Gastric distension during NIV is not a common complication: when a full-face mask is used, gastric distension occurs only when the opening pressure of the upper esophageal sphincter is overcome: this pressure, usually greater than 25-30 cm H_2O [5], is rarely reached in COPD patients, particularly during non-invasive pressure support ventilation (NIPSV). Some masks allow the passage of a nasogastric tube, which protects from the risk of aerophagia, even at pressures $\geq$ 25 cm H_2O.

Assisted mechanical ventilation can be easily applied through a face mask in COPD patients, but the present trend is to use pressure support ventilation, which is more comfortable and causes fewer complications [6]. When NIV is applied, the PEEP is generally set at 3-5 cm H_2O, in order to offset auto-PEEP, at least in part, and the pressure support started at 10-12 cm H_2O. The mask is placed comfortably on the patient's face, and only after a few breaths is it then secured with a progressive increase of the fit, avoiding excessive facial pressure; when no leaks are present, the level of pressure support is increased to obtain a respiratory rate less than 30 breaths/min with a tidal volume of at least 7 ml/kg. FfiOz is set to obtain $SaO_2 > 90\%$ and the trigger is set at -1 cm H_2O, with a peak pressure below 25 cm H_2O.

Ventilator setting during NIV

The criteria of NIV delivery depend upon the severity of the disease: if NIV is applied early in respiratory failure, it is generally possible to discontinue it for periods of 10-20 min, after an initial period of continuous administration (3-6 h, in our experience). When patients are sicker, NIV is continuously applied for 12-24 h and stopping for very short periods is only allowed when the clinical conditition starts to improve.

Clinical response is assessed in terms of gas exchange, pH, respiratory rate, and mental status; when steady improvement is present, short periods of stopping NIV can be progressively increased. Aggressive physiotherapy is crucial during the periods of NIV discontinuation. Needless to say, facilities for immediate endotracheal intubation must always be available.

Clinical outcome

In one of the first papers on NIV use in intensive care units (ICU) [7], good results were obtained in a small number of COPD patients, suggesting that endotracheal intubation could be avoided. In a case-control study, Brochard et al. [3] suggested that this approach could reduce both the need for endotracheal intubation and the time of hospital stay, with economic advantages.

In the first randomized, prospective study, Bott et al. [8] compared NIV with conventional treatment in 60 COPD patients with acute respiratory failure. NIV was given by nasal mask; this group had a significant reduction in $paCO_2$ and dyspnea score, and the survival rate was significantly greater in the group treated with NIV (90% vs. 70%, $p < 0.01$).

The efficacy of NIV in patients with an acute exacerbation of COPD has been recently investigated in a European prospective randomized multicenter study, co-ordinated by Brochard [9]. In this study we evaluated 85 COPD patients, and excluded cardiogenic pulmonary edema, pneumonia and postoperative acute respiratory failure patients. Patients were randomly assigned to receive conventional treatment (i.e., oxygen therapy plus drugs) or conventional treatment plus NIV (set at initial value of 20 cm H_2O, ZEEP). NIV significantly improved gas exchange within 1 h of treatment. The patients assigned to NIV had a significantly lower a intubation rate (26% vs. 74%, $p < 0.001$), a lower complication rate (14% vs. 45%, $p < 0.01$), shorter hospital stay (23 ± 17 vs. 35 ± 33, $p < 0.02$), and reduced mortality rate (9% vs. 29%, $p < 0.02$). NIV was applied for a mean duration of 4 ± 4 days. It is interesting that the mortality rate was similar for intubated patients from both groups (27% vs. 32%).

Kramer et al. [10] assessed NIV by nasal mask in 26 COPD patients, randomly comparing NIV with conventional treatment. Despite a slow reduction in $paCO_2$, not significantly different in the control group, the authors reported a significant reduction in intubation rate, with a significant and stable improvement in paO_2, heart rate, and respiratory rate in the NIV group. Lofaso et al. [11] showed that CO_2 rebreathing could occur with BiPAP ventilators when PEEP is not used or when the expiratory time is too short. This can partially explain the limited paCO changes noted by Kramer et al. [10].

NIV contraindications

Although NIV is a useful alternative to conventional mechanical ventilation in the ICU setting, it is not entirely free from contraindications. NIV should be particularly avoided in patients with cardiovascular instability such as hypotension and/or life-threatening arrhythmia, in patients with severely impaired mental status, who require an ETT to protect the airways from aspiration (e.g., coma, absent cough reflexes, acute abdominal disease with septic encephalopathy and abdominal distension, impaired swallowing reflexes, or impaired respiratory drive), and in patients with facial deformities or recent surgery of the face and neck. Pneumonia or recent myocardial infarction should not be considered as a formal contraindication for NIV, but these patients do not do so well and require high levels of positive pressure [12, 13]. In our experience, treatment with NIV is not contraindicated in patients who are edentulous or who have a beard, although fitting the facial mask is more difficult. In these circumstances, a nasal mask should bc considered first.

NIV in patients with hypoxemic acute respiratory failure

Because good results were obtained in patients with acute exacerbations of COPD, NIV is now being assessed as a more-simple alternative to conventional ventilation with an ETT in patients with hypoxemic acute respiratory failure.

NIV has also been assessed for mechanical ventilation of patients who refuse endotracheal intubation, a problem more frequently found in patients with end-stage diseases complicated by potentially reversible respiratory failure [14].

In hypoxemic patients with acute respiratory failure, NIV is used to: 1) administer PEEP at a level generally lower than 10 cm H_2O; 2) decrease the spontaneous work of breathing needed to produce a physiological tidal volume and correct the rapid shallow breathing that characterizes acute respiratory failure. These results can be obtained with NIV, preventing respiratory fatigue and endotracheal intubation.

NIV can be administered by a nasal or a full-face mask, with the exclusion criteria and general approach similar to that already described in the COPD section. The experience of ourselves and others is that a face mask is better for patients with severe hypoxemia, since they are usually tachypneic and breathing through the mouth [5].

Clinical outcome

One of the first uses of NIV in acute respiratory failure patients was reported by Meduri et al. [7] in 1989. In this study the authors used PSV (pressure support ventilation) and PCV by face mask in four patients with non-cardiogenic pulmonary (2 patients) or cardiogenic pulmonary edema (2 patients), obtaining excellent results in three patients. Subsequently Pennock et al. [15] reported a 50% successful treatment of a large group of patients with acute respiratory failure due to different causes. Promising results were obtained in those patients with postoperative acute respiratory failure.

The first prospective randomized study was recently published by Wysocki et al. [16]. NIV was not superior to the conventional treatment, when used systematically in non-COPD acute respiratory failure. Note that this study was designed to assess NIV to avoid endotracheal intubation, and not as an alternative treatment for acute respiratory failure.

We performed a prospective randomized trial comparing NIV with conventional treatment in 64 ICU patients with hypoxemic respiratory failure requiring mechanical ventilation. NIV reduced the ICU length of stay and the number of infectious complications associated with intubation [17], although approximately 30% of patients randomized to NIV required endotracheal intubation.

Interesting results were also obtained in two pilot studies by Tognet et al. [18] and our group [19] for the treatment of patients with hematological malignancies, complicated by acute respiratory failure. The investigators [20] emphasized the poor outcome of granulocytopenic patients undergoing mechanical ventilation for acute respiratory failure, which represents a common feature of patients with hematological malignancy, caused by the combination of extreme susceptibility to opportunistic infections and the direct pulmonary toxicity of chemotherapy. NIV could be a useful approach in this condition, since it can be used early and easily, with fewer complications. NIV also offers important ethical advantages in patients with hematological malignancies, as it allows the treatment of patients who refuse endotracheal intubation, but not ventilatory support, thus allowing intensive treatment and respecting the patient's wishes.

Conclusions

Although NIV has only recently been introduced for treating patients with acute respiratory failure, some consensus already exists. Particularly in COPD patients, NIV is a useful approach both to avoid endotracheal intubation (reducing the additional morbidity and mortality from intubation) and to give ventilatory support [8, 9]. A trial of NIV should always be considered (when no formal contraindication exists), particularly if the COPD patients are seen early in their deterioration.

In other patients with acute respiratory distress, despite encouraging preliminary results, several aspects still remain controversial. Large prospective randomized multicenter studies are needed to obtain a general consensus.

Table 1. Field of application for non-invasive ventilation (NIV) in intensive care units (ICU)

COPD exacerbation
Hypoxemic ARF
Status asthmaticus
Cystic fibrosis
AIDS
Cardiogenic pulmonary edema
ARF in immunocompromised patients

(*COPD* chronic obstructive pulmonary disease, *ARF* acute respiratory failure, *AIDS* acquired immunodeficiency syndrome)

Table 2. NIV complications

Nasal bridge necrosis
Aerophagia
Air leaks
Claustrophobia
Ocular irritation

References

1. Torres A, Aznar R, Gatell JM et al (1990) Incidence, risk and prognosis factors of nosocomial pneumonia in mechanically ventilated patients. Am Rev Respir Dis 142:523-528
2. Burns HP, Dayal VS, Scott A et al (1979) Laryngotracheal trauma: observation on its pathogenesis and its prevention following prolonged OT intubation in the adult. Laryngoscope 89: 1316-1325
3. Brochard L, Isabey D, Piquet J et al (1990) Reversal of acute exacerbations of chronic obstructive lung disease by inspiratory assistance with a face mask. N Engl J Med 323: 1523-1530
4. Appendini L, Patessio A, Zanaboni S et al (1994) Physiologic effects of positive endexpiratory pressure and mask pressure support during exacerbations of chronic obstructive pulmonary disease. Am J Respir Crit Care Med 149:1069-1076
5. Meduri GU (1996) Non invasive positive-pressure ventilation in patients with chronic obstructive pulmonary disease and acute respiratory failure. Curr Opin Crit Care 2: 35-46
6. Vitacca M, Rubini F, Foglio K et al (1993) Non-invasive modalities of positive pressure ventilation improve the outcome of acute exacerbations in COPD patients. Intensive Care Med 19: 456-461
7. Meduri GU, Conoscenti CC, Menashe P, Nair S (1989) Non-invasive face mask ventilation in patients with acute respiratory failure. Chest 95:865-870
8. Bott J, Carroll MP, Conway JH et al (1993) Randomized controlled trial of nasal ventilation in acute ventilatory failure due to chronic obstructive airways disease. Lancet 341:1555-1558
9. Brochard L, Mancebo J, Wysocki M et al (1995) Efficacy of non-invasive ventilation for treatment of acute exacerbations of chronic obstructive pulmonary disease. N Engl J Med 333: 817-822
10. Kramer N, Meyer TJ, Meharg J et al (1995) Randomized, prospective trial of noninvasive positive pressure ventilation in acute respiratory failure. Am J Respir Crit Care Med 151: 1799-1806
11. Lofaso R, Brochard L, Touchard D et al (1995) Evaluation of carbon dioxide rebreathing during pressure support ventilation with airway management system (BiPAP) devices. Chest 108:772-778
12. Meduri GU, Turner RE, Aboul-Shala N (1996) Non invasive positive pressure ventilation via face mask: first-line intervention in patients with acute hypercapnic and hypoxemic respiratory failure. Chest 109:179-193
13. Pennock BE, Kaplan PD, Carlin BW et al (1991) Pressure support ventilation with a simplified ventilatory support system administered with a nasal mask in patients with respiratory failure. Chest 100:1371-1376
14. Meduri GU, Fox RC, Abo-Shala N et al (1994) Non invasive mechanical ventilation via face mask in patients with acute respiratory failure who refused endotracheal intubation. Crit Care Med 22:1584-1590
15. Pennock BE, Crawshan L, Kaplan PD (1994) Non invasive nasal mask ventilation for acute respiratory failure. Chest 105:441-444
16. Wysocki M, Tric L, Wolff MA et al (1995) Non-invasive pressure support ventilation in patients with acute respiratory failure. A randomized comparison with conventional therapy. Chest 107:761-768
17. Antonelli M, Conti G, Rocco M et al (1998) A comparison of noninvasive positive-pressure ventilation and conventional mechanical ventilation in patients with acute respiratory failure. N Engl J Med 339:429-435
18. Tognet E, Mercatello A, Coronel B et al (1992) Respiratory distress treated by positive pressure ventilation through a facial mask in haematological patients. Intensive Care Med 18[Suppl 2]:S121
19. Conti G, Marino P, Cogliati A et al (1998) NIPSV by nasal mask in patients with haematologic malignancies complicated by acute respiratory failure. Intensive Care Med (in press)
20. Lloyd-Thomas AR, Dhaliwal HS, Lister TA, Hinds CJ (1986) Intensive therapy for life-threatening medical complications of haematological malignancy. Intensive Care Med 12: 317-324

Detection of Respiratory Muscle Fatigue: Diagnostic Tests in Intensive Care Unit

R. BRANDOLESE

Skeletal muscle fatigue in general and respiratory muscle fatigue in particular can be defined as an inability to perform a predictable task or to generate an adequate level of force [1]. The fatigued respiratory muscles are therefore unable to maintain a satisfactory arterial $PaCO_2$ with a normal alveolar ventilation. Respiratory muscle fatigue is characterized by specific features: the respiratory muscles are essential for life and therefore respiratory fatigue is life threatening; moreover, respiratory fatigued muscles become restored with the rest by means of external mechanical support.

Fatigue may occur as a failure at any one of several sites: the activation of central respiratory motoneurons (central fatigue), neurotransmission through the axonal branches, neuromuscular transmission at the neuromuscular junction and the contractile process with uncoupled excitation-contraction which involves calcium release, calcium metabolism and insufficient energy production [2]. Even if different mechanisms may intervene in determining fatigue from one muscle to another it is well established that fatigue occurs owing to an imbalance between the energy supply and the energy demand [3].

Respiratory muscle failure is often the reason for which a patient requires the institution or continuation of the mechanical ventilation. It is well recognized that respiratory failure occurs when the work of breathing increases beyond the endurance capacity of the respiratory muscles. Cohen et al. [4, 5] described the visual manifestations of respiratory fatigue as tachypnea, a decreased tidal volume, respiratory alternans, abdominal paradox respiration. All these patterns are of little utility because they are very subjective and may vary from one patient to another.

Four categories of patients are liable to develop respiratory muscle fatigue: 1) premature and newborn babies, 2) patients with respiratory muscle weakness, 3) patients presenting shock in which there is an inadequate blood flow to the respiratory muscles, 4) asthmatics and COPD during acute exacerbation of their chronic airway obstruction.

Muscle contraction during fatigue

The total time that muscle contraction may be held is inversely related to the force that the muscle has to generate [6]. This time is called "time limit" and its relation to the developed force is expressed by the following equation:

$$Tlim = 1 / F/Fmax$$

Where F is the force generated and Fmax is the maximal force the muscle can develop. Tlim tends to infinite when F is 15-17% of Fmax. Roussos and Macklem first demonstrated inspiratory muscle fatigue in humans [7]. They found that transdiaphragmatic pressure (Pdi) above which fatigue occurred was about 40% of maximum value of Pdi when the duration of inspiratory time was half of the entire respiratory cycle. These findings were confirmed by Bellemare and Grassino by measuring Tlim and Pdicritic in human subjects for different breathing patterns coupled with different percentage of Pdi/Pdimax ratio. The product of pressure and time is called tension time index (TTdi). An inverse relationship was demonstrated for TTdi and Tlim: a TTdi below 0.15 places the diaphragm in a non fatigue zone, whereas a TTdi over 0.15 indicates that the diaphragm will be, in time, fatigued and unable to generate the requested force [8-10].

The progressive weakening of a muscle becoming fatigued can be assessed by measuring its maximal force. Maximal Pdi or maximal pressure at airway opening (Pimax), obtained by Müller manoeuvre against a closed airway, well reflect maximum developed force [11]. There is evidence that during unsuccessful weaning procedure muscle fatigue develops and Pimax decreases [12]. If the respiratory muscles are put at rest by ventilating the patient, Pimax is able to ameliorate [13]. However Pimax is not the only parameter that has to be taken into account during weaning trials because fatigue is concerned more with endurance than strength. Consequently it is important that the muscle is able to maintain, in time, the targeted force.

Maximal inspiratory pressure

The measurement of maximal inspiratory mouth pressure (Pimax) is the simplest test for investigating subjects with suspected respiratory muscle fatigue. It is easily performed by Müller manoeuvre during which the patient makes inspiratory efforts against a closed airway at functional residual capacity (FRC). Usually the best value of three measurements is recorded [14, 15]. For a given lung volume Pimax is higher in young than in older subjects and the maximal force developed by males is higher than that generated by females. Moreover, smaller individuals develop smaller forces because force is obtained by multiplying the pressure by the surface area over which the pressure acts; in the smaller subjects the surface is smaller and consequently the force is decreased but the pressure tends to be preserved. There is a consistent variability of Pimax in the same subject and the mean coefficient of variation for Pimax is 25% so that an abnormal value of Pimax has to be less than 50% of the predicted value. Repetitive measurements of Pimax are a useful tool to guide weaning from mechanical ventilation or continuation of external mechanical support. The following formula gives the Pimax corrected for age and sex:

$$\text{Pimax, cm } H_2O \text{ (male)} = 143 - 0.55 \text{ age}$$

$$\text{Pimax, cm } H_2O \text{ (female)} = 104 - 0.51 \text{ age}$$

Patients with Pimax of 20-30 cm H_2O are at high risk of developing ventilatory insufficiency and similar values are often associated with chronic alveolar hypoventilation [16]. COPD patients, during acute exacerbation of chronic airway obstruction present significant reduction of Pimax reaching values as low as 8-10 cm H_2O (personal unpublished data). Therefore institution of mechanical ventilation is mandatory in these patients in which the mechanical workload is usually higher than the maximal inspiratory pressure that they are able to generate. Despite its broad clinical application Pimax is nonspecific and cannot be used to differentiate lack of effort, muscle weakness, fatigue, and neural disease. Moreover Pimax measurements depend strongly on the patient cooperation so that this measurement may be difficult or impossible to obtain in patients who present a heavy status of their disease.

Force-frequency curve

By stimulating muscles at different frequencies and measuring the forces developed at the correspondent frequencies, the force-frequency curve of the muscles is constructed [17] (Fig. 1). The force-frequency curve obtained in a fatigued muscle shows a decrease in force developed at any frequency of stimulation [18]. After a period of rest the force during high frequency stimulation returns to baseline values. On the contrary, the force elicited by low frequency takes hours to recover. The mechanism for "low frequency fatigue" is due to failure in excitation-contraction coupling, while high frequency fatigue is attributed to failure of neuromuscular transmission [19, 20]. Aubier stimulated at different frequencies the diaphragm and plotted the different elicited Pdi against the respective frequencies of stimulation obtaining the pressure-frequency curve of the diaphragm before and after fatigue [18]. This author proposed his method to detect fatigue or recovery in patients with compromised function of their diaphragm.

There are some problems in application of force-frequency technique to the diaphragm. Nerve stimulation in humans is painful, arm movements are elicited

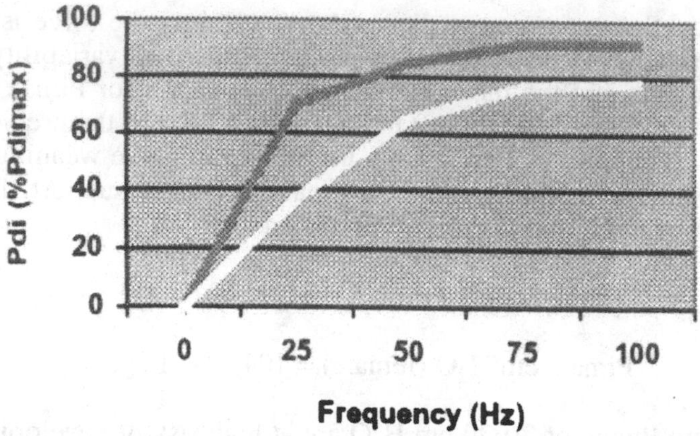

Fig. 1. Representative pressure-frequency curves of Pdi expressed as percentage of Pdimax in a normal subject (upper curve) and in COPD patient whose diaphragm was fatigued (lower curve)

because stimulation of nerves closed to the point of phrenic stimulation and finally liable isometric contraction of the diaphragm is more difficult to obtain in patients than in normal subjects.

Sniff pressure

Miller et al. proposed a test in order to evaluate muscle performance (force) reading it on tracings of mouth pressure, esophageal pressure and transdiaphragmatic pressure by means of a sniff manoeuvre during maximal voluntary contraction against an occluded airway at FRC [21]. Sniff technique determines an activation of all inspiratory muscles, it is easily performed and can be considered a valid substitute of traditional maximal inspiratory pressure (Pimax) [22]. In a clinical study [23] involving 61 patients affected by neuromuscular diseases and COPD, the measurement of sniff Pes was found to be a useful test of inspiratory strength and easier to perform than Pimax manoeuvre. In this study sniff Pes well correlated with Pimax values; patients with low sniff Pes had, too, a low Pimax. In the same study sniff pressure (Pmouth, Pes, Pdi) was compared with the same pressures developed during static manoeuvre. Pdimax was 40-150 cm H_2O while sniff Pdi resulted 80-220 cm H_2O. Sniff manoeuvres are reproducible within subjects and therefore sniff technique is a useful tool to monitor the force of inspiratory muscles.

Rate of muscle relaxation

The rate of relaxation (loss of tension) after cessation of an isometric contraction exhibits an exponential decay curve [24] (Fig. 2). A fatigued muscle shows a prolonged relaxation rate because the reuptake of the calcium previously released is slow [25]. The rate of decay is measured as the peak rate of pressure decay over the first half of the relaxation time (maximum relaxation rate MRR) and as the time constant (TC) of the monoexponential decay observed in the second half of the relaxation curve. Relaxation is measured on Pmouth, Pes, and Pdi tracings [26-28]. The rate of decay on Pmouth tracing represents the rate of decay of all inspiratory muscles, while relaxation rate of the diaphragm is measured on Pdi swing. MRR is linearly related to TTdi and returns to the normal value after 2-5 min postfatigue time [29]. MRR is pressure-dependent, therefore usually it is normalized by dividing it by the peak pressure [30]. TC has a small intersubject variability in non fatigued muscles, therefore it is a good index to assess the impending muscle fatigue: a TC of Pdi of less than 65 ms indicates a non fatigue status, a value greater tha 75 ms shows that fatigue is present or impending [31]. Posture has little or no influence on the measurement [32].

Electromyografic changes during fatigue

By stimulating the neuromuscular junction the muscle fibre membrane is depolarized and then repolarised. Membrane potential changes can be recorded by surface electrodes placed close to muscle fibres: this type of recording is called electromyogram (EMG). It is possible to sum the power of the total EMG output in order to obtain an integrated EMG or the power may be analysed in relation to the different frequencies (power spectrum analysis). The power spectrum analysis of the diaphragm is a further method to investigate the presence of muscle fatigue [33]. The EMG power spectrum rapidly changes after application of fatiguing loads. The high frequency power (H) decreases whereas low (L) frequency power increases indicating the occurrence of fatigue [34]. The EMG power spectrum has been used to detect fatigue in various clinical conditions: weaning from mechanical ventilation, respiratory muscle training in quadriplegic patients [35], and during exercise in patients with chronic airway obstruction [36]. EMG power spectrum analysis remains a complex diagnostic test which requires the presence of qualified operators and therefore this technique cannot be routinely performed in intensive care unit.

Evaluation of inspiratory muscle endurance

TTdi (tension time diaphragm index) in normal subjects, quiet breathing, is about 0.02. This value is obtained by multiplying the diaphragmatic pressure ex-

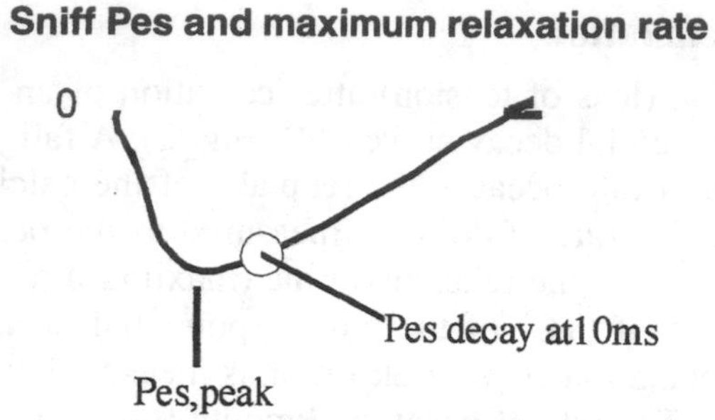

Fig. 2. Schematic enlargement of Sniff Pes swing derived from an original Sniff Pes tracing in a COPD patient just before institution of mechanical support. % Pes decay at 10 ms from Pes peak represents maximum relaxation rate. The time course of Pes decay is very slow indicating respiratory muscle fatigue

pressed as a percentage of maximal developed Pdi pressure by 0.4 which is the ratio between the inspiratory time (TI) and total duration time of one respiratory cycle (TTOT). TTdi = Pdi/Pdimax x TI/TTOT. When the TTdi is 0.15-0.18 the endurance time will be smaller than 1 h [37].

Bellemare and Grassino demonstrated that COPD patients, quiet breathing, have higher Pes and Pdi pressure swings than normal subjects; these patients have lower Pdimax so that their TTdi can be 0.05-0.12. The latter value is, just in baseline condition, close to the threshold fatigue area (0.15-0.18) [8, 9]. If they are compelled to breath by increasing TTdi they develop fatigue. We have shown (unpublished data) that COPD patients during acute exacerbation of chronic airway obstruction breathed through fatigue zone as depicted in the Bellemare-Grassino diagram (Fig. 3).

Zocchi et al. evaluated the endurance of the accessory respiratory muscles breathing against inspiratory threshold loads of various magnitudes and found that the product Pmouth/Pimax x TI/TTOT was related to endurance. Endurance longer than 1 h was achieved with a TTrc = 0.30. Higher TTrc values were related exponentially to endurance time [38].

The TTrc is easy to measure, it needs the measurements of Pes swing or Pmouth during breathing against resistances, is a noninvasive method and may be used to evaluate respiratory force reserve in patients at risk to develop fatigue [39].

Ultrasonography of the diaphragm

To assess the function of the diaphragm it is necessary to know the pressure that it is able to generate, its position and motion. The pressure across the diaphragm

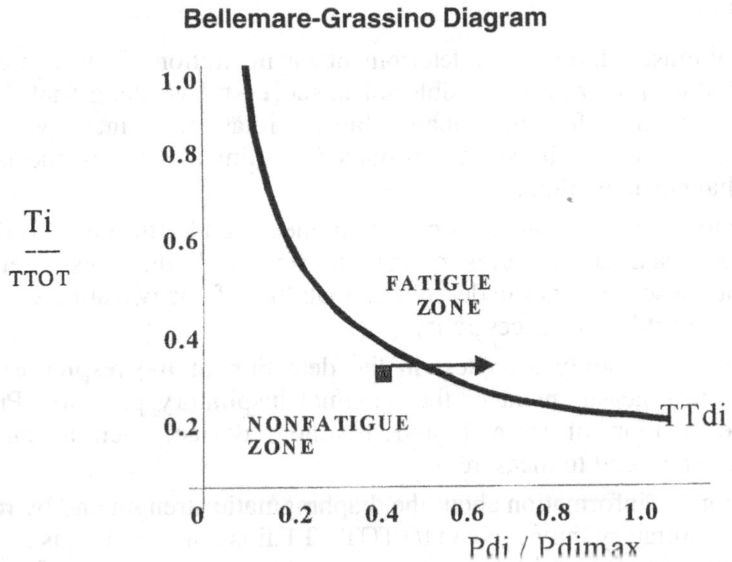

Fig. 3. Relationship between inspiratory duty cycle (TI/TTOT) and critical diaphragmatic pressure (Pdi/Pdimax). Fatigue develops for all breathing patterns falling to the right part of the diagram (fatigue zone) but not for those to the left. Pdi/Pdimax decreases as TI/TTOT increases. (Adapted from Bellemare-Grassino)

is measured relatively noninvasively by means of an esophageal and gastric balloon connected to a differential pressure transducer in order to sum the esophageal and gastric pressure according to the following equation:

$$Pdi = Pga - (-Pes)$$

Recently, ultrasonography of the diaphragm was introduced in clinical practice in order to evaluate diaphragm thickness, configuration, and displacement without use, obviously, of ionizing radiation [40]. The pressure that the diaphragm develops can be related to the stress developed by the contracting muscle and several measured dimensions as expressed by the following formula:

$$Pdi = s \; tdi \; w/A \; span$$

in which it is shown that Pdi is directly proportional to the diaphragm thickness (tdi). Cohn [41, 42], in a group of healthy subjects, measured diaphragm thickness and maximal airway pressure (Pimax). The maximal airway pressure was highly correlated with the diaphragm thickness, even if the range of Pimax was large. This extent can be attributed to the different values of the thickness revealed in different human subjects [41, 42].

Conclusion

Respiratory muscle fatigue is a determinant for institution of mechanical ventilation and almost always responsible for unsuccessful weaning trial. Moreover fatigue is a common feature to many clinical situations in intensive care unit. Consequently it should be strictly evaluated in clinical settings and become a standard diagnostic method.

Respiratory muscle fatigue is objectively measured by means of EMG, pressure swings, maximal pressures, relaxation rate and TTdi. Roussos et al. suggested that muscle fatigue underlay the inability of many patients to resume spontaneous ventilation successfully.

The most commonly used test in the detection of the respiratory muscle function is the measurement of the maximal inspiratory pressure (Pimax). It provides estimation of strength and a simple device, such as an aneroid manometer, is needed to measure it.

Pdimax gives information about the diaphragmatic strength and by relating it to Pdi and inspiratory duty cycle (TI/TTOT), TTdi is obtained that is an index of developed fatigue. Pdi and Pdimax measurements require the use of esophageal and gastric balloons, differential pressure transducers. The performed Pdimax and Pimax are conditioned by the collaboration-motivation of the subject and are unable to differentiate central from peripheral muscle fatigue.

Maximum relaxation rate of the inspiratory muscle is easy to measure and appears to be a splendid indicator of impending muscle fatigue. However the absolute values of MRR measurements vary considerably among normal subjects so that an isolated determination is unable to detect if fatigue is present.

Sniff test is noninvasive and needs simple a device such as a catheter inserted into a nostril.

Pressure-frequency curve is not easily performed in the clinical practice.

Electromyography of the diaphragm and other respiratory muscles is not recommended for general use, it needs the presence of an expert and is more adapted to laboratory investigations than in intensive care.

We can conclude that the ideal test to evaluate respiratory muscle fatigue, yet, has not been developed and further studies will be necessary in order to better evaluate the respiratory muscle fatigue in the clinical settings.

References

1. Edwards RHT (1981) Humans function and fatigue. In: Porter R, Welanhuman J (eds) Muscle fatigue: physiological mechanisms. Pitman Medical, London, pp 1-18
2. Sieck GC, Fournier M (1990) Changes in diaphragm motor unit EMG during fatigue. J Appl Physiol 68(5):1927-1926
3. Roussos Ch, Macklem PT (1982) The respiratory muscles. N Engl J Med 307:786-797
4. Cohen CA, Zagelbaum G, Gross D et al (1982) Clinical manifestations of inspiratory muscle fatigue. Am J Med 73:308-316
5. Moxham J (1984) Respiratory muscle fatigue - aspects of detection and treatment. Bull Eur Physiopath Respir 20:437-444
6. Grassino A, Macklem PT (1984) Respiratory muscle fatigue and ventilatory failure. Ann Rev Med 35:625-647
7. NHLBI Workshop Summary (1990) Respiratory muscle fatigue. Am Rev Respir Dis 142: 474-480
8. Bellemare F, Grassino A (1982) Effect of pressure and timing of contraction on human diaphragmatic fatigue. J Appl Physiol 1190-1195
9. Bellemare F, Grassino A (1982) Evaluation of human diaphragmatic fatigue. J Appl Physiol 53(5):1196-1206
10. Bellemare F, Wigth D, Lavigne C, Grassino A (1983) Effect of tension and timing of contraction on blood flow of the diaphragm. J Appl Physiol 54(6):1597-1606
11. Black LF, Hyatt RE (1969) Maximal respiratory pressures: normal values and relationship to age and sex. Am Rev Respir Dis 99:696-702
12. Tobin MJ, Perez W, Guenther SM et al (1986) The pattern of breathing during successful and unsuccessful trial of weaning from mechanical ventilation. Am Rev Respir Dis 134:1111-1118
13. Tobin MJ, Guenther SM, Perets W (1987) Konno-Mead analysis of rib cage abdominal motion during successful and unsuccessful trial of weaning from mechanical ventilation. Am Rev Respir Dis 135:1320-1328
14. Wen AS, Woo MS, Keen TG (1997) How many manoeuvres are required to measure maximal inspiratory pressure accurately. Chest Mar 111(3):802-807
15. Cook CD, Mead J, Orzalesi MM (1983) Static volume pressure characteristics of the respiratory system during maximal efforts. J Appl Physiol 19:1016-1022
16. Decramer JM, Demedts M, Rochette F (1980) Maximal transrespiratory pressures in obstructive lung disease. Bull Eur Physiopath Respir 16:479-490
17. Edwards RTH (1978) Physiological analysis of skeletal muscle weakness and fatigue. Clin Sci Mol Med 54:463-470
18. Aubier M, Farkas G, De Troyer A et al (1981) Detection of diaphragmatic fatigue in man by phrenic stimulation. J Appl Physiol 50:538-544
19. Moxham H, Morris A, Spiro S et al (1981) Contractile properties and fatigue of the diaphragm in man. Thorax 36:164-168
20. Joned D (1981) Muscle fatigue due to changes beyond the neuromuscular junction. In: Porter R, Welanhuman J (eds) Human muscle fatigue: physiological mechanisms. Pitman Medical, London, 82:178-196
21. Miller J, Moxham J, Green M et al (1985) The maximal sniff in the assessment of diaphragmatic function in man. Clin Sci 69:91-97
22. Laroche CM, Mier AK, Moxham J, Green M (1988) The value of sniff esophageal pressures in the assessment of global inspiratory muscle strength. Am Rev Respir Dis 138:598-603
23. Ejdra F, Dekuijezen PN, Van Herwaarde CL, Folgerin HG (1993) Difference between sniff mouth pressure and static maximal inspiratory pressures. Eur Respir J 6(4):541-546
24. Esau SA, Bye PT, Pardy RL (1983) Changes in rate of relaxation of sniff pressure with diaphragmatic fatigue in humans. J Appl Physiol 55:731-735
25. Kyroussis D, Mills G, Hamnegard CH et al (1994) Inspiratory muscle relaxation rate assessed from sniff nasal pressure. Thorax 49(11):1127-1133

26. Mador MJ, Kufel TJ (1992) Effect of inspiratory muscle fatigue on inspiratory muscle relaxation rates in healthy subjects. Chest 102(6):1767-1773
27. Kyroussis D, Polkey MI, Keilty SE et al (1996) Exhaustive exercise slows inspiratory muscle relaxation rate in chronic obstructive pulmonary disease. Am J Respir Crit Care Med 153(2): 787-793
28. Kouporis N, Vianna LG, Mulvey DA et al (1989) Maximal relaxation rates of esophageal, nose, and mouth pressure during a sniff reflect inspiratory muscle fatigue. Am Rev Respir Dis May 139(5):1213-1217
29. Levy RD, Esau SA, Bye PT, Pardy RL (1984) Relaxation rate of mouth pressure with sniffs at rest and with inspiratory muscle fatigue. Am Rev Respir Dis 130:38-41
30. Nava S (1998) Monitoring respiratory muscles. Monaldi Arch Chest Dis 53(6):640-643
31. Rochester DF, Arora NS (1983) Respiratory muscle failure. Med Clin North Am 54(5): 573-597
32. Koulouris N, Tsintris K, Mauroudis P (1992) Effect of posture on maximal relaxation and contraction rate of respiratory muscle in man. Am Rev Respir Dis 145:A256
33. Gross D, Grassino A, Ross D, Macklem PT (1979) EMG pattern of diaphragmatic fatigue. J Appl Physiol 46:1-7
34. Robertson CH, Paget MA, Johnson RL (1977) Distribution of blood flow oxygen consumption and work output among the respiratory muscles during unobstructed hyperventilation. J Clin Invest 59:43-50
35. Gross D, Ladd H, Riley E et al (1980) The effect of training on strength and endurance of the diaphragm in quadriplegia. Am Med J 68:27-35
36. Cohen CA, Zagelbaum G, Gross D (1980) Clinical manifestation of inspiratory muscle fatigue. Am J Med 73:308-316
37. Roussos C, Macklem PT (1977) Diaphragmatic fatigue in man. J Appl Physiol 43:189-197
38. Zocchi L, Fitting J, Rampulla C (1993) Endurance of human intercostal and accessory muscles. Am Rev Respir Dis 147(4):857-864
39. Similowski T, Straus C, Attali V et al (1998) Cervical magnetic stimulation as a method to discriminate between diaphragm and rib cage muscle fatigue. J Appl Physiol 84(5):1692-1700
40. McCool D, Hopping FC (1995) Ultrasonography of the diaphragm. In: Roussos Ch (ed) Thorax, II ed, part B, vol 85. Dekker, New York, USA, Chapt 44:1295-1311
41. Cohn DB, Benditt JO, McCool FD (1992) Two dimensional ultrasound assessment of diaphragm thickness. Am Rev Respir Dis 145:A255
42. Cohn DB, Benditt JO, Sheman CB et al (1993) Diaphragm thickness: An index of respiratory muscle strength. Am Rev Respir Dis 147:A694

Inspiratory Capacity, Exercise Tolerance, and Respiratory Failure in Chronic Obstructive Pulmonary Disease

J. Milic-Emili, O. Diaz

During the last half-century many studies have investigated the correlation of exercise tolerance to routine lung function in patients with obstructive pulmonary disease. In virtually all of these studies the degree of airway obstruction was assessed in terms of the forced expired volume in 1 sec (FEV_1) and the forced expiratory vital capacity (FVC). Since, in most studies only a weak correlation was found between exercise tolerance and degree of airway obstruction, it has been concluded that other factors than lung function impairment (e.g., deconditioning and peripheral muscle dysfunction) play a predominant role in limiting exercise capacity in patients with chronic airway obstruction. Recent work, however, suggests that in patients with chronic obstructive pulmonary disease (COPD) the inspiratory capacity is a more-powerful predictor of exercise tolerance than FEV_1 and FVC.

Dyspnea and exercise limitation are the predominant complaints of patients with COPD, and are commonly the reason for seeking medical attention. Yet, routine assessment of lung function is in general based almost entirely on FEV_1 and FVC, although there is ample evidence that in COPD patients these tests correlate poorly with both dyspnea and exercise tolerance [1]. Accordingly, it is axiomatic that in COPD the response to any treatment assessed in terms of changes in FEV_1 and FVC should differ from that based on exercise tolerance or on subjective measures of dyspnea and quality of life. In COPD it is hyperinflation that plays a central role in eliciting dyspnea, decreased exercise tolerance, and ventilatory failure [1-4]. Hyperinflation is commonly assessed through measurement of the functional residual capacity (FRC) with body plethysmography, which is complex, expensive, and, in patients with severe COPD, may lead to overestimation of the actual FRC because the transmission of alveolar pressure to the mouth during the panting maneuver is delayed by increased airway resistance [5, 6]. However, the increase of FRC in patients with obstructive pulmonary disease is necessarily accompanied by a reduction in IC, as shown in Figure 1 from reference 6. In contrast to FRC, measurement of IC is simple, cheap, and reliable. Thus, IC testing provides a useful tool for the indirect assessment of pulmonary hyperinflation in COPD patients. In such patients a reduction of IC implies hyperinflation with concomitant dyspnea and decreased exercise tolerance, and implies a poor prognosis [3, 4, 7].

IC and exercise tolerance

The maximal ventilation that a subject can achieve plays a dominant role in determining exercise capacity, and may be limited by the highest flow rates that can be generated. Most normal subjects and endurance athletes do not exhibit tidal expiratory flow limitation (FL) even during maximal exercise [8]. In contrast, in COPD patients tidal expiratory FL is frequently present at rest [1, 2, 7], as first suggested by Hyatt [9]. Tidal FL promotes dynamic hyperinflation (DH) with a concomitant decrease in IC, as shown in Figure 1. Diaz et al. [7] have recently shown that, in most COPD patients who have FL at rest, the IC is lower than normal, while in the patients who do not have FL at rest it is within normal limits (Fig. 2).

In normal subjects there is a substantial expiratory flow reserve both above and below the FRC, as evidenced by the fact that the maximal expiratory flow rates available are much higher than the flow rates used during resting breathing (Fig. 1, *left*). As a result, in normal subjects the tidal volume during exercise can increase both at the expense of the inspiratory and expiratory reserve volumes [2]. In contrast, in COPD patients who exhibit FL at rest, the flows available below FRC are insufficient to sustain even resting ventilation (Fig. 1, *right*). Consequently, in such patients the maximal tidal volume during exercise (V_{Tmax}), and hence the exercise tolerance, should be limited by their reduced IC. Recent studies have shown that in COPD patients there is a much stronger correlation of maximal O_2 uptake ($\dot{V}O_{2max}$) to IC than to FEV_1 and FVC [3, 7], as shown in Figure 3.

Since reduced exercise capacity in COPD patients shows only a weak link to lung function impairment measured in terms of FEV_1 and FVC [1, 3, 10], it has been argued that factors other than lung function impairment (e.g., deconditioning and peripheral muscle dysfunction) are the predominant contributors to reduced exercise tolerance [11-13]. The recent studies based on assessment of IC, however, have shown that lung function impairment is probably the major contributor to reduced exercise tolerance, at least in COPD patients who have FL at rest [7].

As shown in Figure 3, in ambulatory COPD patients the lowest observed values of IC amount to about 40% of predicted. When the IC is reduced below this limit (< 40% predicted), the patients are home-bound or require mechanical ventilation. Thus, a low IC heralds respiratory failure [7].

Assessment of IC also provides useful information in terms of bronchodilator treatment. The effect of bronchodilators in patients with obstructive lung disease is commonly assessed in terms of the change in FEV_1 seen after bronchodilator administration relative to control values. According to the American Thoracic Society's recommended criteria, a change in FEV_1 of more than 12% represents a significant response [14]. Although some COPD patients may not exhibit a significant change in FEV_1 after bronchodilator administration, they nevertheless claim improvement in symptoms [15]. Since pulmonary hyperin-

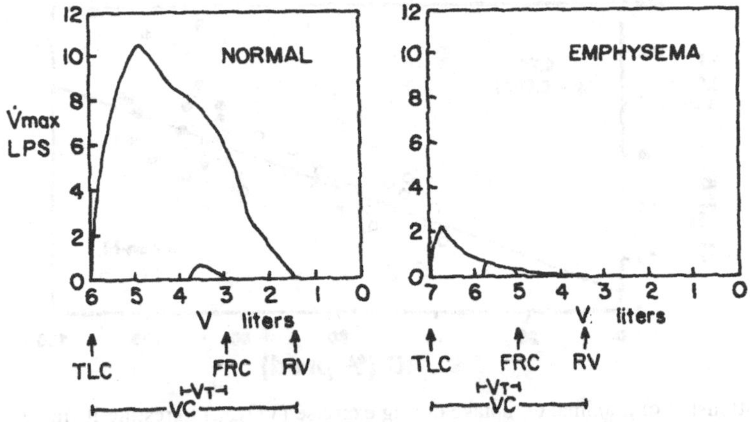

Fig. 1. Flow-volume curves during forced and quiet expiration in a normal subject (*left*) and a patient with severe emphysema (*right*) (*TLC* total lung capacity, *FRC* function residual capacity, *RV* residual value, *VC* vital capacity, *VT* tidal volume during quiet breathing). While in the normal subject there is considerable flow reserve over the resting tidal volume range, in the patient the tidal expiratory flow rates are maximal, i.e., expiratory flow limitation is present. The latter causes increased FRC with concomitant reduction of inspiratory capacity (IC = TLC-FRC) (modified from reference [6], with permission)

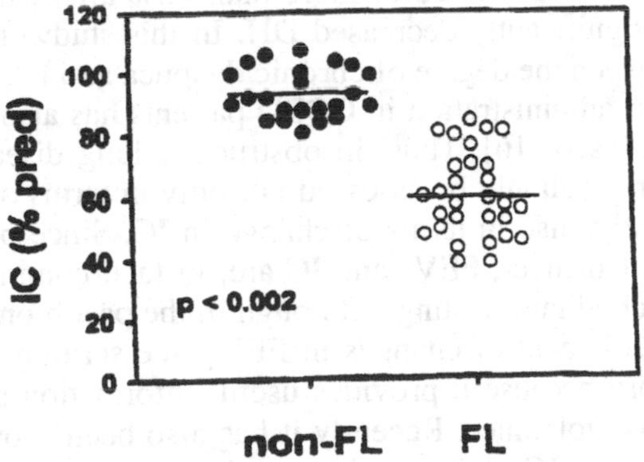

Fig. 2. Inspiratory capacity (*IC*), expressed as percentage predicted, in 52 ambulatory with chronic obstructive pulmonary disease (COPD) patients: 23 without (*non-FL*) and 29 with (*FL*) expiratory flow limitation at rest. Note that in most FL patients IC was decreased while in the non-FL patients IC was within normal limits (modified from reference [7], with permission)

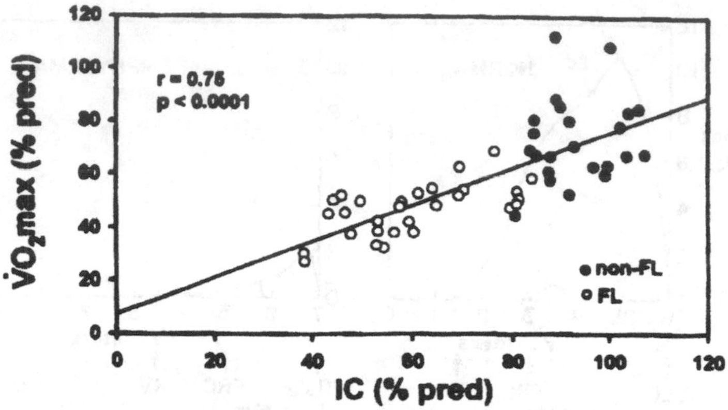

Fig. 3. Relationship of maximal O_2 uptake during exercise ($\dot{V}O_{2max}$) to resting IC in 52 COPD patients with (FL) and without (non-FL) tidal expiratory flow limitation at rest. Same patients as Figure 2 (modified from reference [7], with permission)

flation plays an important role in determining the intensity of dyspnea [1], it is likely that in such patients there is a decrease in the degree of DH (decreased FRC and increased IC) after bronchodilator administration. Tantucci et al. [4] have recently shown that in many COPD patients with little or no change in FEV_1, there was an increase in IC of more than 12% after salbutamol administration, reflecting significantly decreased DH. In this study, a negative correlation was found between the degree of chronic dyspnea and IC. An increase in IC after bronchodilator administration in COPD patients has also been reported by Pellegrino and Brusasco [16]. Thus, in obstructive lung disease the benefit of bronchodilator therapy should be assessed not only in terms of change in FEV_1 but, more importantly, also in terms of change in IC. Since performance of IC precedes the FVC maneuver, FEV_1 and IC are, in fact, commonly recorded together during bronchodilator testing. Although in the past bronchodilator testing was focused on assessment of changes in FEV_1, the scrutiny of changes in IC should be mandatory because it provides useful information pertaining to both dyspnea and exercise tolerance. Recently it has also been shown that in COPD patients the increase in IC after anticholinergic therapy best reflected the improvements in exercise endurance [17]. Assessment of IC has also provided useful information on the effects of surgical treatment (single lung transplantation) in COPD patients [18].

In conclusion, measurement of the IC is useful for monitoring the status and progress of COPD patients, and for assessment of the efficacy of their treatment. It is time for IC, the Cinderella of lung function testing, to take pride of place with her two stepsisters, FEV_1 and FVC.

References

1. Eltayara L, Becklake MR, Volta CA, Milic-Emili J (1996) Relationship between chronic dyspnea and expiratory flow-limitation in patients with chronic obstructive pulmonary disease. Am J Respir Crit Care Med 154:1726-1734
2. Koulouris NG, Dimopoulou I, Valta P et al (1997) Detection of expiratory flow limitation during exercise in COPD patients. J Appl Physiol 82:723-731
3. Murariu C, Ghezzo H, Milic-Emili J, Gauthier H (1998) Exercise limitation in obstructive lung disease. Chest 114:965-968
4. Tantucci C, Duguet A, Similowski T et al (1998) Effect of solbutamol on dynamic hyperinflation in chronic obstructive pulmonary disease patients. Eur Respir J 12:799-804
5. Shore SA, Milic-Emili J, Martin JG (1982) Reassessment of body plethysmographic technique for the measurement of thoracic gas volume in asthmatics. Am Rev Respir Dis 126: 515-520
6. Bates DV, Macklem PT, Christie RV (1971) Respiratory function in disease. Saunders, Philadelphia, p 35
7. Diaz O, Villafranca C, Ghezzo H et al (2000) Exercise tolerance in COPD patients with and without tidal expiratory flow limitation a rest. Eur Respir J 16:269-275
8. Mota S, Casan P, Drobnic F et al (1999) Expiratory flow limitation during exercise in competition. J Appl Physiol 86:611-616
9. Hyatt RE (1961) The interrelationship of pressure, flow and volume during various respiratory maneuvers in normal and emphysematous patients. Am Rev Respir Dis 83:676-683
10. Jones NG, Jones G, Edwards RHT (1971) Exercise tolerance in chronic airway obstruction. Am Rev Respir Dis 103:477-491
11. Maltais F (1996) Oxidative capacity of the skeletal muscle and lactic acid kinetics during exercise in normal subjects and in patients with COPD. Am J Respir Crit Care Med 153: 228-293
12. Hamilton N, Killian KJ, Summers E, Jones NL (1995) Muscle strength symptom intensity, and exercise capacity in patients with cardiorespiratory disorders. Am J Respir Crit Care Med 152:2021-2031
13. Gosselink R, Troosters T, Decramer M (1996) Peripheral muscle weakness contributes to exercise limitation in COPD. Am J Respir Crit Care Med 153:976-980
14. American Thoracic Society (1987) Standards for the diagnosis and care of patients with chronic obstructive pulmonary disease (COPD) and asthma. Am Rev Respir Dis 136:225-244
15. Guyatt GH, Townstead M, Pugsley SO et al (1987) Bronchodilators in chronic air-flow limitation. Effects on airway function, exercise capacity, and quality of life. Am Rev Respir Dis 135:1069-1074
16. Pellegrino R, Brusasco V (1997) Lung hyperinflation and flow limitation in chronic airway obstruction. Eur Respir J 10:543-549
17. O'Donnell DE, Lam M, Webb KA (1999) Spirometric correlates of improvement in exercise performance after anticholinergic therapy in chronic obstructive pulmonary disease. Am J Respir Crit Care Med 160:542-549
18. Murciano D, Pichot M, Boczkowki J et al (1997) Expiratory flow limitation in COPD patients after single lung transplantation. Am J Respir Crit Care Med 155:1036-1041

Chest Roentgenology in the Intensive Care Unit

M. MAFFESSANTI, M. PRAVATO, M. RATTI

Thoracic hardware

The management of the critically ill patient in the Intensive Care Unit (ICU) requires different life support and monitoring devices, many of which, at the chest level, can determine iatrogenic injuries, worsen the patient's conditions and overlap with the main pathology.

Chest X-ray (CXR) in the ICU is a basic tool to examine the above-mentioned conditions; it must be adequately executed with a proper technique; it should also be reported in presence of the ICU physician to ameliorate the radiological interpretation and to obtain the best clinical management [1].

The main monitoring and support devices are the following: endovascular catheters [central venous catheter (CVC) and Swan-Ganz catheter (SGC)], tracheal tubes and cannulas, pleural tubes and esophageal feeding tubes.

Endovascular catheters

Central venous catheter (CVC)

Purpose

It aims to monitor the central venous pressure; fluids and drugs can be administered through this device.

Normal positioning

The CVC is inserted through a peripheral venous approach: right or left internal jugular vein, right or left subclavian vein. The right jugular approach is the safest, because the catheter runs straightforward along the anonymous vein and the superior vena cava (SVC) towards the right atrium where it should not enter [2].

Problems and radiological aspects

Different problems may occur during the positioning procedures, i.e., *misplacements* and *complications* [3].

Misplacements

Misplacements may occur within the right veins (innominate and SVC) or in different, particularly in smaller vessels or within the cardiac chambers. In the first case (looping, knotting), an incorrect evaluation of the central venous pressure may occur and in case of fluid and drugs administration the vessel itself may be damaged (dissection) with severe consequences (phlebitis and thrombosis). Misplacements within other vessels may be in the superior intercostal vein, to the left, in the internal mammary veins, in the azygos and within the pericardiophrenic veins.

The recognition of such conditions on the radiograph requires a thorough knowledge of the mediastinal and vascular anatomy. A typical aspect may be observed in case of misplacement of the *CVC in the right internal mammary vein*: in the frontal projection, a dense ring indicating the anterior bending of the catheter where it enters the mammary vein can be observed; moreover, its final portion does not run straightforward, being slightly angulated medially. When such misplacement is suspected, a lateral projection is required.

Another misplacement can be a *left impending catheter*, which is a catheter with its tip impinging perpendicularly against the right wall of the SVC; in this case, the catheter can act as a sting forth and back with the respiratory movements or, for the jugular catheters, with movements of the patient's neck.

Coiling of the catheter may be responsible of flow turbulences with subsequent vascular thrombosis; a *broken catheter* may release fragments that can be located radiologically and rescued during a radioscopic interventional procedure [2-4].

In case of a *misplaced catheter within a cardiac chamber*, various complications may occur such as arrhythmias, endothelial damage and cardiac perforation.

Complications

The catheter may be responsible for a *vascular damage*, either intimal dissection or complete perforation. Such conditions may be easily testified radiologically by the introduction of few ml of contrast medium [5].

A *pneumothorax* may be the consequence of a subclavian catheter; it can worsen in the patients under mechanical ventilation; therefore it must always be carefully checked on the films, in particular in cases of subclavian catheters. In supine patients, the pneumothorax may appear as a localized paramediastinal hyperlucent stripe or as a diffuse hyperlucency over the whole lung.

Swan-Ganz catheter (SGC)

Purpose

It aims to argue the left atrial pressure throughout the measurement of the PCWP (pulmonary capillary wedge pressure).

Normal positioning

The SGC is inserted through the same veins as the CVC. It is a multiple-way catheter, one of which is connected with an inflatable balloon that makes the catheter to flow downstream towards the right heart and the pulmonary arteries. At rest, the catheter's tip should lie within the right or left main pulmonary artery; at work, the catheter is advanced within a smaller vessel where the balloon is inflated to produce a temporary obstruction and the PCWP is measured.

Problems and radiological aspects

Misplacements occur when, at rest, the tip results more than 2 cm lateral to the hilum, because that means that it is in too small an arterial branch and may cause a lung infarction or an arterial rupture; on the contrary, a tip too proximal within the main pulmonary artery or the right ventricle may be responsible for arrhythmias, cardiac endothelial damage or perforation [1, 6].

Tracheal tubes and cannulas

Purpose

These devices are frequently employed to support the ventilation, to keep the airways open and to ensure an adequate respiratory performance.

Normal positioning

The *endotracheal tube* carries an inflatable balloon which should be inflated up to the tracheal diameter to hold the tube in place; the tube is connected to a mechanical device in order to ensure an adequate ventilation with regular gas exchanges.

The tip of the tracheal tube should project on the film not less than 2 and no more than 6 cm above the carina or at the level of the third or fourth dorsal vertebral body [7].

Problems and radiological aspects

Too proximal a tube may get out spontaneously or after neck's movements, while a *too distal a placement*, typically into the right main stem bronchus or the intermediate bronchus, may be responsible for contralateral atelectasis. Both the above-mentioned conditions are well documented on the films. If the *balloon* is *inflated over the tracheal diameter* both immediate and delayed problems may occur, i.e., tracheal tearing with consequent pneumothorax, pneumomediastinum, mediastinal abscess and mediastinitis; the latter complications can be suspected when hyperlucencies are recognized over the mediastinum or when displacement of the tracheal tube within a mediastinal enlargement occurs. Tracheal ischaemia with subsequent tracheomalacia are delayed problems, sometimes happening after discharge of the patient from the ICU unit; they can be recognized as modifications of the size of the trachea, particularly stenosis [8].

Another complication is the *esophageal misplacement of the tracheal tube*: in these cases chest X-ray shows the tube aside to the left from the trachea which can be pushed apart by the inflated balloon; a gastric dilatation and air within the esophageal lumen may appear. Finally, esophageal rupture may occur and should be suspected when a mediastinal enlargement containing air occurs [9].

Pleural drainages

Purpose

These devices are used to drain pneumothorax and pleural effusions of different origins.

Normal positioning

The drainage are inserted in a posterior or anterior position to drain respectively effusions or pneumothorax. In the first case, the tube is connected to a bag, while in the second case it is connected to an aspiration device. On the films, their course must be straight or gently curved with the extremity always projecting on the lung [1].

Problems and radiological aspects

Pleural drainage misplacement may occur within the soft tissues, the lung parenchyma, the fissures or in the mediastinum; it can be suspected when the tip projects against the soft tissues or the mediastinum, or when the drainage is ineffective. When there is a doubt on the plain films, especially when a parenchymal or scissural misplacement is suspected because of a sharp angulation of the tube, CT can be performed to work out the doubt.

A tube within the soft tissues (possible in obese patients) may appear correctly positioned if it projects against the lung; nevertheless the drainage is not efficient; in these cases, additional films in different oblique positions can easily overcome the problem. For the unsolved cases, CT represents once again the working out tool [10, 11].

Esophageal feeding tubes

Purpose

The critically ill patient nutrition may request the use of an esophageal-gastric feeding tube: fluids and drugs can also be administered through it.

Normal positioning

The tube is positioned through a nasal approach and its extremity has to reach the gastric lumen. On chest CXR the tube should project against the esophageal course ending in the left upper abdomen.

Problems and radiological aspects

The radiograph is a useful tool for detecting esophageal misplacement or even the more severe (and rare) tracheal-bronchial misplacement, responsible for bronchial damage and chemical pneumonia. In the first case, the film shows the tip of the tube within the mediastinum instead than in the abdomen; in the second case, the film can show an extra-esophageal position of the tube, a pleural effusion, a pneumomediastinum with mediastinal enlargement and parenchymal opacities [12].

Pulmonary edema (PE)

PE is a clinical condition produced by modifications of the intravascular pressures or by an increased permeability of the membranes with liquid pouring into the interstitium from the intravascular compartment to the extravascular one (interstitium) and eventually within the lung (alveoli). Under normal conditions, if the barrier is intact, there is just a small amount of fluid moving from the bloodstream to the interstitial space under the effect of the hydrostatic and oncotic pressures (Starling law) with a minimal unbalance so that the interstitium is always a little "ahead of fluids"; the excess is physiologically removed by the lymphatics. Any modification of the feedback between fluid production (i.e., when the hydrostatic pressure rises), its return to the bloodstream (i.e., when the oncotic pressure is low) or any impairment of the alveolar-capillary membrane (i.e., when an injury damages it) can be responsible for the edema.

Hydrostatic pulmonary edema

Definition

This type of edema is the consequence of a raised pulmonary capillary pressure, i.e., after acute left ventricle failure; for this reason this edema is also called *cardiogenic edema.*

Pathophysiology

Cardiogenic edema occurs when the extravascular water increases over the level of the lymphatic drainage [3]. A low protein fluid is produced, a transudate almost entirely represented by albumin. At the beginning the fluid remains restricted within the bronchovascular interstitium and tends to move toward the hilum, following the oncotic pressure gradient (that increases towards the centre) and the gravitational pressure (higher in the lower regions of the lungs). When the pressure reaches a critical level (higher than 22 mmHg), the fluid tends to invade the alveoli and the *interstitial edema* becomes *alveolar edema*. In this phase the patient has the different symptoms related to the gas exchange impairment [13].

Radiological aspects

CXR is useful for the diagnosis and monitoring of the interstitial modifications before the patient becomes symptomatic and to recognize and quantify the typical alveolar opacities of the second stage.

The *interstitial modifications* are the following:

1. *hilar haze*: blurring of hilar vessels;
2. *bronchial haze*: blurring of the bronchial walls with *peribronchial cuffing*;
3. *thickening of the interlobular septa*: this is shown by the well known *Kerley lines* (type A, B and C). Type-A Kerley lines are long and irregularly oblique in the perihilar regions. Type-B Kerley lines are thin and short (2-3 cm), typically perpendicular to the costal pleura. Type-C Kerley lines are seen as a reticular aspect in the paramediastinal portions of the lungs in the PA view;
4. *thickening of the fissures* for accumulation of fluid within the subpleural connective tissue.

The *alveolar edema* becomes evident at CXR as multiple and confluent, mostly gravitational opacities which tend to become more and more homogeneous as the edema increases. An air bronchogram within the opacities is rare because also the bronchi are filled up with fluid; more frequently, there is an associated pleural effusion [13].

Outcome

All the radiographic signs can show quite rapid modifications either during the worsening of the edema or (more slowly) when there is a regression of it after therapy.

Oncotic edema

Definition

This kind of edema is due to a decreased oncotic pressure, due to hypovolemia as in renal failure, hyper hydration, malnutrition, etc.; these conditions act as coagents in the accumulation of fluids within the extravascular compartment.

Pathophysiology

The fluid is also a *transudate* as in the cardiogenic edema; however, the accumulation of the fluid more often is "central", according to Milne due to the preserved thoracic "pump" in these patients compared to the cardiac patients [13, 14].

Radiological aspects

CXR shows an *increased mediastinal transverse diameter* due to the enlargement of the venous compartment (particularly the SVC) which represents the first reservoir of the intravascular excess of volume. Fluid overload is well quantified on the PA films through the measurement of the vascular pedicle, which is enlarged because of the SVC enlargement [7].

Its width is calculated measuring the distance between the SVC to right principal bronchus crossing and the perpendicular line on aortic arcus at the level of the left subclavian artery [1].

This width is important for therapeutical and prognostic purposes for critically ill patients monitoring and it also relates with all possible course complications.

Permeability edema

Definition

In this condition, haemodynamic factors play a secondary role; edema is due to an alveolar capillary membrane alteration with subsequent fluid and protein pouring directly into the alveoli.

Pathophysiology

The adult respiratory distress syndrome is a prototype of this kind of injury edema. ARDS is an heterogeneous syndrome due to the release of endogenous (septic and trauma shock, haemorrhagic pancreatitis, major burns, gastric aspiration, etc.) or exogenous toxic agents (heroin overdose, poison ingestion, toxic gas inhalation, etc.). Noxious substances reach the capillary vessels in different organs, including the lung, and damage the membranes; in turn, the damage produces an increase in its permeability so that a fluid with a high concentration of proteins and cells (exudate) floods the alveoli [7, 13].

Radiological aspects

During the very early initial phase, chest X-ray does not show opacities; in this phase, that lasts only minutes or hours, only diffuse microatelectasis can be visible at the pathological observation; the only visible sign is a *diffuse reduction of the lung volumes*, better recognized on *subsequent films*. Within 12-24 h, there is an impairment of the clinical parameters with cyanosis, oxygen-resistant hypoxemia and respiratory failure. In this stage, the radiograph is positive: the modifications range from a slight pulmonary diffuse haziness to multiple, *not confluent bilateral parenchymal patchy opacities* spreading from the apex through the lung base, often with air bronchogram. Usually, neither pleural effusion nor heart enlargement are identifiable or flow redistribution (quite common in the cardiac edema). Different aspects are related to the severity and evolution of this condition [3, 7].

Outcome

The progression of the disease is not identical in all patients; some of them recover with "restitutio ad integrum" within a few days: in these subjects, a progressive reduction in the number and density of the parenchymal opacities is observed. In other patients, focal areas of interstitial fibrosis and honeycomb aspects can be observed (end-stage lung). Sometimes, during the recovery, one or more episodes of relapsing disease occur, due for example to the release of a new amount of toxins: when this happens, CXR shows a worsening of the opacities. From the pathological point of view, cylindrical or cubic pneumocytes coat the alveolar walls, and interstitial and alveolar inflammation and fibrosis of variable degree occur; these manifestations are responsible for a reticular aspect on the radiograph in the 20% of patients [13].

The radiological evaluation of the chest during the acute phase of the disease should be made taking in account the parameters of ventilation (particularly PEEP) that can produce alveolar overinflation with an only apparent amelioration of the radiological opacities [7, 15].

Parenchymal opacities:

Lung contusion

Definition

It represents a frequent event, typically the consequence of deceleration traumas (for instance high speed accidents, high heights falls, etc.) [16]. Radiologically, a peripheral pulmonary contusion can be observed, associated or not with other signs of minor or major thoracic injuries.

Pathophysiology

The reaction of the lung to the trauma is due to different factors that cause an immediate and diffuse bronchial and alveolar stress with passage of air and blood within the pulmonary parenchyma [3]. While haemorrhage and microatelectasis are the immediate consequences of the trauma (within 4-6 h), during the following 24 h a progressive deterioration of the pulmonary function can be observed.

Radiological aspects

Within 4-24 h after the trauma, *confluent opacities* can be recognized; they can be located in one or both lungs, close to the site of the trauma or away from it (i.e., on the opposite side) [17]. The CT aspects vary according to the involved lung compartment: linear opacities can be observed along the bronchovascular pathways; in the other cases (the majority) one or more parenchymal opacities with faint margins and of variable size, according to the trauma extent, can be observed. CT permits a better detection and overall evaluation of the contusive focuses, if compared with conventional radiography: however, its usage is rarely required, almost in uncomplicated cases. When suspected on the radiographs, CT can demonstrate areas of pulmonary laceration within the densities, which can be of clinical relevance when mechanical ventilation is planned [18] (see also below).

Outcome

The opacities tend to regress in a period of a few (3-7) days, when no complications occur [16]. When the opacities do not regress spontaneously, a complication should be suspected, such "ab ingestis" pneumonia, a bacterial infection or a pulmonary embolism [17].

Pulmonary laceration

Definition

It's an interruption of the parenchymal lung structures of a traumatic origin; the visceral and parietal pleural layers are preserved.

Pathophysiology

The interruption of the continuity of the parenchymal tissue allows the extravasation of blood from lacerated alveoli and bronchi. The alveolar disruption associated to the elastic retraction create a cavity of variable size, with thin walls, single or loculated, sometimes showing an air-fluid level within it (pneumatocele) [10]. Air can also migrate along the bronchial and vascular structures causing mediastinal emphysema.

When blood collects within the cavity, a real pulmonary haematoma that often does not communicate with the bronchial airways occur [10].

Radiological aspects

With conventional radiography, pulmonary *laceration* appears as a *spherical or elliptical pseudo-cystic cavity*, sometimes with an air-fluid level within it. When the cavity is filled up with blood (*haematoma*), it appears as a *round, dense opacity with sharp margins* [17]. Both lesions can be missed radiologically when a contusive focus hides them; the diagnosis with CT is easier: both hyperlucent lacerated parenchyma and hyperdense haemorrhagic haematoma.

Outcome

In the most favourable cases, both pneumatocele and haematoma tend to regress spontaneously between a few weeks and a few months. Sometimes, a fibrotic scar or a dense "coin lesion" can persist when haematoma organizes [3].

Pulmonary collapse and atelectasis

Definition

It is a consolidation of previously aerated lung, either a lobe, a segment or a subsegment. Acquired pulmonary collapse typically occurs in the ICU patients as a consequence of a thoracic trauma, after abdominal surgery, in smokers, obese, COPD patients, etc. or just for the supine decubitus [19].

Pathophysiology

In a majority of cases, pulmonary collapse is determined by endobronchial mucus or coagulated blood that are not removed also because of a reduced mucociliary clearance, a defective cough reflex and surfactant reduction; more rarely, it can be due to an endobronchial lesion such as the rupture of a bronchus [1]. In case of airways obstruction, a real lobar, segmental or subsegmental atelectasis occurs, very often in the region of the lower lobes [1].

Another kind of pulmonary collapse occurs when the airways are open, but the lung is compressed by a pleural effusion or a pneumothorax [10]. The pulmonary collapse from pleural origin tends to involve the lower lobes selectively. In case of massive pneumothorax, a complete pulmonary atelectasis may occur, with the lung completely collapsed towards the hilum.

Radiological aspects

The radiological manifestations vary according to the site and extension of the obstruction or the compression. *Left lower lobe atelectasis (the most frequent) determines an increased opacity of the left cardiac region on the AP projection with a concomitant disappearance of the diaphragmatic profile*; the opacity can be associated to an air bronchogram [1].

Outcome

Obstructive atelectasis in the ICU patients can be resolved by removing the secretions through fiberoptic bronchoscopy, in which case a reduction of the opacity and a re-expansion of the lung may be observed in the subsequent films [1].

Compressive collapse is reversible after removal of the determining cause.

Aspiration pneumonia (ab ingestis)

Definition

It is the pathological consequence of the inhalation of acid material into the airways; it may occur after surgery or in patients with impaired swallowing.

Pathophysiology

The effect of the acid fluid is that of a direct damage over the lungs. The segments most frequently injured in the supine patients are the posterior segments of the upper lobes.

Radiological aspects and outcome

CXR shows *alveolar, confluent, spotty areas of consolidation mostly in the middle and lower paramediastinal regions*, according to the patient position during the aspiration. These focuses show quite low variation with time, according to their nature of opacities from injury edema, and no variation with the decubitus of the patient [20].

Bacterial pneumonia

Definition

It is an acute infection of the pulmonary parenchyma, involving the alveolar spaces and interstitium.

Pathophysiology

The most frequent contaminating mechanisms are represented by the aspiration of upper respiratory airways secretions, an haematogenous or lymphatic or direct spread from contiguous infections. Predisposing factors are viral respiratory infections, alcoholism, advanced age, debilitation, unconsciousness, dysphagia, immunodeficiency, immunosuppressive therapies, etc. Pulmonary involvement may be lobar, segmental or patchy, depending upon the aggressiveness of the infective agent and host vulnerability.

Radiological aspects and outcome

Diagnostic imaging (CXR and CT) gives support to the clinics showing the typical radiological aspects of *swiftly confluent parenchymal opacities usually with associated air bronchogram.*

Often the process tends to be confined to one lobe, while the simultaneous involvement of two or more lobes has a poorer prognosis. The *fissures* limit the extension of the process beyond the lobe; the fissures can be concave or convex depending upon the quantity of edema and inflammation and the association of atelectasis. The *imaging* is *not specific* and usually it is not useful to determine the etiologic agent, but together with the clinics may be useful to restrict the clinical choices and to get a correct diagnosis: a quick onset and receding of the opacities in an infective patient, for example, are more typical of a pulmonary edema than of an inflammatory process; in cases of infectious origin, radiology may be helpful to monitor the regress of the process [1]. CT has an only limited role in this pathology.

References

1. Maffessanti M, Berlot G, Bortolotto P (1998) Chest roentgenology in the intensive care unit: an overview. Eur Radiol 8:69-78
2. Maffessanti M, Bortolotto P, Kette F (1988) Malposizioni e complicanze in seguito a cateterismo venoso centrale in rapporto alla sede d'accesso. Radiol Med 75:609-612
3. Goodman LR, Putman C (1983) Intensive care radiology: imaging of the critically ill. Saunders, Philadelphia
4. Gerlock AM, Mirfakraee M (1987) Retrieval of intravascular foreign bodies. J Thorac Imaging 2:52-60
5. Tocino IM, Watanabe A (1986) Impending catheter perforation of superior vena cava: radiographic recognition. AJR 146:487-490
6. Dunbar RD (1984) Radiologic appearance of compromised thoracic catheters, tubes and wires. Radiol Clin North Am 22:699-722
7. Maffessanti M, Bortolotto P, Berlot G (1991) L'esame radiologico del torace nella terapia intensiva. Radiol Med 82:107-117
8. Rollins RJ, Tocino I (1987) Early radiographic signs of tracheal rupture. AJR 148:695-698
9. Smith GM, Reed JC, Choplin RH (1990) Radiographic detection of esophageal misplacement of endotracheal tubes. AJR 154:23-26
10. Pistolesi GF, Procacci C (1990) Vademecum alla tomografia assiale computerizzata del torace. Piccin, Padova
11. Baldt MM, Bankier AA, German PS et al (1995) Complications after emergency tube thoracostomy: assessment with CT. Radiology 195:539-543
12. Miller KS, Tomlinson JR, Sahn SA (1985) Pleuropulmonary complications of enteral tube feeding. Chest 88:230-233
13. Maffessanti M, Pirronti T, Pistolesi M et al (1988) Diagnosi radiologica dell'edema polmonare. In: Aggiornamento professionale continuativo SIRMN (ed) Radiologia Toracica quattro. Apollonio, Brescia, pp 47-62
14. Milne ENC, Pistolesi M, Miniati M et al (1985) The radiologic distinction of cardiogenic and non cardiogenic edema. AJR 144:879-894
15. Zimmermann JE, Goodman LR, Shahvari MBG (1979) Effect of mechanical ventilation and positive end-expiratory pressure (PEEP) on chest radiograph. AJR 133:811-815
16. Heller M, Jend HH, Genant HK (1986) Computed tomography of trauma. Thieme, New York
17. Canini R, De Florio L, Ghini G et al (1992) I traumi del torace. Radiol Med 84[Suppl2]: 188-201
18. Toombs BD, Lester RG, Ben Menachem Y et al (1981) Computed tomography in blunt trauma. Radiol Clin North Am 19:17-35
19. Henschke CI, Yankelevitz DF, Wand A et al (1996) Accuracy and efficacy of chest radiography in the intensive care unit. Radiol Clin North Am 34:21-31
20. Lipchik RJ, Kuzo RS (1996) Nosocomial pneumonia. Radiol Clin North Am 34:47-58

METABOLISM, KIDNEY, FLUID AND VOLUME

Metabolic Changes with Surgery - Lessons to be Learned

F. CARLI

Activation of the stress response

The host response to injury – surgical, traumatic, or infectious – is characterized by various endocrine, metabolic, and immunologic alterations. If the inciting injury is minor and of limited duration, wound healing and restoration of metabolic and immune homeostasis readily occur. More significant insults lead to further deterioration of the host regulatory processes which, without appropriate intervention, often precludes a full restoration of cellular and organ function or results in death. The spectrum of cellular metabolic and immunologic dysfunction resulting from injury suggests a complex mechanism for identifying and initially quantifying the injurious event. This initial response is inherently inflammatory, inciting the activation of cellular processes designed to restore or maintain function in tissues while also promoting the eradication or repair of dysfunctional cells. The classic response to injury comprises multiple axes. These hormone response pathways are activated by mediators released by the injured tissue, neural and nociceptive input originating from the site of injury, or baroreceptor stimulation from intravascular volume depletion [1].

While the classic neuroendocrine response to injury has been extensively investigated, many characteristics of the inflammatory response associated with injury remain unexplained. Even after the normalization of macroendocrine hormone function after the primary injury, the persistence of systemic inflammation, the progression of organ dysfunction, and even late mortality indicate the presence of other potent mediators influencing the injury response. These mediators usually are small proteins or lipids that are synthesized and secreted by immunocytes. These molecules, collectively referred to as cytokines, are indispensable in tissue healing and in the immune response generated against microbial invasion. Unlike classic hormonal mediators such as catecholamines and glucocorticoids that are produced by specialized tissues and exert their influence predominantly by endocrine routes, cytokines are produced by diverse cell types at the site of injury and by systematic immune cells. Cytokine activity is primarily exerted locally via cell-to-cell (paracrine) interactions.

During systemic inflammation, the response mounted by the host to injury and infection manifests the collective activities of circulation and tissue-fixed immunocytes and endothelial cell populations. In the normal host, programmed cell death (apoptosis) is the principal mechanism by which senescent or dysfunctional cells, including macrophages and PMNs are systematically disposed of without activating other immunocytes or the release or proinflammatory contents.

The inflammatory milieu disrupts the normal apoptotic machinery in dysfunctional or ageing cells, consequently delaying the disposal of activated macrophages and PMNs. Several proinflammatory cytokines delay the normal temporal sequence of macrophage and PMN apoptosis in vitro. The prolonged survival of inflammatory immunocytes may perpetuate and augment the inflammatory response to injury and infection, precipitating multiple organ failure and eventual death in severely injured and critically ill patients.

In addition to modulating coagulation and vasomotor activities, mediators elaborated by the vascular endothelium in response to injury are well-documented contributors to the inflammatory process. In a paracrine fashion, local mediators such as TNF-α, IL-1, endotoxin, thrombin, histamine, and IFN-γ are capable of stimulating or activating the endothelial cell during local tissue injury. The ability to attract leukocytes and produce inflammatory mediators makes endothelial cells important participants in the immune response to injury.

Cytokines

Cytokines are a group of low-molecular-weight proteins which includes the interleukins and interferons [2]. They are produced by activated leucocytes, fibroblasts and endothelial cells as an early response to tissue injury and have a major role in mediating immunity and inflammation. The cytokines act on surface receptors on many different target cells and their effects are produced ultimately by influencing protein synthesis within these cells. They have local effects of mediating and maintaining the inflammatory response to tissue injury, and also initiate some of the systemic changes which occur. The cytokine cascade activated in response to injury consists of a complex network with diverse effects on all aspects of physiological regulatory mechanisms. Cytokines are pivotal determinants of the host response after injury, and their immunobiologic sequelae can have important applications in the comprehensive care of the surgical patient.

After major surgery, the main cytokines released are interleukin (IL)-1, tumour necrosis factor (TNF)-α and IL-6. The initial reaction is the release of IL-1 and TNF from activated macrophages and monocytes in the damaged tissues. This stimulates the production and release of more cytokines, in particular IL-6, the main cytokine responsible for inducing the systemic changes known as the acute phase response. The latter is a 26 kDa protein that is normally present at undetectable concentrations. Within 30-60 min of the start of surgery, IL-6 concentration increases; the change in concentration becomes significant after 2-4 h. Cytokine production reflects the degree of tissue trauma, so cytokine release is lowest with the least invasive and traumatic procedures, for example, laparoscopic surgery. The largest increase in IL-6 occurs after major procedures such as joint arthroplasty and major vascular and abdominal surgery. After these operations, cytokine concentrations are maximal for about 24 h and remain elevated for 48-72 h postoperatively.

The acute phase response is characterized by the production in the liver of acute phase proteins. These proteins act as inflammatory mediators, anti-proteinases, scavengers and tissue repairs agents. They include C-reactive protein, fibrinogen, α_2-macroglobulin and other anti-proteases. Production in the liver of other proteins such as albumin and transferin is decreased during the acute phase response. Cytokines IL-1 and IL-6 can stimulate secretion of ACTH from isolated pituitary cells in vitro. In surgical patients, cytokines may augment pituitary ACTH secretion and subsequently increase the release of cortisol. A negative feedback exists, so that glucocorticoids inhibit cytokine production. The cortisol response to surgery is sufficient to depress IL-6 concentrations.

Protein catabolism

The typical features of altered protein metabolism in surgical and critically ill patients include accelerated muscle protein breakdown and stimulated amino acid oxidation, accompanied by a decrease in whole body protein synthesis. The extent of protein losses following trauma depends on a variety of factors: nutritional status of the host, underlying disease process, type of anaesthesia, and severity of injury.

The cumulative nitrogen losses after elective abdominal operations range between 40 and 80 g nitrogen; complications that delay the use of the gastrointestinal tract may result in nitrogen losses up to 150 g [3]. Patients after multiple injury and during septic shock lose more than 200 g nitrogen, while nitrogen losses after severe burns can exceed 300 g. The clinical importance of this catabolic pattern can be appreciated more readily when one remembers that 1 g nitrogen is the equivalent of approximately 30 g hydrated lean tissue. Therefore, a loss of 50 g nitrogen as seen after uncomplicated cholecystectomy is equivalent to 1500 g lean tissue. Since nitrogen balance studies reflect only net gain or loss of protein from the body, negative nitrogen balance can occur if protein breakdown and oxidation increase and synthesis remains the same, or if breakdown and oxidation rates remain unchanged and the rate of protein synthesis decreases. The use of isotopically labelled, nonradioactive amino acids allows quantification of the changes in whole body protein synthesis and breakdown in surgical patients. Studies employing this methodology have improved our understanding of the mechanisms underlying the alterations in protein metabolism following injury and sepsis.

The catabolic response to surgical trauma probably has evolved to confer a maximum chance of survival due to the increased supply of energy-generating substrates. Because protein represents both structural and body components, erosion of lean tissue may lead to devastating nutritional consequences such as delayed wound healing, compromised immune function, fatigue and diminished muscle strength causing prolonged convalescence and increased morbidity. Thus, several strategies have been designed to minimize protein losses in surgical and critically ill patients.

The effect of anaesthesia and analgesia on the stress response to surgery

Since pain is regarded as a potent trigger for the catabolic response to surgery, specific analgesic techniques have been used to modify protein catabolism. High-dose opioid anaesthesia using morphine or fentanyl suppresses most endocrine and metabolic responses to surgery leading to a reduction of nitrogen losses, but is rarely used for procedures of short or immediate duration because of the occurrence of profound respiratory depression postoperatively [4]. The new, shorter acting opioids, alfentanil and sufentanil similarly prevent the intraoperative stress response, also when administered in smaller doses. The immediate postoperative metabolic changes, however, are unaffected or even more pronounced [5]. Based on the hypothesis that intra- and postoperative block of the surgical stress response might favourably influence postoperative morbidity, it seems, from a metabolic point of view, questionable whether patients can clinically benefit from this anaesthesia concept.

Clonidine

The centrally acting α-2 agonist clonidine has become popular as a premedication because of its sedative, anxiolytic and analgesic properties. Recognized neuroendocrine effects of clonidine include inhibition of sympathoadrenal activity and ACTH secretion with subsequent decrease in plasma cortisol and nitrogen excretion [6]. Clonidine, however, also exerts a dose-dependent inhibitory effect on the β-cells of the pancreas resulting in a decrease in insulin secretion and hyperglycaemia [7].

Epidural blockade

There is clear evidence that a symmetrical sensory block, achieved by local anaesthetics and extending from T4 to S5 dermatones, attenuates the metabolic and endocrines response to abdominal surgery, particularly to procedures below the umbilicus [8]. In upper abdominal or thoracic surgery, it is not possible to completely prevent pituitary hormone responses, even with extensive anaesthetic epidural local blockade. Most of the explanations for this failure to completely abolish the stress response centre around inadequate or incomplete afferent somatic and sympathetic neural blockade which allows pituitary activation and hence cortisol release from the adrenal cortex under the influence of ACTH, while efferent blockade of nerves to the adrenal medulla and the liver inhibits hyperglycaemic responses. Epidural blockade of nociceptive and non-nociceptive pathways such as the sympathetic nervous system has been found to decrease postoperative breakdown and amino acid oxidation [9], and to prevent the fall in muscle protein synthesis after surgery, as long as the block is maintained well into the postoperative period [10]. In contrast, epidural administration of opioids did not effectively inhibit the metabolic and endocrine changes induced by surgical trauma [8]. It has to be noted that most of the studies reporting anticatabolic effects of epidural blockade with local anaesthetics were performed in patients receiving isocaloric and isonitrogenous nutrition. Epidural blockade did not favourably influence protein economy when perioperative calorie intake was low or absent, supporting the contention that the protein-sparing influence of epidural blockade requires adequate energy and nitrogen supply [11].

Due to superior pain control during mobilization, epidural analgesia with local anaesthetics facilitates a more rapid return of mobility after surgery when compared to intravenous opioids. Since prolonged bed rest has been associated with significant muscle wasting and a decrease in whole body protein synthesis, early postoperative ambulation and mobilization might well contribute to the anticatabolic effort of epidural analgesia [12].

Surgery

The catabolic response to surgery is influenced by the type of the surgical procedure. Laparoscopic abdominal surgery (cholecystectomy, colonic resection, appendectomy) leads to reduced injury response in inflammatory mediators (IL-6, CRP, TNF) and immune functions (leucocytosis, wound infection), whereas the endocrine and metabolic alterations are less modified when compared with similar open procedures [13]. Other postoperative responses, such as pulmonary dysfunction, impairment of muscle exercise performance, hypoxaemia and intestinal paralysis appear to be improved by the use of laparoscopic techniques.

Nutrition

The rationale for providing protein and energy substrates to surgical patients is to maintain or replenish lean body mass. The nitrogen-conserving effect of nutrition is directly related to both nitrogen and energy intake. *Hypocaloric* dextrose infusion alone did not affect negative nitrogen balance in traumatized or infected patients, while *hypercaloric* isonitogenous total parenteral nutrition (TPN) restored nitrogen balance [14]. *Isocaloric* isonitrogenous provision of energy and substances in injured patients attenuated protein losses via an increase in whole body protein synthesis, but the elevated rate of protein catabolism continued unaltered [15]. It seems that only a combined high energy and anabolic substrate supply can reverse part of the catabolic response to trauma and infection. This nutritive regimen, however, has been shown to exert a number of disadvantageous effects, in particular acute hyperglycaemia [16]. Plasma glucose concentrations above 250 mg/dl have been associated with poor clinical outcome after cardiopulmonary resuscitation and cerebral ischaemia. The glucose-induced increment of CO_2 production may create substantial difficulties to wean patients from the respirator. In addition, impaired phagocytic capacity of polymorphonuclear leukocytes and dysfunction of the complement system have been frequently described. Furthermore, hypercaloric feeding techniques requiring central venous cannulation increase the risk of infection in the postoperative period.

A number of prospective randomized trials have been undertaken to evaluate the impact of perioperative nutrition or clinical outcome of surgical patients. It was concluded that a week or more of *parenteral* nutritional support in moderately malnourished patients (approximately 15% weight loss) decreased the risk for postoperative complications by 10% [17]. In contrast, intravenous nutrition in well nourished patients caused a 10% *increase* in the overall risk of complications after surgery. *Enteral* feeding through needle catheter jejunostomy also failed to show any beneficial effects in most elective surgical patients [18]. Trauma patients receiving early enteral feeding, however, had fewer complications than parenterally fed control subjects [19].

Clearly, current nutritional support modalities are less effective in preventing protein loss and improving clinical outcome than previously believed, and in fact may be harmful. According to the lessons learned from outcome studies, future investigations will have to aim at identifying surgical patient subgroups, i.e. patients at metabolic risk such as diabetics, malnourished and elderly subjects, who might benefit from nutritional therapy.

Preoperative fasting

Elective surgery is routinely performed after overnight fast to ensure an empty stomach and to minimize the risks of aspiration, when general anaesthesia is induced. The restriction of food before elective surgery is usually set from midnight on the day before the operation. Fasting periods before abdominal surgery can amount to a much longer time (up to 40 hours), because bowel preparation on the preoperative day does not allow any oral food intake. Therefore, fasting periods before abdominal operations are often long enough to substantially deplete carbohydrate reserves and change the metabolic situation of the patient. The rationale for fasting before surgery has been questioned recently, as it was shown that preoperative glucose infusion normalized impaired insulin sensitivity after surgery [20]. Although early postoperative restoration of insulin function is crucial for the normalization of impaired glucose homeostasis, it remaines unclear if this improvement also exerts a positive influence upon protein catabolism. Data in the literature regarding the impact of pre- and intraoperative glucose administration on protein metabolism are conflicting, but the majority of studies conducted so far did not show any modifying effect on plasma concentrations of amino acids and nitrogen balance [21]. Since an integrated analysis of the effects of feeding on the kinetics of protein metabolism in the immediate perioperative period has not yet been performed, this issue warrants further investigation.

Specific nutrients and anabolic agents

Recent attention has focused on the effects of specific nutrients, in particular on the parenteral use of glutamine, the most abundant amino acid in the free amino acid pool of the body. The major portion of this amino acid pool is located within skeletal muscle. Skeletal muscle intracellular concentrations fall dramatically during catabolic illness [22]. Previously, intravenous provision of glutamine to critically ill patients had not been possible because of its instability in aqueous solutions. When added to standard parenteral nutrition, however, glutamine was able to promote nitrogen retention in patients following major abdominal surgery [22]. In a group of critically ill patients recovering from bone marrow transplantation, glutamine-supplemented TPN improved nitrogen balance, diminished clinical infection, and shortened hospital stay [23]. In septic patients, most of whom required ventilatory support, glutamine significantly reduced survival at six months as well as total intensive care unit and hospital costs per survivor [24]. Based on the available data, glutamine must be considered an important dietary amino acid in a number of clinical settings.

The fact that even vigorous nutritional support failed to entirely curtail protein catabolism after trauma and during sepsis has led to the investigation of various pharmacological approaches.

The use of naturally occurring hormones such as insulin is appealing because insulin is the body's key endocrine regulatory factor to promote protein anabolism. Combined infusions of insulin and glucose significantly ameliorated protein losses in critically ill patients [25, 26]. In order to overcome insulin resistance, insulin has to be administered in high doses. At the same time provision of excessive amounts of glucose is required to maintain normoglycaemia. This issue causes potential metabolic concern because high carbohydrate intake causes fatty infiltration of the liver and stimulates carbon dioxide production.

The anabolic effects of recombinant human growth hormone (rGH) have been long established in surgical and critically ill patients. Patients receiving a hypocaloric diet and low doses of rGH following major abdominal surgery exhibited less weight and nitrogen losses than patients in a control group [27]. Respiratory muscle strength also was enhanced in rGH-treated patients after gastrectomy or colectomy, and weaning from the respirator was facilitated [28]. Kinetic studies showed that the anabolic effects of rGH were caused by an increase in protein synthesis and an attenuation of endogenous protein oxidation after surgery [29]. Despite these beneficial effects of rGH treatment upon the catabolic response to surgical trauma, there has been concern recently about the therapeutic use of rGH during critical illness, because treatment of septic patients with rGH was associated with an increased mortality rate [30].

Conclusions

Despite profound advances in anaesthesia care, feeding techniques, and drug development, the catabolic response to injury still represents a metabolic phenomenon in surgical patients that deserves the attention of clinicians and researchers. Although there is evidence that single pharmacological interventions are able to modulate protein catabolism, nitrogen losses following surgery cannot be completely suppressed and organ function promptly restored. I believe that a multimodal approach combining analgesic, anaesthetic and surgical strategies with the provision of specific nutrients and anabolic agents holds great promise for not only reducing the loss of body protein, but also for accelerating recovery, shortening the length of hospitalization, and reducing convalescence, resulting in a major improvement in clinical outcome. Furthermore, the use of tracer methodologies will further increase our understanding of the pathophysiological changes induced by tissue trauma and will help to identify subgroups of patients who might particularly benefit from our therapeutic efforts.

References

1. Lowry SF (1993) Hormone and cytokine regulation of injury metabolism. In: Vincent JL (ed) Yearbook of intensive care and emergency medicine. Springer, Berlin Heidelberg New York, pp 3-9
2. Sheeran P, Hall GM (1997) Cytokines in anesthesia. Br J Anaesth 78:201-219
3. Kinney J, Elwyn DH (1983) Protein metabolism and injury. Ann Rev Nutr 3:433
4. Giesecke K, Klingstedt C, Ljungqvist O, Hagenfeldt L (1994) The modifying influence of anesthesia on postoperative protein catabolism. Br J Anaesth 72:697
5. Schriker T, Carli F, Schreiber M et al (2000) Propofol/sufentanil anesthesia suppresses the metabolic and endocrine responses during, not after lower abdominal surgery. Anesth Analg 90:450
6. Mertes N, Goetters C, Kuhlmann M, Zander JF (1996) Postoperative alpha 2 adrenergic stimulation attenuates protein catabolism. Anesth Analg 82:258
7. Metz SA, Halter JB, Robertson RP (1978) Induction of defective insulin secretion and impaired glucose tolerance by clonidine. Selective stimulation of metabolic alpha adrenergic pathways. Diabetes 27:554
8. Kehlet H (1998) Modification of responses to surgery by neural blockade. In: Cousins MJ (ed) Neural blockade in clinical anesthesia and management of pain. Lippincott-Raven, Philadelphia, p 129
9. Carli F, Webster J, Pearson M et al (1991) Protein metabolism after abdominal surgery: effect of 24-H extradural block with local anesthetic. Br J Anaesth 67:729
10. Carli F, Halliday D (1997) Continuous epidural blockade arrests the postoperative decrease in muscle protein fractional synthetic rate in surgical patients. Anesthesiology 86:1033
11. Schricker T, Wykes L, Carli F (2000) Epidural blockade improves substrate utilization after surgery. Am J Physiol (in press)
12. Ferrando AA, Lane HW, Stuart CA et al (1996) Prolonged bed rest decreases skeletal muscle and whole body protein synthesis. Am J Physiol 270:E627
13. Kehlet H, Nielsen HJ (1998) Impact of laparoscopic surgery on stress response, immunofunction, and risk of infectious complications. New Horizons 6:S80
14. Nordenström J, Askanazi J, Elwyn DH et al (1983) Nitrogen balance during total parenteral nutrition. Ann Surg 197:27
15. Shaw JHF, Wolfe RR (1989) An integrated analysis of glucose, fat, and protein metabolism in severely traumatized patients. Ann Surg 209:63
16. Schriker T, Lattermann R, Schreiber M et al (1998) The hyperglycemic response to surgery: pathphysiology, clinical implications and modification by the anaesthetic technique. Clin Intens Care 9:118
17. Klein S, Kinney K, Jeejeeboy K et al (1997) Nutrition support in clinical practice: review of published data and recommendations for future research directions. J Parenter Enteral Nutr 21:133
18. Hesline MJ, Latkany L, Leung D et al (1997) A prospective randomized trial of early enteral feeding after resection of upper GI malignancy. Ann Surg 266:567
19. Kudsk KA, Croce MA, Fabian TC et al (1992) Enteral versus parenteral feedings: effects on septic morbidity after blunt and penetrating abdominal trauma. Ann Surg 215:503
20. Nygren J, Thorell A, Soop M (1998) Perioperative insulin and glucose infusion maintains normal insulin sensitivity after surgery. Am J Physiol 275:E140
21. Sieber FE, Smith DS, Traystman RJ, Wollman H (1987) Glucose: a reevaluation of its intraoperative use. Anesthesiology 67:72
22. Stehle P, Zander J, Mertes N et al (1989) Effect of parenteral glutamine peptide supplements on muscle glutamine loss and nitrogen balance after major surgery. Lancet 1:231
23. Zigler TR, Young IS, Benfell K et al (1992) Clinical and metabolic efficacy of glutamine-supplemented parenteral nutrition following bone marrow transplantation: a randomized, double-blind controlled trial. Ann Intern Med 116:821

24. Griffiths RD, Jones C, Palmer TEA (1997) Six month outcome of critically ill patients given glutamine supplemented parenteral nutrition. Nutrition 13:295
25. Woolfson AMJ, Heatley RV, Allison SP (1979) Insulin to inhibit protein catabolism after surgery. N Engl J Med 300:14
26. Sakurai M, Aarsland A, Herndon DN et al (1995) Stimulation of muscle protein synthesis by long-term insulin infusion in severely burned patients. Ann Surg 222:283
27. Jiang ZM, He GZ, Zhang SY et al (1989) Low dose growth hormone and hypocaloric nutrition attenuate the protein-catabolic response following major operation. Ann Surg 210:513
28. Knox JB, Wilmore DW, Demling RH et al (1996) Use of growth hormone for postoperative respiratory failure. Am J Surg 171:576
29. Carli F, Webster JD, Halliday D (1997) Growth hormone modulates amino acid oxidation in the surgical patient: leucine kinetics during the fasted and fed state using moderate nitrogenous and caloric diet and recombinant human growth hormone. Metabolism 46:23
30. Takala Y, Ruokonen E, Webster N et al (1999) Increased mortality associated with growth hormone treatment in critically ill patients. N Engl J Med 341:785

Monitoring of Substrates in Catabolic Patients

G. Biolo

Critically ill patients are characterized by a number of metabolic alterations involving proteins [8, 16, 64, 66], carbohydrates [62] and lipids [54] which may rapidly lead to a condition of protein-energy malnutrition [49], especially in patients who already show symptoms and signs of altered nutritional status. These metabolic changes represent a common response in almost every acute illness. The greatest alterations are observed following severe trauma, sepsis or large burns. A milder response is observed during localized infections, myocardial infarction, elective surgery, etc.

Protein and amino acid metabolism

Severely ill patients may lose up to 20% of body protein, much of which originates from skeletal muscle [27]. Although catabolism of muscle protein may be useful in the acute phase to provide substrates for protein synthesis in visceral tissues (i.e., liver, gut, immune cells, wound tissue, etc.), severe depletion of lean body mass may adversely affect morbidity and mortality of patients and delay the recovery from illness. In some patients weakness of respiratory muscles may be so great as to impair pulmonary ventilation and contribute to the respiratory insufficiency often associated with critical illness. Other clinical manifestations of acute protein catabolism include impaired immune response to infections, decreased coagulation capacity, impaired wound healing and reduced gut function.

Net protein catabolism is the result of the balance between the absolute rates of protein synthesis and breakdown. Net balance of body proteins is measured from the difference between nitrogen intake and total nitrogen loss, whereas the absolute rates of protein synthesis and breakdown can be directly measured in vivo using isotopically labelled amino acids. This technique may be used to measure the kinetics of protein at the whole-body level or in distinct tissues such as skeletal muscle. Evidence indicates that loss of lean body mass in severe stress conditions results mainly from a sustained increase of the rate of protein breakdown in skeletal muscle [8, 68]. Depressed protein synthesis may also contribute to the catabolic response. However, despite the fact that both total muscle RNA [32-35] and specific myofibrillar protein mRNA [24] levels were drastically reduced in trauma and sepsis, studies utilizing stable isotopes have often reported increased rates of whole-body and muscle protein synthesis in patients [8, 68]. It may be hypothesized that increased availability of intracellular amino acids derived from proteolysis may directly stimulate protein synthesis, possibly with a post-transcriptional mechanism.

The hydrolysis of intracellular proteins to their constituent amino acids is a highly regulated process which recent studies have revealed to be far more complex than previously believed [11, 46]. Three major pathways have been identified. The most thoroughly characterized in skeletal muscle are the ATP-independent lysosomal proteases, cathepsin B, L, H and D. Skeletal muscle also contains Ca^{++}-dependent protease, μ- and m-calpain. The third proteolytic system is the ATP-dependent pathway requiring the presence of a specialized protein named ubiquitin. Under normal physiological conditions, lysosomes are predominantly involved in the degradation of extracellular and membrane-associated proteins. In contrast, the ubiquitin-dependent system is quantitatively the most important degradative system of myofibrillar proteins in skeletal muscle [46]. Recent evidence in both animals and humans indicates that the ubiquitin-dependent system also plays a major role in muscle wasting in acute catabolic states [3, 45, 46]. Although contradictory results have been obtained on the precise role of cathepsins and calpains, it appears that these proteolytic systems may be important in the chronic phase after trauma and sepsis [32-35].

Glutamine metabolism

Glutamine is the most abundant free amino acid in tissue pools. Intracellular free glutamine concentration is greater than that of essential amino acids by factors of 50 to 200. In skeletal muscle glutamine is largely synthesized from glutamate and free ammonia and then released into the bloodstream to be utilized as a major fuel for rapidly dividing cells (enterocytes, reticulocytes, lymphocytes, etc.) [47] and as a precursor for gluconeogenesis, nucleotide synthesis, ammonia excretion and glutathion formation [39]. Severely ill patients, regardless of the type of disease, are characterized by a severe depletion of the intracellular glutamine pool [2] and increased glutamine requirement in the gut, liver, kidney, immune system and wound tissue. Mechanisms of intramuscular glutamine depletion in trauma patients involve an increased glutamine efflux and/or a decreased rate of glutamine de novo synthesis [4]. The very negative impact of glutamine depletion on the clinical outcome of critically ill patients is indirectly demonstrated by the fact that glutamine supplementation may improve immune response, gut functions and nitrogen balance as well as decrease infectious complications, duration of hospitalization and, ultimately, mortality [30, 40, 55, 60, 61, 70].

Carbohydrate metabolism

In acute illness plasma glucose levels are often increased, and may achieve very high levels in patients with diabetes mellitus, impaired glucose tolerance or obesity, which may require high doses of insulin to obtain metabolic control. An increased hepatic glucose production [62] and a decreased insulin-mediated glucose utilization [14, 59] in skeletal muscle and adipose tissue are the main causes of hyperglycemia. Furthermore, these patients are characterized by a very high rate of glycolysis with accelerated production of pyruvate [29] in the immune system, wound tissue, lung, skeletal muscle, etc. Since pyruvate oxidation to acetyl-CoA by the pyruvate dehydrogenase is a rate limiting reaction, the excess of pyruvate is reduced to lactate (by the lactate dehydrogenase) or aminated to alanine (by the alanine aminotranferase). Such excess of lactate and alanine (with the addition of glycerol deriving from an accelerated hydrolysis of triglycerides in the adipose tissue) is taken up by the liver to drive the increased gluconeogenesis and glucose release into the bloodstream observed in acutely ill patients. Lactate production is further accelerated during hypoxia or tissue hypoperfusion. By these mechanisms lactate concentrations may achieve very high levels when the gluconeogenic capacity of the liver is overwhelmed by peripheral lactate production.

Lipid metabolism

Endogenous lipids represent the main source of energy in critical illness [1, 17], especially when nutritional support is inadequate. In the adipose tissue, triglycerides are hydrolyzed at a high rate to release free fatty acids (FFA) and glycerol into the bloodstream [54]. In peripheral tissues FFA are oxidized to produce energy, whereas in the liver they are in part reesterified to triglycerides and released into the bloodstream as very low density lipoprotein (VLDL). In critical illness, FFA production exceeds FFA utilization, resulting in increased plasma FFA levels which are proportional to the severity of the injury. VLDL clearance is also impaired. Such increase in plasma lipid concentrations plays an important role in determining other metabolic abnormalities such as insulin resistance. Despite the increased FFA flux to the liver, ketone body synthesis is relatively impaired even during insufficient nutritional support.

Energy metabolism

Critically ill patients are often defined as hypermetabolic because of a rise in body temperature and an increased energy requirement. Basal energy expenditure is increased proportionally to the severity of the injury [18], i.e., by 10-20% following localized infections, myocardial infarction or elective surgery and up to 50% after severe trauma, sepsis or large burns. Critically ill patients are characterized by simultaneous accelerations of opposite metabolic pathways such as glycolysis-gluconeogenesis, lipolysis-reesterification of fatty acids and protein synthesis-degradation [67]. This increased rate of substrate cycling is in part responsible for the increase in basal energy expenditure observed in critical illness.

Mediators

The role of different mediators of the metabolic response to critical illness has not been completely clarified. In the last few years, attention has focused on hormones, cytokines, prostaglandins and intracellular glutamine concentration. The so-called counter-regulatory hormones (glucagon, catecholamines and glucocorticoids) are elevated following trauma and sepsis. Evidence indicates that glucagon stimulates gluconeogenesis and essential amino acid catabolism in the liver [8], glucocorticoids also stimulate gluconeogenesis and have acute proteolytic effects in different tissues [8] possibly through the activation of the ubiquitin-dependent system [8]. Catecholamines play a key role in the stimulation of glycogenolysis, glycolysis and lipolysis. In contrast to the catabolic effects of catecholamines on carbohydrates and lipids, these hormones appear to be able to increase muscle protein synthesis through the activation of the $beta_2$ receptor [19]. However, catecholamines do not seem to regulate protein metabolism in critically ill patients because 3-day infusion of either a non-selective beta-blocker (propranolol) or a selective $beta_1$ blocker (metoprolol) did not change whole-body protein kinetics in burned patients [38]. Conversely, anabolic hormones appear to be less efficient in critical illness. Critically ill patients show reduced plasma levels of insulin-like growth factor-1 and resistance to the metabolic effects of insulin and growth hormone, which may contribute to protein catabolism in these patients [14, 51, 59].

Recent findings indicate that cytokines, proteins secreted by mononuclear cells as part of the inflammatory reaction, may mediate some of the metabolic dysfunction observed in patients with trauma and sepsis [22, 43, 53]. In the liver, interleukine 6 is involved in the stimulation of synthesis of the positive acute phase proteins (fibrinogen, plasminogen, PAI-1, fibronectin, C-reactive protein, ceruloplasmin, aptoglobin, ferritin, complement proteins, etc.) and in the inhibition of synthesis of the negative acute phase proteins (albumin, transferrin, alpha-fetoprotein, tyroxine-binding globulin, insulin-like factor-1, etc.). Tumor necrosis factor and interleukine 1 can potentially mediate most of the metabolic alterations seen in critical illness. These cytokines can increase glucocorticoid and catecholamine secretion, accelerate gluconeogenesis, protein degradation and energy expenditure and decrease protein synthesis, lipoprotein lipase activity and VLDL clearance, ketone body synthesis, etc. However, the exact role of cytokines in the metabolic derangement seen in critical illness has not been substantiated in clinical studies. The possible role of prostaglandins as mediators of protein catabolism was based on in vitro studies but has not been confirmed in vivo [68].

A currently attractive hypothesis is that the intracellular concentration of glutamine may play a role in regulating the rates of protein synthesis and degradation. Glutamine is the most abundant free amino acid in tissue pools. Muscle glutamine levels decline markedly in many catabolic disease states [2], and it has been reported that changes in tissue glutamine concentrations correlate with protein turnover. Furthermore, there is evidence that glutamine may both stimulate protein synthesis and inhibit protein degradation in vitro. In addition, administration of glutamine or of its precursor, alpha-ketoglutarate and ornithine alpha-ketoglutarate, may restrain protein catabolism in patients [20, 36, 63]. Haussinger et al. [37] postulated that a decrease in cellular hydration may lead to tissue protein catabolism. Evidence indicates that cell shrinkage is a catabolic signal, whereas cell swelling is anabolic. Cellular hydration is regulated by the intracellular concentrations of ions and metabolites. After severe trauma, the intramuscular glutamine depletion may contribute to cell dehydration by decreasing the osmotically active glutaminc gradient between the intracellular and the extracellular space. Thus, it has been hypothesized that modification of cellular hydration may be the link between intracellular glutamine content and protein catabolism in diseased states.

Metabolic therapy

An optimal nutritional support has been shown to decrease morbidity in critically ill patients [41]. Unfortunately, current forms of artificial nutrition are usually ineffective to induce anabolism (positive nitrogen balance) in severely catabolic patients. Therefore, a number of therapeutic approaches have been developed in an attempt to improve the protein anabolic efficacy of conventional nutrition.

Currently, great interest is devoted to the concept that some metabolites present also in the diet, such as arginine, glutamine, alpha-ketoglutarate, ornithine alpha-ketoglutarate, carnitine, n-3 and n-6 fatty acids, nucleotides, taurine, etc., may improve the metabolic response to critical illness when given at pharmacological doses. These metabolites may have direct metabolic effects or may act through the modulation of the hormonal or inflammatory response to illness [9, 13, 31, 44, 52, 56, 69].

The positive effects of glutamine supplementation have been described in the previous sections. Arginine plays a critical role in the urea cycle and in the biosynthesis of creatine phosphate, nitric oxide and polyamines. Numerous studies have demonstrated that arginine supplementation can improve wound healing, stimulate the immune system and reduce protein catabolism in trauma and septic patients [23]. Arginine is also a potent secretagogue for several hormones, such as growth hormone, prolactine, insulin and IGF-1. Thus, at least some of the metabolic effects of arginine could be mediated by hormone secretion. The role of arginine in regulation of immune function mainly involves stimulation of T lymphocyte proliferation and functions. The postulated mechanisms of action for the immunomodulating effects of arginine involve synthesis of nitric oxide, polyamines and cytokines and stimulation of prolactine and growth hormone secretion. Recent evidence shows positive effects on outcome of patients following a combined administration of arginine, nucleotides and n-3 fatty acids [12, 13].

Carnitine is a metabolite, normally present in the diet, which regulates important aspects of intermediary metabolism. Carnitine is essential for β-oxidation of long-chain fatty acids because it promotes their transport across the mitochondrial membrane. Furthermore, carnitine infusion improved insulin-mediated glucose utilization in humans and reduced nitrogen loss in vivo [10, 58, 60]. Patients with trauma and sepsis exhibit decreased intracellular carnitine concentrations with increased acylcarnitine/free carnitine ratio. It is known that intracellular free carnitine may buffer excessive acyl-CoA production which, in stress conditions, frequently derives from accelerated FFA oxidation. Free carnitine may react with acyl-CoA to form acylcarnitine and regenerate free-CoA. However, other factors may contribute to the low carnitine levels of these patients, such as decreased dietary intake and increased urinary excretion. An imbalance of intracellular carnitine is potentially one of the factors which may adversely affect substrate metabolism in stress conditions, including protein and amino acids. We have shown that carnitine supplementation may restrain whole-body nitrogen loss in severely traumatized humans, possibly acting at extramuscular sites [60].

Insulin is probably the most important regulator of protein metabolism. This hormone stimulates protein synthesis [5] and inhibits protein degradation in selected tissues. Insulin deficiency in type 1 diabetes rapidly results in severe protein loss. Postprandial insulin secretion is a fundamental mediator of protein anabolism after a meal. Nonetheless, the potential anabolic action of exogenous insulin administration in critically ill patients still needs to be definitively demonstrated. Patients with trauma and sepsis exhibit resistance to the hypoglycemic action of insulin, which may extend to the anabolic effect on protein metabolism.

Early studies demonstrated that growth hormone (GH) could increase nitrogen retention in many physiological and pathological conditions [25, 26, 28, 48, 65]. GH promotes protein synthesis by increasing cellular uptake of amino acids and accelerating nucleic acid transcription and translation, thereby enhancing cell proliferation. GH shows both direct and indirect effects via stimulation of insulin-like growth factor-1 (IGF-1) synthesis. GH is a potent anabolic agent in both physiological and pathological conditions. Further, the protein catabolic effect of glucocorticoid can be prevented by the concomitant administration of GH. Administration of either GH or IGF-1 to critically ill patients resulted in reduced whole-body protein catabolism. Recently, Ramirez et al. [50] tested the effects of biosynthetic GH treatment on wound healing in massively burned children using a prospective randomized placebo controlled study design. They found that GH administration accelerated skin graft donor-site wound healing by 25%, resulting in a significant decrease in the overall time (from 46 to 32 days) to totally close the burn wound. However, GH administration in stress conditions may worsen insulin resistance, while IGF-1 may excessively decrease blood glucose levels. The combined treatment with GH and IGF-1 in humans produced significantly greater nitrogen retention and resulted in higher blood glucose concentration than IGF-1 alone. Despite such a large number of studies showing positive effects of GH administration, a recent double-blind randomized clinical study demonstrated an increased mortality in critically ill patients receiving GH therapy [57]. A potential side effect of GH administration involves the hormone effects on glutamine metabolism. We have recently observed that an anabolic effect of GH administration on protein metabolism was associated with a marked decrease of glutamine release from muscle into the bloodstream, which was largely accounted for by a suppression of glutamine de novo synthesis in muscle tissue [6]. By this mechanism, growth hormone administration in trauma patients may decrease systemic glutamine availability in extramuscular tissues leading to potentially negative effects in the intestinal mucosa and in the lymphatic and wound tissues. We may hypothesize that this potentially harmful side effect could be prevented by a simultaneous administration of growth hormone and exogenous glutamine supplementation.

Recent evidence indicates that some drugs, which are clinically used for their cardiovascular effects, may have protein anticatabolic effects. Pentoxifylline and amrinone, which are phosphodiesterase inhibitors, reduced protein catabolism in septic rats, possibly by inhibiting TNF secretion from activated macrophages [7, 15, 21, 42]. Furthermore, pentoxifylline administration improved survival after a lethal dose of endotoxin in mice. We have recently shown that pentoxifylline administration in chronically uremic patients acutely reduced whole-body protein turnover. Agonists of the beta$_2$ receptor of catecholamine, such as clenbuterol and salbutamol, which are clinically used for the treatment of asthma, may stimulate protein synthesis in skeletal muscle.

Conclusions

Critically ill patients are characterized by a number of metabolic abnormalities which lead to increased energy requirement and accelerated protein catabolism. An optimized nutritional support can prevent the excessive depletion of energy stores of patients but does not interfere with the accelerated proteolysis. Anabolic therapy with growth hormone reduces muscle protein catabolism but may increase mortality of patients possibly by decreasing glutamine synthesis and interfering with the immune response. Positive effects on outcome of patients have been observed with the administration of pharmacological doses of immunomodulating nutrients such as glutamine or the combination of arginine, n-3 fatty acids and nucleotides.

References

1. Askanazi J, Carpentier YA, Elwyn DH et al (1980) Influence of total parenteral nutrition on fuel utilization in injury and sepsis. Ann Surg 191:40-46
2. Askanazi J, Carpentier YA, Michelsen CB et al (1980) Muscle and plasma amino acids following injury. Ann Surg 192:78-85
3. Biolo G, Bosutti A, Toigo G et al (2000) Contribution of the ubiquitin-proteasome pathway on overall muscle proteolysis in severely traumatized patients. Metabolism (in press)
4. Biolo G, Fleming RYD, Maggi SP et al (2000) Inhibition of muscle glutamine formation in hypercatabolic patients. Submitted for publication
5. Biolo G, Fleming RYD, Wolfe RR (1995) Physiologic hyperinsulinemia stimulates protein synthesis and enhances transport of selected amino acids in human skeletal muscle. J Clin Invest 95:811-819
6. Biolo G, Iscra F, Bosutti A et al (2000) Growth hormone decreases glutamine production and stimulates muscle protein synthesis in hypercatabolic patients. Submitted for publication
7. Biolo G, Toigo G, Ciocchi B et al (1996) Pentoxifylline acutely decreases proteolysis in uremic patients. Clin Nutr 15[Suppl]:11
8. Biolo G, Toigo G, Ciocchi B et al (1997) Metabolic response to injury and sepsis: Changes in protein metabolism. Nutrition 13[Suppl]:52-57
9. Biolo G, Toigo G, Fiotti N et al (1997) Amino acid infusion acutely increases circulating tumor necrosis factor in humans. Clin Nutr16[Suppl]:27
10. Bohles H, Segerer H, Fekl W (1983) Improved N-retention during L-carnitine-supplemented total parenteral nutrition. JPEN 8:9-13
11. Bosutti A, Biolo G, Toigo G et al (1999) Molecular regulation of protein catabolism in trauma patients. Clin Nutr 18:103-105
12. Bower RH, Cerra FB, Bershadsky B et al (1995) Early enteral administration of a formula (Impact) supplemented with arginine, nucleotides, and fish oil in intensive care unit patients: Results of a multicenter, prospective, randomized, clinical trial. Crit Care Med 23:436-439
13. Braga M, Gianotti L, Vignali A et al (1998) Artificial nutrition after major surgery: Impact of route of administration and composition of diet. Crit Care Med 26:24-30
14. Brandi LS, Santoro D, Natali A et al (1993) Insulin resistance of stress: Sites and mechanisms. Clin Sci 85:525-535
15. Breuille D, Farge MC, Rose R et al (1993) Pentoxifylline decreases the body weight loss and muscle protein wasting characteristic of sepsis. Am J Physiol 265:E660-667
16. Carli F, Webster J, Ramachandra V et al (1990) Aspects of protein metabolism after elective surgery in patients receiving constant nutritional support. Clin Sci 78:621-628
17. Carpentier YA, Simoens C, Siderova V et al (1997) Recent developments in lipid emulsions: Relevance to intensive care. Nutrition 13:S73-78
18. Chiolero R, Revelly JP, Tappy L (1997) Energy metabolism in sepsis and injury. Nutrition 13:S45-51
19. Choo JJ, Horan MA, Little RA et al (1992) Anabolic effects of clanbuterol on skeletal muscle are mediated by β_2-adrenoreceptor activation. Am J Physiol 263:E50-E56
20. Cynober LA (1999) The use of alpha-ketoglutarate salts in clinical nutrition and metabolic care. Clin Nutr Metab Care 2:33-37
21. Doherty GM, Jensen JC, Alaxander HR et al (1991) Pentoxifylline suppression of tumor necrosis factor gene transcription. Surgery 111:192-200
22. Edwards PD, Moldawer LL (1998) Role of cytokines in the metabolic response to stress. Curr Op Clin Nutr Metab Care 1:187-190

23. Efron DT, Barbul A (1998) Modulation of inflamation and immunity by arginine supplements. Curr Op Clin Nutr Metab Care 1:531-538
24. Fong Y, Minei JP, Marano MA et al (1991) Skeletal muscle amino acid and myofibrillar protein mRNA response to thermal injury and infection. Am J Physiol 261:R536-R542
25. Frost RA, Lang CH (1998) Growth factors in critical illness: Regulation and therapeutic aspects. Curr Op Clin Nutr Metab Care 1:195-204
26. Fryburg DA, Gelfand RA, Barrett EJ (1991) Growth hormone acutely stimulates forearm muscle protein synthesis in normal humans. Am J Physiol 260:E499-507
27. Gamrin L, Essen P, Forsberg AM et al (1996) A descriptive study of skeletal muscle metabolism in critically ill patients: Free amino acids, energy-rich phosphates, protein, nucleic acids, fat, water, and electrolytes. Crit Care Med 24:575-583
28. Garibotto G, Barreca A, Russo R et al (1997) Effects of recombinant human growth hormone on muscle protein turnover in malnourished hemodialysis patients. J Clin Invest 99:97-105
29. Gore DC, Jahoor F, Hibbert JM et al (1996) Lactic acidosis during sepsis is related to increased pyruvate production, not deficits in tissue oxygen availability. Ann Surg 224:97-102
30. Griffiths RD, Jones C, Palmer TE (1997) Six-month outcome of critically ill patients given glutamine-supplemented parenteral nutrition. Nutrition 13:295-302
31. Grimble RF (1988) Modification of inflammatory aspects of immune function by nutrients. Nutr Res 7:1297-1317
32. Guarnieri G, Biolo G (1998) Pharmacological nutrition in ICU patients. In: Guarnieri G, Iscra F (eds) Metabolism and artificial nutrition in the critically ill. Springer-Verlag, Milano
33. Guarnieri G, Toigo G, Situlin R et al (1987) Proteinase activity, as well as DNA, RNA and protein content in human skeletal muscle in malnutrition and disease states. Klin Ernaehr 29:3-12
34. Guarnieri G, Toigo G, Situlin R et al (1988) Cathepsin B and D activity in human skeletal muscle in disease states. In: Hoerl WH, Heidland A (eds) Proteases II, potential role in health and disease. Plenum Press, New York, London, pp 243-256
35. Guarnieri G, Toigo G, Situlin R et al (1985) Muscle-biopsy studies on protein metabolism in traumatized patients. In: Dietze G, Grunert T, Kleinberg A et al (eds) Clinical nutrition and metabolic research. Research Proc. 7th Congr. ESPEN, Munich, Basel Karger 1986:28-39
36. Hammarqvist F, Wernerman J, Von Der Decken A et al (1991) Alpha-ketoglutarate preserves protein synthesis and free glutamine in skeletal muscle after surgery. Surgery 109:28-36
37. Haussinger D, Roth E, Lang F et al (1993) Cellular hydration state: An important determinant of protein catabolism in health and disease. Lancet 341:1330
38. Herndon DN, Nguyen TT, Wolfe RR et al (1994) Lipolysis in burned patients is stimulated by the $beta_2$ receptor for catecholamines. Arch Surg 129:1301-1305
39. Hong RW, Rounds JD, Helton WS et al (1992) Glutamine preserves liver glutathione after lethal hepatic injury. Ann Surg 215:114-119
40. Houdijk APJ, Rijnsburger ER, Jansen J et al (1998) Randomised trial of glutamine-enriched enteral nutrition on infectious morbidity in patients with multiple trauma. Lancet 352:772-776
41. Jolliet P, Pichard C, Biolo G et al (1999) Enteral nutrition in intensive care patients: A practical approach. Clin Nutr 81:47-56
42. Koch T, Neuhof H, Duncker HP et al (1993) Influence of pentoxifylline analogue on the granulocyte - mediated pulmonary mediator release and vascular reaction. Circ Shock 40:83-91
43. Lang CH, Dobbrescu C, Bagby GJ (1992) Tumor necrosis factor impairs insulin action on peripheral glucose disposal and hepatic glucose output. Endocrinology 130:43-52
44. Lin E, Kotani JG, Lowry SF (1998) Nutritional modulation of immunity and the inflammatory response. Nutrition 14:545-550
45. Mansoor O, Beaufrere B, Boirie Y et al (1996) Increased mRNA levels for components of the lysosomal Ca^{2+} activated, and ATP-ubiquitin-dependent proteolytic pathways in skeletal muscle from head trauma patients. Proc Natl Acad Sci USA 93:2714-2718
46. Mitch WE, Goldberg AL (1996) Mechanism of muscle wasting: The role of the Ubiquitin-Proteasome Pathway. New Engl J Med 335:1897-1905

47. Newsholme EA, Crabtree B, Ardawi MSM (1985) The role of high rates of glycolysis and glutamine utilization in rapidly dividing cells. Biosci Rep 5:393-400
48. Pichard C, Kyle U, Chevrolet JC et al (1994) Recombinant growth hormone effect on muscle function in ventilated chronic obstructive pulmonary disease. JPEN 18:S35-46
49. Plank LD, Connolly AB, Hill CL (1998) Sequential changes in the metabolic response in severely septic patients during the first 23 days after the onset of peritonitis. Ann Surg 228: 146-158
50. Ramirez RJ, Wolf SE, Barrow RE et al (1998) Growth hormone is safe and efficacious in the treatment of severe pediatric burns. Ann Surg 228:439-446
51. Roth E, Valentini L, Semsroth M et al (1995) Resistance of nitrogen metabolism to growth hormone treatment in the early phase after injury in patients with multiple injuries. J Trauma 38:136-145
52. Rudolph FB, Van Buren CT (1998) The metabolic effects of enterally administered ribonucleic acids. Curr Op Clin Nutr Metab Care 1:527-530
53. Sakurai Y, Zhang XJ, Wolfe RR (1996) TNF directly stimulates glucose uptake and leucine oxidation and inhibits FFA flux in conscious dogs. Am J Physiol 270:E864-872
54. Samra JS, Summers LKM, Frayn KN (1996) Sepsis and fat metabolism. Br J Surg 83:1186-1196
55. Stehle P, Mertes N, Puchstein CH et al (1989) Effect of parenteral glutamine peptide supplements on muscle glutamine loss and nitrogen balance after major surgery. Lancet 1:231-233
56. Stepleton PP, Charles RP, Redmond HP et al (1997) Taurine and human nutrition. Clin Nutr 16:103-108
57. Takala J, Ruokonen E, Webster NR et al (1999) Increased mortality associated with growth hormone treatment in critically ill patients. N Engl J Med 341:785-792
58. Tao RC, Peck GK, Yoshimura N (1981) Effect of carnitine on liver fat and nitrogen balance in intravenously fed growing rats. J Nutr 111:171-177
59. Thorell A, Nygren J, Ljungqvist O (1999) Insulin resistance: A marker of surgical stress. Curr Opin Clin Nutr Metab Care 2:69-78
60. Toigo G, Biolo G, Situlin R et al (1997) Modulation of protein metabolism in acutely-ill patients: Effects of carnitine and glutamine dipeptides. In: Tessari P, Soeters PB, Pittoni G, Tiengo A (eds) Amino acid and protein metabolism in health and disease: Nutritional implications. Smith-Gordon, London, pp 251-258
61. Van Der Hulst RR, Van Kreel BK, Von Meyenfeld MF et al (1993) Glutamine and the preservation of gut integrity. Lancet 341:1363-1365
62. Webber J (1998) Abnormalities in glucose metabolism and their relevance to nutrition support in the critically ill. Curr Opin Cli Nutr Metab Care 1:191-194
63. Wernerman J, Hammarqvist F, Vinnars E (1990) Alpha-ketoglutarate and postoperative muscle catabolism. Lancet 335:701
64. Wernerman J, Hammarqvist, Gamrin L et al (1996) Protein metabolism in critical illness. Baillière's Clinical Endocrinology and Metabolism 10:603-615
65. Wilmore DW (1999) Deterrents to the successful clinical use of growth factors that enhance protein anabolism. Curr Op Clin Nutr Metab Care 2:15-21
66. Wolfe RR, Goodenough RD, Burke JF et al (1983) Response of protein and urea kinetics in burn patients to different levels of protein intake. Ann Surg 197:163-171
67. Wolfe RR, Herndon DN, Jahoor F et al (1987) Effect of severe burn injury on substrate cycling by glucose and fatty acids. N Engl J Med 317:403-408
68. Wolfe RR, Jahoor F, Hartl WH (1989) Protein and amino acid metabolism after injury. Diab Metab Rev 5:149-164
69. Ziegler TR, Leader LM, Jonas CR et al (1997) Adjunctive therapies in nutritional support. Nutrition 13:S64-72
70. Ziegler TR, Young LS, Benfell K et al (1992) Clinical and metabolic efficacy of glutamine-supplemented parenteral nutrition after bone marrow transplantation. A randomized, double-blind, controlled study. Ann Intern Med 116:821-828

Renal Dysfunction in the Perioperative Period

O. VARGAS HEIN, C. SPIES, W.J. KOX

Relevance

The incidence of acute renal failure (ARF) in hospitalized patients is 2-5% [1, 2]. For postoperative ARF an incidence of up to 30% has been described [3]. In the perioperative period renal dysfunction is more frequent in cardiac and vascular surgery [1, 3]. Also, the patient's previous health status regarding renal, cardiovascular and pulmonary function influences the incidence and severity of renal dysfunction postoperatively [2]. As important as the patient's history is the preoperative status (preoperative renal failure, cardiac failure). If the patient undergoes an emergency operation, the incidence of ARF becomes up to 10-fold higher in comparison to elective surgery [4, 5]. These patients often require support postoperatively in the intensive care unit (ICU). ARF develops in the ICU in up to 25% of patients [6, 7]. ARF in these patients is often part of Multiple-Organ-Dysfunction-Syndrome (MODS). The mortality increases with the number of organs failing. MODS alone has a mortality rate of up to 15% [6, 7]. If ARF is part of MODS then the mortality increases to over 50% [2]. Nevertheless, ARF has been independently associated with postoperative mortality [8]. If postoperative ARF occurs isolated, mortality is reported to be 10% [4].

Pathophysiology

Postoperative ARF can be due to prerenal, intrarenal and postrenal causes. Renal ischaemia, as a prerenal cause, is the prevalent factor for postoperative ARF. Surgery and anaesthesia can lead to hormonal disequilibrium, inflammation and infection, hypoxemia, volume depletion and redistribution, haemodynamic insufficiency, decreased cardiac function and electrolyte abnormalities. These factors are associated with inadequate renal perfusion followed by renal ischaemia and finally acute tubular necrosis [2, 3, 5, 8]. Risk factors for intrarenal causes are the treatment with nephrotoxic drugs such as aminoglycosides, anti-inflammatory drugs, exposure to radiocontrast dye, thrombosis and haemolysis [9]. Postrenal causes like obstructive nephropathy account for only a small percentage of postoperative ARF. In contrast to ischaemia of the heart and brain, renal ischaemia is clinically silent and at the beginning compensated. It becomes clinically apparent when decompensation begins and damage is already established.

Risk factors

To identify patients who are at risk, the association of preoperative risk factors with postoperative ARF were studied. Results published so far have been controversial [3]. The main problem is the definition of ARF. Novis et al showed in a review of 28 studies where 30 risk factors were used, that not even two of these studies used the same criteria for ARF (Table 1) [3]. They found that poor preoperative renal function (most commonly diagnosed by elevated serum creatinine and urea) is the strongest significant predictor for postoperative ARF. Also advanced age and congestive heart failure were highly predictive for postoperative ARF [3]. Other risk factors like diabetes, arteriosclerosis, hypertension and liver failure should not remain unmentioned [4].

Different types of surgery

As noted above, the incidence of postoperative ARF is also strongly dependent on the surgery performed and the acute preoperative status of the patient. The incidence of postoperative ARF for the above mentioned publication from Novis et al is listed in Table 2 [3]. Sural et al analysed 140 patients in two centres over a period of 5 years who developed ARF postoperatively [10]. In these patients 67.1% had perioperative hypotension and 63.6% sepsis [10]. The incidence of ARF for the different types of surgery is listed in Table 2.

Cardiac surgery

The incidence in the literature for developing postoperative ARF after cardiac surgery is reported to be 1-5% with a mortality rate of 50-100% [11]. The most important cause is renal ischaemia. If cardio-pulmonary-bypass (CPB) is applied, the incidence of ARF increases up to 14 % [12]. CPB reduces renal blood flow by 30% [4]. Many studies were performed to find out adequate perfusion pressure and flow (pulsatile vs. nonpulsatile). Conflicting results have been obtained regarding the elevation of mean arterial pressure (MAD) over 50-60 mmHg or changing from non-pulsatile to pulsatile flow [12]. Other studies showed that duration of CPB > 140 minutes was a significant risk factor associated with postoperative renal failure [13]. During CPB an inflammatory reaction may occur and remain throughout the duration of CPB [14]. It is of major importance that the activation of coagulation together with other pathways leads to microcirculatory failure and organ failure due to fibrin-layers and thrombosis

Table 1. Definitions of ARF

Urea increase
Urea increase or anuria for 24 hours
Urea increase or dialysis
Urea and creatinine increase
Creatinine rise of 20% or more for 48 hours
Creatinine to > 20 µmol/l for 2 days consecutively
Creatinine increase > 0.5 mg/dl or > 3 mg/dl
Creatinine increase with oliguria
Low creatinine clearance
Decreased urinary output
Dialysis

Abbr.: ARF acute renal failure
Modified from reference Nr.: 3

Table 2. ARF incidence (%) for the different types of surgery

	Sural (10)	Kresse (1)	Novis (3)
Open heart surgery	32.9	39.9	36
Vascular surgery		18.4	43
Abdominal surgery		18.9	7
Gastrointestinal surgery	16.4		
Pancreatic surgery	9.3		
Obstetrical surgery	3.6		
Urological surgery	3.5		
Traumatology		10.1	
Cancer surgery		12.1	
Others	2.8		14

[12]. Hypothermia seems not to worsen CPB induced renal ischaemia [12]. Acid-base-management also did not show any influence on renal function [15]. Unequivocally is the importance of adequate perioperative haemodynamics and fluid status. Predictive for postoperative ARF in cardiac surgery were perioperative haemodynamic instability and preoperative renal dysfunction which were considered to be more important than CPB related factors [13, 15, 16].

Vascular surgery

Another high-risk group for postoperative ARF are patients undergoing aortic vascular surgery. A clear distinction must be made between elective and emergency aortic surgery. Mortality rates associated with ruptured aortic aneurysm are as high as 75-90% [17, 18]. If these patients survive the haemorrhagic shock sepsis with MODS including ARF are common problems. Elective surgery has a mortality rate of 2-11% [18]. The incidence of postoperative ARF in patients undergoing aortic surgery is 5-25%, depending also on the location of the aneurysm besides the already mentioned need for emergency surgery. ARF is the main cause of postoperative morbidity in this group of patients [4,19]. Hypotension and the number of transfusions required as well as preoperative renal dysfunction are predictors for ARF in this group [19]. Another important factor is the duration of cross-clamping. ARF after procedures with cross-clamping is as high as 50%, especially in suprarenal and thoracic clamping [12]. The pathogenesis for renal injury is thought to be ischaemia/reperfusion damage [12]. Another uncommon but disastrous cause of ARF during aortic surgery is bilateral renal artery embolism from cholesterol plaques or thrombi. In this case, a sudden anuria after declamping is observed clinically without resolution after 3 to 4 weeks [4].

Treatment

Postoperative acute renal dysfunction can present with different clinical and laboratory features. Important clinical problems caused by renal dysfunction are fluid overload, hyperkalemia, hyponatremia, acidosis and azotemia. Depending on the patient's clinical course (co-morbidity), the laboratory findings (creatinine and urea) and the severity of the above mentioned clinical conditions, renal replacement therapy (RRT) should be started. But, before starting any diuretics or RRT hypovolemia should be ruled out as the cause of inadequate perfusion pressure. Furosemid, dopamine, mannitol and corticosteroids are the drugs most often used in renal dysfunction for kidney protection. Dopamine infusion has been shown to increase renal blood flow and decrease renal vascular resistance, thereby increasing renal output and natriuresis. However, this effect might be due to increased cardiac output and not induced through dopaminergic renal receptors. Even if urine output is increased there is no or little effect on azotemia [20]. Dopamine has been applied for renal protection during cardiac surgery, showing no protective effect in preventing postoperative renal dysfunction [20]. In addition, if induced natriuresis produces intravascular volume depletion and hyponatremia ischaemic injury to the kidneys could be amplified [12]. Mannitol has been used widely for renal tubular protection during CPB. Mannitol increases renal blood flow by increasing prostaglandin release and promoting intravascular volume retention [12]. In the kidney it promotes glomerular filtration rate acting as an osmotic diuretic. Clinical studies relating to the protective effects of mannitol in patients with postoperative renal dysfunction suggest a significant decrease in the need for CRRT [12, 21]. In contrast, side effects like volume depletion after volume overload and hyperosmolarity have to be taken into account against the postulated benefits [12]. Furosemide, a loop diuretic, is the most widely used diuretic in the treatment of renal dysfunction. It increases urine output and can convert an oliguric ARF to a non-oliguric state, if administered early. Even if non-oliguric ARF is prognosticly better than oliguric ARF its influence on outcome is not clear [12]. Similarly to dopamine and mannitol no protective effect has been proven with furosemide [22]. Regarding renal protective strategies, especially during CPB, corticosteroids should be discussed. Corticosteroids are recommended for improvement of circulatory function after CPB as it was suggested by Wan et al. [14]. Corticosteroids act through membrane stabilisation and reduction of an overwhelming inflammatory reaction [14].

In critically ill patients where ARF is most frequent due to MODS, RRT is nowadays started as early as possible during the course of the disease [1]. Indications for RRT are mentioned in Table 3 [23]. 15% of the patients with postoperative ARF after cardiac surgery require dialysis [13]. RRT can be performed as an intermittent haemodialysis (IHD) or as continuous renal replacement veno-venous haemofiltration (CRRT) technique. Azotemia, electrolyte, metabolic and volume control can be achieved with both techniques [24]. However, IHD is performed over a short time of a few hours and induces rapid shifts in solutes and volume [24]. In critically ill patients this is not well tolerated and haemodynamic instability with possible deleterious effects for renal recovery can be one of the sequelae [24]. CRRT, instead, is performed over 24 hours with a continuous and slow volume shift and is well tolerated in ICU patients [24]. Therefore, in critically ill patients CRRT is the method of choice. In haemodynamic stable patients who develop ARF or patients with chronic renal failure on dialysis IHD can be performed postoperatively [1, 24]. The outcome (mortality < 60%) in postoperative patients with ARF under CRRT is mostly dependent on co-morbidities such as MODS [1]. It has been suggested that an early start of CRRT could influence outcome positively [1]. If the patient survives ARF secondary to acute tubular necrosis then long-term renal function recovery can be expected in 52-72% of the cases [25].

In conclusion, due to the increased morbidity and mortality, it is essential to recognize patients who are at risk from developing postoperative ARF. To detect this group of patients, screening tests for renal dysfunction should be performed in patients undergoing cardiovascular surgery. During the perioperative period

Table 3. Indications for RRT

Oliguria (urine output < 200 ml/12 hours)
Anuria (urine output < 50 ml/12 hours)
Severe acidemia (pH < 7.1) due to metabolic acidosis
Azotemia (urea > 30 mmol/l)
Hyperkalemia (K > 6.5 mmol/l)
Severe dysnatremia (Na > 160 or < 115 mmol/l)
Hyperthermia (core temperature > 39.5°C)
Clinically significant organ edema

Modified from reference Nr.: 23

monitoring and treatment strategies should aim at achieving haemodynamic stability. The treatment of renal dysfunction, particularly the early initiation of RRT compared to pharmaceutical approaches in the critically ill patient seems to be advantageous.

References

1. Kresse S, Schlee H, Deuber HJ et al (1999) Influence of renal replacement therapy on outcome of patients with acute renal failure. Kidney Int 56(Suppl 72):75-78
2. Corwin HL, Bonventre JV (1988) Acute renal failure in the intensive care unit. Part 1. Intensive Care Med 14:10-16
3. Novis BK, Roizen MF, Aronson S et al (1994) Association of Preoperative Risk Factors with Postoperative Renal Failure. Anesth Analg 78:143-149
4. Kellerman PS (1994) Perioperative Care of the Renal Patient. Arch Intern Med 154:1674-1688
5. Urzua J, Lema G, Canessa R et al (1999) Renal Preservation in the Perioperative Period. Int Anesthesiol Clin 37(2):111-123
6. Mangano CM, Diamondstone LS, Ramsay JG et al (1998) Renal Dysfunction after Myocardial Revascularization: Risk Factors, Adverse Outcomes, and Hospital Resource Utilization. Ann Intern Med 128(3):194-203
7. Guerin C, Girard R, Selli JM et al (2000) Initial versus Delayed Acute Renal Failure in the Intensive Care Unit. A multicenter prospective epidemiological study. Am J Respir Crit Care Med 161(3):872-879
8. Bowen Fortescue E, Bates DW, Chertow GM (2000) Predicting acute renal failure after coronary bypass surgery: Cross-validation of two risk-stratification algorithms. Kidney Int 57:2594-2602
9. Chertow GM, Lazarus JM, Christiansen CL et al (1997) Preoperative renal risk stratification. Circulation 95(4):878-884
10. Sural S, Sharma RK, Singhal M et al (2000) Etiology, prognosis and outcome of post-operative acute renal failure. Ren Fail 22(1):87-97
11. Chertow GM, Levy EM, Hammermeister KE et al (1998) Independent association between acute renal failure and mortality following cardiac surgery. Am J Med 104(4):343-348
12. Aronson S, Blumenthal R et al (1998) Perioperative Renal Dysfunction and Cardiovascular Anesthesia: Concerns and Controversies. J Cardiothorac Vasc Anesth 12(5):567-586
13. Suen WS, Mok CK, Chiu SW et al (1998) Risk factors for development of acute renal failure (ARF) requiring dialysis in patients undergoing cardiac surgery. Angiology 49(10):789-800
14. Wan S, Leclerc JL, Vincent JL (1997) Cytokine responses to cardiopulmonary bypass: lessons learned from cardiac transplantation. Ann Thorac Surg 63(1):269-276
15. Badner NH, Murkin JM, Lok P (1992) Differences in Ph management and pulsatile/nonpulsatile perfusion during cardiopulmonary bypass do not influence renal function. Anesth Analg 75:696-701
16. Valentine S, Barrowcliffe M, Peacock J (1993) A comparison of effects of fixed and tailored cardiopulmonary bypass flow rates on renal function. Anesth Intensiv Care 21:304-308
17. Barrat J, Prajasingam R, Sayers RD et al (2000) Outcome of acute renal failure following surgical repair of ruptured abdominal aortic aneurysms. Eur J Endovasc Surg 20(2):163-168
18. Cao P, De Rango P (1999) Abdominal aortic aneurysms: current management. Cardiologia 44 (8):711-7
19. Godet G, Fleron MH, Vicaut E et al (1997) Risk factors for acute postoperative renal failure in thoracic or thoracoabdominal aortic surgery: a prospective study. Anesth Analg 85 (6):1227-1232

20. Perdue PW, Balser JL, Lipsett PA et al (1998) "Renal Dose" Dopamine in Surgical Patients. Ann Surg 227(4):470-473
21. Sirivella S, Gielchinsky I, Parsonnet V. (2000) Mannitol, furosemide, and dopamine infusion in postoperative renal failure complicating cardiac surgery. Ann Thorac Surg. 69(2):501-506
22. Lassnigg A, Donner E, Grubhofer G et al (2000) Lack of renoprotective effects of dopamine and furosemide during cardiac surgery. J AM Soc Nephrol 11(1):97-104
23. Bellomo R, Ronco C (1999) Continuous renal replacement therapy in the intensive care unit. Intensive Care Med 25:781-789
24. Bellomo R, Ronco C (1998) Continuous versus intermittent renal replacement therapy in the intensive care unit. Kidney Int 53(Suppl 66):125-128
25. Liano F, Pascual J (1998) Outcomes in Acute Renal Failure. Sem Nephrol 8(5):541-550

Patient Selection, Timing and Stopping of Continuous Renal Replacement Therapy

P. Rogiers

Acute renal failure (ARF) occurs frequently, and the mortality remains very high despite the introduction of dialysis more than 25 years ago. In a recent prospective, multidisciplinary study of 1,086 patients with ARF, the overall hospital mortality rate was 66% [1].

Many factors interfere with the outcome of patients with ARF, such as severity of both acute and underlying illness, nephrology consultation, dialytic therapy, nutrition, and new pharmacological agents. In this chapter we will mainly focus on dialytic therapy and more specifically on continuous renal replacement therapy (CRRT).

In a study of Mehta et al. [2] it was shown that delay in nephrology consultation occurred in 28% of intensive care unit (ICU) patients with ARF, and this delay was associated with increased mortality, a larger number of failing organs, and a longer ICU stay.

Different scores are often used in publications. We shouldn't forget however that the often quoted acute physiology and chronic health evaluation (APACHE) II score was not intended to predict survival of patients with ARF requiring dialysis [3]. Newer more-specific scores have recently been developed, such as the Liaño score [4] and the APACHE III score.

Dialytic therapy

Several important questions regarding dialysis in ARF are under current evaluation. Does the use of biocompatible membranes affect outcome? What is the optimal dose of dialysis in the ARF setting? Are intermittent and continuous renal replacement therapies equal or is one superior to the other? What is the role of extracorporeal removal of inflammatory mediators?

Role of the membrane biocompatibility

It has been shown in an animal study that dialysis with bio-incompatible membranes can induce an inflammatory response of complement and neutrophil activation that can result in renal injury [5]. In patients various prospective randomized studies have shown beneficial effects of dialysis with biocompatible membranes, such as shortening of the duration of ARF, decrease in hospital stay, and even an increase in survival [6-8]. However, recently these positive results could not be reproduced in other studies [9, 10]. Even in animals, Kränzlin et al. [11] could not demonstrate any superiority of biocompatible membranes. In a more-recent prospective, randomized, multicenter trial, Jörres et al. [12] were not able to demonstrate any differences in outcome for patients with dialysis-dependent ARF between those treated with cuprophan membranes and those treated with polymethyl-methacrylate membranes.

Dose of dialysis

One of the first publications about dialysis in ARF was the paper of Teschan et al. 'Prophylactic haemodialysis in the treatment of acute renal failure', published in the *Annals of Internal Medicine* in 1960 [13]. They applied prophylactic hemodialysis in the treatment of 15 patients with ARF. Hemodialysis was performed during 6 h on a daily basis, before the nonprotein reached 200 mg/dl. This resulted in a dramatic improvement of the patient's condition, wound healing, and infection control. Since then, retrospective studies demonstrated that dialysis is better than no dialysis [14, 15]. Using the Cleveland Clinic Severity of Illness Score, Paganini et al. [16] showed a link between dialysis dose and outcome of ARF in critically ill patients. Interestingly, the dose of dialysis did affect outcome in patients with an intermediate score. In this subgroup of patients, higher dialysis delivery was associated with reduction in morbidity compared to low-dose dialysis. At the two ends of the severity of illness score, changing dialysis dose had no effects, meaning that mild ARF recovers regardless of therapy and severe ARF in very sick patients recovers seldom because of the severity of associated disease. Schiffl et al. [17] recently compared daily and alternate-day dialysis in critically ill patients with ARF. Overall mortality was dramatically improved from 47% in the alternate-day group to 21% in the daily dialysis group.

CRRT: patient selection

We should bear in mind that critically ill patients who develop ARF in the ICU are completely different from patients with chronic end-stage renal disease and should thus be treated differently. ARF in the ICU is seldom a unique finding, but rather part of a multiple organ function syndrome with, very often, respiratory failure needing artificial ventilation and vasoplegia due to sepsis, needing vasopressor therapy, or cardiac failure with inotropic support. Continuous therapies have several theoretical advantages compared to intermittent hemodialysis in critically ill patients. One of the most-important points in this respect is the hemodynamic stability. Initiation of intermittent hemodialysis and/or fluid removal frequently leads to a fall in blood pressure, often resulting in an increase of the dose of vasopressors. This can lead to further impairment of organ function. It has been shown that blood pressure drops during intermittent hemodialysis can result in fresh ischemic lesions, further preventing renal recovery [18, 19]. CRRT, however, does not decrease arterial blood pressure and can even be applied in hemodynamically unstable patients. This can even result in hemodynamic improvement [20] and a decrease of vasopressor therapy [21]. Improved hemodynamic stability during CRRT may have a beneficial effect on the preservation and recovery of renal function [22, 23].

Moreover, most of these patients are very catabolic, resulting in a need for high urea clearances. This can be performed by continuous veno-venous hemofiltration (CVVH) or continuous veno-venous hemodiafiltration (CVVHDF). With the use of modern machines with automatic control of fluid balance, 3-4 roller pumps, double-lumen venous catheters, commercially available substitution fluids, and high-flux membranes, excellent fluid control and urea clearances can be achieved. For the same Kt/V continuous techniques achieve a better metabolic control than intermittent hemodialysis [24]. Fluid removal can be performed very smoothly at a rate of 100-200 ml/h, thereby allowing enough caloric intake enterally and/or parenterally [25]. This will reduce edema caused by hypo abuminemia and sepsis-induced capillary leak syndrome.

Therefore, CVVH has become a widely accepted procedure and even, at least in some parts of Europe, the golden standard for treatment of ARF in critically ill patients [26, 27]. A recent prospective survey of 21 hospitals in Australia showed that 100% of ICU patients treated for ARF received CRRT [28]. Jacob et al. [29] performed a survey of 15 studies comparing intermittent (522 patients) and continuous (651 patients) renal replacement therapy. They were not able to find differences between the two techniques, although a strict meta-analysis was not possible due to major design problems.

The question is if we really need to prove if one technique is superior to the other. Both techniques have their advantages and disadvantages and can be applied together in different clinical situations in well-organized centers, with well-trained intensivists and nephrologists who are willing to co-operate. Therefore, it seems reasonable to recommend intermittent hemodialysis in stable, uncomplicated ARF, e.g., stable hemodynamic situations, absence of respiratory failure, or the need for immediate correction of hyperkalemia. On the other hand CRRT should be preferred in hemodynamically unstable patients, in case of artificial ventilation, in sepsis syndromes with the need for large amounts of fluid administration and removal, in cases of parenteral nutrition, and in patients at risk of cerebral edema. A considerable influx of water in the brain has been noticed after intermittent hemodialysis, responsible for the so-called dysequilibrium syndrome [30]. This may lead to life-threatening elevations of intra-cranial pressure in patients with cerebral edema, liver failure, trauma, or neurosurgery. Continuous hemofiltration gradually decreases plasma osmolarity and thus does not have these side effects. Therefore, in patients at risk of cerebral edema, ARF should be treated with a continuous technique [31].

CRRT: timing

In the past decade a lot of progress has been made in the materials and machines that are available for the treatment of ARF. The question of timing, however, has been somewhat neglected until now. Indeed, no clear rules or criteria are defined when to start dialysis or CRRT in ARF in unstable, critically ill patients. Therefore, we notice that almost every hospital has developed its own habits and even in a single center there can be different attitudes between various physicians. It is known that this can result in conflicts between nephrologists and intensivists [32]. There is however a growing consensus among physicians not to wait until all the physiological parameters have deteriorated so far that definite organ failure and death are inevitable. The earlier application of CRRT can result in control of fluid balance, acid-base status, and urea clearance necessary for homeostasis of the organism. This can only be achieved when nephrologists, intensivists, and critical care nurses collaborate in such a way that the only goal is the care and cure of the patient.

Experimentally, early intervention has been shown to be more beneficial than late intervention in sepsis [33]. This brings us to the last issue. Is there a role of hemofiltration in the early treatment of severe sepsis, even before the onset of ARF? Both experimentally and clinically many studies describe the removal of inflammatory mediators with hemofiltration. Despite this removal, plasma levels seldom decrease. This is because the inflammatory mediators have a high endogenous clearance that exceeds the clearance of hemofiltration. Also because of the very short plasma half-life of these mediators, from 6-17 min [34], hemofiltration can only remove a small fraction of the total amount of inflammatory mediators. Recently the clinical application of high-volume hemofiltration has received more attention. In a prospective cohort analysis by Oudemans-van Straaten et al. [35] the observed mortality was lower than predicted in 306 patients with ARF treated with high-volume hemofiltration. In another prospective randomized study of 425 patients with ARF, Ronco et al. [36] used three different ultrafiltration rates, 20, 35, and 45 ml/kg per hour. Survival was significantly lower in the group with the lowest ultrafiltration rate than in the two other groups. Increasing the ultrafiltration rate from 35 to 45 ml/kg per hour did not change the mortality.

In all of these studies the diagnosis of ARF is based upon rise in plasma creatinine or the development of oliguria. This brings a delay in recognition of early renal injury and does not allow accurate assessment of the degree of renal damage. From the animal experiments we know that to prevent further renal damage therapy must be started within the first 24 h [37].

CRRT: stopping

When the hemodynamic instability is over and vasoactive drugs are stopped, when the patients is no longer on artificial ventilation, when the capillary leak syndrome and edema have disappeared, then it is time to stop CRRT and to switch to intermittent hemodialysis, in case of persistent renal failure. This will allow the conscious patient to sit up and to be more mobile. Another advantage is that continuous anticoagulation can be stopped. This policy will avoid keeping patients in the ICU longer than needed. These patients should rather go to nephrology wards, where they are treated under the supervision of nephrologists.

References

1. Guerin C, Girard R, Selli J-M et al (2000) Initial versus delayed acute renal failure in the intensive care unit. A multicenter prospective epidemiological study. Am J Respir Crit Care Med 161:872-879
2. Mehta R, Farkas A, Pascual M et al (1995) Effect of delayed consultation on outcome from acute renal failure in the ICU. J Am Soc Nephrol 6:A471
3. Parker R, Himmelfarb J, Tolkoff-Rubin N et al (1998) Prognosis of patients with acute renal failure requiring dialysis: results of a multicenter study. Am J Kidney Dis 32:432-443
4. Liaño F, Pascual J (1996) Epidemiology of acute renal failure: a prospective, multicenter, community-based study. Kidney Int 50:811-818
5. Schulman G, Fogo A, Gung A et al (1991) Complement activation retards resolution of acute ischemic renal failure in the rat. Kidney Int 40:1069-1074
6. Schiffl H, Lang SM, Konig A et al (1994) Biocompatible membranes in acute renal failure: prospective case controlled study. Lancet 344:570-572
7. Hakim RM, Wingard RL, Parker RA (1994) Effect of the dialysis membrane in the treatment of patients with acute renal failure. N Engl J Med 331:1338-1342
8. Himmelfarb J, Tolkoff RN, Chandram P et al (1998) A multicenter comparison of dialysis membranes in the treatment of acute renal failure requiring dialysis. J Am Soc Nephrol 9:257-266
9. Jones CH, Newstead CG, Goutcher E et al (1997) Continuous dialysis for ARF in the ICU: choice of membrane does not influence survival. J Am Soc Nephrol 8:126A
10. Mehta R, Mc Donald B, Gabbai F et al (1996) Effect of biocompatible membranes on outcomes from acute renal failure in the ICU. J Am Soc Nephrol 7:1457A
11. Kränzlin B, Gretz N, Kirschfink M et al (1996) Dialysis in rats with acute renal failure: evaluation of three different dialyser membranes. Artif Organs 20:1162-1168
12. Jörres A, Gahl GM, Dobis C et al (1999) Hemodialysis-membrane biocompatibility and mortality of patients with dialysis-dependent acute renal failure: a prospective randomised multicentre trial. Lancet 354:1337-1341
13. Teschan PE, Baxter CR, O'Brien TF et al (1960) Prophylactic hemodialysis in the treatment of acute renal failure. Ann Intern Med 53:992-1016
14. Kleinknecht D, Jungers P, Chanard J et al (1972) Uremic and non-uremic complications in acute renal failure: evaluation of early and frequent dialysis on prognosis. Kidney Int 1: 190-196
15. Fisher RP, Griffen WO Jr, Reiser M et al (1996) Early dialysis in the treatment of acute renal failure. Surg Gynecol Obstet 123:1019-1023

16. Paganini EP, Tapolyai M, Goormastic M et al (1996) Establishing a dialysis therapy patient outcome link in intensive care unit acute dialysis for patients with acute renal failure. Am J Kidney Dis 28[Suppl 3]:81-89
17. Schiffl H, Lang SM, König et al (1997) Dose of intermittent hemodialysis and outcome of acute renal failure: a prospective randomized study. J Am Soc Nephrol 8:290A
18. Conger JD (1990) Does hemodialysis delay recovery from acute renal failure? Semin Dial 3:146-148
19. Kelleher SP, Robinette JB, Miller F et al (1987) Effect of hemorrhagic reduction in blood pressure on recovery from acute renal failure. Kidney Int 31:725-730
20. Davenport A, Will EJ, Davidson AM (1993) Improved cardiovascular stability during continuous modes of renal replacement therapy in critically ill patients with acute hepatic and renal failure. Crit Care Med 21:328-338
21. Bellomo R, Baldwin I, Ronco C (1998) Preliminary experience with high-volume hemofiltration in human septic shock. Kidney Int 54[Suppl 66]:182-185
22. Bellomo R, Mansfield D, Rumble S et al (1993) A comparison of conventional dialytic therapy and acute continuous hemdiafiltration in the management of acute renal failure in the critically ill. Ren Fail 15:595-602
23. van Bommel EFH, Bouvy ND, So KL et al (1995) Acute dialytic support for the critically ill: intermittent hemodialysis versus continuous arteriovenous hemodiafiltration. Am J Nephrol 15:192-200
24. Clark WR, Müller BA, Alaka KJ et al (1994) A comparison of metabolic control by continuous and intermittent therapies in acute renal failure. J Am Soc Nephrol 4:1413-1420
25. Boulain T, Delpech M, Legras A et al (1996) Continuous venovenous hemodiafiltration in acute renal failure associated with multiple organ failure: influence on outcome. Clin Intensive Care 7:4-10
26. Ronco C (1994) Continuous renal replacement therapies in the treatment of acute renal failure in intensive care patients. I. Theoretical aspects and techniques. Nephrol Dial Transplant 9[Suppl 4]:191-200
27. Ronco C (1994) Continuous renal replacement therapies for the treatment of acute renal failure in intensive care patients. Clin Nephrol 4:187-198
28. Silvester W (1997) Prospective study of renal replacement therapy for acute renal failure in 21 hospitals in state of Victoria, Australia. Blood Purif 15:147
29. Jacob SM, Frey FJ, Uehlinger DE (1996) Does continuous renal replacement therapy favourably influence the outcome of the patients? Nephrol Dial Transplant 11:1250-1255
30. Ronco C, Bellomo R (1996) Acute renal failure in patients with kidney transplants: continuous versus intermittent renal replacement therapy. Ren Fail 18:461-470
31. Davenport A (1995) The management of renal failure in patients at risk of cerebral edema/hypoxia. New Horiz 3:717-724
32. Bellomo R, Cole L, Reeves J et al (1997) Renal replacement therapy in the ICU: the Australian experience. Am J Kidney Dis 30:80-83
33. Mink SN, Li X, Bose D et al (1999) Early but not delayed continuous arteriovenous hemofiltration improves cardiovascular function in sepsis in dogs. Intensive Care Med 25:733-743
34. Grooteman MPC, Groeneveld ABJ (2000) A role for plasma removal during sepsis? Intensive Care Med 26:493-495
35. Oudemans-van Straaten HM, Bosman RJ, van der Spoel JI et al (1999) Outcome of critically ill patients treated with intermittent high-volume hemofiltration: a prospective cohort analysis. Intensive Care Med 25:814-821
36. Ronco C, Bellomo R, Homel P et al (2000) Effects of different doses in continuous veno-venous hemofiltration on outcomes of acute renal failure: a prospective randomized trial. Lancet 355:26-30
37. Star R (1998) Treatment of acute renal failure. Kidney Int 1998 54:1817-1831

Fluid and Electrolyte Dynamics in the Body

F. SCHIRALDI, S. DEL GAUDIO, E.G. RUGGIERO

In the critically ill we often observe some dysregulation of the fluid/electrolyte balance; far from being an innocent bystander, the intensivist could sometimes be responsible for that, due to overzealous corrections, drugs interferences, or "cosmetic" approach to the problem. In this short review, we will try to recall some basic principles that could help to improve the therapeutic strategies.

Applied physiology background

Because of the requirement for osmotic equilibrium between the cells and the extracellular fluid, any alteration in extracellular osmolality is accompanied by an identical change in intracellular osmolality, with a concomitant change in cell volume and possibly in cell function [1]. Putting it in another way, extra and intra-cellular fluids have different compositions, but almost equal solute concentrations: because water diffuses from the compartment with lower concentrations to the other, what makes the water move across the membranes is a "temporary" difference between solute concentrations, i.e. an osmotic gradient (think of extracellular glucose in diabetic emergencies).

It is useful to start from some simple physiological statements, which regulate the transmembrane watery fluxes in human subjects.

Total body water (TBW) is calculated as 60% of body weight in normal adult subjects, but can vary from 50% in older groups to 75% in the newborn [2].

Intracellular fluids (ICF) are responsible for 2/3 of TBW, while extracellular fluids (ECF) occupy 1/3 of TBW. Intravascular fluids are 1/4 of ECF, that is only 1/12 of TBW.

Normally, the major osmotic solutes in the ECF are potassium, magnesium, phosphates and protein, while in the ECF they are sodium and its chloride and bicarbonate anions.

Plasma osmolality (Posm) is normally between 280 and 295 mOsm/kg of water, while urine osmolality (Uosm) can vary from 300 to 1200 mOsm/kg [3].

Hyperosmolality is present when Posm exceeds 295 mOsm/kg, which is followed by a water shift from ICF to ECF, thirst stimulation and antidiuretic hormone (ADH) release.

The solutes must be divided, from a physiological point of view, into osmotically active (mostly confined to the extracellular or intracellular spaces) and osmotically inactive (urea, ethanol), being free to cross the cellular membranes [4].

Therefore it is useful to conceptualize clinically the osmolality as the tonicity (i.e. the accumulation of osmotically active solutes in ECF is hypertonicity, which is invariably a hyperosmolar syndrome; while if urea accumulates in blood due to renal insufficiency, osmolality may increase but tonicity could be normal or even reduced) [5].

This distinction underlines that hypertonicity usually implies ICF volume depletion and neurological impairment, while hyperosmolality sometimes does not. The distinction between osmolality and tonicity also is useful to tailor the intravenous fluid therapy: an isoosmotic solution can be "not isotonic" (5 per cent dextrose in water is isoosmotic but hypotonic: as glucose is metabolized, what remains is electrolyte-free water). This explains why the serum sodium concentration, pseudohyponatremia excluded, is a more valid measure of body fluid tonicity, than is the plasma osmolality.

The cornerstones of effective osmolality (tonicity) regulation are strictly linked to the control of extracellular sodium concentration, which is determined by:
- salt and water intake
- ADH secretion
- aldosterone release
- atrial natriuretic peptide
- intrarenal haemodynamics.

The main involved receptors are firstly the osmotically sensitive and finally, if circulating volume depletion is superimposed, the volume receptors [6].

The intimate relationship between osmotic sensors and water balance is clearly underlined by the following mathematical coupling:

$$\Delta \text{ Uosm} = 95 \, \Delta \text{ Posm}$$

This relationship indicates a remarkable gain in the osmoregulatory mechanism for vasopressin, since a 1 mOsm/kg change in plasma osmolality is able to produce a 95 mOsm/kg change in urine osmolality.

However, once the urine is maximally concentrated, further increases in vasopressin secretion are incapable of limiting urinary water losses any further, so that the last defence is only the thirst.

Not to be forgotten, stretch receptors in the left atrium and baroreceptors in the great vessels are the "haemodynamic" modulators of similar responses.

Main clinical aspects of pathologic osmoregulation

Hypernatremia

Human beings ordinarily regulate sodium balance by changes in sodium excretion via the kidneys, but rarely a reduced sodium excretion leads to hypernatremia and hyperosmolar syndromes. Moreover it is quite rare, and easy to exclude, a net hypertonic sodium gain, which could only be due to wrong clinical interventions or accidental sodium loading. In the end, in the clinial field a mismatch between water intake and renal/extrarenal water losses must exist to produce effective hyperosmolality [7] (Table 1).

Table 1. Net water losses

Pure water
insensible losses
hypodipsia
diabetes insipidus
– post-traumatic
– due to tumours or granulomatous diseases
– idiopathic
– infectious diseases
nephrogenic diabetes insipidus
– tubulo-interstitial renal diseases
– hypercalcemia, hypokalemia
– drugs (lythium, demeclocycline, amphotericin B...)
Hypotonic fluid
diuretics
osmotic diuresis
post-ATN
gastrointestinal losses
burns

Whatever could be the causes of hypertonicity, there is a common cellular/metabolic response to the hyperosmolar syndromes. As the water tends to diffuse down its concentration gradient from the ICF to the ECF, ultimately a decrease in cell volume will ensue with cell shrinkage and possibly metabolic derangements. The brain is particularly susceptible to alterations in cell volume: decreases in brain volume can lead to disruption of bridging blood vessels and likelihood of intracranial haemorrhage [8]. There are some adaptive mechanisms: following exposure to hyperosmolar solutions, neurons undergo rapid changes in their cytoplasmic make up in order to minimize osmotically induced cell dehydration [9-12]. The quite complex compensatory mechanisms are due to:

- the increased flow of cerebrospinal fluid (CSF) into the cerebral interstitium;
- the selective increase in potassium transporters, followed by chloride and sodium, which counteracts nearly two thirds of the cellular water losses;
- the generation of the so-called "idiogenic osmoles" (aminoacids, methylamines, polyols), which ultimately lead the cellular volume to normal.

These osmoprotective processes must be taken into account when the therapeutic approach starts (see therapy) [13-15] (Fig. 1).

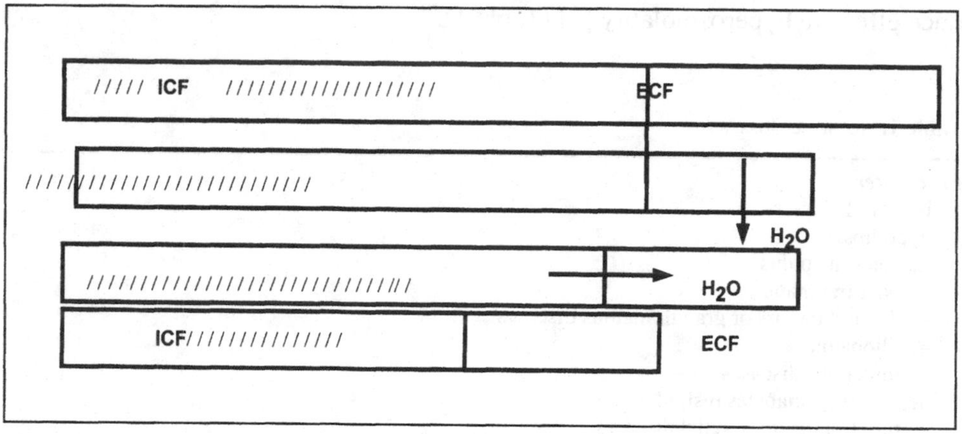

Fig. 1. Timing of hypertonic dehydration

Hyponatremia

Pseudohyponatremia is easy to understand as a laboratory misinterpretation, due to hypertriglyceridemia or paraproteinemia.

Translocational hyponatremia results from a shift of water from cells to extracellular fluid, driven by solutes confined in the extracellular compartment (hyperglycemia or osmotically active drugs): it is usually a self-limited temporary disorder.

True dilutional hyponatremia is invariably a nickname for water excess. It is due to impaired renal excretion of water or high plasma concentration of ADH despite the presence of hypotonicity [16]. An excessive water intake is not capable, by itself, i.e. without renal impairment, of provoking clinically relevant dilutional hyponatremia. The main causes are summarized in Table 2.

Table 2. Causes of true hyponatremia

↓ ECF	↑ ECF	SIADH
Renal Na losses	Heart failure	Cancer
diuretics	Cirrhosis	CNS disorders
adrenal insufficiency	Nephrotic syndrome	Drugs
tubulopathies		Pulmonary disease
Extrarenal losses		↑ pressure vent.
Gastrointestinal		Postoperative
"Third space"		Hypothyroidism?

Hypernatremia and hyponatremia represent a very challenging task for the intensivist: both share the need to be corrected with a "religious" respect of the timing, i.e. taking into account any pathophysiologic adjustment the subject has been performing meanwhile.

To do that, one must tailor the management not only to the laboratory findings but also to a clinically very close observation.

Laboratory findings

The laboratory diagnosis of hyperosmolar syndromes could be misleading, if the reader did not take into account the interplay among TBW deficit, electrolyte concentrations and the temporary intra-extracellular shift of water and electrolytes.

An *effective osmolality* > 320 mOsm/kg is the better guide to the diagnosis of hyperosmolar syndrome. Plasma sodium, potassium, phosphate and magnesium levels may be low, normal or high (due to different timing of the blood sampling), but they do not reflect total body losses, even if significant lowering of the potassium and magnesium pools is common [17].

Because of renal underperfusion the urea/creatinin ratio in blood is frequently high (> 40), due to both renal and prerenal insufficiency.

Elevation of muscle enzymes may be occasionally observed and suggests rhabdomyolysis, which per se could lead to renal failure [18, 19]. It could be quite troublesome the evaluation of plasma sodium if any hyperglycemia is present: during the first 24-48 hours of hyperglycemia there is a water shift from ICF to ECF and the sodium concentration will be diluted proportionally (1.6 mEq/L less per 100 mg/dl of raised glucose concentration); after prolonged osmotic diuresis, the sodium concentration will rise due to the ICF/ECF contraction: therefore one must be very careful in approaching a patient affected by any hyperosmolar syndrome if there is any concomitant hypernatremia.

The measurement of the *urine osmolality* and its response to ADH may be extremely helpful in establishing the cause of hypernatremia; with ADH release, the urine osmolality should be very high in hypernatremic states (Uosm > 800 mOsm/kg or urinary gravity > 1022) if ADH release and renal response are intact [20, 21]. Concentrating ability should be normal in patients with sodium overload, enhanced watery losses or hypodipsia without DI, so that initial Uosm should exceed 800 mOsm/kg and there should be no response to any ADH administration [22-24] (Table 3).

Table 3. Urine osmolality and response to ADH in hypernatremia

Urine osmolality	**Response to ADH**
< 300 mOsm/kg	
° Central DI	++
° Nephrogenic DI	–
300-800 mOsm/kg	
° Volume depletion in central DI	++
° Partial central DI	+
° Osmotic diuresis	–
> 800 mOsm/kg	
° Na overload	–
° Primary hypodipsia	–

The lab help in hyponatremias is firstly focused on the exclusion of the pseudohyponatremias and translocational forms. If a true hyponatremia is confirmed, the main point is to understand the water balance of the patient, i.e. the extracellular fluids status, the central venous pressure, intrathoracic fluids or more invasive information.

Management

The therapy of hyperosmolar syndromes must address underlying medical conditions, as usual in fluid, acid-base and electrolyte disorders.

Moreover, because of the dangerous effects of hypertonicity on CNS and of the associated dehydration on haemodynamics, treatment must be tailored on the basis of a careful monitoring of the patient. On the basis of the present knowledge, the priorities of the treatment could be as follows:

1. restore perfusion, if compromised, with plasma substitutes rapidly enough to correct shock and stabilize the circulatory system (if needed, invasively monitoring the patient);

2. estimate theoretical total fluid deficits as either:
   H_2O DEFICIT = 0.6 x weight (kg) x (Na/140 – 1) or
   H_2O DEFICIT = 0.6 x weight (kg) x (285 – Posm)/Posm;
3. give half the calculated deficit in 12-24 hours, aiming for a decrement in plasma osmolality of approximately 1 mOsm/L per hour. Chronic hypertonicity should be treated slowly, whereas acute changes require more urgent treatment;
4. hypotonic fluids should be administered, but do not forget that the so-called "normal" saline is relatively hypotonic if injected in a very hypertonic environment! Anyhow it is easy to produce slightly hypotonic solutions, substituting sterile water with equivalent amounts of normal saline in a percentage of 10-50%;
5. plasma electrolyte levels should be frequently monitored. Due to osmotic diuresis there is usually a "covert" deficit of potassium, magnesium and phosphate, that the rehydration will discover. As a general rule, if the diuresis is > 1 ml/m′, potassium (10-20 mEq/h) and magnesium (4 mEq/h) infusions should be started simultaneously with the fluid replacement. ECG monitoring is mandatory;
6. the gastrointestinal tract should be the first route of water replacement in chronic hyperosmolality;
7. if a central venous catheter is being employed, do not simply rely on the absolute value of the central venous pressure (CVP), but always titrate the CVP variations against the first fluids infusions.

Hyperosmolar syndromes are a difficult challenge to the intensivist, as they usually still carry high percentages of mortality, especially if elderly people or children are involved. A very close clinical monitoring and a critical interpretation of the laboratory findings, associated with careful nursing, could improve the prognosis, even if the treatment of the underlying disorders is always mandatory. Haemodynamic invasive monitoring is rarely requested.

Regarding the management of hyponatremias, an "evergreen" definition was given by T. Berl in 1990, something like: damned if we treat damned if we don't... [25]. That provocative sentence was obviously linked to the early clinical reports of pontine mielinolysis due to overzealous corrections of hyponatremias. The following experiences confirmed that the timing of the therapy should always respect the timing of the ongoing disorder: this is sometimes very difficult to achieve, particularly when a life-threatening cerebral edema must be faced [26, 27]. Even if there is still no consensus about the optimal treatment of symptomatic hyponatremia, some suggestions could be followed to improve the therapeutic approach:

- water restriction to induce negative water balance is indicated in asymptomatic (chronic) hyponatremias;

- loop diuretics associated with dietary sodium supplements can be used in the inappropriate secretion of ADH;
- hyponatremias associated with ECF depletion require slightly hypertonic saline plus colloids if the intravascular compartment is reduced too;
- if there is any contemporary hyperkalemia, think of adrenal insufficiency;
- the patients with cerebral impairment should be treated by a two-step strategy: rapid correction of half the calculated deficit (never raising Na plasmatic concentration more than 1 mmol/L/hour), followed by a slower-paced management (< 0.5 mmol/L/hour) up to a near-normal (130-135 mmol/L) blood value, closely monitoring the CNS.

References

1. Lang F, Ritter M, Volkl M (1993) The biological significance of cell volume. Renal Physiol Biochem 16:48-56
2. Snyder NA, Feigal DW, Arieff AI (1987) Hypernatremia in elderly patients: a heterogeneous, morbid and iatrogenic entity. Ann Int Med 107:309-314
3. Kinne RKH, Ruhfus B, Tinel H et al (1995) Renal organic osmolytes: signal transduction pathways and release mechanisms. In: De Santo NG, Capasso G (eds) Acid base and electrolyte balance. IISS 237-242
4. Daugirdas JT, Kronfol NO (1989) Hyperosmolar coma: cellular dehydration and the serum sodium concentration. Ann Intern Med 110:855-857
5. Lewis SA, Donaldson P (1990) Ion channels and cell volume regulation: chaos in an organized system. News in Physiological Sciences 5:112-118
6. Schrier RW (1988) Pathogenesis of sodium and water retention in high output and low output cardiac failure, nephrotic syndrome, cirrhosis and pregnancy. N Engl J Med 319:1065-1073
7. Vin-Christian K, Arieff AI (1993) Diabetes insipidus, massive polyuria and hypernatremia leading to permanent brain damage. Am J Med 94:341-345
8. Arieff AI, Guisado R (1976) Effects on the central nervous system of hypernatremic and hyponatremic states. Kidney Int 10:104-111
9. Lien YHH, Shapiro JI, Chan L (1990) Effects of hypernatremia on organic brain osmoles. J Clin Invest 85:1427-1433
10. Elisaf M, Litou H, Siamopoulos KC (1989) Survival after severe iatrogenic hypernatremia. Am J Kidney Disease 14:230-234
11. Cserr HF, De Pasquale, Patlak CS (1987) Regulation of brain water and electrolytes during acute hyperosmolality in rats. Am J Physiol 253:F 522-F526
12. Haussinger D, Roth E, Lang F, Gerok V (1993) Cellular hydration state: an important determinant of protein catabolism in health and disease. Lancet 341:1330-1333
13. Ayus JC, Krothapalli R, Freiberg M (1990) Role of hypercatabolism in mortality associated with chronic hypernatremia in rats. Kidney Int 36:263-266
14. Levine SN, Sanson TH (1989) Treatment of hyperglycaemic hyperosmolar non-ketotic syndrome. Drugs 38:462-472
15. Rose BD (1986) New approach to disturbances in the plasma sodium concentration. Am J Med 81:1033-1040
16. Weisberg LS (1989) Pseudohyponatremia: a reappraisal. Am J Med 86:315-318
17. Adrogué H, Madias NE (2000) Hypernatremia. N Engl J Med 342:1493-1499
18. Lustman CC, Guerin JJ (1991) Hyperosmolar non ketotic syndrome associated with rhabdomyolysis and acute kidney failure. Diabetes Care 14:146-147

19. Wang LM, Tsai ST (1994) Rhabdomyolysis in diabetic emergencies. Diabetes Research Clinical Practice 26(3):209-214
20. Richardson DW, Robinson AG (1985) Desmopressin. Ann Intern Med 103:228-233
21. Bartter FC, Schwartz WB (1967) The syndrome of inappropriate secretion of antidiuretic hormone. Am J Med 42:790-806
22. Chanson P, Jedynak CP, Dabrowski G et al (1988) Management of early postoperative diabetes insipidus with parenteral desmopressin. Acta Endocrinol 117:513-519
23. Jamison RJ (1987) The renal concentrating mechanism. Kidney Int 32[Suppl21]:S43-50
24. Bichet DG (1994) Nephrogenic diabetes insipidus. Semin Nephrol 14:349-356
25. Berl T (1990) Treating hyponatremia: damned if we do and damned if we don't. Kidney Int 37:1006-1018
26. Lauriat SM, Berl T (1997) The hyponatremic patient: practical focus on therapy. J Am Soc Nephrol 8:1599-1607
27. Adrogué H, Madias NE (2000) Hyponatremia. N Engl J Med 342:1581-1589

Monitoring of Blood Volume

N. BRIENZA

Normovolaemia is a critical feature of haemodynamic wellness. Achieving normovolaemia, however, is complicated by the difficulty of accurately assessing volume status in critically ill patients. Commonly used variables for assessing volume status are indirect parameters such as filling pressures (central venous pressure and capillary filling pressure). Their accuracy in estimation of intravascular volume is affected by numerous factors, and absolute pressure values can often be misleading. In a classic report by Shippy et al. [1], data of commonly monitored variables were compared with blood volume measurements (obtained by indicator dilution method with ^{125}I-labeled human serum albumin) during early resuscitation, in critical periods in intensive care unit and after fluid therapy. Although in blood volume and monitored variables such as mean arterial pressure, heart rate, cardiac index, central venous pressure and wedge pressure were altered, there was no correlation between the extent of blood volume changes and the monitored variables during resuscitation or throughout critical illness. After administration of fluid load, blood volume and commonly monitored variables improved in the right direction, but the correlation coefficients were not good.

Central venous pressure and wedge pressure are not determined by the volume inside the vessels alone, but by numerous other factors, such venous compliance, cardiac function and intrathoracic pressure [2]. In normal heart, left ventricular filling pressure is a few mmHg higher than right ventricular filling pressure such that the latter may be used to reflect cardiac preload. However, assessment of cardiac filling from central venous pressure is strongly affected by the physiological determinants of right ventricle performance. The high diastolic compliance of the right ventricle may produce small changes in filling pressure in the presence of large changes in end-diastolic volume [3] and filling pressure of right ventricle changes little over the normal physiologic range of end-diastolic volumes [4]. Central venous pressure may not accurately reflect right ventricular end-diastolic volume, and may not predict left ventricular filling pressure in presence of left ventricular dysfunction, pulmonary hypertension and/or right ventricular dysfunction. Moreover, wedge pressure itself may be invalidated as a measure of ventricular preload due to variability and changes in left ventricular distensibility. A reduction in diastolic left ventricular compliance will change wedge pressure without any change in diastolic volume. Furthermore, since the pressure/volume relationship of the left ventricle is steeper than that of the right ventricle, any small variation in ventricular volume can induce disproportionately greater variation in wedge pressure. Thus, changes in cardiac filling pressure do not indicate changes in indices of cardiac volume, especially in cardiac patients [5].

What is preload? Basically it the is considered to be the myocardial fibre length. According to Frank Starling, the longer the fibre is, the larger is the force that it will generate. The preload would then be ideally measured by a technique able to record fibre length, such as sonomicrometry. It is, however, impossible to measure this variable, so it must be substituted by some other parameter which is directly related to sarcomere length. End-diastolic volume of the ventricle is a more practical measure of the configuration of myocardial sarcomeres. In the 1980s, a pulmonary artery catheter equipped with a fast-response thermistor with a bedside microprocessor was developed. This technique allowed bedside monitoring of right ventricular volumes providing more information on right ventricular preload than central venous pressure. Martyn et al. [6] showed that right ventricular end diastolic volume measured by this technique was a useful clinical tool for assessing preload and volume replacement. This holds true during mechanical ventilation with and without PEEP when cardiac preload decreases while filling pressures increase [7]. Moreover, right volume measurement allows evaluation of right ventricular performance in both acute and acute on chronic respiratory failure [8, 9]. However, nowadays, in association with the recent debate concerning the safety of invasive haemodynamic monitoring with Swan Ganz catheter, right ventricular volume monitoring is less widely used.

An alternative approach to the Swan Ganz catheter for blood volume monitoring is the recently developed transpulmonary indicator dilution technique, requiring a catheter for indicator injection into the right atrium, and a catheter for sampling in the femoral artery. As with Swan Ganz catheter, measurement of cardiac output is based on thermodilution, the only difference being the arterial sampling site of the signal. As arterial catheter is equipped with a fiberoptic-thermistor tip, intravascular volume status can be assessed by a dye dilution method. The rationale behind this blood volume determination lies in the use of indocyanine green as pure intravascular tracer. Once injected at a known concentration, indocyanine green will dilute in the intravascular volume and, by measuring the dye dilution curve, volume will be measured as the product of cardiac output and mean transit times [10]. The measurement of mean transit time of the first pass from injection to sampling sites, i.e. from right atrium to descending aorta, will allow calculation of intrathoracic blood volume (ITBV).

Total circulating blood volume measurement relies on the same principle. However, in order to get an accurate estimate of total blood volume, at least 30 minutes of blood sampling are commonly needed, while fiberoptic measurements of total blood volume are recorded for 5 minutes only. Therefore, total blood volume measured at 5 minutes can include only the fast vascular compartments, i.e. vascular compartments of total circulation where indocyanine green dilutes in the first 5 minutes. Therefore, even though a close correlation between TBV at 5 minutes and total blood volume is observed, fiberoptically measured blood volume is significantly lower than total blood volume [11].

Filling of central circulation can be assessed by intrathoracic blood volume (ITBV). Several reports demonstrate that ITBV is much more reliable than wedge pressure as indicator of left ventricular preload. This holds true in mechanically ventilated patients in whom central venous pressure or wedge pressure lead to an overestimation of circulatory volume status while ITBV seems to be a reliable tool to assess volume status [12-14]. In cardiac surgery patients, not only central venous pressure and capillary wedge pressure, but also right atrial and right ventricular end diastolic volumes were not considered suitable as preload parameters when compared to ITBV and global end diastolic blood volumes measured by transpulmonary dilution technique [15].

Indocyanine green dilution is the basis of a newly developed technique that measures circulating blood volume by pulse dye-densitometry (PDD) with probes attached to the nostril and the finger. Blood dye concentration correlates well with values obtained by PDD. Moreover, when comparing PDD values with those obtained by measuring human serum albumin – standard procedure for central blood volume measurement – mean bias averaged 4% in healthy volunteers [16]. When applied in patients undergoing general anaesthesia, pulse-spectrophotometry provided reliable measures of blood volume [17]. This technique shares the same pitfall as the transpulmonary dilution method, since it measures the fast component or circulating blood volume (or active blood volume) and not total blood volume. However, it is less invasive, can be repetitively applied within short period of time without blood sampling and constitutes an important step forward in blood volume monitoring.

More recently, a simpler approach using single arterial thermodilution without indicator has been used to measure ITBV [18]. The principle underlying this estimation is that global end-diastolic volume is directly correlated with ITBV and can be calculated by thermodilution. The results of the above study show that determination of ITBV by single thermodilution agrees closely with corresponding values from the double indicator technique (mean bias, 7.6 ± 57.4 ml/m^2) [18].

A further new, rapid, and simple method that allows reliable assessment of circulating blood volume uses sampling of hydroxyethyl starch (HES), a high molecular weight marker, 5 minutes after its injection. More specifically, blood samples are drawn before and 5 minutes after injection of 100 ml HES. After HES hydrolysis, the resulting glucose concentrations are measured and compared before and after HES injection [19]. With this method, a marked intravascular hypovolaemia despite highly positive fluid balance was demonstrated after cardiopulmonary bypass [20].

Nowadays, the possibilities of measuring blood volume are numerous. Even though appreciating that marked imbalance in circulating blood volume, hypovolaemia as well as hypervolaemia contribute to significant increases in mortality [21, 22], during haemodynamic evaluation it should not be forgotten that blood volume and other preload indicators are only some of the factors affecting cardiac output. When cardiac output changes parallel blood volume changes, there is no doubt that a preload problem exists. However, blood volume must not be considered to be synonymous with cardiac output and it should not substitute for it.

References

1. Shippy CR, Appel PL, Shoemaker WC (1984) Reliability of clinical monitoring to assess blood volume in critically ill patients. Crit Care Med 12(2):107-112
2. Jacobson Ed (1968) A physiologic approach to shock. N Engl J Med 278:348-360
3. Janicki JS, Weber KT (1980) The pericardium and ventricular interaction, distensibility and function. Am J Physiol 238:H494-H503
4. Tyberg JV, Taichman GC, Smith ER et al (1986) The relationship between pericardial pressure and right atrial pressure: an intraoperative study. Circulation 73:428-432
5. Buhre W, Weyland A, Schorn B et al (1999) Changes in central venous pressure and pulmonary capillary wedge pressure do not indicate changes in right and left heart volume in patients undergoing coronary artery bypass surgery. Eur J Anaesthesiol 16:11-17
6. Martyn JAJ, Snider MT, Farago LF et al (1981) Thermodilution right ventricular volume: a novel and better predictor of volume replacement in acute thermal injury. J Trauma 21: 619-624
7. Brienza A, Dambrosio M, Bruno F et al (1988) Right ventricular ejection fraction measurement in moderate acute respiratory failure (ARF). Effects of PEEP. Int Care Med 14:478-482
8. Dambrosio M, Fiore G, Brienza N et al (1996) Right ventricular myocardial function in ARF patients. Int Care Med 22:722-780
9. Dambrosio M, Cinnella G, Brienza N et al (1996) Effect of positive end-expiratory pressure on right ventricular function in COPD patients during acute ventilatory failure. Int Care Med 22:923-932
10. Zierler KL (1962) Theoretical basis of indicator-dilution methods for measuring flow and volume. Circ Res 10:393-407
11. Hoeft A, Schorn B, Weyland A (1994) Bedside assessment of intravascular volume status in patients undergoing coronary artery bypass surgery. Anesthesiology 81:76-86
12. Lichtwark-Aschoff M, Zeravik J, Pfeiffer UJ (1992) Intrathoracic blood volume accurately reflects circulatory volume status in critically ill patients with mechanical ventilation. Int Care Med 18:142-147
13. Brienza N, Dambrosio M, Cinnella G et al (1996) Effetti della PEEP sui volumi ematici intratoracico e totale valutati con sistema COLD in pazienti con insufficienza respiratoria acuta. Studio preliminare. Minerva Anestesiologica 62(7/8):235-242
14. Borelli M, Benini A, Denkewitz T et al (1998) Effects of continuous negative extrathoracic pressure versus positive end-expiratory pressure in acute lung injury patients. Crit Care Med 26:1025-1031
15. Godje O, Peyerl M, Seebauer T et al (1998) Central venous pressure, pulmonary capillary wedge pressure and intrathoracic blood volumes as preload indicators in cardiac surgery patients. Eur J Cardiothorac Surg 13(5):533-539

16. Iijima T, Iwao Y, Sankawa H (1998) Circulating blood volume measured by pulse dye-densitometry: comparison with (131)I-HSA analysis. Anesthesiology 89:1329-1335
17. He YL, Tanigami H, Ueyama H et al (1998) Measurement of blood volume using indocyanine green measured with pulse-spectrophotometry: its reproducibility and reliability. Crit Care Med 26(8):1446-1451
18. Sakka SG, Ruhl CC, Pfeiffer UJ (2000) Assessment of cardiac preload and extravascular lung water by single transpulmonary thermodilution. Int Care Med 26(2):180-187
19. Tschaikowsky K, Meisner M, Durst R et al (1997) Blood volume determination using hydroxyethyl starch: a rapid and simple intravenous injection method. Crit Care Med 25: 599-606
20. Tschaikowsky K, Neddermeyer U, Pscheidl E et al (2000) Changes in circulating blood volume after cardiac surgery measured by a novel method using hydroxyethyl starch. Crit Care Med 28:336-341
21. Shoemaker WC, Bryan BC, Quigley L et al (1973) Body fluid shifts in depletion and post-stress states and their correction with adequate nutrition. Surg Gynecol Obstet 136:371-374
22. Paret G, Cohen AJ, Bohn DJ et al (1992) Continuous arteriovenous hemofiltration after cardiac operations in infants and children. J Thorac Cardiovasc Surg 101:1225-1230

Volume Replacement - Crystalloids vs Colloids vs Colloids Controversy

A. GULLO

The integrity of the intravascular compartment and its blood volume are essential prerequisites for maintenance of the body's homeostasis. Maintaining the body's physiological condition involves a balance between intracellular, extra cellular and interstitial sectors. This balance can be acutely altered in such clinical instances as trauma; haemorrhages during surgery; generalised inflammatory reaction resulting in increased capillary endothelium, as in sepsis with multiple-organ failure; hypovolemia, occurring frequently in patients in intensive care where reduced circulating blood volume results from enclosed thoracic and abdominal trauma; cerebral lesions and in cardiac and vascular surgery and in patients with severe burns. A modest fall in blood volume may trigger compensation mechanisms, such as vasoconstriction, to redistribute the blood supply to the vital organs.

The process of hypovolemia and the resulting impoverishment of blood supply to various organs, such as the kidneys and the gastrointestinal tract, causes rapid deterioration in the patient's general condition and progression towards ischemic damage, although in the initial stages compensation mechanisms may be able to maintain normal arterial blood pressure levels with the patient in a state of compensatory shock [1].

If the physician does not promptly intervene and if the intensive care treatment is not adequate, important changes take place to the body's homeostasis and decompensatory shock develops [2].

In such a scenario the marked decrease of blood flow from the heart and the resulting insufficient supply of oxygen essential for tissue metabolism may result in irreversible damage. This is because reduced perfusion and the resulting decrease of oxygenation causes severe ischemia in the gastrointestinal mucosa [3], a condition that plays a key role in the development of organ failure

A fall in pH is an important prognostic factor with critically ill patients [4-7]. Measuring circulating blood volumes is an ideal perioperative and intensive care practice but difficult to carry out routinely and at the patient's bedside [8].

Monitoring of volemia involves techniques providing indirect indications of volume replacement in critically ill patients.

Monitoring central venous pressure, catheterisation of the pulmonary artery to check capillary pressure and measurements of cardiac capacity and diuresis are the standard tests used for guidance in the administration of fluids and the transfusion of blood and blood derivatives. Although, however, such tests are able to provide important information for the choice of the treatment, they are not able to provide an exact estimate of the volume of circulating blood [9].

It is important to note that the relationship between red blood cell volume, plasmatic volume and circulating blood is difficult to establish as can vary also normal physiological conditions and can be masked by selective vasoconstriction taking place in different regions and with different degrees of intensity.

A series of biohumoral cascade reactions may also be triggered in the above clinical situations, capable of irreversibly undermining physiological compensation mechanisms.

While a number of different techniques are now available for measuring intravascular blood volumes, they are infrequently used both because of their technical complexity and because of the complexity of the clinical conditions of critically ill patients. Fluid treatment, although it is now considered a routine, is nevertheless a very controversial subject as regards the choice of fluids and their method of administration.

For several decades now a heated debate has being going on over the use of crystalloids as against colloids and over which of the available colloids is the most suitable.

While the use of saline solutions is preferable as these physiological solutions, the fact remains that in certain situations where there is sudden hypovolemia, colloids and also blood derivatives like plasma and albumin may be indicated to ensure sufficient cardiac capacity and to provide tissues with sufficient quantities of oxygen for their metabolism.

Volume replacement in critical care practice

Trauma involves the loss of part of the circulating blood volume; the amount of consequent damage to the tissues may determine a significant transfer of fluids from one compartment to another with repercussions on the various regulatory mechanisms. In the initial stages of hypovolemia, compensation mechanisms are set on that facilitate the re-entry of fluids into the intravascular compartment, through their active re-absorption by way of the capillaries. This situation causes a shift in fluids that is greater than necessary.

The clinical conditions which determine a reduction in volemia and the passage of fluids and electrolytes from the intracellular and interstitial sectors towards the intravascular department, may occur abnormally and undermine the balance between the various parts of the organism.

The resulting state of alarm is capable, in its turn, of triggering a mediator cascade. The consequent inflammation may cause generalised increase of capillary permeability and worsen of the clinical condition of patients suffering from hemorrhagic-hypovolemic 'shock'.

In such a situation prompt action is needed to support the flow of fluids, taking into account both the volume of blood to be replaced and the amount of fluids that have been inappropriately shifted from one compartment to the other [10]. After head trauma primary cerebral damage follows as a consequence of the direct damage caused by trauma. Later on contusions and lacerations of cerebral tissue determine secondary cerebral damage. Because of the progression of oedema in the cerebral parenchyma and the involvement of the glia, there is an increase in endocranial pressure with severe stress on cerebral tissues and rapid development of apoptosis. The restoration of cerebral perfusion is thus a major priority and for this reason indications arise both for hyperosmolal solutions and colloid treatment, while bearing in mind that the restoration of systemic arterial pressure is theoretically desirable, but could have a deleterious effect on the patient's condition, especially in rapidly evolving lesions.

Sepsis and its progression towards septic shock is a complex clinical condition. Most commonly it is secondary to bacterial infection with consequent release into the circulation of endotoxins capable of triggering a generalised response on the part of the body as a whole. The difficulties in understanding the most important pathophysiological aspects underlying the development of shock lies in the problem of understanding the immune system's response, with our current understanding being somewhat limited. It has been shown, however, that endotoxinemia is able to subvert the normal workings of the regulatory mechanism both in the micro-circulation (vasoparalysis) and in the vital organs and systems (mediator explosion); their dysfunction may have different degrees of severity and depends on the functional reserves of the body. However, it is generally agreed that endotoxinemia is capable of subverting the normal state.

Progression of sepsis to septic shock can cause substantial hemodynamic instability due to the effect of myocardial depression and increased permeability of vascular epithelium, as well as vasoparalysis resulting from the endotoxinemia. In addition to this, hypovolemia may be well compensated initially but may then progress towards a condition of absolute hypovolemia with severe systemic repercussions. At this stage the condition of the patient becomes more and more critical as the increased capillary permeability causes plasmatic exemia with a loss of solutes, particularly albumin, which is deposited in the interstice, significantly impoverishing the intravascular compartment.

Sepsis reduces liver synthesis of albumin with a resultant fall in the osmotic colloid pressure values. This condition leads to impairment of the circulatory function and altered perfusion of the main tissues due to an increased production of lactic acid, considered an important vital apparatus deterioration index, with consequent and progressive dysfunction of one organ after another [11, 12].

It is therefore a matter of high priority to restore haematic stability, bearing also in mind that the reduction of oedema can favour the functional recovery of various organs. A rational use of fluids, particularly volume expanders, is therefore essential.

Burns are clinical states that can have both local and systemic consequences. The severity of the lesion depends on its depth and extension. Tissue perfusion impaired by the inflammatory response of the endothelium with increased permeability and a marked reduction in the plasmatic component that, because of subversion of Starling's forces, is the cause of significant sequestration and dispersion of fluids. The resulting tissue oedema and the ischemic distress cause a condition of hypovolemic shock [13, 14].

The priority is to support circulation; the crystalloids, the synthetic colloids, plasma and albumin are the key elements for volume replacement and can be used in association to restore volume and improve organs perfusion. In practice this is a much debated issue. In particular albumin and plasma have very limited indications, as their use is not always justified. The debate therefore focuses on the controversy between crystalloids and colloids.

Crystalloids vs colloids vs colloids controversy

The intravenous administration of various kinds of fluids is indicated for the maintenance or restoration of volemia in the perioperative period and in situations of important volume deficit. Crystalloids, plasma, albumin, or synthetic colloids such as gelatines, dextrans, and hydroxyethil starch are the possible options. For reasons of simplicity, and as the subject of fluid therapy primarily interests anaesthesiologists, surgeons, intensive care specialists and doctors in general, it may be useful to make some short reference to the main physiological and pharmacological properties of the fluids that are most commonly used in clinical practice and to discuss the indications for and results the use of the various solutions available today. In the course of this short paper some experimental and clinical experience will be described, together with a cost benefit analysis of the different fluids, particularly hypertonic solutions and the most recently used colloids such as hydroxyethil starch.

The use of hypertonic solutions, both experimentally and in clinical practice, began in the early nineteen eighties, thanks to some groups of researchers [15, 16], in the treatment of haemorrhagic hypovolemic shock. This experience paved the way to experimental studies and at least 60 clinical trials [17] on the use of 7.5% NaCl solutions in the treatment of various types of shock (including hypovolemic, cardiogenic and septic) and the use of these solutions to maintain volemia during major surgery. These authors showed that in the case of animals in a state of shock on removal of intravascular volume, the bolus administration of a 7.5% solution of NaCl (at a volume of 4 ml per kg of body weight) was able to restore arterial blood pressure and cardiac flow and prolong survival.

In particular, the administration, of hypertonic solutions creates an osmotic gradient that enables passage of fluids from the various regions of the body to the intravascular compartment. On the other hand, in the case, of animals treated with isotonic saline solution the hemodynamic response failed with a consequent significant decrease of survival rate. After this experience the same researchers were able to show the hemodynamic effectiveness of hypertonic solutions in patients treated in the intensive care department. Other authors [18-22] later obtained comparable results and the rapid improvement in cardiovascular indices was attributed to the effect of the expansion of volemia, microcirculation vasodilation and a direct cardiac inotropic effect [23, 24].

The above research testifies to the effectiveness of hypertonic solutions in clinical practice although researchers suggest some caution in their use in certain populations, such as paediatric patients, particularly subjects with severe organ function impairment and those suffering from chronic and debilitating diseases.

Hypertonic solutions are recommended for post-trauma hypotension, particularly in penetrative trauma and cranial-encephalic trauma. Such treatment is indicated in the course of elective surgery, their use produces hemodynamic stability and a saving in the fluids administered. Lastly these types of solutions do not cause changes to the coagulation cascade, do not determine clinically significant hypernatremia, and, of course, do not trigger allergic reactions. However, despite much reassuring data, the use of hypertonic solutions in intensive care, in perioperative medicine and, in general, in the treatment of critically ill patients requires further information that must also be collected with multicentric trials. Their main objective will be to establish the real advantages and the types of patients who will benefit from the administration of hypertonic saline solutions.

As for colloids, Gronwall's observations [25] of 1957 are still valid, i.e. the molecular weight must ensure an adequate colloid effect; the colloid-osmotic pressure and viscosity must be the same as that of plasma and such elements must be pure, have no antigenic activity and specific procedures of product preparation and storage must be followed. Hydroxyethil starch and its compounds are synthesised derivatives of amilopectin, formed from a chain of dipolysaccharide polymers. The composition of the hydroxyethil ether linked to the glucose units is degraded by serous amylases [26-28]. The pharmacokinetics of hydroxyethil starch is influenced by its molecular weight and the ratio between the number of hydroxyethil groups and the number of glucose molecules. Furthermore, particles of less than 50Kd are filtered by the kidneys within 48 hours, while larger molecules undergo a process of hydrolysis by the amylases and are excreted in the urine and the bile or are englobed by the reticuloendothelial system. The currently used solutions have a molecular weight of 450 Kd and a high molar replacement ratio of 0.7 (HES 450/0.7) with a half-life of approx. 17 days (Table 1).

Table 1.

Starch-colloids	Volume effect %	PM	PCO (mmHg)	SM	Half-life
6% HES	100	450,000	30	0.7	17 days
Pentastarch	140	280,000	40	0.5	8-12 h
Pentafraction	140	350,000	40	0.5	8-12 h
HES	140	200,000	40	0.5	8-12 h

Recent studies confirmed the clinical benefits of this type of colloid [27, 28] and the low incidence of adverse reactions [29-31]; however, they were not able to demonstrate the superiority of one solution over another. The most recent clinical trials suggest the validity of colloids is on a par with that of crystalloids in terms of volume replacement in the perioperative period and under emergency conditions [32-35], however, the crystalloids versus colloids debate does not involve a specific colloid, and the properties and effects of different colloids are influenced by their physical and chemical characteristics, molecular weight, half life, colloid-osmotic pressure, and they have different side effects and cost.

Boldt et al. [28] recently demonstrated the favourable effects of hydroxyethil starch. They compared the effect of 10% solution of hydroxyethil starch with a colloid-osmotic pressure of 66 mmHg, with a 20% albumin infusion with a colloid osmotic pressure of 78 mmHg.

All patients were subjected to monitoring of hemodynamics, transport and consumption of oxygen and pH, which was shown to correlate with mortality rate [36]. Fluids, blood and inotropic drugs were administered to optimise hemodynamic parameters. The cardiac index, oxygen transport and oxygen consumption significantly increased in patients treated with hydroxyethil starch.

Septic patients treated with hydroxyethil starch were found to have a better PaO_2/FiO_2 ratio, and an improved respiratory function. The patients treated with hydroxyethil starch scored significantly low in the APACHE system, indicating an improvement in clinical condition and a lower mortality risk. Septic patients treated with albumin recorded lower pH, suggesting reduced splanchnic perfusion. There has been a recent resurgence in the debate on the use of different fluids [37, 38]. In particular, Schierhout and Roberts carried out systematic analysis of randomised trials on the use of crystalloids and colloids. The most significant results indicate that the crystalloids are preferable to colloids in relation to the onset of pulmonary oedema.

Mortality rate was found to be 4% higher in the traumatised patients treated with colloids as against those treated with crystalloids. The same criticisms of the use of colloids over crystalloids were made by the Cook group [38] who stated that the results were not conclusive, and that further studies on homogenous groups of patients are required.

Other researchers [39] maintain that Schierhout and Roberts reach conclusions that cannot be accepted. In fact, frequently data are not perfectly comparable and may lead to mistaken conclusions.

Whyncoll et al. [40] criticise Schierhout and Roberts when they assert that the use of colloids is associated with a 4% increase in mortality over the crystalloids, in their view, such a difference is not statistically significant, and they state that colloids are much more expensive than crystalloids and should therefore not be used outside prospective, controlled and randomised trials.

Schierhout and Roberts conclude the debate with a letter in the BMJ [41] in which they insist on their preference for the use of crystalloids over colloids, in agreement with the American Trauma College that recommends the use of crystalloids over colloids in traumatised patients needing volume replacement, implicitly recognising the choice of fluids to be administered.

The same authors emphasise that, although they made explicit reference to the role of colloids in general, research should be continued to assess the effectiveness of specific colloids, as data on the use of this type of fluid may appear negative or at least controversial.

Conclusion

Crystalloids are the fluids of choice for circulating blood volume replacement, and their properties make them particularly useful for correcting water and electrolyte deficits in the interstitial compartment.

In conditions of severe hypovolemia with hypotension and in cases of shock, physiological solutions are not indicated as they are not useful for restoring microcirculation.

Hypertonic saline solutions may be useful for volume replacement but must always be associated with the administration of other available fluids.

Albumin is not considered to be a first choice preparation for volume replacement. It should only be used in particular circumstances (i.e. where there are contraindications for other solutions or where their further use may not be advisable). Gelatines are a good alternative to the other fluids and have a longer volume replacement effect than saline solutions.

Hydroxyethil starch, in its various formulations, has a number of advantages vis-a-vis the other solutions now used in clinical practice. In particular, molecules have specific properties which result in: their remaining in circulation for a longer time, with consequent greater hemodynamic effects; a significant reduction in side effects, particularly anaphylaxis; their power to modify the endothelium and their ability to reduce the inflammatory and biohumoral effects which can often be devastating.

The question of blood volume replacement in the critically ill patient is still controversial. In clinical practice, however, each of the solutions available in hospitals and ambulances may be useful for elective or emergency treatment.

The availability of a wider range of treatment options may be necessary in order to use the most appropriate volume replacement therapy, and particularly in situations of hemodynamic instability and worsening hypotension which cannot be controlled otherwise.

In the perioperative period and in intensive care it is essential, to carefully monitor hemodynamic parameters and oxygenation indices as blood volume stabilization is frequently necessary in clinical practice. The availability of different crystalloid and colloid solutions in their various formulations, and in particular hydroxyethil starch, seem to offer the best guarantee of successful treatment. The debate is still open on the costs and benefits of each choice. It is reasonable to suppose that further pathophysiological and clinical studies in such an important branch of medicine as volume replacement will help to select the most effective treatment option.

Even though Mitchell [42] reported a negative correlation between survival and a positive fluid balance in critically ill patients, there is no standard treatment for blood volume restoration. The best preparation for the restoration of volume, whether crystalloid or colloid, or an association between these, should have the following characteristics: the ability to quickly replace the lost blood volume, regain normal hemodynamics and oxygen transportation improve the blood flow of microcirculation and restore the biohumoral balance. In addition, it must also possess the physical, chemical and metabolic qualities needed to remain in circulation for as long as possible, and to well tolerated and easily metabolised. It may perhaps be possible to reach a crystalloids versus colloids versus colloids consensus as the different conditions of patients, individual responses and the complexity of the clinical pictures may require ad-hoc treatment. The physician's primary duty must be "primum non nocere" – first and foremost do no harm.

References

1. Hillman K, Bishop G, Bristow P (1996) Focus on: physiology and pathophysiology of fluids and electrolytes. Fluid resuscitation. Curr Anesth Crit Care 7:187-191
2. Fiddian-Green RG (1993) Goals for the resuscitation of shock. Crit Care Med 21:25-31
3. Wardrop CAJ, Holland BM, Jacobs S, Jones JC (1992) Optimisation of the blood for oxygen transport and tissue perfusion in critical Care. Postgrd Med 68:2-6
4. Doglio GR, Pusajo JF, Egurolla MA et al (1991) Gastric mucosal pH as a prognostic index of mortality in critically ill patients. 19:1037-1040
5. Fiddian-Green RG, Baker S (1987) Predictive value of the stomach wall pH for complications after cardiac operations: comparison with other monitoring. Crit Care Med 15:153-156
6. Gys T, Hubens A, Neels H et al (1988) Prognostic value of gastric intramural pH in surgical intensive care patients. Crit Care Med 16:1222-1224
7. Schielder M, Cutler BS, Fiddian Green RG (1987) Sigmoid intramural pH for prediction of ischaemic colitis during aortic surgery. Arch Surg 122:881-886
8. Jones JG, Wardrop CAJ (2000) Measurements of blood volume in surgical and intensive care practice. British Journal of Anaesthesia 84:226-235
9. Shippy CR, Appel PL, Shoemaker WC (1984) Reliability of clinical monitoring to assess blood volume in critically ill patients. Crit Care Med 12:107-112
10. Haljamae H (1999) Use of fluid in trauma. Int J Intensive Care 6:20-30
11. Vincent JL (1995) The 'at risk patient population'. In: Sibbald WJ, Vincent JL (eds) Clinical trials for the treatment of sepsis. Springer, Heidelberg, pp 13-34
12. Christ F, Camble J, Gartside IB, Kox WJ (1998) Increased microvascular water permeability in patients with septic shock, assessed with venous congestion plethysmography (VCP). Intensive Care 24:18-27
13. Kinsky MP, Guha Sc, Button BM, Kramer GC (1998) The role of interstitial Starling forces in the pathogenesis of burn edema. J Burn Care Rehab 19:1-9
14. Lund T, Onarheim H, Reed RK (1992) Pathogenesis of edema formation in burn injuries. World J Surg 16:2-5
15. Velasco IT, Ponticri V, Rocha M et al (1980) Hyperosmotic NaCl and severe hemorrhagic shock. Am J Physiol 239:H664-H673
16. De Fellipe JJ, Timoner J, Velasco IT et al (1980) Treatment of refractory hypovolaemic shock by 7,5% sodium chloride injections. Lancet 2:1002-1004
17. Poli de Figueredo LF, Kramer GC et al (1999) Safety concerns and contraindications of hyperosmolar small – volume resuscitation. In: Kreimeier U, Christ F, Messmer K (eds) Small-volume hyperosmolar volume resuscitation. Heidelberg, Springer
18. Nakayama S, Silbey L, Gunther R et al (1984) Small-volume resuscitation with hypertonic saline resuscitation (2400 mosm/l) during haemorrhagic shock. Circ shock 13:149-159
19. Smith GJ, Kramer GC, Perron P et al (1985) A comparison of several hypertonic solutions for resuscitation of bled sheep. J Surg Res 39:517-529
20. Kramer GC, Perron PR, Lindsey DC et al (1986) Small-volume resuscitation with hypertonic saline dextran solution. Surgery 100:239-247
21. Poli de Figueiredo LF, Peres Ca, Attalah AN et al (1995) Hemodynamic improvement in hemorrhagic shock by aortic balloon occlusion and hypertonic saline solutions. Cardiovasc Surg 3:679-686
22. Rocha e Silva M, Negraes G, Soares A et al (1986) Hypertonic resuscitation from severe hemorrhagic shock: patterns of regional circulation. Circ Shock 19:165-175
23. Kreimeier U, Bruckner U, Niemczyk S, Messmer K (1986) Hyperosmotic saline dextran for resuscitation from traumatic–hemorrhagic hypotension: effect on regional blood flow. Circ Shock 32:83-99
24. Rocha e Silva M, Velasco IT, Noguiera da Silva RI et al (1987) Hyperosmotic sodium salts reverse severe hemorrhagic shock: other solutes do not. Am J Physiol 253:H751-H762
25. Gronwall A (1957) Dextran and its use in colloidal infusion solutions. Almquist and Wiksell, Uppsala

26. Taylor RJ, Ronald G, Pearl G (1996) Crystalloid vs colloids vs colloids: all colloids are not created equal. Anesth Analg 83:209-212
27. Camu F, Ivens D, Christiaens F (1995) Human albumin and colloid fluid replacement: their use in general surgery. Acta Anaesthesiologica (Belg) 46:3-18
28. Boldt J, Heesen M, Muller M et al (1996) The effects of albumin vs hydroxyethil starch solution on cardiorespiratory and circulatory variables in critically ill patients. Anaesth Analg 83:254-261
29. Imm A, Carlson RW (1993) Fluid resuscitation in circulatory shock. Crit Care Clin 9:313-331
30. Strauss RG, Stansfield C, Henriksen RA, Villhauer PJ (1988) Pentastarch may cause fewer effects on coagulation than hetastarch. Transfusion 28:257-260
31. Prough DS, Kramer G (1994) Medium starch, please. Anesth Analg 79:1034-1035
32. Velanovich V (1989) Crystalloids vs colloid fluid resuscitation: a metaanalysis of mortality. Surgery 10:65-71
33. Vermeulen LC Jr, Ratko TA, Erstad BL et al (1995) A paradigm for consensus: the university hospital consortium guidelines for the use of albumin, nonprotein colloid, and crystalloid solution. Arch Int Med 155:373-379
34. Rady M (1994) An argument for colloid resuscitation for shock. Acad Emerg Med 1:572-579
35. Hippala S, Linko K, Mylila et al (1995) Replacement of major surgical blood loss by hypooncotic or conventional plasma substitutes. Acta Anaesthesiologica Scand 39:228-235
36. Doglio Gr, Pusajo JF, Egurriola MA et al (1991) Gastric mucosal pH as a prognostic index of mortality in critically ill patients. Critical Care Med 19:1037-1040
37. Schierhout G, Roberts I (1998) Fluid resuscitation with colloid or crystalloid solutions in critically ill patients: a systematic review of randomized trials. Br Med J 316:961-964
38. Choi PTL, Gordon Yip, Quinonez LG, Cook DJ (1999) Crystalloids vs colloids in fluid resuscitation. A systematic review. Crit Care Med 27:200-210
39. McAnult GR, Ground RM (1998) Fluid resuscitation with colloid or crystalloid solutions. Br Med J 317:278
40. Whyncoll DLA, Beale RJ, McLuckie S (1998) Crystalloids vs colloids. Br Med J 317: 278-279
41. Schierhout G, Roberts I (1998) Crystalloid vs colloid solution. Br Med J 317:278
42. Mitchell JP, Schuller D, Calandrino FS, Schuster DP (1992) Improved outcome based on fluid management in critically ill patients requiring pulmonary artery catheterization. Am Rev Resp Dis 145:990-998

PERIOPERATIVE MEDICINE

PHARMACOLOGY OF THE PERIOPERATIVE PERIOD

Sedatives - Pharmacological Advances and Clinical Use

N.G. Volpe

Many therapeutic and diagnostic procedures used in medicine can cause distress and anxiety. Indeed, many efforts have been made in the history of medical and surgical disciplines to find physical and pharmacological means to allay anxiety, produce unconsciousness and to relieve pain. Light sedation provides a calm and relaxed patient without loss of consciousness. This ensures that protective reflexes are maintained, respiration is efficient and verbal contact is immediate. Deeper sedation will involve some degree of reduced or loss of consciousness with the potential risk of reduction in effectiveness of protective reflexes and the loss of airway control. Incremental techniques of intravenous sedation may cause the patient to fluctuate between these two states. The Royal College of Surgeons of England has defined conscious sedation as follows: *"Sedation is a technique in which the use of a drug, or drugs, produces a state of depression of the central nervous system enabling treatment to be carried out, but during which communication is maintained such that the patient will respond to command throughout the period of sedation"* [1].

Verbal contact is the crucial factor in drawing the dividing line between the two very different entities of conscious sedation and deep sedation or anaesthesia. Adequate monitoring of consciousness and cardiorespiratory function is mandatory whenever pharmacological sedation is used as well as experience in cardiopulmonary resuscitation.

The aim of this review is to examine the pharmacology of many compounds used in medicine to produce sedation, and the progress made in the last few years in the techniques and substances used to provide a state of reduced anxiety during diagnostic or surgical procedures.

Pharmacological methods of sedation

Administration of pharmacological compounds with sedative properties can be performed by oral, inhalation, intravenous, transmucosal and rectal administration.

Light levels of inhalational sedation are often used in dental practice in the technique of relative analgesia where the patient breathes low to moderate concentrations of nitrous oxide in oxygen through a nasal mask to provide sedation as an adjunct to dental surgery under local anaesthesia. This has been shown to alleviate fear, reduce pain and improve patient cooperation [2]. Concentrations of nitrous oxide higher than 35% induce alterations in laryngeal reflex activity in 20% of patients breathing a mixture of nitrous oxide in oxygen [3]. Subanaesthetic concentrations of volatile anaesthetic agents are also used to supplement regional anaesthesia, particularly for ambulatory procedures in dental practice [4]. All inhalational techniques, however, necessitate the use of close fitting masks or mouthpieces to ensure adequate drug intake and reduced environmental pollution and many patients find this unpleasant and uncomfortable.

Intravenous and oral administration of sedative drugs is more suited to routine use than the inhalational route and is much more extensively practised. It is easier to administer, does not involve the use of bulky equipment, does not cause environmental pollution and is much more acceptable to the patient. It should always be delivered slowly, either by incremental doses or by continuous infusion with the aim to tritrate the dose to the individual patient in view of obtaining the desired effect.

The ideal sedative is the compound that *"would provide reliable sedation or sleep with airway maintenance and minimal effect on the circulation or respiration and recovery would be rapid with no residual drowsiness"* [5]. Furthermore, it should be compatible with other anaesthetic drugs, non-toxic, free of hypersensitivity problems and, ideally, hydrosoluble and stable in solution.

Three main groups of drugs are used in an attempt to meet these criteria, namely, tranquillisers, intravenous anaesthetic agents and opioids.

Tranquillisers

The benzodiazepines provide the main drugs in this group.

Benzodiazepines

All benzodiazepines possess anxiolytic, hypnotic, anticonvulsant, muscle relaxant and amnesic properties. They act on specific receptor sites throughout the central nervous system and produce their effect by potentiating inhibitory interneurones, which use gamma-amino-butyric acid (GABA) as neurotransmitter. GABA receptors are widely distributed throughout the CNS and are responsible for both pre- and post-synaptic inhibition. The facilitation of the entry of Clorine ions into the cells induces hyperpolarization of the post-synaptic membrane causing inhibition of neuronal activity [6]. The benzodiazepine GABA channel system has been demonstrated in myocardial papillary muscle. It has the effect of decreasing myocardial contractility and shortening the duration of the action potential [7]. The different scenarios in which these drugs are used depend more on their pharmacokinetic properties than their primary pharmacodynamic effect. Their administration is followed by a dose dependent cerebral depression ranging from light sedation to sleep. Diazepam and midazolam are the most widely used compounds for intravenous sedation whereas lorazepam and temazepam are mostly used via the oral route.

The main pharmacokinetic parameters of midazolam, diazepam and lorazepam are illustrated in Table 1 [8].

Table 1.

	t½α (min)	Vl (l/kg)	t½α (h)	Vdα (l/kg)	Cl (ml/min)
Diazepam	9-130	0.31-0.41	31.3-46.6	0.9-1.2	26-35
Midazolam	3-38	0.17-0.44	2.1-2.4	0.8-1.14	202-324
Lorazepam	3-10	0.30-072	14.3-14.6	1.14-1.30	70-80

t½α, distribution half-life; Vl, volume of central compartment, t½α, elimination half life; Vdα, apparent volume of distribution; Cl, total plasma clearance

Diazepam has many of the desirable features of an intravenous sedative. It provides good sedation and amnesia, it causes minimal depression of the cardiovascular and respiratory systems and is a good anticonvulsant, increasing protection against local anaesthetic toxicity. It has been shown that a small intravenous dose of 2.5-5 mg of diazepam was effective in producing sedation in patients undergoing surgery under regional anaesthesia [9]. Anterograde amnesia with this technique has also been reported.

As an intravenous sedative, diazepam has several important disadvantages including pain on injection with subsequent thrombophlebitis, wide biological variations in patient response and delayed recovery [10]. Like many other benzodiazepines, diazepam is insoluble in water and the original intravenous preparation was solubilised in propylene glycol, ethanol and sodium benzoate in benzoic acid. Reformulation in a soy bean emulsion has virtually eliminated the venous problem with no alteration in the therapeutic effect [11]. Delayed recovery and patient variation in response remain the major problems with diazepam, no matter how formulated. The drug has a long elimination half-life between 20 and 70 hours and there is a second peak effect some 4-6 hours after initial intravenous administration due to enterohepatic recirculation of the drug excreted in the bile and reabsorbed by the intestinal mucosa [10].

Midazolam, an imidazobenzodiazepine derivative, was marketed in Europe at the beginning of the 1980s. Its unique structural formula offers many advantages over the other benzodiazepines. Its fused imidazole ring makes the drug highly basic and therefore soluble in water and also allows rapid hepatic metabolism [12]. Midazolam has an elimination half-life of approximately 2 hours and its plasma clearance is 10 times higher than that of diazepam. There is no evidence of active metabolites or of enterohepatic recirculation. Its water solubility makes midazolam non-irritant to the venous wall and pain on injection is rare. The respiratory depression induced by midazolam is dose-dependent and care has to be used when administered to patients with compromised respiratory function. It has been shown in patients with COPD that the depression of respiration induced by a dose of midazolam of 0.2 mg/kg occurs earlier and lasts longer that in patients without a history of chronic respiratory dysfunction [13]. Many comparative studies have been reported with midazolam and diazepam for sedation. All have shown that midazolam provides equivalent or better quality of sedation with an average dose of 0.1 mg/kg. Greater amnestic effect and faster onset of sedation have been reported after administration of midazolam in many studies [14-16]. Recovery and fitness to discharge seem to be faster after administration of midazolam.

It has also been shown that midazolam administration in surgical patients delays the need for postoperative analgesia [17]. This effect is thought to be the result of synergistic effect between the two drugs rather than due to a direct analgesic activity of midazolam. The pharmacological effects of midazolam and of other benzodiazepines can be reversed by the administration of flumazenil.

Propofol

Propofol (2,6-diisopropylphenol) is a chemically inert phenol derivative, which is a short acting anaesthetic agent with rapid onset of action [18]. Besides its use to induce and maintain anaesthesia, propofol has also been successfully used for conscious sedation [19]. Its rapid metabolism makes propofol suitable for use either as a bolus or in continuous infusion. The recovery from propofol anaesthesia or sedation is fast and complete in a very short period of time. It causes both respiratory and cardiovascular depression. Propofol should be used only by physicians experienced in advanced life support techniques.

Ketamine

The sedative, analgesic and dissociative properties of this phencyclidine derivative have encouraged its use for analgesia, sedation and induction of general anaesthesia. Its lack of respiratory depression is a distinctive advantage over opioids and benzodiazepines [20]. The ketamine used in clinical practice consists of a racemic mixture composed of equal amounts of 2 optical isomers. Recent studies have shown that the molecular target of ketamine action is the N-methyl-D-aspartate (NMDA) glutamate receptor. Ketamine exerts a non competitive antagonistic action. It has also been shown that ketamine can bind to opioid receptors and its pharmachological effects are not reversed by naloxone

[21]. In contrast to other intravenous agents used for sedation and anaesthesia, ketamine has also shown analgesic effects at low doses. In adults dreams and hallucinations frequently accompany recovery from the pharmacological effects of ketamine. This effect can be minimised by the concurrent administration of benzodiazepines [22].

A recent comparative study has shown that the combination of ketamine with propofol results in better sedation than that produced by propofol alone in a group of patients undergoing ophthalmic surgery under retrobulbar block [23]. The authors reported a faster onset and a better quality of sedation without unwanted side effects such as hallucinations or respiratory depression. Another study in which ketamine had been used for conscious sedation reported that all patients but one showed anterograde amnesia [24]. Ketamine has also been shown to be effective in addition to midazolam and propofol for office based plastic surgical procedures in 1264 patients. Oxygen saturation below 90% was noted in 1% of the patients and antiemetic medications were needed in 2% of this population [25]. The excellent safety profile and the beneficial pharmacological actions together with the better explanation of its molecular interactions make ketamine an interesting compound to be used in sedation for various surgical and invasive procedures.

α_2-adrenoceptor agonists

These compounds exhibit a variety of pharmacological effects that make them useful in association with other drugs for the administration of sedation and general anaesthesia. The potent sedative and hypnotic effect of these compounds is mediated by their action on a single type of receptor [26]. α_2-adrenoceptor agonists act on pre and post-synaptic adrenoceptors by inhibiting noradrenaline release. The inhibition of release of the neurotransmitter causes a reduction of excitatory phenomena in the central nervous system, especially in the locus coeruleus [27].

Clonidine and dexmedetomidine are the only 2 compounds of this class that have been used in clinical practice to provide sedation and anxiolysis. Several studies have shown that the administration of these 2 compounds in association with other sedative or analgesic drugs for premedication before general anaesthesia has resulted in an enhancement of sedation and a reduction in the dose of the drugs used to provide general anaesthesia. In a study on 28 male patients undergoing orthopedic surgery it has been shown that the administration of clonidine as a premedicant has induced a 15% reduction in the induction dose of propofol and a 52% reduction in additional propofol boluses [28]. The reduction in anaesthetic drug requirement for induction and maintenance of general anaesthesia has been confirmed in healthy volunteers and in patients undergoing surgery. In one study on healthy volunteers the administration of dexmedetomidine has been shown to decrease in a dose dependent manner the requirement of isoflurane needed to induce and maintain general anaesthesia [29].

The use of these drugs in sedation and anaesthesia has shown some undesirable effects. The most important are bradycardia and hypotension. Both these effects can be prolonged and of variable severity.

Further studies are needed to establish the definitive role of these compounds in sedation, anaesthesia and the treatment of acute and chronic pain.

Conclusions

The advances in neurophysiological knowledge have opened a new chapter in the search for pharmacological compounds with sedative properties. It has also allowed a better use of drugs already available. New pharmacological strategies have been elaborated in order to provide safer and more effective techniques for sedation.

References

1. Royal College of Surgeons of England. Report Working Party (1993) Guidelines for sedation by non-anaesthetists. London: Royal College of Surgeons of England
2. Roberts GJ (1983) Relative analgesia in clinical practice. In Anaesthesia and Sedation in Dentistry, Monographs in Anaesthesiology 12. Editors MP Coplans and RA Green, Elsevier, Amsterdam, 231-279
3. Rubin J, Brock-Utne JG, Greenberg M et al (1977) Laryngeal incompetence during experimental relative analgesia using 50% nitrous oxide in oxygen. British Journal of Anaesthesia 49:1005-1008
4. Parbrook GD, Still DM, Parbrook EO (1989) Comparison of I.V. sedation with midazolam and inhalational sedation with isoflurane in dental outpatients. British Journal of Anaesthesia 63:81-86
5. McClure JH, Brown DT, Wildsmith JAW (1983) Comparison of the I.V. administration of midazolam and diazepam as sedation during spinal anaesthesia. British Journal of Anaesthesia 55:1089-1093
6. Horton RW (1989) Amino acid neurotransmitters. In: Webster RA, Jordan CC (Eds) Neurotransmitters, drugs and disease. Blackwell Scientific Publications Oxford, pp 165-181
7. Mestre M, Carriot T, Belin C et al (1985) Electrophysiological and pharmacological characterization of peripheral benzodiazepine receptors in a guinea-pig heart preparation. Life Science 35:953-962
8. Volpe N, Pelosi G (1996) Guida tascabile di farmacocinetica per Anestesisti Rianimatori. Adis International Limited, p 31
9. Gjessing J, Tomlin PJ (1977) Intravenous sedation and regional anaesthesia. Anaesthesia 32: 63-69
10. Calvey NT, Williams NE (1997) Principles and Practice of Pharmacology for Anaesthesia. 3rd edn. Oxford: Blackwell Science
11. Thorn-Alquist AM (1977) Parenteral use of diazepam in an emulsion formulation. A clinical study. Acta Anaesthesiologica Scandinavica 21:400-404
12. Reves JG, Fragen RJ, Vinik HR Greenblatt DJ (1985) Midazolam: pharmacology and uses. Anesthesiology 62:310-24
13. Morel D, Forster A, Bachmann M, Suter PM (1982) Changes in breathing patterns induced by midazolam in normal subjects. Anaesthesiology 57:A481

14. Berggren L, Eriksson I, Mollenholt P, Wichbom G (1983) Sedation for fibreoptic gastroscopy: a comparative study of midazolam and diazepam. British Journal of Anaesthesia 55:289-296
15. Barker I, Butchart DGM, Gibson J et al (1986) I.V. sedation for conservative dentistry. A comparison of midazolam and diazepam. British Journal of Anaesthesia 58:371-377
16. Whitwam JG, Al-Khudhairi D, McCloy RF (1983) Comparison of midazolam and diazepam in doses of comparable potency during gastroscopy. British Journal of Anaesthesia 55:773-777
17. Gilliland HEM, Prasad BK, Mirakhur RK, Fee JPH (1996) An investigation of the morphine-sparing effects of midazolam. Anaesthesia 51:808-811
18. Glen JB, Hunter SC (1984) Pharmacology of an emulsion ICI 35 868. British Journal of Anaesthesia 56:617-626
19. Rudkin GE, Osborne GA, Finn BO et al (1992) Intraoperative patient-controlled sedation. Comparison of patient-controlled propofol with patient-controlled midazolam. Anaesthesia 47:376-381
20. White PF, Way WL, Trevor AJ (1982) Ketamine - its pharmacology and therapeutic uses. Anesthesiology 56:119-136
21. Hurstveit O, Maurset A, Øye I (1995) Interaction of the chiral forms of ketamine with opioid, phencyclidine and muscarinic receptors. Pharmacol Toxicol 77:355-359
22. Grant IS, Nimmo WS, McNicol LR, Clements JA (1983) Ketamine disposition in children and adults. British Journal of Anaesthesia 55:1107-1110
23. Frey K, Sukhani R, Pawlowski J et al (1999) Propofol versus propofol-ketamine sedation for retrobulbar nerve block: comparison of sedation quality, intraocular pressure changes, and recovery profiles. Anesthesia and Analgesia 89:317-321
24. Gruber RP, Morley B (1999) Ketamine-assisted intravenous sedation with midazolam. Benefits and potential problems. Plastic and Reconstructive Surgery 104:1823-1825
25. Friedberg BL (1999) Propofol-ketamine technique: dissociative anesthesia for office surgery (a 5 year review of 1264 cases). Aesthetic and Plastic Surgery 23:70-75
26. Maze M, Tranquilli W (1991) Alpha-2 adrenoceptor agonists: defining the role in clinical anesthesia. Anesthesiology 74:581-605
27. Chiu TH, Chen MJ, Yang YR et al (1995) Action of dexmedetomidine on rat locus coeruleus neurones: intracellular recording in vitro. European Journal of Pharmacology 285:261-268
28. Guglielminotti J, Descraques C, Petitmarie S et al (1998) Effects of premedication on dose requrements for propofol: comparison of clonidine and hydroxyzine. British Journal of Anaesthesia 80:733-736
29. Khan ZP, Munday IT, Jones RM et al (1999) Effects of dexmedetomidine on isoflurane requirements in healthy volunteers. 1: Pharmacodynamic and pharmacokinetic interactions. British Journal of Anaesthesia 83:372-380

Advances in Clinical Pharmacology of the Muscle Relaxants

C. Melloni

Atracurium and vecuronium marked a first revolution in the daily practicc of anesthesia in the mid 1980s, paving the way for two distinct approaches to research and practice; the first was slightly more innovative; it was guided by the Wellcome Foundation, later Glaxo Wellcome, which explored the class of benzylisochinolines compounds, characterized by spontaneous degradation via Hoffman reaction (atracurium first and cisatracurium lately) or degradation by plasma enzymes, like pseudocholinesterase, with mivacurium an outstanding example of this class.

The second, more traditional in the pharmacological approach and followed by the Organon Teknika Company, strove to modify the structure of the aminosteroidal compounds, producing drugs with progressively faster onset, starting with the parent compound vecuronium, passing through rocuronium, and resulting now in the new drug rapacuronium, eventually the first muscle relaxant able to compete with succynilcholine for fast onset and short duration of action. Continuing in the search for the "Holy Grail" of the neuromuscular blockers, a fast onset with short duration of action drug, interest focused on the two drugs mivacurium and rapacuronium, especially because of the increase in the practice of day surgery, day anesthesia is broadening its spectrum, thus encompassing slightly more-invasive procedures, where control of the airway is mandatory.

Mivacurium is characterized by a large clearance and a rate of hydrolysis of 70-88% that of succinylcholine [1, 2]. Lacroix et al. [3] estimated that the clearances for the two pharmacologically more-active isomers of mivacurium (*cis-trans* and *trans-trans*) are 92 and 53 ml/kg per min respectively, values clearly resulting in more-rapid spontaneous recovery than other available nondepolarizing relaxants, with a recovery index (the time for recovery of TI from 25-75% of control) of only about 6 min. Once some evidence of spontaneous recovery has taken place (TI of 5-10% of control), the TOF ratio will usually return to a value > 0.70 in under 20 min, and the average time from TI 95% to TOF 70% is only about 3 min [4]; more recently it has been shown that, in a given patient, recovery form an intubating dose of 0.3 mg/kg, administered as two boluses of 0.15 mg/kg 30 s apart, indicates the time course of spontaneous recovery after discontinuation of an infusion of mivacurium. More precisely the time from induction to 5% recovery of T1 and the times to recovery of TOF ratios 0.70 and 0.90% are strictly correlated, so that each patient becomes his own indicator of recovery. For instance, if it takes a patient 24 min to recover to 5% of baseline strength or approximately one palpable twitch after 0.3 mg/kg mivacurium, it is likely to take 24 min to spontaneously recover to a TOF ratio of 90% after a mivacurium infusion that had been dosed to maintain a 95% depression of T1, i.e., only one palpable twitch in the TOF, is discontinued. If a patient takes either more or less time to recover from the initial bolus, final recovery from infusion will be longer or shorter, accordingly.

The clinical implications are evident: the sicker the patients are and the longer the procedures and the corresponding infusion of mivacurium, the predictability of final recovery once initial recovery is determined would allow for precise control over the need of reversal and avoid the problem of residual curarization, especially so because interpatient variability of the speed of recovery from mivacurium-induced neuromuscular block is considerable and is related to its rapid metabolism by plasma cholinesterase.

The elimination half-lives of its potent *cis-trans* and *trans-trans* isomers are 1.8-2.5 min and 1.5-2.4 min, respectively [5, 6]. Individual patient clearance of the *cis-trans* and *trans-trans* isomers of mivacurium is related to the patient's plasma cholinesterase activity: the rate of infusion of mivacurium required to maintain a stable depth of neuromuscular block depends therefore on a patient's plasma cholinesterase activity [7, 8]; patients with greater plasma cholinesterase activity require more mivacurium. The wide range of normal plasma cholinesterase activities accounts for at least some of the interpatient variability in terms of recovery of neuromuscular function after mivacurium-induced neuromuscular block, and accounts for the fact that in some patients with acquired or inherited deficits of this enzyme its duration of action could be greatly increased, as was the case with suxamethonium.

I should emphasize again that, according to the quoted clinical work of Savarese et al. [1] and Lien et al. [4, 5], even in case of unexpected long duration, the anesthesiologist will at least appreciate the length of the block in the early phase of the intervention, noting the interval of time required from the initial dosage to the initial recovery, and without sophisticated monitoring, therefore anticipating the need for reversal or adopting a different strategy, i.e., continuing the mechanical ventilation and sedation.

There has been much debate about whether it is required, or even advisable, to pharmacologically antagonize residual mivacurium-induced neuromuscular block. The anticholinesterase neostigmine will inhibit plasma cholinesterase, as well as acetylcholinesterase; therefore, the administration of anticholinesterase may actually slow the clearance of this otherwise rapidly metabolized relaxant, resulting in a slowed recovery of neuromuscular function [9]. Recent studies have demonstrated increases in the plasma concentrations of the potent isomers of mivacurium after the administration of either neostigmine or edrophonium, in the presence of an ongoing infusion of the relaxant [10, 11].

Despite these data, however, cholinesterase inhibitors do not prolong a mivacurium-induced block in rats [12], and both edrophonium [13, 14] and neostigmine [15-17] shorten the time required for recovery from mivacurium-induced neuromuscular block. Some patients are more likely to require antagonism of residual mivacurium-induced block than others; these are likely to be patients who will have a slower spontaneous recovery of neuromuscular function, either because of decreased but normal, or markedly decreased, plasma cholinesterase activity. If mivacurium-induced block is not routinely antagonized pharmacologically, a significant number of patients may be admitted to the post-anesthesia care unit with unacceptably high levels of neuromuscular block, if enough time is not allowed for adequate spontaneous recovery. A strong case can be made that routine reversal of mivacurium is often unnecessary; at best, cholinesterase-accelerated recovery will speed return to control of neuromuscular function by about 7-8 min, and it is debatable if this interval constitutes a real benefit in daily practice, even considering the cost of the reversal drugs and their potential side effects. It should also be noted that the antagonist of choice if reversal is deemed advisable is probably edrophonium, not neostigmine [18].

Despite its singular pharmacokinetic profile, mivacurium has achieved only a modest niche in the anesthesiologist's neuromuscular armamentarium, most probably because the potential for triggering histamine release [19], causing systemic hypotension and the inconvenience of its slow onset even at 2 ED95, so that the impatient anesthesiologist can not uniformly obtain good intubating conditions.

The Organon answer to some of the problems demonstrated by mivacurium is ORG 9487, a steroidal-based blocker of low potency with a very rapid onset of 60-90 s and a duration of action of 15-20 min [20]. The pharmacokinetic profile of ORG 9487 suggests that it will probably be classified as a short-acting drug. It has a clearance of 8.5-11.0 ml/kg per min and a MRT of only 33-44 min [21].

Following a single 1.5 mg/kg bolus, recovery of twitch height to 25% of control T1 has been reported to be [22] as short as 10.5 min and as long as 18 min.

However, duration of action was dose dependent, reaching 50 min with the higher dosages; moreover if administered as a 1-h infusion, ORG 9487 changed its time course characteristics gradually from that of a short-acting neuromuscular blocking agent to that of a relaxant with an intermediate duration of action, and it has been demonstrated that the prolongation of action of the muscle relaxant could largely be attributed to its degradation to ORG 9488, its desacetyl metabolite, a muscle relaxant of its own of weak potency, but longer duration of action [23].

The clinical niche of rapacuronium remains undetermined; while providing faster onset at higher dosages, duration of action could be longer, even if reversal with glycopyrrolate and neostigmine 0.05 mg/kg is capable of rapidly antagonizing the neuromuscular blocking properties of the drug [24, 25].

However, return to a T1/tc ratio of 75% is not indicative of complete return of force, since to attain a TOF 0.70 or higher 25-30 min are required, either attempting reversal after 2 min from the injection of the full dose of rapacuronium, or allowing a spontaneous recovery of T1 25%.

Kopman [26] was the first to note an inverse correlation between the potency of nondepolarizing muscle relaxants, as defined by the dose producing 95% twitch depression and, by extension, by plasma concentration, and their speed of onset. The explanation lies, most probably, in the fact that a large bolus dose with many molecules produces a gradient of muscle relaxant from plasma to neuromuscular junction; the drug reaches the neuromuscular junction traversing the local capillaries and binds to the receptor; some reaches the neuromuscular junction by equilibration with extracellular fluid adjacent to the receptor (the biophase). Assuming that a given degree of paralysis results from binding of a fixed number of receptors, the higher plasma concentration produced by a less-potent relaxant increases the magnitude of this gradient, so that more molecules of a less-potent relaxant are available in plasma to fill the biophase and receptors in a given period. This concept is analogous to the effect of a high versus a low tissue-blood partition coefficient: a depot with a high partition coefficient takes longer to fill than one with a low partition coefficient; due to the lower coefficient more drug remains at the receptor or at the effector site.

The other factor that influences the time course of the concentrations of the muscle relaxant at the effect site is its time course in plasma. A more-rapid decrease in plasma concentration of a muscle relaxant, i.e., a shorter distribution half-life, as might result from either a larger clearance or a larger distributional clearance, would hasten the time at which the concentration peaked at the effect site and would also decrease the magnitude of the peak concentration at the effect site, possibly necessitating a larger dose. In turn, the peak effect of equipotent doses would occur earlier with a larger clearance. Thus the finding that rapacuronium clearance in the volunteers in the Wright study [27] (8.55-10.25 ml/kg per min) is larger than that of vecuronium (5.1 ml/kg per min) and rocuronium (2.89 ml/kg per min) may also contribute to the rapid onset of the rapacuronium effect. However, rapacuronium clearance is markedly less than that of the potent isomers of mivacurium, suggesting that differences in clearance are not sufficient to explain speed of onset.

A second explanation for the fast onset of rapacuronium lies in its rapid equilibration between plasma concentration and effect compartment; its Keo of 0.45/min is much larger than that of rocuronium (0.15-0.18) and vecuronium (0.12), differing by an order of 2.5-3.5 times. As a consequence of the rapid Keo for rapacuronium, the laryngeal muscles equilibrate more rapidly than do the adductor pollicis muscles; this indicates either that, compared with the adductor pollicis, the laryngeal muscles have a greater blood flow volume per gram of tissue or their partition coefficient is smaller. In any case, a fast onset at the laryngeal muscles will allow for a better relaxation of the tracheal muscles, allowing a faster intubation with better intubating conditions. From this point of view, rapacuronium is more similar to succinylcholine and offers significant advantages in comparison with rocuronium, which possesses a longer duration of action.

Another advantage of rapacuronium lies in the fact that its dynamic behavior does not seem to differ between adults and children or infants. ED 50s were similar between neonates, children, and adults: ED 50 (mg/kg) neonates 0.32 [28, 29], infants 0.32 [28] or 0.28 [29], children 1-12 years 0.40 [28] or 0.39 [29]. Duration of action was also similar.

A significant disadvantage, especially in comparison with cisatracurium and vecuronium, has been reported by [30]. The drug causes a dose-dependent release of histamine and, albeit not histamine related, an increase in heart rate and decrease in mean arterial pressure. How much of this effect could be attributed to a direct vasodilator effect of the drug is uncertain at present.

It is probable that more work will soon elucidate the position of rapacuronium among the muscle relaxants currently available. The wide spectrum of onsets, duration of action, metabolism, and minimal side effects exhibited by the array of neuromuscular blockers in clinical use today will allow the choice of the proper drug at the right moment, tailoring the drug to the patient and procedure.

References

1. Savarese JJ, Ali HH, Basta SJ, et al (1988) The clinical neuromuscular pharmacology of mivacurium chloride (BW B1090U): a shortacting nondepolarizing ester neuromuscular blocking drug. Anesthesiology 68:723-732
2. Cook RD, Stiller RL, Weakly JN et al (1989) In vitro metabolism of mivacurium chloride (BW 1090U) and succinylcholine. Anesth Analg 68:452-456
3. Lacroix M, Donati F, Varin F (1997) Pharmacokinetics of mivacurium isomers and their metabolites in healthy volunteers after intravenous bolus administration. Anesthesiology 86: 322-330
4. Lien CA, Belmont MR, Abalos A et al (1999) The nature of spontaneous recovery from mivacurium-induced neuromuscular block. Anesth Analg 88:648-653
5. Lien CA, Schmith VD, Embree PB et al (1994) The pharmacokinetics and pharmacodynamics of the stereoisomers of mivacurium in patients receiving nitrous oxide/opioid/barbiturate anaesthesia. Anaesthesiology 80:1296-1302
6. Head-Rapson AG, Devlin JC, Parker CIR et al (1994) Pharmacokinetics of the three isomers of mivacurium and pharmacodynamics of the chiral mixture in hepatic cirrhosis. Br J Anaesth 73:613-618
7. Ali HH, Savarese JJ, Embree PB et al (1988) Clinical pharmacology of mivacurium chloride (BW B1090U) infusion: comparison with vecuronium and atracurium. Br J Anaesth 61: 541-546
8. Hart PS, McCarthy GJ, Brown R et al (1995) The effect of plasma cholinesterase activity on mivacurium infusion rates. Anesth Analg 80:760-763
9. Kao YJ, Le N (1996) The reversal of profound mivacurium induced neuromuscular blockade. Can J Anaesth 43:1128-1133
10. Hart PS, Wright PMC, Brown R et al (1995) Edrophonium increases mivacurium concentrations during constant mivacurium infusion, and large doses minimally antagonize paralysis. Anesthesiology 82:912-918

11. Szenohradszky J, Lau M, Brown R et al (1995) The effect of neostigmine on twitch tension and muscle relaxant concentration during infusion of mivacurium or vecuromum. Anesthesiology 83:83-87
12. Fleming NW, Lewis BK (1994) Cholinesterase inhibitors do not prolong neuromuscular block produced by mivacurium. Br J Anaesth 73:241-243
13. Kopman AF, Mallhi MU, Justo MD et al (1993) Antagonism of mivacurium-induced neuromuscular blockade in human, edrophonium dose requirements at threshold train-of-four: Count of four. Anesthesiology 81:1394-1400
14. Brandom BW, Taiwo OO, Woelfel SK et al (1996) Spontaneous versus edrophonium-induced recovery from paralysis with mivacurium. Anesth Analg 82:999-1002
15. Bevan JC, Tousignant C, Stephenson C et al (1996) Dose responses of neostigmine and edrophonium as antagonists of mivacurium adults and children. Anesthesiology 84:354-361
16. Devcic A, Munshi CA, Gandhi SK et al (1995) Antagonism of mivacurium neuromuscular block: neostigmine versus edrophonium. Anesth Analg 81:1005-1009
17. Baurain MI, Dernovoi BS, d'Hollander AA et al (1994) A comparison of neostigmine-induced recovery with spontaneous recovery from mivacurium-induced neuromuscular block. Br J Anaesth 73:791-794
18. Naguib M, Abdulatif M, Al-Ghamdi A et al (1993) Dose-response relationships for edrophonium and neostigmine antagonism mivacurium-induced neuromuscular block. Br J Anaesth 71:709-714
19. Naguib M, Samarkandi AH, Bakhamees HS (1995) Histamine-release haemodynamic changes produced by rocuronium, vecuronium, mivacurium, atracurium, and tubocurarine. Br J Anaesth 75:588-592
20. Wierda JMKH, van den Broek L, Proost JH et al (1993) Time course of action of endotracheal intubating conditions of ORG 9487, a new short-acting steroidal muscle relaxant; a comparison with succinylcholine. Anesth Analg 77:579-584
21. van den Broek L, Wierda JMKH (1994) Pharmacodynamics and pharmacokinetics of an infusion of ORG 9487, a new short-acting steroidal neuromuscular blocking agent. Br J Anaesth 73:331-335
22. Kahwaji R, Bevan DR, Bikhazi G et al (1997) Dose ranging study in younger adults and elderly patients of ORG 9487, a new rapid onset, short duration muscle relaxant. Anesth Analg 84:1011-1018
23. Schiere S, Proost JH, Schuringa M et al (1999) Pharmacokinetics and pharmacokinetic-dynamic relationship between rapacuronium (ORG 9487) and its desacetyl metabolite (ORG 9488). Anesth Analg 88:640-647
24. Deepika K, Keenan CA, Bikhazi GB et al (2000) Comparative study of recovery parameters of rapacuronium bromide after early and late reversal. Anesth Analg 90:S399
25. Bartkowski R, Witkowski TA, Epstein RH (2000) Recovery from rapacuronium, early vs. late reversal. Anesth Analg 90:s389
26. Kopman AF (1989) Pancuronium, gallamine, and d-tubocurarine compared: is speed of onset inversely related to drug potency? Anesthesiology 70:915-920
27. Wright PMC, Brown R, Lau M et al (1999) A pharmacodynamic explanation for the rapid onset/offset of rapacuronium bromide. Anesthesiology 90:16-25
28. Kaplan RF, Fletcher JE, Hannallah R et al (1996) The ED 50 of ORG 9487 in infants and childen. Anesthesiology 85:A1059
29. Kaplan RF, Fletcher JE, Hannallah RS et al (1999) The potency (ED 50) and cardiovascular effects of rapacuronium (DRG 9487) during narcotic-nitrous oxide-propofol anaesthesia in neonates, infants and children. Anesth Analg 89:1172-1176
30. Levy JH, Pitts M, Thanopoulos A et al (1999) The effects of rapacuronium on histamine release and haemodynamics in adult patients undergoing general anaesthesia. Anesth Analg 89:290-295

Recommendations on the Appropriate Use of the Muscle Relaxant

P. MASTRONARDI, T. CAFIERO, P. DE CILLIS

Recommendations on the appropriate use of the muscle relaxants (MR) are strictly related to the good knowledge of pharmacokinetics, pharmacodynamics, interaction with specific receptors, and monitoring of the neuromuscular junction (NMJ). The first recommendation regards the choice of the MR to be used. This choice must be based on:

- the tracheal intubating conditions; when the indicators of difficulty [1-4] lead us to predict that intubation is fairly easy to perform it is advisable to use nondepolarizing blocking drugs (ND); in cases of difficult intubating conditions it may be wiser to provide relaxation by using succinylcholine;
- duration of the operative procedure, since a large number of MR are now available, including long-, intermediate-, and short-acting drugs.

The new MR and their organ-based degradation and elimination, are summarized in Table 1. Steroidal compounds like vecuronium [5, 6] and rocuronium [7, 8] rely on hepatic and renal mechanisms of metabolism and elimination; so that in the presence of decreased hepatic and/or renal function, preexisting or deriving from general anesthesia, the efficacy and the duration of muscle relaxation can be altered. Furthermore, the MR with steroidal structure can undergo degradation to active metabolites on the NMJ: someone with a potency of blockade ranging from 50 to 80% of the parent drug, as the 3-hydroxyl metabolite of vecuronium, for which the major route of elimination is the kidney [9]. The new benzylisoquinolinium compounds, in contrast, have organ-based metabolism (chemical reaction of Hofmann elimination that is not affected by biological disorders) with no metabolites active on NMJ. Mivacurium represents an exception because it is hydrolyzed by plasma cholinesterase; so that it depends either on the hepatic function for the production of that enzyme or on the genetic predisposition in producing normal functioning enzyme. It can be assumed that for mivacurium the same recommendations suggested for succinylcholine are valid, i.e., preoperative screening. Benzylisoquinolinium substances do not undergo organ-based elimination and, furthermore, of the new ND they are the drugs whose parameters are the least likely to be altered in the elderly. As a logic consequence, the ND which do not undergo organ-based elimination with no active metabolites must be preferred.

Table 1. Metabolism of the newer nondepolarizing drugs

	OBM	NOBM	AM	IM
Atracurium		X		X
Cisatracurium		X		X
Mivacurium	X*			X
Rocuronium	X		X**	
Vecuronium	X		X	

OBM organ-based metabolism; *NOBM* non-organ-based metabolism; *AM* active metabolites; *IM* inactive metabolites; *NMJ* neuromuscular junction
* At least for synthesis and production of pseudocholinesterase
** Some metabolites seem to have intrinsic, even if weak, activity on NMJ

Another relevant aspect is the involvement of MR in anaphylactic or anaphylactoid reactions during general anesthesia. Several recent studies and earlier ones have pointed out that drugs like vecuronium and rocuronium with no histamine-releasing property [11] are still involved in severe anaphylactic reactions. It has been hypothesized that vecuronium induces the inhibition of the histamine-N-methyl-transferase [12], an enzyme responsible for the metabolic inactivation of histamine. This transient block of the histamine metabolism, lowering the histamine elimination, may be deleterious if, concomitantly, other drugs with histamine-releasing property are administered or surgical manipulations of organs such as bowel, lung, or liver are performed inducing displacement of the contents of mast cell granules containing histamine. The histamine accumulation may induce dangerous systemic reactions. The involvement of vecuronium is well known and recent articles show that rocuronium is involved in anaphylactic reactions. A case of anaphylaxis has been reported in which an involvement of cisatracurium has been hypothesized [13], even if clinical studies in humans have shown that with doses eight times the ED_{95} (0.4 mg/kg) statistically significant changes in histamine plasma concentrations and in hemodynamics were not found [14]. Therefore it is mandatory, especially in high-risk patients, to use the ND with no histamine-releasing properties or those statistically less involved in anaphylactic reactions during general anesthesia such as cisatracurium. In other cases when the duration of the surgical procedure does not permit using cisatracurium it may be convenient to avoid drugs which induce transient inhibition of metabolic inactivation of histamine, such as vecuronium and those potentially involved in anaphylactic reactions during general anesthesia without, to date, a valid hypothesis on its mechanism.

It is surprising that when it is impossible to use cisatracurium, it is advisable to administer a ND like atracurium or mivacurium, involved in anaphylactic reactions but with a well-known mechanism. The explanation of this paradox is that it is possible to decrease or even abolish the histamine release because the mechanism of histamine release is well known. The principal factors affecting the histamine release are mainly related to the dose and the speed of injection [15, 16]; the dose can be managed only by administering the lowest dose compatible with a proper action, even if a longer onset time is obtained. The speed of injection is a much more likely to influence the histamine release. Reducing the speed of injection of MR with histamine releasing propertias (time > 60-70 s) or using an infusion pump for injecting the MR, it is possible to avoid the release of histamine or other compounds produced ex novo such as leukotrienes. This phenomenon can be explained by the fact that the slower injection reduces the concentration at the basophil and mast cells.

For appropriate use of MR it would be advisable to consider the different pharmacological interactions. Many drugs used in anesthesia and intensive care can alter the pharmacokinetics of MR. Certainly it is well understood that the supplemental doses or the infusion rate must be decreased in the presence of potent inhaled anesthetics. The most-frequent interactions between ND and other drugs or pathophysiological conditions are summarized in Table 2. For many interactions illustrated in Table 2 the mechanism is discussed or unknown, whilst there is clinical evidence for other interactions; it is necessary to emphasize that the response to MR is affected by several factors, so it is not surprising that the clinical responses obtained during muscle relaxation were different from those expected. Some of the interactions are precede anesthesia and they can be evaluated with a complete clinical examination in the preoperative period. Many others may be underestimated or may occur during general anesthesia (acid-base imbalance). The pharmacological interactions are difficult to manage. It is enough to bear in mind steroids, deliberately not listed in Table 2 owing to the existing controversies [17-20]. Steroids are thought to be able to potentiate or decrease the activity of MR and to be involved in myopathy in intensive care units (ICU); so that the use of steroids in the preoperative period must alert the anesthesiologist to the possibility of a different response to MR.

Other recommendations can be deduced from the type of postjunctional receptors: two isomeric forms exist; the first "mature" to which the whole physiology of neuromuscular transmission (NMT) is referred and the second "immature" or extrajunctional receptor (EJR). The latter type of receptors, equivocally called extrajunctional, as they are produced only outside the NMJ, is formed in fetal life and at birth tends to disappear rapidly and is replaced by the "mature" post-junctional receptors. Muscle cells possess the genes for synthesizing both types of receptors [21] and the proliferation of the EJR restarts in several pathophysiological conditions [22]. As a general rule, muscular inactivity stimulates the mechanism of synthesis of EJR and, for this reason, the EJR is present in the newborn and it reappears, due to the lesion of motoneuron, during septic shock, burns, muscular hypercatabolic state, or many other diseases. Also in very old age, characterized by reduced muscular activity, the growth of EJR may be stimulated. The two isomers are structurally similar; they are made up of five subunits arranged as a pentameric complex with four subunits (2α, β, δ) which are exactly equal in both receptors. The difference between the two receptors is due

Table 2. Interference among muscle relaxants (MR), drugs, and particular physiopathological conditions

Drugs	Action	Clinical conditions	Action
Volatile anesthetics	P	↑α1-acid glycoprotein	D
Antibiotics	P	Hypercalcemia	D
Anticholinesterase	D	Hypercapnia	P
Antiepileptics		Hypermagnesemia	P
acute use	P	Hyperparathyroidism	D
chronic use	D	Hypocalcemia	P
Antirheumatics	P	Hypothermia	P
Cytostatics	P	Lesion of motoneuron	D
Clorpromazine	P	Malnutrition	P
Dantrolene	P	Myasthenia	P
Lithium	P	Burns	D

P potentiate, *D* decrease

to the fifth unit: type e in the mature form and type γ in the EJR form. So they act functionally in different pharmacological, electrophysiological, and metabolic ways [23]. The half-life of EJR is within 24 h, whilst that of "mature" receptor is about 2 weeks. The very important electrophysiological feature is the difference in the duration of channel opening, which in the EJR is four to ten times longer than that of the mature receptors. This electrophysyological phenomenon induces a prolonged channel opening with a great ionic movement, especially with efflux of K^+; this response by the EJR together with their particular sensitivity to succinylcholine may be the explanation for those severe reactions reported in burned patients after administration of succinylcholine. The EJR is synthesized early after the clinical event has occurred and the complete restoration of "mature" receptors needs up to 24 months, in the burned patient. For this reason it is advisable in those patients to avoid the use of succinylcholine for a long time, even though the natural healing from the clinical illness has been completed. The EJR proliferation explains also the resistance to ND in the presence of burns, immobilization, or other pathological diseases. As regards the use of the MR in ICU, the main recommendations are related to the necessity of associated adequate sedative and/or analgesic techniques in order to avoid the risk of unpleasant situations in which the critically ill patient is paralyzed but experiencing consciousness and pain! Other very important recommendations include the choice of the MR and the modality of managing it. The choice of MR must be guided by pharmacological considerations mentioned in the initial part of this manuscript.

- ND should not have organ-based metabolism because the critically ill patient in ICU may suffer from renal and/or hepatic failure;

- ND should not undergo enzymatic inhibition or induction, especially on the wide family of the cytochrome P_{450}, caused by concurrent administration of other drugs – it must be remembered that the critically ill patient is under aggressive treatment with several drugs;
- ND should not produce active metabolites on NMJ; the delayed recovery due to the use of vecuronium in the presence of renal failure in ICU owing to the production and accumulation of the 3-hydroxy metabolite should be remembered;
- ND should not be involved in unleashing anaphylaxis; this would be a tragic adverse reaction in the critically ill patient – it must be underlined that cisatracurium is the ND least involved in this kind of reactions;
- ND should not induce directly or as concomitant factor, a clinical pathological condition like polyneuromyopathy in ICU, which is characterized by adverse effects like muscle weakness, atrophy, tetraplegia, areflexia, and paresis. These effects are more frequently associated with the steroidal ND in ICU [25-27], than benzylisoquinolinium compounds like atracurium and cisatracurium.

From these considerations it can be deduced, as logic consequence, the necessity of monitoring the neuromuscular transmission (NMT). In addiction to a general knowledge of the guidelines, precise practise requires the use of a peripheral nerve stimulator to adjust relaxant dosage to the individual patient. It represents the sole chance for correct use of MR in the critically ill patient, especially to maintain a light degree of muscular response, and it would seem the best solution to some of the described problems. The other advantages deriving from monitoring of NMT are described later. Important recommendations have to be formulated on the modality of administration of MR both in anesthesia and in ICU. The use of MR as repeated boluses is the most-common and economic method of injecting MR. However, the best method is by continuous infusion, since the pharmacokinetic features of the new MR with short or intermediate duration of action allow it. The infusion of MR, as for all other drugs, is the most physiological way to assure the constancy of the necessary plasma concentrations. MR should be titrated to match the needs of the patient, avoiding "peaks and valleys" in drug concentrations corresponding to over- or underdosage. The ideal recommendation is to administer MR by means of continuous infusion together with monitoring of NMT. In this way it is possible to achieve muscle relaxation with a neuromuscular block of about 90%, which is optimal for all surgical procedures, but in the presence of a muscular response of 10% allows a more-rapid and preventable recovery of NMT. The rates of infusion that allow, after an initial bolus dose, to hold the neuromuscular blockade at about 90% in adult patients are shown in Table 3. We have often referred to the monitoring of NMT and so we do recommend the "routine" use of it as well as the monitoring of arterial pressure, electrocardiography, oximetry, and end tidal CO_2. Only from monitoring of NMT can we obtain useful information for the adequate use of MR with sufficient level of blockade for the different purposes

Table3. Rates of infusion for achieving a neuromuscular blockade of 90% in adults

MR	**Rate** (μg/kg per min, mean ± SD)
Atracurium	7.9 ± 0.4
Cisatracurium	1.5 ± 0.4
Mivacurium	8.3 ± 0.7
Rocuronium	9.5 ± 1.8
Vecuronium	1.2 ± 0.3

during surgery or for the ventilatory support in ICU. These include: titration of dosage for the necessary neuromuscular blockade; correct timing for performing the tracheal intubation; recognizing the possibility of a pharmacological antagonism of neuromuscular blockade; detection of recovery of NMJ function.

It is obvious that outside these indications you have to rely on clinical empirical principles which are not similarly recommended. The availability of recording equipment of small dimension and capable of measuring the muscle acceleration, determined on the muscle fibers supplied by the superficial stimulated nerve, is an easy, manageable and very useful method of monitoring NMT. This kind of equipment allows a useful performance of the nerve stimulation with the concurrent possibility of viewing the elicited responses. The same equipment also records the local temperature of muscle, which is important because hypothermia can affect the pharmacokinetic parameters of MR. The superficial nerves that can easily be stimulated are the ulnar, median, tibial, posterior tibial, lateral popliteus, and orbicularis; so in any positions or conditions we can monitor the NMT, even if not all muscles react to a given dose with the same intensity and in the same time. The abductor of the thumb, for instance, is more sensitive than the orbicularis [28]. It is only necessary that the skin is clean, dry, and greaseless and the limb is not affected by pathology. The main parameters of stimulation are: single twitch (ST), train-of-four (TOF), tetanic nerve stimulation (TNS), post-tetanic count (PTC), and double-burst stimulation (DBS). Even though each parameter of stimulation has a distinct validity as regards the given information, knowledge of the ST and even more of the TOF allows the management of muscle relaxation with absolute safety. The remaining parameters of monitoring are reserved for the detection of more-precise information gaining experience with monitoring of NMT. Further recommendations are related to constant frequency of stimulation during the same monitoring, stimulus generated as rectangular wave and not as another kind of wave, maintenance of a time interval at least of 10-12 s between a TOF and the next one in order to obtain reliable responses during monitoring, not absolutely trusting the ST during recovery because it can return to 100% in the presence of a residual neuromuscular block; therefore TOF is the most-reliable method of monitoring. The administration of MR without monitoring NMT is like "to shoot without taking aim"!

As a simple example of how monitoring of NMT could change the use of muscle relaxation, we remember that it has become easier and more reliable to use MR in some diseases. The use of monitoring of NMT during general anesthesia in patients with myasthenia has permitted a purposeful muscle relaxation for the necessary degree of neuromuscular blockade with a drastic reduction of postoperative stay in ICU.

The last recommendations regard the use of anticholinesterase. For correct use of anticholinesterase it must be borne in mind that several factors affect the recovery time of neuromuscular blockade. These include: neuromuscular blockade at the moment of antagonism; pharmacological features of ND; modality of administration of ND (continuous infusion allows more-rapid recovery times); dosage of anticholinesterase; pharmacological interferences; pathophysiological conditions (neuromuscular disease, hydroelectrolytic or acid-base imbalance).

The anticholinesterase, as is well known, induces inhibition, with reversible binding of acetylcholine, but can also interact with presynaptic receptors, increasing the acetyl release, and with the postjunctional receptors. The anticholinesterase can exert a "ceiling effect", so there is a dose-related response to a point and after that any further increase of dosage does not produce any effect. The concurrent events due to the anticholinesterase are various and when they occur, they worsen the quality of life in the postoperative period. They are bradycardia, bronchospasm, hypersecretion, increased intestinal peristalsis, nausea, vomiting, and interference with the NMJ. The most-commonly used cholinesterase inhibitor is neostigmine; it must be administered in a proper dose of 0.05 mg/kg (range 0.04-0.07 mg/kg) and the peak effect needs 5-7 min. Hence, after having given neostigmine in the proper dose you have to wait for the necessary latency without anxiety. What is the right moment for administering the anticholinesterase? Surely when monitoring evidences a certain response to the ST or when one (T1), two (T2) or, preferably, three (T3) responses to TOF stimulation can be felt; without monitoring it is advisable to administer the cholinesterase inhibitor only in the presence of clinical signs showing an initial spontaneous neuromuscular recovery. When can you consider that the neuromuscular recovery has definately occurred? When the TOF ratio (T4/T1) is major or equal to 0.75, a value that indicates the presence of inspiratory strength and valid vital capacity, with the ability of the patient to hold his head up for some seconds. Without monitoring several tests have been proposed, and among them the most-reliable test is to hold the head, for 5 s at least, raised at 90° over the thorax, with the patient in the supine position. This test shows the ability of the patient to obtain a patent airway and to swallow. Considering the side effects of anticholinesterase which need the constant association with a vagolytic, it is advisable to recommend avoiding as much as possible their use to achieve neuromuscular recovery, giving preference to those ND like cisatracurium and atracurium that do not have organ-based metabolism and assure constant neuromuscular recovery, because they have no active metabolites and therefore no residual blockade.

References

1. Frerk CM (1991) Predicting difficult intubation. Anaesthesia 46:1005-1010
2. Mallampati SR (1983) Clinical sign to predict difficult tracheal intubation (hypothesis). Can Anaesth Soc J 30:316-321
3. Samsoon GLT, Young JRB (1987) Difficult tracheal intubation: a retrospective study. Anaesthesia 42:487-492
4. Mathew M, Hanna LS, Andrete J (1989) Preoperative indices to anticipate a difficult tracheal intubation. Anaesth Analg 68:S187
5. Bencini AF, Scaf AHJ, Sohn YJ et al (1986) Hepatobiliary disposition of vecuronium bromide in man. Br J Anaesth 58:988-993
6. Bencini AF, Scaf AHJ, Sohn YJ et al (1986) Disposition and urinary excretion of vecuronium bromide in anesthetized patients with normal renal function or renal failure. Anesth Analg 65:245-251
7. Magorian T, Wood P, Caldwell JE et al (1991) Pharmacokinetics, onset, and duration of action of rocuronium in humans: normal vs. hepatic dysfunction. Anesthesiology 75:A1069
8. Wierda JMHK, Kleef UW, Lambalk LM et al (1991) The pharmacodynamics and pharmacokinetics of ORG 9426: a new nondepolarizing neuromuscular blocking agent in patients anaesthetized with nitrous oxide, halothane and fentanyl. Can J Anaesth 38:430-435
9. Marshall IG, Gibb AJ, Durant NN (1983) Neuromuscular and vagal blocking actions of pancuronium bromide, its metabolites, and vecuronium bromide (ORG NC45) and its potential metabolism in the anaesthetized cat. Br J Anaesth 55:703-714
10. Savarese JJ, Ali HH, Basta SJ et al (1988) The clinical neuromuscular pharmacology of mivacurium chloride (BW B1090U): a short-acting nondepolarizing ester neuromuscular blocking drug. Anesthesiology 68:723-732
11. Laxenaire MC (2000) Anaphylaxis and NMBAs. In: EuroSIVA Meeting on Intravenous Anaesthesia, Vienna, pp 49-51
12. Futo J, Kupferberg JP, Moss J (1990) Inhibition of histamine n-methyltransferase (HNMT) in vitro by neuromuscular relaxants. Biochem Pharmacol 39:415-420
13. Toh KW, Deacock SJ, Fawcett WJ (1999) Severe anaphylactic reaction to cisatracurium. Anesth Analg 88:462-464
14. Doenicke A, Soukup J, Hoernecke R et al (1997) The lack of histamine release with cisatracurium: a double-blind comparison with vecuronium. Anesth Analg 84:623-630
15. Basta SJ (1992) Modulation of histamine release by neuromuscular blocking drugs. Curr Opin Anaesth 5:572-578
16. Scott RPF, Savarese JJ, Ali HH et al (1985) Atracurium: clinical strategies for preventing histamine release and attenuating the hemodynamic response. Br J Anaesth 52:550-556
17. Durant NN, Briscoe JR, Katz RL (1984) The effect of acute and chronic hydrocortisone treatment on neuromuscular blockade in the anesthetized cat. Anesthesiology 61:144
18. Parr SM, Robinson BJ, Rees D et al (1991) Interaction between betamethasone and vecuronium. Br J Anaesth 67:447-451
19. Parr SM, Galletly DC, Robinson BJ (1991) Betamethasone-induced resistance to vecuronium: a potential problem in neurosurgery? Anesth Intensive Care 19:103-105
20. Schwartz AE, Matteo RS, Ornstein E et al (1986) Acute steroid therapy does not alter nondepolarizing muscle relaxant effects in humans. Anesthesiology 65:326-327
21. Hall Z, Merlie JB (1993) Synaptic structure and development: the neuromuscular junction. Cell 72:99-121
22. Martyn JAJ (1995) Basic and clinical pharmacology of the receptor: implication for the use of neuromuscular relaxants. Keio J Med 44:1-13
23. Martin JAJ, White DA, Gronert GA et al (1992) Up-and-down regulation of skeletal muscle acetylcholine receptors. Anesthesiology 76:822-841
24. Segredo V, Caldwell JE, Matthay MA et al (1992) Persistent paralysis in critically ill patients after long-term administration of vecuronium. N Engl J Med 327:524-528

25. Kupfer Y, Namba T, Kaldawi E et al (1992) Prolonged weakness after long-term infusion of vecuronium bromide. Ann Intern Med 117:484-486
26. Op de Coul AA, Verheul GA, Leyten AC et al (1991) Critical illness polyneuromyopathy after artificial respiration. Clin Neurol Neurosurg 93:27-31
27. Gooch JL, Suchyta MR, Balbierz JM et al (1991) Prolonged paralysis after treatment with neuromuscular junction blocking agents. Crit Care Med 19:1125-1128
28. Donati F, Meistelman C, Plaud B (1990) Vecuronium neuromuscular blockade at the diaphragm, the orbicularis oculi, and adductor pollicis muscles. Anesthesiology 73:870-875

Muscle Relaxants: Side Effects and Complications

V. VILARDI, M. SANFILIPPO, A. CIARLONE

Neuromuscular drugs are the cornerstones of general anesthesia [1]
The side effects of the neuromuscular blocking agents (NMBAs) have been studied by several authors [2-4]. Furthermore, their complications can be masked by other drugs used in general anesthesia. Recently, Berg et al. [5] observed an association between the action of pancuronium bromide and some postoperative complications. The association between the "postoperative residual curarization" (PORC) and the use of non-depolarizing muscle relaxants (MRs) has less importance than pharyngolaryngeal obstructive effects of analgesics and volatile agents. These drugs are responsible for PORC other than chemical and neurophysiological changes of respiratory drives. PORC is the result of muscle relaxants, halogenated agents, and morphine acting together. The side effects of MRs can be drastically reduced by the use of anticholinesterases drugs and neuromuscular monitoring, as suggested by Viby-Mogensen, Baillard et al., and Tramèr and Fuchs-Buder [6-9].

The chemical division of basic benzylisoquinolinic compounds and steroid agents and the correlation with histamine-releasing potency of the former [10] has recently been revised by introducing rapacuronium, which seems to have an high incidence of histamine release. In contrast, the chlorfumarate GW280430A, an asymmetrical mixed-onium compound, seems to have less histamine release and greater cardiovascular stability, because of the onium group on the molecule [11].

Rapacuronium results in vasodilation due to a direct relaxant effect on vascular smooth muscle, possibly mediated through the inhibition of voltage-gated L-type calcium channels [12]. Bronchospasm after rapacuronium, observed by Levy et al. [13], can be consequent to a "light" anesthesia or to a pre-existing respiratory disease.

Additional mechanisms for bronchospasm may also include antagonizing interaction at M_2 selective muscarinic receptors [14]. However, antagonizing M_3 selective muscarinic activity results in bronchial relaxation and decreases salivary secretions [14]. Rapacuronium seems to cause an increase in plasma histamine levels (> 5 ng/ml) at 2-3 mg/kg [13]. Rapacuronium is also associated with an increase in heart rate (17%) and cardiac index (15%), and with a decrease in mean arterial pressure (11%) and systemic vascular resistance (18%) [15]. Rapacuronium's low potency may explain its rapid onset, because more molecules are required to achieve the desired effect [16]. This results in a large gradient into the site of action [16]. Other potential causes for its rapid onset include high lipophilicity that promotes diffusion to the neuromuscular junction [17], or its effects on Ca^{2+} channels to increase muscle blood flow or to decrease contractility [18].

A vagolytic effect of rapacuronium could explain the increase in heart rate noted by Sparr et al. [19]. According to studies on animals, there is no evidence that rapacuronium, like pancuronium, inhibits uptake of norepinephrine [20]. Tachycardia, erythema, and bronchospasm have also been reported [19, 21, 22]. The incidence of bronchospasm seems to be high, reaching 10.7% [23]. The heart rate is significantly increased after a dose of 2.5 mg/kg rapacuronium in humans [24].

It appears that this aminosteroid may liberate histamine or leukotrienes. It would be a retrograde step to introduce an aminosteroid neuromuscular blocking drug with significant histamine release properties [25, 26] in spite of the opinions of Levy et al. [13].

Side effects

Histamine release

The anaphylactoid reactions occurring during anesthesia are of immune origin, due to specific Ig E antibodies. MRs remain the most-common cause of anaphylaxis [27]. Laxenaire et al. [27] considered MRs responsible for 61.6% of the 692 cases of anaphylaxis. In this study, the MRs implicated in anaphylaxis included vecuronium (n = 130), atracurium (n = 107), suxamethonium (n = 106), pancuronium (n = 41), rocuronium (n = 41), mivacurium (n = 18), and gallamine (n = 9). In the 70% of the patients who were allergic to one MR, cross sensitivity was found with the other relaxants [27].

Fisher and Baldo [28] reported 477 episodes of clinical anaphylaxis during anesthesia, of which 283 were due to MRs. Their data have been confirmed from France, United States, New Zealand, and United Kingdom [29-38].

The use of pancuronium appears to be safe as well as vecuronium [39, 40], whereas concerns about vecuronium have been raised [31]. Atracurium also seems to have an incidence of reactions disproportionate to its market share [40].

Three clinical mechanisms of histamine release of have been described [10].

1. Antigen mediated. The MR combines with specific IgE molecules which are fixed to the surface of mast cells, stimulating the release of vasoactive endogenous substances (the complement cascade is not involved).

2. Non-immunological mechanism. The MR combines with IgG or IgM antibodies activating the complement cascade.
3. Direct chemical action of the drug on the mast cells which does not involve any interaction with antibodies. The latter mechanism occurs most frequently following the use of non-depolarizing MRs [10]. Suxamethonium has long been suggested to produce the highest incidence of histamine release of the chemical type, due in part to the common use in the clinical practice [41]. This direct chemical effect does not require prior sensitization.

The clinical features of anaphylaxis can be responsible for cardiovascular collapse, bronchospasm, rash, urticaria, erythema, angioedema, pulmonary edema, and gastrointestinal symptoms [28]. H_1 and H_2 receptors are activated by histamine [42]. The increased heart rate and cardiac index were thought to be due to increased baroreceptor activity and increased sympathetic stimulation as adrenaline and noradrenaline concentrations were also increased [42]. The bronchodilator effect may be mediated through a subtype of the H_2 receptor [43], the so called H_3 receptor [44]. This modulates cholinergic neurotransmission at parasympathetic ganglia and post-ganglionic neurones in human bronchi [45, 46]. In addition, histamine may stimulate irritant (H_1) receptors within the lungs at concentrations that otherwise would not directly cause bronchospasm [47].

The action on H_2 receptors is increased by prostaglandins and leukotrienes. Coronary vasoconstriction is observed with a high concentration of platelet-activating factor [42]. Different methods of MR administration do not offer a great advantage in avoiding histamine release.

Cardiovascular effects (Table 1)

Cardiovascular effects are commonly mediated by histamine release and its plasma concentration (Fig. 1). Sometimes, tachycardia and hypotension are not associated with histamine release. The blocking effects on cholinergic muscarinic receptors M_1, M_2, M_3, M_4 (on ganglia, peripheral nervous terminals, and smooth muscle) can interfere with the heart rate [48]. The ratio ED_{50} (muscular action/vagolytic action) is 34 and 63 for pancuronium and vecuronium, respectively [48]. This may explain the parasympatholytic effect of pancuronium and bradycardia induced by vecuronium [48]. The prior administration of low doses of analgesics can amplify the vecuronium effect on autonomic ganglia [48, 49].

The vagolytic effect of pancuronium can be accompanied by a sympathicomimetic or antimuscarinic presynaptic effect and subsequent norepinephrine release [48]. Pipecuronium, vecuronium and rocuronium develop a reduced potency in blocking cardiac M_2 muscarinic receptors in comparison with pancuronium [50, 51]. The cardiovascular stability of pipecuronium seems to be controversial [52, 53].

Tachycardia observed in children after a dose of 3 times ED_{95} rocuronium [54] is probably due to a parasympathilytic effect. The cardiovascular side ef-

Table 1. Comparative cardiovascular effects of non-depolarizing relaxants[a, b]

Effects	Pan	Vec	Atr	Miv	Dox	Pip	Roc
Ganglionic block	1	1	1	1	1	1	1
Vagal block	2	1	1	1	1	1	1-2
Increased catechol effect	2	1	1	1	1	1	1
Histamine release	1	1	2	2	1-2	1	1

Pan pancuronium, *Vec* vecuronium, *Atr* atracurium, *Miv* mivacurium, *Dox* doxacurium, *Pip* pipecuronium, *Roc* rocuronium.
[a] 1 = none or minimal, 2 = slight to moderate, 3 = marked
[b] Modified from Silverman [3]

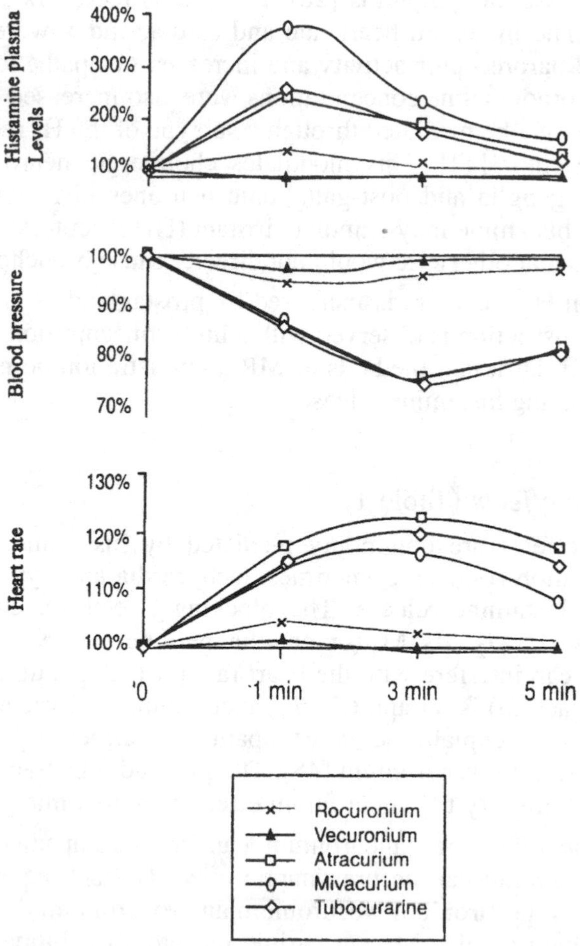

Fig. 1. Plasma histamine levels and cardiovascular parameters before and after i.v. administration of 0.6 mg/kg rocuronium, 0.1 mg/kg vecuronium, 0.6 mg/kg atracurium. 0.2 mg/kg mivacurium, and 0.5 mg/kg tubocurarine. $p < 0.01$ vs. control values; $p < 0.05$ vs. rocuronium and vecuronium; $p < 0.05$ vs. mivacurium. The control values have been considered as 100%. Adapted from Naguib et al. [25]

fects of benzylisoquinolinic compounds are due to histamine release [25]. The main effect is observed 1-2 min after administration [25].

Central nervous system effects

Direct effects of MRs on the central nervous system have not been shown yet [55]. The high degree of ionization and low lipophilicity of MRs do not allow passage of the blood-brain barrer (BBB) [56]. The intrathecal injection of MRs in rats can be responsible for convulsion and excitement [57]. The increased permeability of BBB to MRs in critically ill patients occurs have been [55]. Hyperexcitability and convulsions leading to death have been shown in animals receiving an infusion of atracurium, pancuronium, or vecuronium, probably because of an increase of intracellular calcium level [57]. The BBB osmotic disruption in pigs has increased significantly the pancuronium concentrations in the cerebral spinal fluid [58].

Respiratory effects

Histamine, leukotrienes, and prostaglandins may enhance the respiratory side effects of MRs [42]. Interactions of MRs with M_3 muscarinic receptors on airway has been studied in anesthetized dogs [59] and guinea pigs [60]. In the lung, blockade of pre-junctional M_2 muscarinic receptors potentiates vagally induced bronchoconstriction [59, 61]. Conversely, blockade of M_3 muscarinic receptors on airway smooth muscle inhibits vagally induced bronchoconstriction [62].

Gallamine, atracurium, and low concentrations of pancuronium are M_2 receptors blockers [59, 61]. Higher concentrations of pancuronium block M_3 receptors [61], while vecuronium does not appear to have either M_2 or M_3 blocking properties [59].

Mivacurium chloride is a more-potent antagonist at M_3 than M_2 receptors, and should not potentiate irritant-induced bronchoconstriction in the clinical range [60]. Pipecuronium is an M_2 receptor antagonist and can potentiate reflex-induced bronchoconstriction only at larger doses [60].

During lung injury, pancuronium increases pulmonary arterial pressure, especially when there is hypoxemia [63]. On the isolated human bronchial rings, pipecuronium has shown an inhibiting effect on pilocarpine-stimulated prejunctional M_2 muscarinic receptors [64]. Rocuronium has neither pre- nor postjunctional inhibitory effects on muscarinic receptors [64]. Because the distribution and the relative abundance of receptors may vary between species [65, 66], the results of animal studies cannot be extrapolated to human airways [64].

The different effects of MRs on bronchial smooth muscle have to be carefully considered in case of tracheal intubation during "light" anesthesia [13]. Bronchospasm caused by "light" anesthesia may be enhanced by muscarinic bronchial effects of MRs.

The lung first pass uptake of MRs does not contribute to a difference in potency and/or onset time of d-tubocurarine, rocuronium, vecuronium, rapacuronium, and Org 7616 [67]. The vecuronium-induced partial neuromuscular block attenuated the ventilatory response to hypoxemia without influencing the response to hypercapnia [68].

The technique of priming of MRs to reduce their onset time must be avoided. Several cases of pulmonary aspiration of gastric content with this technique have been reported [69, 70].

Intraocular pressure

MRs do not influence intraocular pressure. The choroidal blood flow may be locally influenced by the re-uptake of noradrenaline. Pancuronium inhibits noradrenaline re-uptake, increasing its release. Vecuronium does not interact with the extraneuronal re-uptake of noradrenaline. MRs can be safely used even in penetrating ophthalmological injuries [71, 74].

Miscellaneous

Rapacuronium and rocuronium produce an injection site reaction, with an incidence of topical reaction of 2.5% after rapacuronium and severe burning pain after rocuronium [75-78] with spontaneous movements [79]. The low pH of 4 does not explain local pain, because other chininogen-type substances might be involved.

A very high incidence of erythema at the injection site has been observed after mivacurium (80%) in fast-running infusion [80-82]. Other authors did not report any topical reaction [83, 85]. Erythema is probably due to histamine release. A decrease of postoperative nausea and vomiting after benzylisoquinolinic compounds has been recently observed. These drugs might have an antagonist effect, as ondansetron, on $5HT_{3a}$ receptors [86].

Complications

Post operative residual curarization

The use of vecuronium and atracurium has drastically reduced the incidence of PORC [87], although this complication may still occur. Residual effects of NMBAs and volatile anesthetics interfere with ventilatory control by different mechanisms [88]. Subparalyzing doses of NMBAs can depress the hypoxic ventilatory control due to an interaction with the carotid body chemoreceptors [88].

Inhaled anesthetics cause a dose-dependant reduction of resting ventilation and minute ventilation during hypercarbia and hypoxia, due to a general depression of central neuronal control, including the respiratory neurons of the brainstem [88]. The hypoxic chemosensitivity of the carotid body chemoreceptors is minimally affected by inhaled anesthetics [88]. Residual neuromuscular block causes impaired regulation of ventilation during hypoxia and impaired pharyngeal function and airway protection, and is a risk factor for the development of postoperative pulmonary complications [88]. To assure normal vital muscle function and normal ventilatory regulation, an adductor pollicis (train-of-four) (TOF) ratio of 0.90 should ideally be achieved [88]. Inhaled halogenated anesthetics depress ventilation at anesthetic and subanesthetic levels. The carotid body chemoreceptor function is, however, well maintained at subanesthetic end-tidal concentrations of volatile inhaled anesthetics [88].

Residual curarization is present more frequently than supposed [6]. Clinically significant residual block after routine use of vecuronium, without the use of a nerve stimulator and without reversal, was found in a great number of patients [6, 7]. Good evidence-based practice dictates that much more attention should be paid by anesthetists to the problem of residual curarization. First, long-acting NMBAs should not be used [5, 89]. Second, the block should be antagonized at the end of the procedure, but reversal should not be initiated before two and preferably three or four responses to TOF stimulation are present [6]. Third, the normal vital muscle function, including normal pharyngeal function, requires the TOF ratio at adductor pollicis to recover ≥ 0.90 [6].

Postoperative pulmonary complication (POPC)

This complication is represented by pneumonia and or atelectasia confirmed by X-rays, with fever, cough, and stethoscopic rales [5]. A significant risk for development of postoperative pulmonary complications has been observed after pancuronium in elderly patients undergoing abdominal surgery [5]. Short- or intermediate-acting MRs have drastically reduced this risk [5].

Minor complications

In volunteers receiving subparalyzing doses of mivacurium, diplopia and lack of tongue control have been reported [90].

Myopathies

These complications have been observed more frequently in critically ill patients. Corticosteroids and MRs appear to trigger some types of myopathies [91]. These drugs should be avoided or administered at the lowest doses possible to critically ill patients. Sepsis, denervation, and muscle membrane inexitability may be additional factors [91].

Acute myopathy has been described after MRs in cases of near-fatal asthma [92], and its incidence increased with each additional day of muscle relaxation [92]. A downregulation of the acetylcholine receptors at the neuromuscular junction can account for some of the muscle weakness of the myopathies observed in intensive care patients [93].

References

1. Raeder JC (2000) Anaesthesiology into the new millennium. Acta Anaesthesiol Scand 44:3-8
2. Agoston S, Bowman WC (eds) (1990) Muscle relaxants. Elsevier Science Publishers BV (Biomedical Division), Amsterdam
3. Silvermann DG (1994) Neuromuscular block in perioperative and intensive care. Lippincott, Philadelphia
4. Harper NJN, Polland BJ (1995) Muscle relaxants in anaesthesia. Arnold, London
5. Berg H, Viby-Mogensen J, Roed J et al (1997) Residual neuromuscular block is a risk factor for postoperative pulmonary complications. A prospective, randomised, and blinded study of postoperative pulmonary complications after atracurium, vecuronium and pancuronium. Acta Anaesthesiol Scand 41:1095-1103
6. Viby-Mogensen J (2000) Postoperative residual curarization and evidence-based anaesthesia. Br J Anaesth 84:301-303
7. Baillard C, Gehan G, Reboul-Marty J et al (2000) Residual curarization in the recovery room after vecuronium. Br J Anaesth 84:394-395
8. Tramèr MR, Fuchs-Buder T (1999) Omitting antagonism of neuromuscular block: effect on postoperative nausea and vomiting and risk of residual paralysis. A systematic review. Br J Anaesth 82:379-386
9. Viby-Mogensen J (1999) Why, how and when to monitor neuromuscular function. Minerva Anestesiol 65:239-244
10. Hunter JM (1993) Histamine release and neuromuscular blocking drugs. Anaesthesia 48: 561-563
11. Boros EE, Mook RA, Boswell GE et al (1999) Structure-activity relationship of the asymmetrical mixed-onium chlorofumarate neuromuscular blocker GW280430A and some congeners in rhesus monkeys. Anesthesiology 91:A1022
12. Yamaguchi K, Huraux C, Szlam F, Levy JH (1998) Vascular effects of ORG 9487 in human mammary arteries, a new short acting muscle relaxant (abstract). Anaesth Analg 86:SCA109
13. Levy JH, Pitts M, Thanopoulos A et al (1999) The effects of rapacuronium on histamine release and hemodynamics in adult patients undergoing general anesthesia. Anesth Analg 89:290-295
14. Hou VY, Hirshmann CA, Emala CW (1998) Neuromuscular relaxants as antagonists for M_2 and M_3 muscarinic receptors. Anesthesiology 88:744-750
15. McCourt KC, Elliot P, Mirakhur RK et al (1999) Haemodynamic effect of rapacuronium in adults with coronary artery or valvular disease. Br J Anaesth 83:721-726
16. Wierda JMKH, Beaufort AM, Kleef UW et al (1994) Preliminary investigations of the clinical pharmacology of three short-acting non-depolarizing neuromuscular blocking agents, ORG 9453, ORG 9489, and ORG 9487. Can J Anaesth 41:213-220
17. Wierda JMKH, Proost JH, Muir A, Marshall RJ (1993) Design of drugs for rapid onset. Anaesth Pharmacol Rev 1:57-63

18. Tian L, Mehta MP, Prior C, Marshall IG (1992) Relative pre- and post-junctional effects of a new vecuronium analogue, ORG 9426, at the rat neuromuscular junction. Br J Anaesth 69: 284-287
19. Sparr HJ, Mellinghoff H, Blobner M, Nöldge-Schomburg G (1999) Comparison of intubating conditions after rapacuronium (ORG 9487) and succinylcholine following rapid sequence induction in adult patients. Br J Anaesth 82:537-541
20. Muir AW, Sleigh T, Marshall RJ et al (1998) Neuromuscular blocking and cardiovascular effects of ORG 9487, a new short-acting aminosteroidal blocking agent, in anaesthetized animals and in isolated muscle preparations. Eur J Anaesthesiol 15:467-479
21. Onrust SV, Foster RH (1999) Rapacuronium bromide. A review of its use in anaesthetic practice. Drugs 58:887-918
22. Kahwaji R, Bevan DR, Bikhazi G et al (1997) Dose-ranging study in younger adult and elderly patients of ORG 9487, a new rapid-onset, short-duration muscle relaxant. Anaesth Analg 84:1011-1018
23. Donati F (2000) Neuromuscular blocking drugs for the new millennium: current practice, future trends – comparative pharmacology of neuromuscular blocking drugs. Anaesth Analg 90:S2-6
24. Miguel R, Witkowski T, Nagashima H et al (1999) Evaluation of neuromuscular and cardiovascular effects of two doses of rapacuronium (ORG 9487) versus mivacurium and succinylcholine. Anesthesiology 91:1648-1654
25. Naguib M, Samarkandi AH, Bakhamees HS et al (1995) Histamine-release haemodynamic changes produced by rocuronium, vecuronium, mivacurium, atracurium and tubocurarine. Br J Anaesth 75:588-592
26. Goulden MR, Hunter JM (1999) Rapacuronium (ORG 9487): do we have a replacement for succinylcholine? Br J Anesth 82:489-492
27. Laxenaire MC et le Groupe d'études des réactions anaphylactoïdes peranesthésiques (1999) Épidémiologie des réactions anaphylactoïdes peranestésiques. Quatrième enquête multicentrique (juillet 1994-décembre 1996). Ann Fr Anesth Reanim 18:796-809
28. Fisher M, Baldo BA (1994) Anaphylaxis during anaesthesia: current aspects of diagnosis and prevention. Eur J Anaesth 11:263-284
29. Moneret-Vautrin DA, Laxenaire MC, Hummer-Siegel M et al (1990) Myorelaxants. In: Laxenaire MC, Moneret-Vautrin DA (eds) Le risque allergique en anesthesia – reanimation. Masson, Paris, pp 52-58
30. Galletly DC, Treuren BC (1985) Anaphylactoid reaction during anaesthesia. Seven years experience of intradermal testing. Anaesthesia 40:329-333
31. Laxenaire MC, Moneret-Vautrin DA, Widmer S et al (1990) Sugstances anesthetiques responsables de chocs anaphylactiques. Enquete multicentrique francaise. Anaesthetic drugs responsible for anaphylactic shock. French multi-center study. Ann Fr Anesth Reanim 9:501-506
32. Leynadier F, Sansarriq M, Didier JM, Dry J (1987) Prick tests in the diagnosis of anaphylaxis to general anaesthetics. Br J Anaesth 59:683-689
33. Moscicki RA, Sockin SM, Corsello BF et al (1990) Anaphylaxis during induction of general anaesthesia: subsequent evaluation and management. J Allergy Clin Immunol 86:325-332
34. Thacker MA, Gibbs JM (1984) A hypersensitivity screening clinic following untoward reactions to anaesthesia. N Z Med J 97:232-234
35. Sage D (1981) Intradermal drug testing following anaphylactoid reactions during anaesthesia. Anaesth Intensive Care 9:381-386
36. Assem ESK (1990) Anaphylactic anesthetic reactions. Anaesthesia 45:1032-1038
37. Facon A, Grzybowski M, Divry M et al (1988) L'allergie aux agents anesthésiques: Analyse de 96 observations récentes. Cah Anesthesiol 36:97-100
38. Vervloet D, Nizankowska E, Arnaud A et al (1983) Adverse reactions to suxamethonium and other muscle relaxants under general anaesthesia. J Allergy Clin Immunol 71:552-559
39. Watkins J (1988) Anaesthetic reactions. In: Watkins J, Levy CJ (eds) Guide to immediate anaesthetic reactions. Butterworths, London, pp 13-31

40. Fisher MM (1991) Anaphylaxis to anaesthetic drugs: aetiology, recognition and management. Curr Anaesth Crit Care 2:182-186
41. Watkins J (1985) Adverse anaesthetic reactions. Anaesthesia 40:797-800
42. McKinnon RP, Wildsmith JAW (1995) Histaminoid reactions in anaesthesia. Br J Anaesth 74:217-228
43. Fleish JH, Calkins PJ (1976) Comparison of drug induced responses of rabbit trachea and bronchus. J Appl Physiol 41:66
44. Arrang JM, Garbarg M, Lancelot JC et al (1987) Highly potent and selective ligands for histamine H_3 reeceptors. Nature 327:117-123
45. Ichinose M, Barnes PJ (1989) Inhibitory histamine H_3 receptors on cholinergic nerves in human airways. Eur J Pharmacol 163:383-386
46. Ichinose M, Stretton CD, Schwartz JC, Barnes PJ (1989) Histamine H_3 receptors inhibit cholinergic bronchoconstriction in guinea pig airways. Br J Pharmacol 97:13-15
47. Gold WM (1977) Neurohumoral interactions in airways. Am Rev Respir Dis 115:127-137
48. Vilardi V, Nocente M, Sanfilippo M, Cavalletti MV (1995) Il miorilassante ideale tra sogno e bisogno. Acta Anaesth Ital 46:215-231
49. Morton CPJ, Drummond GB (1992) Bradycardia and vecuronium: comparison with alcuronium during cholecystectomy. Br J Anaesth 68:619-620
50. Appadu BL, Lambert DG (1994) Studies on the interaction of steroidal neuromuscular blocking drugs with cardiac muscarinic receptors. Br J Anaesth 72:86-88
51. Durant NN, Marshall IG, Savage DS et al (1979) The neuromuscular and autonomic blocking activities of pancuronium, ORG NC 45, and other pancuronium analogues, in the cat. J Pharm Pharmacol 31:831-836
52. Thompson IR (1994) Are 'clean' muscle relaxants better? Can J Anaesth 41:459-464
53. Stanley JC, Carson JW, Gibson FM et al (1991) Comparison of the haemodynamic effects of pipecuronium and pancuronium during fentanyl anaesthesia. Acta Anaesthesiol Scand 35: 262-266
54. Fuchs Buder T, Tassonyi E (1996) Intubating conditions and time course of rocuronium induced neuromuscular block in children. Br J Anaesth 77:335-338
55. Vilardi V, Conti G, Sanfilippo M et al (1996) I miorilassanti in terapia intensiva. E.M.C. Anestesia-Rianimazione, Roma, p 11
56. Naguib M, Magboul MMA (1998) Adverse effects of neuromuscular blockers and their antagonists. Middle East J Anesthesiol 14:341-373
57. Szenohradszky J, Trevor A, Bickler P et al (1993) Central nervous system effects of intrathecal muscle relaxants in rats. Anaesth Analg 76:1304-1309
58. Werba A, Gilly H, Weindlmayr-Goettel M et al (1992) Porcine model for studying the passage of non depolarizing neuromuscular blockers through the blood-brain barrier. Br J Anaesth 69:382-386
59. Vettermann J, Beck KC, Lindahl SGE et al (1988) Actions of enflurane, isoflurane, vecuronium, atracurium, and pancuronium on pulmonary resistence in dogs. Anesthesiology 69:88-95
60. Okanlami OA, Fryer AD, Hirshman C (1996) Interaction of nondepolarizing muscle relaxants with M_2 and M_3 muscarinic receptors in guinea pig lung and heart. Anesthesiology 84: 155-161
61. Fryer AD, Maclagan J (1987) Pancuronium and gallamine are antagonists for pre- and postjunctional muscarinic receptors in the guinea pig lung. Naunyn Schmiedebergs Arch Pharmacol 335:367-371
62. Roffel AF, Meurs H, Elzinger CRS, Zaagsma J (1990) Characterization of the muscarinic receptor subtype involved in phosphoinositide metabolism in bovine tracheal smooth muscle. Br J Pharmacol 99:293-296
63. Du H, Orii R, Yamada Y et al (1996) Pancuronium increases pulmonary arterial pressure in lung injury. Br J Anaesth 77:526-529
64. Zappi L, Song P, Nicosia S et al (1999) Do pipecuronium and rocuronium affect human bronchial smooth muscle? Anesthesiology 91:1616-1621

65. Zappi L, Song P, Nicosia S et al (1997) Inhibition of airway constriction by opioids is different down the isolated bovine airway. Anesthesiology 86:1334-1341
66. TenBerge REJ, Zaagsma J, Roffel AF (1996) Muscarinic inhibitory autoreceptors in different generations of human airways. Am J Respir Crit Care Med 154:43-49
67. Beaufort TM, Proost JH, Houwertjes MC et al (1999) The pulmonary first-pass uptake of five nondepolarizing muscle relaxants in the pig. Anesthesiology 90:477-483
68. Eriksson LI, Lenmarken C, Johnson A (1992) Attenuated ventilatory response to hypoxaemia at vecuronium-induced partial neuromuscular block. Acta Anaesthesiol Scand 36:710-715
69. Shorten GD, Brande BM (1997) Pulmonary aspiration of gastric contents after a priming dose of vecuronium. Paediatr Anaesth 7:167-169
70. Musichs J, Walts LF (1986) Pulmonary aspiration after a priming dose of vecuronium. Anesthesiology 64:517-519
71. Vilardi V, Sanfilippo M, Pelaia P, Gasparetto A (1983) The effects of vecuronium on intraocular pressure during general anesthesia. In: Clinical experiences with norcuron. Symposium, Geneva, 21-22 April 1983. Excepta Medica, Amsterdam, pp 163-166
72. Esente S, Passani F, Vaccari LG et al (1984) Anaesthesia and ocular hypotension. A multicentric investigation. Reprint from cataract surgery and visual rehabilitation. Proceedings of the Third International Congress on Cataract Surgery and Visual Rehabilitation, Florence (Italy), 9-12 May 1984. Kugler, Amsterdam, pp 11-14
73. Sanfilippo M, Vilardi V, Martini O, Gasparetto A (1985) Impiego del besilato di atracurio nell'anestesia generale per oftalmochirurgia. Acta Anaesth Ital 36:29-33
74. Sanfilippo M, Vilardi V, Moreno E et al (1985) Il bromuro di pipecuronium in anestesia generale per oftalmochirurgia: effetti sul tono endoculare. Acta Anaesth Ital 36:45-50
75. Organon (1999) Raplon™ (rapacuronium bromide) prescribing information. West Orange, New Jersey, USA
76. Morthy SS, Dierdorf SF (1995) Pain on injection of rocuronium bromide. Anaesth Analg 80:1067
77. Lockey D, Coleman P (1995) Pain during injection of rocuronium bromide. Anaesthesia 50:474
78. Steegers MAH, Robertson EN (1996) Pain on injection of rocuronium bromide. Anaesth Analg 83:203
79. Borgeat A, Kwiatkowsky D (1997) Spontaneous movements associated with rocuronium: Is pain on injection the cause? Br J Anaesth 79:382-383
80. Phillips BJ, Hunter JM (1992) Use of mivacurium chloride by constant infusion in the anephric patient. Br J Anaesth 68:492-498
81. Cheng M, Lee C, Yang E, Cantley E (1988) Comparison of fast and slow bolus injections of mivacurium chloride under narcotic-nitrous oxide anesthesia (abstract). Anesthesiology 69:A877
82. Savarese JJ, Ali HH, Basta SJ et al (1989) The cardiovascular effects of mivacurium chloride (BW B1090U) in patients receiving nitrous oxide-opiate-barbiturate anesthesia. Anesthesiology 70:386-394
83. Goldberg ME, Larijani GE, Azad SS et al (1989) Comparison of tracheal intubating conditions and neuromuscular blocking profiles after intubating doses of mivacurium-chloride or succinylcholine in surgical outpatients. Anaesth Analg 69:93-99
84. Weber S, Brandom BW, Powers DM et al (1988) Mivacurium chloride (BW B1090U) - induced neuromuscular blockade during nitrous oxide-isoflurane and nitrous oxide-narcotic anesthesia in adult surgical patients. Anaesth Analg 67:495-499
85. Wrigley SR, Jones RM, Harrop-Griffiths AW, Platt MW (1992) Mivacurium chloride: a study to evaluate its use during propofol-nitrous oxide anaesthesia. Anaesthesia 47:653-657
86. Kyeong TM, Wu CL, Yang J (2000) Nondepolarizing neuromuscular blockers inhibit the serotonin-type 3A receptor expressed in Xenopus oocytes. Anesth Analg 90:476-481
87. Vilardi V, Sanfilippo M, Nocente M et al (1994) Muscle relaxants and postoperatory period. In: Gasparetto A, Pinto G, Mattia C et al (eds) Il post operatorio immediato. Aspetti anestesiologici e rianimativi. Univ. St. La Sapienza Roma, pp 21-34

88. Eriksson LI (1999) The effects of residual neuromuscular blockade and volatile anesthetics on the control of ventilation. Anaesth Analg 89:243-251
89. Bevan DR, Smith CE, Donati F (1988) Postoperative neuromucular blockade: a comparison between atracurium, vecuronium, and pancuronium. Anesthesiology 69:272-276
90. Kopman AF, Ng J, Zank LM et al (1996) Residual postoperative paralysis. Pancuronium versus mivacurium, does it matter? Anesthesiology 85:1253-1259
91. Hund E (1999) Myopathy in critically ill patients. Crit Care Med 27:2544-2547
92. Awadh Behbehami N, Al-Mane F, D'yachkova Y et al (1999) Myopathy following mechanical ventilation for acute severe asthma. The role of muscle relaxants and corticosteroids. Chest 115:1627-1631
93. Martyn JAJ, Vincent A (1999) A new twist to myopathy of critical illness. Anesthesiology 91:337-339

Opioid Pharmacology

C. HARRISON, D.G. LAMBERT

Opium (from the Greek word for juice - opion) comes from the seeds of the poppy *Papaver somniferum*. Evidence of early civilisations cultivating poppy seeds can be found from around 4000 BC and by 2000 BC knowledge of opium was widespread throughout Europe, the Middle East and North Africa, where it was considered a cure for all ailments. Opium was considered important in Greco-Roman pharmacy, and was used to alleviate pain as well as insomnia, coughs, bowel problems and a variety of other conditions. In Europe the use of opium declined with the collapse of the Roman Empire, but re-appeared with the return of the crusaders in the 12th and 13th centuries. By the sixteenth century opium had an established role as a medicine in Europe, and became increasingly popular in the 18th century.

There existed two arguements in the 18th century as to the mode of action of opium. The first of these was the idea that opium caused the blood to become rarefied or thinned, an action due to absorption and circulation of the drug. The second argument was that it was acting on nerves to where it was applied and was distributed by 'consent' and this explained the fast mode of action of the drug.

In 1806 Friedrich Sertürner isolated a major active constituent of opium and named it morphine after Morpheus, the Greek god of dreams. By the early 1820s morphine was commercially available in Western Europe in standard measures of strength, and was widely used in the 19th century to combat pain, often given as an injection. The identification of stereo-specific binding sites for opioids was made in 1973 [1-3] and so began the field of opioid receptor pharmacology.

Endogenous opioids and their receptors

From the demonstration of stereo specific opioid binding sites, it was postulated that receptors did not exist only for application of exogenous substances, but there were endogenous substances that produced 'morphine - like' effects. Indeed a substance was isolated from mammalian brain that produced contractions of mouse vas deferens and guinea pig myenteric plexus [4]. This work led to the identification of two related opioid peptides, termed met- and leu-enkephalins, which were isolated from porcine pituitary [5]. Soon afterwards it was noted that the C fragment of lipotropin (a fat-mobilizing hormone) displayed opioid activity [6], and was later termed β-endorphin. A third endogenous opioid peptide, termed dynorphin was isolated from porcine pituitary in 1979 [7].

Due to the presence of multiple endogenous ligands it was suggested that there might be multiple opioid receptor subtypes. Evidence for this came from the work of Martin et al., who in 1976, suggested μ- (from morphine) and κ- (from ketocyclazocine) opioid receptors using cross-tolerance studies in dogs [8]. A σ receptor (from SKF10-047) was also identified, but this was later found to be non-opioid [9]. The identification of the δ- (from vas deferens) opioid receptor was reported in 1977, following the identification of the enkephalins [10].

Some 22 years after the isolation of the first endogenous opioid ligand, two peptides were discovered that displayed high affinity and selectivity for the μ-opioid receptor [11]. This group of opioid peptides was synthesised by amino acid substitution of the peptide Tyr-Pro-Trp-Gly-NH_2, a peptide with opioid related activity, to yield two peptides termed endomorphin-1 and endomorphin-2.

In the original paper describing endomorphins [11], endomorphin-1 displayed high affinity (K_i = 0.36 nM) and selectivity for μ-opioid receptor (4000 and 15000 fold preference over δ and κ receptors respectively). This was mirrored by endomorphin-2, with a K_i = 0.69 nM and a 13000 fold and 15000 selectivity over δ and κ receptors respectively. Both peptides were more potent than DAMGO in vitro and produced analgesia in mice. Endomorphin-1 and -2 were originally isolated from bovine brain, and have subsequently been found to occur in human brain at higher levels than that found in bovine brain [12]. It has been proposed that the endomorphins could in fact be endogenous ligands at the μ-opioid receptor.

Although it has been demonstrated that endomorphins produce in vivo effects consistent with opioids, such as analgesia and hypotension/bradycardia [11, 13-16], a basic understanding of the cellular effects of endomorphin is critical to the further understanding of the physiological role of these peptides. The receptor selectivity for endogenous opioid peptides is shown in Table 1.

In addition, other opioid peptides cleaved from endogenous precursors exist; these include morphiceptin and haemorphin-4 cleaved from casein and haemoglobin respectively [17] and others shown in Table 1. Opioid peptides have also been isolated from amphibian skin – dermorphin and deltorphin – which are selective for μ and δ-opioid receptors [18]. As well as the three main types of opioid receptor, others have been proposed [18]. In addition, a receptor specific for the active metabolite of morphine, morphine-6-glucoronide (M6G), has also been proposed [19, 20].

Table 1. Endogenous opioid peptides, their precursors and receptor selectivity

Peptide	Precursor	Receptor selectivity	Other active products (opioid)
Dynorphin	Pro-opiomelanocortin	κ	Dynorphin B Dynorphin A (1-8) α/β neoendorphin
Enkephalin	Pro-enkephalin	δ	Metorphamide
β-endorphin	Pro-endorphin (from β-lipotropin)	μ and δ	–
Endomorphin-1/2	?	μ	–

Alternative nomenclature

The International Union of Pharmacology subcommittee on opioid receptors has proposed an alternative classification of opioid receptors, these being OP_1 (δ), OP_2 (κ) and OP_3 (μ) [21], based on the order in which they were cloned and where OP = opioid peptide. However, this nomenclature has not been widely adopted by the scientific community, and throughout the remainder of this article we will use the traditional μ-, δ-, and κ-terminology.

Cloned opioid receptors

The first opioid receptor to be cloned and sequenced (and hence formally identified) was the δ subtype, cloned simultaneously by two independent groups [22, 23]. Soon after, both the κ- [24] and μ- [25] opioid receptors were formally identified. Following this it was shown definitively that opioid receptors belonged to the G protein receptor family, which contains many members, sharing common structural features [26]. All consist of seven transmembrane spanning domains, rich in hydrophobic amino acids, an extracellular N terminus with multiple glycosylation sites, an intracellular C terminus in which there are potential phosphorylation sites (serine and threonine residues), and cysteine residues which form a disulphide bridge between the first and second extracellular loop of the receptor [27].

Each of μ-, δ-, and κ-opioid receptors has approximately 60% homology with each other, the greatest homology being in the transmembrane regions (73-76%) and the intracellular loops (86-100%). The greatest diversity is at the N and C termini and the extracellular loops [27]. Each sub-type of opioid receptor is able to differentially bind opioid ligands and all three subtypes are able to mediate analgesia, and share common second messenger systems.

Opioid receptor subtypes and ligands

Numerous subtype selective agonists and antagonists have been developed for each of the opioid receptor subtypes; some are in use clinically and others are used for research purposes. Some ligands are based upon the simplification of morphine, for example fentanyl, used clinically in the induction and maintenance of anaesthesia. Thebaine is an alkaloid, structurally related to morphine that is also found in opium. Although this compound is relatively inactive, commonly used non-selective antagonists such as naloxone, naltrexone and diprenorphine are derived from this compound. Commonly used ligands are shown in Table 2, which shows peptide analogues and synthetic ligands.

Table 2. Commonly used subtype selective agonists and antagonists

Receptor	Selective agonists	Selective antagonists	Clinical ligand
μ	DAMGO	CTOP	Morphine, fentanyl
δ	DPDPE, DSLET, DADLE	Naltrindole	None
κ	Spiradoline, enadoline, U50488	NorBNI	None

DAMGO = [D-Ala^{2},Me-Phe^{4}Gly-ol]-enkephalin; DPDPE = [D-Pen^{2,5}]-enkephalin; DSLET = [D-Ser^{2},Leu^{5}]-enkephalyl-Thr; DADLE = [D-Ala^{2},D-Ala^{5}]-enkephalin; CTOP = D-Phe-Sys-Tyr-D-Trp-Orn-Thr-Pen-Thr NH_2; NorBNI = nor-binaltorphimine

From evidence based on differing affinities and actions of subtype selective ligands, it has been proposed that each opioid receptor subtype exists as multiple isoforms. These include μ_1, μ_2 [28] and μ_3 [29], δ_1 and δ_2 [30, 31] and κ_1, κ_2 and κ_3 [32, 33]. It is possible that μ_1 opioid receptors mediate supraspinal analgesia whilst μ_2 opioid receptors mediate spinal morphine analgesia, and it may be the μ_2 site that is responsible for respiratory depression [28].

To date, there is no molecular biological evidence to support the idea of subtype division, since only one example of each of the $\tilde{\mu}$, $\tilde{\delta}$ and κ-opioid receptors has been cloned from any one species. However, the possibility of post-translational modification or interaction with receptor activity modifying proteins (RAMPs) [34] remain a possibility. It is possible that opioid receptors may exist as complexes, composed of distinct but interacting μ-, δ- and possibly κ-opioid receptors. It has been proposed that there are two δ binding sites; δ_{ncx} which is not associated with any other opioid receptors, and is pharmacologically the δ_1 receptor, and δ_{cx} which is the δ receptor complexed with μ receptors [30, 35]. Opioid receptors have also been shown to exist of heterodimers between κ- and δ-opioid receptors [36] which display binding and functional properties distinct from either receptor. Indeed, receptor dimerization of GPCRs as been shown to modulate ligand affinity and efficacy [37].

Splice variants of the pharmacological μ_1-opioid receptor have been isolated, these being MOR1 and MOR1B, where MOR1B is seven residues shorter than MOR1 [38]. In addition, further alternative isoforms of MOR1 have been proposed, including MOR1C, MOR1D, MOR1E [39] and MOR1F [40]; again the differences occur in the C terminal tail of the receptor and it is interesting to note that some of the variants displayed a differential regional distribution. Three mRNA variants of the κ-opioid receptor [41] have also been isolated. It remains to be seen what the full biological role of these splice variants are.

Signal transduction

In general opioids inhibit adenylyl cyclase, close voltage sensitive Ca^{2+} channels and enhance an outward K^+ conductance.

Adenylyl cyclase is the enzyme responsible for the generation of cAMP from ATP. Each of μ-, δ-, and κ-opioid receptors have been shown to couple negatively to adenylyl cyclase to cause a reduction in cAMP formation [42-44]. Functional consequences of cAMP inhibition may be diverse but opioids may reduce neuronal excitability by modulating the hyperpolarization activated cation current, I_h [45] and this may be one of the mechanisms by which opioids produce analgesia. Opioids have been shown to have an inhibitory effect on N, P/Q, R and T types of Ca^{2+} channels [18, 46-48]. Since it is accepted that neurotransmitter release is a Ca^{2+} dependent process, inhibition of Ca^{2+} channels at nerve terminals may lead to a reduction in neurotransmitter release. All three types of opioid receptor have been shown to activate inwardly rectifying K^+ channels [49-51]. The result of this activation will be movement of the membrane potential to a more negative value and thus reducing the likelihood of an action potential producing depolarization.

The combined effect of these actions of opioids (closure of VOCCs, activation of K_{ir} and inhibition of cAMP formation) would be to bring about a reduction in neurotransmitter release and if this occurs in the pain pathway, analgesia.

Opioid receptor location

The distribution of opioid receptors within the body differs depending upon receptor type, although there is some overlap. It should be noted however, that the majority of localization studies have been performed on rat brain, and there are species differences in the anatomy of opioid receptors [21]. The μ-opioid receptor has the widest distribution, being found in brain areas such as the caudate putamen, cortex, thalamus, nucleus accumbens, amygdala, globus paladus, locus ceruleus and periaqueductal grey, pons and medulla [21, 52, 53]. Receptors can also be found in the superficial layers of the dorsal horn of the spinal cord, as well as in peripheral sites such as the gut and vas deferens. Δ-opioid receptor can be found in the olfactory cortex, caudate putamen, hippocampus and nucleus accumbens as well as in the dorsal horn. [21, 52, 53]. Like the μ-opioid receptor it is also found in the periphery, such as the *vas deferens* (from which it was first identified). With regard to the κ-opioid receptor, there appear to be great species differences in distribution. However, this receptor is found in the amygdala, hypothalamus, thalamus, caudate putamen, nucleus accumbens, cortex, hippocampus, pons/medulla and brainstem [21, 52, 53].

Information from knockout animals

It is possible to genetically manipulate animals (usually mice) so that they do not express any of a certain type of opioid receptor (homozygotes) or approximately 50% reduction in receptor number (heterozygotes). These 'knockout mice' then can be used for pharmacological and behavioral studies of opioid receptor function. For example, mice lacking the μ-opioid receptor gene do not display morphine induced analgesia and do not display symptoms of opioid withdrawal, but have no major differences in the number and distribution of δ- and κ-opioid receptors [54, 55]. Δ-opioid receptor knock-out mice have shown that the κ-opioid receptor gene is involved in the perception of chemical visceral pain, and is necessary for other actions of the agent U50-4088H including hypolocomotion and aversion [56]. Intriguingly, in mice lacking the δ-opioid receptor gene, there is retention of DPDPE induced supraspinal analgesia, although there is loss of morphine tolerance [57]. The reasons behind the analgesic effect of DPDPE remain to be clarified.

Nociceptin receptors

In 1994 several groups identified a receptor with considerable homology (~60%) to opioid receptors [see 58]. Although the homology between the nociceptin receptor and opioid receptors is almost equal to the homology between μ̃, δ̃ and κ-opioid receptors, it does not bind traditional opioid ligands, and so became known as the orphan receptor. However, the endogenous ligand for this receptor was isolated a year after the discovery of the receptor [59, 60] and named orphanin F/Q (due to its terminal amino acids) or nociceptin (due to its ability to produce a pro-nociceptive response). Nociceptin/OFQ is a heptadecapeptide cleaved from pro-nociceptin and shows similarity to dynorphin-A [see 58]. The 'orphan' receptor has been given numerous names, ORL-1 (opioid receptor like), NCR (nociceptin receptor), OP_4 or is still sometimes referred to as the orphan receptor.

NCR is distributed widely throughout the CNS, in the cortex, hippocampus, hypothalamus, PAG, locus ceruleus and spinal cord (laminae I, II and X), indeed areas where classical opioid receptors are found. An exception to this is the caudate putamen, in which NCR is absent [61]. On the whole, spinal actions of nociceptin are to produce analgesia, whilst supraspinally NCR produces hyperalgesia [see 58]. At a cellular level, actions of NCR are similar to those of opioids, inhibition of adenylyl cyclase, activation of K_{ir}, closure of VOCCs and a reduction in neurotransmitter release [see 58]. Nociceptin can also produce anxiolytic-like actions, modulation of spontaneous locomotor activity, stimulation of food intake, hypotension and bradycardia and inhibition of gastrointestinal transit, but in contrast to classical opioids, it does not produce rewarding effects [see 58]. There is much debate at present as to whether this receptor is opioid, and much depends on what criteria are use to classify opioid receptors (e.g. genetics, pharmacology).

Non-analgesic and peripheral actions of opioids

In addition to producing analgesia, opioids are able to produce modulatory effects on a variety of functions. For example opioid receptors are found on most immune cells, and it is known that B and T cells produce and secrete enkephalin [62]. T lymphocytes may also act as vectors, delivering β-endorphin to inflamed tissue and thus allowing highly specific opioid control of peripheral analgesia [63]. Indeed, this localised release of opioid peptides may mediate analgesia following conditions such as joint injury [64], and it has been demonstrated that inflammation causes an increase in the number of peripheral opioid receptors [65].

With respect to cardiovascular modulation, opioid receptors are found both in brain areas involved in cardiovascular regulation, especially the hypothalamic nuclei and also at peripheral sites such as the heart, blood vessels, kidney, sympathetic ganglia and adrenal medulla. Responses to opioid agonists differ according to subtype, dose and can produce both tachycardic and bradycardic responses as well as either hypo- or hypertension [66]. See also section on endomorphins above.

Another action of ,opioids is effects on gastro-intestinal function. All three types of opioid receptor are found in longitudinal muscle, myenteric plexus, intestinal smooth muscle and gastrointestinal nerves within the enteric nervous system. Opioids may affect gastrointestinal motility, transit secretion and absorption [67]. μ-opioids in particular slow gastric emptying [68]; this may be seen as either an unwanted side effect (constipation) or a beneficial effect (treatment of diarrhoea).

References

1. Pert CB, Snyder SH (1973) Properties of opiate receptor binding in rat brain. Proc Natl Acad Sci USA 70:2243-2247
2. Simon EJ, Hiller JM, Edelman I (1973) Stereospecific binding of the potent narcotic analgesic [^{3}H]etorphine to rat brain homogenates. Proc Natl Acad Sci USA 70:1947-1949
3. Terenius L (1973) Stereospecific interaction between narcotic analgesics and a synaptic plasma membrane fraction of the guinea-pig ileum. Acta Pharmacol Toxicol 32:317-320
4. Hughes J (1975) Isolation of an endogenous compound from the brain with pharmacological properties similar to morphine. Brain Res 88:295-306
5. Hughes J, Smith TW, Fothergill LA et al (1975) Identification of two related peptides from the brain with potent opiate agonist activity. Nature 258:577-579
6. Bradbury AF, Smythe DG, Snell CR (1976) C fragment of lipotropin has a high affinity for brain opiate receptors. Nature 260:793-795
7. Goldstein A, Tachibana S, Lowney LI et al (1979) Dynorphin-(1-13), an extraordinarily potent opioid peptide. Proc Nat Acad Sci USA 76:6666-6670
8. Martin WR, Eades CG, Thomson JA et al (1976) The effects of morphine and nalorphine like drugs in the non-dependent and morphine dependent chronic spinal dog. J Pharmacol Exp Therap 197:517-532
9. Manallack DT, Beart PM, Gundlach AL (1986) Psychotomimetric σ-opiates and PCP. Tr Pharmacol Sci 7:448-451
10. Lord JAH, Waterfield AA, Hughes J, Kosterlitz HW (1977) Endogenous opioid peptides; multiple agonists and receptors. Nature 267:495-499
11. Zadina JE, Hackler L, Ge LJ, Kastin AJ (1997) A potent and selective endogenous agonist for the μ-opioid receptor. Nature 386:499-502
12. Hacker L, Zadina JE, Ge LJ, Kastin AJ (1997) Isolation of relatively large amounts of endomorphin-1 and endomorphin-2 from human brain cortex. Peptides 18:1635-1639
13. Stone LS, Fairbanks CA, Laughlin TM et al (1997) Spinal analgesic actions of the new endogenous opioid peptides of endomorphin-1 and endomorphin-2. Neuroreport 8:3131-3135
14. Goldberg IE, Rossi GC, Letchworth SR et al (1998) Pharmacological characterization of endomorphin-1 and endomorphin-2 in mouse brain. J Pharmacol Exp Ther 286:1007-1013
15. Champion HC, Zadina JE, Kastin AJ, Kadowitz PJ (1997) The endogenous μ-opioid receptor agonists, endomorphin-1 and 2 have vasodilator activity in the hindquarters vascular bed of the rat. Life Sci 61:PL409-415
16. Czapla MA, Champion HC, Zadina JE et al (1998) Endomorphin-1 and 2, endogenous μ-opioid receptor agonists, decrease systemic arterial pressure in the rat. Life Sci 62:PL175-179
17. Yang YR, Chiu TH, Chen CL (1999) Structure activity relationships of naturally occurring and synthetic opioid tetrapeptides acting on locus ceruleus neurons. Eur J Pharmacol 372: 229-239
18. Corbett A, McKnight AT, Henderson G (1999) Opioid receptors. In: Tocris Cookson Ltd. sponsored receptor and ion channel nomenclature supplement (Elsiver Trends Journals)
19. Paul D, Standifer KM, Inturrisi CE, Pasternak GW (1989) Pharmacological characterization of morphine-6-beta-glucuronide, a very potent morphine metabolite. J Pharmacol Exp Therap 251:477-483
20. Brown GP, Yang K, Ouefelli O et al (1997) [^{3}H]morphine-6-β-glucuronide binding in brain membranes and a MOR-1 transfected cell line. J Pharmacol Exp Therap 282:1291-1297
21. Dhawan BN, Celsselin F, Raghubir R et al (1996) International Union of Pharmacology: 12. Classification of opioid receptors. Pharmacol Rev 48:567-592
22. Kieffer B, Befort K, Gaveriaux-Ruff C, Hirth CG (1992) The delta-opioid receptor: isolation of cDNA by expression cloning and pharmacological characterization. Proc Nat Acad Sci USA 89:12048-12052
23. Evans CJ, Keith DE, Morrison H et al (1992) Cloning of a delta-opioid receptor by functional expression. Science 258:1952-1955

24. Yasuda K, Raynor K, Kong H et al (1993) Cloning and functional comparison of kappa-opioid and delta-opioid receptors from mouse-brain. Proc Natl Acad Sci USA 90:6736-6740
25. Thompson RC, Mansour A, Akil H, Watson SJ (1993) Cloning and pharmacological characterization of a rat μ-opioid receptor. Neuron 11:903-913
26. Birnbaumer L, Yatani A, Vandongen AMJ et al (1990) G-protein coupling of receptors to ionic channels and other effector systems. Br J Cl Pharmacol 30:S13-S22
27. Law PY, Loh HH (1999) Regulation of opioid receptor activities. J Pharmacol Exp Therap 289:607-624
28. Pasternak GW, Wood PJ (1986) Multiple mu opiate receptors. Life Sci 38:1889-1898
29. Cruciani RA, Dvorkin B, Klinger HP, Makman MH (1994) Presence in neuroblastoma cells of a mu(3) receptor with selectivity for opiate alkaloids but without affinity for opioid peptides. Brain Res 667:229-237
30. Traynor JR, Elliott J (1993) Delta opioid receptor subtypes and cross-talk with mu-opioid receptors. Tr Pharmacol Sci 14:84-86
31. Sofuoglu M, Portoghese PS, Takemori AE (1991) Differential antagonism of delta-opioid agonists by naltrindole and its benzofuran analogue (NTB) in mice - evidence for delta-opioid receptor subtypes. J Pharmacol Exp Therap 257:676-680
32. Pasternak GW (1993) Pharmacological mechanisms of opioid analgesics. Clin Neuropharmacol 16:1-18
33. Cheng J, Standifer KM, Tublin PR et al (1995) Demonstration of κ3-opioid receptors in the SH-SY5Y human neuroblastoma cell line. J Neurochem 65:170-175
34. Foord SM, Marshall FH (1999) RAMPS; accessory proteins for seven transmembrane receptors. Tr Pharmacol Sci 20:184-187
35. Rothman RB, Bykov V, Jacobson AE et al (1992) A study on the effect of [D-Ala-^{2}Leu^{5}Cys^{6}] Enkephalin on δ_{cx} and δ_{ncx} opioid receptor binding sites in vitro and in vivo. Peptides 92:691-694
36. Joarden B, Devi LA (1999) G protein coupled receptor heterodimerization modulates receptor function. Nature 399:697-700
37. Onaran HO, Gurdal H (1999) Ligand efficacy and affinity in an interacting 7tm receptor model. Tr Pharmacol Sci 20:274-278
38. Zimprich A, Simon T, Hollt V (1995) rMOR1 and rMOR1B: comparison of both rat μ-opioid receptor variants with respect to second messenger coupling. Analgesia 1:886-889
39. Pan YX, Xu J, Bolan E et al (1999) Identification and characterization of three new alternatively spliced mu-opioid receptor isoforms. Mol Pharmacol 56:396-403
40. Pan ZZ (1998) M-opposing actions of the κ-opioid receptor. Tr Pharmacol Sci 19:94-98
41. Wei LN, Hu XL, Bi J, Loh H (2000) Post-transcriptional regulation of mouse kappa-opioid receptor expression. Mol Pharmacol 57:401-408
42. Smart D, Hirst RA, Hirota K et al (1997) The effects of recombinant rat μ-opioid receptor activation in CHO cells on phospholipase C, $[Ca^{2+}]_i$ and adenylyl cyclase. Br J Pharmacol 120: 1165-1171
43. Hirst RA, Hirota K, Grandy DK, Lambert DG (1997) Coupling of the cloned rat κ-opioid receptor to adenylyl cyclase is dependent on receptor expression. Neurosci Lett 232:119-122
44. Hirst RA, Smart D, Devi LA, Lambert DG (1998) Effects of C-terminal truncation of the recombinant δ-opioid receptor on phospholipase C and adenylyl cyclase coupling. J Neurochem 70:2273-2278
45. Ingram SL, Williams JT (1994) Opioid inhibition of I-h via adenylyl-cyclase. Neuron 13: 179-186
46. Seward E, Hammond C, Henderson G (1991) M-opioid-receptor-mediated inhibition of N-type calcium-channel current. Proc R Soc Lond 244:129-135
47. Soldo BL, Moises HC (1998) M-opioid receptor activation inhibits N and P type Ca channel currents in magnocellular neurons of the rat supraoptic nucleus. J Physiol 513:787-804
48. Piros IT, Hales TG, Evans CJ (1996) Functional analysis of cloned receptors in transfected cell lines. Neurochem Res 21:1277-1285

49. Christie MJ, North RA, Surprenant A, Williams JT (1987) M-and δ-opioid receptors both belong to a family of neurotransmitter receptors which increase an inwardly rectifying potassium conductance. J Physiol 390:P199
50. Henry DJ, Grandy DK, Lester HA et al (1995) K-opioid receptors couple to inwardly rectifying potassium channels when coexpressed in Xenopus oocytes. J Pharmacol Exp Therap 47:551-557
51. Han SH, Cho YW, Kim CJ et al (1999) M-opioid agonist induced activation of G protein coupled inwardly rectifying potassium current in rat periaqueductal gray neurons. Neurosci 90:209-219
52. Mansour A, Khachaturian H, Lewis ME et al (1988) Anatomy of CNS opioid receptors. Tr Neurolog Sci 11:308-314
53. George SR, Zastawny RL, Briones-Urbrina R et al (1994) Distinct distribution of mu, delta and kappa opioid receptor mRNA in rat brain. Biochem Biophys Res Comm 205:1438-1444
54. Matthes HWD, Maldonado R, Simonin F et al (1996) Loss of morphine-induced analgesia, reward effect and withdrawal symptoms in mice lacking the μ-opioid receptor gene. Nature 383:819-823
55. Kitchen I, Slowe S, Mattehes HWD, Kieffer B (1997) Quantitative autoradiographic mapping of μ-, δ-, and κ-opioid receptors in knockout mice lacking the μ-opioid receptor gene. Brain Res 778:73-88
56. Simonin F, Valverde O, Smadja C et al (1998) Disruption of the κ-opioid receptor gene in mice enhances sensitivity to chemical visceral pain, impairs pharmacological actions of U50-4088H and attenuates morphine withdrawl. EMBO J 17:886-897
57. Zhu YX, King MA, Schuller AGP et al (1999) Retention of delta-like analgesia and loss of morphine tolerance in delta opioid receptor knockout mice. Neuron 24:243-252
58. Calò G, Guerrini R, Rizzi A et al (2000) Pharmacology of nociceptin and its receptor: a novel therapeutic target. Br J Pharmacol 129:1261-1283
59. Meunier JC, Mollereau C, Toll L et al (1995) Isolation and structure of the endogenous agonist of opioid receptor-like ORL(1) receptor. Nature 377:532-535
60. Reinscheid RK, Northacker HP, Bourson A et al (1995) Orphanin-FQ - a neuropeptide that activates an opioid-like G-protein-coupled receptor. Science 270:792-794
61. Darland T, Grandy DK (1998) The orphanin FQ system: an emerging target for the management of pain? Br J Anaesth 81:29-37
62. Sanders VM (1995) The role of opioid peptides in immune function. In: Tseng LF (ed) The pharmacology of opioid peptides. Harvard Academic Publishers, USA
63. Webster NR (1998) Opioids and the immune system. Br J Anaesth 81:835-836
64. Schaible HG, Grubb BD (1993) Afferent and spinal mechanisms of joint pain. Pain 55:5-54
65. Zhou LI, Zhang Q, Stein C, Schafer M (1998) Contribution of opioid receptors on primary afferent versus sympathetic neurons to peripheral opioid analgesia. J Pharmacol Exp Ther 286: 1000-1006
66. Paakkari P, Feuerstein G (1995) Opioid peptides in cardiovascular and respiratory regulation. In: Tseng LF (ed) The pharmacology of opioid peptides. Harvard Academic Publishers, USA
67. Burks TF (1995) Opioid peptides in gastrointestinal functions. In: Tseng LF (ed) The pharmacology of opioid peptides. Harvard Academic Publishers, USA
68. Crighton IM, Martin PH, Hobbs GJ et al (1998) A comparison of the effects of intravenous tramadol, codeine and morphine on gastric emptying in human volunteers. Anaes Analg 87: 445-449

New Narcotics

G. Savoia, G. Scibelli, M. Loreto

Analgesia is absence of pain. Throughout surgery, numerous nociceptive stimuli are produced which in conscious patients are cause of pain.

In 1960 Gray proposed the famous triad of anaesthesia which includes narcosis, muscle-relaxants and depression of the reflexes or according to modern thoughts abolition of conscience, control of the reflexes and muscle-relaxation (Fig. 1) [1].

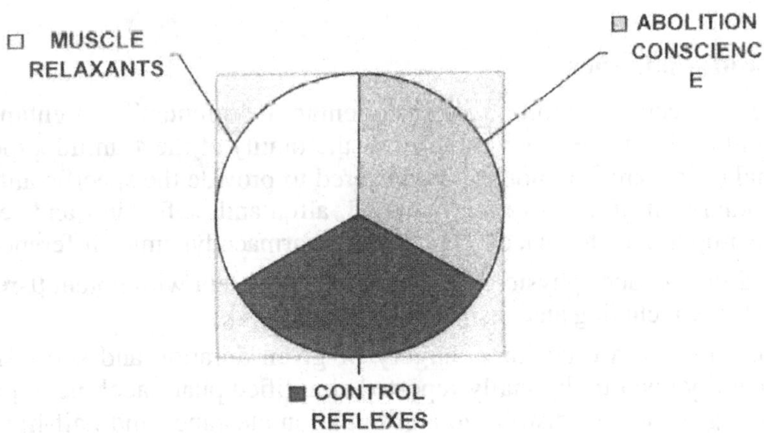

Fig. 1. The components of anaesthesia

The control of the reflexes is certainly the most difficult component to value.

The suppression of perception and the pain memory can be obtained with intravenous and inhalation anaesthetics, the motor responses with muscle-relaxants respectively (Fig. 2) [2].

Nociceptive stimuli induce neurovegetative (sweating, lachrymation, hemodynamic alterations: Δ AP: arterial pressure and Δ HR: heart rate) and hormonal responses. The stimulated reflexes are related to type of surgery, used drugs and properties (load, capacity).

PAINFULL STIMULI						
	Sensitive-response	Motor-response	Neurovegetative response			
/			Δ AP Δ HR	Sweating	Lachrymation O pupil	Hormonal increase
Hypnotics	+ + +					
Inhalation anaesthetics	+ + +	+ +	+ +	+ +	+ +	+ +
Analgesics	+		+ +	+ + +	+ + +	+ +
Neuroleptics			+ +	+ +	+ +	+ +
Muscle relaxants		+ + +				

Fig. 2. Responses to painful stimuli and action of drugs on the control of the reflex responses

The role of analgesics in the control of the reflexes to pain is more important in anaesthesia, even if volatile anaesthetics contribute efficacy to the control of these components too [2].

New opioid analgesics

The pure μ-receptor opioid agonists: fentanyl, sufentanil, alfentanil and remifentanil (the last one a new member in the family of the 4-anilidopiperidine opioid-analgesics) are commonly administered to provide the specific anti-nociceptive component of anaesthesia. Fentanyl, alfentanil, sufentanil and remifentanil have important pharmacokinetics and pharmacodynamic differences [3].

These drugs produce physiological changes consistent with potent μ-receptor agonist activity including analgesia and sedation [3, 4].

The selection of a drug for a surgery of given duration and seriousness is based generally upon traditionally reported simplified pharmacokinetic parameters including volume of distribution, elimination clearance and half-life [5, 6].

The context-sensitive half-time is the time required for drug concentration to decrease by half of its value, after a given time of drug infusion (determined by computer simulation). It is not a fixed value, but a curve representing the half-time as a function of the time of drug infusion. Each drug exhibits a characteristic context-sensitive half-time curve that is the better comparative predictor of drug concentration decay (Fig. 3) [7].

The curve of fentanyl increases rapidly in spite of clinically apparent rapid recovery rate. Therefore it has a clinically unreasonable half-time. Fentanyl does not appear to be the drug of choice for continuous administration [5]. Alfentanil shows a very unusual curve: the context-sensitive half-time rapidly increases and reaches a plateau approximately at 60 minutes after 3 hours' infusion (this property is related to its small distribution volume).

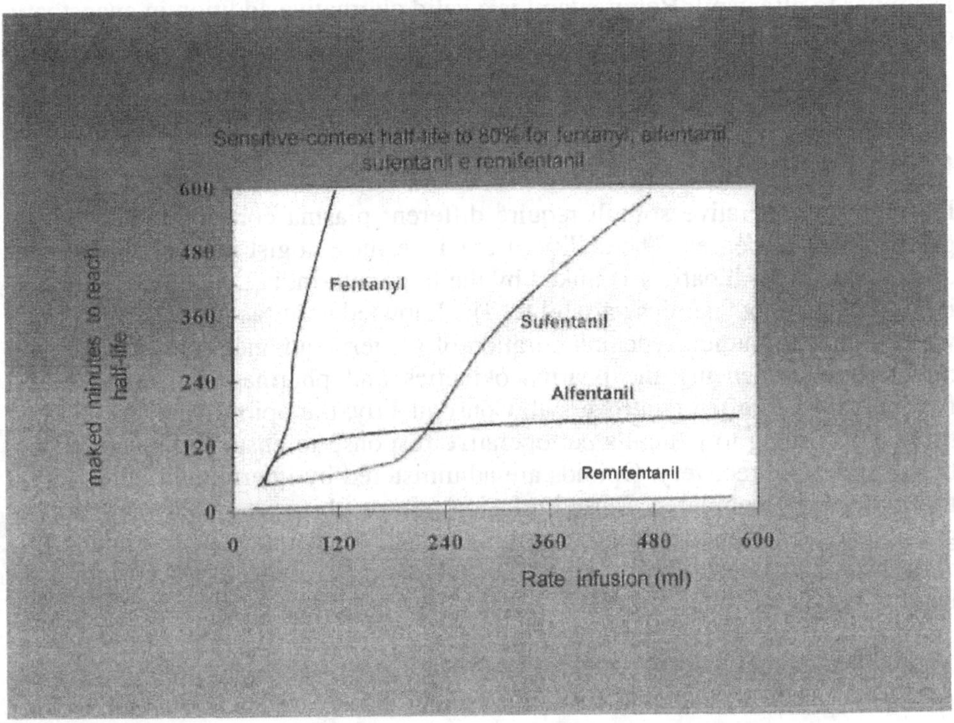

Fig. 3. Context-sensitive half-life of fentanyl, sufentanil, alfentanil and remifentanil [7]

Sufentanil can be used for long lasting invasive surgery; it shows a shorter context sensitive half-time than alfentanil, up to 10 hours of infusion too [5].

Remifentanil is an ultrashort μ-receptor agonist opioid: it is unique among the currently marketed agents because of its ester structure and undergoes a widespread extrahepatic metabolism by blood and tissue non specific esterases (the drug is named EMO: esterase metabolised opioid), resulting in an extremely rapid clearance rate of approximately 3 L/min (180 L/hr).

Because of its unique metabolic pathway and rapid clearance, remifentanil represents a new pharmacokinetic class of opioid [8].

Like other drugs of this class, remifentanil is lipophilic and is widely distributed in body tissues with a steady-state distribution volume of approximately 30 L. Unlike other fentanyl-related agents the decrease of its therapeutic effects mainly depends on metabolic clearance rather than on redistribution. Therefore the time required for decreasing percentage plasmatic concentrations after infusion is independent of infusion time. The context-sensitive half-time is very short (3 minutes) and this is perhaps the most compelling evidence of the drug's pharmacokinetic singularity. The onset time is very rapid at 1 to 2 minutes and is similar to alfentanil. Remifentanil is a valid alternative addition in anaesthetic drug protocols [9-11].

Clinical utilization

Different perioperative stimuli require different plasma concentrations to suppress patient responses. The ability of the anaesthesiologist in selecting an adequate dose for each patient is linked by the large interindividual pharmacokinetics and pharmacodynamics variability. The knowledge of factors (age, sex, body weight, cardiac output, type and duration of surgery and anaesthesia, lean body mass, etc.) influencing the pharmacokinetics and pharmacodynamics is still fragmentary and often controversial. Consequently, the opioid dose needs to be titrated according to patient's perioperative response to ensure adequate anaesthesia and rapid recovery. Opioids are administered by intermittent bolus injection ordered by computer-assisted infusion pumps; this system allows us to target a specific plasmatic drug concentration and to maintain or to change this concentration as needed, in spite of the fluctuation of plasma concentration related to bolus injection (Tables 1, 2, 3) [5, 12].

Table 1. Drug's equivalent doses for intravenous PCA

Opioid	Dose-demand (mcg)	IV-Continuous infusion mcg/kg/hr	mg 70 kg/die
Sufentanil	6	0.1	0.2
Fentanyl	34	0.46	0.8
Alfentanil	212	4.96	8.3

Table 2. Guidelines for opioids' continuous epidural infusion

Opioid	Bolus (mg)	Concentration (mg/ml)	Infusion rate (mg/h)
Fentanyl	0.05-0.1	0.005-0.025	0.02-0.15
Sufentanil	0.025-0.05	0.001	0.05-0.1
Alfentanil	1	0.25	0.2

Table 3. Target manual infusion for intravenous opioids

Opioid	Blood target concentration (ng/ml)	Bolus (μg/kg)	Infusion rate (μg/kg/min)
Fentanyl A	1	3	0.020
Fentanyl B	4	10	0.070
Alfentanil A	40	20	0.25
Alfentanil B	160	80	1.00
Sufentanil A	0.15	0.15	0.003
Sufentanil B	0.50	0.50	0.010
Remifentanil A	1	0.25	< 0.025
Remifentanil B	10-20	1-2	> 0.025

A: analgesia target; B: anaesthesia target

The alfentanil is widely and appropriately used for surgery longer than 6-8 hours when a rapid decrease of opioid concentration is required at the end of the infusion. Although sufentanil has a longer distribution and elimination half-life than alfentanil, recovery from sufentanil infusion may be more rapid than alfentanil infusions for surgery shorter than 6-8 hours [5].

Remifentanil may be used within a wide range of safety and effectiveness. In major surgery remifentanil combines the properties of intraoperative control of stress responses and rapid recovery. The rapid termination of remifentanil action warrants modifications of the current practice related to early postoperative pain control [13]. Remifentanil may be used as a sedative during monitored analgesia or as a postoperative analgesic in spontaneously breathing patients [14]. Remifentanil may increase patient's safety by eliminating the risk of delayed respiratory depression but its correct use requires major changes in our prescribing habits, especially conceming the problem of development of tolerance which is very rapid when we use it [15].

The adverse effects of this class of drug include respiratory depression, nausea, vomiting, stiffness, bradycardia and pruritus [16]. Because remifentanil does not release histamine, it shows fewer haemodynamic adverse effects than other analgesics such as morphine.

The short-acting opioids, fentanyl and alfentanil, may be used without significant effects on postoperative recovery, particularly if they are administered in association with propofol for induction and with or without propofol for maintenance. Their use may reduce the need for propofol and decrease postoperative pain levels. Initial reports on the use of remifentanil suggest that it produces stable anaesthesia when used by infusion with propofol, but postoperative pain may be a problem due to its rapid clearance [11, 13].

The use of morphine and its analogues may significantly delay recovery (Fig. 4) [16]. When morphine is used in day surgery, it may delay or prevent the discharge. In paediatric day surgery, morphine significantly increased PONV, both in hospital and after discharge home. In major surgery the need for morphine for postoperative analgesia results in adverse effects, like drowsiness and PONV [16].

It is essential that pain is expected and planned for; analgesic strategies usually include a variety of drugs given at different stages of patient's recovery ("balanced analgesia") [6, 17-19].

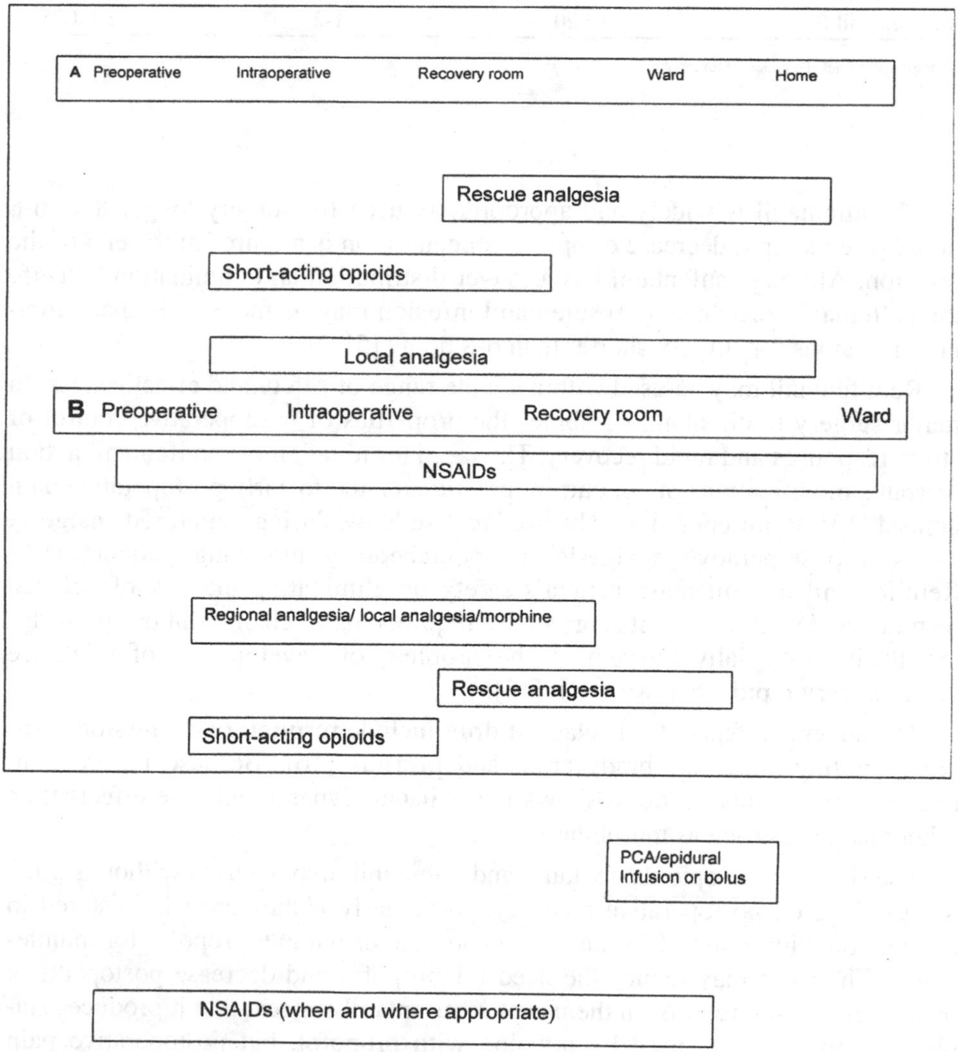

Fig. 4. Analgesia strategies for A) day surgery and B) in patient surgery

Morphine is strongly emetic. The addition of droperidol (doses of 3-10 mg/60 mg morphine) in PCA reduces PONV but increases sedation, so the addition of cyclizine and ondansetron has been studied. Cyclizine (100 mg/60 mg morphine) was effective, but produced a sedation like droperidol (3 mg/60 mg morphine). Ondansetron (8 mg/60 mg morphine) was more effective than droperidol (5 mg/60 mg morphine). Further studies need to determine the best doses and concentrations of these drugs.

The use of non-steroidal anti-inflammatory drugs (NSAIDs) as analgesics may reduce the required dose of morphine, but they have not showed significant effects on recovery [6, 16] (Fig. 4).

In order to achieve a comprehension of clinical aspects of perioperative opioids use, we have performed a metanalysis of the last years' literature on this argument, extracted by medline. We have considered only the papers that respond completely to the following parameters:

- double-blind evaluation;
- randomization;
- correct comparison between two different perioperative analgesic regimes.

The summary of this metanalysis is printed in Table 4.

Our experience on the perioperative use of remifentanil

The object of our study was to evaluate the analgesic efficacy and safety of remifentanil. We recruited 50 patients (22 F; 28 M; age: 63 ± 21 years; bw 72 ± 17 kg; ASA I-III) subjected to abdominal surgery. After informed consent, the patients were pretreated with midazolam 2 mg e.v. + atropina 0.01 mg/kg (if HR < 70 bpm), and the induction was achieved with continuous infusion of remifentanil 0.2 mcg/kg/min (solutions of 50 mcg/ml, infusion velocity 20 ml/h) for 5 minutes; finally cisatracurium 0.2 mg/kg and propofol 1 mg/kg were given in 60 seconds. Maintenance was effected with a mixture of O_2/air, end-tidal Sevorane 1-1.5% and remifentanil 0.2 mcg/kg/min ± 0.02 mcg/kg/min until steady-state was achieved.

All patients received 15 minutes before the end-operation ketorolac 30 mg i.v. and infiltration of the wound with ropivacaina 0.75%; they were randomized in two groups of 25 patients each; group A were given remifentanil 0.05 mcg/kg/min and group B remifentanil 0.1 mcg/kg/min for 24 hr; all patients were monitored with ECG, HR, AP, RR (respiratory rate), SaO_2, $EtCO_2$, integrated VAS and Ramsey sedation score. The HR was stable in the preoperative, the AP decreased < 20% with respect to baseline values in 8 patients, while respiratory depression appeared in all patients. Intraoperative analgesia was optimal with a remifentanil infusion rate of 0.21 ± 0.03 mcg/kg/min while the postoperative analgesia was inadequate in all patients of group A (integrated VAS 0-240 > 80) who required a rescue dose of morphine 2-3 mg i.v.; in group B the analgesia was good (integrated VAS < 50) in 80% of the patients and only 20% asked for morphine. Postoperative monitoring showed stability of the RR (> 10/min), SaO_2 > 94%, and Ramsey score 1 in 100% of group A, while it was 2-3 in 16 patients and 4 in 9 patients of group B. The chosen infusion rate avoids muscle rigidity and respiratory depression, and allows good analgesia only at postoperative higher infusion rates, but it requires a strict surveillance of respiratory parameters and sedation level in a protected intensive area.

Conclusions

According to reports in Table 4 and to more recent recommendations conceming treatment of intraoperative and postoperative pain, it is necessary to include opioids in perioperative planning to ensure the best level of analgesia, which is different in day-surgery or hospital regime.

The use of new analgesics with very short context-sensitive half-time may enable an intraoperative plan of reducing the recovery time from awakening.

Therefore, a comparison between remifentanil, sufentanil and alfentanil administered by the intravenous route has been made. As regards awakening it is possible to choose several strategies to assure the continuity of the analgesia:

a) to continue infusion of remifentanil ≤ 0.1 mcg/kg/min until the appearance of analgesic effects of other opioids administered at the end of surgery;
b) to continue i.v. patient controlled analgesia (IV-PCA) by using classical drugs such as morphine (bolus demand 1-2 mg; lock-out interval 5-7 minutes) or sufentanil (bolus demand 5-10 mcg; lock-out interval 5-7 minutes);
c) continuous e.v. prolonged infusion in a controlled place (ICU);
d) to commence multimodal programs including fans, weak opioid and/or α-2 agonists, before surgery-end.

In the literature a major controversy of the last years has concerned the superiority of "balanced" or "integrated" anaesthesia technique (intravenous hypnotic anaesthesia + continuous segmentally peridural anaesthesia) and intravenous anaesthesia technique [6, 12, 18].

The integrated techniques should allow a better postoperative outcome through a reduced influence of pulmonary infections, better control of pain and comfort of the patients, a shorter recovery in ICU or in ward. It is controversial too whether these advantages are due to the techniques of perioperative epidural analgesia with opioids and local anaesthetics or to the intraoperative epidural local anaesthetics [4, 7, 16]. Epidural opioids should be limited to the immediate perioperative period to avoid delays of canalization, in association with local anaesthetics by continuous infusion. Opinions about the better technique differ between continuous epidural infusion or patient controlled analgesia by epidural route to assure a gold standard for perioperative analgesia.

Table 4. Perioperative analgesia: intravenous and epidural route

Ref.	No. of patients	Surgery	Operative analgesia Intraop	Operative analgesia Postop	μ-Receptor opioid and dose	Comparison drug and dose	Route	Results
20	234 (116-R 118-A)	Major abdominal	Yes		Remifentanil 1 mcg/kg/min-loading dose; 0.5 mcg/kg/min continuous infusion It was discontinued in the immediate postoperative period	Alfentanil 25 mcg/kg-loading dose; 1 mcg/kg/min continuous infusion It was discontinued in the immediate postoperative period	I.v.	More patients receiving alfentanil had one or more responses to surgery (72% vs 57%). The incidence of adverse events in both groups was 82% and 75% of patients respectively. Adverse events associated with remifentanil were rapidly controlled by dose reductions. The incidence of intra-operative hypotension and bradycardia was higher in the remifentanil group.
21	201 (102-R 99-A)	Undefined	Yes		Remifentanil	Alfentanil	I.v.	Fewer remifentanil patients responded to skin closure (11% and 22%, $p < 0.05$) and had stress responses to surgical stimuli (52.9% and 65.7%, $p < 0.05$); than patients who received alfentanil. More patients in the alfentanil group required extra analgesia compared with the remifentanil group ($p < 0.05$). Time to respond to verbal command, times to spontaneous respiration (median 5 min vs 8 min), adequate respiratory rate (median 6 min vs 9 min), and tracheal extubation (median 6 min vs 9 min) were significantly shorter

								for alfentanil in comparison with remifentanil ($p < 0.05$). Remifentanil patients, however, showed significantly better recovery of psychomotor and psychometric function between 30 and 90 min after surgery ($p < 0.05$). The incidences of hypotension intraoperatively and shivering postoperatively were significantly higher with remifentanil. The pharmacological profile of remifentanil suggests that rapid recovery will occur after its use. This study of 200 outpatients shows that the differences suggested from kinetic studies are not always borne out in clinical practice.
22	35	Total abdominal hysterectomy	Yes	Remifentanil 2 mcg/kg-single dose over 60 sec at induction + Remifentanil 0.25 mcg/kg/min in continuous infusion for maintenance + 0.25 mcg/kg/min at skin incision until removal	Remifentanil 2 mcg/kg-single dose over 60 sec at induction + Remifentanil 0.25 mcg/kg/min at maintenance + saline placebo at skin incision until removal of the uterus	Alfentanil 50 mcg/kg-single dose over 60 sec at induction + Alfentanil 0.5 mcg/kg/min at maintenance + saline placebo at skin incision until removal of the uterus	I.v.	Awakening times were significantly shorter ($p < 0.05$) in the remifentanil population compared with the alfentanil population, but discharge times were similar. More patients received naloxone to reverse opioid effects in the alfentanil population (60%) than in the remifentanil population (20%) ($p < 0.05$). Doubling of the remifentanil infusion to 0.5 microgram/kg/min before the major stress event improves suppression of responses and

				of the uterus			lowers intraoperative use of remifentanil without prolonging recovery times. Remifentanil allows faster awakening times than alfentanil, but preemptive administration of postoperative analgesics is recommended to facilitate discharge.
23	18	Major abdominal	Yes	Sufentanil 1 mcg/kg + 0.7 mcg/kg/hr up to the end of surgery	Fentanyl 7 mcg/kg + 5 mcg/kg/hr up to the end of surgery	I.v.	With both regimens, the sympathoadrenal stress response to major abdominal surgery was nearly completely suppressed, resulting in stable haemodynamics during the operations. S and A were equally well suited as analgesic components of total IV anaesthesia with propofol.
24	27 (PCEA: 12 PCA: 15)	Abdominal	Yes	Sufentanil PCA 10 mcg + 5 mcg lockout interval 15 min and max 40 mcg/4 hr	Sufentanil PCEA 20 mcg + 5 mcg lockout interval 15 min and max 40 mcg/4 hr	I.v. (PCA) epidural (PCEA)	There appears to be no clinical advantage of epidural (PCEA) over IV (PCA) sufentanil for analgesia after major abdominal surgery
25	20	Abdominal	Yes	Alfentanil-PCEA 1 mg + 0.2 mg/hr + infusion PCA	Alfentanil-PCA Sodium chloride with catheter + infusion PCA	i.v. epidural	The epidural administration of alfentanil reduces intravenous alfentanil requirements during NO_2-O_2-anesthesia; the results indicate a spinal mechanism of action of epidural alfentanil
26	32	Abdominal	Yes	Alfentanil-EPI Increments of 250 mcg and lockout of 10 min for 16 hr	Alfentanil-IV Increments of 250 mcg lockout of 5 min for 16 hr	Epidural e.v.	Alfentanil EPI-PCA was no more effective than IV PCA and it was associated with the same incidence of oxyhemoglobin desaturation (SpO_2 85% in

										69% of EPI group vs 56% in IV group).
27	45	Abdominal	Yes		Sufentanil EPI 15 pg-bolus + 5 pg/hr infusion	Sufentanil IV 15 pg-bolus + 5 pg/hr infusion	Fentanyl EPI 60 mcg bolus + 20 mcg /hr infusion		I.v. epidural	S-IV and S-EPI are almost equipotent; IV administration of an equipotent initial dose is hazardous because of the risk of respiratory depression. The higher degree of sedation observed with S-IV during entire treatment may be a point in favor of the EPI route. The equianalgesic dose of epidural S was found to be approximately four times less than the EPI F dose in pain treatment after abdominal surgery.
28	20	Abdominal	Yes		Sufentanil EPI	Sufentanil IV			I.v.	The plasma concentrations of sufentanil were comparable between the 2 groups. The initial transfer of S from the epidural space to the systemic circulation appeared to be very rapid while the transfer into the CSF is lower, though it varied interindividually.
29	41	Abdominal gynaecologic		Yes	Sufentanil 25 mcg in 10 ml saline	Sufentanil 40 mcg in 10 ml saline	Sufentanil 55 mcg in 10 ml saline	Sufentanil 70 mcg in 10 ml saline	Epidural	In the patients recovering from lower abdominal surgery, a single 40-55 mcg epidural bolus of S provides 3-3.5 hr of effective analgesia, and larger doses are not warranted.
30	40	Abdominal surgery		Yes	Sufentanil 50 mcg	Sufentanil 25 mcg + clonodine 1 mcg/kg			Epidural	The duration of complete pain relief was significantly longer in those who received the mixture, and oxygen saturation and arterial blood pressure were reduced after

								S alone but remained stable after S + C.
31	20	Abdominal surgery		Yes	Sufentanil 75 mcg	Sufentanil 75 mcg + Adrenaline 75 mcg	Epidural	The addition of adrenaline significantly prolonged the duration of analgesia provided by epidural S. It was accompained by less hypercapnia and less reduction in respiratory rate. The diminished vascular uptake of S shown by the lower plasma concentration in group S + adrenaline might explain the lessened respiratory impairment.
32	40	Abdominal surgery	Yes	Yes	Sufentanil 5 mcg/hr in continuous infusion + Sufentanil bolus 50 mcg in postoperative	Morphine 0.5 mg/hr in continuous infusion + Morphine bolus 5 mg in postoperative	Epidural (L2-3)	The quality of pain relief was similar in each group. The incidence of nausea and vomiting, pruritus, and drowsiness was similar in the two groups. Forced vital capacities were statistically better during the first 1-4 hr with S.
33	20	Myocardial revasculariz-ation	Yes		Flunitrazepam + Nalbuphine-2.5 mg/kg continuous infusion	Flunitrazepam + Fentanyl 7.5 mg/7 kg continuous infusion	I.v.	All hormone concentrations significantly increased in the nalbuphine group, whereas they did not exceed the baseline values in the F group. Post-operatively, 5 of 10 patients given N complained of recall, pain, or unpleasant dreams during or after the procedure. Flunitrazepam-N cannot be recommended for anesthesia in patients undergoing coronary artery surgery.

34	171	Upper abdominal (99 patients) Lower abdomminal (72 patients)		Yes	Bupivacaine 0.167%	Bupivacaine 0.167% + Sufentanil-2 mcg/ml (5 mcg/hr)	Bupivacaine 0.167% + Sufentanil-4 mcg/ml (10 mcg/hr)	Sufentanil-4 mcg/ml (10 mcg/hr)	Epidural	The infusion of S without bupivacaine was less effective than S-B mixtures after upper abdominal surgery while indistiguishable in analgesic affectivness after either upper or lower abdominal surgery.
35	96 (S+B: 50 M: 46)	Major abdominal		Yes	Sufentanil 2 mcg/ml + Bupivacaine 0.25% (PCEA) bolus dose 0.05 ml/kg, lockout 10 min		Morphine 1 mg/ml (PCA) bolus dose 2 mg, lockout 10 min		I.v. epidural (thoracic)	Postoperative pain intensities (VAS) were lower with PCEA (median = 1) compared to PCA (median = 2; $p > 0.001$) while heart rate, mean arterial pressure, PaO_2 and $PaCO_2$ were comparable at all points in time.
36	40	Abdominal	Yes	Yes	Sufentanil 0.5 mcg/kg in 10 ml-20 min (at induction) + 0.25 mcg/kg/hr infusion during 12 hr (5 ml/hr)		Clonidine 4 mcg/kg in 10 ml-20 min (at induction) + 2 mcg/kg/hr infusion during 12 hr (5 ml/hr) Postoperatively Sufentanil boluses (5 mcg)-PCA		I.v. epidural	Epidural clonidine improved intraoperative hemodynamic stability when compared with epidural sufentanil. Both substances provided reliable postoperative analgesia. A longer lasting residual analgesic effect was demonstrated after the use of epidural clonidine. Both substances showed different but potentially worrying side effects.
					Sufentanil boluses for ↑ AP, HR (0.035 mcg) intraoperatively or postoperatively-PCA (5 mcg)					
37	40	Cesarean section	Yes		Sufentanil-PCEA (212.7 ± 9.5 mcg/24 hr)		Placebo (128.4 ± 10.8 mcg/24 hr)		Spinal-epidural	A background infusion in PCEA with S does not offer major advantages in terms of sleep quality or S consumption, except for a lower pain score during the initial hours. Side effects may be more pronounced owing to increased drug administration.

38	16	Maxillo-facial	Yes		Fentanyl Bolus dose of 12 mcg/kg + 6 mcg/kg/hr	Sufentanil Bolus dose of 1 mcg/kg + 0.5 mcg/kg/hr	I.v.	The faster elimination of S than F observed after the end of a continuous infusion was related to its higher clearance, while Vd were not statistically different. When compared with a single bolus S administered by continuous infusion has longer elimination and a larger Vd.
39	20 (I group: 10 II group: 10)	Coronary artery bypass	Yes		I: Remifentanil 5 mcg/kg at induction 3 mcg/kg/min for maintenance	II: Remifentanil 2 mcg/kg at induction 1 mcg/kg/min for maintenance	I.v.	Heart rate, MAP, and $PaCO_2$ did not change over time in either group. Transcranial doppler sonography was used to monitor remifentanil-induced changes in cerebral perfusion. We found that large doses of remifentanil reduced cerebral flow velocity despite constant perfusion pressure. This may implicate a central mechanism for cerebral hemodynamics.
40	20	Abdominal	Yes		Fentanyl 7 mcg/kg (3 mcg/kg/hr)	Sufentanil 1 mcg/kg (0,4 mcg/kg/hr)	I.v.	Sufentanil was similar to fentanyl in attenuating the haemodynamic and hormonal responses to surgical stimulation. In two patients in the fentanyl group and three in the sufentanil group, myocardial lactate production was observed temporarily, indicating myocardial ischaemia caused by surgical stress

A: alfentanil; B: bupivacaine; F: fentanyl; M: morphine; N: nalbuphine; R: remifentanil; S: sufentanil

References

1. Torri G (1992) L'anestesia generale e le sue componenti. In: Temi di anestesia - Il controllo della moderna anestesia bilanciata. Centro Scientifico, Torino, pp 3-4
2. Torri G (1992) Il controllo dei riflessi alla stimolazione nocicettiva. In: Temi di anestesia - Il controllo della moderna anestesia bilanciata. Centro Scientifico, Torino, pp 8-9
3. Rushton AR, Sneyd JR (1997) Opioid analgesics. Br J Hosp Med 52;4:105-106
4. Incze F (1998) Advances in anesthesiology in the 90's. Orv Hetil 139;17:1003-1010
5. Meert TF (Reprint 1996) Pharmacotherapy of opioids-present and future developments. Pharmacy World & Science 18;1:1-15
6. Lemmens HJM (Reprint 1995) Pharmacokinetic-pharmacodynamic relationships for opioids in balanced anesthesia. Clinical Pharmacokinetics 29;4:231-242
7. Gepts E (1997) New concepts in pharmacokinetics and pharmacodynamics. Acta Anaesth Belg 48:199-204
8. Dumont L, Picard V, Marti RA, Tassonvi E (1998) Use of remifentanil in a patient with chronic hepatic failure. Br J Anaesth 81;2:265-267
9. Wilhelm W, Huppert A, Brun K et al (1997) Remifentanil (ed). Anaesthesia 52;4:291-293
10. Scholz J, Steinfath M (1996) Is remifentanil an ideal opioid for anesthesiologic management in the 21st century? Anasthesiol Intensivmed Notfallmed Schmerzther 52;4:592-607
11. Egan TD (1995) Remifentanil pharmacokinetics and pharmacodynamics. A preliminary appraisal. Clin Pharmacokinet 52;4:80-94
12. Rockemann MG, Feeling W, Goertz AW et al (1997) Intravenous and epidural patient-controlled analgesia (PCA). Anasthesiologie Intensivmedizin Notfallmedizin Schmerztherapie 32;7:414-419
13. Kovac AL, Azad SS, Steer P et al (1998) Use of remifentanil in patients breathing spontaneously during monitored anesthesia care and in the management of acute postoperative care. Anesthesiology 85;7:1124-1126
14. Vinik HR, Kissin I (1998) Rapid development of tolerance to analgesia during remifentanil infusion in humans. Anesth Analg 86;6:1307-1311
15. Wiebalck A, Zenz M (Reprint 1997) Neurophysiological aspects of pain. Anaesthesist 46; [Suppl 3]:147-153
16. Kovac AL, Azard SS, Steer P et al (1997) Severe bradycardia after remifentanil [letter]. Anesthesiology 85;7:1019-1020
17. Millar JM (2000) Factors influencing recovery. In: Anaesthesia rounds - Recovery from Anaesthesia. Oxfordshire Astrazeneca, pp 9-15
18. Langlade A, Briard C, Bouguet D et al (1994) PCA and postoperative pain. Cahiers d'Anesthesiologie 42;2:183-189
19. Camu F (2000) Why should I change my practice of anesthesia? Opioids. Minerva Anestesiol 66:268-272
20. Schuttler J, Albrecht S, Breivick H et al (1997) A comparison of remifentanil and alfentanil in patients undergoing major abdominal surgery. Anaesthesia 52;4:307-317
21. Cartwright DP, Kvalsvik O, Cassuto J et al (1997) A randomized, blind comparison of remifentanil and alfentanil during anesthesia for outpatient surgery. Anesth Analg 85;5:1014-1019
22. Kovac AL, Azad SS, Steer P et al (1997) Remifentanil versus alfentanil in a balanced anesthetic technique for total abdominal hysterectomy. J Clin Anesth 85;7:532-541
23. Kietzmann D, Hahne D, Crozier TA et al (1996) Comparison of sufentanil-propofol anaesthesia with fentanyl-propofol anaesthesia in patients undergoing major abdominal surgery. Anaesthesist 45;12:1151-1157
24. Badaoui R, Carpentier F, Thouvenin T et al (1996) Comparison of postoperative analgesia with patient-controlled intravenous or epidural sufentanil after colic surgery. Cahiers d'Anesthesiologie 44;6:489-493
25. Haakvanderlely F, Burm AGL, Vankleef JW et al (Reprint 1994) The effect of epidural administration of alfentanil on intraoperative intravenous alfentanil requirements during nitrous-

oxide oxygen alfentanil anesthesia for lower abdominal surgery. Anaesthesia 49;12:1034-1038
26. Chauvin M, Hongnat JM, Mourgeon E et al (Reprint 1993) Equivalence of postoperative analgesia with patient-controlled intravenous or epidural alfentanil. Anesth Analg 76;6:1251-1258
27. Geller E, Chrubasik J, Graf R, Chrubasik S (1993) A randomized double-blind comparison of epidural sufentanil versus intravenous sufentanil or epidural fentanyl analgesia after major abdominal surgery. Anesth Analg 76, 6:1243-1250
28. Taverne RHT, Ionescu TI, Nuyten STM (1992) Comparative absorption and distribution pharmacokinetics of intravenous and epidural sufentanil for major abdominal surgery. Clin Pharmacokinet 23;3:231-237
29. Graf G, Sinatra R, Chung J et al (1991) Epidural sufentanil for postoperative analgesia dose-response in patients recovering from major gynecologic surgery. Anesth Analg 73;4:405-409
30. Vercauteren M, Lauwers E, Meert T et al (1990) Comparison of epidural sufentanil plus clonidine with sufentanil alone for postoperative pain relief. Anaesthesia 45;7:531-534
31. Verborgh C, Van Der Auwera D, Noorduin H, Camu F (1988) Epidural sufentanil for post-operative pain relief: Effects of adrenaline. Europ J Anaesthesiol 5;3:183-191
32. Dyer RA, Anderson BJ, Michell WL, Hall JM (1990) Postoperative pain control with a continuous infusion of epidural sufentanil in the intensive care unit: a comparison with epidural morphine. Anesth Analg 71;2:130-136
33. Weiss BM, Schmid ER, Gattiker RI (1991) Comparison of nalbuphine and fentanyl anesthesia for coronary-artery bypass-surgery-hemodynamics, hormonal response, and postoperative respiratory depression. Anesth Analg 73;5:521-529
34. Black AMS, Wolf A, McKenzie IM et al (1994) Epidural infusions of sufentanil with and without bupivacaine: Comparison with diamorphine-bupivacaine. Europ J Anaesthesiol 11; 4:285-299
35. Rockemann MG, Seeling W, Schirmer U et al (1996) Epidural and intravenous patient controlled analgesia after intraabdominal surgery - a comparison. Anasthesiologie und Intensivmedizin 37;6:332-638
36. De Kock M, Famenne F, Deckers G, Scholtes JL (1995) Anesth Analg 81, 6:1154-1162
37. Vercauteren MP, Coppejans HC, Tenbroecke W et al (1995) Epidural sufentanil for postoperative patient-controlled analgesia (PCA) with or without background infusion-a double-blind comparison. Anesth Analg 80;1:76-80
38. Rockemann MG, Seeling W, Schimer U et al (1996) Epidural and intravenous patient controlled analgesia after intraabdominal surgery - A comparison. Anasthesiologie und Intensivmedizin 37;6:332-338
39. Chrubasik J, Chrubasik S, Ren YG et al (Reprint 1994) Epidural versus subcutaneous administration of alfentanil for the management of postoperative pain. Anaesth Analg 78;6:1114-1118
40. Ostapkovich ND, Baker KZ, Fogarty-Mack P et al (1998) Cerebral blood flow and CO_2 reactivity is similar during remifentanil/N_2O and fentanyl/N_2O anaesthesia. Anaesthesiology 89; 2:358-639

TARGET-CONTROLLED INFUSION (TCI)

Target-Controlled Infusion: Definition, Methods, and Limits

F. Cavaliere, M. A. Pennisi, R. Proietti

Rationale for TCI

The acronym TCI, standing for Target Controlled Infusion, refers to a system by which a drug is given intravenously with a pump controlled by a computer; a TCI system aims to get a target plasma concentration chosen by the user [1]. The importance of getting a steady plasma concentration of a drug lies in the link between that concentration and the concentration near the effector, in the assumption that the intensity of the pharmacological effect is proportional to the latter. Since the 1980s, TCI has been largely employed for controlling intravenous infusion of anaesthetics, analgesics, and sedatives since it is particularly suitable to quickly achieve and then maintain satisfactory degrees of anaesthesia, analgesia, and sedation. However, in last years, the use of this technique has been extended to many other drugs, such as antiarrhythmics, antineoplastics, and antibiotics [2-4], all sharing the common property that their pharmacokinetics can be described by a multicompartment model.

The difficulty of achieving steady blood levels of a drug characterized by a multicompartment pharmacokinetic model without using TCI is exemplified by propofol, which has been one of the first drugs to which TCI technique was applied. Propofol pharmacokinetics can be described by a 2- or 3-compartment model; Figure 1 shows the scheme of a 3-compartment model [1]. Propofol given intravenously enters the compartment 1 or central compartment, in which the concentration is equal to that measured in plasma. Propofol leaves compartment 1 because it is removed by the emunctory systems, such as the liver and the kidney, or because it diffuses into one of the two peripheral compartments, 2 and 3, which differ from each other by the rate of diffusion that is faster for compartment 2. Propofol can as well diffuse from compartments 2 and 3 to the compartment 1 so that the net flux of the drug among the compartments is ruled by the amounts of the drug contained in each of them. At any instant the rates at which propofol diffuses from any compartment or is removed by the emunctory systems can be calculated by multiplying a specific constant by the amount of the drug contained in the compartment from which propofol diffuses or is removed. Each pharmacokinetic model is characterized by a complete set of such constants; for instance, K_{12} relates to the rate of diffusion from compartment 1 to 2, K_{21} to the rate of diffusion from compartment 2 to 1, and so on. K_{10} relates to

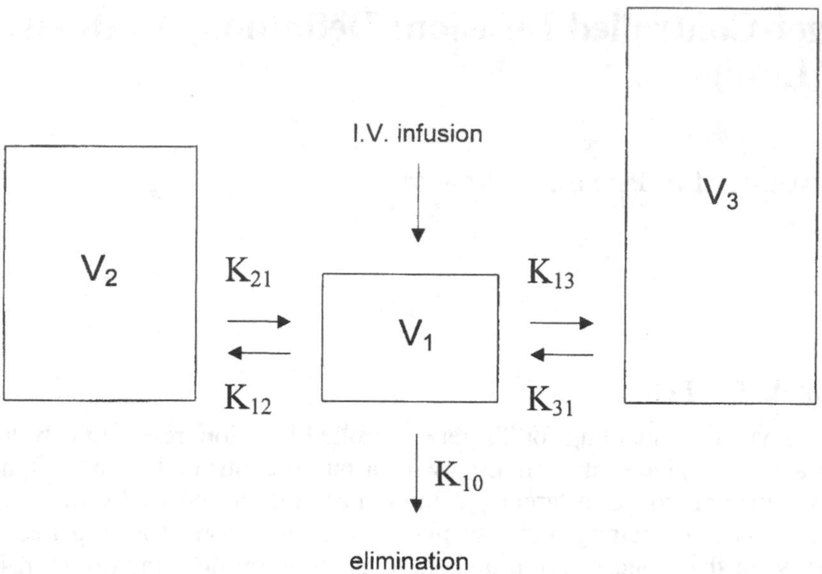

Fig. 1. The scheme of a 3-compartment pharmacokinetic model. V_1 is the central compartment, V_2 and V_3 are the peripheral ones

the rate of removal from compartment 1 by the emunctory systems. The volume of the central compartment, V_1, is also peculiar to each model and is usually expressed by the product of a constant times the weight of the patient.

Figure 2 shows the 6-hour trend of plasma concentration during an intravenous infusion of propofol at the constant rate of 6 mg/kg/h in a subject weighing 50 kg after an initial i.v. bolus of 1 mg/kg. The trend was calculated by an apposite software on the base of a 3-compartment phamacokinetic model developed by Gepts et al. [5]. Propofol concentration increases progressively and stabilizes only about 2 hours following the beginning of the infusion. The difficulty in getting steady plasma levels of propofol with a conventional infusion is caused by the changing rate of diffusion from plasma to tissues. Initially, propofol diffuses from the compartment 1 to compartments 2 and 3 at a faster rate because very small amounts of drug are present in peripheral compartments; as far as these amounts grow, the rate of diffusion to the peripheral compartments decreases since the efflux from compartment 1 is balanced by the diffusion in the opposite direction. A few schemes of intravenous infusion have been suggested for propofol in order to balance the effects of the diffusion among the compartments. Figure 2 shows the 6-hour trend of plasma concentration calculated by the aforementioned software on the base of the scheme proposed by Tackley et al., i,e, an initial bolus of 1 mg/kg is given, followed by an infusion at the rates of 10 mg/kg/h for 10 minutes, 8 mg/kg/h for 10 minutes and then 6 mg/kg/h [6].

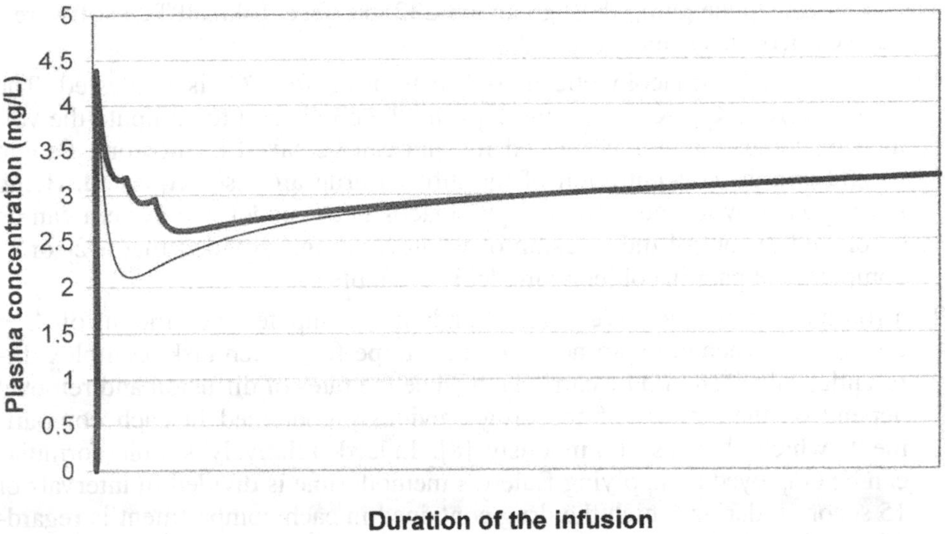

Fig. 2. a) Thin curve: Plasma concentration trend during an infusion of propofol lasting 6 hours, at the rate of 6 mg/kg/h after an initial bolus of 1 mg/kg. The trend was calculated on the base of a 3-compartment pharmacokinetic model by Gepts et al. [5]. b) Thick curve: Plasma concentration trend during an infusion of propofol lasting 6 hours, performed according to Tackley et al. [6]. An initial bolus of 10 mg/kg was given; the infusion was started at the rate of 10 mg/kg/h for 10 minutes, followed by the rate of 8 mg/kg/h for 10 minutes, and then by the rate of 6 mg/kg/h till the end of the infusion. The trend was calculated on the base of a 3-compartment pharmacokinetic model by Gepts et al. [5]

Plasma concentration is steady enough around a value of 3 mg/L, which is usually associated with an adequate level of anaesthesia. The major limit of such schemes is that they do not allow the anaesthetist to change the rate of infusion in order to deepen or lighten the anaesthetic level; in that case plasma concentration is indeed no more stable and follows an unpredictable trend. Target controlled infusion aims to overcome this problem by computing the amount of drug contained in each compartment as long as the infusion is performed on the base of a pharmacokinetic model; the computer is therefore able to regulate the rate of infusion in order to balance the variable amount of propofol that at any time leaves the central compartment.

A system for TCI

Basically, a TCI system includes a computer, a software, and a pump. We developed a system that we called "Visual TCI" [7], in which the software was written in Visual Basic 3 and a Vial Anaesthesia Pump was employed; the computer was connected to the pump through an RS-232 interface. Like all TCI softwares, Visual TCI performs some basic tasks:

1. initially, the pharmacokinetic model to be used for TCI is requested. The constants K_{12}, K_{21}, K_{13}, K_{31}, and K_{10} and the coefficient to compute the volume of compartment 1 are asked for and can be saved in memory. Patient weight and the concentration of the infused drug are also requested. Being not supplied by a predetermined pharmacokinetic model, the system can be employed to control the infusion of whatever drug, provided that a 2- or 3-compartment pharmacokinetic model is available;
2. a routine is performed every 15 seconds that computes the amount of drug contained in each compartment. In order to perform such task, complex differential calculi should be carried out since the rates of diffusion and removal depend on the amount of the drug previously contained in each compartment, which changes continuously [8]. Indeed, relatively simple formulas can be employed by applying Eulero's method: time is divided in intervals of 15 seconds, during which the drug contained in each compartment is regarded as constant. The use of Eulero's method does not cause any significant error in comparison with the use of differential equations [9];
3. a second routine, performed every 30 seconds, computes the amount of the drug that must be given by the pump in order to balance the drug leaving the central compartment. Data are transmitted to the pump by means of two programs. The first, directly controlling the pump, has been supplied by Vial, but only accepts input from the keyboard; the second is Starkey, a commercially available program that transmits data from Visual TCI to the former program as they were supplied through the keyboard;
4. a routine lets the operator change the plasma concentration target;
5. further routines calculate the amount of drug given, the time elapsed from the start of the infusion and the time needed to recover patient's consciousness after stopping the infusion;
6. during TCI several data are supplied to the user, including the estimated concentration of the drug in plasma, the amount of drug contained in each compartment, the duration of the infusion, the estimated arousal time;
7. at the end of TCI, data concerning the infusion can be stored in a file. They include the amount of drug infused and the rate of infusion in each 15-second interval, as well as the correspondent amount of the drug contained in each compartment.

Limits of TCI

What degree of precision can be achieved by a TCI system or, in other words, does the plasma concentration estimated by the system really correspond to the true concentration of the drug in plasma? The parameter commonly employed to evaluate the performance of a system for TCI is the Predictive Error (PE), defined as:

$$PE = 100 \times (Cm - Cs) / Cs$$

where Cm is the measured concentration and Cs that estimated by the system. The limits by now accepted in literature have been defined as: i) mean PE should not exceed 30 and ii) the largest values of PE observed should not exceed 50-60 [10]. Such criteria, which reflect the performances of most TCI systems, allow a rather wide band of oscillation among the values set up by the operator and the real concentration of the drug in plasma. However a further analysis of the sources of error in TCI should be performed since systematic errors that cause nearly constant PE values in the single patient are less harmful than random errors. The former affects the plasma concentration chosen by the operator, but once a correct level of anaesthesia is achieved, the correspondent level of drug in plasma is maintained constant by the system; the latter simply prevents the system from achieving its target.

Different sources of errors can affect TCI:

1. *sources of errors related to the patient*:
   a) influence of age [11] and abnormal anthropometric parameters; for instance, according to some authors, the lean body mass should be utilized instead of the weight in obese patients [12];
   b) conditions like disprotidemia that affect the volume of the central compartment;
   c) decreased drug removal caused by hepatic or renal failure;
2. *sources of errors related to the system*:
   a) Eulero's simplified equations vs differential equations;
   b) oscillations of plasma concentration caused by infusion performed during discrete time intervals alternate to pauses could theoretically affect drug diffusion to peripheral compartments;
3. *sources of errors related to blood sampling*:
   a) plasma concentration to calculate PE should be assessed in arterial samples rather than in venous ones and cycling in drug infusion should be considered;
4. *sources of errors related to the pharmacokinetic model.*

The errors related to the patient are probably the main source of error in TCI, while errors related to the system do not play a major role; particularly no significant difference was observed by comparing computational methods employing Eulero's simplified equations vs differential equations [9].

Usually more than one pharmacokinetic model is reported in literature for one drug and often they differ appreciably. Sometimes a 2-compartment model can be used as well as a 3-compartment one, but also models with the same number of compartments can differ appreciably as far as the values of constants K and, particularly, of V_1 are concerned. Pharmacokinetic models are the description of the trend of plasma concentration in a sample of patients or of healthy subjects and therefore cannot be applied to a single patient without errors [13]. Nevertheless some models could theoretically be more suitable to TCI than others and this hypothesis was investigated by a few authors that compared some pharmacokinetic models during TCI for propofol infusion. Some failed to point out appreciable systematic differences linked to the pharmacokinetic model [14], others found that a higher degree of precision was associated with some pharmacokinetic models [15, 16]. Figure 3 shows the estimated plasma concentration of propofol during an infusion at 6 mg/kg/h lasting 6 hours in a subject weighing 50 kg; 9 different pharmacokinetic models were compared. The figure emphasizes that the highest estimated values were nearly double the lowest ones. Furthermore, curves did not usually cross each other, suggesting that differences among the pharmacokinetic models were poorly affected by the interval of time elapsed from the start of the infusion. We obtained similar results by studying 11 patients undergoing cardiac surgery for myocardial revascolarization who underwent TCI for propofol infusion aimed at a plasma concentration of 2.5 mg/L for one hour prior to cardiopulmonary bypass commencement. Anaesthesia was induced with sodium thiopentone, maintained with sufentanyl, and supplemented with isoflurane if need be. Visual TCI was employed and one of two pharmacokinetic models, by Gepts [5] and by Tackley [6] were randomly assigned to each patient. Propofol concentration was assessed by HPLC in plasma 5, 10, 20, 40, and 60 minutes after TCI commencement. At the end of the infusion, the data relative to the infusion, including the amount of propofol given every 15 seconds, were recorded; such record was successively utilized to compute the plasma concentrations estimated with 13 pharmacokinetic models [6, 17-20]. The results showed a picture very similar to the theoretical one, in which the values estimated by the models showed large differences. Two models, by Gepts et al. [5] and by Tackley et al. [6], predicted the plasma concentrations of propofol more effectively than the others. Besides, ANOVA pointed out that significant differences among PEs were related to the model applied, but not to the time at which samples were collected. Such findings suggest that the estimated volume of the central compartment could play a major role in differences among pharmacokinetic models. Such estimate is particularly important since the main body of calculations performed by TCI concerns the amounts and not the concentrations of the drug in the compartments. Plasma concentration is then obtained by dividing the amount of drug contained in compartment 1 by the estimated volume; as a consequence differences among the estimated volumes can affect PE systematically. By comparing the coefficients utilized for such estimation it is possible to observe that in the models taken into account during the study the highest value is about double the lowest one. Such differences can be at least partly explained because the pharmacokinetic models reported in literature have

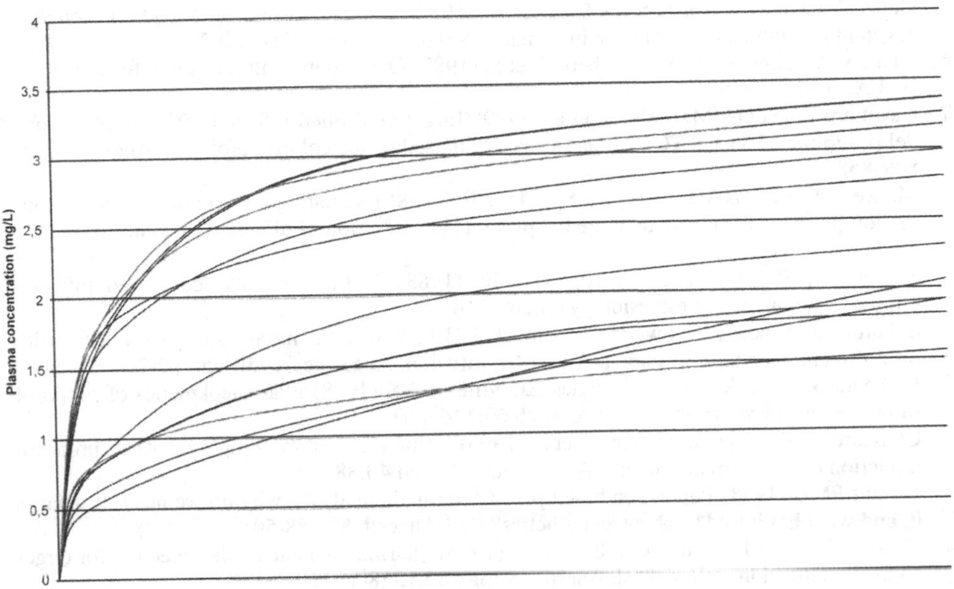

Fig. 3. The trends of plasma concentration and of peripheral compartment contents estimated by different pharmacokinetic models during the intravenous infusion of Propofol lasting 6 hours at the rate of 6 mg/kg/h in a man weighing 50 kg

been obtained with different techniques (bolus vs infusion), sampling (arterial or venous samples), and analyses (whole blood or plasma).

In conclusion, TCI is a powerful technique for managing the intravenous infusion of drugs. Potential clinical and scientific applications are not limited to anaesthesia, but spread to many other clinical fields. However a preliminary evaluation of the precision of the technique and the selection of the best pharmacokinetic model should be performed prior to applying TCI to a new drug.

References

1. Gepts E (1998) Pharmacokinetic concepts for TCI anaesthesia. Anaesthesia 53[Suppl 1]:4-12
2. Woodnutt G, Berry V (1999) Two pharmacodynamic models for assessing the efficacy of amoxicillin-clavulanate against experimental respiratory tract infections caused by strains of Streptococcus pneumoniae. Antimicrob Agents Chemother 43:29-34
3. Bugnon D, Potel G, Xiong YQ et al (1997) Bactericidal effect of pefloxacin and fosfomycin against Pseudomonas aeruginosa in a rabbit endocarditis model with pharmacokinetics of pefloxacin in humans simulated in vivo. Eur J Clin Microbiol Infect Dis 16:575-580
4. Wallace MS (1997) Concentration-effect relations for intravenous lidocaine infusions in human volunteers: effects on acute sensory thresholds and capsaicin-evoked hyperpathia. Anesthesiology 86:1262-1272

5. Gepts E, Camu F, Cockshott ID, Douglas EJ (1987) Disposition of propofol administered as constant rate intravenous infusion in humans. Anesth Analg 66:1256-1263
6. Tackley RM, Lewis GT, Prys-Roberts C et al (1987) Open loop control of propofol infusions. Br J Anaesth 59:935
7. Cavaliere F, Pennisi MA, Meo F et al (1999) Target controlled infusion (TCI): applicazione del programma "Visual TCI" all'anestesia ed alla sedazione col Propofol. Min Anestesiol 65: 849-858
8. Maitre PO, Ausems ME, Vozeh H, Stansky DR (1988) Evaluating the accuracy of using population pharmacokinetic data to predict plasma concentration of alfentanil. Aesthesiology 68: 59-67
9. Shafer SL, Siegel LC, Cooke JE, Scott JC (1988) Testing computer-controlled infusion pumps by simulation. Aesthesiology 68:261-266
10. Schuttler J, Kloos S, Schwilden H, Stoeckel H (1988) Total intravenous anaesthesia with propofol and alfentanil by computer-assisted infusion. Anaesthesia 43[Suppl]:2-7
11. Kirkpatrick T, Cockshott ID, Douglas EJ, Nimmo WS (1988) Pharmacokinetics of propofol (diprivan) in elderly patients. Br J Anaesth 60:146-150
12. Chassard D, Berrada K, Bryssine B et al (1996) Influence of body compartments on propofol induction dose in female patients. Acta Anaesth Scand 40:889-891
13. Wright PMC (1998) Population based pharmacokinetic analysis: why do we need it; what is it; and what has it told us about anaesthetics? Br J Anaesth 80:488-501
14. Coetzee JF, Glen JB, Wium CA, Boshoff L (1995) Pharmacokinetic model selection for target controlled infusions of propofol. Anesthesiology 82:1328-1345
15. Hans P, Coussaert E, Contraine F et al (1997) Predictive accuracy of continuous propofol infusions in neurosurgical patients: comparison of pharmacokinetic models. J Neurosurg Anesthesiol 9:112-117
16. Glen JB (1998) The development of "Diprifusor": a TCI system for propofol. Anaesthesia 53 [Suppl 1]:13-21
17. Marsh B, White M, Morton N, Kenny GNC (1991) Pharmacokinetic model driven infusion of propofol in children. Br J Anaesth 67:41-48
18. Servin F, Desmonts JM, Haberer JP et al (1988) Pharmacokinetics and protein binding of propofol in patients with cirrhosis. Anesthesiology 69:887-891
19. Adam HK, Briggs LP, Bahar M et al (1983) Pharmacokinetic evaluation of ICI 35868 in man. Br J Anaesth 55:97-103
20. Kay NH, Sear JW, Uppington J et al (1986) Disposition of propofol in patients undergoing surgery. Br J Anaesth 58:1075-1079

Target-Controlled Infusion: Clinical Use in Anesthesia and Intensive Care

P. Mastronardi, T. Cafiero, P. De Vivo

Target-controlled infusion (TCI) has been recently introduced. Although it is in its infancy, a lot of clinical experience has shown its use both in anesthesia and intensive care.

The clinical evaluation of TCI in comparison with the manual-controlled infusion cannot be based on patient outcome because in modern anesthesia, mortality and morbidity are very rare events. Therefore it is necessary to rely on the evaluation of recovery time, quality of recovery, variations of physiological parameters (blood pressure, heart rate, breathing, etc.) and other pre-established clinical purposes for the various applications of TCI. Among the proposed infusion techniques, TCI is the most studied by research groups around the world. Nevertheless, TCI has been proposed for the administration of other analgesic and hypnotic drugs. When TCI is used for all intravenous drugs in anesthesia, it will become an integrated part of all anesthetic techniques either for total intravenous anesthesia (TIVA) or for inhalation anasthesia.

In one of the early clinical studies [1], TCI was used to administer alfentanil comparing the computer-assisted technique with intermittent bolus administration. In the group treated with TCI there was a lower incidence of hemodynamic instability, muscle rigidity, and necessity to administer naloxone compared with intermittent boluses. As previously anticipated, the largest clinical studies [2, 3] have been on propofol TCI. These studies indicated that in the group treated with TCI, propofol consumption was higher than in the group treated with manual-controlled infusion, reducing the occurrence of spontaneous movements during anesthesia. A significant preference for TCI was expressed by anesthesiologists, even if it was their first experience with this kind of infusion technique. During the induction of anesthesia, properly selecting the propofol target infusion, it is possible to achieve either a rapid induction (initial target of 10 μg/ml) [4], as like after a starter bolus dose of propofol 2.5 mg/kg, or a smoother and more-gradual induction with a target of 4 μg/ml. The latter target seems to be the best choice in elderly patients and in those with ASA status ≥ III class. The target of 4 μg/ml can be achieved with two different techniques: initial target plasma concentration of 6 μg/ml followed by a reduction to 4 μg/ml when this latter concentration in the biophase has been reached, or directly with a target of 4 μg/ml, awaiting the equilibration with the biophase, which is obtained within

15 min versus 4 min with the other technique. Groups of patients, ASA I or II, premedicated with a benzodiazepine (temazepam) were given propofol by TCI with three different target values (3, 4, and 5 μg/ml), and the induction was considered successful when verbal contact had been lost within 3 min. With similar cardiorespiratory tolerability in the three groups, 40, 75, and 90% successes were recorded [5].

The synergism between propofol and benzodiazepines is well known and, obviously, it is well documented during the induction of anesthesia using TCI. In a randomized study [6] 45 patients, ASA I or II, were divided into three groups and allocated to receive propofol TCI (target 4 μg/ml) with three different protocols as regards the pre-anesthetic medication: 1) no drugs, 2) diazepam 10 mg p.o. 1 h prior to induction, and 3) diazepam 10 mg plus alfentanil 10 μg/kg. In the studied groups induction was successfully achieved in 37, 87, and 93% of patients, respectively. In the remaining patients of each group, the propofol TCI has been continued with two further target values (6 and 8 μg/ml) until complete induction. The mean target value in the three groups was 5.2, 4.9, and 4.4 μg/ml, respectively. The induction with propofol by TCI can also be used in patients with poor cardiocirculatory compliance, starting with initial target plasma concentration of 1-1.5 μg/ml and then adjusting the target by incremental doses of 0.5 μg/ml every 4-5 min. At the cost of a more-prolonged induction, a good hemodynamic stability was achieved. For the maintenance of anesthesia using propofol TCI, as well as for the minimal alveolar concentration (MAC) during inhalation anesthesia, the effective concentration 50 (EC_{50}) has been determined in patients pre-medicated with temazepam [6]. The EC_{50} is the plasma concentration of propofol capable of preventing the motor response to a given stimulus in 50% of patients and is equal to 6 μg/ml. This value is reduced to 4.5 μg/ml in association with 67% nitrous oxide. As the MAC, the EC_{50} can also vary as a function of both clinical factors (age, temperature) and pharmacological factors (concurrent administration of anesthetics or other drugs with depressant activity on the CNS). This means that for the maintenance of balanced anesthesia, when the association with other drugs is unavoidable, the requirement of propofol as a hypnotic component is strictly related to the administration of drugs for achieving the other components of anesthesia.

A low target value of propofol administered by TCI can be used in the maintenance of anesthesia in association with remifentanil which is a "context-insensible" opioid, because even after prolonged infusions it has a context-sensitive half-time of 3-5 min [7]. Remifentanil, therefore, can be administered as a continuous infusion at an adequate rate, in order to occupy a high percentage of receptors, without any delay in the recovery time. The very rapid pharmacokinetics of remifentanil implies the significant reduction of the target plasma concentration of propofol. The decrease in target plasma concentration of propofol due to the concurrent administration of opioids induces a shorter recovery time [8]. The awakening can be generally achieved with a target plasma concentration of about 1.5 μg/ml (range 1-2) even if many factors can affect the recovery time (plasma or biophase concentrations of other CNS depressant drugs, analgesics, pain stimulations).

Furthermore in general anesthesia, TCI is finding new and wider fields of application for sedation, either during local anesthesia or o performing diagnostic or therapeutic procedures without local anesthesia. Co-sedation, with a bolus dose of midazolam (2 mg) with propofol TCI has also been studied; two groups of patients, ASA I or II, undergoing surgery under local anesthesia, in a double-blinded randomized study were allocated to receive either midazolam or normal saline bolus. It has been shown that a low dose of midazolam with the same level of sedation allows a reduction of one-third of the target plasma concentration of propofol in comparison with the control group. Furthermore, there is an evident synergism, potentiating the amnestic activity and decreasing the incidence of side effects, together with a complete correlation with bispectral index (BIS) [9, 10]. Recently the definition of "patient-monitored sedation" (PMS) has been proposed [11], to describe the anesthetic technique based on propofol TCI with a target value of 1 µg/ml, which could be augmented 0.2 µg/ml by the patient, simply by pushing a button with a lockout of 2 min. If for 6 min consecutively there of were no requirements the patient during the initial 20 min of infusion, an automatic decrement of 0.2 µg/ml occurred. After this first period the delivery system reduced the target every 12 min. The mean value of target for an optimal sedation was 0.8-0.9 µg/ml, associated with a good hemodynamic stability without oversedation and necessity for oxygen. In 8 of 36 patients, an oxygen saturation below 92% was found for short periods without prolonging the recovery room stay.

TCI and, especially, the use of the target in the biophase will optimize patient-controlled sedation (PCS) in the near future. The interest in TCI intensive care unit (ICU) patients is also increasing. In 1994 and 1999 [12, 13] experiences have been reported of for pharmacokinetics and pharmacodynamics of midazolam administered by TCI in ICU patients. These articles have shown an inter-individual significant variability and no close correlation between plasma concentrations and sedation score: 200 µg/ml of midazolam can correspond to a sedative level of Ramsey score of 3 to 5! Using propofol TCI it has been demonstrated that the EC_{50} for sedation corresponds to a target concentration of 0.47 µg/ml [14], with a value ranging from 0.3-5. Differences in several studies can also be related to the fact that the wide spread use of TCI is based on the pharmacokinetic model of Marsh [15]. It is not cthe ideal model in critically ill patients, even if a better modulation of sedation is achieved in comparison with manual-controlled infusion. It is expected that soon we will be able to modulate the proper sedation level for the various needs of patients in ICU by means of more-suitable pharmacokinetic software.

Anesthetic drugs that permit the plasma and biophase to rapidly come into equilibrium allow titration of the analgesic or hypnotic effects on the basis of plasma concentrations. Therefore, apart from propofol and alfentanil, remifentanil can also be used by TCI, which can also optimize the safety and manageability of this opioid. Although the pharmacokinetics and pharmacodynamics are known, the manual-controlled infusion of remifentanil can give intrapatient and interpatient variability in opioid plasma concentrations, with poor correlation with the patients' requirements. The same rate of infusion determines plasma concentrations, which are different in a 90-kg patient than a 58-kg patient, or in a 45-year-old patient in comparison with a 68-year-old patient! Remifentanil TCI allows drug administration to better fit the patient requirements. The formulated pharmacological model for remifentanil [16] is sufficiently complete because it considers the age, height, weight, and body surface. The remifentanil TCI, if managed properly during surgery, can be used for the transition to early postoperative analgesia [17]. Also the patient can be involved in the management of infusion [18]. The remifentanil infusion for intra-operative analgesia is progressively reduced to a plasma concentration of 0.1 μg/ml, until the recovery of spontaneous breathing, patients are extubated, and transferred to the post-anesthesia care unit (PACU). In PACU patients can increase the target concentration to 0.2 μg/ml with a lockout of 2 min; without any requirement for 30 min, a decrease in target concentration to 0.1 μg/ml occurred. With method, analgesia with a VAS ≤ 30 can be achieved with a remifentanil target concentration of 2.0 μg/ml, generally associated with arterial oxygen saturation never below 95% and a respiratory rate of 9 breaths/min; with nausea and vomiting in 27 and 10% of cases, respectively.

There have now been numerous studies evaluating analgesia in the postoperative period [19-23], nevertheless pharmacokinetic knowledge in the postoperative period is not supported by valid research. In the early 1990s the research group of Hill was concerned with computer-assisted opioid infusion [24, 25], and the author indicated that opioid TCI was a safe and efficacious method for analgesia [26, 27]. Recently, alfentanil TCI has been compared with morphine patient-controlled administration in the postoperative period after cardiac surgery [20], without evidence of substantial differences between the methods as regards sedation, nausea, vomiting, and hemodynamic response. TCI, besides anesthesia for surgery, can offer several advantages to patients. Some clinical experience shows that alfentanil and remifentanil TCI can determine adequate analgesia in the postoperative period. Unfortunately we have to emphasize that there have been very few double-blinded randomized studies regarding this field of application, and the algorithm to fit the target to the various pain stimulation in the postoperative period or during ICU stay does not exist. The different pain stimulation and various clinical therapeutic maneuvers need rapid changes of the target with a short response in the biophase. For this reason alfentanil and, espccially, remifentanil can be useful drugs due to their rapid pharmacokinetics, allowing short onset and offset times.

The TCI technique for many aspects is analogous to inhalation vapor delivery using a calibrated vaporizer. The pharmacokinetic models of infusion make drug administration easy in relation to the drug concentration in plasma or the in biophase rather than to the drug dosage per kilogram of body weight. The more-widespread use TCI will soon allow an increase in casuistic and clinical studies. So that it will be possible to abolish any gaps of knowledge noted in this pioneering phase from clinical experience in all fields of anesthesia and intensive care.

References

1. Ausems ME, Vuyk J, Hug CC et al (1988) Comparison of a computer-assisted infusion versus intermittent bolus administration of alfentanil as a supplement to nitrous oxide for lower abdominal surgery. Anesthesiology 68:851-861
2. Struys M, Versichelen L, Thas O et al (1996) Comparison of computer-controlled propofol administration with two manual infusion methods. Br J Anaesth 76[Suppl 2]:87
3. Russel D, Wilkes MP, Hunter SC et al (1995) Manual compared with target-controlled infusion of propofol. Br J Anaesth 75:562-566
4. Specialised Data System (1997) PK-SIM version 3.09. Jenkintown, Pa., USA
5. Chaudhri S, White M, Kenny GNC (1992) Induction of anaesthesia using a target-controlled infusion system. Anaesthesia 47:551-551
6. Struys M, Versichelen L, Rolly G (1998) Influence of pre-anaesthetic medication on target propofol concentration using a "diprifusor" TCI system during ambulatory surgery. Anaesthesia 53[Suppl 1]:68-71
7. Davidson JAH, MacLeod AD, Howie JC et al (1993) Effective concentration 50 for propofol with and without 67% nitrous oxide. Acta Anaesthesiol Scand 37:458-464
8. Egan TD, Lemmens HJM, Fiset P et al (1993) The pharmacokinetics of the new short-acting opioid remifentanil (GI87084B) in healthy adult male volunteers. Anesthesiology 79:881-887
9. Vuyk J, Mertens MJ, Olofsen E et al (1997) Propofol anesthesia and rational opioid selection. Determination of optimal EC50-EC95 propofol-opioid concentrations that assure adequate anesthesia and a rapid return of consciousness. Anesthesiology 87:1549-1562
10. Servin FS, Marchand-Maillet F, Desmonts JM et al (1998) Influence of analgesic supplementation on the target propofol concentrations for anaesthesia with "Diprifusor" TCI. Anaesthesia 53:72-76
11. Mastronardi P, De Vivo P, Scanni E et al (1998) Farmaci e modalità di somministrazione. Minerva Anestesiol 64:515-520
12. Irwin MG, Thompson N, Kenny GNC (1997) Patient maintained propofol sedation. Anaesthesia 52:525-530
13. Zomorodi K, Donner A, Somma J et al (1998) Population pharmacokinetics of midazolam administered by target controlled infusion for sedation following coronary artery bypass grafting. Anesthesiology 89:1414-1429
14. Somma J, Donner A, Zomorodi K et al (1998) Population pharmacodynamics of midazolam administered by target controlled infusion in SICU patients after CABG surgery. Anesthesiology 89:1430-1443
15. Barr J, Egan TD, Feeley T et al (1994) The pharmacokinetics and pharmacodynamics of computer-controlled propofol infusions in ICU patients. Clin Pharmacol Ther 55:185
16. Marsh B, White M, Morton N et al (1991) Pharamacokinetic model driven infusion of propofol in children. Br J Anaesth 67:41-48
17. Minto CF, Schnider TW, Egan TD et al (1997) Influence of age and gender on the pharmacokinetics and pharmacodynamics of remifentanil. I. Model development. Anesthesiology 86:10-23
18. Browdle TA, Camporesi EM, Maysick L et al (1996) A multicenter evaluation of remifentanil for early postoperative analgesia. Anesth Analg 83:1292-1297

19. Schraag S, Kenny GNC, Mohl U et al (1998) Patient-maintained remifentanil target-controlled infusion for the transition to early postoperative analgesia. Br J Anaesth 81:365-368
20. Van den Nieuwenhuyzen MCO, Engbers FHM, Burm AGL et al (1995) Computer-controlled infusion of alfentanil versus patient-controlled administration of morphine for postoperative analgesia: a double-blind randomized trial. Anesth Analg 81:671-679
21. Irwin MG, Jones RDM, Visram AR et al (1996) Patient-controlled alfentanil. Target-controlled infusion for postoperative analgesia. Anaesthesia 51:427-430
22. Checketts MR, Gilhooly CJ, Kenny GNC (1998) Patient-maintained analgesia with target-controlled alfentanil infusion after cardiac surgery: a comparison with morphine PCA. Br J Anaesth 80:748-751
23. Van den Nieuwenhuyzen MCO, Engbers FHM, Burm AGL et al (1999) Target-controlled infusion of alfentanil for postoperative analgesia. Contribution of plasma protein binding to intrapatient and interpatient variability. Br J Anaesth 82:580-585
24. Hill HF, MacKie AM, Jacobsen RC (1990) Infusion-based patient-controlled analgesia systems, In: FerranteFM, Ostheimer GW, Covino BG (eds) Patient-controlled analgesia. Blackwell Scientific, Boston, pp 214-222
25. Hill HF, Saeger L, Bjurstrom R et al (1990) Steady-state infusions of opioids in human volunteers. I. Pharmacokinetic tailoring. Pain 43:57-67
26. Hill HF, Jacobson RC, Coda BA et al (1991) A computer-based system for controlling plasma opioid concentration according to patient need for analgesia. Clin Pharmacokinet 20:319-330
27. Hill HF, MacKie A, Coda B et al (1992) Evaluation of the accuracy of a pharmacokinetically-based patient-controlled analgesia system. Eur J Pharmacol 43:67-75

PERIOPERATIVE MEDICINE IN CARDIAC SURGERY

Decision Making in Patients Undergoing CABG

G. Clementi

Every patient has to be considered in relation to the strategy from induction of anaesthesia to the delicate phase of recovery. Sometimes is difficult to establish which one is the target to be reached.

Intraoperative haemodynamic abnormalities are associated with mortality, stroke, or perioperative myocardial infarction (PMI) in patients undergoing coronary artery bypass grafting. In a recent paper Reich et al. [1] reported the results of a large observational study: multivariate logistic regression identified independent predictors of perioperative mortality, stroke, and PMI. Among 2149 patients, there were 50 mortalities, 51 strokes, and 85 PMIs. In the precardiopulmonary bypass (pre-CPB) period, pulmonary hypertension was a predictor of double mortality rate while bradycardia and tachycardia were predictors of three-fold and two-fold higher mortality, respectively.

In the post-CPB period, tachycardia was a predictor of triple mortality rate, diastolic arterial hypertension was a predictor of stroke (OR, 5.4) and pulmonary hypertension was a predictor of PMI (OR, 7.0). Increased pulmonary arterial diastolic pressure post-CPB was a predictor of myocardial infarction (OR, 2.2). Oxygen consumption is usually increased in critically ill patients, but the concept of supply-dependent oxygen consumption has been seriously questioned on the grounds of mathematical coupling and inadequate oxygen consumption measurement. Higher oxygen delivery is associated with increased survival and reduced incidence of organ dysfunction, but it is unclear whether or not this is cause and effect. It may be that the ability of the patient to respond to haemodynamic manipulations with an increase in DO_2 is simply a marker of sufficient physiological reserve likely to produce survival. The ability of a patient to increase oxygen consumption in response to dobutamine has been shown to predict survival [2].

Optimal haemodynamic values during surgery improve outcome in high-risk patients. The maintenance of cardiac output and tissue oxygen delivery depends more on appropriate management of the preload than on the use of inotropes.

Common use of cardiokinetics have been discussed recently because of the risk of desensitization. Desensitization from a clinical perspective has been shown to be important in CHF, a chronic disease in which serum norepinephrine concentrations are elevated and are accompanied by profound and selective b1AR downregulation. Mild uncoupling of the b2AR is apparent in CHF, but occurs to a lesser extent than with b1ARs. In order to prevent or disrupt agonist-induced activation of myocardial bARs resulting in receptor desensitization and CHF, cardiologists now often administer low-dose bAR antagonists to patients with CHF [3].

One can also increase preload so that patients have significantly better visceral perfusion than those at normal preload with addition of inotropes. This higher preload does not adversely affect pulmonary function. When inotropes are indicated, the selection of individual drugs may be important. There appears to be no place for the use of low-dose dopamine for the management of renal dysfunction, but a recent study suggested that fenoldopam may produce beneficial increases in renal blood flow [4]. Whether or not this translates into improved renal outcome remains to be seen. Dopamine may also impair mesenteric tissue oxygenation, and its role in critical care management has been questioned. Adrenaline, despite potential advantages in terms of good inotropic function and peripheral vasoconstriction, has also been shown to impair intestinal mucosal perfusion. One might intuitively assume that ischaemia is bad for vital organs like the heart, regardless of how long it lasts, and that repeated periods of ischaemia are worse. This intuitive belief was in accord with experimental results until the early 1980s. However in 1986, Murry et al. [5] showed that 4 periods of ischaemia for 5 minutes each, separated by 5 minutes of reperfusion, were able to protect the heart (i.e. limit infarct size) during a subsequent 40-min occlusion. They termed this "preconditioning with ischaemia", which later became "ischaemic preconditioning" (IP). The good news for anaesthesiologists is that volatile agents that we routinely use seem to provide a significant protective effect, not only on the myocardium, but also on the vascular endothelium. If endothelium in other vascular beds shows similar degrees of protection, then the use of volatile anaesthetics may provide important protection for a far wider variety of tissues. Over the next few years we can look forward to more detailed explanations of the pathways of anaesthetic preconditioning, as well as of the extent to which other tissues share the beneficial effects observed in the myocardium. Considerable effort will no doubt be expended to develop pharmacological means to maximize protection, perhaps seeking other drugs that can provide the similar kind of protection provided by volatile anaesthetics [6].

Although an important part of the strategy to reduce the systemic inflammatory response, modulation of circuit components (e.g. heparin binding to circuit components) will not be considered here. Attempts to block endothelial cell activation using adhesion molecule-specific agents are in their early investigative stages. Likewise, specific complement inhibitors are undergoing active investigation. Currently, the agents most actively investigated as inhibitors of the systemic inflammatory response are aprotinin and the glucocorticoids.

Aprotinin is a serine protease inhibitor. Its action to prevent excessive bleeding occurring as part of the systemic inflammatory response is due, in part, to its effects on free plasmin present when pathological fibrinolysis is present (e.g. following cardiopulmonary bypass). It does not interfere to any major extent with plasmin bound to the fibrin binding site as part of the normal fibrinolytic cascade. In addition, it blocks the effect of kallikrein to activate the complement cascade and preserves platelet surface adhesive glycoproteins which have been demonstrated to be lost as a result of platelet activation by the cardiopulmonary bypass apparatus thus preserving platelet function. Aprotinin is also associated with vasodilatation due to a direct vascular effect and due to its ability to inhibit conversion of arachidonic acid to the potent vasoconstrictor thromboxane. This may facilitate passage of white blood cells and prevent vascular occlusion by abnormal clumps of white blood cells generated during the systemic inflammatory response. Aprotinin inhibits expression and activity of adhesion molecules on endothelium, thus preventing white blood cells from becoming sticky and adhering to the endothelium. Aprotinin reduces the cytotoxic effects of activated neutrophils on the endothelium and reduces tissue injury produced by lipid peroxidation. Clinically, these effects have been translated into reduced bleeding, improved myocardial performance, reduced pulmonary artery pressures, improved renal perfusion, and reduced adverse neurological events.

Corticosteroids reduce complement activation, and prevent proinflammatory cytokine release which has been associated with improved haemodynamic stability. The production of interleukin-10, an antiinflammatory cytokine, is increased following steroid administration. The coronary blood flow is normally around 225 ml/min but has the potential to vary over a wide range. The aim of this variation, naturally, is to match the coronary blood flow with the myocardial oxygen demand. Epidural anaesthesia with local anaesthetics given for surgical or other medical reasons necessarily provides a sympathetic blockade that allows significant manipulation of critical physiological parameters.

The effects vary depending on a multitude of factors, in particular: the location and extension of the blockade; patients with normal versus diseased coronary arteries. The myocardium and the coronary arteries and arterioles are densely innervated by sympathetic fibres. The sympathetic tone in the coronary circulation normally plays an important role in blood flow regulation both at rest and during exercise, and works in parallel with arteriolar metabolic vasodilatation.

On the other hand, new opioids are available for deep control of stress- and pain-induced haemodynamic impairment. Remifentanil is a short-acting opioid that is commonly used by infusion when given for maintenance of anaesthesia. The quick offset of intraoperative infused remifentanil may result almost in immediate postoperative pain.

Several attempts have been made to use remifentanil to allow fast-track open heart operations. The combination propofol-remifentanil has a substantial role in the haemodynamic managed, safely conducted anaesthesia utilizing EMO (esterase-metabolized opioid) based TIVA (total intravenous anaesthesia).

Sebel et al. investigated the histamine concentration after remifentanil and concluded that a bolus of 2-30 μg/kg is not associated with alteration in histamine concentration [7]. Unlike morphine, the first opioid used in cardiac surgery [8], the decrease in arterial blood pressure observed with remifentanil is not secondary to histamine release.

The main advantage of this kind of anaesthesia is the possibility to extubate the patients as soon as possible, thereby reducing the rate of respiratory complication and LOS (length of stay) while improving the protection of the heart [9].

The interest in cardiac surgery is related to the new techniques of warm extra-corporeal circulation in which total intravenous anaesthesia is preferred.

Royston et al. used this drug in association with propofol to induce and control anaesthesia in CPBG operations [10]. Another advantage is related to the low pulmonary extraction which allows use during CPB [11].

The use of alpha agonists improves the level of analgesia by lowering the haemodynamic instability in the weaning phase [12].

Caution must be used during induction in TIVA because opioids cause muscle rigidity at high doses, and this side effect can complicate anaesthesia induction. In addition the initial arterial concentrations of propofol after IV administration are inversely related to cardiac output. This implies that cardiac output may be a determinant of the induction-required dose of propofol [13] and cardiac output can also be lowered by coinduction with drugs that depress contractility, e.g. midazolam, remifentanil and pentothal, provoking dangerous hypotension during this delicate phase of anaesthesia.

To prevent PMI during laryngoscopy one can reach MAC or MIC BAR (blocking adrenergic response) or associate beta blockers and Ca^{++} antagonists to the induction of anaesthesia [14]. Recently, off-pump techniques have been increasing because of the increasing evidence that CPB continues to be associated with an unacceptable incidence of adverse neurologic events. The cause of these complications is likely a combination of embolic phenomena and hypoperfusion. Whereas elevated perfusion pressures during CPB (> 70 mmHg) may help decrease the incidence of hypoperfusion in some patient groups. This beneficial effect may be offset by increased embolic loads, bleeding complications, compromised myocardial protection and operating conditions. Before becoming routine practice, groups of patient who benefit will need to be differentiated from those harmed by higher perfusion pressure. To date, these appears to be patients with severe atherosclerotic disease (aortic arch or cerebrovascular) or chronic hypertension. Patients who have diabetes or are elderly are at higher risk for adverse neurologic outcome, but whether they will benefit or suffer from the use of higher perfusion pressure during CPB is unknown. Likewise, the optimum perfusion pressure for the remaining patient population has yet to be determined. Currently, there is no rationale for the routine use of perfusion pressures greater than 70 mmHg.

References

1. Reich DL, Bodian CA, Kroll M et al (1999) Haemodynamic predictors of CABG complications. Anesth Analg 89:814-822
2. Polonen P, Roukone E, Hipelainen A (2000) Prospective, randomized study of goal-oriented haemodynamic therapy in cardiac surgical patients. Anesth Analg 90:1052-1059
3. Mathur SV, Swan SK, Lambrecht LJ et al (1999) The effects of fenoldopam, a selective dopamine receptor agonist, on systemic and renal heamodynamics in normotensive subjects. Crit Care Med 27(9):1832-1837
4. Schwinn DA, Leone BJ, Spahan DR et al (1991) Desensitization of myocardial adrenergic receptors during cardiopulmonary bypass: evidence for early uncoupling and late downregulation. Circulation 84:2559-2567
5. Murry CE, Jenning RB, Reimer KA et al (1986) Preconditioning with ischaemia: a delay of lethal cell injury in ischaemic myocardium. Circulation 74:1124-1136
6. Novalija E, Fujita S, Kampine JP et al (1999) Sevoflurane mimics ischaemic preconditioning effects on coronary flow and nitric oxide release in isolated hearts. Anesthesiology 91: 701-712
7. Sebel PS, Hoke J, Westmoreland C et al (1995) Histamine concentrations and haemodynamic response after remifentanil. Anesth Analg 80:990-993
8. Lowestein E, Hallowell P, Levine FH et al (1969) Cardiovascular response to large doses of intravenous morphine. N Engl J Med 281:1389-1393
9. Prakash O, Jonson B, Meij S (1977) Criteria for early extubation after intracardiac surgery in Adults. Anesth Analg 56:703-708
10. Royston D, Kirkham A, Adt M et al (1996) Extubation following CABG using remifentanil based total intravenous anaesthesia (TIVA). Anesthesiology 85(3A):A239
11. Duthie DJR, Stevens JJWM, Doyle AR et al (1997) Remifentanil and pulmonary extraction during and after cardiac anaesthesia. Anesth Analg 84(4):740-744
12. Jage J, Olthoff D, Rohrbach A et al (1997) Clonidine diminishes sympathetic activity after balanced anaesthesia with remifentanil in patients with abdominal hysterectomy - A double blind, placebo-controlled study. Anesthesiology 87(3A):A790
13. Upton RN, Ludbrook GL, Grant C et al (1999) Cardiac output is a determinant of the initial concentrations of propofol after short-infusion administration. Anesth Analg 89:545-552
14. Atlee JL, Dhamee MS, Olund TL et al (2000) The use of esmolol, nicardipine, or their combination to blunt haemodynamic changes after laryngoscopy and tracheal intubation. Anesth Analg 90:280-285

Perioperative Period in the Elderly

P.J.A. VAN DER STARRE

The problem of medical management of the elderly is reported as a major issue from the 1980s, since in earlier years old age was more or less a contraindication for elective major surgery. Particularly in cardiac surgery mean age has increased considerably, from 52 years in the 1980s to 62 years today. In fact it is expected that in the year 2010 22% of the population will be older than 65 years.

It is interesting to observe that in the three major randomized studies published on outcome after coronary bypass surgery [1-3], patients older than 65 years were excluded. In 1988 Acinapura et al. [4] reported a significantly higher mortality in elderly patients (> 70 years) of 7% vs. younger patients (2%) undergoing coronary surgery, but it was striking that the mortality rate did not correlate with different cardiac complications, but that it was attributable to non-cardiac organ failure.

Because of the increased number of complications in the elderly patients compared to the younger ones postoperative hospital length of stay also increases, leading to higher costs. Still, surgery appears to be favourable over medical treatment in the elderly, since 6-year survival in non-operative patients is reported as 64%, and in operative patients 79% [5].

Co-morbidity

In elderly patients (> 65 years) we have to consider the following co-morbidity:
- diabetes mellitus
- cerebrovascular disease
- peripheral vascular disease
- ischaemic heart disease and hypertension
- renal dysfunction

and combinations of these forms of associated diseases.

Diabetes mellitus

Diabetes is the most common endocrine disease and affects 5-10% of the population of 60-80 years [6]. They have an increased risk of morbidity and mortality associated with surgery, including:

- high susceptibility of infection
- hypoglycemia
- hyperglycemia
- cardiovascular autonomic dysfunction and neuropathy

It is for this reason that it is recommended to manage the levels of blood glucose perioperative as closely to normal as possible. This is mostly performed by a continuous infusion of glucose-insulin-potassium, and the continuation with the original therapy when normal feeding is re-established.

Cerebral and peripheral vascular disease

The most devastating complication of cardiac surgery in the elderly is stroke. It is reported in at least 3% of elderly patients, with adverse outcome leading to coma and death [7]. The strongest independent predictor is proximal aortic atherosclerosis, followed by a history of neurological disease. This supports the hypothesis that most strokes are caused by emboli liberated during surgical manipulation of the aorta. It leads to a substantial increase in mortality and hospital length of stay.

A history of neurological disease suggests impaired cerebral blood flow and autoregulation. The use of cardiopulmonary bypass, including unstable systemic blood flow and blood pressure, might induce hypoperfusion of the brain.

Both forms of adverse outcome may be prevented by extensive preoperative evaluation, intraoperative monitoring (TEE!), and perioperative prevention of hypotension and low cardiac output. A less devastating but still disabling complication is long-term postoperative cognitive dysfunction. This is reported in 10% of the patients 3 months following surgery, and in 5% after one year [8]. It is supposed to be due to micro-emboli which cause cerebral ischaemia, particularly during rewarming after hypothermia, when the increase of cerebral metabolic rate of oxygen is not met by an increase in cerebral blood flow. The systemic inflammatory response, induced by surgery and extracorporeal circulation, is more expressed in the elderly, which may contribute to this phenomenon.

Modern surgical techniques like off-pump surgery might improve outcome in this respect, as well as early extubation postoperatively. Perfusion improvements including heparin-coated circuits and the use of special filters could contribute to a better cerebral outcome in the elderly.

Ischaemic heart disease and hypertension

During ageing the cardiovascular reserve diminishes gradually, mainly due to atherosclerosis and consequently progressive ischaemia. Chronic hypertension causes left ventricular hypertrophy and an increased stiffness of the myocardium. As a result the reactive increase of cardiac output as compensation for surgical stress or hypotension is reduced.

Renal dysfunction

Perioperative renal dysfunction is reported in as high as 30% of the patients in complicated cardiac surgery, and is associated with a mortality of 20-50% [9].

Preoperative risk factors for the development of acute renal failure are:

- volume depletion
- hypertension
- congestive heart failure
- diabetes mellitus
- advanced age

It is clear that the kidneys of the elderly patient undergoing cardiac surgery are vulnerable, because mostly more than one of these risk factors are present. An extensive preoperative evaluation including the measurement of creatinine clearance is obligatory to obtain a clear indication of the patients renal status.

Perioperatively the maintenance of an adequate preload, cardiac output and distribution of blood flow in the kidneys are the main tools to prevent deterioration of renal function.

In addition the prevention of prolonged mechanical ventilation might be useful, since it is recognized that positive-pressure ventilation decreases intravascular volume with subsequent decreases of renal blood flow.

Infection and sepsis

Two of the often cited complications of surgery in the elderly are infection and sepsis, attributing to the higher mortality rate. The most appealing mechanisms are:

- diabetes mellitus, with an impaired polymorphonuclear leucocyte function;
- translocation of endotoxinen in the digestive tract, due to poor blood flow in the splanchnic circulation;
- infection from the urinary tract.

These explanations could lead to the assumption that in this group of patients preoperative optimization including selective decontamination of the digestive tract (SDD) should prevent these serious infectious complications.

Conclusions

Cardiac surgery in the elderly is today a routine procedure, but it carries a higher mortality rate than in younger patients, mainly due to non-cardiac complications.

To improve the results three forms of approach are to be considered:

1. preoperative evaluation and optimization, including the treatment of hypovolemia and malnutrition, and the start of decontamination of the digestive tract (SDD) in selected cases;
2. intraoperative maintenance of adequate volume status and cardiac output, and the application of special surgical and perfusion techniques;
3. prevention of prolonged postoperative mechanical ventilation and sedation [10];
4. adequate control of pain, to prevent further stress and consequent mental disorder [11].

References

1. Murphy ML, Hultgren HN, Detre K et al (1977) Treatment of chronic stable angina: a preliminary report of survival data of the randomized Veterans Administration Cooperative Study. N Engl J Med 297:621
2. European Coronary Surgery Study Group (1979) Coronary artery bypass surgery in stable angina pectoris: survival at two years. Lancet 1:889
3. CASS Principal Investigators and Their Associates (1983) A randomized trial of coronary artery bypass surgery; survival data. Circulation 68:939
4. Acinapura J, Rose DM, Cunnungham JN et al (1988) Coronary artery bypass in septuagenarians. Analysis of mortality and morbidity. Circulation 78[Suppl I]:179
5. Gersh BJ, Kronmal RA, Schaff H et al (1985) Comparison of coronary artery bypass surgery and medical therapy in patients 65 years of age or older: a nonrandomized study from the CASS registry. N Engl J Med 313:217
6. Dunnet JM, Holman RR, Turner RC, Sear JW (1988) Diabetes mellitus and anaesthesia. Anaesthesia 43:538
7. Roach GW, Kanchuger M, Mora Mangano C et al (1996) Adverse cerebral outcomes after coronary bypass surgery. N Engl J Med 335:1857
8. Moller JT, Cluitmans P, Rasmussen LS et al (1998) Long-term postoperative cognitive dysfunction in the elderly. Lancet 351:857
9. Aronson S, Blumenthal R (1998) Perioperative renal dysfunction and cardiovascular anesthesia: concerns and controversies. J Cardiothorac Vasc Anesth 12:567
10. Gravlee GP (edn) (1998) On ageing, fast-tracking, and derailment in CABG patients. J Cardiothorac Vasc Anesth 12:379
11. Parikh SS, Chung F (1995) Postoperative delirium in the elderly. Anesth Analg 80:1223

Inflammatory Response to Cardiopulmonary Bypass Cardiac Operations

The Role of Anaesthesia and Steroid Treatment

M. Ranucci, G. Clementi

Anaesthetic management

The role of anaesthetic management, considered in terms of techniques and drug administration, has been outlined for many years as one of the key points inducing major changes in the stress-mediated response to cardiac operations.

Fifteen years ago Slogoff [1] demonstrated that inside the same operating theatre, and using the same pharmacological approach, an anaesthetist was able to induce a perioperative myocardial infarction (POMI) with a ten-fold rate difference compared to his colleagues. Among other factors, stress response is one of the major causes of POMI: recently, Mangano proposed the use of beta-blockers to prevent myocardial ischaemia in high-risk patients [2]. Applying a target value of a heart rate below 55 and systolic arterial pressure below 100, he demonstrated a reduction in mortality and POMI rate.

A well known link exists between myocardial ischaemia and stress-mediated inflammatory response: ischaemia induces lactates release and a decrease in cellular pH, consequently activating host defence response and cytokine release.

Cytokines are a rapidly increasing group of proteins serving as chemical messengers between cells: in innate immunity the effector cytokines are mostly produced by mononuclear phagocytes and natural killer cells; in specific immunity cytokines are produced by activated T lymphocytes (IL-1, IL-6 and TNF). The release of cytokines to counteract bacteremia or endotoxemia can result in catastrophic host responses: TNF, IL-1 and other proinflammatory cytokines act with detrimental effects on many organs during cardiac surgery, both at a local (myocardium) or systemic (kidney, lung, brain) level. IL-6 impairs cardiac function with a consequent negative inotropic effect [3].

The effects of different anaesthetic techniques on the cytokine response during many different surgical procedures have been the topic of many researches, as more and more anaesthetic drugs or techniques became available.

During cardiac operations there is an increased release of IL-6, IL-10, IL-1 and granulocyte-colony stimulating factor, both in cardiopulmonary bypass (CPB) and off-pump procedures. IL-8 release is increased mainly during CPB.

The extent and duration of IL-6 response reflect the severity of the inflammatory changes following a surgical trauma [4].

Pain is one of the key events generating and maintaining the inflammatory response. Stress and hyperalgesia generate the induction of an acute phase response by macrophages and monocytes locally increasing TNF, IL-1 and IL-6; on the other hand, IL-1 and TNF induce hyperalgesia [3], therefore triggering a vicious feedback.

It is therefore not surprising that endogenous or exogenous drugs modulating the pain response may induce changes in the inflammatory response. IL-6 release can be reduced for 7 days after surgery by low-dose ketamine given prior to CPB [5]; exogenous morphine downregulates the activity of immunocompetent cells such as lymphocytes, natural killer cells, granulocytes and macrophages; endogenous morphine increases after the cytokine response elicited by CPB [6].

Regional anaesthesia does not attenuate the acute phase response to cardiac surgery as neuronal blockade does not influence the inflammatory response [7].

Even if, on a theoretical basis, the anaesthetic management could modify the cytokine response and the following postoperative complications, there is still little evidence to support that major changes in anaesthetic management may modify the inflammatory response to cardiac operations with or without CPB: regional anaesthesia or high-dose opioid anaesthesia compared to inhalation anaesthesia do not differ in terms of cytokine release. Brix-Christensen recently demonstrated that during coronary operations the cytokine production was not modified by the type of anaesthesia [8].

Rather than the anaesthetic management, the use of sympathetic modulators such as beta-blockers [2] or alpha adrenergic agonists [9] may induce a beneficial effect respectively in terms of cardiac and pulmonary outcome.

To increase the complexity of this pattern, we must consider that cytokine release should be seen as a balance between proinflammatory and antiinflammatory proteins. IL-10 inhibits the synthesis of many proinflammatory cytokines (TNF, IL-1, IL-6) and attenuates the systemic inflammatory response by suppressing cell mediated immuno response and facilitating antibody production [10].

Gilliand and coworkers could demonstrate that the release of IL-10 is actually modified by the anaesthetic management in non-cardiac surgery [10].

In the cardiosurgical environment, other factors, more related to the homeostatic management rather than anaesthetic drug administration may possibly play a role in modulating the cytokine response.

Kidney filters both proinflammatory and antiinflammatory cytokines but, due to the lower molecular weight, the proinflammatory cytokines are more readily filtered than the antiinflammatory ones [11]. Therefore, maintaining a good renal function during cardiac operations could be beneficial in terms of cytokine balance.

The role of monitoring techniques in this setting is still a matter of debate. No data presently exist to support the fact that an intraoperative monitoring with pulmonary artery catheters (PACs), through a possible more accurate control of cardiac function, may modify the stress-mediated response: as a matter of fact, still there is a strong debate even on the quality of the outcome whether or not using a PAC.

Some authors consider this technique as associated with a higher mortality, greater length of stay, and higher total costs [12], others affirm that a haemodynamic-targeted strategy ($SvO_2 > 70\%$ and lactates < 2 mmol/lt) significantly improves the outcome and reduces mortality [7].

Finally, the role of CPB modifications (heparin-coated materials, leukocyte filtration) in modulating the inflammatory response during cardiac operations is still debated, and besides encouraging biochemical studies no clear evidence of a clinical benefit does presently exist.

Steroid treatment

Immunomodulation by steroids during cardiac surgery has been subjected to a number of studies.

Steroid pretreatment modifies the cytokine response to cardiac surgery [13] but its role in inducing an improvement of clinical outcome is still debated and may be related not only to the dose but even to a correct timing [13, 14].

The majority of the studies focused on steroid treatment in cardiac surgery consider a loading dose of 30 mg/kg of methylprednisolone (MP) at the induction of anaesthesia, even if the use of dexamethasone (1 mg/kg) has been proposed.

Endotoxin translocation has been one of the topics of these studies. Andersen and coworkers [15] failed in demonstrating a limitation of endotoxin release during cardiac operations in a group of patients treated with MP, conversely finding that endotoxemia was more relevant in this group during CPB. Karlstad and coworkers, four years later, confirmed that there were no significant changes in endotoxin levels related to MP use [16]. Conversely, in 1994, Inaba and coworkers demonstrated that MP suppresses endotoxin-like activity during CPB [17].

Complement activation is limited by steroid treatment according to Andersen. This effect seems to be related not only to the alternate pathway activation, but even to a classical pathway inhibition: patients treated with MP have a limited release of both C3a and C4a after protamine administration [18].

A general agreement exists with respect to the role of steroids in modulating the cytokine response to CPB. IL-6 release during CPB is limited in patients treated with MP according to Inaba. In a very recent paper, Kawamura and coworkers [19] studied the influence of MP on cytokine balance during cardiac surgery. Serum IL-6 and IL-8 concentrations increased less after declamping the aorta in the MP group. Conversely, and most importantly, the antiinflammatory

IL-10 concentrations were not affected by steroid treatment, and the same happened for the other antiinflammatory IL-1 levels.

Toft and coworkers [20] studied the effects of MP on the oxidative burst activity of granulocytes during cardiac surgery, not finding any significant effect.

As a result of these and other studies, it seems generally accepted that steroids limit the release of proinflammatory cytokines without affecting antiinflammatory cytokines, therefore positively modifying the balance between the two different cytokine groups.

Whether or not this action results in an improvement of the clinical outcome is still debated, and as a consequence the steroid pre-treatment is not generally accepted in cardiac surgery. According to Toft and coworkers, MP induces a less positive fluid balance and prevents postoperative hyperthermia, without modifying the time on ventilator or the stay in the Intensive Care Unit (ICU).

Yared and coworkers [21] applied a dexamethasone protocol to cardiac patients, demonstrating a lower incidence of shivering.

Pulmonary function has been the topic of some studies considering steroids in cardiac surgery. In 1998 Chaney and coworkers stressed the action of MP on pulmonary function after cardiac operations with CPB [22]. Surprisingly, they found out that patients in the MP group had a larger increase in postoperative A-a oxygen gradient and intrapulmonary shunt, with no difference in static lung compliance and dead space. Patients in the MP group suffered a prolonged tracheal intubation and did not demonstrate any difference in ICU stay.

The apparent discrepancy between the well-defined limitation of the inflammatory response and the lack of a clear clinical advantage is common to many studies involving cardiac surgery with CPB and antiinflammatory strategies. The main problems of these studies are a) a limited amount of patients enrolled and b) the low rate of severely ill patients. In the majority of the cardiac surgery patients the cytokine changes previously described are not associated with clinical detectable sequelae. This, in part, is the result of the well functioning body's control mechanism restoring the immunological homeostasis. Nevertheless, some patients develop an inflammatory mediated organ failure, and there is some evidence that the longer or more complex is the surgery, and the worse is the patient's profile, the greater is the inflammatory response and the complications rate.

Due to all the above reasons, more clinical studies are required enrolling either large numbers of low-risk patients or smaller cohorts of high-risk patients to better elucidate the clinical role of steroids in cardiac surgery.

References

1. Slogoff S, Keats AS (1985) Does perioperative myocardial ischaemia lead to postoperative myocardial infarction? Anesthesiology 62:107-114
2. Mangano DT, Layug EL, Wallace A et al (1996) Effect of atenolol on mortality and cardiovascular morbidity after non cardiac surgery. N Engl J Med 335:1713-1720
3. Sheeran P, Hall GM (1997) Cytokines in anaesthesia. Br J Anaesth 78:201-219
4. Crickshank AM, Fraser WD, Burns HJG et al (1990) Response of serum interleukin-6 in patients undergoing elective surgery of varying severity. Clinical Science 79:161-165
5. Roytblat L, Talmor D, Rachinsky M et al (1998) Ketamine attenuates the interleukin-6 response after cardiopulmonary bypass. Anesth Analg 87:266-271
6. Brix-Christensen V, Tonnesen E, Sanchez RG et al (1997) Endogenous morphine levels increase following cardiac surgery as a part of the inflammatory response? Int J Cardiol 62: 191-197
7. Poloner P, Roukone E, Hipelainen A (2000) Prospective, randomized study of goal oriented haemodynamic therapy in cardiac surgical patients. Anesth Analg 90:1052-1059
8. Brix-Christensen V, Tonnesen E et al (1998) Effects of anaesthesia based on high vs. low doses of opioids on the cytokine and acute-phase protein responses in patients undergoing cardiac surgery. Acta Anaesthesiol Scand 42:63-70
9. Procaccini B, Clementi G, Varrassi G (1993) Effetti della clonidina vs trinitroglicerina sul bilancio di ossigeno miocardico e sullo scambio gassoso polmonare durante e dopo intervento di rivascolarizzazione miocardica. Minerva Anestesiol 235-245
10. Gilliand HE (1997) The choice of anaesthetic maintenance technique influences the antiinflammatory cytokine response to abdominal surgery. Anesth Analg 85:1394-1398
11. Gormley SMC, Armstrong MA, McMurray TJ et al (1998) Comparison of plasma and urinary pro and antiinflammatory cytokine changes during cardiac surgery. Br J Anaesth 81:639P
12. Ramsey RS, Sullivan SS, Lory Dey L et al (1998) Clinical and economic effects of pulmonary artery catheterization in non emergent coronary artery bypass graft surgery. J Cardiothor Vasc Anesth 14:113-118
13. Lodge AJ, Chai PJ, Daggett CW et al (1999) Methylprednisolone reduces the inflammatory response to cardiopulmonary bypass in neonatal piglets: timing of dose is important. J Thorac Cardiovasc Surg 117:515-522
14. Tennenberg SD, Bailey WW, Cotta LA et al (1986) The effects of methylprednisolone on complement-mediated neutrophil activation during cardiopulmonary bypass. Surgery 100:134-142
15. Andersen LW, Baek L, Thomsen BS et al (1989) Effect of methylprednisolone on endotoxemia and complement activation during cardiac surgery. J Cardiothorac Anesth 5:544-549
16. Karlstad MD, Patteson SK, Guszca JA et al (1993) Methylprednisolone does not influence endotoxin translocation during cardiopulmonary bypass. J Cardiothorac Vasc Anesth 7:23-27
17. Inaba H, Kochi A, Yorozu S (1994) Suppression by methylprednisolone of augmented plasma endotoxin-like activity and interleukin-6 during cardiopulmonary bypass. Br J Anaesth 72:348-350
18. Loubser PG (1997) Effect of methylprednisolone on complement activation during heparin neutralization. J Cardiovasc Pharmacol 29:23-27
19. Kawamura T, Inada K, Nara N et al (1999) Influence of methylprednisolone on cytokine balance during surgery. Crit Care Med 27:545-548
20. Toft P, Christiansen K, Tonnesen E et al (1997) Effect of methylprednisolone on the oxidative burst activity adhesion molecules and clinical outcome following open heart surgery. Scand Cardiovasc J 31:283-288
21. Yared JP, Starr NJ, Hoffmann-Hogg L et al (1998) Dexamethasone decreases the incidence of shivering after cardiac surgery: a randomized, double-blind, placebo controlled study. Anesth Analg 87:795-799
22. Chaney MA, Nikolov MP, Blakeman B et al (1998) Pulmonary effects of methylprednisolone in patients undergoing coronary artery bypass grafting and early tracheal extubation. Anesth Analg 87:27-33

Fast Track Cardiac Surgery

The Italian Multicenter Study on Steroids in Coronary Bypass Surgery

B. Biagioli, G. Grillone

The evolution of cardiac surgery in the last decade has been particularly exciting for its broadening of the indications related to age, the seriousness of the pathology and the patients treated, not to mention the regard paid to containment. The approach which goes by the name "Fast Track cardiac surgical pathways" is most certainly, along with the mini-invasive techniques, a fundamental component in this procedure.

Through their knowledge of perioperative physiopathology, anaesthetists have had the great opportunity of taking part in this evolution, defining protocol and implementing measures with the aim of reducing costs and thereby allowing for better use of resources. This objective was not achieved by merely stripping down procedures, but through a determined attempt to reduce the morbidity and mortality rates related to the modifications in surgical and anaesthetic trauma and as such can even be considered a measure of quality control [1].

The anaesthetic treatment that goes by the name of "Fast Track cardiac anaesthesia", the focal point of the aforementioned "Fast Track cardiac surgical pathways" would allow for extubation within 1 to 6 hours after surgical intervention. The attainment of this objective respecting physiopathological feedback is both the aim and at the same time the control of a therapeutic process whose approach is multi-disciplinary [2].

The first question that we might ask, together with Cheng, is the following:

Is Fast Track cardiac anaesthesia safe?

There are numerous observational studies in this regard that are inevitably compared to the Pre-Fast Track cohort study. London et al. [3] in particular did not reveal a rise in the post-operative mortality and morbidity rates. In a prospective randomized controlled trial, Cheng et al. [4] recently demonstrated that early extubation did not increase postoperative cardio-respiratory or sympathoadrenal stress, morbidity or mortality rates.

The next question then is:

How early should patients be extubated?

Many authors agree on the fact that while it may be possible to extubate the patient while on the operating table, this practice is not advisable for many hospital centres, indeed the risk of hypothermia, bleeding and circulatory instability may even thwart our attempts to reduce costs as they would necessitate further time in the operating room [6, 7]. There is, however, consensus on the fact that extubation can safely occur within 1 to 6 hours after surgical intervention [4]. On the other hand, early extubation has not necessarily been proven to lead to early discharge from the ICU or the hospital. Even the use of short-acting anaesthetics, while facilitating extubation, does not seem to affect the aforementioned discharges [5].

Some centres, after having acquired experience in this type of approach, have then broadened it to include patients in compromising pre-operative conditions, without increased risk. As such, a conviction arises as to the possibility of establishing a pathway for cardiac surgery patients that excludes the necessity of ICU and allows them to pass directly from the recovery room into the post-cardiac surgical unit where the level of care is less intense [6].

In order to opt for a less intense alternative in addition to having a quicker discharge from the ICU, the recovery of the patient's mental state after extubation is a key point and this too has been demonstrated as occurring faster after early extubation [7].

Is CPB a SIRS model?

A great deal of evidence shows the ability of CPB to set off a generalized inflammatory response characterized by large fluid shifts, temperature changes, coagulation disturbances, increased concentrations of catecholamines and stress hormones, neutrophil attachment, transmigration of neutrophils into the interstitial space and release of large amounts of free radicals. This syndrome, tied to blood contact with extraneous surfaces and inevitable conditions of regional ischaemia-reperfusion during extracorporeal circulation, is often responsible for an increased waste of energy, metabolic and circulatory instability, and may evolve into multi-organ failure [8]. The steroids pretreatment modifies the inflammatory response to cardiac surgery but its role in inducing an improvement of clinical outcome is still under debate [9, 10]. The possible inflammatory response reduction combined with early extubation are supposed to be the base of a management plan aimed at improving surgical and anaesthesiological efficiency [11-16].

We undertook a prospective, controlled, clinical trial to evaluate morbidity outcomes and the safety of Fast Track anaesthetic management and steroids pretreatment. In order to achieve the substantial number of participants necessary to properly analyze data results, five Italian cardiac anaesthesia centres collaborated in the undertaking of this study; to obtain a more balanced comparability of the groups, only low-risk CABG patients were selected.

Patient selection, anaesthesiological and postoperative management

Patients were selected according to the following criteria:

- *preoperative phase*: adequate left ventricular function (FE < 40%), creatinine < 1.6 mg/dl, elective intervention, not a redo operation, Ht > 38%, non-BPCO, diabetics not engaged in therapy, no active gastropathic disorder, no colelitiasis or colecystectomy, Higgins score < 3;
- *operative phase*: CEC not complicated and of a duration of < 150 min, low or absent dosage of inotropic drugs at CEC off, no alterations in ECG ischaemic (complete revascularization), CEC conducted in moderate hypothermia (not < 32°C), utilization of blood bank < 3 units;
- *postoperative phase*: haemodynamics stable and adequate, no significant arrhythmia, complete warming (axillar temp > 36°C), adequate peripheral perfusion (peripheral pulse at least 3 out of 4), adequate diuresis (> 1 ml/kg/h), bleeding < 100 ml/h after 2 hrs, neurologically unharmed, pH > 7.35 and $PaCO_2$ < 50 mmHg in vs. or with p. supp < 10 cm H_2O with FiO_2 < 50%, PaO_2 > 70 mmHg.

Patients were randomized into two groups - the first treated with steroids and the second not treated (control group). By the end of the study, however, there were far more patients enrolled in the control group because of the drop-out rate in the treated group.

The verification of stable conditions in each phase determines the course or the interruption at any moment of the study's protocol.

The pre-anaesthesia is done with phenobarbital 100 mg the evening before the operation; morphine 0.1 mg/kg and scopolamine 0.5 mg the morning of surgery; metoclopramide 10 mg, ranitidine 50 mg before entering the O.R.; induction is done with fentanyl 5 y/kg, diazepam 0.3 mg/kg, and pancuronium 0.1 mg/kg; isoflurane < 1% + O_2/NO_2 50%, and atracurium 0.01 mg/kg/min are used to maintain state; and fentanyl 10-15 y/kg is administered before the sternotomy. At CEC on, the isoflurane is suspended and tiopentone 5 mg/kg is used, and propofol 4-6 mg/kg/h is begun. In the ICU sedation is maintained with propofol 1-3 mg/kg/h and morphine 1-6 mg/h.

Anaesthetic management differed, however, in that the treated group was administered metilprednisolone (MPS) 1 gr before entering the OR and another 125 mg at CEC off. In the ICU an additional bolus of MPS 125 mg/6 h was administered.

As this study is a collaborative effort, the anaesthesiological protocol permits each Centre to vary its procedure with regards to pharmaceutical type and dosage while remaining within the constraints of anaesthesiological conduct aimed at early extubation.

Results and discussion

The 349 patients enrolled in this study were divided in two groups: the 1st treated with steroids (147 patients) and the 2nd (control group) did not receive any steroid medication (202 patients). The mean age of the two groups was similar, 62 years (44-75) for the steroid group and 65 years (41-75) for the control group. The surgical time was longer for the control group (304 min) than for the steroid group (285.6 min), with $p > 0.05$. 4 patients from the 1st group and 9 pts from the 2nd underwent single CABG; 38 patients from the 1st group and 54 patients from the 2nd underwent double CABG; 78 from the 1st group and 86 patients from the 2nd underwent triple CABG; finally, 22 patients from the 1st group and 51 patients from the 2nd underwent quadruple or more CABG. We found no statistical differences in age, gender or number of grafts performed between the groups. The haemodynamic parameters monitored: cardiac rate, mean arterial pressure, left atrial pressure, central venous pressure were similar in the two groups and at the times considered. A relevant difference was noted in the trend of central temperature: at T0 (ICU admission) this parameter was the same for both groups; at T1 (extubation time) and T2 (3 hours after extubation) the central temperature was higher in the control group, $p > 0.05$. These results in addition to a lower systemic vascular resistance in the control group might be related to a higher inflammatory response in comparison to the treated group.

Differences were also noted in the number of complications both during and after surgery. The complications under examination in this study were as follows: resternotomy, myocardial infarction, inotropic support, atrial fibrillation, coma and encephelopathy, A/V block necessitating pacemaker, creatinine > 2, dialysis, $PaO_2 < 50$ and $PaCO_2 > 60$, OT intubation > 24 h, and transfusion.

The perioperative incidence was lower in the group with steroids (11.6%) than in the control group (13.9%). This difference increased in the incidence of postoperative complications with 13 patients (10%) in the steroid group and 34 (16.4%) in the control group being affected. The complications which decreased remarkably in the steroid group were resternotomy for bleeding (1.4 vs. 5%) and atrial fibrillation (1.4 vs. 5.4%). These results might be explained by the hypothesis that the systemic side effects of cytokines were limited reducing inflammatory response, and as such improve myocardial performance, vascular microcirculation and coagulation [4, 5]. The hyperadrenergic status and the pericarditis were described as risk factors predisposing to atrial fibrillation after CPB [6]. The results of the complications, while intriguing, necessitate further examination as the outcome of patients was basically similar in the two groups: in the steroid group both the mechanical ventilation hours and ICU-stay hours were slightly less.

At the time of discharge, patients were presented with a questionnaire enquiring about their state upon awaking; the need for analgesics; ability to collaborate; satisfaction with the entire procedure. Answers were limited to Yes = 1; No = 2; I don't know = 3. Patients in the steroid group showed significantly less pain upon waking necessitating fewer analgesics, 10.88% vs. 20.20%. In conclusion, our results suggest that by decreasing inflammatory reaction with steroids administration, it might be possible to accelerate recovery rendering the patient more autonomous and able to collaborate and with diminished postoperative pain.

References

1. Cheng DCH, Karski J, Peniston C et al (1996) Early tracheal extubation after coronary artery bypass graft surgery reduces costs and improves resource use: A prospective randomized controlled trial. Anesthesiology 85:1300-1310
2. Cheng DC (1998) Fast Track cardiac surgery pathways: Early extubation, process of care, and cost containment. Anesthesiology 88:1429-1433
3. London MJ, Shroyer AL, Coll JR et al (1998) Early extubation following cardiac surgery in a veterans population. Anesthesiology 88:1447-1458
4. Cheng DCH, Karski J, Peniston C et al (1996) Morbidity outcome in early versus conventional tracheal extubation following coronary artery bypass graft (CABG) surgery: A prospective randomized controlled trial. J Thorac Cardiovasc Surg 12:755-764
5. Butterworth J, James R, Prielipp RC et al (1998) Do shorter-acting neuromuscular blocking drugs or opioids associate with reduced intensive care unit or hospital length of stay after coronary artery bypass grafting? Anesthesiology 88:1437-1446
6. Westaby S, Pillai R, Parry A et al (1993) Does modern cardiac surgery require conventional intensive care? Eur J Cardiothorac Surg 7:313-318
7. Chong JL, Grebenik C, Sinclair M et al (1993) The effects of a cardiac surgical recovery area on the timing of extubation. J Cardiothorac Vasc Anaesth 7:137-141
8. Herskowitz A, Mangano DT (1966) Inflammatory cascade a final common pathway for perioperative injury? Anesthesiology 85:957-960
9. Lodge AJ, Chai PJ, Daggett CW et al (1999) Methylprednisolone reduces the inflammatory response to cardiopulmonary bypass in neonatal piglets: timing of dose is important. J Thorac Cardiovasc Surg 117:515-522
10. Tennenberg SD, Bailey WW, Cotta LA et al (1986) The effects of methylprednisolone on complement-mediated neutrophil activation during cardiopulmonary bypass. Surgery 100: 134-142
11. Kevin HT, Bradley CA, Gauldie J et al (1995) Steroid inhibition of cytokine-mediated vasodilation after warm heart surgery. Circulation 92[Suppl II]9:347-353
12. Wan S, Le Clerc JL, Vincent JL (1997) Inflammatory response to cardiopulmonary bypass. Chest 112:676-692
13. Frering B, Philip I, Rolland C et al (1994) Circulating cytokines in patients undergoing normothermic CPB. J Thor Cardiovasc Surg 108:636-641
14. Hall R, Smith MS, Rocker G (1997) The systemic inflammatory response to cardiopulmonary bypass pathophysiological, therapeutic, and pharmacological considerations. Anesth Analg 85:766-782
15. Hennein HA, Ebba H, Rodriguez JL (1994) Relationship of the proinflammatory cytokines to myocardial ischemia and dysfunction after uncomplicated coronary revascularisation. J Thor Cardiovasc Surg 108:626-635
16. Bharucha DB, Kowey PR (2000) Management and prevention of atrial fibrillation after cardiovascular surgery. Am J Card 85:20D-24D

ORGANIZATION, TECHNIQUES, DECISION MAKING

Postoperative Morbidity - What the Anaesthetist Needs to Know

F. CARLI

Despite advances in anaesthesia care and surgical techniques, major surgery is still beset with undesirable consequences among which the most important are infection, thrombo-embolic and cardiorespiratory complications, cerebral dysfunction, gastrointestinal paralysis, pain, fatigue and prolonged convalescence. Although postoperative morbidity can be related to some imperfections of surgery and anaesthesia, complications do occur regardless of surgical skills and drug regimens. One could ask the simple question: why is a successful operation followed by an unsuccessful postoperative period? Clearly, the key pathogenic factor in postoperative morbidity is the surgical stress response with subsequent demands on organ function.

Postoperative morbidity

Cardiovascular complications

Perioperative cardiac morbidity is the leading cause of death after anaesthesia and surgery. It is generally defined as the occurrence of myocardial ischaemia, unstable angina, congestive heart failure, serious dysrhythmias or cardiac death. Cardiac complications occur in 2-4% of patients undergoing major surgery, with greater incidence (up to 20%) in those patients with preoperative risk factors [1]. In spite of intraoperative monitoring and cardiovascular support therapy, cardiac complications occur during the postoperative period, particularly within the first four postoperative days. A recent study [2] reported that in a selected population cardiovascular complications are not uncommon during the first 24 hours after surgery. At times this can be fatal. Cardiovascular complications are uncommonly associated with symptoms, making clinical detection difficult. The pathogenesis of postoperative cardiac morbidity is multifactorial and includes sympathetic stimulation, tachycardia, increased cardiac work, altered coagulation and hypoxaemia.

Pulmonary complications

Postoperative pulmonary complications (atelectasis, pneumonia) can be related to postoperative impairment of pulmonary function in addition to other perioperative factors. On direct measurements, lung volumes are decreased by 30-40%. Compliance is decreased because of the decrease in FRC [3]. Work of breathing is also increased. These changes are present immediately after operation, evolve slowly over 2-3 days, and return to normal in young patients after five days, while it takes longer in elderly [4]. The extent and duration are greatest for operations of the thorax and upper abdomen, and progressively decrease for operations situated more distally and more superficially. Increased pulmonary hydrostatic pressure, decreased plasma oncotic pressure, and increased capillary permeability may all occur in the surgical patient. All these states will cause increased pulmonary extravascular water and deterioration of lung function. The incidence of pulmonary complications varies between 1-4% following non-thoracic surgery and 20-30% after thoracic surgery [5].

Thromboembolic complications

The formation of deep vein thrombosis (DVT) is dependant on interactions between endothelial injury, venous stasis and a hypercoagulable state. Within minutes of venous obstruction, in the presence of surgical injury, leukocytes and platelets adhere to the endothelium with formation of clots. During total hip arthroplasty, the time of maximal thrombogenesis occurs when the femoral component is inserted. Thrombogenesis is most pronounced after a cemented prosthesis is inserted [6]. The duration and extent of femoral venous occlusion occurring during hip arthroplasty are related to the genesis and timing of intraoperative pulmonary embolism. Amplifying factors are concomitant diseases and immobilization. The incidence of DVT varies between 10-20% for hip arthroplasty and 18-50% for knee arthroplasty.

Gastrointestinal dysfunction

Postoperative gastrointestinal complications are related to disturbances of motility resulting in ileus, nausea and vomiting. The frequency varies between 20 and 50%. The development of these sequelae is related to the operative site, the intensity of surgical trauma, the use of anaesthetic agents and opioids. Inhibitory sympathetic efferents are activated by surgery and pain. Nausea and vomiting result from direct neurogenic stimulation of the vomiting center. Surgery promotes breakdown of gut mucosal barrier function, leading to translocation of endotoxins [7].

Confusional states and delirium

Cerebral dysfunction is a common postoperative complication associated with poor functional recovery and longer duration of hospital stay. Specific risks are: age greater than 70 years [8], poor preoperative cognitive function, alcohol abuse, altered serum electrolyte concentrations, use of psychoactive medications, hypoxaemia, and sleep disturbances. The incidence varies between 2 and 15% in patients over 50 years.

Fatigue

Fatigue is a common complication and patient complaint after surgery. It is not clear what is the physiologic explanation of fatigue. Early fatigue may be related to postoperative sleep disturbances, inflammatory mediators and increased protein breakdown. Late fatigue appears to be related more to cardiorespiratory deconditioning, loss of body weight, and loss of muscle mass and function [9]. Preliminary investigations using a quality of life questionnaire (SF36) at three and six weeks after major abdominal surgery indicate that patients are physically tired and unable to perform up to 25% of the daily chores [10]. In contrast, the mental component remains intact (score after surgery greater than before surgery) indicating that they had overcome successfully the psychological burden of surgery. The greater the magnitude of surgery and the preoperative fatigue score are, the more fatigued patients are after surgery.

Features of perioperative pathophysiology

Preoperative organ dysfunction

Medical and surgical dysfunctions before surgery interfere with the healing process. Correction of anaemia, normalization of blood pressure, optimization of respiratory function in high-risk patients before surgery, and control of diabetes can decrease postoperative complications. Several clinical guidelines and indices have been developed to assess cardiovascular, respiratory and nutritional risks. The scoring system, while of use in quantifying the risk, does not influence postoperative morbidity per se, unless it is implemented as a tool for correcting the dysfunction [11].

Stress response

The surgical stress response contributes to organ dysfunction, loss of body protein and increased demands of physiological reserve. The body is alerted to the surgical insult by two afferent signals: neuronal and inflammatory afferent responses. Neuronal responses are activated through nociceptive pathways. Inflammation is associated with the production of cytokines, prostanoids, complement and other inflammatory factors that act locally to facilitate host defence and repair. Both neuronal and inflammatory systems modulate endocrine and metabolic responses which might be detrimental to the body and are implicated in the development of postoperative morbidity. The magnitude of the response is related to the intensity of surgery. Development of hyperglycaemia, increased secretion of catabolic hormones, hypermetabolism, breakdown of body proteins, fluid retention, altered coagulation and fibrinolysis are some of the changes associated with surgical stress. The distinguishable feature of debility after surgery is muscle wasting, a consequence of disuse and accelerated muscle protein breakdown. The increased protein breakdown serves to mobilize amino acids for synthesis of new protein tissue in wounds, for proliferation of macrophages, and other cellular components involved in human healing, and for synthesis of acute phase proteins and glucose in the liver. Although we can block, to some extent, the neurogenic component, our ability to inhibit detrimental activation of the inflammatory responses is limited by our restricted understanding.

Hypothermia

Anaesthesia contributes considerably to hypothermia if patients are not insulated or actively warmed. The patient's core temperature often falls 1.0-1.5°C during the first hour of anaesthesia. In the subsequent few hours, core temperature decreases at a slower rate. Approximately 90% of body heat loss is through the skin surface, with radiation and convection contributing more than evaporative or conductive losses. Although hypothermia confers some neuroprotective effects in specific surgery, the consequences of hypothermia are detrimental to the body. Among the complications induced by mild hypothermia are impaired coagulation, sympathetic hyperactivity with increased oxygen demand and vasoconstriction leading to myocardial ischaemia, impaired resistance to surgical wound infection and loss of body nitrogen.

Haemorrhage and blood transfusion

The use of perioperative blood transfusion correlates with an increased risk of infective complications and probably recurrence after cancer surgery, as a result of the content of white cells and non-cellular transfusion components [12]. Toxic mediators such as histamine and myeloperoxidase can be released from leucocytes and platelets during storage. On the other hand there are several risks associated with a haemoglobin concentration of less than 9-10 g/dl in patients with coronary artery disease or comorbid conditions.

Immunosuppression

Major surgery causes immunosuppression with reduced delayed hypersensitivity response to recall antigen stimulation, T-cell-dependent antibody response, IL-2 production and HLA-DR antigen expression, IFN-γ production and T cell blastogenesis. In contrast, neutrophil and macrophage functions are activated with increased release of oxygen radicals, TNF, and chemotaxis. Perioperative blood transfusion enhances postoperative immunosuppression. Perioperative immunological changes increase susceptibility to infective complications [13, 14].

Pain

Pain is a common feature of surgery. It amplifies the metabolic response, autonomic reflexes, ileus and nausea and delays mobilization and feeding. The effect of improved pain relief alone on postoperative outcome is controversial [15], particularly with opioids whether used parentally or via epidural route.

Hypoxaemia

Postoperative episodic hypoxaemia and sleep disturbances appear to be related phenomena in patients following major non-cardiac surgery [16]. Postoperative constant hypoxaemia is thought to result from a pulmonary shunt due to diaphragmatic dysfunction. Postoperative episodic hypoxaemia is primarily due to pain to stress-induced sleep disturbances. Hypoxaemia occurs most often on the second and third nights after major surgery. There is considerable evidence that late postoperative hypoxaemia is involved in the pathogenesis of cardiac [17], cerebral and wound complications [18] after major surgery.

Sleep disturbances and brain dysfunction

Sleep disturbances (alterations in REM sleep) are associated with sympathetic activation, haemodynamic instability, swing in blood pressure and heart rate, and increased urinary excretion of catecholamines. They are related to the degree of surgical trauma and, thereby, to the surgical stress response. Cortisol, sympathetic discharge and cytokines can lead to abnormal sleep [19]. In addition, opioids can exacerbate sleep disturbances by altering the ventilatory pattern. Postoperative impairment in cognitive function and delirium can be related to hypoxaemia. Low oxygenation values throughout the night correlate with confusion.

Ileus

Ileus is a neurogenic stress response [20]. The large bowel, especially the descending colon, takes the longest time to recover normal motility after surgery. Increased sympathetic activity and nociceptive stimulation inhibit gut function and motility. Ileus is recognized as abdominal distension which results in third space loss of fluids and electrolytes. Increased intracolonic pressure may decrease colonic blood flow and affect the integrity of bowel anastomosis by decreased perfusion and pressure effects. Breakdown of mucosal barrier function leads to bacterial overgrowth, translocation of endotoxins and development of organ failure [7].

Wound

The surgical wound is not only the site of tissue disruption but also a site of inflammation and repair. The cellular processes involved in wound healing are critically dependent on adequate perfusion and delivery of oxygen, glucose and other essential nutrients. Inadequate perfusion may result in tissue ischaemia or delayed wound healing. Contused tissue, fractures, tissues around an abscess or site of infection can be considered a wound because resolution of inflammation depends on the same basic cellular processes as does healing of an external wound. With the proliferation of minimally invasive techniques, operative incisions can be limited in size, and consequently, patients recover more rapidly as a result of reduced tissue destruction.

Semistarvation

Food is commonly withheld from the patient during the perioperative period. If food deprivation is prolonged, the complications of starvation will compound the effects of surgical illness such as loss of body proteins, presence of ileus and anastomotic weakness. The presence of food in the gut lumen is known to be a major stimulus for mucosal cell growth. Mucosal atrophy is observed in the absence of enteral nutrition [21], in periods of parenteral feeding or in defunctionalized intestinal segments. The presence of nutrients in the gut stimulates the elaboration of trophic hormones for the intestinal mucosa, particularly glutamine and butyrate.

Immobility

Bed rest and immobility contribute to loss of muscle mass and strength. Immobility may result in progressive atelectasis, respiratory insufficiency, and pulmonary sepsis. If immobility is prolonged, bed pressure sores may develop over bony prominences. Bed rest predisposes to orthostatic intolerance and instability during standing. Postoperative hypoxaemia is more pronounced in the supine position.

References

1. Mangano DT (1990) Perioperative cardiac morbidity. Anesthesiology 72:153-184
2. Badner NH, Knil RL, Brown JE et al (1998) Myocardial infarction after noncardiac surgery. Anesthesiology 88:572-578
3. Wahba RWM (1991) Perioperative functional residual capacity. Can J Anaesth 38:384-400
4. Watters JM, Clancey SM, Moulton SB et al (1993) Impaired recovery of strength in old patients after abdominal surgery. Ann Surg 218:380-393
5. Ballantyne C, Carr DB, de Ferranti S et al (1998) The comparative effects of postoperative analgesic therapies on pulmonary outcome: cumulative meta-analyses of randomized, controlled trials. Anesth Analg 86:598-612
6. Sharrock NE, Go G, Harpel PC et al (1995) Thrombogenesis during total hip arthroplasty. Clin Orthop 319:16-27
7. Deitch EA (1989) Simple intestinal obstruction causes bacterial translocation in man. Arch Surg 124:699-701
8. Parikh SS, Chung F (1995) Postoperative delirium in the elderly. Anesth Analg 80:1223-1232
9. Christensen T, Kehlet H (1993) Postoperative fatigue. World J Surg 17:220-225
10. Carli F, Klubien K, De Angelis R et al (1998) An intensive versus graded perioperative management program for recovery after colorectal surgery: preliminary results on quality of life. Reg Anesth Pain Med 23:11
11. Culen DJ, Apolone G, Greenfield S et al (1994) ASA physical status and age predict morbidity after three surgical procedures. Ann Surg 220:3-9
12. Nielsen HJ (1995) The effect of histamine type-II receptor antagonists on post-traumatic immune competence. Dan Med Bull 44:162-174
13. Wakefield CH, Carry PD, Foulds S et al (1993) Polymorphonuclear leukocyte activation. An early marker of the postsurgical sepsis response. Arch Surg 128:390-395
14. Windsor ACJ, Klava A, Somers SS et al (1995) Manipulation of local and systemic host defense in the prevention of perioperative sepsis. Br J Surg 82:1460-1467
15. Kehlet H (1994) Postoperative pain what is the issue? Br J Anaesth 72:375-378
16. Rosenberg J (1995) Late postoperative hypoxemia. Mechanisms and clinical implications. Dan Med Bull 42:40-46
17. Rosenberg J, Pedersen MH, Ramsing T, Kehlet H (1992) Circadian variation in unexpected postoperative death. Br J Surg 79:1300-1302
18. Jonsson K, Jensen JA, Goodson WH III et al (1991) Tissue oxygenation, anemia and perfusion in relation to wound healing in surgical patients. Ann Surg 214:605-613
19. Rosenberg-Adamsen S, Kehlet H, Dodds C, Rosenberg J (1996) Postoperative sleep disturbances - mechanisms and clinical implications. Br J Anaesth 76:552-559
20. Livingston E, Passaro E (1990) Postoperative ileus. Dig Dis Sci 35:121-132
21. Clarke RM (1976) Evidence for both luminal and systemic factors in the control of rat intestinal epithelial replacement. Clin Sci Mol Med 50:139

Basic Concepts of Closed-Loop Anesthesia Delivery Systems

F. GIUNTA, A. FERRARI, F. FORFORI

With the introduction of the closed-loop anesthesia systems with the breath-by-breath gas monitoring, the clinical depth of anesthesia is expressed by the end-tidal anesthetic concentration. Several studies found a strong relationship between end-tidal and arterial partial pressure. The end-tidal agent value is the only clinical value that is available and reliable to close the loop.

Mathematical models of pharmacokinetics offer a feedback control for the target-controlled infusion (TCI) system, delivering the appropriate dose of the drug to reach and to maintain the target concentration. Closed-loop delivery of muscle relaxant can be obtained by train-of-four (TOF) guard value. The closed-loop anesthesia delivery system now needs some more-precise clinical targets: the proposal is the control of the drug delivery based on the electroencephalographic (EEG) signal or similar [i.e., bispecral index (BIS)] and on the auditory evoked potential (AEP). These two systems are specific for some aspects of anesthesia, but they don't seem to cover the whole process of anesthesia.

The clinical observation that the depth of anesthesia depends on variations of the anesthetic concentration in the inspired gases implicates the attainment of an equilibrium between alveolar and effector site concentration.

The concept of MAC (minimum alveolar concentration) is the expression of the response of 50% of the anesthetized patients (ED_{50}) at a certain alveolar concentration of anesthetic, so that at the equilibrium they do not move in response to a noxious stimulus (surgical incision). This parameter, expression of the anesthetic potency, simplifies the conduction of inhalational anesthesia by means of a constant alveolar concentration of anesthetic.

The principles and the pharmacokinetic theories [1, 2] that determine the variations of the alveolar concentration of anesthetics were studied by Eger et al. [3, 4] and have been validated by the modern systems of anesthesia with breath-by-breath monitoring. Eger and Guadagni [5] elaborated a theoretical model to predict the temporal variability of the distribution in different groups of organs (vascular-rich group, muscle group, fatty group) and the influence that this distribution has on the inspiratory concentration of the anesthetic, with the purpose of maintaining a constant alveolar concentration. What Eger elaborated, beginning with an indefinite and unreliable inspiratory fraction (FI), is now confirmed by the breath-by-breath gas monitoring systems that are clinically available.

The concept of MAC can be defined as a "pharmacological target obtained empirically". MAC is a value that corresponds to a certain anesthetic effect and is also strictly related to the arterial agent concentration. MAC is not useful before the achievement of a steady state, so it is not related to the kinetics of the first minutes of inhalation anesthesia. In the formulation of the MAC concept, it is assumed that the alveolar partial pressure of the anesthetic vapor is transmitted without modifications to the arterial blood and from there to the site of action.

Automatic feedback controlled totally closed circuit systems have been developed for quantitative practice of inhalation anesthesia, with the complete closed-loop control of gas supply (O_2, N_2O, anesthetic) by means of an end-expired gas signal (Table 1).

Table 1. Closed-loop control of anesthesia

Now available	Actual proposal	Near feature
Physioflex (end-tidal concentration)	TIVA	TIVA – inhalational anesthesia
Muscle relaxant (TOF)	(TCI - mathematical model)	(BIS - AEP)

(*TIVA* total intravenous anesthesia, *TCI* target-controlled infusion, *BIS* bispecral index, *AEP* auditory evoked potentials)

In the past few years many studies have been carried out in order to establish the exact relationship between the end-expired and the arterial partial pressure of the anesthetic. According to the findings of Cromwell and Eger [6] on patients breathing subanesthetic concentrations of isoflurane, no significant differences were found between the two values. Later other studies highlighted a significant difference in the two values, the ratio ranging from 0.66 to 0.86 [7-9].

Such a difference seems to be due to several factors: 1) resistance to the transfer of the anesthetic agent through the alveolar capillary membrane; 2) shunt; 3) alveolar dead space.

The resistance to the transfer of the anesthetic agent through the alveolar capillary membrane, and therefore a non-uniform distribution within the alveoli [9], can play an important role, especially for anesthetic agents with a high molecular weight [2]. A smaller contribution comes from the shunt and the alveolar dead space. In normal subjects the alveolar dead space is small, but it can become relevant in cases of ventilation/perfusion (V/Q) mismatching and during anesthesia. There is no evidence that this is due to the pulmonary hypotension, which is in turn responsible for the development of West's zone 1. Another explanation could be the existence of relatively unperfused areas. Therefore if the end-expired partial pressure differs from the arterial pressure, the MAC will not correspond to this value and consequently to the partial pressure at the site of action.

Nevertheless, in the absence of the arterial anesthetic partial pressure or of the pressure at the site of action, the end-expired partial pressure is the only clinically useful value to establish the uptake of the anesthetic and its comparison with the MAC can give information on the depth of anesthesia. In fact MAC plays a dual role: it is well related to the arterial agent concentration (with the above-mentioned pathophysiological exceptions) and it is a value of the clinical response (ED_{50}).

Another field of development is total intravenous anesthesia (TIVA); its development offers positive benefits not only to the patient but also to the medical staff in term of operative room pollution. TIVA has recently become popular because of the introduction of new fast-acting intravenous drugs and the understanding of the pharmacokinetic/pharmacodynamics of these drugs, and because of the development of a computer-controlled system for the intravenous administration of anesthetic (Table 1).

Nevertheless, there is a clear difference in the basic concept of achieving the desired objectives by using TIVA or inhalational anesthetics [10]. The receptor specificity of the drugs involved in TIVA involves a single druging act at its own receptor site to obtain specific effects rather than a widespread cellular effect caused by volatile anesthetics [10].

For some drugs there is a close relationship between blood concentration and effect, so that with exact knowledge of the pharmacokinetic properties of such drugs it is possible to titrate the infusion to achieve the desired clinical effects. The target for TIVA should be that blood concentration which maintains the optimal receptor site binding.

TCI is a recent evolution of TIVA. It is as alternative to manually controlled infusion that allows attainment and maintenance of a steady-state blood concentration of various intravenous drugs [11, 12]. The system incorporates real-time pharmacokinetic models that deliver the appropriate dose of the drug to achieve and to maintain the target concentration. The system does not sample the blood, but it uses population kinetics to provide the best estimate blood concentration [13].

Although the TCI system allows attainment of the exact target blood concentration, it is not possible to know if this is satisfactory for each patient. There is no doubt that significant and uncertain questions still exist in the delivery of anesthetics, including 1) the blood concentration is not the site of the drug effect [14], 2) the drug concentration at the site of action is not measurable [15], 3) a large inter-individual variability has been found studying population pharmacology (i.e., pharmacokinetics may be modified by diseases, drugs, or by the same surgical operation) [16].

Nevertheless, TCI provides the anesthetist with direct control of blood concentration giving: 1) a better control and predictability of the effect achieved, adequate for the surgical requirements, 2) a constant blood concentration, and 3) avoiding peak blood concentrations to reduce risks associated with over-dosage and side effects.

However the control of the blood concentration does not automatically imply control of the anesthetic depth. General anesthesia is usually a mix between amnesia, analgesia, hypnosis, and muscle relaxation. Induction and recovery are like a voyage from consciousness to unconsciousness and back, and during this period unexpected awareness or recall (implicit or explicit) may occur. Such experience may be very unpleasant either for the patients, ranging from an unpleasant sensation to a post-traumatic stress disorder (sleep disturbance, dreams, depression, and panic) or for the anesthesiologist, who may risk medical malpractice litigation. Conscious recall of intra-operative events is only "the tip of an iceberg" [17], and the incidence of unconscious perception may be much higher than that reported [18].

For long time anesthesiologists have been looking for a device able to measure the depth of anesthesia and to avoid awareness and recall during surgery. The depth of anesthesia has been clinically judged by the observation of somatic and autonomic reflexes, but often these measures are not specific, and not well related to the depth of anesthesia. A relevant and additional problem comes from the synergic action of other drugs as opioids.

Moreover, no correlations between the hemodynamics and probability of recall were found [19]. Therefore we need new and more-precise monitor devices to control the anesthetic process (hypnosis, analgesia, and muscle relaxation). Devices measuring the lower esophageal contractility and surface electromyography were dismissed, while the AEP, the EEG, and now the BIS (from EEG) can today help anesthesiologists to monitor hypnosis for an appropriate level of anesthesia, in order to avoid awareness or recall and to allow a quick recovery.

The EEG still remain the golden standard to monitor hypnosis [20]. However, the interpretation requires a neurologist and computerization of this technique is necessary when it is used continuously in the operating room, so that it is not easy to use in this setting.

A new technique of processing EEG data, BIS analysis, has been recently developed. This patent technology processes EEG data on real time using an algorithm incorporating BIS analysis in combination with other EEG features, such as the level of burst suppression and component of the power spectrum, providing a non-invasive, direct measure of the effect of anesthetic-hypnotic drug on the brain [21, 22].

BIS index is a single numeric value ranging from 0 to 100. The awake state is around 100 while the deep hypnotic state is around 40, and in the middle there are different forms of sedation from the light to the deep.

The BIS index offers an excellent correlation with the state of unconsciousness or hypnosis, but it does not provide any information on the analgesic state or the movement of the patient. A decrease in BIS index value can predict unconsciousness, but can not predict whether the patient will move or not under surgical stimuli.

If we ensure adequate analgesia, the BIS allows us to titrate volatile anesthetic and hypnotics to the appropriate level of anesthesia, providing faster and predictable patient awakening, earlier discharge from the post-anesthesia care unit, and a significant reduction in anesthetic drug utilization, preventing overdosage [23, 24].

Another measure of the depth of anesthesia is the AEP. AEPs were used to monitor central nervous system (CNS) effects during induction and recovery from anesthesia. This non-invasive technique has been used in clinical practice to record the changes in the electrical potentials that occur within the CNS of the patient in response to an external auditory stimulus. The principle of these techniques is based on repetitive stimulation with the corresponding signal of interest time-locked to the stimulus [25]. Their low voltage combined with high background noise requires the use of amplifier and computer averaging equipment. From the several waves originated during the progress of the stimulus in the CNS, Pa and Nb waves, which occur between 20 and 80 ms (middle latency response), best reflect cortical activity [26, 27]. It was observed that changes in the amplitude and latency of these waves is highly related to a transition from consciousness to unconsciousness [28, 29].

AEP index (mathematical derivative of the morphology of the AEP waveform) is more sensitive than BIS index for distinguishing a relatively rapid transition from unconsciousness to consciousness [30] and is more stable than BIS index during hypothermia [31].

Recently since muscle relaxants have become generally used in anesthesia, there is the necessity to monitor adequately the degree of neuromuscular blockage during and above all after the anesthesia.

TOF nerve stimulation [32] represents the golden standard. It is simply to use and it allows titration of the neuromuscular blockage to clinical requirements. Assessing the response of a single patient to the muscle relaxant drug used, it indicates to the anesthetist the optimal time for tracheal intubation and indicates awareness more easily. Leading the administration of muscle relaxant antagonist, it favors the recovery of the patient by avoiding residual neuromuscular blockage in the recovery room.

Although the use of TOF does not exclude completely significant clinical residual paralysis [33], it allows accurate monitoring and titration of neuromuscular function during anesthesia, reducing postoperative complications [34] and so improving outcome.

In 1924 Haggerd observed that "the toxic effects of a substance depends on its quantity in the body, that is the total dose. The idea of total dosing, besides universally known for the ingested or injected substances, it is not well known for the inhalation substances; this concept is often skipped, considering the physiological response to gas and vapours only in terms of duration of the exposure and concentration of gas or vapour in the inspired mixture".

In the past the anesthetist could only control the inspired concentration of agent, and the use of high-flow anesthesia reflects this attitude. The exact dose of the inhalation agent can be determined only with closed circuit anesthesia, which is the best application of pharmacokinetic principles. This quantitative method allows the delivery of a known quantity of anesthetic to exactly balance the patient uptake and the possible leakage; however if this amount is enough to justify the immediate clinical cardiovascular effects, its time course (in other words the total dosage of agent) can explain the long-term actions, such as the effects on hypoxic pulmonary vasoconstriction and vasodilatation induced by sevoflurane.

The "ideal" target of any kind of anesthesia is the concentration at the site of action and the CNS, and some models have been developed to correlate arterial to brain concentration. The future challenge will be therefore be the possibility to control the brain concentration by applying these models.

The study of the concentration at the site of action (CNS) cannot ignore the patient response to the dosage (ED_{50}, ED_{95}). During the years we have moved from having as a guide of the anesthetic state, blood pressure, heart rate, respiratory frequency, then TOF and Et-concentration (this one still the only clinical value to establish the uptake of volatile anesthetic and then in relation to the MAC able to indicate the depth of anesthesia) to the EEG, and recently to BIS and AEP. Today the cardio-respiratory parameters may no longer represent a guide to the anesthetic depth.

These devices allow easy separation of components of anesthesia (hypnosis, analgesia, and muscle relaxation) and allow careful monitoring. However, it is not possible to measure "anesthesia" as there is no golden standard model available to define the state of anesthesia. Perhaps in the future when we can define exactly what "anesthesia" is we will be able to measure in detail the individual response to a drug and to quantify it as a cellular effect. Hence we will be able to tailor to the patient any specific pharmacological effect that circumstance require, but that day will we still be anesthetists?

References

1. Kety SS (1950) The physiological and physical factors governing the uptake of the anaesthetic gases by the body. Anesthesiology 11:517-526
2. Kety SS (1951) The theory and application of the exchange of inert gas at the lungs and tissue. Pharmacol Rev 3:1-41
3. Eger EI II, Saidman LJ, Brandstater B (1965) Minimum alveolar anaesthetic concentration: a standard of anaesthetic potency. Anaesthesiology 26:756
4. Eger EI II (1974) MAC, anaesthetic uptake and action. Williams and Wilkins, Baltimore
5. Eger EI II, Guadagni NP (1963) Halotane uptake in man at constant alveolar concentration. Anaesthesiology 24:299-304
6. Cromwell TH, Eger EI, Stevens WC, Dalan WM (1971) Forane uptake, excretion and blood solubility in man. Anaesthesiology 35:401-408
7. Frei FJ, Zbinoten DA, Thompson DA et al (1991) Is the end-tidal partial pressure of isoflurane a good predictor of its arterial partial pressure? Br J Anaesth 66:331-339
8. Dwyer RC, Fell JPH, Howard PJ et al (1991) Arterial washing of halotane and isoflurane in young and elderly patients. Br J Anaesth 66:572-579
9. Landon MJ, Matson AM, Royston BD et al (1993) Components of the inspiratory-arterial isoflurane partial pressure differences. Br J Anaesth 70:605-611
10. Camu F, Kay B (1991) Why total intravenous anaesthesia (TIVA)? In: Kay B (ed) Total intravenous anaesthesia. Elsevier Science, Amsterdam
11. Jacobs JR, Williams EA (1993) Algorithm to control "effect compartment" drugs concentration in pharmacokinetic model-driven drug delivery. IEEE Trans Biomed Eng 40:993-999
12. Schuttler J, Schwilden H, Stoeckel H (1983) Pharmacokinetics as applied to total intravenous anaesthesia. Anaesthesia 38[Suppl]:53-56
13. Kenny NC (1997) The development and future of TCI. Acta Anaesthsiol Belg 48:229-232
14. Shafer SL (1993) Towards optimal intravenous dosing strategies. Semin Anaesth 12:222-234
15. Schnider TW, Minto CF, Stanski DR (1994) The effect compartment concept in pharmacodynamic modelling. Anaesth Pharmacol Rev 2:204-213
16. Moerman N, Bonke B, Oosting J (1993) Awareness and recall during general anaesthesia. Facts and feelings. Anaesthesiology 79:454-464
17. Schwender D, Klasing S, Daunderer M et al (1995) Awareness during general anaesthesia. Definition, incidence, clinical relevance, causes, avoidance and medico-legal aspects. Anaesthetist 44:743-754
18. Sebel PS (1997) Awareness during general anaesthesia. Can J Anaesth 44:124-130
19. Shafer SL (1996) Drug concentrations, EEG signals and clinical signs: what really predicts depth of anaesthesia? Annual Meeting of The Society for Intravenous Anaesthesia (SIVA), New Orleans
20. Rampil IJ, Matteo RS (1987) Changes in EEG spectral edge frequency correlate with the haemodynamic response to laryngoscopy and intubation. Anaesthesiology 67:139-142
21. Struys M, Versichelen L, Mortier E et al (1998) Comparison of spontaneous frontal EMG, EEG power spectrum and bispectral index to monitor propofol drug effect and emergence. Acta Anaesthesiol Scand 42:628-636
22. Smith WD, Dutton RC, Smith NT (1996) Measuring the performance of anaesthetic depth indicators. Anaesthesiology 84:38-51
23. Gan TJ, Glass PS, Windsor A et al (1997) Bispectral index monitoring allows faster emergence and improved recovery from propofol, alfentanil and nitrous oxide anaesthesia. BIS Utility Study Group Anaesthesiology 84:808-815
24. Song D, Joshi JP, White PF (1997) Titration of volatile anaesthetics using bispectral index facilitates recovery after ambulatory anaesthesia. Anaesthesiology 87:842-848
25. Kalkman CJ (1994) Monitoring the central nervous system. Anesth Clin North Am 12: 173-176
26. Thornton C, Barrowcliffe MP, Konieczko KM et al (1989) The auditory evoked response as an indicator of awareness. Br J Anaesth 63:113-115

27. Pockett S (1999) Anaesthesia and the electrophysiology of auditory consciousness. Conscious Cogn 8:45-61
28. Davies FW, Mantzardis H, Kenny GNC, Fisher AC (1996) Middle latency auditory evoked potentials during repeated transition from consciousness to unconsciousness. Anaesthesia 51:107-113
29. Thornton C, Sharpe RM (1998) Evoked response in anaesthesia. Br J Anaesth 51:107-113
30. Doi M, Gajraj RJ, Mantzaridis H et al (1997) Effects of cardiopulmonary by-pass on electroencephalographic variables. Anaesthesia 52:1048-1055
31. Gajraj RJ, Mantzaridis H, Kenny GNC (1998) Analysis of EEG bispectrum, auditory evoked potentials and the EEG power spectrum during repeated transition from consciousness to unconsciousness. Br J Anaesth 80:46-52
32. Ali HH, Utting JE, Gray C (1970) Stimulus frequency in the detection of neuromuscular blocks in human. Br J Anaesth 42:967
33. Fruergaard K, Viby-Mogensen J, Berg H, El Mahdy AM (1998) Tactile evaluation of the response to double burst stimulation decreases, but does not eliminate the problem of postoperative residual paralysis. Acta Anaesthesiol Scand 42:1168
34. Berg H, Viby-Mogensen J, Roes J et al (1997) Residual neuromuscular block is a risk factor for postoperative pulmonary complications. A prospective, randomised, and blinded study of postoperative pulmonary complications after atracurium, vecuronium and pancuronium. Acta Anaesthesiol Scand 41:1095

Clonidine Smoothing Anesthesia

J. RUPREHT

"When the dust settles, we shall see whether we are riding a horse or an ass" is the end sentence of the splendid medical intelligence article about α_2-adrenoceptor agonists published by Maze and Tranquilli in Anesthesiology back in 1991 [1]. Their aim was to define the role of these drugs in clinical human anesthesia, where the use was promising but only sporadically applied, which contrasted with the nearly universal use of α_2-agonists for analgesia and sedation in veterinary anesthesia. Maze and Tranquilli [1] concluded that the full potential of α_2-agonists was not realised in 1991 and that a fundamental impact on anesthetic practice would only be possible by the appearance of more-selective and potent compounds than clonidine or medetomidine which were registered for use in humans.

By 1996 a chapter "The α_2 adrenoceptor agonists and anaesthesia" had already entered the leading textbook "International Practice of Anaesthesia" and the message was that clinical application of the α_2-agonists was increasing rapidly as anesthetic adjuvants and that dexmedetomidine was more likely to become the most-appropriate adjunct agent in human anesthesia. More disadvantageous side effects were described, along with treatment when they occurred, but the authors Peden and Prys-Roberts [2] clearly stated that additional studies in older and sicker patients were warranted before the widespread clinical use of α_2-agonists. This chapter ends with a statement of intelligent doubt "It remains to be seen whether the α_2-agonists can fulfil their promise as adjuncts to human anaesthesia".

Whereas there was much hope in 1992 that the highly specific α_2-agonist dexmedetomidine would become a powerful new adjunct to anesthesia, according to an editorial [3], the limitations of developing the drug into an anesthetic in its own right became quit clear. Side effects like nausea, hypotension, and headache were most unwelcome, but the fact that recovery from anesthesia including α_2-agonists was no faster than after a conventional combination of drugs was disappointing. Moreover, dexmedetomidine was studied in very healthy patients and the lack of experience in sicker patients continued.

By the year 2000, dexmedetomidine has been developed and recommended for use as a sedative, anxiolytic, and accessory analgesic in intensive care.

Progress in its application during anesthesia appears to have been limited and it is difficult to judge where one stands now in regard to the phenomenon of tolerance to effects of the drug and the feasibility of antagonizing its effects in human anesthesia. The disappointing progress is illustrated by the decision of the FDA to approve the agent only as a sedative for patients in the intensive care [4] and, unexpectedly, by refusal, so far, of the European Union to register the agent for general clinical use (information from Abbott).

Clonidine is approved and helpful in anesthesia

Clonidine exhibits much lower selective affinity for the α_2-receptor than dexmedetomidine but has been in clinical use as an antihypertensive for over 30 years, and is thus more predictably useful. Its α_2-agonistic effects are predominantly of central nervous system origin. The antihypertensive adult daily dose of 0.2-0.3 mg is well absorbed after oral administration and 60% is excreted unchanged in the urine. The hypotensive effect lasts about 8 h after intake. The elimination half-life is about 8.5 h. The parenteral form is called Catapressan, in Europe.

Physiological responses

Clonidine stimulates α_2-inhibitory neurons in the medullary vasomotor center thus diminishing sympathetic outflow and causing centrally induced hypotension and bradycardia. After an intravenous injection it causes transient peripheral vasoconstriction. Following prolonged intake, an abrupt discontinuation of medication causes rebound hypertension. The appreciated feature of clonidine-induced hypotension is the unaffected function of cardiovascular homeostatic reflexes and maintained renal blood flow and glomerular filtration [5].

Respiratory effects are minor following higher doses, but clonidine does not depress the ventilatory response to CO_2 in man [6]. The sympathoinhibitory effect of clonidine is based probably on both the diminished central sympathetic tone and the decreased presynaptic peripheral activity of α_2-receptor. Release of growth hormone is inhibited and the cortisol release in response to surgical stress is attenuated. Release of insulin is inhibited by the direct effect of clonidine on the Langerhan's cells, but this effect is quite short lived.

Dry mouth results from direct effect on the salivary glands. There is also reduced vagally mediated gastric and bowel motility, and clonidine has been successfully used in cases of watery diarrhea. Clonidine causes enhanced platelet aggregation, but the clinical significance of this effect has not been established.

Anxiolysis is caused by decreased central turnover of noradrenaline, a clonidine effect which is subject to tolerance after prolonged use. Similarly, the sedative effect of clonidine is pronounced during initial intake but disappears with time. The powerful analgesic action of clonidine is undisputed, but the mechanism has remained a subject of debate [7]. It appears that enhancement of noradrenergic descending inhibitory pathways and of inhibited substance P release play a role [8].

Anesthesiological applications of clonidine

In contrast to widespread and very efficient routine use of α_2-agonists in veterinary anesthesia [1], there is now an immense body of evidence that these agents can indeed be useful adjuncts in human anesthesia. The reasons why approval for use has not been forthcoming are unknown and would be difficult to justify. However, clonidine has been around and, if appropriately used, is a most-beneficial tool in the anesthetist's hands.

Decreased anesthetic requirements were described when clonidine was used in conjunction with neuroleptanaesthesia [9] in 1979; "smoothing out" of the entire perioperative hemodynamic profile was reported. Clonidine diminishes requirements for anesthetic agents and opiate agents on the basis of its intrinsic analgesic and anesthetic properties. During anesthesia, 45% less fentanyl and 40% less isoflurane are sufficient when 5 μg/kg clonidine is administered. This reduced anesthetic requirement may consequently but unreliably result in shorter recovery from anesthesia. Hemodynamic perturbations during anesthesia are minimal. Nevertheless, this should not be taken for granted, because one must identify the patients who are not suitable candidates for hypotension and bradycardia accompanying the actions of clonidine. Very recently renewed recommendations to use clonidine as adjunct to general anesthesia have been published, substantiated by a remarkable decrease of MAC-isoflurane [10].

Improved postoperative analgesia follows perioperative use of clonidine. Less opiate drugs are required with fewer side effects. No studies have been published about postoperative vigilance and ability of the patient to fast-track following an ambulatory surgical procedure. Clonidine does smooth the perioperative course, but is not a short-acting drug and may result in more-sluggish recovery.

Clonidine has been advocated as an adjunct to caudal and epidural mixtures, decreasing the need for local analgesic and the opiate component of the mixtures. The combination of clonidine and bupivacaine results in a significantly better and longer duration of analgesia than when each drug is administered separately. Cardiovascular changes and the incidence of side effects were not more than with alternative epidural mixtures [11]. The main advantage lies in a decreased chance of a respiratory depression and improved muscle strength [12].

Intensive care indications for clonidine are numerous, the drug being useful in management of central sympathetic hyperactivity, in the prevention of delirium tremens, in supplementing ever-increasing doses of opiates, in supplementing other sedatives, and in dealing with withdrawal states. The safety of clonidine in severe neuro-trauma has not been established [13].

Tourniquet hypertensive response is a very tenuous and not easily soluble disturbance during surgical procedures involving ischemia of an extremity. Practice has shown that this tourniquet pain starts after some 30-45 min of limb ischemia, irrespective of the type of surgical anesthesia, local, regional, or general. Tourniquet ischemic pain starts earlier and is more intense in rheumatic patients. Misery for an awake patient may be intractable, whereas hemodynamic deregulation may be unacceptable for an anesthetized patient. It is noteworthy that pethidine is more effective in the prevention of tourniquet pain and hypertension than other opiate agents. Clonidine, however, completely prevents tourniquet pain and hypertension if administered at least 30 min beforehand, the dose being 1-2 μg/kg intravenously in a slow injection.

Chronic pain treatments frequently deal with a component of intractable ischemic pain. Addition of clonidine to other modalities of this pain treatment greatly enhances the beneficial effect, decreasing the occurrence of unwanted side effects at the same time. The advantage is quite clear, because clonidine lacks direct addictive and respiratory depressant action [7].

In conclusion, the available knowledge and experience with the α_2-agonist activity of clonidine should more frequently be used to smooth the course of anesthesia. It is true that inclusion of clonidine in the anesthetic method may call for more judgement and more vigilance during the procedure, but the smoother course of anesthesia by far outweighs the effort. Clonidine is an excellent drug for premedication in selected patients and before certain surgical procedures, acting as a reliable background stabilizing agent during anesthesia. Care must certainly be taken to exclude patients in whom bradycardia and hypotension are unwarranted. Also, the ever-increasing ambulatory surgery and fast-track demands of recovery call for more studies on the quality of recovery from anesthetic techniques including clonidine.

References

1. Maze M, Tranquilli W (1991) Alpha-2 adrenoceptor agonists: defining the role in clinical anaesthesia. Anesthesiology 74:581-605
2. Peden CJ, Prys-Roberts C (1996) The alpha-2 adrenoceptor agonists and anaesthesia. In: Prys-Roberts C, Brown BR Jr (eds) International practice of anaesthesia. Butterworth-Heinemann, Oxford 1;19:1-13
3. Peden CJ, Prys-Roberts C (1992) Dexmedetomidine – a powerful new adjunct to anaesthesia? (editorial) Br J Anaesth 68:123-125
4. Bhana N, Goa KL, McClellan KJ (2000) Dexmedetomidine. Drugs 59:263-268
5. Stoelting RK (1991) Antihypertensive drugs. In: Stoelting RK (ed) Pharmacology and physiology of anaesthetic practice, 2nd edn. Lippincot, Philadelphia, pp 311-323
6. Sperry RJ, Bailey PL, Pace NL et al (1990) Clonidine does not depress the ventilatory response to CO_2 in man. Anesth Analg 70:S383
7. Maze M, Fujinaga M (2000) Alpha-2 adrenoceptors in pain modulation. Editorial views. Anesthesiology 92:234-236
8. Ono H, Mishima A, Ono S et al (1991) Inhibitory effects of clonidine and tizanidine on release of substance P from slices of rat spinal cord and antagonism by alpha-adrenergic receptors antagonists. Neuropharmacology 30:585-589
9. Kaukinen S, Kaukinen L, Eerola R (1979) Postoperative use of clonidine with neuroleptanaesthesia. Acta Anaesthesiol Scand 23:113-120
10. El-Kerdawy HMM, Van Zalingen EE, Bovill JG (2000) The influence of the alpha-2 adrenoceptor agonist, clonidine, on the EEG and on the MAC of isoflurane. Eur J Anaesth 17:105-110
11. Carabine UA, Milligan KR, Moore J (1992) Extradural clonidine and bupivacaine for postoperative analgesia. Br J Anaesth 68:132-135
12. Luz G, Innerhofer P, Oswald E et al (1999) Comparison of clonidine 1 $\mu g\ kg^{-1}$ with morphine 30 $\mu g\ kg^{-1}$ for post-operative caudal analgesia in children. Eur J Anaesth 16:42-46
13. Spies D, Bubisz N, Neumann T et al (1996) Therapy of alcohol withdrawal syndrome in intensive care unit patients following trauma. Crit Care Med 24:414-422

Anaphylactic and Anaphylactoid Reactions During Anesthesia

M.M. FISHER

The systemic inflammatory response is due to the release and formation of mediators that interact with defense and endothelial cells. Although the interactions are usually beneficial, in some circumstances, e.g., septic shock, adult respiratory distress, and anaphylaxis, it is believed an exaggerated or prolonged effect produces a response detrimental to the host. In anesthesia release of endogenous mediators produces a spectrum of effects. The most-common example is the non-immunological release of histamine in response to drugs or surgical and anesthetic stimuli, producing effects which are usually minor, transient, and of confined to the skin and blood vessels [1]. Massive release of histamine in response to an antigen-antibody reaction leads to the activation of longer-acting mediators producing a sustained effect.

Histamine is the major mediator that has been studied in anesthesia. Histamine is released in response to a variety of stimuli, such as antigen-antibody reactions, drugs and physical stimuli. There is a marked variability in release in individuals. There is a correlation between the quantity of histamine released due to drugs or given by infusion and the cardiovascular, cutaneous, and subjective symptoms, but not to bronchospasm [1, 2]. This may be related to the histamine-induced release of endogenous catecholamines protecting the subject from bronchospasm. The adverse effects of histamine in anesthesia can be blocked by pretreatment with H_1 and H_2 blockers [3-5]. The degree of histamine release in response to a particular drug is related to its ability to produce minor but not severe reactions, and potent releasers, such as morphine, are not as commonly associated with severe reactions as weak histamine releasers, such as suxamethonium. However Lorenz et al. [6] described a group of patients they called the 'super responders' who showed severe non-immunological reactions to atracurium.

Host factors in mediator release

Responsiveness

A number of important host factors influence the clinical effects of mediator release. These factor relate to the individual's histamine releasability and histamine responsiveness.

The considerable variability of histamine release to individual drugs and stimuli is reflected in both plasma levels of histamine and in histamine release from individual mast cells, with mastocytosis being an example of exaggerated responses. Patients with allergy, atopy, and asthma may have increased histamine releasability and responsiveness. In patients who are at the extremes of age, immunosuppressed, or shocked, anaphylaxis is rare.

In shock the natural catecholamine response inhibits the release of and opposes the actions of histamine. Patients on β-blockers manifest anaphylaxis with bradycardia rather than tachycardia, and the anaphylactic reaction is more difficult to treat as an increased dose of β-stimulants is required.

Recent work has suggested that the clinical manifestations of anaphylaxis may be associated with impairment of the renin/angiotensin system. Fifty patients with anaphylaxis to *Hymenoptera* venom had lower levels of renin, angiotensin I and II, and angiotensinogen than healthy controls. The levels correlated inversely with the severity of symptoms and were returned to normal by immunotherapy [7]. A failure of a protective mechanism is an attractive hypothesis to explain the lack of correlation between antibody levels, histamine responsiveness, and histamine releasability and the severity of reactions [8].

Atopy and allergy

All studies have shown an increased incidence of allergy, atopy, or asthma in patients who have anaphylactic reactions under anesthesia. When compared to non-reacting cohorts, three to five times the incidence is observed [9], although a French study where reactors were matched for age, gender, and social class, and atopy was measured by antigen testing, did not show a difference between reactors and non-reactors [10]. This increase in incidence in allergy and asthma is not an indication that these are significant risk factors. The majority of patients in all series who develop anaphylaxis do not have such a history, and the majority of patients with such a history have uneventful anesthetics. History of asthma, atopy, and allergy is a poor predictor of anaphylactic reactions [11].

Previous exposure

In anaphylaxis to thiopentone more than five uneventful exposures is usual [12]. A history of previous exposure in found in less than 50% of patients who are allergic to neuromuscular blocking drugs (NMBDs), even when IgE antibodies are demonstrated [13]. It is likely that the antibody which binds NMBDs is formed in response to exposure to some antigen other than anesthetic drug, even with previous exposure to NMBDs.

Clinical expressions of mediator release

The clinical effects of mediator release have variable expression, depending on the mediator released, the quantity, and the timing. As a general principal the effects are on smooth muscle producing bronchoconstriction in the airway and vasodilatation in the peripheral blood vessels, increased capillary leakage and increased secretions of exocrine glands.

Very high blood levels of histamine or mast cell tryptase generally correlate with the severity of the reaction and suggest an immunological cause [14, 15]. Minor skin changes are the most-common signs of histamine release [1] but do not suggest a risk of anaphylaxis with subsequent anesthetics. The role of direct histamine release in major reactions is less clear. Histamine can be the only mediator in severe reactions, especially in β-blocked patients with cardiac disease, but direct release is usually transient. Persistently high levels have not been recorded during severe reactions, but late hemodynamic improvement with the use of H_2 blockers suggest this may occur. Persistent severe reactions involve the release of the other mediators. It should be assumed that all reactions lasting greater than 10 min are immune mediated.

Anaphylaxis during anesthesia

Incidence

An incidence of anaphylaxis during anesthesia is difficult to determine and probably different in different countries. The largest anesthesia study is a multicenter French study which showed an incidence of 1:6,000 [16]. To accurately establish an incidence of severe anaphylaxis with 5% confidence limits, about 30 million patients would have to be studied [17]. Therefore incidences of reactions for specific drugs are likely to be even less meaningful and specific numbers difficult to obtain.

The reactions investigated in our clinic from 1974 to 2000 are shown in Table 1.

Table 1. Patients investigated 1974-1999

	General anesthesia	Local anesthesia	Total
Severe anaphylasis	684	6	690
Not anaphylactoid	182	262	444
Trivial	125	125	
Delayed	49	49	
Preoperative	79		
Histamine release	74		
Total	1,193	268	1,481

Drugs producing anaphylaxis

The drugs producing anaphylaxis over a 24-year period are shown in Table 2.

Table 2. Life-threatening clinical anaphylaxis during anesthesia 1974-1999

***n* = 690**	
Induction agents (*n* = 88)	
Thiopentone	46
Alfathesin	29
Propanidid	6
Methohexitone	1
Propofol	5
Midazolam	1
Induction agent and relaxant (n = 4)**	
Thiopentone/suxamethonium	2
Thiopentone/alcuronium	1
Thiopentone/atracurium	1
NMBDs (*n* = 410)	
Reaction to single drug (*n* = 392)	
Suxamethonium	131
Alcuronium	125
Atracurium	39
Rocuronium	24
d-Tubocurarine	23
Vecuronium	19
Gallamine	16
Pancuronium	12
Cisatracurium	2
Mivacurium	1
Reaction to both relaxants given at same anesthetic (*n* = 9)	
Suxamethonium/atracurium	1**
Suxamethonium/gallamine	2**
Suxamethonium/alcuronium	4**
Suxamethonium/vecuronium	1**
Suxamethonium/d-tubocurarine	1**
Reactions to two NMBDS on separate occasions (*n* = 9)	
α-Tubocurarine alcuronium	3
Decamethonium/suxamethonium	1
Pancuronium/alcuronium	1
Gallamine/alcuronium	1
Suxamethonium/pancuronium	1
Alcuronium/vecuronium	1
Rocuronium/vecuronium	1
Colloid solutions (*n* = 38)	
Haemaccel	28
Dextran 70	6
Dextran 40	1
SPPS	1
NSA	1
Plasma	1
Local anesthetics (*n* = 6)	
Prilocaine/lignocaine	1***
Bupivacaine	2
Lignocaine	2
Ropivicaine/lignocaine	1

Other drugs ($n = 30$)		**Narcotics ($n = 16$)**	
Protamine	10	Morphine	8
Contrast media	4	Fentanyl	4
Neostigmine	1	Omnopon	1
Atropine	2	Pethidine	3
Platelets	2		
Ondansetron	1		
Latex	4		
Gortex	1		
Patent blue	1		
Fragmin	1		
Ergometrine	1		
Blood	2		
Antibiotics ($n = 48$)			
Cephalothin	14		
Cephamandole	1		
Cephazolin	10		
Cefotaxime	3		
Cefotetan	5		
Penicillin	2		
Ampicillin	5		
Flucloxacillin	4		
Vancomycin	2		
Ampi/fluclox	1**		
Amoxycillin	1		
No drug determined ($n = 50$)			

(*NMBDs* neuromuscular blocking drugs)

* Patients referred to author for investigation. Includes patients from New Zealand, Australia, and Europe

** Both drugs received prior to reaction and positive skin and or RAST tests

*** Two reactions on separate occasions

Neuromuscular blocking drugs

NMBDs are the commonest causes of anaphylactic reactions in all large series. Suxamethonium is the most-common culprit everywhere except Australia, where alcuronium was commonest, and rocuronium is currently the most common. Pancuronium and vecuronium appear inherently safer than other NMBDs. Usage is the major factor in rate of reactions. However examination of the incidence of positive skin tests to NMBDs in reactors (Table 3) suggests that some NMBDs are higher risk than others due to the prevalence of sensitivity. Cross-sensitivity occurs in 60% of reactors, with the most-common pairings of suxamethonium and gallamine, alcuronium and d-tubocurarine, and pancuronium and vecuronium [17, 18]. Cisatracurium and atracurium are antigenically identical [19].

Table 3. Percentage of patients allergic to NMBDs allergic to individual drugs by skin testing

	Number tested	% positive
Alcuronium	321	48%
Suxamethonium	322	44%
d-Tubocurarine	264	42%
Atracurium	201	33%
Gallamine	163	29%
Vecuronium	197	13%
Pancuronium	315	12%
Rocuronium	100	31%
Mivacurium	100	21%

Induction agents

Thiopentone remains a significant cause of life-threatening allergy and is often suspected in delayed reactions, although a cause and effect relationship is hard to establish. Two studies suggest the incidence is in the order of 1:20,000. Multiple uneventful exposures usually occur before the abnormal reaction, but rarely it may occur on the first exposure. There is variable cross-sensitivity with other barbiturates.

Cremophor-based drugs

Previously used anesthetic drugs althesin and propanidid and initially Propofol were dissolved in Cremophor EL and had a very high incidence of anaphylaxis. The precise roles in anaphylaxis of the active drug and the solvent were not elucidated.

Propofol

After changing the solvent to intralipid, life-threatening reactions to Propofol still occurred, but to a lesser extent. The exact incidence is unknown. Positive skin tests and radioimmunoassay tests have been documented [20]. There is no evidence in the literature to support the relationship between allergy to eggs and allergy to the solvent causing anaphylaxis.

Others

Reactions to ketamine, midazolam, etomidate, and methohexitone have been described, but these reactions are extremely rare.

Opioids

Reactions to morphine, codeine phosphate, pethidine, omnopon, and fentanyl have all been described, but these are also rare. Fewer than 20 cases have been reported in the literature [21].

Antibiotics

Antibiotics account for between 2 and 6% of reported anaphylactic reactions, with cephalosporins being the most-common culprits. The incidence is increasing in Australia and France. Cross-reactivity between cephalosporins is unusual, as the antigenicity is usually related to side chains rather than the β-lactam group. Cross-sensitivity to penicillin through the β-lactam group is probably overestimated, and there is no evidence of cross-sensitivity between penicillin and second-, third-, and fourth-generation cephalosporins [22]. Cephalexin has a common side chain with ampicillin with some cross-over in allergy, while ceftazidine (without the common side chain) does not [23]. A recent study has shown up to 25% of patients undergoing major surgery had non-immune non-histamine-mediated reactions to antibiotics [24].

Protamine

Reactions to protamine may involve a number of mechanisms, including IgE, IgG, and complement [25-27]. Two different types of reaction may occur, a classical anaphylactic reaction and a syndrome producing pulmonary hypertension and right heart failure [28]. A prolonged and persistent capillary leak post bypass has been attributed to protamine and plasma products, although no direct cause and effect has been shown [28]. Fish allergy and vasectomy have been suggested as predisposing factors to protamine anaphylaxis, but there is no convincing association.

Colloids and blood products

All synthetic colloids have been shown to produce clinical anaphylaxis and their is no major evidence that one particular colloid has a higher incidence than another. As previously described, these reactions are rare during shock and there is little evidence that IgE is involved in the reactions. Pretreatment with high molecular weight dextrans reduces the incidence of reactions to dextrans [29], but anaphylaxis has occurred with pretreatment and after pretreatment, but are infrequently reported to our unit.

Latex

Allergy to latex is becoming more of a problem to both health care workers and to patients. Multiple glove changes are now required, with the institution of universal precautions in hospitals and in dental clinics. This has led to a 5-17% risk of latex allergy in health care workers, mostly showing signs of contact dermatitis (type IV). Other workers show evidence of bronchospasm at work which reverses when leaving the hospital environment. Latex allergy in the general population is more common in those who have atopy, who reportedly have a 4.4 times incidence. Children with spina bifida or congenital urological abnormalities have a 20-65% chance of having a latex allergy, which may arise from repeated surgical exposure and multiple catheterization required for the treatment. In the general population the incidence of latex allergy is thought to be very low: one report quotes 0.37%. Cross-reactivity between latex and foods such as kiwi fruit, banana, avocado, and chestnut have been found [30].

As well as type IV reaction, type I hypersensitivity reactions also occur and a large number of case reports show life-threatening reactions to latex from urinary catheters [31], surgical gloves [32], anesthetic equipment, rubber-stoppered vials [30], and balloons on thermodilution catheters [33]. The onset of anaphylaxis is usually delayed from the start of anesthesia by 15 mins and gets progressively worse over the next 5-10 min, and so is difficult to distinguish from reactions to other drugs. Most have positive prick tests [32] and elevated mast cell tryptase level [34], suggesting an IgE-mediated reaction. Latex allergy is an increasing problem in anesthetics.

Local anesthetics

Anaphylactic reactions to local anesthetics are extremely rare. Of the 260 patients referred to our unit with a history of allergy to local anesthetics, only 4 had severe anaphylaxis to local anesthetics, 4 reacted to additives, and 4 had delayed reactions. The commonest "reactions" seen were psychological in 102 patients [35]. Some of the reactions may be related to the additives in local anesthetics [36], but this is difficult to prove as the tests for preservatives are unreliable; where this cannot be excluded, these solutions should be avoided. In three other published studies, only 10 of 443 patients with a history of local anesthetic allergy had positive skin tests to local anesthetics [36].

Clinical features of anaphylaxis

Reactions occur most commonly immediately after induction. Table 4 shows the first clinical feature noted in 672 patients. The most-common first features in the last few years have been difficulty in inflation and desaturation, due to loss of waveform or desaturation.

Table 4. First clinical feature noted during anaphylactic reactions in 672 patients

Symptom	Number
Subjective	13
Cough	44
No pulse	174
No bleeding	2
Swelling	8
Difficult to inflate	159
ECG abnormality	14
Rash	31
Flush	107
Urticaria	13
Other	21
Desaturation	78
Total records	672

(*ECG* electrocardiogram)

The clinical features in 672 patients are shown in Table 5.

Table 5. Clinical features of anaesthetic anaphylaxis in 689 patients

	Number of cases	Sole feature	Worst feature
Cardiovascular collapse	596	75	543
Bronchospasm	257	33	121
Transient	102		
Asthmatics	96	9	
Cutaneous signs			
Rash	94		
Erythema	303		
Urticaria	53		
More than one	32		
Angioedema	165	9	21
Generalized edema	42	1	
Pulmonary edema	17	2	3
Gastrointestinal	39	1	

Cardiovascular manifestations are the most-common feature, and the full constellation of symptoms does not occur in every patient. Cardiovascular collapse is associated with vasodilatation and supraventricular tachycardia. It is the only feature in approximately 10% of cases, which may lead to the reaction being attributed to other causes.

Asthmatics during anaphylaxis invariably get broncospasm. This is the most-difficult feature to treat when severe. The pulmonary edema is a low-pressure membrane edema due to leaky capillaries and is associated with a volume deficit.

Treatment

There is a wide spectrum of severity of reaction and efficacy of response to treatment. Some patients respond to crystalloid and steroids, both of which are ineffective in severe cases, and others die in spite of excellent early management. There are no controlled trials of treatment in humans.

Non-specific measures

1. Stop the administration of the suspected antigen and give 100% oxygen.
2. Call for help and stop surgery if able.
3. Large-bore IV access.
4. Secure the airway.
5. Adrenaline should be given IV if ECG and blood pressure are monitored, but IM for less-severe reactions and if no monitoring is available. The route of adrenaline administration is controversial. IV adrenaline may produce cardiac arrhythmias, infarction, and severe hypertension, particularly if the diagnosis is incorrect or in unmonitored patients. While adrenaline should not be withheld until the patient is monitored, IM adrenaline may be a safer route and effective early.
6. External cardiac massage if patient is pulseless.
7. Intermittent positive pressure ventilation (IPPV) if necessary.

Specific treatment

Cardiovascular collapse

Treatment should involve sympathomimetic vasoconstrictor drugs and IV fluids. What evidence there is favors the use of colloid solutions in preference to crystalloid [37, 38] and adrenaline as the sympathomimetic with both vasoconstrictor and bronchodilator effects. German workers suggest that colloid fluid alone is preferable to using adrenaline, because of the risk of adverse effects [37]. In our studies, sympathomimetic drugs appear to enable more-rapid stabilization. Adrenaline usually stops the progression of angioedema [38, 39]. In monitored patients with severe reactions 3-5 ml of 1 in 10,000 IV adrenaline should be given followed a rapid infusion of 1-2 l of colloid solution [38]. In over 90% of patients this will produce a rapid response. In β-blocked patients it may be advisable to use drugs with mainly an α effect, such as noradrenaline or metaraminol. In refractory cases noradrenaline should be tried, and we now have seen a number of refractory cases where there was improvement with H_2 blockers [40].

Anaphylactic shock only rarely involves the heart as a target organ, although patients with cardiac disease may develop cardiac failure and are more likely to develop arrhythmias. If the heart becomes a target organ, severe global myocardial depression requiring balloon counterpulsation occurs [41].

Bronchospasm

If bronchospasm occurs it is often the most-difficult problem to treat. IV adrenaline is the first-line drug. Continuous nebulization of B_2 agonists, such as salbutamol, and steroids (e.g., 1 g of methylprednisolone) should be given. Volatile anesthetic agents may be of benefit. Isofluorane is the agent of choice when an adrenaline infusion is running. Ketamine may produce a dramatic response, especially in children.

The main aim of ventilation is to maintain oxygenation and to avoid barotrauma. Slow-rate (less than 6 breaths per min) hand ventilation may be better at this than IPPV. Providing the pH is greater than 7.0 and oxygenation is adequate, then the absolute level of carbon dioxide is unimportant. Pneumothorax is a major concern in this situation, and if there is any sudden deterioration then chest drains should be inserted. If all else fails and mechanical ventilation is impossible, barotrauma has occurred and cardiac arrest is imminent, then consideration should be given to cardiopulmonary bypass if available.

Angioedema

In angioedema if dyspnea is progressing then intubating the patient's trachea is mandatory. Adrenaline usually stops the process and H_1 blockers should be given. When a leak occurs around the endotracheal tube in a patient who is awake and spontaneously breathing, the patient can be extubated.

Pulmonary edema

Pulmonary edema in this situation is best controlled by positive endexpiratory pressure (PEEP) until capillary leakage is controlled and the saturation improved. Diuretics are not useful in this situation, as it is a low-pressure edema and the patient has a volume deficit. In rare reactions following cardiopulmonary bypass, large volumes of high-protein edema fluid may occur. This needs invasive monitoring and massive fluid replacement, and on using PEEP the fluid may leak through the lung surface into the thoracic cavity tamponading the lungs and heart, leading to the insertion of chest drains [42].

Diagnosis

The diagnosis of anaphylaxis during anesthesia is important, not only to prevent subsequent reactions, but also for epidemiological and medicolegal reasons. The goals of diagnostic testing are to determine the cause of the event, the drug responsible for the event, detect other drugs which may produce a similar event and which drugs are safe drugs to use in future anesthetics.

The history is important. If a patient develops severe bronchospasm, erythema, and cardiovascular collapse after a single injection of Propofol and all the investigations are negative, it is still important to assume anaphylaxis occurred and give a written warning.

Minor reactions restricted to the skin, self-limiting reactions, reactions that respond rapidly to treatment, and delayed reactions are difficult to investigate. The available tests provide little help, perhaps because they are not IgE mediated and the studied tests detect IgE. We have not been able to document a single patient in whom a minor reaction has preceded a severe reaction.

Investigation of an anaphylactic reaction

The investigation during or shortly after the reaction aims to establish if the reaction is immunologically mediated. The agent may be identifiable at the time with radioimmunoassys (RIAs) for drug-specific antibodies.

Histamine assays

Raised concentrations of plasma histamine implicate histamine in the reaction High levels do not establish the cause, but concentrations above 20 nmol/l suggest that histamine is involved and very high levels suggest that the reaction is anaphylactic [14, 15]. Histamine assays have limited value, as the rise is usually transient and sampling must occur when resuscitation is a priority.

IgE levels

Alterations in serum total IgE levels after a reaction have been suggested as evidence that IgE is involved in such reactions, but the evidence is unconvincing. Drug-specific IgE measured during the reaction usually correlates with subsequent measurements [15].

Complement levels

Changes in serum complement levels and activation of the classical and alternative pathways have been demonstrated after clinical anaphylaxis particularly, due to Althesin, contrast media, and protamine [43-45]. These changes have also been shown in IgE-mediated reactions, where they may represent activation secondary to shock or an independent process. Complement activation may occur without clinical manifestations, especially after cardiopulmonary bypass when heparin-protamine complexes may activate complement [46]. In investigations of suspected anaphylaxis, complement levels have limited value, do not detect the drug responsible, and only confirm that some immunological event has occurred.

Mast cell tryptase

Measurement of mast cell tryptase (MCT) is an important advance in the diagnosis of anaphylactoid reactions during anesthesia. Tryptase is a protease in mast cell granules and is released during their activation [47]. In anaphylactic reactions the levels are elevated for 1-5 h after the onset of the reaction [48], enabling resuscitation to occur before the need for blood sampling. The assay is robust, easy to transport, and requires no special handling of the blood samples. It is not affected by hemolysis and reliable samples can be obtained at postmortem examination [49, 50]. Although in reactions to anesthetic drugs, mast cell tryptase appears to be highly specific and sensitive for anaphylaxis, severe reactions may occur where there is evidence of IgE involvement by skin testing or RIA and tryptase levels are not elevated. Laroche et al. postulate an allergic mechanism where the mediators of anaphylaxis are released from basophils that do not contain tryptase [15]. Tryptase is also released during direct histamine release.

Table 6 shows the incidence of positive skin and RIA tests associated with elevated MCT. Although the association of elevated MCT levels and positive tests is high, the severity of reactions means that skin testing is still necessary when MCT levels are not elevated [51].

Table 6. Relationship between IgE and elevated mast cell tryptase (MCT) in anesthetic anaphylaxis

Group	Total patients	No. skin test positive/ no. performed	RIA no. positive/ no. performed	IgE detected
MCT not elevated in appropriately timed sample	143	6/87	4/81	7/137
MCT elevated	158	108/113	72/101	125/158
p value (chi-squard)	< 0.0001	< 0.0001	< 0.0001	

(*RIA* = radioimmunoassay)
Modified from [51]

Investigations after a reaction

Skin testing

Skin testing is performed 4-6 weeks after the reaction, but only detects reactions due to IgE and possibly IgG. It is the best investigation to determine the drug responsible in all studies published. Two forms of skin testing are used – intradermal and prick testing. Intradermal tests involve diluting the drug and injecting it into the dermis; in prick testing the undiluted drug is introduced into the dermis by pricking the patient's skin. It is usual to use controls such as histamine and/or high concentrations of an opioid to determine that the histamine response and release is normal. The great advantages of skin tests are that they have the highest yield of positive results, and can be performed by anyone, and cross-sensitivity determined by skin testing usually enables safe subsequent anesthesia [17, 51, 52]. Prick testing causes less trauma to the skin, and is easier, cheaper, and safer. It is more likely to be tolerated by and successfully completed in children. Intradermal tests may produce more false positives and so may be slightly safer in that respect. The two tests have a greater than 90% agreement for the drug implicated [53, 54], but agreement in determining cross-sensitivity with NMBDs is less reliable.

Skin tests are of little value in reactions to colloids, contrast media, and blood products. Local anesthetic allergy is so rare that the aim is to exclude allergy. Skin testing alone is inadequate and so without a clear-cut history suggestive of anaphylaxis and a positive wheal and flare reaction to local anesthetic at 1:100 dilution of 0.5%, local anesthetic the dose should be increased to 2 ml of undiluted local. Before skin testing, challenging the patient with 2 ml of saline often reproduces the symptoms.

Deaths have occurred during skin testing (although not to anesthetic drugs). In over 1,200 intradermal tests we have had only 3 easily treatable reactions, but resuscitation facilities should always be present.

RIA tests

Use of these tests in over 300 patients has shown the following.

1. RIA tests detect the responsible drugs less often than skin tests.
2. A combination of RIA tests and skin tests will increase the detection of responsible drugs by about 5%. There is generally agreement between the tests for the drugs responsible, but a 50% disagreement for tests to other NMBDs when a battery of tests is performed.
3. Cross-sensitivity as determined by RIA is greater than by skin testing, due to both false-positive RIA and false-negative skin tests.
4. Recently we have shown that a RIA for morphine is a more-reliable detector of antibodies to NMBDs than specific assays [55].

Other tests

Leukocyte and basophil histamine release tests have been used in specialized laboratories and give similar results to RIA.

Preoperative testing

Preoperative testing of either all or perceived high-risk patients has been suggested. We preoperatively tested 79 patients because of a family history of a reaction, multiple allergies, or alleged environmental chemical sensitivity syndrome, and found 2 weakly positive skin tests. French studies showing a high incidence of positive skin tests in the population in some regions present a challenge to anesthetists. To prick test patients preoperatively with the drugs drawn up for use may be a valid, and virtually cost free, method of preventing anaphylaxis in areas where the apparent risk is high. Adoption of the practice makes the anesthetist who does not pretest a patient who reacts, medicolegally vulnerable.

Desensitization and blocking

Thomas et al. [56] used the monoquaternary compound tiemmonium to block allergy to NMBDS by binding to the quaternary receptor. French workers have used other monoquaternary compounds to block reactions [57]. H_1 and H_2 antihistamines in combination with steroids and ephedrine should also at least modify and possibly block reactions, but this has not been convincingly demonstrated in anesthesia.

Documentation

Allergic patients should be encouraged to wear a warning device stating the drugs implicated by the testing and be given a letter stating which drugs were given, what happened, which tests were performed, the results of those tests, and the conclusion. Subsequent anesthetists should add details of subsequent anesthesia. Anesthetic allergy has been shown to persist for up to 27 years, and few patients lose their sensitivity [58].

With this method of testing and follow-up, we have seen five subsequent allergic reactions in 320 subsequent exposures. Of 69 patients who were diagnosed as not anaphylactic, 68 have had uneventful subsequent anesthesia and 1 had a second prolonged block.

References

1. Lorenz W, Doenicke A, Schoning B et al (1982) Definition and classification of the histamine-release response to drugs in anaesthesia and surgery: studies in the conscious human subject. Klin Wochenschr 60:896-913
2. Kaliner M, Sigler R, Summers R et al (1981) Effects of infused histamine: analysis of the effects of H-1 and H-2 histamine receptor antagonists on cardiovascular and pulmonary responses. J Allergy Clin Immunol 68:365-371
3. Moss J, Rosow CE, Savarese JJ et al (1981) Role of histamine in the hypotensive action of d-tubocurarine in humans. Anesthesiology 55:19-25
4. Philbin DM, Moss J, Akins CW et al (1981) The use of H1 and H2 histamine antagonists with morphine anesthesia: a double-blind study. Anesthesiology 55:292-296
5. Hosking MP, Lennon RL, Gronert GA (1988) Combined H1 and H2 receptor blockade attenuates the cardiovascular effects of high-dose atracurium for rapid sequence endotracheal intubation. Anesth Analg 67:1089-1092
6. Lorenz W, Sitter H, Stinner B et al (1991) Controlled clinical trials and cross-sectional studies with plasma histamine measurements and histamine receptor antagonists: solving the problem of pre-operative H1 + H2 prophylaxis by asking new questions? Agents Actions [Suppl 33]:197-229
7. Hermann K, Ring J (1995) Association between the renin angiotensin system and anaphylaxis. Adv Exp Med Biol 377:299-309
8. Hermann K, von Eschenbach CE, von Tschirschnitz M et al (1993) Plasma concentrations of arginine vasopressin, oxytocin and angiotensin in patients with Hymenoptera venom anaphylaxis. Regul Pept 49:1-7
9. Laforest M, More D, Fisher M (1980) Predisposing factors in anaphylactoid reactions to anaesthetic drugs in an Australian population: the role of allergy, atopy and previous anaesthesia. Anaesth Intensive Care 8:454-459
10. Charpin D, Benzarti M, Hemon Y et al (1988) Atopy and anaphylactic reactions to suxamethonium. J Allergy Clin Immunol 82:356-360
11. Fisher MM, Outhred A, Bowey CJ (1987) Can clinical anaphylaxis to anaesthetic drugs be predicted from allergic history? Br J Anaesth 59:690-692
12. Clark MM, Cockburn HA (1971) Anaphylactoid response to thiopentone. Case report. Br J Anaesth 43:185-189
13. Fisher MM, Munro I (1983) Life-threatening anaphylactoid reactions to muscle relaxants. Anesth Analg 62:559-564
14. Laroche D, Vergnaud MC, Sillard B et al (1991) Biochemical markers of anaphylactoid reactions to drugs. Comparison of plasma histamine and tryptase. Anesthesiology 75:945-949
15. Laroche D, Dubois F, Lefrancois C et al (1992) Marquers biologiques precoces des reactions anaphylactoides peranesthesiques. Ann Fr Anesth Reanim 11: 613-618
16. Laxenaire MC, Moneret-Vautrin DA, Widmer S et al (1990) Substances anesthesiques responsables de chocs anaphylactiques. Enquete multicentrique francaise. Anaesthetic drugs responsible for anaphylactic shock. French multi-center study. Ann Fr Anesth Reanim 9: 501-506
17. Fisher MM, Baldo BA (1993) The incidence and clinical features of anaphylactic reactions during anaesthesia in Australia. Ann Fr Anesth Reanim 12:97-104
18. Moneret-Vautrin DA, Laxenaire MC, Hummer-Siegel M et al (1990) Myorelaxants. In: Laxenaire MC, Moneret-Vautrin DA (eds) Le risque allergique en anesthesie-reanimation. Masson, Paris, pp 52-58
19. Fisher MM (1999) Atracurium and cisatracurium as antigens. Anaesth Intensive Care 27: 369-370
20. Laxenaire MC, Mata Bermejo E, Moneret Vautrin DA et al (1992) Life-threatening anaphylactoid reactions to propofol (Diprivan). Anesthesiology 77:275-280
21. Fisher MM, Harle DG, Baldo BA (1991) Anaphylactoid reactions to narcotic analgesics. Clin Rev Allergy 9:309-318

22. Anne S, Reisman RE (1995) Risk of administering cephalosporin antibiotics to patients with histories of penicillin allergy. Ann Allergy Asthma Immunol 74:167-170
23. Audicana M, Bernaola, I, Urrutia S et al (1994) Allergic reactions to betalactams: studies in a group of patients allergic to penicillin and evaluation of cross-reactivity with cephalosporin (abstract). Allergy 49:108
24. Kuenneke M, Celik I, Stinner B et al (1996) Cardiovascular adverse effects of antimicrobials in complex surgical cases. Eur J Surg 162:24-28
25. Weiss ME, Nyhan D, Zhikang P et al (1989) Association of protamine IgE and IgG antibodies with life-threatening reactions to intravenous protamine. N Engl J Med 320:886-892
26. Sharath MD, Metzger WJ, Richerson HB et al (1985) Protamine-induced fatal anaphylaxis. Prevalence of antiprotamine immunoglobulin E antibody. J Thorac Cardiovasc Surg 90:86-90
27. Lakin J, Blocker T, Strong D et al (1978) Anaphylaxis to protamine sulphate mediated by a complement dependent IgG antibody. J Allergy Clin Immunol 61:102-106
28. Horrow JC (1985) Protamine: a review of its toxicity. Anesth Analg 64:348-361
29. Messmer K, Ljungstrom KG, Gruber UF et al (1980) Prevention of dextran-induced anaphylactoid reactions by hapten inhibition (letter). Lancet 1:975
30. Kam PCA, Lee MSM, Thompson JF (1997) Latex allergy: an emerging clinical and occupational health problem. Anaesthesia 52:570-575
31. Zerin JM, McLaughlin K, Kerchner S (1996) Latex allergy in patients with myelomeningocele presenting for imaging studies of the urinary tract. Pediatr Radiol 26:450-454
32. Laxenaire MC, Moneret Vautrin DA (1994) L'allergie au latex. Chirurgie 120:526-532
33. Gosgnach M, Bourel LM, Ducart A et al (1995) Pulmonary artery catheter balloon: an unusual cause of severe anaphylactic reaction. Anesthesiology 83:220-221
34. Volcheck GW, Li JT (1994) Elevated serum tryptase level in a case of intraoperative anaphylaxis caused by latex allergy. Arch Intern Med 154:2243-2245
35. Fisher MM, Bowey CJ (1997) Alleged allergy to local anaesthetics. Anaesth Intensive Care 25: 611-614
36. Kajimoto Y, Rosenberg ME, Kytta J et al (1995) Anaphylactoid skin reactions after intravenous regional anaesthesia using 0.5% prilocaine with or without preservative – a double-blind study. Acta Anaesthesiol Scand 39:782-784
37. Waldhausen E, Keser G, Marquardt B (1987) Der Anaphlaktishe schock. Anaesthesist 36:150-158
38. Fisher MM (1977) Blood volume replacement in acute anaphylactic cardiovascular collapse related to anaesthesia. Br J Anaesth 49:1023-1026
39. Fisher MM (1986) Clinical observations on the pathophysiology and treatment of anaphylactic cardiovascular collapse. Anaesth Intensive Care 14:17-21
40. De Soto H, Turk P (1989) Cimetidine in anaphylactic shock refractory to standard therapy. Anesth Analg 69:260-269
41. Raper RF, Fisher MM (1988) Profound reversible myocardial depression after anaphylaxis. Lancet 1:386-388
42. Olinger GN, Becker RM, Bonchek LI (1980) Noncardiogenic pulmonary edema and peripheral vascular collapse following cardiopulmonary bypass: rare protamine reaction? Ann Thorac Surg 29:20-25
43. Best N, Teisner B, Grudzinskas JG et al (1983) Classical pathway activation during an adverse response to protamine sulphate. Br J Anaesth 55:1149-1153
44. Cogen FC, Norman ME, Dunsky E et al (1979) Histamine release and complement changes following injection of contrast media in humans. J Allergy Clin Immunol 64:299-303
45. Watkins J, Appleyard TN, Thornton JA (1976) Immune mediated reactions to althesin (alphaxalone). Br J Anaesth 881-886
46. Best N, Sinosich MJ, Teisner B et al (1984) Complement activation during cardiopulmonary bypass by heparin-protamine interaction. Br J Anaesth 56:339-341
47. Enander I, Matsson P, Nystrand J et al (1991) A new radioimmunoassay for human mast cell tryptase using monoclonal antibodies. J Immunol Methods 138:39-46

48. Schwartz LB, Yunginger JW, Miller J et al (1989) Time course of appearance and disappearance of human mast cell tryptase in the circulation after anaphylaxis. J Clin Invest 83:1551-1555
49. Yunginger JW, Nelson DR, Squilace DL et al (1991) Laboratory investigation of deaths due to anaphylaxis. J Forensic Sci 36:857-865
50. Fisher MM, Baldo BA (1993) The diagnosis of fatal anaphylactic reactions during anaesthesia: employment of immunoassays for mast cell tryptase and drug-reactive IgE antibodies. Anaesth Intensive Care 21:353-357
51. Fisher MM, Baldo BA (1998) Mast cell tryptase in anaesthetic anaphylactoid reactions. Br J Anaesth 80:26-29
52. Leynadier F, Sansarricq M, Dry J (1987) Reproducibility of intradermal tests after anaphylaxis caused by muscle relaxants (in French). Presse Med 16:523-525
53. Leynadier F, Sansarricq M, Didier JM et al (1987a) Prick tests in the diagnosis of anaphylaxis to general anaesthetics. Br J Anaesth 59:683-689
54. Fisher MM, Bowey CJ (1997) Intradermal versus prick testing in the diagnosis of anaesthetic anaphylactic reactions. Br J Anaesth 79:59-63
55. Fisher MM, Baldo BA (2000) Immunoassays in the diagnosis of anaphylaxis to neuromuscular blocking drugs: the value of morphine for the detection of IgE antibodies in allergic subjects. Anaesth Intensive Care 28:167-170
56. Thomas H, Eledjam JJ, Machebouef M. et al (1988) Rapid preoperative immunotherapy in a patient allergic to muscle relaxants. Eur J Anaesth 5:385-389
57. Moneret-Vautrin DA, Kanny G, Gueant JL et al (1995) Prevention by monovalent haptens of IgE dependent leucocyte histamine release to muscle relaxants. International archives of allergy and immunology 107:172-175
58. Fisher MM, Baldo BA (1992a) Persistence of allergy to anaesthetic drugs. Anaesth Intensive Care 20:143-146

Combined Epidural and General Anesthesia in High-Risk Patients

G. GALIMBERTI, D. CARISTI, F. RUBULOTTA

Epidural (EA) and spinal (SA) anesthesia are well-established regional procedures in hospitals around the world. In recent years, besides continuous spinal anesthesia (CSA), combined anesthesia (CA), such as epidural-general anesthesia (CEGA) and spinal-epidural anesthesia (CSE), becoming increasingly popular particularly in high-risk patients.

Regional anesthesia has been used alone or with light general anesthesia in various surgical and non-surgical procedures, such as abdominal, urological, vascular, and orthopedic surgery, or during labor or cesarean section. The rationale for using a combination of two techniques is to associate the advantages of each technique, minimizing specific disadvantages.

CSE for example combines the best features of spinal blockade such as rapid onset, deep blockade, low drug dose with the possibility of prolonging indefinitely anesthesia, and analgesia due to the epidural blockade. Both EA and SA affect the cardiovascular system, leading to hypotension and bradycardia particularly in high-risk patients. Thus, it is very important to titrate the total dose of the anesthetic solution into the subarachnoid space and to increase the sensitive level by using epidural top-up (2-3 ml of local anesthetic solution). SA, either single shot or continuous, allows shorter onset, smaller amount of local anesthetic, and lower local anesthetic plasma concentration than EA. Nevertheless, despite intravenous pre-load and the use of vasopressor drugs, it is often difficult to maintain cardiovascular homeostasis when high levels of spinal block are induced, specially in elderly, high-risk patients or in pregnant women. CSE by using a small initial dose for the SA and afterwards titrating the epidural block until the desired level of anesthesia, avoids excessive sympathetic block and intercostal paralysis. These advantages make CSE specially appropriate for high-risk patients.

The contraindications of CA are the same as for regional anesthesia alone, including low platelet count (< 100,00 mm^3), impairment of the clotting system, severe heart disease (i.e., aortic stenosis, cardiogenic shock), skin infection at the injection site or sepsis, endocranial hypertension, and psychiatric or neurological disease.

Another important issue in the high-risk patient is the prediction of outcome after surgery. Surprisingly, after 150 years of modern anesthesia, one is still unable to assess accurately the impact of the anesthetic technique on patient outcome [1]. Surgery and anesthesia induce a strong change in body homeostasis and are strictly associated with a postoperative morbidity and mortality, according to surgical procedure, duration of anesthesia, American Society of Anesthesiologists (ASA) physical status, age, anesthetic technique, and elective versus emergency procedure [2]. Large trials were conducted to estimate outcome and identify risk factors for different groups of patients [3-7]. Moreover, several studies were performed to show if the choice of anesthesia technique influences patient outcome, concluding that anesthetic-related factors have no significant impact on patient outcome, while knowledge of patients factors (age, sex, and preoperative status) and the type of surgery performed (emergent or major) are all that is necessary to predict outcome [8, 9]. In recent years there has been an increased interest in modifying anesthetic techniques to improve outcome [7, 10]. CA has been one of these techniques and has been shown to exert a favorable effect on several aspects of operative outcome. CA is effective in reducing the incidence of respiratory and cardiovascular complications and improving the postoperative outcome in high-risk patients undergoing major surgery [11]. Data collected in controlled studies showed that CA, as compared to general anesthesia (GA), reduces mortality, intra- and postoperative blood losses, and thus the need for homologous blood transfusions and deep venous thrombosis, duration of postoperative intensive care stay, and incidence in postoperative infections and the overall postoperative complications rate [12-16]. Therefore we performed a prospective trial comparing the outcome of a particular CA (CEGA) with GA in high-risk patients undergoing major surgery.

Our experience

We enrolled 153 high-risk patients (ASA ≥ 3) to compare the incidence of morbidity and mortality after GA or CA. Patients were enrolled after informed written consent in agreement with the Helsinki Declaration and approval by the regional ethics committee. Patients were randomized to receive either CEGA or GA and were investigated from surgery to discharge. The criteria for entry into this study were: 1) age greater than 18 years; 2) ASA ≥ 3; 3) elective major abdominal and urological surgery lasting more 180 min; 4) no contraindications to the insertion of an epidural catheter (i.e., septicemia, preoperative coagulopathy, localized infection, and neurological diseases). The patients were scheduled preoperatively to receive postoperative care in an intensive care unit (ICU). Premedication consisted of diazepam per os (0.1 mg/kg) 60 min before surgery.

On arrival in the operating room, an intravenous catheter and a radial arterial line were inserted and electrocardiograph (ECG) and pulse oximetry monitoring commenced. In the CEGA group, after a quick volemic refilling with 500-1,000 ml of crystalloids, an 20-gauge epidural catheter was inserted through a 18-gauge Tuohy needle into the epidural space of thoracic spine (usually T11-T12).

Following a 2-ml test dose of lignocaine 2% (40 mg) without epinephrine, a further dose of 5-10 ml of isobaric bupivacaine (0.5%) or ropivacaine (0.75%) was administered alone or associated with opioids such as fentanyl 0.05-0.10 mg or morphine 2-3 mg (morphine: fentanyl equivalency ratio = 100:1) [16]. Starter local anesthetic dose was calculated according to the patient's weight, age, and surgical level required, and was performed immediately before the induction of GA. Further boluses of 0.5% isobaric bupivacaine were injected intraoperatively every 60-90 min, using a sufficient dose to achieve and maintain surgical analgesia (usually 50% of the first dose). Both groups of patients were treated intraoperatively according to the preoperative status and the usual dictates of "good anesthesia care" with provision for patients' amnesia, hemodynamic stability, optimal pulmonary ventilation, and muscle relaxation. GA was induced by administering 1-3 μg/kg fentanyl, 1-2 mg/kg propofol or 2-4 mg/kg thiopentone. Intubation was performed employing succinylcholine 1 mg/kg or 0.08 mg/kg vecuronium bromide, and ventilation was controlled throughout surgery. GA was maintained with isoflurane in N_2O-O_2 (50%:50%) or air-O_2, fentanyl, and 0.04 mg/kg vecuronium bromide every 40-60 min. Other monitoring included end-tidal CO_2 ($EtCO_2$), end-tidal concentrations of isoflurane, urine output, blood loss, pre- and postoperative hemoglobin levels, and pH on transfer to the ICU.

Intraoperative blood loss was estimated from the increase in weight of swabs and towels and the content of suction bottles; postoperative blood loss for the following 24 h was calculated from the vacuum drainage bottles and the increase in weight of operative wound dressings [12]. Intraoperative maintenance fluids were given at 5-10 ml/kg per hour and blood loss was initially replaced with polygeline (Eufusin, Emagel) and autologous blood predeposited. Hypertension (systolic blood pressure ≥ 20% basal value) was treated with intravenous urapidil and hypotension (systolic blood pressure ≤ 20% basal value) with blood volume expansion and/or intravenous metaraminol 1 mg or ephedrine 5 mg if associated with bradycardia (heart rate ≤ 60 beats/min). We considered mean arterial pressure (MAP), heart rate (HR), and $EtCO_2$ at four particular times: basal (in the operating room before induction of GA), 30 min and 60 min after the first bolus of epidural anesthetics, performed immediately before the induction of GA, and at awakening.

Postoperative analgesia was maintained for 48-72 h after surgery in all patients by epidural infusion of a mixture of local anesthetic and opioids (usually 0.125% bupivacaine or 0.1% ropivacaine plus 3-5 mg morphine per day) in CE-GA patients and by an intravenous infusion of ketorolac tromethamine (1 mg/kg per day) and pethidine (1.5-3 mg/kg per day) in GA patients. The target of postoperative pain relief was to maintain the visual analogical score (VAS) below 3 for at least three consecutive measurements. Clinical outcome was defined as previously described by Yeager et al. [11]. Major clinical outcome variables analyzed were mortality and morbidity. Mortality was defined as a death which occurred in the hospital while a patient was recovering from the original surgical procedure. Major morbidity was defined as the appearance of organ failure or reoperation for a complication related to the original surgical procedure. Variables analyzed for cost utilization were duration of postoperative stay in ICU (time until patients were discharged from the ICU) and total hospital stay (time until patients were discharged from the hospital).

Data (mean ± SD) were examined by factorial and repeated variance analysis (ANOVA-test) and by non-parametric test for paired and unpaired groups (Mann-Whitney test), by chi-squared with continuity correction. Significance of all values was assessed at $p < 0.05$.

Results

A total of 153 patients were enrolled in this study, 82 in the CEGA group and 71 in the GA group. Demographic data are listed in Table 1. There were no significant differences between groups as regard to age, sex, weight, height, ASA, surgical procedure, average duration of the operation, blood loss, intraoperative fluid balance, and postoperative mortality. Table 2 shows the hemodynamic trend in the patient groups.

Table 1. Patient demographic data (mean ± SD

Parameter	GA (n = 71)	CEGA (n = 82)	Significance
Age (years)	76.8 ± 9.2	78.4 ± 8.5	NS
Sex (M/F)	42/29	45/37	NS
Weight (kg)	79.5 ± 6.7	76.7 ± 6.5	NS
Height (cm)	173.2 ± 11.2	174.6± 10.1	NS
ASA (3/3-5)	58/13	65/17	NS
Time surgery (min)	293.38 ± 64.45	291.78 ± 72.85	NS

(*NS* not significant) (*ASA* atrial septal aneurysm)

In GA-ASA > 3 group, basal with MAP and 60-min MAP were lower than in others and 60-min MAP was also associated with a significant decrease in $EtCO_2$ ($p < 0.03$). Heart rate was lower in urological surgery in both groups, but significantly higher in GA-ASA > 3 ($p < 0.02$). Between GA and CEGA groups, there were no significant differences as regard to MAP. The variation of MAP in realtion to ASA physical status and anesthetic technique is shown in Figure 1.

There were statistically significant variations of MAP during the various stages of surgery in the CEGA group and GA group (Fig. 1), although patients did not need therapeutic treatment (variation ≤ 20% from basal value). The vari-

Table 2. Hemodynamic trends in the patient groups (mean ± SD)

Parameter	CEGA ASA 3 (*n* = 53)	CEGA ASA > 3 (*n* = 29)	GA ASA 3 (*n* = 46)	GA ASA > 3 (*n* = 25)	*p*
MAP basal (mmHg)	108.90 ± 15.36	110.53 ± 12.24	106.78 ± 14.64	*98.53 ± 16.61	0.01
MAP 30 min	94.35 ± 13.06	93.45 ± 13.48	96.81 ± 12.54	85.46 ± 12.13	NS
MAP 60 min	88.88 ± 16.12	89.46 ± 13.28	97.67 ± 13.72	*84.02 ± 13.14	0.03
MAP at awakening	94.05 ± 11.06	92.12 ± 11.92	94.24 ± 13.02	83.87 ± 14.69	NS
HR basal (beats min)	66.53 ± 14.65	68.72 ± 15.27	71.36 ± 15.34	*80 ± 17.22	0.01
HR 30 min	64.85 ± 12.58	64.51 ± 14.74	66.23 ± 11.57	*78.18 ± 10.62	0.01
HR 60 min	65.81 ± 14.28	65.14 ± 13.51	64.58 ± 14.72	*76.71 ± 12.47	0.01
HR at awakening	70.34 ± 12.56	72 ± 13.85	79.35 ± 17.77	78.42 ± 13.63	NS
$EtCO_2$ basal (kPa)	4.48 ± 0.41	4.52 ± 0.36	4.48 ± 0.42	4.46 ± 0.42	NS
$EtCO_2$ 30 min	4.31 ± 0.38	4.37 ± 0.32	4.41 ± 0.33	4.38 ± 0.37	NS
$EtCO_2$ 60 min	4.11 ± 0.42	4.13 ± 0.38	4.15 ± 0.42	4.12 ± 0.27	NS
$EtCO_2$ at awakening	4.37 ± 0.31	4.38 ± 0.37	4.41 ± 0.45	4.39 ± 0.39	NS

* GA - ASA > 3 group versus other group
(*MAP* mean arterial pressure, *HR* heart rate, *$EtCO_2$* end-tidal CO_2)

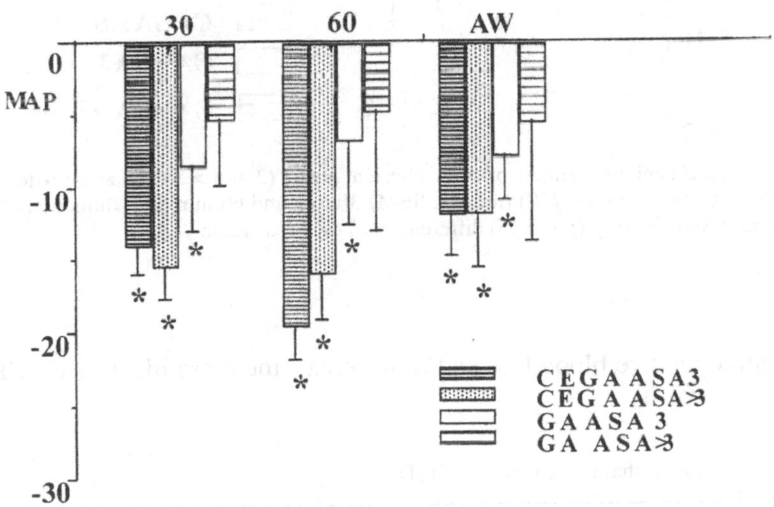

Fig. 1. Histograms depicting effects of ASA physical status (3 and > 3) and anesthetic technique [combined epidural - general anesthesia (CEGA) and (GA)] on mean arterial pressure (*MAP*) (mean ± SEM) 30 min and 60 min after induction of GA and at awakening. *Significantly ($p <$ 0.05) different from the basal value

ation in heart rate was statistically significant between 60 min after induction of anesthesia and at awakening ($p = 0.0001$). There were no statistically significant variations among the other steps.

Between GA and CEGA groups there was a significant difference in heart rate only at awakening, with the CEGA patients having a lower heart rate than those undergoing GA ($p < 0.05$). The variation of heart rate in relation to ASA physical status and anesthetic technique is shown in Figure 2.

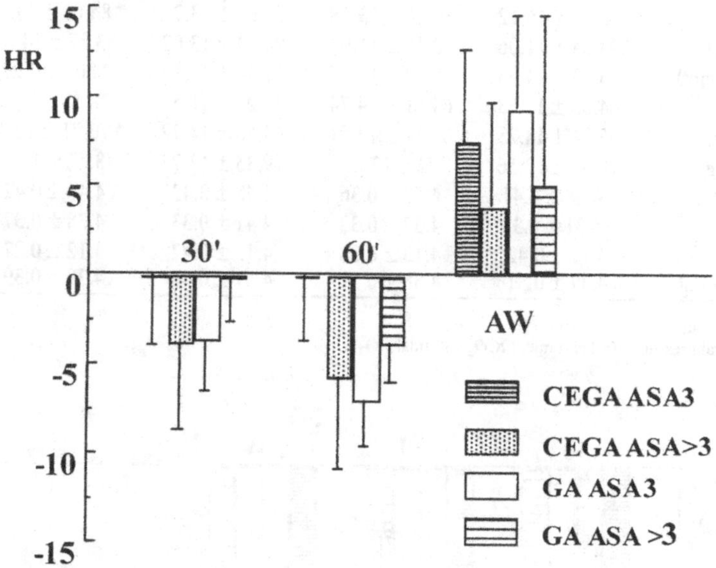

Fig. 2. Histograms depicting effects of ASA physical status (3 and > 3) and anesthetic technique (CEGA and GA) on heart rate (*HR*) (mean ± SEM) 30 min and 60 min after induction of GA and at awakening. *Significantly ($p < 0.05$) different from the basal value

The intraoperative blood loss and fluid replacement are illustrated in Table 3.

Table 3. Intraoperative characteristics: mean (SD)

	GA ($n = 71$)	CEGA ($n = 82$)	Significance
Time surgery (min)	220.48 (78.32)	208.71 (68.76)	NS
Crystalloids (ml)	862.25 (187.94)	753.62 (176.63)	NS
Colloid (ml)	174.82 (102.68)	157.77 (97.39)	NS
Blood (ml)	225.5 (164.7)	176.2 (132.5)	NS
Blood loss (ml)	855.3 (265)	782.1 (241)	NS
Diuresis (ml/h)	83.25 (42.23)	93.6 (53.17)	$p = 0.0088$
MAC/h isoflurane	0.670 (0.41)	0.41 (0.23)	$p < 0.0001$
IV opioids (mg/h)	4.32 (3.1)	1.38 (0.6)	$p < 0.0001$

MAC: minimum alveolar concentration

Twenty-four patients (15.68%) required a postoperative ICU stay. The number of patients in the CEGA group requiring a ICU stay (5 patients) was significantly different from that of the GA group (19 patients) and the ICU and hospital stay was less ($p < 0.001$) (Table 4).

Table 4. Postoperative characteristics: mean ± SD

	GA ($n = 71$)	CEGA ($n = 82$)	Significance
Admission in ICU	19/71	5/82	$p = 0.001$
ICU stay (days)	3.17 ± 2.78	0.8 ± 0.52	$p = 0.001$
Hospital stay (days)	15.72 ± 7.28	12.15 ± 6.58	$p = 0.001$
Non-survivor/survivor	7/64	8/76	NS

Sparing of isoflurane (0.41 vs. 067) and opioids (1.38 vs. 4.32 mg/h of morphine) was really significant in the CEGA group ($p < 0.0001$).

Discussion

The anesthetic technique employed during surgery is an important determinant of perioperative morbidity. GA is advocated for its cerebral protection, but is also associated with greater perioperative blood pressure lability, vasoactive drug use, and ICU stay. GA is associated with increased risk in patients with cardiac disease because hypertension or hypotension may lead to undetected cerebral or coronary ischemia. Regional anesthesia has been advocated as a mean of reducing perioperative complications in carotid artery surgery, its advantages being primarily related to hemodynamic stability, shorter hospital stay, and improved neurological monitoring. The incidence of ventricular dysrhythmias following carotid endoarterectomy is greater among patients receiving GA. Is still important to underline that the incidence of death, myocardial infarction, and stroke is independent of anesthetic technique used. CEGA allows early extubation and a decreased need for systemic narcotics in the postoperative period. CEGA, in high-risk patients undergoing aortic reconstruction, it is also associated with a lower incidence of respiratory complications than GA. CEGA during open heart surgery attenuates the stress response and thereby provides a better quality of postoperative pain control than GA.

Epidural postoperative pain treatment has the advantage of diminishing post-surgical bleeding as compared to pain treatment with parenteral analgesics, on average 25-35% [17]. Epidural analgesia alone may prevent most of the endocrine-metabolic changes following lower abdominal and gynecological operations and procedures on the lower extremities. Thus, there are many theoretical reasons favoring the use of CEGA. These include a dampening of the hormonal response to stress [11, 18, 19], improved myocardial blood flow and reduced myocardial oxygen consumption [20, 21], improved postoperative lung function [22] and postoperative analgesia. On the other hand, EA is associated with rare but serious complications due to insertion of the epidural catheter, such as headache, backache, neurological injuries, epidural abscess, and hematoma, particularly during vascular surgery for the intraoperative anticoagulation required [10]. Furthermore, CEGA may be associated with severe hypotension with increased requirement for fluids and intravenous vasopressors. Therefore, in order to justify the combination of EA with GA there must be good evidence that improved outcome may outweigh the risks associated with EA [23].

In our experience both techniques, CEGA and GA, allowed a good intraoperative hemodynamic stability during surgery in high-risk patients. In particular MAP values were always lower in the CEGA group than the GA group, but the patients never needed vasoconstrictor drugs; MAP reduction was always $\leq 20\%$ from basal value. Furthermore, heart rate and MAP values at awakening were not statistically significantly different from the basal level underlining the good relief of postoperative pain either by epidural analgesia or by antinflammatory and opioid intravenous drugs [11, 24].

Although no statistically significant differences were found in intraoperative blood losses, fluid balance, and colloid infusion between CEGA and GA groups, GA patients required more intraoperative blood transfusion and more blood and colloids in the ICU. Theoretically, local anesthetics should increase bleeding by their inhibitory effects on platelets aggregation [25, 26] and on the clotting tendency, as measured by factor VIII capacity and factor VIII-related antigen [27, 28]; the fibrinolytic system is also stimulated, so that patients with CEGA would be more susceptible to develop bleeding problems. Thus platelets are activated in surgery releasing vasoactive substances such as thromboxane (TXB2), serotonin (5-HT), and beta-thromboglobulin (beta-TG); platelets become temporarily hypoaggregable during surgery, followed by a postoperative hyperaggregability, and CEGA does not significantly modify this stress response [29]. Also intraoperative blood losses are similar in CEGA and GA groups despite the pharmacological sympathectomy, hypotension, use of vasopressors and anesthetic drugs such as fentanyl, morphine, nitrous oxide, vecuronium, and isoflurane. These agents have not been implicated as affecting intraoperative bleeding [30]. Positive pressure ventilation has been shown to increase intrathoracic pressure and central venous pressure with decreased venous return to the heart [31, 32] from the periphery and increased peripheral venous pressure [33]. Increased peripheral venous pressure has been shown to increase blood losses during surgery [34].

Recovery of postoperative pulmonary function in the CEGA group was earlier than in the GA group and CEGA patients requiring ICU for postoperative respiratory failure also needed a shorter period of mechanical ventilation. In fact,

CEGA has been associated with less sedation [35], earlier ambulation [36], higher pulmonary flow rates [37, 38], and improved oxygenation [39].

Davies et al. [10] found a wide spectrum of postoperative complications in both groups (CEGA vs. GA), but the GA group was not associated with an increased incidence of cardiovascular and respiratory complications, there was no difference in the duration of time in either the ICU and total hospital stay between groups, and consequently the cost of patient treatment would be comparable between groups. Other studies [11, 15] show that ICU stay and total hospital stay are significantly higher in the GA group compared to the CEGA group due to a prolonged endotracheal intubation and mechanical ventilation with a major incidence of infective complications and a well-documented inhibition of the immune system during surgical stress. The debate about the anesthetic technique in high-risk patients continues.

With regard to the clinical implications of our study, it should be stressed that the costs for the ICU stay (the mean ICU cost per day for surgical patients was US$ 1,501) were 3.8 times the costs for the non-ICU stay [10]. So, although the anesthesia costs are generally a small portion of the overall costs associated with a surgical patient's hospital stay (≤ 5%), we think that a greater cost saving may be obtained by improving operating room efficiency as well as those processes of care that reduce the length of hospital stay.

In summary, our experience in high-risk patient supports previous findings that the combination of EA and GA in high-risk patients undergoing major surgery seems to be an optimal strategy in reducing ICU stay, total hospital stay, and care costs.

References

1. Myles PS, Williams NJ, Powell J (1994) Predicting outcome in anaesthesia: understanding statistical methods. Anaesth Intensive Care 22:447-453
2. Hines R, Barash PG, Watrous G, O'Connor T (1992) Complications occurring in the Postanesthesia Care Unit: a survey. Anesth Analg 74:503-509
3. Vacanti C, Van Houten RJ, Hill RC (1970) A statistical analysis of the relationship of physical status to postoperative mortality in 68.388 cases. Anesth Analg 49:564-566
4. Marx GF, Mateo CV, Orkin LR (1973) Computer analysis of postanesthetic deaths. Anesthesiology 39:54-58
5. Farrow SC, Fowkes FGR, Lunn JN et al (1982) Epidemiology in anaesthesia. II. Factors affecting mortality in hospital. Br J Anaesth 54:811-816
6. Holland R (1987) Anaesthetic mortality in New South Wales. Br J Anaesth 59:834-841
7. Bode RH, Lewis KP, Zarich SW (1996) Cardiac outcome after peripheral vascular surgery. Anesthesiology 84:3-13
8. Cohen MM, Duncan PG, Tate RB (1988) Does anesthesia contribute to operative mortality? JAMA 260:2859-2863
9. Tiret L, Hatton F, Desmonts JM (1988) Prediction of outcome of anaesthesia in patients over 40 years: a multifactorial risk index. Stat Med 7:947-954

10. Davies MJ, Silbert BS, Mooney PJ et al (1993) Combined epidural and general anaesthesia versus general anaesthesia for abdominal aortic surgery: a prospective randomised trial. Anaesth Intensive Care 21:790-794
11. Yeager MP, Glass DD, Neff RK, Brinck-Johnsen T (1987) Epidural anesthesia and analgesia in high risk surgical patients. Anesthesiology 66:729-736
12. Modig J (1988) Regional anaesthesia and blood loss. Acta Anaesthesiol Scand 32:44-48
13. Ryan P, Schweitzer SA, Woods RJ (1992) Effect of epidural and general anaesthesia compared with general anaesthesia alone in large bowel anastomoses. Eur J Surg 158:45-49
14. Tuman KJ, McCarthy RJ, March RJ et al (1991) Effects of epidural anesthesia on coagulation and outcome after major vascular surgery. Anesth Analg 73:696-704
15. Her C, Kizelshteyn G, Walker V et al (1990) Combined epidural and general anaesthesia for abdominal aortic surgery. J Cardiothorac Anesth 4:552-557
16. Koch SM (1997) Critical care catalog. In: Civetta JM, Taylor RW, Kirby RR (eds) Critical care, 3rd edn. Lippincott-Raven, Philadelphia, pp 2255-2281
17. Rawal N (1995) Acute pain service in Europe – a 17 nation survey. Reg Anesth 20:85
18. Madsen SN, Brandt MR, Engquist A et al (1977) Inhibition of plasma cyclic AMP, glucose and cortisol response to surgery by epidural analgesia. Br J Surg 64:669-671
19. Stenseth R, Bjella L, Berg EM et al (1994) Thoracic epidural analgesia in aortocoronary bypass surgery. II. Effects on the endocrine metabolic response. Acta Anaesthesiol Scand 38: 834-839
20. Kirnö K, Friberg P, Grzegorczyk A et al (1994) Thoracic epidural anesthesia during coronary artery bypass surgery: effects on cardiac sympathetic activity, myocardial blood flow and metabolism, and central hemodynamics. Anesth Analg 79:1075-1081
21. Klassen GA, Bramwell RS, Bromage PR (1980) Effect of acute sympathectomy by epidural anaesthesia on the canine coronary circulation. Anesthesiology 52:8-15
22. Mankikian B, Cantineau JP, Bertrand M (1988) Improvement of diaphragmatic function by a thoracic extradural block after upper abdominal surgery. Anesthesiology 68:379-386
23. Blake DW (1995) The general versus regional anaesthesia debate: time to re-examine the goals. Aust N Z J Surg 65:51-56
24. Cousins MJ (1984) Intrathecal and epidural administration of opioids. Anesthesiology 61: 276-310
25. Modig J, Karlstrom G (1987) Intra- and postoperative blood loss and haemodynamics in total hip replacement when performed under lumbar epidural versus general anaesthesia. Eur J Anaesthesiol 4:345-355
26. Gibbs NM (1991) The effect of anaesthetic agents on platelet function. Anesth Intensive Care 19:495-520
27. Keith I (1977) Anaesthesia and blood loss in total hip replacement. Anaesthesia 32:444-450
28. Thornburn J, Louden JR, Vallance R (1980) Spinal and general anaesthesia in total hip replacement: frequency of deep vein thrombosis. Br J Anaesth 52:1117-1121
29. Naesh O, Hindberg I, Friis J (1994) Platelet activation in major surgical stress: influence of combined epidural and general anaesthesia. Acta Anaesthesiol Scand 38:820-825
30. Shir Y, Raja SN, Frank SM, Brendler CB (1995) Intraoperative blood loss during radical retropubic prostatectomy: epidural versus general anaesthesia. Urology 45:993-999
31. Hodgson DC (1964) Venous stasis during surgery. Anaesthesia 19:96-99
32. Nanas S, Magder S (1992) Adaptations of the peripheral circulation to PEEP. Am Rev Respir Dis 146:688-693
33. Morgan BC, Martin WE, Hornbein TF (1966) Hemodynamic effects of intermittent positive pressure respiration. Anesthesiology 27:584-590
34. Di Stefano VJ, Klein KS, Nixon JE (1974) Intraoperative analysis of the effect of body position and body habitus on surgery of the low back. A preliminary report. Clin Orthop 99:51-56
35. Hole A, Terjesen T, Breivik H (1980) Epidural versus general anaesthesia for total hip arthroplasty in elderly patients. Acta Anaesthesiol Scand 24:279-287

36. Rawal N, Sjostrand U, Christofferson E (1984) Comparison of intramuscular and epidural morphine for postoperative analgesia in the grossly obese: influence on postoperative deambulation and pulmonary function. Anesth Analg 63:583-592
37. Pflug AE, Murphy TM, Butler SH (1974) The effects of postoperative peridural analgesia on pulmonary therapy and pulmonary complications. Anesthesiology 41:8-17
38. Shulman M, Sandler AN, Bradley JW (1984) Posthoracotomy pain and pulmonary function following epidural and systemic morphine. Anesthesiology 61:569-575
39. Catley DM, Thornton C, Jordan C (1985) Pronounced episodic oxygen desaturation in the postoperative period: its association with ventilatory pattern and analgesic regimen. Anesthesiology 63:20-28

Critical Point in Perioperative Medicine: Anaesthesia for Day Surgery

P.F. WHITE

Ambulatory surgery accounts for over 60% of all elective operative procedures performed in North America. With the recent growth in office-based surgery, this percentage may increase to 70% as we begin the new millennium. When surgery is performed outside the conventional hospital environment, it can offer a number of advantages for patients, healthcare providers, third-party payers, and even hospitals [1]. Patients benefit from day-surgery because it decreases separation from their home and family environment, decreases their likelihood of contracting hospital-acquired infections and reduces postoperative complications. Compared to traditional hospital admissions, there is less preoperative lab testing and also a reduced demand for postoperative medications following ambulatory surgery. Unlike inpatient surgery, ambulatory surgery does not depend upon the availability of a hospital bed and may permit the patient greater flexibility in selecting the time of their operation. Furthermore, there is greater efficiency in the utilization of the operating and recovery rooms in the ambulatory setting, contributing to a decrease in the overall patient charges compared to similar in-hospital care. As a result, hospitalization for many procedures is now considered inappropriate. In fact, it has become difficult to convince insurance and healthcare agencies that there are indeed some patients who benefit from overnight admission prior to most elective operations.

Patient preparation

Several studies have now convincingly demonstrated that a variety of clear liquids can be safely ingested up to two hours before surgery without increasing residual gastric volume. Furthermore, the intake of oral fluids may actually dilute gastric secretions and stimulate gastric emptying, resulting in lower residual gastric volumes. An additional advantage of liberalizing NPO policies is that patients find preoperative fluid restriction unpleasant, and permitting oral fluids results in reduced anxiety, as well as decreased feelings of thirst and hunger [2]. For example, if a patient is scheduled for an ambulatory procedure later in the day, they can be instructed to ingest coffee, tea or juice on the morning of surgery and thereby avoid the anxiety and discomforts associated with caffeine withdrawal and fasting-induced hypoglycemia. Aggressive preoperative hydration will decrease drowsiness, dizziness, thirst, as well as fatigue and nausea after ambulatory surgery [3].

Outpatients should also be instructed to take all their chronic oral medications with a small amount of water up to one hour before the procedure. For patients "at risk" of pulmonary aspiration (e.g. morbidly obese, diabetics), preoperative administration of H_2-antagonists and metoclopramide can reduce both residual gastric volume and acidity. Most patients scheduled to undergo elective operations will experience some degree of anxiety. In addition, intraoperative "awareness" during general anaesthesia is a common concern of patients undergoing elective surgery. Despite the widespread use of premedication for inpatients, outpatients have been traditionally denied pharmacological anxiolysis because of the mistaken belief that sedative premedicant drugs would significantly delay discharge following ambulatory surgery. With the availability of shorter-acting benzodiazepines and sympatholytic drugs (e.g. β-blockers, α_2-agonists), it is now possible to provide reliable preoperative sedation, amnesia and anxiolysis without a clinically significant delay in recovery times even after short ambulatory procedures. In fact, midazolam (1-3 mg intravenously (IV)) or diazepam emulsion (2.5-7.5 mg IV) has recently been reported to improve patient outcome following minor ambulatory procedures [4].

Use of local, regional and general anaesthetic techniques

Ambulatory surgery may potentially be conducted using a wide variety of general, regional or local anaesthetic techniques. The choice of anaesthetic technique depends upon both surgical and patient factors. Increasingly important is the use of intravenous (i.v.) sedation to supplement local anaesthetic-based techniques, as part of a so-called monitored anaesthesia care (MAC) technique [5]. For many procedures, general anaesthesia remains the most popular technique with both patients and hospital staff. Although central neuroaxis blockade (e.g. spinal and epidural anaesthesia) can delay discharge secondary to the residual sympathectomy, peripheral nerve block procedures can actually facilitate the recovery process. Therefore, an increasing percentage of cases are being performed using a combination of peripheral neural blockade and intravenous sedation. The availability of sedative, anaesthetic, analgesic and muscle relaxant drugs with a rapid onset of action, short and highly predictable duration of effect, lack of accumulation, and minimal side effects, has made brief surgical procedures safer and more pleasant for outpatients, and will permit even longer and more complex operations to be performed under general anaesthesia on an ambulatory basis in the future. Newer anaesthetic drugs (e.g. desflurane, remifentanil, rapacuronium) and devices (e.g. EEG-BIS monitor) are also facilitating "fast-tracking" (i.e. "bypassing" the PACU) after ambulatory procedures [6, 7].

Intravenous agents are used for induction of anaesthesia in both adults and older children. Propofol has recently become the IV induction agent of choice for outpatient anaesthesia. Its use is associated with a rapid emergence (as a result of its rapid redistribution and short elimination half-life) and a very low incidence of postoperative side effects. Use of propofol is frequently associated with a degree of euphoria on emergence and a low incidence of postoperative nausea and vomiting (PONV), in particular when it is combined with the ultra-short-acting opioid analgesic remifentanil [8, 9]. Combining propofol with low-dose ketamine has become an increasingly popular technique for ambulatory plastic surgery.

In spite of the increased interest in IV anaesthetic techniques, inhaled agents remain the most popular drugs for maintenance of general anaesthesia. The newer halogenated ether compounds (e.g. sevoflurane, desflurane) have significantly lower blood: gas solubility characteristics, thereby permitting a more rapid onset and termination of their clinical effects. In addition, these less-soluble volatile agents provide a greater degree of intraoperative haemodynamic stability secondary to their enhanced titratability. Desflurane has rapidly gained popularity for maintenance of anaesthesia during ambulatory surgery because it possesses the lowest blood:gas solubility of all volatile anaesthetics, and is associated with the most rapid awakening. Sevoflurane is also associated with faster awakening times and fewer postoperative side effects than halothane and isoflurane. Because it is non-irritating to the airway, sevoflurane can also be used for induction of anaesthesia as an alternative to propofol in both adult and paediatric outpatients. Although propofol infusions are used during the maintenance period to improve the "quality of recovery" from general anaesthesia (e.g. reduce PONV), their use has not been shown to permit a faster recovery or earlier discharge than either sevoflurane or desflurane. When these newer volatile anaesthetics are combined with a low-dose remifentanil infusion (0.04-0.08 $\mu g \cdot kg^{-1} \cdot min^{-1}$), emergence from anaesthesia is extremely rapid, facilitating the fast-tracking process [9, 10]. Of the available opioid analgesics, the newer more potent, rapid and shorter-acting drugs offer advantages in the ambulatory setting.

Muscle relaxants are also an essential component of a "balanced" anaesthetic technique and facilitate laparoscopic surgery. The availability of shorter-acting nondepolarizing muscle relaxants, mivacurium and rapacuronium, has decreased the need for reversal agents even after brief ambulatory procedures. Avoidance of neostigmine-glycopyrrolate will result in a decreased incidence of uncomfortable postoperative side effects. The availability of more rapid and shorter-acting nondepolarizing muscle relaxants facilitate tracheal intubation and provides for a more predictable spontaneous recovery, while avoiding uncomfortable side effects associated with succinylcholine (e.g. myalgias). Although face masks and oral airways are still frequently employed during brief, superficial ambulatory procedures, the use of tracheal intubation remains popular in the day-surgery setting because it minimizes the risk of airway complications.

The laryngeal mask airway (LMA) and the cuffed oropharyngeal airway (COPA) devices are increasingly being employed in situations where either a face mask or tracheal tube would have been used in the past [11]. These newer airway devices have advantages including a clearer, "hands-free" airway when compared to a face mask and oral airway, reduced requirement for anaesthetic agents, a lower incidence of postoperative sore throat, decreased acute haemodynamic changes during induction and emergence, and avoidance of muscle relaxants and reversal agents compared to the use of a tracheal tube. Therefore, the use of "minimally-invasive" airway devices will also facilitate the fast-tracking process.

The flexibility of ambulatory surgery can be greatly enhanced by the use of local anaesthetic infiltration and peripheral nerve block techniques as adjuvants to general anaesthetics or in combination with intravenous sedative-analgesics as part of monitored anaesthesia care (MAC) technique. The use of MAC avoids the common side effects of general anaesthesia, the need for postanaesthesia nursing care decreases, and residual analgesia is provided in the early postoperative period. For upper and lower extremity procedures, as well as localized (superficial) procedures, peripheral nerve block techniques are extremely useful. Recent comparative studies suggest that intraoperative conditions are similar to general anaesthesia central neuroaxis blockade; however, the use of a peripheral nerve block technique with intravenous sedation is associated with an improved recovery profile [12, 13]. In general, subarachnoid blockade is preferable to epidural anaesthesia because it is more readily performed and produces more rapid and consistent effects, thereby decreasing operating room (OR) costs and the need for adjunctive drugs. Although the risk of postdural puncture headache (PDPH) has limited the popularity of this technique in younger patients, the availability of fine pencil-pointed needles has significantly reduced the incidence of PDPH. The primary limiting factor to the more widespread use of central neuroaxis block in the outpatient setting relates to the secondary effects of the residual block (e.g. delayed ambulation, postural hypotension, inability to void). The use of low-dose local anaesthetic-opioid combinations (e.g. 25 mg lidocaine and 25 μg fentanyl or 5 μg sufentanil) for subarachnoid blockade will facilitate the recovery process [14].

Many outpatients find the use of local anaesthetic techniques highly acceptable alternatives to both general and regional anaesthesia when adequate sedation, amnesia and anxiolysis is provided by adjuvant drugs [4, 5]. The availability of rapid and short-acting intravenous sedative-anxiolytic and analgesic drugs can enhance patient comfort during these procedures. Midazolam (2 mg, IV) combined with propofol (25-75 mg • kg^{-1} • min^{-1}) has been shown to significantly increase sedation, amnesia and anxiolysis during procedures performed under local anaesthesia without delaying recovery [15]. Low-dose infusions of propofol can achieve satisfactory levels of sedation, are rapidly adjustable, and permit a rapid recovery and early discharge in both adults and children. The rapid, short-acting esterase-metabolized opioid analgesic remifentanil (0.25 μg •

kg^{-1} and/or 0.05-0.1 $\mu g \cdot kg^{-1} \cdot min^{-1}$) is a valuable adjuvant to midazolam and propofol during MAC. Patients who require large doses of midazolam (6-12 mg) or manifest enhanced sensitivity to benzodiazepine-induced CNS depression can be administered flumazenil (0.25-1.0 mg IV) to reverse residual sedation and amnesia, and thereby facilitate the early recovery process [16].

Fast-tracking concepts

Ambulatory anaesthesia is administered with the goal of rapidly and safely establishing satisfactory conditions for the performance of therapeutic or diagnostic procedures, while ensuring a rapid, predictable recovery with minimal postoperative sequelae. If the careful titration of short-acting drugs permits a safe transfer of patients directly from the operating room suite to the less labour-intensive Phase II (step-down) recovery area, potential cost savings to the institution could be achieved. Bypassing the Phase I recovery (i.e. PACU) has been termed "fast-tracking" after ambulatory surgery [17]. With a more rapid recovery, fewer patients remain deeply sedated in the early postoperative period and the duration of time they are "at risk" for airway obstruction and haemodynamic instability is decreased, along with the need for intensive nursing care. The adoption of fast-tracking criteria may permit an institution to use fewer nurses in the recovery areas [17]. While the availability of more rapid and shorter-acting anaesthetic drugs has clearly facilitated the early recovery process, the prophylactic use of nonopioid analgesics (e.g. local anaesthetics, nonsteroidal anti-inflammatory drugs, acetaminophen) and antiemetics (e.g. droperidol, metoclopramide, 5-HT_3 antagonists, dexamethasone) reduces postoperative side effects and enhances immediate and late recovery after ambulatory surgery. The use of the more costly drugs is economically justified only if improvements in recovery and work patterns can be demonstrated [18]. Anaesthetic practices have advanced to the point where cost savings from variations in drug use are only apparent when system-wide improvements are made in the efficacy of resource utilization (including personnel, space, time, consumables and capital investments [19].

Postoperative analgesia and emesis

The ability to effectively control postoperative pain and emesis may make the difference between performing a given procedure on an inpatient or ambulatory basis. For routine antiemetic prophylaxis, the most cost-effective combination consists of low-dose droperidol (0.625 mg) and dexamethasone (4 mg) [20]. Higher risk patients may benefit from the addition of a 5-HT_3 antagonist. A multi-modal (or "balanced") approach to providing analgesia is also recommended after ambulatory surgery [21-23]. Following outpatient surgery, pain should be controllable with oral analgesics (e.g. ibuprofen, acetaminophen with codeine) before patients are discharged from the facility. Although the potent rapid-acting opioid analgesics are commonly used to treat moderate-to-severe pain in the early recovery period, these compounds increase the incidence of PONV and contribute to a delayed discharge after ambulatory surgery [24, 25]. Recently, there has been an increased use of potent non-steroidal anti-inflammatory agents (e.g. diclofenac, ketorolac), which can effectively reduce the requirements for opioid analgesics after ambulatory surgery and can lead to an earlier discharge [26]. Other less expensive oral non-steroidal analgesics (e.g. ibuprofen, naproxen) have compared favourably to ketorolac [27]. The new Cox-2 antagonists (e.g. parecoxib) may be useful in situations where postoperative bleeding is a major concern (e.g. tonsillectomy, plastic surgery). However, acetaminophen is a more cost-effective alternative if given in appropriate dosages (40-60 mg/kg) [28].

Use of local anaesthetic techniques for intraoperative analgesia or as adjuncts to general anaesthesia, can provide supplemental analgesia during the early postoperative period. Simple wound infiltration or instillation has been shown to improve postoperative analgesia following a variety of lower abdominal, extremity and even laparoscopic procedures. Following laparoscopic procedures, abdominal pain can also be minimized by the use of a local anaesthesia at the portals and topically applied at the surgical site. Shoulder pain is also common following laparoscopic surgery, and this has recently been reported to be effectively treated with subdiaphragmatic instillation of local anaesthetic solutions. Following arthroscopic knee surgery, instillation of 30 ml 0.5% bupivacaine into the joint space reduces postoperative opiate requirements and permits earlier ambulation and discharge. The addition of morphine (1-2 mg), ketorolac (15-30 mg), or even clonidine (0.1-0.2 mg) to the intraarticular solution can further reduce pain after arthroscopic surgery. Future growth in the complexity of surgical procedures that can be performed on an ambulatory basis will require further improvements in our ability to provide effective postoperative pain relief outside the surgical facility (e.g. subcutaneous PCA, transcutaneous iontophoresis).

Conclusions

Ambulatory anaesthesia has become recognized as an anaesthetic subspecialty, with the institution of formal postgraduate training programs. Expansion of the speciality of ambulatory anaesthesia and surgery is likely to continue with the growth in minimally-invasive (so-called keyhole) surgical procedures. The rate of expansion of ambulatory anaesthesia will probably vary depending upon local needs, the level of ancillary home healthcare services, and economic considerations. Many recently developed drugs have pharmacological profiles which are ideally suited for use in the ambulatory setting. Newer anaesthetic drugs (e.g. desflurane, sevoflurane, remifentanil, rapacuronium) and monitoring devices (e.g. BIS monitor) can facilitate fast-tracking in the ambulatory setting [30, 31]. Use of non-pharmacological techniques should also be considered for prevention of postoperative pain and emesis [32, 33]. Given the changing pattern of healthcare reimbursement, it is incumbent upon all practitioners to carefully examine the impact of new drugs and devices on the quality of ambulatory anaesthesia care they are providing to the patient. Future studies on new drugs and techniques for ambulatory anaesthesia need to focus not only on subjective improvements for the patient during the immediate perioperative period, but also on the overall cost-effectiveness of the care being provided [34]. These studies must compare the increased cost of newer treatments with the potential financial savings resulting from earlier hospital discharge, reduced consumption of supplemental drugs, improvements in patient satisfaction, and earlier return to work. The future challenge that all practitioners must face is to provide high-quality ambulatory anaesthesia care in a wide variety of venues [35].

References

1. White PF (1997) Ambulatory anesthesia and surgery - Past, present and future. In: White PF (ed) Ambulatory anesthesia and surgery. WB Saunders, London, pp 1-34
2. Hutchinson A, Maltby JR, Reid CRG (1988) Gastric fluid volume and pH in elective inpatients. Part I: Coffee or orange juice versus overnight fast. Can J Anaesth 35:12-15
3. Yogendran S, Asokumar B, Chung F (1995) A prospective randomized double-blind study of the effect of intravenous fluid therapy on adverse outcomes after outpatient surgery. Anesth Analg 80:682-686
4. Van Vlymen JM, Sa Rego MM, White PF (1999) Benzodiazepine premedication: can it improve outcome in patients undergoing minor ambulatory procedures? Anesthesiology 90: 740-747
5. Sa Rego MM, Watcha MF, White PF (1997) The changing role of monitored anesthesia care in the ambulatory setting. Anesth Analg 85:1020-1036
6. Song D, Joshi GP, White PF (1997) Titration of volatile anesthetics using bispectral index facilitates recovery after ambulatory anesthesia. Anesthesiology 87:842-848
7. Song D, Joshi GP, White PF (1998) Fast-track eligibility after ambulatory anesthesia: a comparison of desflurane, sevoflurane, and propofol. Anesth Analg 86:267-273
8. Philip BK, Scuderi PE, Chung F et al (1997) Remifentanil compared with alfentanil for ambulatory surgery using total intravenous anesthesia. Anesth Analg 84:515-520
9. Song D, White PF (1999) Remifentanil as an adjuvant during desflurane anesthesia facilitates early recovery after ambulatory surgery. J Clin Anesth 11:364-367
10. Song D, Whitten CW, White PF (2000) Remifentanil infusion facilitates early recovery for obese outpatients undergoing laparoscopic cholecystectomy. Anesth Analg 90:1111-1113
11. Van Vlymen JM, Fu W, White PF (1999) Use of the cuffed oropharyngeal airway as an alternative to the laryngeal mask airway with positive pressure ventilation. Anesthesiology 90: 1306-1310
12. Song D, Greilich N, Tongier K et al (1999) Recovery profiles of outpatients undergoing unilateral inguinal herniorrhaphy: a comparison of three anesthetic techniques. Anesth Analg 88:S30
13. Li S, Coloma M, White PF et al (2000) A comparison of the costs and recovery profiles of three anesthetic techniques for ambulatory anorectal surgery. Anesthesiology (in press)

14. Vaghadia H, McLeod DH, Mitchell GW et al (1997) Small-dose hypobaric lidocaine-fentanyl spinal anesthesia for short duration outpatient laparoscopy. A randomized comparison with conventional dose hyperbaric lidocaine. Anesth Analg 84:59-64
15. Taylor E, Ghouri AF, White PF (1992) Midazolam in combination with propofol for sedation during local anesthesia. J Clin Anesth 4:213-216
16. Ghouri AF, Ramirez Ruiz MA, White PF (1994) Effect of flumazenil on recovery after midazolam and propofol sedation. Anesthesiology 81:333-339
17. White PF, Song D (1999) New criteria for fast-tracking after outpatient anesthesia: a comparison with the modified Aldrete's scoring system. Anesth Analg 88:1069-1072
18. Kain ZN, Gaal DJ, Kain TS et al (1994) A first-pass cost analysis of propofol versus barbiturates for children undergoing magnetic resonance imaging. Anesth Analg 79:1102-1106
19. White PF, White LD (1994) Cost-containment in the operating room. J Clin Anesth 6: 351-356
20. White PF, Watcha MF (1999) Postoperative nausea and vomiting: prophylaxis versus treatment. Anesth Analg 89:1337-1339
21. Kehlet H (1994) Postoperative pain relief - What is the issue? [Editorial] Br J Anaesth 72:387-440
22. Eriksson H, Tenhunen A, Korttila K (1996) Balanced analgesia improves recovery and outcome after outpatient tubal ligation. Acta Anaesth Scand 40:151-155
23. Michaloliakou C, Chung F, Sharma S (1996) Preoperative multimodal analgesia facilitates recovery after ambulatory laparoscopic cholecystectomy. Anesth Analg 82:44-51
24. Tang J, Watcha MF, White PF (1996) A comparison of costs and efficacy of ondansetron and droperidol as prophylactic antiemetic therapy for outpatient procedures. Anesth Analg 83: 304-313
25. Tang J, Wang B, White PF et al (1998) Effect of timing of ondansetron administration on its efficacy, cost-effectiveness, and cost-benefit as a prophylactic antiemetic in the ambulatory setting. Anesth Analg 86:274-282
26. Coloma M, White PF, Huber PJ et al (2000) Effect of keterolac on recovery after anorectal surgery: intravenous vs local administration. Anesth Analg 90:1107-1110
27. Souter AJ, Fredman B, White PF (1994) Controversies in the perioperative use of nonsteroidal anti-inflammatory drugs. Anesth Analg 79:1187-1190
28. Korpela R, Konvenoja P, Meretoja OA (1999) Morphine-sparing effect of acetaminophen in pediatric day-care surgery. Anesthesiology 91:442-447
29. White PF, Smith I (1993) Impact of newer drugs and techniques on the quality of ambulatory anesthesia. J Clin Anesth 5:3S-13S
30. White PF, Song D (1999) Criteria for fast-tracking outpatients after ambulatory surgery. J Clin Anesth 11:78-79
31. Song D, Whitten CW, White PF (2000) Remifentanil infusion facilitates early recovery for obese outpatients undergoing laparoscopic cholecystectomy. Anesth Analg 90:1111-1113
32. Chen L, Tang J, White PF et al (1998) The effect of location of transcutaneous electrical nerve stimulation on postoperative opioid analgesic requirement: acupoint versus nonacupoint stimulation. Anesth Analg 87:1129-1134
33. White PF (199) Are nonpharmacologic techniques useful alternatives to antiemetic drugs for the prevention of nausea and vomiting? Anesth Analg 84:712-714
34. Watcha MF, White PF (1997) Economics of anesthetic practice. Anesthesiology 86:1170-1196
35. White PF (2000) Ambulatory anesthesia advances into the new millennium. Anesth Analg 90: 1234-1235

PERIOPERATIVE MANAGEMENT OF OBESE PATIENTS

Challenges for Perioperative Management of Obese Patients: How to Manage the Airways

G. FROVA, D. TUZZO, O. BAROZZI

Obesity is increasing worldwide. In Italy, as in France and Germany, the prevalence of obese citizens is approximately 15% among the middle-aged population [1], i.e., about five million people; therefore, more frequently than in the past, anesthetists have to deal with the difficulties expected in these patients and to plan their management accordingly [2].

Obesity is, in general terms, the condition in which the increase of body fat is no more compatible with a full physic and mental health and a normal expectancy of life [3], but the precise limits between normality and obesity are somewhat arbitrary and are based on definitions expressed in values of body mass index (BMI), which measures the ratio between weight and height:

$$\text{BMI} = \text{body weight in kg/height}^2 \text{ in meters}$$

or of relative weight (RW), the ratio between actual and ideal weight, where the ideal weight is obtained by subtracting 100 in adult males and 105 in adult females from the patient's height in centimeters [4]. For clinical purposes, a subject is considered non-obese when the BMI is under 25; between 25 and 30 he is overweight and over 30 he is considered truly obese.

BMI is strongly correlated with morbidity and mortality, with these two rates sharply rising when the BMI is over 30; overweight patients have a mortality rate 3.9 times greater than normal-weight patients [5].

In the obese, the body fat increase leads to many unfavorable alterations in physiological functions, which influence the whole anesthesiological management, but, in particular, the amount of fat as well as its anatomical distribution heavily interfere with airway management. Face mask ventilation and intubation maneuvers are often difficult, and many of the coexisting pathological conditions concur to dramatically reduce the safety margin of the procedures intended to secure the airway. Moreover, the possibility of using loco-regional techniques is frequently limited or impractical in these patients.

Probably, difficulty in airway management is at least partially responsible for the increased perioperative morbidity and mortality observed in obese patients.

Obesity and vital functions

In obese patients oxygen consumption and carbon dioxide production are increased, because of the excess of metabolically active adipose tissue and the increased workload on musculature [6]. Thoracic compliance is strongly reduced by the chest wall and intrabdominal fat deposits, as well as pulmonary parenchymal compliance, because of the increase of intrapulmonary blood content. This causes increase of the work of breathing, leading to rapid and shallow breathing and thus to the reduction of the efficiency of breathing and of expiratory reserve volume, functional residual capacity, and vital capacity.

A ventilation/perfusion mismatch and large intrapulmonary blood shunt are commonly observed, with consequent hypoxemia and in the worse cases hypercarbia. These conditions can bring about clinical situations such as Pickwick syndrome or obstructive sleep apnea syndrome (OSAS), beside a high incidence of concomitant respiratory diseases. The changes of pulmonary compliance and volumes and their effects are dramatically worsened by the supine (and even Trendelenburg) position, which is needed intraoperatively, especially at the time of induction of general anesthesia, causing a quick desaturation during apnea phases.

Peculiar gastrointestinal modifications are observed in the obese subject, such as a high incidence of gastroesophageal reflux and of diaphragmatic hiatus hernia. Seventy-five percent of obese subjects, specially pregnant patients, present with delayed gastric emptying and a pH less (< 2.5) and a bigger gastric volume content than the general population [7]. These factors, in association with the increased intrabdominal pressure, are responsible for the higher risk of gastric fluid regurgitation and aspiration, and of more-severe complications.

The morbid obese subject is prone to heart failure. The increased intravascular volume and basal metabolic rate require increased cardiac output and therefore cardiac work. The frequently associated chronic hypertension leads to left ventricular hypertrophy and later to dilatation, with reduced compliance and higher filling pressures. As a consequence, the right sections become hypertrophic and dilated, causing global heart failure. In such instances, arrhythmia, stroke, and coronary disease are frequent, because of concomitant atherosclerosis, dyslipidemia, diabetes, lack of physical activity, and varicose veins.

The described hemodynamic instability influences the pharmacological management of the patient, especially at the time of the induction of general anesthesia, with the aim of creating the best conditions to perform the tracheal intubation. In these patients the high basal metabolic rate is one of the factors causing an earlier quick desaturation during the apnea phase of intubation [8].

Obesity and anesthesia

The use of loco-regional anesthesia in obese patients is controversial. Many authors recommend loco-regional procedures every time they are feasible [3] to avoid likely difficult tracheal intubation and the risk of gastric content aspiration. However, precise identification of anatomical landmarks may be difficult and standard instruments (particularly needles) are often inadequate. On the other hand, the emergency treatment of possible major complications can be very difficult. For example, in the case of central blocks, if the dose of local anesthetic is not adequate to the reduced epidural and subarachnoid spaces, it is not uncommon to observe an unexpected upward extension of the level of anesthetic block, which may affect partially the accessory respiratory musculature, leading to the need for respiratory support. Therefore, risks and benefits should be carefully evaluated case by case on a personalized base.

Pharmacokinetics of anesthetic agents are different in the obese subjects. The changes in volume of distribution as well as in plasma protein binding, the increased renal clearance, and the potentially reduced liver clearance influence the proper dosage of drugs.

At the moment of the induction, the dose of hypnotic agent should be larger to compensate for the increased intravascular volume, muscular mass, and cardiac output. Thiopental at a dose of 7.5 mg/kg ideal weight is recommended [9], whereas an increased propofol dose could cause severe cardiovascular depression given its more-significant hemodynamic effects [10]. Opioid kinetic modifications are not constant and difficult to foresee.

A rapid sequence induction-intubation modality utilizing depolarizing muscle relaxant agents, such as suxamethonium 1.2-1.5 mg/kg, is recommended [11]. Neuromuscular blocking agents are often overdosed during surgery, as a consequence of the low thoracic compliance and/or at the surgeon's request. Atracurium is the drug of choice, given its predictable duration of effect due to its organ function-independent elimination [12].

Among the inhalation agents, the use of nitrous oxide obviously reduces the oxygen inspiratory fraction. Volatile agents may require prolonged time of elimination, because of their supposed wide redistribution in the adipose tissue.

Predicting a difficult airway

The weight is a component of the Wilson score [13], but its importance as a single predictive parameter is very limited. It is a common observation during clinical practice that the risk of mechanical interference with airway management may become evident only if the degree of obesity is particularly marked, but it is difficult to identify the threshold of danger.

The definition of morbid obese, such as a patient with a BMI > 35 [14] or > 40 [15] or when his/her actual body weight is twice the ideal weight [16], and of super-morbid obese, when BMI > 55 [14], not only is not homogeneous, but also describes a condition of high or very high risk of medical complication and it is scarcely useful to clearly define the anatomical component of risk due to difficulty in airway management.

A risk assessment based on BMI alone is probably unreliable and incomplete, because physiological alterations indirectly relevant to airway management (i.e., the oxygen relative deficit, the limitation in ventilation, the increased gastric acidity, and the increased risk of reflux) generally increase with increasing body mass index, but a direct relationship between BMI and airway management difficulty is not clearly demonstrated for the considerable variability between obese patients [17]. Bond [18] found no apparent correlation between BMI and difficulty encountered during laryngoscopy, but, in a large number of BMI > 40 obese patients, Voyagis et al. [15] demonstrated an increased risk of difficult laryngoscopy and a great improvement of positive predictive value of the Mallampati test.

There are many consequences of all these considerations: 1) BMI increase is generically predictive of increase in anesthetic risk; 2) BMI alone is scarcely predictive of difficult airway management; 3) very high BMI may mechanically interfere with airway management; 4) the value of BMI must integrate the evaluation of other parameters of difficulty resulting from a careful and detailed assessment of the patient.

Preoperative airway assessment

A detailed patient history and a careful preoperative evaluation of the upper airway of the morbid obese patient is fundamental for reducing the risk and for correct planning of airway management. The minimum assessment is not different by that recommended by SIAARTI guidelines [19] in normal patients and must include:

- examination of previous anesthetic charts and description of difficulties eventually encountered in previous anesthetics, questioning the patient if some relevant change happened successively (such as developments of symptoms of upper airway obstruction, head and neck surgical intervention or radiotherapy, further weight gain, pregnancy, dental treatments or teeth modification, etc.); the detection of excessive snoring and day-time sleepiness is relatively frequent because approximately 5% of morbid obese patients will have obstructive sleep apnea [20] and are more subject to airway obstruction during deep sedation or anesthesia without tracheal tube. The overweight (BMI) is a component of the obstructive apnea syndrome score (Mallampati class, tonsil size, thyro-mental and hyoid-mental distance), which is a good predictor of actual sleep apnea and of its gravity. The OSA obstructive sleep apnea score may help to identify those patients who should have a definitive diagnosis by polysomnography [21]. Their airway examination is completed with the assessment of bilateral patency of the nostrils;

- thyro-mental distance for the assessment of larynx position and neck and head extension, which are directly related to an easy laryngoscopy; the movements of the neck could usefully be integrated by assessment of flexion and lateral rotation of the head; it is also important to evaluate if a dorsal accumulated mass of fat forces the patient in an fixed position and compromises the possibility of obtaining the best intubation position of the head;
- interincisive distance for the assessment of jaw mobility and mouth opening, parameters which could limit the use of many devices;
- Mallampati test for assessment of the relationship between oro-pharynx and soft tissue content integrated by an accurate assessment of dentition; the Mallampati test and its modified version (pulling of the tongue) is particularly useful in the morbid obese; obesity associated with a disproportionately large base of the tongue is a predisposing factor for difficult laryngoscopy [15].

Difficult ventilation and its management

There are no specific guidelines dealing with the induction of anesthesia in the obese patient, but general opinion is that it is particularly hazardous for the patient, with an increased risk of difficult airway management, difficulty in ventilation, and in tracheal intubation [22].

It is suggested that two skilled anesthetists should be involved in the induction of the anesthesia and routinely the full range of aids for difficult airway management should be available [23]. The minimum necessary equipment is the same described in every anticipated borderline difficulty [19].

The described rapid fall of arterial saturation during apnea after induction of anesthesia in the supine position makes a careful pre-oxygenation obligatory. Four vital capacity breaths of 100% oxygen is the more-appropriate procedure for pre-oxygenation in morbid obese patients [24]. The technique considered the safest is a rapid sequence induction using propofol and suxamethonium, but a preliminary evaluation of potential difficulty in ventilation and intubationis mandatory. If there a severe difficulty in ventilation and/or an impossible intubation is suspected, the safest technique is not general anesthesia but an awake fiberoptic intubation with topical anesthesia.

While these extreme conditions are fortunately rare, grossly obese patients may normally present some variable problems with face mask ventilation [25, 26], since the abundant soft tissue makes upper airway obstruction very common. Features such as fat cheeks, large tongue, excessive pharyngeal soft tissues, and short and large neck [27] interfere with the correct positioning on the face of the mask and a “three hands” mask ventilation is not always successful.

Facial mask ventilation is likely to be difficult also because of reduced pulmonary compliance and increased resistance to insufflation, which limits the effectiveness of ventilation and facilitates gastric distension, which further increase the risk of regurgitation and aspiration of stomach contents. It has been also demonstrated that obesity predisposes to the risk of aspiration due to frequent occurrence of hiatus hernia, and that the volume and acidity of the gastric contents are increased [28].

The limits of use of the face mask during induction continue during the maintenance of anesthesia, and its use is considered inappropriate and hazardous for controlled ventilation; it is particularly important to bear in mind that not only is airway obstruction likely to occur, but tendency to atelectasis and hypoventilation with hypercapnia and hypoxia is very frequent in the obese patients, who should not be allowed to breathe spontaneously [29]. The spontaneous respiration also increases the risk of reflux associated with any degree of upper respiratory obstruction and the consequent increased negative intrathoracic pressures.

The laryngeal mask plays a more-important role in the management of grossly obese patients; it is a good alternative to the facial mask during induction ventilation, particularly if the difficulty in ventilation was not foreseen and airway obstruction is severe. In similar conditions, in a grossly obese patient with bull neck requiring immediate but impossible intubation, the use of Combitube is also described [30].

The utility of laryngeal mask airway (LMA) in emergency ventilation is not discussed, but more controversial is its use in the induction and particularly maintenance of anesthesia in the morbid obese. During induction its safest use requires an adequately deep plane of anesthesia because the gastroesophageal reflux occurs frequently during episodes of “bucking” [31].

During maintenance, the risk of using the LMA is not different from that of the face mask. If we consider the constant necessity of assisted or controlled ventilation in the obese, irrespective of the length of operation and the necessity of using neuromuscular blocking agents, the risk of gastric distension during insufflation and regurgitation is markedly increased.

In the morbid obese the use of LMA as an aid to awake intubation is also described [32, 33] with the same procedure used in patients with anticipated difficult intubation, but in these patients it is safer to prefer direct vision of a fiberscope to the blind insertion of a tracheal tube or of an introducer [34].

Difficult intubation and its management

Difficulties with tracheal intubation may be considerable [25, 26], caused by features such as excessive pharyngeal soft tissues, large and fat tongue, large breasts, short neck, fat gibbus, high and anterior larynx, restricted mouth opening, and limitation of cervical spine and atlo-occipital motility [27]. The reported incidence of difficult intubation in the grossly obese is quoted at around 13%

[11], but the induction of general anesthesia in the obese should always be followed by tracheal intubation [11, 29].

The incidence of awake intubation under topical anesthesia is markedly increased [22, 35] but some authors [18] think that an awake intubation in these patients is the safest method. The standard laryngoscopic intubation may be used in many cases when it is evident that the anticipated difficulty in intubation is not severe and impossiblity of ventilation is not suspected. All appropriate equipment must be immediately available and there must be experience with its fundamental use; an adequate knowledge of the published failed intubation drill [19] is also mandatory.

It is suggested to perform only a single intubation attempt [29] after correct pre-oxygenation. The rapid desaturation of the obese during apnea does not limit the number of attempts, but the time permitted without oxygen provision does. In consequence, the attempt at intubation must be expeditious and a new prolonged oxygenation eventually allows a second attempt with an alternative procedure. It is important to bear in mind that the chance for a first successful attempt will be greater if a correct sniffing position is obtained; this is not easy in the grossly obese [8]; it is necessary in some cases to place folded towels not only under the head, but also under shoulders and nape to obtain a true flexion of the neck on the chest and give the head enough room to permit its hyperestension at the atlo-occipital joint. The fat accumulated on the upper part of the thorax may increase the difficulty of introducing the blade of the laryngoscope in the mouth; the use of an instrument with a short handle may facilitate the maneuver [36].

The use of suxamethonium is considered mandatory [29] for a rapid and complete relaxation. The first attempt should not be performed with the standard stylet alone, but with a procedure habitually used in difficult laryngoscopy, like the tracheal introducer (gum elastic bougie), as suggested by Bond [18] from a large experience with 400 morbidly obese patients; however, the Trachlight was completely useless for obese patients with a body weight > 120% of the standard [37].

If severe difficulty in intubation is envisaged, than an awake fiberscopic intubation should be considered and discussed with the patient [23]. The procedure is sometime more complicated than in the normal-weight patient, because it is not possible to anticipate difficulty in visualizing the vocal cords due to the presence of pharyngeal folds [34].

A simultaneous application of a nasal CPAP continuous positive airway pressure may have a pharyngeal splitting action during fiberoptic intubation, facilitating the visualization of anatomical landmarks [38]; the size of the instrument may be changed [39].

The detection of correct tracheal tube placement in morbidly obese patient with common clinical signs is frequently misleading, and capnography is the most-reliable test used in these patients. The use of the aspiration test is also described, but a recent study on 54 adult obese patients (BMI > 35) demonstrated a high incidence of false-negative results related to reduction of caliber of airways secondary to the marked decrease in functional residual capacity and collapse of the tracheal wall [40].

The extubation is also a hazardous time for these patients and must be performed when the neuromuscular block has completely disappeared or reversed, and with the positioning, before tracheal tube removal, a tube-exchanger or an introducer with a continuous oxygen flow.

Management of cannot intubate-cannot ventilate obese patient

In a normal-weight patient, two different approaches are usually suggested for tracheal access and the oxygen provision after failed intubation, after the progressive decrease in oxygen saturation with face mask and the failure of LMA to resolve the emergency [19]: 1) tracheal puncture and jet oxygenation; 2) cricothyrotomy.

The well-known emotional and technical difficulties of an airway emergency are enormously increased in the grossly obese for various anatomical reasons: 1) the neck is large, short, and fat; 2) the airway is low-lying; 3) the hyperextension of the head is difficult and depends on the quantity of fat accumulated in the nape and intra-suprascapular area; 4) normal shoulder roll is often ineffective; 5) surgical anatomical landmarks are distorted and not easily palpated; 6) the submental fat (double chin) may occasionally reach the base of the neck and frequently cover laryngeal structures; 7) the size of the trachea is not proportional to the patient's body size.

The landmarks for usual cricothyrotomy, hyoid bone, cricoid cartilage and thyroid cartilage (particularly the V-shaped notch popularly called "Adam's apple"), are barely palpable through the fat, and sometimes even experienced physicians occasionally "get lost in the neck" [41], but the feeling of a prominent structure on the midline is often appreciated.

The palpation of landmarks and the procedure may be easier if the head is immobilized in the best hyperetension with traction on the chin taping out the submental fat, and many folded towels are placed separately below every shoulder and scapula, leaving room on the middle for the fat gibbus.

Between the two suggested procedures, it is preferable to use the Seldinger technique and percutaneous cricothyrotomy with a disposable set and 4 ID cannula, entering exactly on the midline and using the aspiration test to identify the airway, while the use of a over-the-needle small catheter (tracheal puncture) is not recommended for the facility of dislodgement and the small size of the cannula. It is essential in every case to have experience and skilled help by trained personnel. An emergent lifesaving procedure can turn to a dangerous operation in inexperienced hands!

Paradigmatic cases

Of 11 cases of morbidly obese patients treated in the last 3 years at the First Department of Anaesthesia and Intensive Care of Brescia Hospital, 3 cases had an interesting airway management. Obviously, decision making in difficult airway management can be subjective and affected by the experience of the operator, but some rules are recognized as a common ground for planning.

Case no. 1: use of LMA in an elective context for ventilation and as an aid for intubation

A 75-year-old female, with weight of 116 kg, height of 160 cm, BMI of 44.6, and RW of 2.1, was scheduled for pielolythotomy.

The patient had a neck fixed in intermediate position; Mallampati class 3 with a relatively small tongue and long neck. The thyromental distance was reduced to 5 cm due to the restricted mobility of the neck. The patient had no history of snoring or obstructive sleep apnea, but a long history of gastric hyperacidity and night acid regurgitation. Some difficulties were encountered in positioning the face mask on her small nose and large cheeks. The patient was very anxious and refused awake intubation. Since difficult ventilation was not suspected, the anesthesiologist agreed with her desire to sleep during the maneuver.

After pre-oxygenation, general anesthesia was induced with 200 mg propofol and 100 mg suxamethonium i.v. and topic anesthesia of the pharynx with 40 mg spray lidocaine 10%. A standard size 4 laryngeal mask was easily inserted and controlled ventilation with oxygen was possible.

Through the LMA tube an Aintree catheter [41] mounted on a 4.5-mm outer diameter fiberscope was inserted in the airway to obtain a clear vision of the tracheal rings.

The catheter was gently pushed inside the airway and then connected to an oxygen flow of 5 l/min after removal of the fiberscope and LMA; when pulse oximetry returned to 99%, an ID 8.0 TT was railroaded along the catheter, and the latter was removed. Surgery was uneventful and the Aintree catheter was reused for a safe extubation.

Tracheal intubation has been considered necessary for a long operation in the obese patient; the small-size tongue, the absence of ventilation abnormalities and of clear symptoms of difficult ventilation let the anesthesiologist agree with the patient's request to be intubated once asleep. The use of fiberscope increased the safety of the intubation through the LMA; the Aintree catheter avoided the necessity of using the LMA Fastrach and of a blind intubation, also permitting an optimal oxygenation during the maneuver. The ventilation was optimally maintained with LMA. The possibility of a prolonged use of LMA without intubation was abandoned due to the risk of regurgitation.

Case no. 2: use of the tracheal introducer after a previous intubation performed by a fiberscope

A 62-year-old male, with a weight of 131 kg, height of 173 cm, BMI of 43.6, and RW of 1.8, was scheduled for laparotomy with a diagnosis of small bowel obstruction. The patient had an interdental distance of 35 mm, small mouth, small tongue, antheriorised larynx, bull fixed neck, voluminous interscapular and nape fat accumulation, Mallampati class 3, and a thyro-mental distance of 6.5 cm.

Six months earlier, the patient underwent thyroidectomy for cancer and he was submitted to a difficult and painful awake fiberoptic intubation because of his very small nose, which did not allow the introduction of a greater than 6.0 ID TT; the larynx was also dislocated by the thyroid cancer.

The actual intubation difficulty was evaluated in the new anatomical situation created by the ablation of the tumor and it was judged as borderline. Intubation in general anesthesia was planned with the aid of an introducer and the patient's consent. After pre-oxygenation, the anesthesia was induced with propofol and suxamethonium. Forcing the larynx toward the right side, the right arytenoid cartilage was seen and the Frova's Cook hollow tracheal introducer was blindly inserted with a flow of oxygen; an 7.5 ID TT was then placed in the trachea at the first attempt.

An expected moderately difficult intubation may successively become an impossible laryngoscopic intubation, as in a toothless patient who has undergone denture implantation. This case highlights the contrary, as the causes of difficulty were partially removed (tracheal dislocation by the tumor, impossible emergency cricothyrotomy). In this context, the anesthetist opted for considering the probable ease of ventilating, encountered at the previous intubation, and concluded that intubation in general anesthesia was possible and probably easier, safer, and better tolerated by the patient.

Case no. 3: use of LMA in airway emergency after extubation

A 58-year-old male, with a weight of 147 kg, height of 170 cm, BMI of 50.6, and RW of 2.1, arrived in a coma at the emergency department where he was oro-tracheally intubated. A curved, large-sized laryngoscopic blade and a styletted tube were used, and it was difficult to visualize his glottis due to the presence of blood in his pharynx due to the oro-facial trauma and to his enormous chest. After 3 days of in the intensive care unit stay and restored reactivity of the patient, it was decided to substitute his oro-tracheal tube with a naso-tracheal one, in order to improve the patient's comfort and nursing before a delayed tracheotomy. The first TT was withdrawn without introducing a tube-exchanger. The subject was impossible to intubate and to ventilate, since larynx and tongue edema had altered local anatomy. An emergency cricothyrotomy was not feasible, because the fat accumulation in the neck did not allow recognition of the airway. Mild desaturation occurred before a size 5 LMA was placed, by which ventilation was easily possible. After re-oxygenation, a long straight Soper blade and a tracheal introducer were used to oro-tracheally place a 6.0 ID TT; then, a fiberoptic naso-tracheal intubation was performed, pushing the instrument beside the deflated cuff of the oral TT and railroading along the fiberscope a 7.5 TT, and withdrawing the oral tube before the removal of the tracheal introducer.

This case emphasizes the importance of considering the anamnestic data on airway management and the possible variations of the local anatomical conditions. Moreover, it underlines the potential life-saving role of the LMA. When a morbidly obese patient is treated in an intensive care setting, the necessity of emergency re-intubation should always be considered and, whenever possible, the extubation should be planned when experienced personnel are available, especially if the previous intubation was problematic.

References

1. Björntorp P (1997) Obesity. Lancet 350:423-426
2. Shenkman Z, Shir Y, Brodsky JB (1993) Perioperative management of the obese patient. Br J Anaesth 70:349-359
3. Oberg B, Poulsen D (1996) Obesity: an anaesthetic challenge. Acta Anaesthesiol Scand 40: 191-200
4. Harrison GG (1983) Height-weight tables. Ann Intern Med 98: 855-859
5. Garrison RJ, Castelli WP (1985) Weight and thirty-year mortality of men of the Framingham study. Ann Intern Med 103:1006-1009
6. Luce MJ (1980) Respiratory complications of obesity. Chest 78:626-631
7. Vaughan RW, Bauer S, Wise L (1995) Volume and pH of gastric juice in obese patients. Anesthesiology 43:686-689
8. Benumof JL (1996) Conventional laryngoscopic orotracheal and nasotracheal intubation (single lumen tube). In: Benumof JL (ed) Airway management. Principles and practice. Mosby, St Louis, pp 261-264
9. Olefsky JM (1994) Obesity. In: Isselbacher KJ, Braunwald E, Wilson JD et al (eds) Harrison's principles of internal medicine. McGraw-Hill, New York, pp 446-452
10. Servin F, Farinotti R, Haberer J-P et al (1993) Propofol infusion for the maintenance of anesthesia in morbidly obese patient receiving nitrous oxide. Anesthesiology 78:657-665
11. Buckley FP (1994) Anaesthesia for the morbidly obese patient. Can J Anaesth 41:R94-R100
12. Weinstein JA, Matteo RS, Ornstein E et al (1988) Pharmacodynamics of vecuronium and atracurium in the obese surgical patient. Anaesth Analg 67:1149-1153
13. Wilson ME, Spiegelhalter D, Robertson JA et al (1988) Predicting difficult intubation. Br J Anaesth 61:211-216
14. Bray GA (1992) Pathophysiology of obesity. Am J Clin Nutr 55:488-494
15. Voyagis GS, Kyriakis KP, Dimitriou V et al (1998) Value of oropharyngeal Mallampati classification in predicting difficult laryngoscopy among obese patients. Eur J Anaesthesiol 15: 330-334
16. Stoelting RK, Diedorf SF, McCammon RL (1988) Metabolism, nutrition and obesity. In: Stoelting RK, Dierdorf SF, McCammon RL (eds) Anesthesia and coexisting disease. Churchill-Livingstone, New York, pp 517-555

17. Brimacombe JR, Brain AIJ, Berry AM (1997) The laryngeal mask airway. Saunders, London, pp 138-139
18. Bond A (1993) Obesity and difficult intubation. Anaesth Intensive Care 21:828
19. SIAARTI (1998) Linee guida per l'intubazione difficile e la difficoltà di controllo delle vie aeree nell'adulto. Minerva Anestesiol 64:361-371
20. Murphy PG (2000) Obesity. In: Hemmings HC Jr, Hopkins PM (eds) Foundations of anaesthesia. Basic and clinical sciences. Mosby, London, pp 703-711
21. Friedman M, Tanyeri H, La Rosa M et al (1999) Clinical predictors of obstructive sleep apnea. Laryngoscope 109:1901-1907
22. Vaughan RW (1982) Anesthetic management of the morbidly obese patient. In: Brown BR et al (eds) Anesthesia and obese patients. Davis, New York, pp 71-94
23. Adams GP, Murphy PG (2000) Obesity in anaesthesia and intensive care. Br J Anaesth 85: 91-108
24. Goldberg ME, Norris MC, Larijani GE et al (1989) Preoxygenation in the morbidly obese: a comparison of two techniques. Anesth Analg 68:520-522
25. Hood DD, Dewan DM (1993) Anesthetic and obstetric outcome in morbidly obese partients. Anesthesiology 79:1210-1218
26. Lee JJ, Larson RH, Buckley JJ et al (1980) Airway maintenance in the morbidly obese. Anesth Rev 7:33-36
27. Brodsky JB (1986) Anesthetic management of the morbidly obese patient. Int Anesthesiol Clin 24:93-103
28. Vaughn RW, Bauer S, Wise L (1975) Volume and pH of gastric juice in obese patients. Anesthesiology 43:686
29. Øberg B, Poulsen TD (1996) Obesity: an anesthetic challenge. Acta Anaesthesiol Scand 40: 191-200
30. Banyai M, Falgers S, Roggla M et al (1993) Emergency intubation with the Combitube in a grossly obese patient with bull neck. Resuscitation 26:271-276
31. Illing L, Duncan PG, Yip R (1991) Gastro-oesophageal reflux during anaesthesia. Can J Anaesth 39:466-470
32. Godley M, Ramachandra AR (1996) Use of LMA for awake intubation for Cesarean section. Can J Anaesth 43:299-302
33. Biro P, Kaplan V, Block KE (1995) Anesthetic management of a patient with obstructive sleep apnea syndrome and difficult airway access. J Clin Anesth 7:417-421
34. Latto IP, Vaughan RS (1997) Difficulties in tracheal intubation, 2nd edn. Saunders, London, pp 178-184
35. Damia G, Mascheroni D, Croci M et al (1988) Perioperative changes in the functional residual capacity in morbidly obese patients. Br J Anaesth 60:574-578
36. Datta S, Briwa J (1981) Modified laryngoscope for endotracheal intubation in obese patients. Anesth Analg 60:120
37. Nishiyama T, Matsukawa T, Hanaoka K (1999) Optimal length and angle of a new lightwand device (Trachlight). J Clin Anesth 11:332-335
38. Rothfleish R, Davis LL, Kuebel DA et al (1994) Facilitation of fiberoptic nasotracheal intubation in a morbidly obese patient by simultaneous use of nasal cpap. Chest 106:287-288
39. Da Broi U, Zauli M, Bonfreschi V et al (1996) Problematiche anestesiologiche in pazienti affetti da malattia di Launois-Bensaude-Madelung. Minerva Anestesiol 62:333-337
40. Lang DJ, Wafai Y, Salem MR et al (1996) Efficacy of the self-inflating bulb in confirming tracheal intubation in the morbidly obese. Anesthesiology 85:246-253
41. Ledereich PS (1998) Tracheotomy in the obese and morbidly obese patient. In: Myers EN, Johnson JT, Murry T (eds) Tracheotomy. Singular Publishing Group, San Diego, pp 145-150

Respiratory Management in Obese Patients

P. PELOSI, N. BOTTINO, P. CAIRONI

Obesity is a metabolic disease in which adipose tissue represents a proportion of body mass tissue greater than normal. Up to 33% of the population in North America, 15% in Europe and in Italy can be considered obese [1]. Many etiologic factors may be implicated in determining this disease, such as genetic, environmental, socioeconomic and individual ones (age, sex, weight, height, etc.). In absence of further pathologic conditions, adipose tissue represents 15-18% of body weight males and about 25% in females.

In clinical practice, several criteria have been proposed to exactly define the obesity condition [2]: the simpler criterion is to compare the actual weight of the patient with his/her "ideal" weight on the base of sex, age and height. From this point of view, a person who presents a weight greater than 120% of his/her "ideal" weight may be considered obese, and greater than 200% of "ideal" weight a pathologic obese. An index of obesity that may be easily obtained during the pre-anaesthesiology visit is the Body Mass Index (BMI, or Quetelet's index). This index is computed as the ratio between the weight, expressed in kilograms, and the height squared, expressed in meters. On the base of BMI, it is possible to divide the population into several classes, from a condition of underweight to a condition of pathologic obesity – obese subjects present a BMI greater than 30 kg/m^2 and morbidly obese patients greater than 40 kg/m^2 – [1]. Moreover, BMI was well correlated with the risk of negative effect on health and with the longevity of obese patients.

Recently, new surgical techniques have been developed for the treatment of obesity, such as ileo-jejunal by-pass or gastric binding. However, since these patients are characterized by several systemic physiopathological alterations, the perioperative management may present some problems, mainly related to their respiratory alterations [3].

Preoperative period

Simple obesity, i.e. uncomplicated by upper or lower airway obstruction leading to hypoventilation syndrome, generally produces only mild effects on pulmonary function [4, 5]. The range of forced vital capacity (FVC), functional residual capacity (FRC) and total lung capacity (TLC) is within the normal values in most of these patients. In morbidly obese patients the FVC is reduced by 25% without any reduction in FRC or TLC.

On the contrary, in a high grade obesity the respiratory system presents characteristic alteration of the pulmonary volume, both static and dynamic ones, and a reduction of the effectiveness of gas exchange. These modifications lead to an arterial hypoxic state also in a rest condition; the inefficiency of respiratory function is not counteracted by an increase of ventilation, that usually is decreased because of also a simultaneous increase of work of breathing. A very obese patient appears to have a reduction of FRC, of TLC and expiratory reserve volume, besides a decrease of dynamic pulmonary volumes, with a restrictive type of spirometry [6].

Concerning respiratory mechanics, the obese patient is characterized by a decrease of the compliance of the respiratory system – that resulted in 35% lower than expected values [7] –, because of a reduction of either lung or chest wall compliance [8]. These alterations of respiratory mechanics are directly owed to the increase and to the distribution of adipose tissue, and their importance in determining the inefficiency of respiratory function parallels the increase of abdominal mass.

Finally, the obese patient is characterized by an enhance of work of breathing because of an increase in intra-abdominal pressure, a reduction of compliance of respiratory system, an increase of airway resistance and of metabolic demands. This enhancement produces an increment of oxygen delivery and, because of the inefficiency of ventilation, an increased retention of carbon dioxide, with hypoxia and hypercapnia as a consequence.

Intraoperative period

Body mass is an important determinant of respiratory function during anaesthesia and paralysis, in supine position, not only in morbidly but also moderate obese patient. In fact, it is well realizable that the obese patient, coming from a respiratory condition that is already physiologically poor, feels much more the morphological and functional variations of the respiratory system due to the induction and the maintenance of anaesthesia and paralysis.

Lung volumes. Lung volumes are well associated with body mass [9]. In morbidly obese patients, the FRC decreases after induction of anaesthesia to approximately 50% of pre-anaesthesia values [10]. Also in healthy subjects the induction of anaesthesia and paralysis constantly leads to a decrease in FRC, and the magnitude of this reduction has been related to several individual factors as age, weight and height. However, the mechanisms leading to FRC decrease during anaesthesia are not completely understood. In particular, some factors such that seem to be involved in this modification may be the occurrence of atelectasis, the blood shift from abdomen to thorax [11] and the distortion of rib cage without diaphragm shift [12]. The formation of atelectasis has been ascribed to a decreased distribution of ventilation in the dependent lung regions during anaesthesia and mechanical ventilation – the paravertebral regions in supine position – [13]. The loss of diaphragmatic tone induced by anaesthetics makes the movement of the diaphragm passively dependent [14]. Because of a gravitational pressure gradient in the abdomen due to the presence of abdominal viscera, the distribution of ventilation is preferentially directed towards the non-dependent lung regions. With increasing body mass, an increase in abdominal mass and intra-abdominal pressure occur [15], with an increased load particularly on the most dependent lung regions and a more important cephalad displacement as a consequence, with a reduction in the passive movements of the dependent part of the diaphragm. It is likely that, when active, the ventilatory muscles counteract the intra-abdominal pressure load towards the diaphragm. Therefore, the removal of ventilatory muscle tone by anaesthesia and muscle paralysis likely plays an important role in determining the reduction in FRC. This preferential alteration of the diaphragm favours the development of atelectasis in the dependent lung regions at a higher grade than in healthy subjects.

Respiratory mechanics. The alterations of respiratory mechanics that occur during anaesthesia and paralysis are well related to the extent of body mass. The decrease of compliance of the respiratory system with the increase of body mass is mainly determined by the reduction in lung compliance, rather than by a reduction in chest wall compliance [9]. The more important factor for the decreased lung compliance probably is the same reduction in FRC, since the intrinsic mechanic characteristics of lung parenchyma – "specific compliance" – are hardly at all changed. Also respiratory resistance is influenced by body mass, mainly because of an increase in lung resistance. This enhance is mainly caused by an increase in the airway resistance component – probably due to a decreased lung volume and/or intrinsic narrowed airways –, whereas the viscoelastic component is only weakly affected by the body mass.

Gas exchange. The arterial hypoxia that characterize the awakened obese patient is worsened during anaesthesia and paralysis [16], since these patients, as normal subjects, are predisposed, with the induction and the maintenance of anaesthesia, to the occurrence of pulmonary atelectasis and shunt, and to an alteration of ventilation/perfusion ratio. The lung collapse often determines an hypoxia that continues for a long time also in the postoperative period. This abnormal condition, as a consequence, makes the obese patient, and much more pathologic obese patient, a subject at high anaesthesiologic risk.

Mechanical ventilation

The increased intraabdominal pressure seems to play a relevant role in the reduction of FRC, which seems to be the prevalent phenomenon, resulting in a decrease in respiratory compliance and oxygenation. This suggests the occurrence of relevant collapse and lung dependent atelectasis [17].

As a consequence of respiratory modifications induced by general anaesthesia and paralysis, the main aim of mechanical ventilation in obese patients is to keep the lung open during the entire respiratory cycle. This counteracts negative effects induced by the increased body mass and the high intraabdominal pressure (airway closure, atelectasis, impaired respiratory mechanics and oxygenation), which persist for a few days in the postoperative period.

To ventilate a lung showing a tendency to collapse we have to provide inspiratory pressure enough to open the collapsed lung regions, and positive end-expiratory pressure (PEEP) enough to maintain the lung open at end-expiration.

Adequate opening pressure can be obtained by applying periodic large, manually performed lung inflations (recruitment manoeuvres) [18, 19], since the use of continuously high tidal volumes (> 13 mL/kg ideal body weight) is ineffective to further improve oxygenation [20].

The use of low tidal volumes (and, as a consequence, low alveolar ventilation) and high inspired oxygen fraction (FiO_2) should be avoided since it has been clearly shown that this may lead to the formation of progressive reabsorption atelectasis [21].

The application of periodic hyperinflations (sighs) may be beneficial, providing inspiratory pressures are enough to re-open the lung and alveolar ventilation is enough to avoid the formation of reabsorption atelectasis [22].

The role of PEEP in anaesthesia is still controversial: in fact, different studies reported different results in oxygenation response in different patient populations and clinical conditions [23-26]. This is likely due to the opposite effects induced by PEEP on oxygenation in different patients. PEEP can resolve atelectasis, if present, and prevent small airways collapse, improving ventilation-perfusion matching and oxygenation. On the other hand, increasing PEEP may lead to negative effects on ventilation-perfusion ratio and pulmonary shunt, if alveolar overstretching and cardiac output reduction or redistribution become the prevalent phenomena. The final effect on oxygenation of PEEP application depends on the balance between positive and negative effects in any given patients. We found that applying 10 cm H_2O of PEEP during anaesthesia and paralysis induce an oxygenation improvement in morbidly obese patients, but not in normal subjects [17]. Moreover, we found that the partitioned Pressure-Volume curves measured at PEEP 0 and 10 cm H_2O roughly follow the same pattern in normal subjects, while in obese patients the P-V curves at 10 cm H_2O PEEP are shifted upward and on the left, suggesting the occurrence of alveolar recruitment (see Fig. 1). This amount of alveolar recruitment was related to the improvement of oxygenation.

More recently, we found that applying a PEEP level of 10 cm H_2O during pneumoperitoneum improves oxygenation and total respiratory system compli-

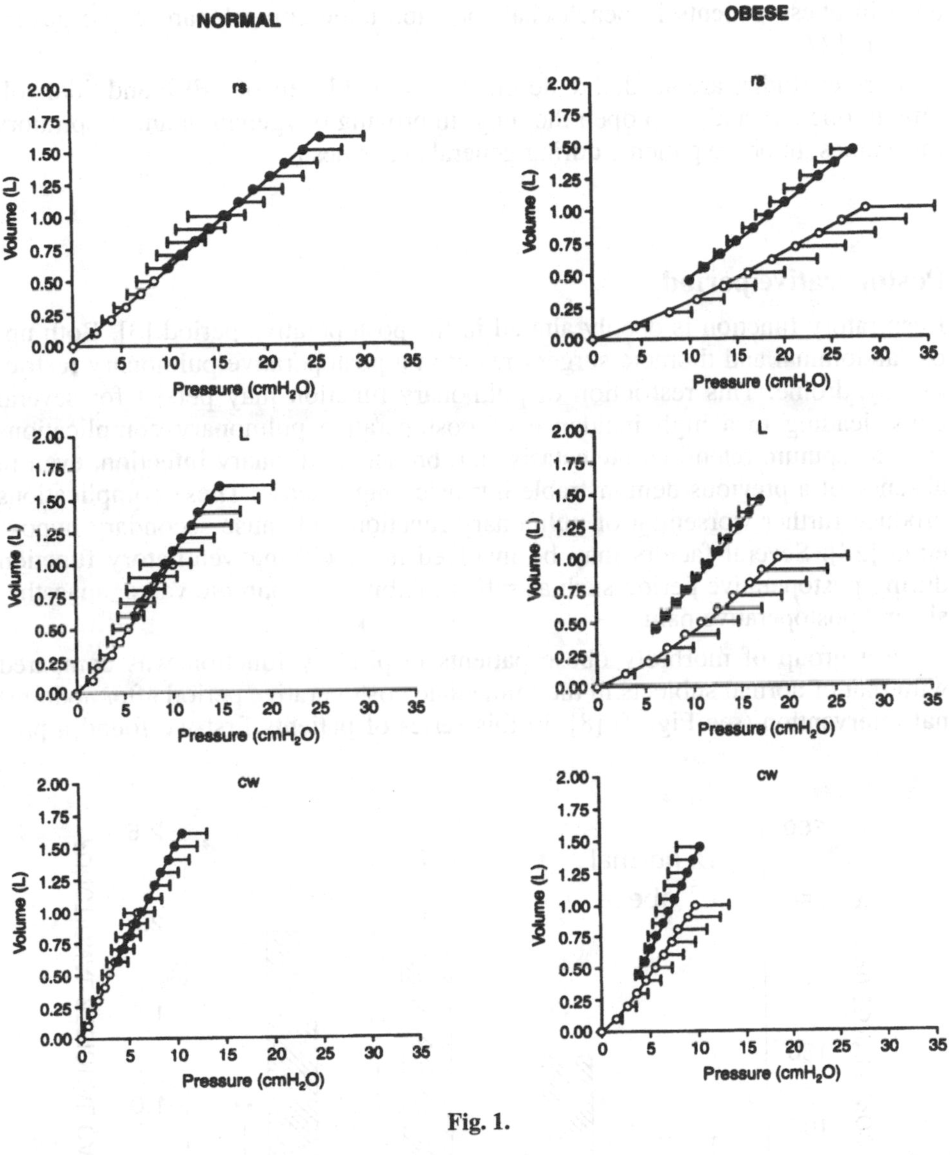

Fig. 1.

Pressure-Volume curves of the total respiratory system (rs), lung (L) and chest wall (cw) in normal subjects (left panel) and obese patients (right panel) at positive end-expiratory pressures of 0 cm H_2O (white circles) and 10 cm H_2O (black circles). Data are presented as mean ± standard deviation. (Modified from [17] with permission)

ance in obese patients in beach chair position undergoing laparoscopic gastric binding [27].

Further studies are needed to define the optimal levels of PEEP and tidal volume to open up and keep open the lung, improving oxygenation and respiratory mechanics, in obese patients during general anaesthesia.

Postoperative period

Respiratory function is deeply altered in the postoperative period [3]. Both upper abdominal and thoracic surgery result in a postoperative pulmonary restrictive syndrome. This restriction of pulmonary function may persist for several days, leading to a high incidence of postoperative pulmonary complications such as sputum retention, atelectasis, and bronchopulmonary infection, even in absence of a previous demonstrable intrinsic lung disease. These complications produce further worsening of pulmonary function and cause secondary hypoxemia [28]. Several factors may be involved in modifying ventilatory function during postoperative period such as reflex inhibition of phrenic valve, anaesthesia and postoperative pain.

In a group of morbidly obese patients respiratory function was compared with that of normal subjects in the immediate postoperative period after abdominal intervention (see Fig. 2) [8]. In this series of patients first we found a pro-

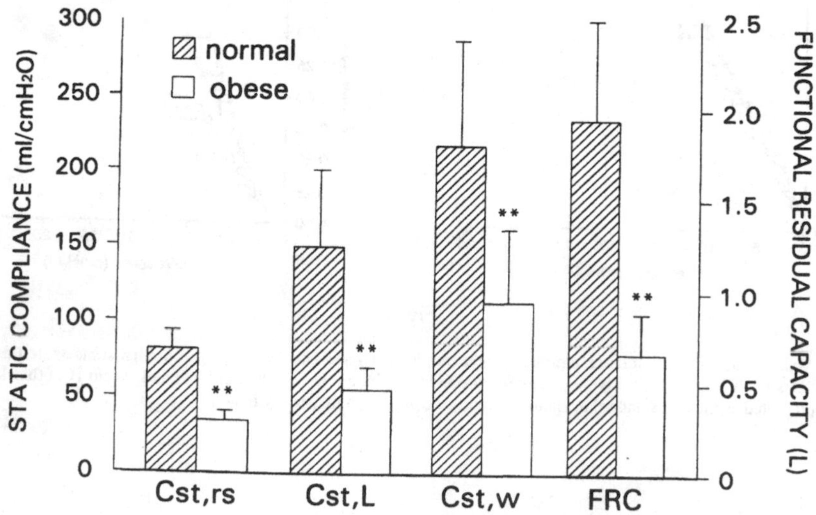

Fig. 2.

Total respiratory system (Cst,rs), lung (Cst,L) and chest wall (C,w) static compliance, and functional residual capacity (FRC) in normal subjects and in obese patients, in the postoperative period. Data are expressed as mean ± standard deviation. ** $p < 0.01$ compared with normal. (Modified from [8] with permission)

nounced reduction in FRC compared to normal subjects, since FRC was about one third of a normal value. Considering the compliance of respiratory system partitioned into its lung and chest wall components, we found that the reduction in respiratory system compliance was caused by a decrease in both lung and chest wall compliance.

Reduced chest wall compliance may be due to an increased adiposity around the ribs, diaphragm and abdomen, limited movements of the ribs caused by thoracic kyphosis and lumbar hyperlordosis from excessive abdominal fat content. Another possible cause is that the decreased total thoracic and pulmonary volume may pull the chest wall below its resting level and therefore to a flatter portion of its Pressure-Volume curve. However, the most likely cause of the reduction in chest wall compliance during postoperative period probably is the increased intra-abdominal pressure which prevents, at least in part, the diaphragm from freely moving and affects the shape of the upper and lower thorax [17]. Other abnormalities in the respiratory function during the postoperative period are a reduction in the effectiveness of gas exchange, strictly dependent on the decreased lung volumes, and an increase in work of breathing, mainly resulting from a reduction in lung and chest wall compliance and high pulmonary resistance [8].

From all these data, we supported the hypothesis that marked derangement in FRC, elastic (reduction in lung and chest wall compliance) and resistive (increase in lung resistance) components of the respiratory system might account for the significant respiratory dysfunction and arterial hypoxemia occurring in the postoperative period.

Postoperative management

All these alterations can explain the higher incidence of postoperative pulmonary complication in obese than in non obese patients [3]. To reduce postoperative pulmonary complication different techniques and treatment have been proposed, such as chest physiotherapy, incentive spirometry, and intermittent positive pressure breathing [29]. Some Authors proposed the use of continuous positive airway pressure (CPAP) or bi-level positive airway pressure (Bi-PAP) administered by non-invasive techniques in the first 24 hours postoperatively [30]. The aim is to give a ventilatory support to more rapidly restore lung volumes to the pre-operative values, improving oxygenation and reducing work of breathing. Moreover, for several days after surgery, patients should remain in semirecubent position (30-45°) [31], to reduce the abdominal pressure on the diaphragm.

The role of a preventive admission of morbidly obese patients undergoing abdominal surgery in the intensive care unit (ICU) in the postoperative period is not yet defined [32]. Some advantages of ICU admission are a gentler weaning from the ventilator and to easily perform chest physiotherapy and non-invasive ventilatory treatment, optimized fluid treatment, and more careful pain control. On the other hand, there are increased costs and more difficulties of organizing the time schedule of the surgical operations.

To define the role of preventive ICU admission in the postoperative morbidly obese patient we compared the incidence of postoperative pulmonary complications and mortality in 38 morbidly obese patients admitted to our ICU after abdominal surgery between 1993 and 1998 with historical controls in which patients were not admitted to the ICU in the postoperative period [28, 33-37].

The patients' characteristics are shown in Table 1.

Table 1. Patients characteristics

No.	38	
Sex	18 males	
Age	37.5 ± 9.9 years	
BMI	48.5 ± 6.6 kg/m^2	
Preoperative PFT and gas analysis		
FVC	3.8 ± 1.0 L (89 ± 13% of expected)	
FEV_1	3.0 ± 0.8 L (86 ± 15% of expected)	
PaO_2	87 ± 10 mmHg	
$PaCO_2$	39 ± 2 mmHg	
pHa	7.41 ± 0.03	
Preoperative clinical characteristics		
	No.	(%)
Smokers	6	(15.8)
Effort dyspnea	2	(5.3)
Hypertension	8	(21.0)
Asthma/nocturnal apnea	4	(10.5)
PFT < 20% expected	9	(23.7)

Data are expressed as mean ± SD

Definition of abbreviation: BMI = body mass index, PFT = pulmonary function tests, FVC = forced vital capacity, FEV_1 = forced expiratory volume

After the end of surgical procedures (20 gastric binding and 18 jejuno-ileal bypass), all the patients were admitted to the ICU for the postoperative treatment, intubated and mechanically ventilated. The fluid treatment was titrated to achieve a diuresis higher than 0.5 mL/hr/kg ideal body weight and antibiotic treatment was given for two-three days after surgery. Patients were mechanically ventilated in synchronized intermittent mechanical ventilation (SIMV) and pressure support to achieve a tidal volume of 13 mL/kg of ideal body weight and $PaCO_2$ within normal range, with a PEEP level set to give the "best oxygenation" (a PaO_2 increase of at least 10 mmHg). Patients were successively weaned from the ventilator at first reducing FiO_2 to obtain a PaO_2 of 90-100 mmHg at FiO_2 40%, and then progressively reducing the ventilatory support. We performed extubation when the following criteria were satisfied: 1) forced vital capacity (FVC) higher than 1 L; 2) spontaneous unassisted tidal volume higher than 400 mL; 3) spontaneous respiratory rate lower than 25 breaths/min; 4) PaO_2 higher than 80 mmHg at 30% FiO_2 during spontaneous breathing.

We evaluated in this population of morbidly obese patients the incidence of postoperative pulmonary complications, defined as the new occurrence of three or more of the following signs or symptoms [29]: cough, positive sputum culture, dyspnea, chest pain or discomfort, fever (temperature higher than 38°C), tachycardia (more than 100 beats/min), and positive chest X-ray (atelectasis, abnormal hemidiaphragm elevation, new pleural effusion, new infiltrate). In Table 2 is shown how the incidence of postoperative pulmonary complications is significantly lower in obese patients admitted to the ICU compared to the population of historical controls which was not admitted to the ICU in the immediate postoperative period.

Table 2. Postoperative pulmonary complications and mortality in obese patients admitted or not to the intensive care unit

[Reference number]	Pts (n°)	BMI (kg/m²)	Age (yrs)	PPC (%)	Mortality (%)
No ICU admission					
[33]	70	–	–	–	5.7
[34]	46	142[a]	34	0	–
[28]	17	147[a]	36	47.0	0
[35]	110	135[a]	35	21.8	0
[36]	102	> 25.0	54	26.5	0
[37]	181	28.5	58	29.3	0
Total	526	–	48	24.6	0.8
ICU admission					
Our experience	38	48.5	37	7.9*	0

Data refer only to average data.
Definition of abbreviations: BMI = body mass index, PPC = postoperative pulmonary complications, [a] weight (kg), * $p < 0.05$ vs No ICU admission

Conclusion

The important alterations in the respiratory function of morbidly obese patients in the perioperative period may play a significant role in determining pulmonary complications in the postoperative period. Adequate ventilatory settings during general anaesthesia and ICU admission in the postoperative period may help to reduce the incidence of postoperative pulmonary complications and, likely, to improve mortality.

References

1. Jack DB (1996) Fighting obesity the Franco-British way. Lancet 347:1756
2. Shenkman Z, Shir Y, Brodsky (1993) Perioperative management of the obese patients. Br J Anaesth 70:349-359
3. Luce JM (1980) Respiratory complication of obesity. Chest 78:626-631
4. Ray CS, Sue DY, Bray G et al (1983) Effects of obesity on respiratory function. Am Rev Respir Dis 128:501-506
5. Rochester DF (1995) Obesity and abdominal distention. In: Roussos C (ed) The Thorax, Part C: Disease, 2nd ed. M. Dekker, New York, pp 1951-1973
6. Zerah F, Harf A, Perlemuter L et al (1993) Effects of obesity on respiratory resistance. Chest 103:1470-1476
7. Eriksen J, Andersen J, Rasmussen JP, Soresen B (1978) Effects of ventilation with large tidal volumes or positive end-expiratory pressure on cardiorespiratory function in anesthetized obese patients. Acta Anaesth Scand 22:241-248
8. Pelosi P, Croci M, Ravagnan I et al (1996) Total respiratory system, lung and chest wall mechanics in anesthetized-paralyzed morbidly obese patients. Chest 109:144-151
9. Pelosi P, Croci M, Ravagnan I et al (1998) The effects of body mass on lung volumes, respiratory mechanics, and gas-exchange during general anesthesia. Anesth Analg 87:645-660
10. Damia G, Mascheroni D, Croci M, Tarenzi L (1988) Perioperative changes in functional residual capacity in morbidly obese patients. Br J Anesth 60:574-578
11. Hedenstierna G, Strandberg A, Brismar B et al (1985) Functional residual capacity, thoracoabdominal dimensions, and central blood volume during general anesthesia with muscle paralysis and mechanical ventilation. Anesthesiology 62:247-254
12. Warner DO, Warner MA, Ritman EL (1995) Human chest wall function while awake and during halotane anesthesia. I. Quiet breathing. Anesthesiology 82:6-19
13. Brismar B, Hedenstierna G, Lundquist H et al (1985) Pulmonary densities during anesthesia: a proposal of atelectasis. Anesthesiology 62:422-428
14. Froese AB, Bryan CH (1974) Effects of anesthesia and paralysis on diaphragmatic mechanics in man. Anesthesiology 41:242-255
15. Pelosi P, Croci M, Ravagnan I et al (1997) Respiratory system mechanics in anesthetized, paralyzed, morbidly obese patients. J Appl Physiol 82:811-8181
16. Hedenstierna G, Svensson J (1976) Breathing mechanics, dead space and gas exchange in the extremely obese, breathing spontaneously and during anesthesia with intermittent positive pressure ventilation. Acta Anesth Scand 20:248-254
17. Pelosi P, Ravagnan I, Giurati G et al (1999) Positive end-expiratory pressure improves respiratory function in obese patients but not in normal subjects during anesthesia and paralysis. Anesthesiology 91:1221-1231
18. Rothen HV, Sporre B, Engber G et al (1993) Reexpansion of atelectasis during general anesthesia: a computed tomography study. Br J Anaesth 71:788-795
19. Rothen HV, Sporre B, Engber G et al (1995) Reexpansion of atelectasis during general anesthesia may have a prolonged effect. Acta Anaesth Scand 39:118-125
20. Bardoczky GI, Yernault JC, Houben JJ, d'Hollander AA (1995) Large tidal volume ventilation does not improve oxygenation in morbidly obese patients during anesthesia. Anesth Analg 81:385-388
21. Rothen HV, Sporre B, Engber G et al (1995) Influence of gas composition on recurrence of atelectasis after a reexpansion maneuver during general anesthesia. Anesthesiology 82: 832-842
22. Pelosi P, Cadringher P, Bottino N et al (1999) Sigh in Acute Respiratory Distress Syndrome. Am J Respir Crit Care Med 159:872-880
23. Wyche MQ, Teichner RL, Kallos T et al (1973) Effects of continuous positive pressure breathing on functional residual capacity and arterial oxygenation during intra-abdominal operations: studies in man during nitrous oxide and d-tubocurarine anesthesia. Anesthesiology 38:68-74

24. Salem MR, Dalal FY, Zygmunt MP et al (1978) Does PEEP improve intraoperative oxygenation in grossly obese patients? Anesthesiology 48:280-281
25. Eriksen J, Andersen J, Rasmussen JP, Sorensen B (1978) Effects of ventilation with large tidal volumes or positive end-expiratory pressure on cardiorespiratory function in anesthetized obese patients. Acta Anaesth Scand 22:241-248
26. Santesson J (1976) Oxygen transport and venous admixture in the extremely obese: influence of anaesthesia and artificial ventilation with and without positive end-expiratory pressure. Acta Anaesth Scand 20:387-394
27. Vannucci A, Francesconi S, Vagginelli F et al (2000) Effect of pneumoperitoneum, surgical positioning and PEEP on PaO_2/FiO_2 ratio and quasi static respiratory compliance in obese patients during laparoscopic gastric binding. In: Braschi A, Gattinoni L, Pesenti A, Raimondi F (eds) Comunicazioni Libere - Simposio Mostra Anestesia Rianimazione e Terapia intensiva, Springer, Milano 2000, A-10
28. Soderberg M, Thomson D, White T (1977) Respiration, circulation and anaesthetic management in obesity. Investigation before and after jejunoileal bypass. Acta Anesth Scand 21: 55-61
29. Celli BP, Rodriguez K, Snider GL (1984) A controlled trial of intermittent positive pressure breathing, incentive spirometry and deep breathing exercise in preventing pulmonary complications after abdominal surgery. Am Rev Respir Dis 130:12-15
30. Joris JL, Sottiaux TM, Chiche JD et al (1997) Effect of Bi-Level positive airway pressure (BiPAP) nasal ventilation on the postoperative pulmonary restrictive syndrome in obese patients undergoing gastroplasty. Chest 111:665-670
31. Vaughan RW, Wise L (1975) Postoperative arterial blood gas measurement in obese patients: effect of position on gas exchange. Ann Surg 182:705-709
32. Marik P, Varon J (1988) The obese patients in the ICU. Chest 113:492-498
33. Postlethwait RW, Johnson WD (1972) Complications following surgery for duodenal ulcer in obese patients. Archives Surg 105:438-440
34. Vaughan RW (1974) Anesthetic considerations in jejunoileal small bowel bypass for morbid obesity. Anesth Analg 53:421-429
35. Fox GS, Whalley DG, Bevan DR (1981) Anaesthesia for the morbidly obese. Experience with 110 patients. Br J Anaesth 53:811-816
36. Hall JC, Tarala RA, Hall JL, Mander J (1991) A multivariate analysis of the risk of pulmonary complications after laparotomy. Chest 99:923-927
37. Brooks-Brunn JA (1997) Predictors of postoperative pulmonary complications following abdominal surgery. Chest 111:564-571

Challenges for Perioperative Management of Obese Patients – How to Manage Complications

J.O.C. AULER JR

As reported in the literature, the excellent results seen with gastroplasty in the treatment of refractory morbid obesity have renewed interest in the anaesthetic management of these groups of patients [1, 2]. Morbid obesity, defined as a body mass index (BMI) greater than 35 kg/m^2, has increased significantly in the last decades, above all in the more developed world, and is nowadays considered an important cause of health complications in early life and premature death [3]. As severe obesity is a life-limiting condition, these patients have been frequently scheduled for abdominal surgery, such as gastroplasty, to treat diet-resistant obesity. Bariatric surgery may be considered an effective method to treat refractory obesity and, according to the National Institutes of Health (NIH) Consensus Conference in 1996, surgery remains the only efficient treatment for severe obese patients, principally for those that have failed on clinical treatments primarily based on caloric intake restriction [4]. Nevertheless, the perioperative mortality rate has been described to be higher in the morbidly obese (6.6%), when compared to non-obese patients undergoing gastrointestinal tract surgery (2.6%) [5]. These findings may be explained because obesity results in multiple pathophysiological disturbances, including cardiovascular, respiratory, endocrine and metabolic, and may cause negative influences in the perioperative outcome [6].

Besides these clinical consequences, overweight may even cause several perioperative logistic problems that require expertise and knowledge of anaesthesiology for a successful outcome Therefore there are several important challenges for perioperative management of obese patients:

1. to select one of the various indices to correct overweight to normal;
2. cardiac and respiratory abnormalities are to be managed during the perioperative period;
3. comprehension of metabolic disarrangement, as well as pharmacokinetic characteristics of obesity, that may cause alterations in drug distribution.

Consistent with these introductory statements, our aim in this chapter is to present some aspects of practical interest for perioperative management of morbid obese patients, discussing the more-frequent problems and suggested management.

Indices to correct overweight to normal

Ideally, any index to define obesity should be independent of height, muscle, and skeletal mass. Apart from defining obesity, the ideal weight obtained by different methods is also important for several reasons, e.g., for using a correct dose of anaesthetic drugs and for adjusting tidal volume during ventilation. In the literature it is possible to find several indices to predict ideal weight; a widely used method is denominated BMI, where BMI = body weight in kilograms/height^2 in meters. Evidently, the purpose of this index is to minimize the effect of height on weight. Normal values of BMI may vary between 22 and 28 according to the country, whereas morbid obesity is accepted to be greater than 35. It was also an attempt to classify the risk of obesity in accordance with BMI; e.g., high-risk obese patients presented BMI over 40 [7]. Subtracting 100 (men) and 105 (women) may also easily obtain the ideal weight by height/tables or simply from the patient's height in centimeters [8]. According to the localisation of the adipose tissue in the body, obesity may be classified as central-android obesity, in which fat is located mainly in the upper body, and peripheral-gynecoid obesity, in which the fatty tissue is distributed predominantly in the inferior body, hips, buttocks and thighs [9]. As a consequence, in upper or android obesity, an increased difficulty in airway access and ventilation, as well as higher incidence of diabetes, hypertension, and cardiovascular disease, is projected when compared to gynecoid obesity [10].

Cardiovascular alterations

The pathophysiological consequences of obesity on cardiac function are complex. Diabetes, excessive obesity, duration of overweight, presence of arterial hypertension and coronary artery disease may be associated with more-severe cardiac dysfunction. In obese patients, circulating blood volume, plasma volume, cardiac output, filling pressures and oxygen consumption increase in proportion to added weight [11]. An increase in pulmonary blood volumes and flows predisposes obese individuals to pulmonary hypertension, which may be accentuated, or even worsened, by hypoxic pulmonary vasoconstriction, which, in turn, occurs due to respiratory changes that cause hypoxemia. Sleep apnea syndrome that is strongly associated with obesity may even accentuate daytime hypoxemia and aggravate pulmonary hypertension [12]. Heart failure occurs often in severe obese patients and seems to be an important cause of death [11]. Although some heart failure is associated with overweight, congestive heart failure is more common with progressive weight gain [13]. Obesity and hypertension are closely associated; surely with increasing body mass the vascular system must increase in size. The reason for increasing arterial pressure may just be a greater driving force necessary to push blood through a larger vascular system, as systemic vascular resistance tends to have a negative correlation with mass gain [14]. Most important health risks linked to obesity, diabetes, hypertension, i.e., coronary heart disease and sudden death, augment progressively with increasing weight. Accordingly, in the absence of clinical symptoms, obese patients require careful cardiovascular investigation before any elective surgery.

Electrocardiograph alterations are common in obese patients: low QRS voltage, leftward shift of the P, and electric signals of left ventricular (LV) hypertrophy and left atrial enlargement [15]. Cardiac arrhythmia and conduction defects may cause sudden death in some obese patients. Myocardial hypertrophy, hypokalemia resulting from diuretics, hypoxemia and coronary heart disease may also explain the high incidence of arrhythmia in these patients [16]. De Divitus et al. [11]found that even in young obese patients LV function is depressed, in spite of the absence of clinical evidence of cardiopathy or other associated diseases. The ventricular function of 16 consecutive morbidly obese people candidates for bariatric surgery, relatively free of cardiac symptoms, was investigated with radionuclide cardiograph preoperatively. In this study, Kral [13] found that 12 of the 16 had right ventricular dysfunction and 5 had important right ventricular dilation. Of 16, 8 presented LV dysfunction, and in 5 ejection fraction was less than 50% [13]. Echocardiography data from the literature have shown that a longer the duration of morbid obesity is associated with higher LV mass, poorer LV systolic function and the greater impairment of LV diastolic filling. Weight loss-induced decreases in LV mass and improvements in LV systolic and diastolic filling are in part due to decrease in LV loading conditions [17]. Obesity causes relaxation and early filling abnormalities, and diastolic filling is compensated by rising atrial contribution. Thus, increasing LV mass is associated with progressive impairment of LV diastolic filling and increase of LV end-systolic wall stress in morbidly obese individuals [18].

Controversy persists concerning the relationship between obesity and coronary artery disease. Several long-term prospective epidemiological studies have suggested a relationship between severe obesity and coronary artery disease. However, even if many studies have demonstrated a correlation between central obesity and coronary artery disease, independent of coexisting coronary risk factors such as systemic hypertension, diabetes mellitus and hypercholesterolemia, others studies have failed to identify obesity as an isolated risk factor for coronary heart disease [19].

In conclusion, severe obesity may result in alterations of cardiac structure and function, even in the absence of systemic hypertension and other coexisting diseases. The elevated cardiac output due to increased circulating volume may predispose to ventricular dilatation, eccentric LV hypertrophy, which produces diastolic dysfunction, and ultimately the excessive wall stress may cause systolic dysfunction. Obese patients require careful cardiac investigation before surgery and complete haemodynamic perioperative monitoring, which means central venous and arterial lines. Depending on previous cardiac function, pulmonary catheter and/or trans-oesophageal echocardiography is indicated.

Respiratory alterations

Obesity imposes profound alterations on the respiratory system and metabolic demands. Obese people present higher oxygen consumption and carbon dioxide production at rest and during exercise; however, the basal metabolic rate, because it is related to body surface area, is usually normal [20, 21]. Metabolic fat activity and higher energy expenditure for locomotion, and a high respiratory minute volume to maintain normocapnia, may explain the increased oxygen consumption. However, obesity may be associated with obstructive sleep apnea and obesity hypoventilation syndrome, which is believed to reduce lung volumes causing hypoxemia and hypercapnia [22]. In the upright position, expiratory reserve volume and functional residual capacity (FRC) are decreased, so tidal volume may reduce within the range of closing capacity, determining ventilation to perfusion alterations or even true right to left shunt with subsequent hypoxemia. In the recumbent position FRC often falls, further aggravating gas exchange [23]. Despite these changes in respiratory variables the usual tests, e.g., force vital capacity, forced expiratory volume in 1 s and peak expiratory flow rate, are usually normal in obesity. Otherwise, Rubinstein et al. [24] found airflow limitation between 50 and 75% of vital capacity in obese people. Besides functional pulmonary alterations, obese patients may also present important respiratory mechanical changes. There is a general consensus that the total respiratory compliance is decreased due to both components, chest and lung compliance, the chest component being the most important. The reduction in chest wall compliance is believed to be caused by fat added around the ribs and thorax. The increased pulmonary blood volume is responsible for the decrease in lung compliance [23]. As we know, the total respiratory system is commonly divided into two components: the chest wall and the lung. Which of these two components, or both, is responsible for the decrease in the total respiratory compliance in anaesthetised morbidly obese patients is another important question. The literature presents discrepancy results. In awake obese patients, investigators, sometimes using different methodology, found decreased chest compliance [25, 26].

In contrast to the above studies, Suratt et al. [27], comparing normal and obese awake subjects, found no correlation between BMI and $C_{st,w}$. On the other hand, in sedated and paralyzed morbidly obese patients, when compared to the normal, Van Lith et al. [28] found that $C_{st,w}$ was low in obese patients. The same results were related by Pelosi et al. [29] in anaesthetised obese patient. These authors attributed the reduction in chest wall compliance to an increase in the adiposity around the ribs, diaphragm and abdomen. Interesting enough, the same group investigated the effects of body mass (BMI) on respiratory mechanics (compliance and resistance) in another group of anaesthetised obese patients and found that the reduction in respiratory compliance along with increased body mass was caused mostly by the lung component. In this study, the chest wall compliance was only weakly dependent on the BMI, causing minimal contribution to the total system compliance variation [30]. Our data on anaesthetised morbidly obese patients showed that the C_{st} decrease could be mainly attributed to the lung component, as $C_{st,w}$ is high in obese compared to normal patients and did not vary during laparotomy [31, 32]. These findings reinforce the theory of cranial displacement of diaphragm muscle during anaesthesia in decreasing FRC, lung compliance and, consequently, total respiratory compliance.

When the abdomen is opened, the intra-abdominal pressure decreases suddenly, moving the relaxed diaphragm position outward from the thorax. During our study, the lung compliance increased significantly during the period of abdomen opening, 48.41 ± 12.60 after anaesthetic induction to 72.20 ± 18.20 ml/cm H_2O, 1 h after abdomen opening, almost 60% rise, decreasing again after the abdomen had been closed. Hedenstierna and Santesson [33] measured $C_{st,w}$ in ten anaesthetised paralysed obese patients and determined that it was normal. Recent data from our research group have found that anaesthetised obese patients presented and low respiratory compliance and higher airway resistance, which was mainly determined by the lung component. Intra-abdominal pressure may play an important role in decreasing lung compliance and increasing lung resistance [31, 32].

Another important point is a lack of consensus of the literature about the ideal value of tidal volume to be settled during anaesthesia, as well as PEEP (positive endexpiratory pressure) uses and indication [34, 35]. Obese patients, due to reduced lung volumes, decreased functional residual capacity and high closing capacity, have a tendency for hypoxemia because of ventilation/perfusion mismatching and increase in the intrapulmonary shunt [36, 2]. Anaesthesia, muscular relaxation and recumbent position may even worsen this situation. Adequate transpulmonary inspiratory pressure and or PEEP to maintain end-expiratory volume, together with high FIO_2 have been recommended to preserve blood oxygenation [2, 36]. The literature has reported different approaches to handle this problem, such as high levels of FIO_2 and tidal volume (V_T), sometimes PEEP and even the prone position [37, 38]. Related to the V_T during anaesthesia for morbidly obese patients, the literature focuses on three principal procedures. First, tidal volume guided by the normal levels of end tidal CO_2 [37]; secondar, high tidal volume (15-20 ml/kg) adjusted according to the calculated ideal weight (for the ideal body weight one can subtract 100 for men and 105 for women from the patients height in cm) [6]; third, some authors just recommend high levels of V_T, but do not mention the exact values [2, 39]. Compared to literature that recommends higher V_T, more than 15 ml per ideal kg, the values of V_T employed in our obese patients were close to 0.62 l (calculated per ideal kg, V_T was approximately 11 ml). Pelosi et al. [29, 35] in different studies have been employed similar V_T values (mean average tidal volume of 10-11 ml per ideal kg). Bardoczky et al. [34] evaluated the effect of large tidal volume (calculated by the ideal body weight) from the baseline, 13 ml/kg, in increments of 3 ml/kg until reaching 22 ml/kg. They concluded that the increase in tidal volume was not accompanied by important improvement in the oxygenation and caused severe hypocapnia. Application of PEEP can improve oxygenation, although this finding may not always be agreed upon in the literature [40].

Eriksen et al. [41] have shown that in obese patients PEEP reduced cardiac index by about 20% and a similar improvement of oxygenation could be achieved with large tidal volumes. On the other hand, Söderberg et al. [42] found that PEEP reduced p_aO_2 in obese patients during anaesthesia. Recently, Pelosi et al. [35] reported mean values of p_aO_2 of 110.2 ± 29.6 mmHg in anaesthetised obese patients utilising FIO_2 of 50%, average tidal volume of 0.683 ± 0.043 l. After 10 cm H_2O of PEEP, they observed a p_aO_2 elevation of 130.0 ± 28.0 mmHg. According to these authors, the decrease in oxygenation is associated with lung volume reduction, suggesting that a significant lung collapse is probably present in the obese patients.

As suggested in the literature, during anaesthesia obese lungs have a tendency to collapse [35]. The opening of collapsed units is a function of transmural pressure, which according to the literature depends on high tidal volume that may cause marked elevation of airway pressure. This may be intrinsically harmful to lung parenchyma, so it may be more rational to use a V_T compatible with acceptable p_aO_2, p_aCO_2 and P-V curves.

Expected difficulties in airway access

Obese patients, especially in the recumbent position, present a rapid fall in arterial oxygen saturation when in apnea, because of a low reserve of oxygen. For this reason, a very well-planned anaesthetic induction and tracheal intubation should be prepared to avoid potential risk of acute hypoxemia. Preoxygenation in the semi-recumbent position is indicated prior to anaesthetic induction and tracheal intubation [43]. The literature presents a lot of discrepancy about this matter. Potential problems in airway access may be expected during anaesthesia in morbidly obese patients. These can be listed as limited range of motion of neck, jaw, short neck, gross tongue that may limit the visualisation of larynx and epiglottis region, or even huge breasts that may interfere with laryngoscope handling. Algorithms for difficult airway should be observed and included, careful inspection of mouth and cervical movements, laryngoscope blades of different sizes, intubation stylets, laryngeal mask and fiberoptic intubation devices should be available. Anticipating airway access difficulties, awake tracheal intubation may also be performed under topical anaesthesia [44]. A useful practice is a prior look utilising a laryngoscope blade inside the mouth. The larynx region could be examined after topical anaesthesia, before anaesthesia induction [45]. Obesity is also associated with hiatal hernia, gastroesophageal reflux, hyperacid gastric fluid and poor gastric emptying. For the outlined reasons, there is an increased risk of aspiration during anaesthetic induction. Routine pretreatment with H_2 antagonists and metoclopramide should be considered.

Endocrine, metabolism, pharmacokinetics and pharmacodynamics

Oxygen and CO_2 demand and alveolar ventilation are elevated in obese patients because metabolic rate is proportional to body weight. The degree of fatty infiltration of the liver is proportionally correlated with body weight, and may be associated with glucose intolerance. Regardless of the state of carbohydrate tolerance, pancreatic islet cell hypertrophy and hyperinsulinaemia may reflect the high prevalence of diabetes mellitus in obese patients [13]. The changes in distribution of drugs in obese patients are consequences of modifications in the compartments and increase in cardiac output. The higher proportion of fat to body weight in severe obesity, with smaller muscle mass and water content, as well as liver fatty infiltration and decreased renal filtration, may explain the variations in volume of distribution, biotransformation and excretion of drugs administered to these patients [46]. Water-soluble drugs are less affected than lipophilic compounds in their distribution. Fat-soluble drugs have an increased volume of distribution and longer elimination. Many drugs are administered according to total weight, assuming that clearance is according to body weight and volume of distribution of compounds is per unit weight and does not vary with a large deviation in body weight. However, because of the changes in body compartments, and possible liver and renal dysfunction, doses should be calculated utilising appropriate indices to correct overweight to normal [2]. Obese patients seem to also have increased biotransformation of inhaled anaesthetic agents when compared to the normal [47].

In conclusion, morbidly obese patients present many characteristics that should be carefully considered in the perioperative period. Once followed attentively, the challenges should be minimised.

References

1. Naslund E, Backman L, Granstrom L et al (1997) Seven-year results of vertical banded gastroplasty for morbid obesity. Eur J Surg 163:281-286
2. Buckley FP (1994) Anaesthesia for the morbidly obese patient. Can J Anaesth 41:94-100
3. McGinnis JM, Foege WH (1993) Actual causes of death in the United States. JAMA 270: 2207-2212
4. Brolin RE (1996) Update: NIH consensus conference. Gastrointestinal surgery for severe obesity. Nutrition 12:403-404
5. Domínguez-Cherit G, Gonzalez R, Borunda D et al (1998) Anaesthesia for morbidly obese patients. World J Surg 22:969-973
6. Shenkman Z, Shir Y, Brodsky JB (1993) Perioperative management of the obese patient. Br J Anaesth 70:349-359
7. Bray GA (1992) Pathophysiology of obesity. Am J Clin Nutr 55:488S-494S
8. Harrison GG (1985) Height-weight tables. Ann Intern Med 103:989-994
9. Ashwell M, Chinn S, Stalley S et al (1982) Female fat distribution – a simple classification based on two circumference measurements. Int J Obes 6:143-152
10. Abraham S, Johnson CL (1980) Prevalence of severe obesity in adults in the United States. Am J Clin Nutr 33[Suppl 2]:306-309

11. De Divitu O, Fazio S, Petitto M et al (1981) Obesity and cardiac function. Circulation 64:477-482
12. Laaban JP, Cassuto D, Orvoen-Frija E et al (1998) Cardiorespiratory consequences of sleep apnoea syndrome in patients with massive obesity. Eur Respir J 11:20-27
13. Kral JG (1985) Morbid obesity and related health risks. Ann Intern Med 103:1043-1047
14. Dustan HP (1985) Obesity and hypertension. Ann Intern Med 103:1047-1049
15. Alpert MA, Terry BE, Cohen MV et al (2000) The electrocardiogram in morbid obesity. Am J Cardiol 85:908-910
16. Drenick EJ, Fisler JC (1988) Sudden cardiac arrest in morbidly obese surgical patients unexplained after autopsy. Am J Surg 155:720-726
17. Alpert MA, Lambert CR, Panayiotou H et al (1995) Relation of duration of morbid obesity to left ventricular mass, systolic function, and diastolic filling, and effect of weight loss. Am J Cardiol 76:1194-1197
18. Alpert MA, Lambert CR, Terry BE et al (1995) Influence of left ventricular mass on left ventricular diastolic filling in normotensive morbid obesity. Am Heart J 130:1068-1073
19. Alpert AM, Hashimi MW (1993) Obesity and the heart. Am J Med Sci 306:117-123
20. Farebrother MJB (1979) Respiratory function and cardiorespiratory response to exercise in obesity. Br J Dis Chest 73:211
21. Vaughan RW (1982) Pulmonary and cardiovascular derangements in the obese patients. In: Brown BR (ed) Anaesthetics and the obese patient. Contemporary anaesthesia practice series. Davis, Philadelphia, p 19
22. Lopata M, Onal E (1982) Mass loading, sleep apnea, and the pathogenesis of the obesity hypoventilation. Am Rev Respir Dis 126:640-645
23. Luce JM (1980) Respiratory complications of obesity. Chest 78:626-631
24. Rubinstein I, Zamel N, DuBarry L et al (1990) Airflow limitation in morbidly obese, nonsmoking men. Ann Intern Med 112:828-832
25. Sharp JT, Henry SK, Sweany WR et al (1964) Total work of breathing in normal and obese men. J Clin Invest 43:728-739
26. Naimark A, Cherniack RM (1960) Compliance of the respiratory system and its components in health and obesity. J Appl Physiol 15:377-382
27. Suratt PM, Wilhoit CS, Hsiao HS et al (1984) Compliance of chest wall in obese subjects. J Appl Physiol 57:403-407
28. Van Lith P, Johnson FN, Sharp JT (1967) Respiratory elastances in relaxed and paralyze states in normal and abnormal men. J Appl Physiol 23:475-486
29. Pelosi P, Croci M, Ravagnan I (1996) Total respiratory system, lung and chest wall mechanics in sedated-paralysed postoperative morbidly obese patients. Chest 109:144-151
30. Pelosi P, Croci M, Ravagnan I et al (1998) The effects of body mass on lung volumes, respiratory mechanics, and gas exchange general anaesthesia. Anesth Analg 87:654-660
31. Auler JOC Jr, Miyoshi E, Fernandes CR et al (2000) Respiratory system resistance during laparotomy in morbidly obese patients. Am J Respir Crit Care Med 161:A693
32. Auler JOC Jr, Miyoshi E, Fernandes CR (2000) Respiratory system compliance during laparotomy in morbidly obese patients. Abstracts of the World Congress of Anaesthesiologists, June 4-9; Montreal, p 34
33. Hedenstierna G, Santesson J (1976) Breathing mechanics, dead space and gas exchanges in the extremely obese, breathing spontaneously and during anaesthesia with intermittent positive pressure ventilation. Acta Anaesthesiol Scand 20:248-254
34. Bardoczky GI, Yernault JC, Houben JJ et al (1995) Large tidal volume ventilation does not improve oxygenation in morbidly obese patients during anaesthesia. Anesth Analg 81: 385-388
35. Pelosi P, Ravagnan I, Giurati G et al (1999) Positive end-expiratory pressure improves respiratory function in obese but not in normal subjects during anaesthesia and paralysis. Anaesthesiology 91:1221-1231
36. Öberg B, Poulsen TD (1996) Obesity: an anaesthetic challenge. Acta Anaesthesiol Scand 40:191-200

37. Dumont L, Mattys M, Mardirosoff C et al (1997) Changes in pulmonary mechanics during laparoscopic gastroplasty in morbidly obese patients. Acta Anaesthesiol Scand 41:408-413
38. Pelosi P, Croci M, Calappi E et al (1996) Prone positioning improves pulmonary function in obese patients during general anaesthesia. Anesth Analg 83:578-583
39. Fox GS, Whalley DG, Bevan DR (1981) Anaesthesia for the morbidly obese. Experience with 110 patients. Br J Anaesth 53:811-816
40. Salem MR, Dalal FY, Zygmunt MP et al (1978) Does PEEP improve intraoperative arterial oxygenation in grossly obese patients? Anaesthesiology 48:280-281
41. Eriksen J, Andersen J, Rasmussen JP (1977) Postoperative pulmonary function in obese patients after upper abdominal surgery. Acta Anaesthesiol Scand 21:336-341
42. Söderberg M, Thomson D, White T (1977) Respiratory, circulation and anaesthetic management in obesity. Investigation before and after jejuno-ileal bypass. Acta Anaesthesiol Scand 21:55-61
43. Berthoud MC, Peacock JE, Reilly CS (1991) Effectiveness of preoxygenation in morbidly obese patients. Br J Anesth 67:464-466
44. Lee JJ, Larson RH, Buckley JJ (1980) Airway maintenance in the morbidly obese. Anesth Rev 7:33-37
45. Buckley PF (1996) Anaesthesia and obesity and gastrointestinal disorders. In: Barash PG et al (eds) Clinical anaesthesia. Lippincott-Raven, Philadelphia, p 975
46. Abernethy DR, Greenblatt DJ (1982) Pharmacokinetics of drugs in obesity. Clin Pharmacokinet 7:108-124
47. Higuchi H, Satoh T, Arimura S et al (1993) Serum inorganic fluoride levels in mildly obese patients during and after sevoflurane anaesthesia. Anesth Analg 77:1018-1021

PERIOPERATIVE MEDICINE IN THE ELDERLY

Gero-Anesthesia: Functional Reserve, Cardiovascular Changes, and Postoperative Complications

S. MURAVCHICK

Functional reserve

The most-important recent advance in our understanding of the anesthetic implications of aging has been recognition of the need to distinguish clearly between processes of aging as opposed to age-related disease. Consequences of altered tissue and organ system structure and function that are universally observed in all elderly individuals and increase in severity or magnitude with advancing years reflect aging. On the other hand, changes in tissue structure or organ system function that are not seen in all members of a geriatric population, or those changes that do not increase in severity with advancing chronological age, are probably due to age-related disease. Even in healthy and fit older individuals, however, maximal levels of organ function decline more rapidly than do basal functional requirements. The difference between maximal and basal function defines the concept of functional reserve. Therefore, normal aging typically produces a progressive loss of organ system functional reserve (Fig. 1).

Many gerontologists consider increased susceptibility to stress- and disease-induced organ system decompensation to be a defining characteristic of geriatric medicine [1]. Therefore, preoperative testing of the elderly patient is most effective when it is clinically directed according to symptoms and complaints referable to age-related cardiopulmonary disease or the erosion of metabolic and immune homeostasis, because it provides the anesthesiologist with a quantifiable assessment of organ system reserve [2]. Organ system functional reserve is, in effect, the "safety margin" of organ capacity available to meet, for example, the additional demands for cardiac output, carbon dioxide excretion, or protein synthesis imposed upon the patient by trauma or disease, or by surgery and convalescence. In elderly surgical patients, demonstration of substantial cardiopulmonary, metabolic, and central nervous system functional reserve appear to be the most-important predictors of ability to successfully undergo surgery [3].

Cardiopulmonary functional reserve can be assessed clinically and quantified using various exercise or aerobic stress tests. However, there are at present no standard techniques for assessment of hepatic, immune, or nervous system functional reserve. Anesthetic requirement falls linearly with increasing age, beginning in young adulthood. The reduction in anesthetic requirement, because it

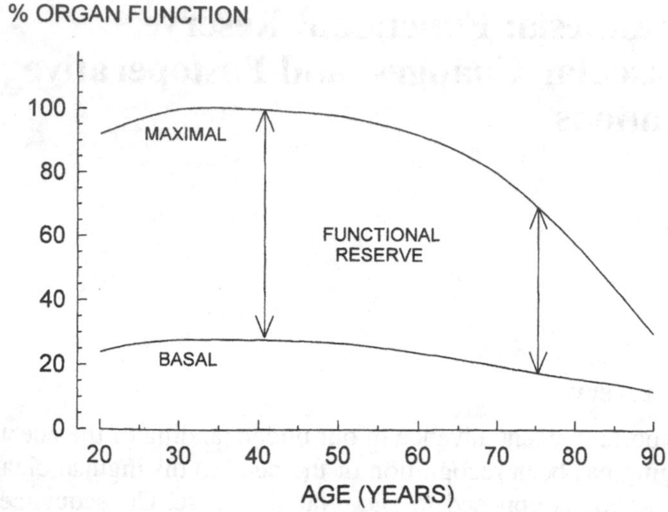

Fig. 1. The difference between maximal achievable levels of organ function and the minimal or basal levels of organ function associated with inactivity is the basis for the concept of organ system functional reserve. Maximal function is far more variable than basal function, but functional reserve is reduced even in older individuals who are physiologically "young"

occurs with all agents, regardless of their chemical structure, is probably due to fundamental neurophysiological changes within the brain, such as reduced neuron density or, more likely, altered concentrations of brain neurotransmitters. Typically, an 80-year-old patient will require only two-thirds to three-quarters of the anesthetic concentration needed to produce comparable effects in a young adult. Anesthetic requirement can be considered a quantifiable measure of the functional reserve of the central nervous system (Fig. 2).

Cardiovascular system

In healthy older individuals, loss of vascular and myocardial elasticity produces significant changes in cardiovascular parameters, but only minor change in hemodynamics. Stiffening of the arterial tree and decreased total vascular cross-sectional area increases afterload by two mechanisms: steady-state systemic vascular resistance increases by about one-third, but frequency dependent impedance to ejection of stroke volume more than doubles because of the increased reflection of aortic pulse waves. Increased hydraulic impedance increases myocardial work at any given blood pressure and eventually produces concentric hypertrophy of the left ventricular myocardial wall. It also results in a progressive rise in systolic blood pressure and a widening of arterial pulse pressure, especially in women (Fig. 3).

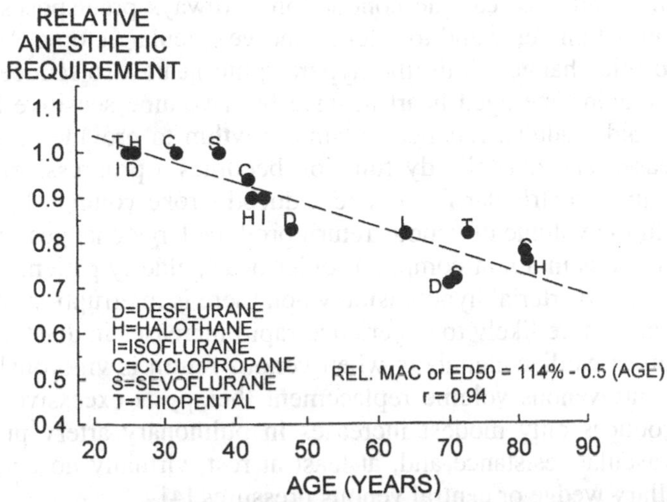

Fig. 2. With increasing age, anesthetic requirement for unsedated human subjects expressed as relative median effective dose (ED_{50}) or its inhalational equivalent, minimum alveolar concentration (*MAC*), is progressively and consistently reduced. Despite many differences in chemical structure and clinical pharmacology, anesthetic requirement declines both for inhalational (C, D, H, I, S) and for intravenous (T) anesthetics, suggesting that this is a physiological process-specific, rather than a drug-specific, phenomenon

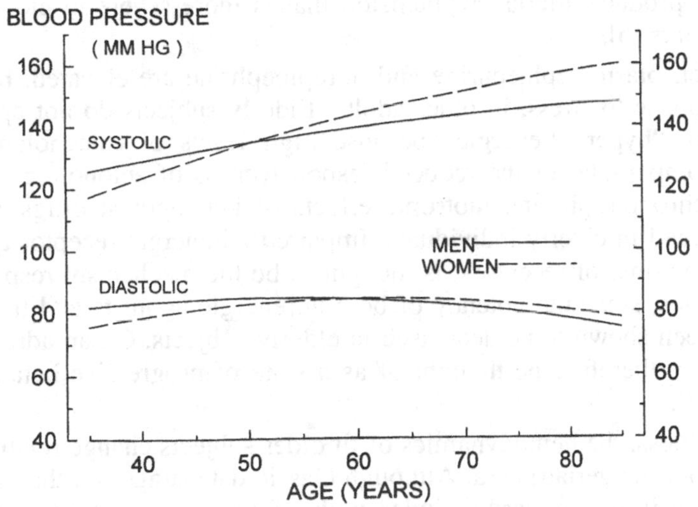

Fig. 3. Data from the Framingham longitudinal study illustrate that the progressive loss of peripheral vascular elasticity and increases in collagen cross linking due to aging increase systolic pressure and widen arterial pulse pressures. These changes are even more dramatic in women (*broken lines*) than in men (*solid lines*)

Fibrotic infiltration of cardiac conduction pathways predisposes the elderly patient to conduction delay and to arterial and ventricular ectopy. Reduced elasticity and fibrotic change within the hypertrophic heart also reduce ventricular compliance, making the aged heart at once both volume sensitive and volume intolerant. In older adults, reliance on sinus rhythm to provide atrial "kick" is greatly increased and diastolic dysfunction becomes a progressively important cause of impaired ventricular filling and reduced stroke volume. Because small fluctuations in the volume of venous return produce large changes in ventricular "preload" pressures in a non-compliant older heart, elderly patients are particularly predisposed to arterial hypotension when there is interruption of venous return, yet are also more likely to experience rapid increases in diastolic pressures and distention of cardiac chambers when venous return is vigorously augmented, or when intravenous volume replacement therapy is excessive. In general, age itself produces only modest increases in pulmonary artery pressures and pulmonary vascular resistance and, at least at rest, virtually no change in pulmonary capillary wedge or central venous pressures [4].

The speed, magnitude, and efficacy of overall autonomic homeostasis is progressively impaired with increasing age. Baroreflex responsiveness, the vasoconstrictor response to cold stress, and beat-to-beat heart rate responses following postural change in elderly subjects, also diminish in effectiveness with advancing age. The autonomic nervous system in the elderly patient is "underdamped", permitting wider variation from homeostatic set points and delayed restabilization during hemodynamic stress [5]. Therefore, anesthetic agents that disrupt end-organ function or reduce plasma catecholamines, or techniques associated with a pharmacological sympathectomy such as spinal or epidural anesthesia, produce arterial hypotension that is more severe in elderly than in young patients [6].

However, plasma epinephrine and norepinephrine are elevated, both at rest and in response to stress, in older adults. Elderly subjects do not appear to be functionally "hyper-adrenergic" because high levels of catecholamines only partially compensate for the reduced responsiveness of autonomic end-organs. Both the chronotropic and inotropic effects of beta-agonist drugs are significantly reduced in elderly individuals. Impaired adrenergic receptor quality, not decline in number of receptors, is thought to be the mechanism responsible for these changes, since the potency of both adrenergic agonists and their antagonists has been shown to be decreased in elderly subjects. On an adrenergic level, aging can therefore be thought of as a state of progressive beta-adrenergic blockade [7].

Nevertheless, the hemodynamics of fit older subjects change relatively slowly throughout the geriatric era. Although classic data suggested that there was a rapid decline in resting cardiac index with advancing age, more-recent studies indicate that normally active, adequately conditioned elderly individuals maintain resting cardiac index at levels almost indistinguishable from their younger counterparts. Cardiac output is reduced in proportion to the decreased skeletal muscle mass and reduced aerobic demands seen in an older subject. At submaximal levels of demand, there are no consistent age-related reductions of velocity of myocardial shortening or ventricular pressure generation. In other words, ventricular pump function appears to be largely a reflection of conditioning and aerobic demand, not chronological age. During exercise, cardiac output in the elderly subject is augmented in part by increased heart rate, but also by a unique additional ability to augment left ventricular diastolic volume in response to rising preload, probably through the Frank-Starling mechanism. In young adults, in contrast, most of the increase in cardiac output that occurs in response to exercise reflects increase in heart rate and the enhancement of ejection fraction by the neural and humoral components of the sympathoadrenal nervous system.

Postoperative complications

For the elderly population at large, the epidemiological patterns of disease encountered throughout the geriatric era are different than those of young adults [8]. For both men and women, the predominant risk factors for cardiovascular mortality are increased systolic blood pressure and hypercholesterolemia. Older subjects with left ventricular hypertrophy or arterial hypertension are at increased risk of cerebrovascular accident and have a two- to threefold increase in the risk of congestive heart failure. Chronic obstructive pulmonary disease and other forms of lung disease, as well as hepatic, renal, and metabolic disorders, also appear to retain nearly proportional representation as causes of death in elderly subjects. Data from the Framingham longitudinal study [9] reveal the complexity of the interaction between intrinsic and extrinsic factors with regard to cardiovascular mortality in an aging population. Systolic blood pressure is directly related to cardiovascular mortality both in men and in women, but cigarette smoking is significantly related to cardiovascular mortality only in women. Subjects of either gender with glycosuria experience an increase in overall mortality, but diabetes mellitus itself is specifically associated with increased mortality only in women. Myocardial re-infarctions occur at the same rate in elderly individuals with either documented or “silent” prior infarction. Nevertheless, overall, the increased probability of mortality in an elderly population primarily reflects progressive age-related increases in the prevalence of cardiovascular disease, both in men and in women (Fig. 4).

Although age can no longer be considered a contraindication to anesthesia and surgery, anesthetic-related mortality is higher in the elderly than in the young adult surgical patient. Nevertheless, aging is associated with a complex interaction of factors that predispose to adverse outcome (Fig. 5). Overt hepatic dysfunction and failure appear in a small but significant fraction of elderly surgical patients, about 4%, but more-subtle degrees of hepatic compromise and limited hepatic functional reserve explain many postoperative metabolic complications and may require supportive therapy and intensive care. The risks of ad-

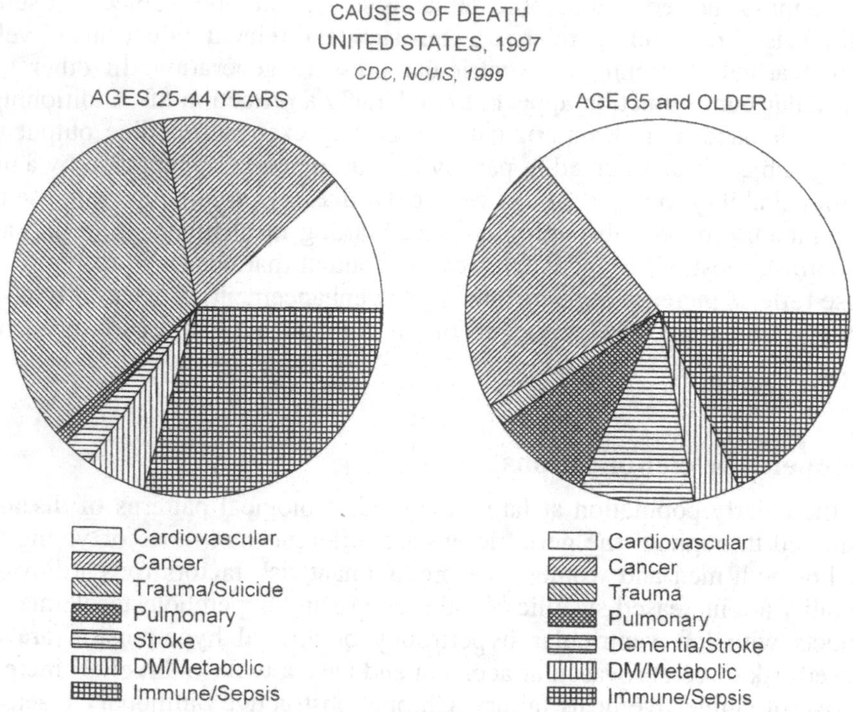

Fig. 4. For the elderly population at large, the epidemiological patterns of disease encountered throughout the geriatric era are significantly different than those of young adults. Increased probability of mortality from cardiovascular disease largely displaces the high rate of trauma and death by suicide and homicide in young adults. In older adults, increases in the incidence of stroke and dementia-related morbidity replace the high rate of death from immune disorders such as human immunodeficiency virus infection seen in younger adults. However, cancer, pulmonary disease, and hepatic, renal, and metabolic disorders retain a nearly proportional representation as causes of death in elderly subjects
(*DM* diabetes mellitus)

verse drug interaction, already high in the elderly, also make a thorough review of the indications and dosage of essential perioperative medication an important part of the preoperative assessment process. Drug interactions are a form of iatrogenic disease due to the additive, synergistic, or antagonistic actions of multiple drugs sharing common sites of action, or to unexpected changes in the duration of drug effects. They occur in elderly patients far more often than in young patients primarily because polypharmacy is most common in older adults and because reduced hepatic and renal functional reserve prolongs both the desired and the unwanted effects of many medications.

Elderly patients account for 30% of all drug prescriptions, approximately twice the rate expected from their representation in the general population, and

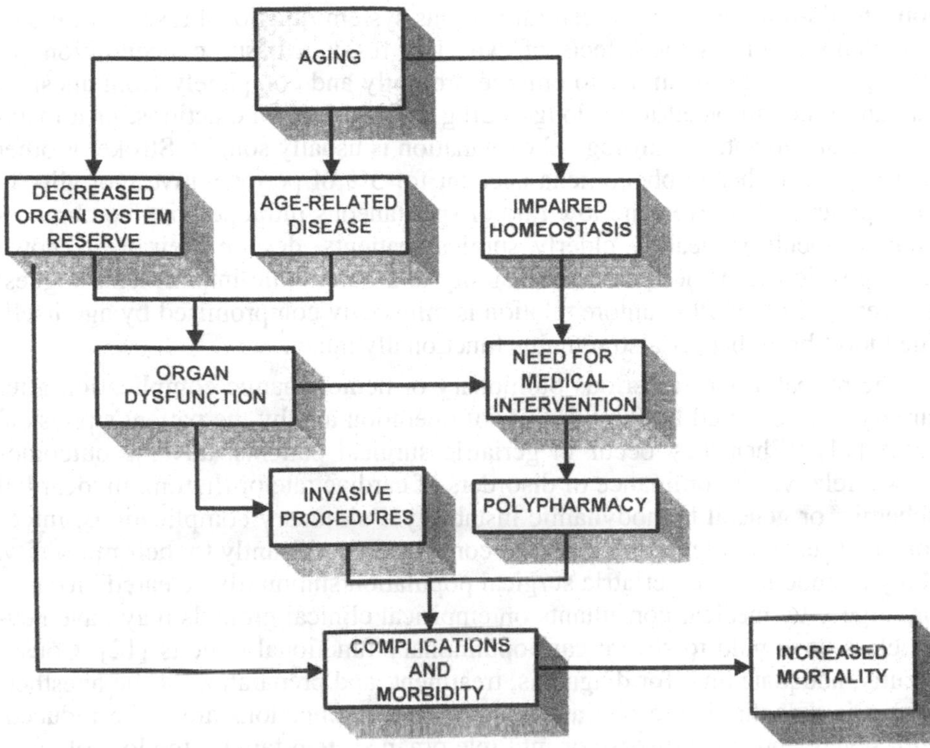

Fig. 5. An increased rate of perioperative complications and a greater likelihood of perioperative mortality in elderly subjects reflects the interaction of the effects of aging on organ system functional reserve and autonomic homeostatic integrity as well as the consequences of age-related disease and its therapy. Increased invasive testing, such as cardiac catheterization, has led to an increase in the rate of both coronary artery bypass grafting and transluminal angioplasty. Polypharmacy and the need for medical intervention further amplify the likelihood of side-effects, drug interactions, and adverse outcome

they consume 40% of all-over-the counter medications. Although it is appropriate to maintain elderly patients perioperatively on all medications needed to effectively control the symptoms of their disorders, especially cardiovascular, neurological, and metabolic disease, some perioperative drug interactions may complicate anesthetic management or make the pharmacokinetics of drugs used perioperatively less predictable. The most-common cause of prolonged depression of consciousness, disorientation, autonomic instability, hyperreflexia, or other manifestations of acute postoperative nervous system dysfunction in elderly patients is, simply stated, residual anesthetic drug effects [10]. In a geriatric surgical population, this form of anesthetic morbidity may be observed more frequently than in younger patients, and may be more persistent, because there is age-related compromise of organ system function that delays drug elimination. In addition, the reduced central nervous system functional reserve of elderly patients amplifies the effects of even low residual tissue concentrations of these potent drugs. If failure to emerge promptly and completely from anesthesia cannot be attributed to prolonged drug effects, drug interactions, or a metabolic derangement, a neurological explanation is usually sought. Stroke or other neurological ischemic phenomena account for 3% of perioperative mortality in older patients. However, the low rate of spontaneous intraoperative cerebrovascular accidents in healthy elderly surgical patients, despite their well-known predisposition to hemodynamic instability and autonomic impairment, suggest that cerebral blood flow autoregulation is minimally compromised by age itself. The blood-brain-barrier also remains functionally intact.

The probability of a serious pulmonary or hemodynamic complication after surgery is determined both by the site of operation and by the patient's physical status [11]. When they occur in geriatric surgical patients, adverse outcomes show a relative predominance of disorders of cardiac rate or rhythm, myocardial ischemia, or general hemodynamic instability. Pulmonary complications, infections and sepsis, and renal failure also contribute significantly to their morbidity. Many members of the geriatric surgical population summarily "cleared" for major surgery by medical consultants on empirical clinical grounds may have nevertheless have mild to severe cardiopulmonary functional deficits [12]. Consequently, adequate time for diagnosis, treatment, and preparation of the anesthetic plan is essential if the rate and severity of complications are to be reduced. With severe end-stage disease or multiple organ system failure, the loss of autonomic homeostasis intrinsic to aging may act as an additional age-related factor that increases perioperative risk. Site of surgery is also a significant determinant of outcome in older adults. However, recent prospective studies of perioperative mortality as a function of physical status (ASA PS) confirm that age-related disease, not aging itself, actually plays the most important role in this relationship (Fig. 6).

Other recent large-scale prospective studies of neurological complications in outpatients suggest that there is less nausea and vomiting in older adults [13] after general anesthesia but a greater likelihood of prolonged postoperative confusion [14]. In fact, even when anesthetic management of the older patient is appropriate and surgical convalescence uncomplicated, after a prolonged general anesthetic full return of cognitive function to preoperative levels may require 5-10 days. Classic and more-recent studies demonstrate consistently that 20-40% of elderly patients are, however, uniquely prone to a more-subtle form of postoperative delirium characterized by shortened attention span, disorientation, and abrupt fluctuations in either mood or in levels of consciousness beginning 1-2 day after surgery and persisting for several days to several weeks. Delirium may, in many cases, simply be due to inadequate pain control [15] or anticholinergic drugs or other agents used intraoperatively that cross the blood-brain-barrier freely and enter the central nervous system in quantities sufficient to cause symptoms. However, the mechanism in other cases is not clear, and delirium in

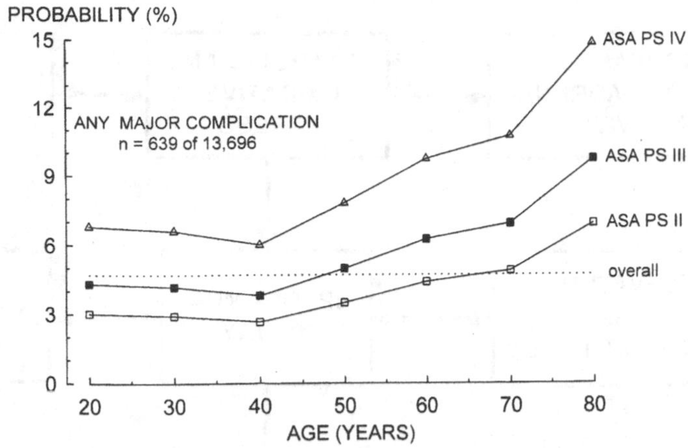

Fig. 6. The probability of a serious perioperative cardiovascular complication such as myocardial infarction, congestive heart failure, arterial hypotension, or persistent arrhythmia increases slightly after young adulthood but is determined primarily by overall physical status, graded according to the American Society of Anesthesiologists Physical Status (ASA PS) system. Therefore, the number and severity of pre-existing disease states have significant predictive value for the likelihood of cardiovascular complications

elderly surgical patients is equally common whether regional or general anesthesia has been used [16]. A history of alcohol abuse, anemia, psychiatric depression, or simply poor functional outcome after surgery are thought to be predisposing factors for adverse psychological outcome in elderly patients, particularly after orthopedic surgery [17].

There is some evidence that idiopathic delirium may also predispose to long-term postoperative cognitive impairment [18]. The neurophysiological or pharmacological explanation for impairment of cognitive function seen in 10-15% of patients 60 years of age or older who have had major procedures and a hospital stay of 4 or more days remains unknown [19]. At least in older adults with reduced central nervous system functional reserve, either the process of general anesthesia itself or the drugs used to produce it may have effects upon the metabolic and neurotransmitter functions of neuronal tissue that can actually produce residual neurological injury, now termed postoperative cognitive dysfunction. Acute stress-related glucocorticoid responses [20] to tissue injury, pain, or the psychosocial consequences of disability may interact to produce or accelerate cognitive decline in those aged adults in whom nervous system tissue and neurotransmitter reserve is severely reduced by neuronal loss and bioenergetic failure at a mitochondrial level (Fig. 7).

Whatever the cause, delayed recovery of postoperative mental function following anesthesia in some older patients prolongs hospital stay and increases

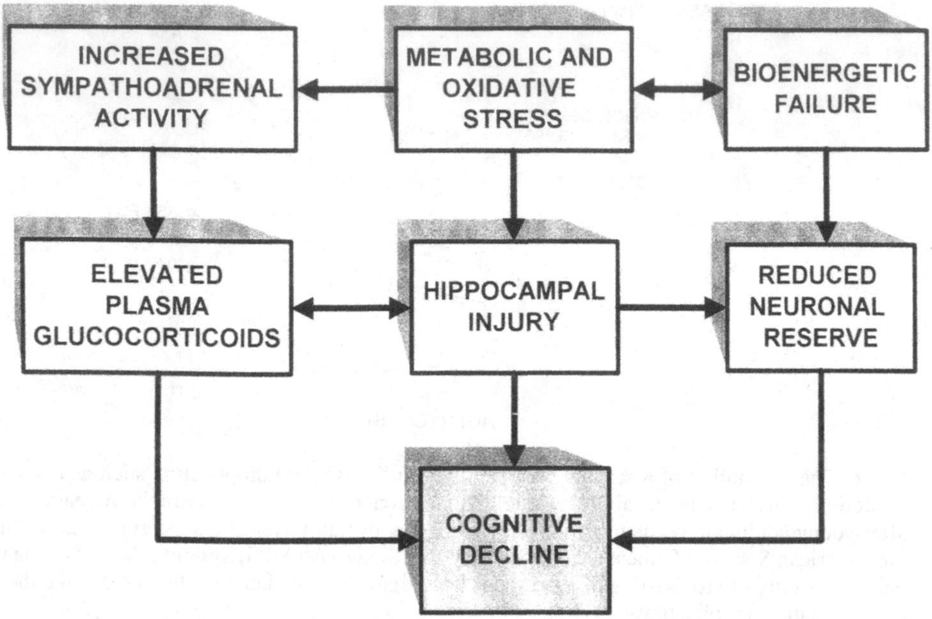

Fig. 7. Cognitive decline after apparently uncomplicated anesthesia and surgery may reflect the complex interaction between stress-related neuroendocrine changes, pre-existing hippocampal injury, and the general bioenergetic decline and loss of neuronal reserve that appears to characterize the aging brain

other forms of adverse outcome, and is therefore a major determinant both of discharge disposition and ultimate full functional recovery. Major neuraxial conduction anesthesia and peripheral nerve and plexus blocks may not necessarily be preferable, because they appear to be associated with an increased risk of nerve palsies, persistent numbness, and other neurological complications in older patients. Neuropraxias due to regional anesthesia occur more often in older than in young adults [21, 22]. Perioperative environmental factors such as chronic medication and drug interaction [23], disorientation due to sensory deprivation, or the disruption of normal routine needed to maintain "implicit" memory [24] may also explain the high incidence of "delirium" in older surgical patients after minor procedures or regional anesthetics.

Currently, there is great interest in the mechanism and the importance of long-term oxidative stress [25] as a cause of increasing damage to mitochondrial DNA and intracellular protein [26] that eventually impairs intracellular bioenergetics [27]. Within mitochondria, increasing levels of oxygen-derived free radicals within the mitochondria appear to disrupt the structural and enzymatic machinery of oxidative phosphorylation. As the ability of aging cells to synthesize the enzymes needed to scavenge these byproducts of aerobic metabolism declines, a "vicious cycle of aging" develops. This might explain the age-related deterioration of maximal organ function and loss of functional reserve that inevitably occurs throughout adulthood even in the most fit older subjects. Consequently, advocates of stress reduction techniques, antioxidant "scavengers" such as vitamin E, and those who propose that severe caloric restriction prolongs life [28] may have found a rational and unifying hypothesis (Fig. 8).

In elderly patients, as in surgical patients of any age, the spectrum of anesthetic options ranges from local anesthesia to general anesthesia. The details of the anesthetic and perioperative plan is determined by the wishes of the patient, the nature of the proposed surgery, the patient's physical status, and by the anticipated extent of tissue injury due to the surgery and the severity and duration of the physiological disruption that it produces. However, in order to be successful and to minimize adverse outcome, the anesthetic plan for any elderly surgical patient must also include a considered judgment regarding the degree of psychological stress associated with awareness, the extent of tissue injury and the risk/benefit ratio for invasive monitoring, the relative risk associated with muscle relaxation and controlled ventilation as opposed to spontaneous ventilation under these circumstances, and the consequences of using many potent drugs in

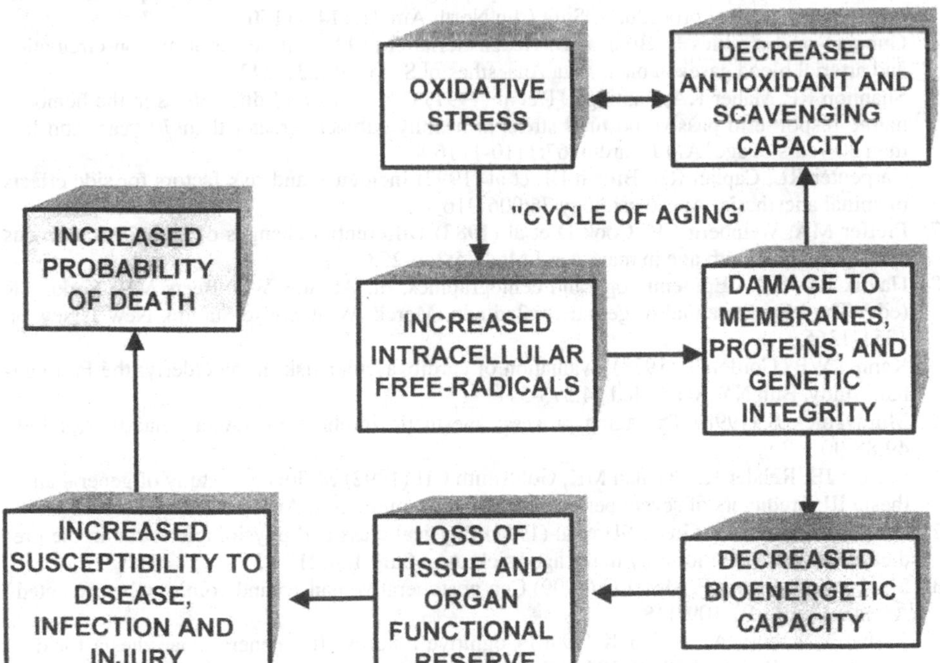

Fig. 8. At a molecular level, a self-perpetuating cycle of aging that progressively impairs mitochondrial bioenergetics could eventually compromise organ system functional reserve to the point that increased susceptibility to disease increases the probability of death with advancing age

the setting of pre-existing polypharmacy common in older adults because of age-related disease. Finally, the skilled anesthetist will be familiar with the effects of aging on anesthetic requirement as measured both from a pharmacodynamic (drug concentration effect) and from a pharmacokinetic (molecular drug disposition over time) perspective [29]. Therefore, there is no "best" anesthetic for elderly patients. Large-scale, prospective, randomized studies of contemporary anesthetic practice fail to suggest any clinically or statistically significant advantage to regional as opposed to general anesthesia. Similarly, there is no evidence to support the preferential selection of a specific general anesthetic agent. The use of pharmacological sympathectomy with epidural local anesthetics to minimize postsurgical pain and stress responses may, however, provide significant reductions in perioperative morbidity.

References

1. Barry PP (1987) Primary care evaluation of the elderly for elective surgery. Geriatrics 42: 77-80
2. Blery C, Charpak Y, Szatan M et al (1986) Evaluation of a protocol for selective ordering of preoperative tests. Lancet 1:139-141
3. Gagner M (1991) Value of preoperative physiologic assessment in outcome of patients undergoing major surgical procedures. Surg Clin North Am 71:1141-1150
4. Gunnarsson L, Tokics L, Brismar B, Hedenstierna G (1996) Influence of age on circulation and arterial blood gases in man. Acta Anaesthesiol Scand 40:237-243
5. Shannon RP, Maher KA, Santinga JT et al (1991) Comparison of differences in the hemodynamic response to passive postural stress in healthy subjects greater than 70 years and less than 30 years of age. Am J Cardiol 67:1110-1116
6. Carpenter RL, Caplan RA, Brown DL et al (1992) Incidence and risk factors for side effects of spinal anesthesia. Anesthesiology 76:906-916
7. Pfeifer MA, Weinberg CR, Cook D et al (1983) Differential changes of autonomic nervous system function with age in man. Am J Med 75:249-258
8. Havlik RJ (1991) Epidemiology and demographics. In: Abrams WB, Beers MH, Berkow R (eds) The Merck manual of geriatrics, 2nd edn. Merck, Whitehouse Station, New Jersey, pp 1351-1365
9. Kannel WB, Gordon T (1978) Evaluation of cardiovascular risk in the elderly: the Framingham study. Bull NY Acad Med 54:573-591
10. Muravchick S (1998) The aging process: anesthetic implications. Acta Anaesthesiol Belg 49:85-90
11. Forrest JB, Rehder K, Cahalan MK, Goldsmith CH (1992) Multicenter study of general anesthesia III; predictors of severe perioperative adverse outcomes. Anesthesiology 76:3-15
12. Lewin I, Lerner AG, Green SH et al (1971) Physical class and physiologic status in the prediction of operative mortality in the aged sick. Ann Surg 174:217-231
13. Sinclair DR, Chung F, Mezel G (1999) Can postoperative nausea and vomiting be predicted? Anesthesiology 91:109-118
14. Tzabar Y, Asbury AJ, Millar K (1996) Cognitive failures after general anaesthesia for day-case surgery. Br J Anaesth 76:194-197
15. Lynch EP, Lazor MA, Gellis JE et al (1998) The impact of postoperative pain on the development of postoperative delirium. Anesth Analg 86:781-758
16. O'Keefe ST, Conchubhair AN (1994) Postoperative delirium in the elderly. Br J Anaesth 73: 673-687

17. Williams-Russo P, Urquhart BL, Sharrock NE, Charlson ME (1992) Postoperative delirium: predictors and prognosis in elderly orthopedic patients. J Am Geriatr Soc 40:759-767
18. Knill RL, Novick TY, Skinner MI (1991) Idiopathic postoperative delirium is associated with longterm cognitive impairment. Can J Anaesth 38:A541
19. Moller JT and the ISOPCD investigators (1998) Long-term postoperative cognitive dysfunction in the elderly; ISPOCD1 study. Lancet 351:857-861
20. O'Brien JT (1997) The "glucocorticoid cascade" hypothesis in man; prolonged stress may cause permanent brain damage. Br J Psychiatry 170:199-201
21. Hampl KF, Heinzmann-Wiedmer S, Luginbuehl I et al (1998) Transient neurologic symptoms after spinal anesthesia. Anesthesiology 88:629-633
22. Martinez-Bourio R, Arzuaza M, Quintana JM et al (1998) Incidence of transient neurologic symptoms after hyperbaric subarachnoid anesthesia with 5% lidocaine and 5% prilocaine. Anesthesiology 88:624-628
23. Jolles J, Verhey FR, Riedel WJ, Houx PJ (1995) Cognitive impairment in elderly people; predisposing factors and implications for experimental drug studies. Drugs Aging 7:459-479
24. Inouye SK, Bogardus ST, Charpentier PA et al (1999) A multicomponent intervention to prevent delirium in hospitalized older patients. N Eng J Med 340:669-676
25. Sohal RS, Weindruch R (1996) Oxidative stress, caloric restriction, and aging. Science 273: 59-63
26. Stadtman ER, Berlett BS (1998) Reactive oxygen-mediated protein oxidation in aging and disease. Drug Metab Rev 30:225-243
27. Ozawa T (1997) Genetic and functional changes in mitochondria associated with aging. Physiol Rev 77:425-464
28. Lee C-K, Klopp RG, Weindruch R, Prolla TA (1999) Gene expression profile of aging and its retardation by caloric restriction. Science 285:1390-1392
29. Vestal RE, Dawson GW (1989) Pharmacology and aging. In: Finch CE, Schneider EL (eds) Handbook of the biology of aging, 2nd edn. Van Nostrand-Rheinhold, New York, pp 744-819

Suggested further reading

Collins KJ, Exton-Smith AN, James MH (1980) Functional changes in autonomic nervous responses with ageing. Age Ageing 9:17-24

Creasey H, Rapoport SI (1985) The aging human brain. Ann Neurol 17:2-10

Fulop T Jr, Worum I, Csongor J et al (1985) Body composition in elderly people. Gerontology 31:6-14

Hayflick L (1990) Biologic and theoretical perspectives of human aging. In: Katlic MR (ed) Geriatric surgery: comprehensive care of the elderly patient. Urban and Schwarzenberg, Baltimore, pp 3-21

Lassen NA, Ingvar DH, Skinhoj E (1978) Brain function and blood flow. Sci Am 239:62-71

McLachlan MSF (1978) The ageing kidney. Lancet II:143-146

Muravchick S (1986) Immediate and long-term nervous system effects of anesthesia in elderly patients. Clin Anaesth 4:1035-1045

Muravchick S (1997) Geroanesthesia: perioperative management of the elderly patient. Mosby-Year Book Medical Publishers, Chicago

Wahba WM (1983) Influence of aging on lung function – clinical significance of changes from age twenty. Anesth Analg 62:764-776

Management of the Hopelessly Ill Patient: To Stop or Not to Start?

Assessment and Decisions in the Perioperative Period

G.M. GURMAN, N. WEKSLER, R. STARIKOV

A 75-year-old male was brought from a retirement home to the emergency department of a county hospital. He had been a heavy smoker (45 pack years) but had quit smoking 5 years earlier, after his cigarettes had caused some fire incidents. These episodes, together with decreased concentration and memory and inability to take care of himself had obliged the family (two sons and a daughter) to admit him to the retirement home. In the past year he had become increasingly demented and required continual supervision. Over the previous six months he also required assistance in performing usual activities such as feeding, washing and changing clothes. He no longer recognized family members and he sat in a chair throughout the day without any communication with those around him.

Three days before his admission to the hospital he refused food and fluids. On the day prior to admission he vomited, developed a fever and subsequently became oliguric and stuporotic.

At the request of the family he was taken to the hospital by ambulance. A referral letter from the family physician reported co-morbidity with hypertension, chronic ischemic heart disease and mild chronic renal failure. His daily medications included enalapril, mononitrate and a mild diuretic.

Physical examination in the emergency room revealed a dehydrated and obtunded patient. The blood pressure was 75/50, the heart rate was 98/min, the temperature was 35.5ºC, and the respiratory rate was 36/min. The examining physician noted guarding of the abdomen, especially in the epigastric area, rebound tenderness and the absence of bowel sounds.

The results of blood tests revealed: a hemoglobin level of 16.9 g/dl, WBC 18 800/ml, BUN 88 mg/dl, creatinine 4.8 mg/dl, sodium 122 mEq/l, potassium 3.0 mEq/l, chloride 98 mEq/l and bicarbonate 17.5 mEq/l.

An infusion of saline was started and oxygen was administered through a nasal cannula. The bladder was catheterized and 50 ml of concentrated urine was drained.

A plain radiograph of the abdomen showed free air under the right diaphragm. A surgical consultant suspected a perforated viscus, probably a duodenal ulcer, and discussed the feasibility of an urgent laparotomy. The anesthesiologist on duty was asked to assess the patient's condition and advise on preparation for surgery.

This case exemplifies a typical doctor's dilemma. The patient's baseline condition warranted a discussion with the family on the relative advantages and disadvantages of surgery compared to conservative management of the acute abdomen.

Matters do not always develop in this way. Palliative treatment of a perforated viscus implies the avoidance of aggressive treatment and a prolonged, difficult and uncomfortable process of dying for this hopelessly ill patient. However, it is not clear whether this approach is acceptable to many in the medical community.

In this paper we will try to present the conflicting opinions among various medical practitioners and discuss the futility of aggressive treatment for patients such as the one presented in the preceding case.

The hopelessly ill patient

We often are in the position of treating patients who are incapable of expressing their wishes, of communicating with the surroundings, or even of taking care of their basic needs. Incompetent patients can be classified into one of the following clinical conditions [1]:

1. *Patients with brain death*. They are considered medically and legally dead and no further treatment is planned;
2. *Patients in a persistent vegetative state*. Withholding aggressive management is a sound solution, but the prior wishes of the patient and/or the family might affect medical decision-making;
3. *Patients with irreversible, severe dementia*. Most of these patients are elderly and suffer from serious medical co-morbid conditions that affect their clinical outcomes. Their mental capacity is deteriorating continuously and they are totally incapable of initiating purposeful activity. They accept nourishment and bodily care passively.

The patient presented at the beginning of this paper belongs to the last category. He could not even enjoy a moderately restricted life, as do patients described as "pleasantly senile". This patient could not participate in a discussion of his own condition or contribute to the decision-making process on the appropriate management of his acute illness. His basic disease, most likely Alzheimer's disease, and the acute abdomen that had been neglected for at least 72 hours, would categorize him as a hopelessly ill patient.

Is treatment of the hopelessly ill patient doomed to be futile?

The concept futility, in the presence of a serious illness, means different things to different people. What is medically unnecessary from the physician's standpoint, may still be important to the family, which often demands that "everything be done". Futile management was once described [2] as care that neither produces a demonstrable positive effect, nor changes the prognosis, nor improves the patient's quality of life. As Jacker and Pearlman pointed out [3], futile treatment is not only at odds with ethical medical traditions but also is a waste of the society's already scarce resources. The American Society of Critical Care Medicine [2] stated that "foregoing therapy should be discussed... when the quality of the patient's life is expected to be unacceptable". The American Thoracic Society provided a statement [4] in which the result of the futile treatment is defined as "survival in a state of permanent loss of conscience (that) may be generally regarded as having no value for such a patient". Finally, preliminary results of a prospective study conducted in the Department of Critical Care of the Soroka Medical Center, Beer Sheva, Israel [5] showed a significant decrease in ICU survival for a group of patients whose pre-admission functional capacity (as expressed by performance of minimal daily activity) was significantly limited.

The decision to withhold aggressive treatment is even more justified in cases in which patients have expressed their will before becoming ill. However, no living will can predict all possible circumstances relating to an acute episode such as a car accident, intra-abdominal emergencies, fulminant pneumonia or accidental poisoning. A patient may express, in writing, a wish not to be resuscitated under certain circumstances in which consciousness is no longer viable, but this living will lose its relevance in an uncooperative and incomprehensible patient whose health status has deteriorated acutely due to unforeseen illness.

The ethical directives of various religious groups are also not universally held, even concerning the most basic life support measures such as artificial nutrition and hydration. Gillick [6] quoted the National Conference of Catholic Bishops' position that withholding the provision of food and water by tube from patients with dementia is *not* immoral. However, Burke [7] opposed this position and demanded that food and water be provided under all circumstances. Kupfer and Tessler [8] stated that not providing "impediments of dying" applies only to medical interventions. In other words, the Orthodox Jewish judicial code permits withholding medical/surgical management in the case of advanced dementia.

What is the most appropriate level of care for our patient?

Wanzer et al. [1] described the following general levels of care:

1. Emergency resuscitation

2. Intensive care and advanced life support
3. General medical care (antibiotics, drugs, surgery, artificial hydration and nutrition, etc.)
4. General nursing care.

In the case previously described, it might be difficult to choose between general medical care and general nursing care. Let us presume the following credible scenario.

Suppose that it was decided, in our patient's case, to operate on him immediately. After rapid rehydration, a laparotomy was performed under general anesthesia and a perforated duodenal ulcer with a generalized purulent peritonitis was diagnosed. Still intubated and ventilated, the patient was transferred to the recovery room. He was unstable hemodynamically and oligo-anuric. The medical team (surgeon and anesthesiologist) decided to continue mechanical ventilation and fluid resuscitation. Ten hours later acute pulmonary edema (overloading? ARDS?) was diagnosed. A pulmonary artery catheter was inserted and the patient was transferred to the general ICU. He was sedated, received vasopressors, total parenteral nutrition and broad spectrum antibiotics and was monitored. The oliguria was reversed, but the patient could not be weaned from the mechanical ventilator. A tracheostomy was performed on the 12th postoperative day. The patient remained comatose until gram-negative septic shock terminated in cardiac arrest, which did not respond to usual resuscitation efforts.

How often do we see cases like this with similar tragic outcomes? Published data are scarce on this specific group of patients, but in our experience dismal outcomes are the rule. Recuperation is almost impossible in the presence of a critically acute medical condition and serious medical co-morbidity and in the absence of patient cooperation in this elderly age group.

In our case, despite the initial decision to restrict the level of care to general medical management (e.g. surgery and postoperative care), critical developments necessitated the patient's transfer to ICU and upgrading of the level of care. In actuality, the outcome of this case could have been predicted from the inception. Even under the best of circumstances, the outcome of treatment could only have been the reinstatement of the patient's pre-crisis status, i.e., the terminal stage of Alzheimer's disease.

Alzheimer's disease is the most common cause of dementia in Western countries. In the USA more than 50 billion dollars per year are spent on the care of 3-4 million individuals affected by this ailment [9]. The final stages of the disease involve wandering, total loss of judgement, reason and cognitive abilities. Patients become rigid, mute, incontinent and bedridden. Help is needed for the simplest tasks. An enormous physical, mental and emotional burden is placed on the family and the nursing staff. Death usually occurs as a result of infection, malnutrition or vital organ failure, on a background of total lack of comprehension or ability to cope with the realities of daily living. The issue at question is whether society can afford to support, financially and morally, heroic attempts to treat hopelessly ill patients in the terminal stage of their illness.

The physician's role in the decision-making process

Several problems are inherent in the decision-making process. Our medical training obliges us to sustain and prolong life. Family pressure is sometimes insurmountable. On the other hand, the provider of care (the insurance company) tries to minimize the cost of the medical management, citing its futility. Last, but not least, fear of legal liability often interferes with the physician's ability to make the best choice for the patient. Still, many are of the opinion that even in the framework of these unusual circumstances, physicians have the right to make value-based decisions as well as medical judgements [10]. Tomlinson and Brody [11] suggested that physicians should retain their moral authority and refuse to play "the vainly heroic part assigned to him or her". Sprung [12] commented that if a treatment is deemed futile not because it will fail technically but because the life saved is deemed not worthy of being saved, a moral and not a medical judgement has been made. This means that doctors have moral duties alongside their medical responsibilities.

However, physicians face not only the ethical implications of foregoing or withholding care and precipitating death. The medico-legal implications are no less critical to a physician's career. The danger of a legal suit is more in evidence in the United States than in Europe, but even the judicial authorities are coming to understand the fact that the doctor cannot always fight death and maintain life at all costs. In some Western European countries, such as France and Belgium, futile therapy is even condemned [13]. In these countries the difference between withholding treatment and euthanasia is evident.

So, in summarizing the various approaches to the medico-legal and ethical decisions concerning the hopelessly ill patient, one should remember Gillon's statement [14] that the "medico-moral decisions I take are those that concern norms and values, good or bad, right or wrong, and what ought to be or ought not to be done in the context of medical practice".

The role of the patient's family

When the patient cannot participate in the decision-making process, it is vital to define the role of the next of kin. In many cases there is no correlation between the patient's previous views and the wishes and position of the family as expressed when the non-competent patient's life is at stake. Nevertheless, the family plays a significant role in the process and it is critically important to learn to communicate with surrogates of hopelessly ill patients.

Ruark and Raffin [15] defined the difficulties of communicating with families: the stress that accompanies bearing bad news, the peak of the physician's emotional fatigue, the need for enough time to explain details and offer explanations. One must bear in mind that eventually, the family will have to decide on the patient's life. This is why the process of developing a special relationship with the family is so critical. Language barriers have to be averted. Simple vocabulary should be used. Requesting the family to summarize what has been said may be a good strategy for the elimination of misunderstandings. Crucial questions should be clearly answered, especially those relating to the patient's comfort, prediction of the timing of death, or the possibility of spending the remaining moments near the dear one's deathbed [16].

Epilogue

The alternate strategy for our patient would have been to avoid surgery. The family might accept the treating team's suggestion to avoid aggressive intervention. Opiates could have been judiciously prescribed for pain relief. The patient would have been transferred from the emergency department to a surgical ward. The patient's children could have been permitted to spend the remaining time with their parent. Death would most likely have been pronounced about 24 hours after admission.

We do think that this clinical approach entails significant medical and moral dilemmas. However, teaching, learning and practicing this humane approach is not effortless. It must be taught in medical school with the active participation of social workers and religious personalities. Similar cases should be discussed frequently with students and residents.

If these strategies are properly understood and implemented by the medical team and other caregivers, then "patients and families may again think of hospitals as sources of comfort to both the living and the dying, instead of places where one must too often struggle to exercise the right to determine one's own fate" [6].

References

1. Wanzer SH, Adelstein SJ, Cranford RE et al (1984) The physician's responsibility toward hopelessly ill patients. N Engl J Med 310:955-959
2. Swisher KN, Ayres SM (1992) Who decides when care is futile? Int Crit Care Digest 11: 59-64
3. Jacker NS, Pearlman RA (1992) Medical futility? Who decides? Arch Intern Med 152:1140-1144
4. American Thoracic Society (1991) Withholding and withdrawing life-sustaining therapy. Am Rev Respir Dis 144:726-731
5. Gurman GM, Roy-Shapira A, Weksler N et al (1999) Prior functional status as a predictor of outcome in critically ill patients. Crit Care Med 27:20
6. Gillick MR (2000) Rethinking the role of tube feeding in patients with advanced dementia. N Engl J Med 342:206-210
7. Burke WJ (2000) Letter to the editor. N Engl J Med 342:1755
8. Kupfer Y, Tessler S (2000) Letter to the editor. N Engl J Med 342:1755-1756
9. Bird TD (1998) Alzheimer's disease and other primary dementias. In: Fauci AS (ed) Harrison's principles of internal medicine. McGraw-Hill, New York, pp 2348-2356
10. Callahan D (1991) Medical futility, medical necessity. The-problem-without-a-name. Hastings Cent Rep 21:30-35
11. Tomlinson T, Brody H (1990) Futility and the ethics of resuscitation. JAMA 264:1267-1280
12. Sprung CL (1990) Changing attitudes and practices in foregoing life-sustaining treatments. JAMA 263:2211-2215
13. Vincent JL (1996) Ethical issues in critical care medicine. Int Care World 13:142-144
14. Gillon R (19985) An introduction to philosophical medical ethics: the Arthur case. BMJ 290:1117-1119
15. Ruark JE, Raffin TA (1998) Initiating and withdrawing life support. Principles and practice in adult medicine. N Engl J Med 318:25-30
16. Brody H, Campbell ML, Faber-Langendoen K, Ogle KS (1997) Withdrawing intensive life-sustaining treatment. Recommendations for compassionate clinical management. N Engl J Med 336:652-657

Pre- and Intraoperative Methods to Reduce Immediate Postoperative Pain

G.M. GURMAN

Anesthesiology has been described as a medical discipline that cares for patients during surgery and endeavors to prevent the pain caused by tissue injury occurring during surgery. However, although advances in pharmacology, pathophysiology, and anesthesia techniques have combined to make anesthesia a safe procedure for the vast majority of patients, many continue to experience significant postoperative pain.

Several explanations have been proposed for our perceived neglect of postoperative pain. One is the lack of knowledge pertaining to the effect of analgesic drugs in the immediate postoperative period. The recent introduction of remifentanil is a good example of the critical need to reduce the level of postoperative pain in the awakening patient, without resorting to long-acting opiates. Fear of the untoward secondary effects of analgesic drugs seems to strongly influence anesthesiologists' decisions relating to the reduction of postoperative pain. Another explanation is that the anesthesiologist who administered anesthesia during surgery often does not go to see patients in the postoperative period, so he/she is not always in a position to assess correctly the patient's need for analgesia during that time. Finally, some clinicians still think that postoperative pain is normal, a natural part of the surgical process, so little needs be done to alleviate this symptom.

However, postoperative pain, a unique entity, with specific physiological and clinical features, should receive appropriate attention and care. The pain is inflammatory in nature, as it is associated with peripheral tissue damage. Sometimes it is accompanied by a pathological phenomena, allodynia, that is characterized by a reduced stimulus threshold and consequent enhancement of pain. Hyperalgesia is another interesting factor that can even affect non-injured tissue, a phenomenon known as secondary hyperalgesia.

Two mechanisms are responsible for the development of inflammatory hyperalgesia, as seen following tissue damage. Hyperalgesia associated with peripheral sensitization is caused by a positive feedback loop that develops when peripheral C fiber terminals release neurotransmitters such as substance P. These neurotransmitters cause inflammatory cells to secrete mediators that in turn reactivate C fiber release of substance P.

Hyperalgesia associated with central sensitization can arise from the death of inhibitory spinal interneurons, the sprouting of new synapses between non-nociceptive neurons, or the sensitization of spinal dorsal horn neurons that receive C fiber input.

The clinical features of postoperative pain are equally important. Upper abdominal surgery produces respiratory complications related to the magnitude of untreated pain and explained by an increase in the abdominal muscle tone [1] and a decrease in diaphragmatic function [2]. Pain also produces cardiovascular effects, such as tachycardia, hypertension, increased cardiac work and stroke volume, mediated by the hypersecretion of catecholamines. Suprasegmental reflex responses result in increased sympathetic tone, producing water retention, hyperglycemia, and increased blood levels of free fatty acids and ketone bodies.

A number of factors may influence the intensity and duration of postoperative pain. Bonica [3] selected the most important of these as: the site and duration of surgery, the physiological makeup of the patient, preoperative preparation, complications related to surgery, anesthetic management before, during, and after surgery, and preoperative treatment aimed at eliminating painful stimuli prior to surgery. Thus, optimal management should cover both the pre- and postoperative periods in order to preempt the appearance of hyperalgesia, the most-important factor in the development of postoperative pain.

Preemptive analgesia

The concept

The term preemptive analgesia (PEA) was introduced for the first time by Wall [4]. It was defined by Woolf and Chong [5] as a therapeutic intervention, which is performed in advance of pain rather than in reaction to it, with the implication that analgesia given before the painful stimulus occurs prevents or reduces subsequent pain. It was established in the 1980s as a method of minimizing postoperative pain and was expected also to reduce the length of hospitalization and the rate of postoperative pulmonary complications, and to facilitate early mobilization of the patient.

McQuay [6] described the physiological basis of PEA as an effect of preventing or reducing the development of any "memory" of the pain stimulus in the nervous system. Preventing pain memory by preventing spinal cord excitability produced by noxious stimuli will lead to a lower level of postnoxious pain and a reduced need for postoperative analgesia.

Based on preliminary clinical studies [7], Wall [4] stated that relatively minor preoperative manipulations may stop the spinal cord from reaching a hyperexcitable state. He called this phenomena cord priming and defined it as prevention, or reduction to a minimum, of central neuron activation by the barrage of afferent activity evoked during surgery, by pre- or intraoperative treatment. It should be emphasized that Wall [4] extended the period of time in which pain can be prevented by including the intraoperative stage. We will refer below to some methods for reducing the degree of immediate postoperative pain by carefully watching the level of anesthesia administered.

The mechanisms of PEA are not well understood. One possible explanation for the interception of nociceptive input is blocking of n-methyl-d-aspartase (NMDA) receptors [8]. Figure 1 presents the "classical" concept of PEA, based on the hypothesis that it prevents or at least reduces the activity-dependent trigger at the spinal level. Based on this hypothetical concept, earlier studies tried to prove the existence of the PEA phenomena, but had contradictory results.

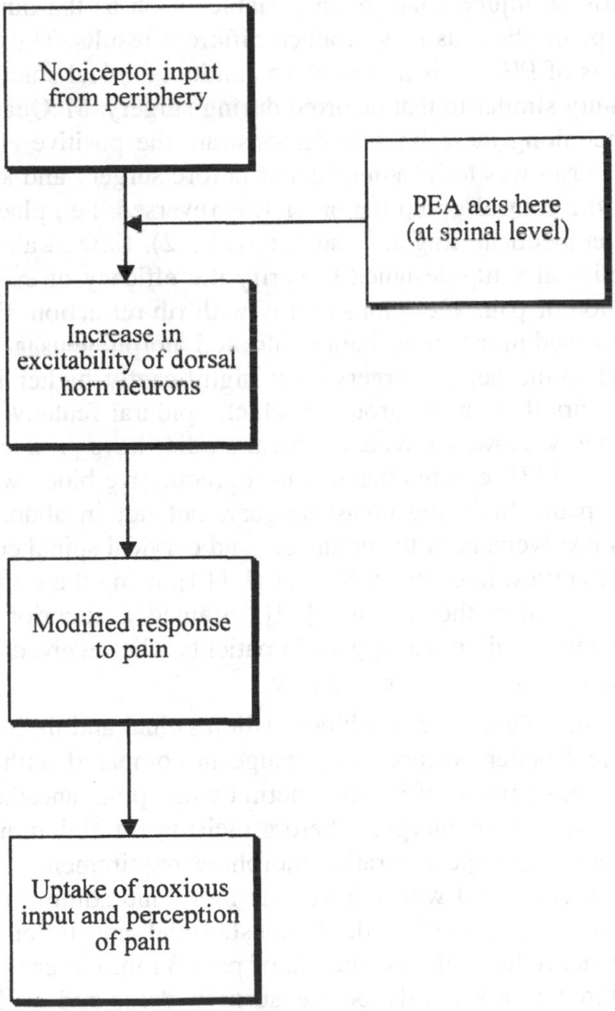

Fig. 1. Prevention of central sensitization by preemptive analgesia (*PEA*)

Experimental and clinical studies

Neurophysiological recordings performed by Dickenson and Sullivan [9, 10] in animals showed that intrathecal injection of opioids before formalin-induced tissue inflammation increased the degree of inhibition of C fibers by 70%, compared with the same opiate dose injected intrathecally after formalin. Similar results have been obtained by Coderre et al. [11], who showed that local infiltration before formalin-induced injury abolished the animal's behavioral response. The results could not be reproduced if the infiltration was performed following formalin-induced inflammation.

Obviously, results obtained from animal studies cannot be automatically translated into clinical guidelines. Experimental tissue inflammation is different from surgical tissue injury. Changes in variables such as the duration, amount and specific type of stimulus may produce different results. Thus, to assess the beneficial effects of PEA, it is important to conduct clinical studies using models of tissue injury similar to that incurred during surgery. McQuay [6] designed a clinical model along these lines to demonstrate the positive effects of PEA. The designated drug was to be administered before surgery and a placebo at its conclusion. In the control group the order was reversed, i.e., placebo given before and the therapeutical drug after surgery (Fig. 2). Katz et al. [12] used this strategy in a clinical setup designed to verify the efficacy of epidural fentanyl for the prevention of pain after thoracotomy with rib retraction. Epidural saline was the placebo used in the study. Pain-controlled morphine usage in the control group (epidural saline before surgery) was significantly higher in the first 24 postoperative hours than in the group in which epidural fentanyl was administered before surgery. However, recent clinical studies have produced conflicting results. Aida et al. [13] reported that epidural preemptive block was reliably effective in orthopedic limb and breast surgery, but not in abdominal surgery. They proposed involvement of the brainstem and cervical spinal cord via the vagus and phrenic nerves. In contrast, Katz et al. [14], using the same protocol for prevention of pain after thoracotomy [12], attained a superior postoperative analgesia after lower abdominal surgery in patients who received epidural bupivacaine injected half an hour before surgery.

Preoperative percutaneous nerve blocks (ilioinguinal and iliohypogastric) also appear to yield better postoperative analgesia compared with no preoperative block, in cases of repair of inguinal hernia with spinal anesthesia [15]. Administration of intravenous morphine before incision for abdominal hysterectomy significantly reduced postoperative morphine requirements in patient-controlled analgesia, compared with intravenous morphine administered when the peritoneum was being closed [16]. A nonsteroidal anti-inflammatory drug, such as diclofenac, reduced the magnitude of pain 30 min after tooth extraction when administered intravenously before surgery compared with intravenous fentanyl [17].

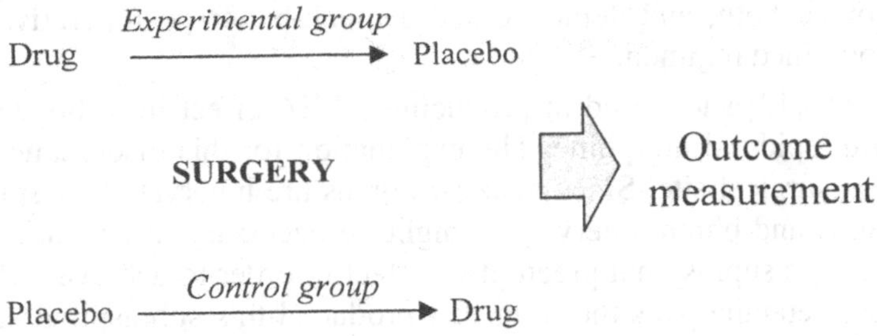

Fig. 2. McQuay design for demonstrating the effect of PEA [6]

Combination regimens, as reported by McQuay et al. [18], also produced superior results to single drug techniques. The median time to the first request for postoperative analgesia was 5 h in orthopedic surgery patients who received opiate premedication combined with a local anesthetic block for orthopedic procedures compared with 9 h in patients who received only opiate premedication. However, this result was not significantly different from the interval of 8 h to first request in patients who received only the local block.

Other studies have produced negative results. These include preoperative compared with postoperative administration of bupivacaine for tooth extraction [19], or alfentanil before or after skin incision for abdominal hysterectomy [20].

In the light of the conflicting results described in this short survey of published studies on the efficacy of PEA, it can be concluded that to date there is no compelling evidence that PEA works in the postoperative period.

Possible explanations for the failure of PEA in some of the studies have been proposed. Eisenach [21], in a recent editorial, hypothesized that tolerance to opioids can develop very quickly after their administration. The acute increase in dose requirements after large doses of opiates supports this possibility. Celerier et al. [22], in the same issue of *Anesthesiology*, suggested a different explanation for PEA failure, as it is used today in clinical practice. They were able to produce postopioid hyperalgesia for a relatively long period after fentanyl administration. The more fentanyl administered, the greater the hyperalgesic effect. Based on a rather well-known phenomena of prevention of morphine tolerance by treatment with NMDA receptor antagonists [23], the authors used ketamine pretreatment, at a dose devoid of analgesic effect, and succeeded in preventing the development of long-lasting hyperalgesia. Thus, it is possible that by blocking NMDA receptors, ketamine intercepts the nociceptive input and increases the threshold for noxious stimuli.

In support of this concept, Aida et al. [24] provided PEA with epidural morphine, low doses of intravenous ketamine (a bolus of 1 mg/kg prior to skin incision and continuous infusion up to 0.5 mg/kg per hour during surgery), or a combination of both, and demonstrated a much-better postoperative analgesia with the combined regimen.

Aida et al. [13] succeeded in producing a PEA effect in orthopedic surgery patients with epidural morphine. The explanation for this discrepancy might be the different surgical site. Since visceral organs are innervated by spinal nerves and the vagus and phrenic nerves, it might be necessary to produce not only a spinal but also a supraspinal preemptive effect in order to achieve a PEA effect. In this case, ketamine was the drug that produced this supraspinal suppression of nociceptive stimuli. This dual blockade proved to be essential in the most-recent study of Aida et al [24], possibly heralding a new stage in the development of PEA as an efficient preoperative method to reduce the magnitude of postoperative pain.

Does the level of general anesthesia affect immediate postoperative pain?

Bonica [3] stated that the type of anesthetic management affects the magnitude of postoperative pain. However, a review of the literature does not provide further practical details relating to this hypothesis. In an early study [25], designed to assess methods for preventing awareness during general anesthesia for cesarean section, we reported the effect on immediate postoperative pain of maintaining cortical electrical activity [measured by spectral edge frequency, a parameter of computerized electroencephalography (EEG)] within the "normal range". We monitored spectral edge frequency (SEF) in 55 patients during maintenance of general anesthesia. The anesthesiologist in charge had no view of the EEG screen, so his/her clinical decisions regarding anesthetic dosage were not influenced by the SEF parameter. According to the postoperative analysis of SEF behavior during general anesthesia, the patients were allocated to two groups that were found to be similar in age, weight, and anesthetic dosage. In the first group, SEF remained between 8 and 12 Hz for more than 50% of the maintenance time, and in the second group SEF was found to be higher than 12 Hz most of the time. The results showed that patients in whom SEF remained in the "normal range" most of the time expressed less-severe pain (on a visual analogue scale) and needed less analgesics in the recovery room.

A similar study was performed on patients who underwent laparoscopic cholecystectomy [26]. In this study, we found that, in toto, SEF remained for most of the procedure between 8 and 12 Hz, so once again we divided our patients into two groups that were similar in terms of demographic and anesthetic dosage variables. In this study we used a cut-off point of 80% to differentiate the groups. In the first group of 22 patients, SEF was kept in the normal range more than 80% of the time anesthesia was administered. In the second group of

18 patients, SEF was maintained within normal limits less than 80% of the time. The anesthesiologist in charge was not aware of the SEF data during the course of the operation. No statistically significant differences were observed between the two groups in the level of postoperative analgesia. However, patients in the group in which SEF was maintained between 8 and 12 Hz more than 80% of the time showed a clear tendency to require less analgesia in the recovery room ($p = 0.06$).

Finally, in a yet unpublished study we repeated the protocol during laparoscopic banding gastroplasty for morbidly obese patients (body mass index above 35). Patients whose SEF was maintained in the normal range for more than 80% complained less of pain in the recovery room and received less morphine during the 1st postoperative hour than the second group. In this study, we also found that in the group with a "normal" SEF more than 80% of the time, the end-tidal isoflurane concentration was significantly higher than in the second group. This finding raises the possibility that the level of general anesthesia can influence the magnitude of postoperative pain.

It seems that in the absence of other clinical or instrumental parameters to assess the depth of anesthesia, SEF or other EEG derivatives can serve as useful tools for maintenance of a constant level of electrical cortical activity during anesthesia. This, in turn, may have a positive effect on the level of immediate postoperative pain.

In conclusion, postoperative pain is still a neglected part of routine anesthetic care. In the absence of a validated method to reduce its magnitude, various techniques have been proposed to prevent, or at least to reduce, patient suffering immediately following surgery. Some of these techniques, such as patient-controlled analgesia, intravenously or epidurally, necessitate continuous supervision and a safe setting.

The concept of PEA now represents an attractive objective for anesthesiologists, adopting a logical physiological and pharmacological approach, based on the presumption that it is better to prevent postoperative pain rather than to treat it. However, the mechanism of action of the proposed techniques for PEA have not been sufficiently elucidated. Aida's "bipolar" approach is promising, but the doses of ketamine used for this purpose may not be completely free of secondary effects.

One of the declared aims of modern anesthesia is to keep patients as stable as possible during surgery. However, to date there is no suitable definition of depth of anesthesia, so it is difficult to establish parameters to assess patient stability. The results of our studies suggest that postoperative pain can be reduced by maintaining a stable level of cortical electrical activity during surgery.

The multidimensional approach to prevention of postoperative pain is consistent with the view expressed by Kissin [27], who pointed out the importance of differentiating between *preventive analgesia* and PEA, reserving the term PEA for the effect related to that part of preventive treatment that begins prior to surgery. This approach can lead to the development of new methods to prevent postoperative pain alongside the improvement of those already practised.

References

1. Duggan J, Drummond GB (1987) Activity of lower intercostal and abdominal muscle after upper abdominal surgery. Anesth Analg 66:852-855
2. Ford GT, Whitelaw WA, Rosenal TW et al (1983) Diaphragm function after upper abdominal surgery in humans. Am Rev Respir Dis 127:431-436
3. Bonica JJ (1983) Current status of postoperative pain therapy. In: Yokota T, Dubner R (eds) Current topics in pain research and therapy. Excerpta Medica, Amsterdam, p 169
4. Wall PD (1988) The prevention of postoperative pain. Pain 33:289-290
5. Woolf CJ, Chong MS (1993) Pre-emptive analgesia - treating postoperative pain by preventing the establishment of central sensitization. Anesth Analg 77:362-379
6. McQuay HJ (1992) Pre-emptive analgesia. Br J Anaesth 69:1-3
7. Woolf CJ (1983) Evidence for a central component of post-injury pain hypersensitivity. Nature 306:686-688
8. Cook AJ, Woolf CJ, Wall PD et al (1987) Dynamic receptive field plasticity in rat spinal cord dorsal horn following C-primary afferent input. Nature 325:151-153
9. Dickenson AH, Sullivan AF (1987) Subcutaneous formalin-induced activity of dorsal horn neurones in the rat: differential response to an intrathecal opiate administered pre or post formalin. Pain 30:349-360
10. Dickenson AH (1991) Recent advances in the physiology and pharmacology of pain: plasticity and its implications for clinical analgesia. J Psychopharmacol 5:342-351
11. Coderre TJ, Vaccarino AL, Melzack R (1990) Central nervous system plasticity in the tonic pain response to subcutaneous formalin injection. Brain Res 535:155-158
12. Katz J, Kavanagh BP, Sandler AN et al (1992) Preemptive analgesia. Clinical evidence of neuroplasticity contributing to postoperative pain. Anesthesiology 77:439-446
13. Aida S, Baba H, Yamakura T et al (1999) The effectiveness of preemptive analgesia varies according to the type of surgery: a randomized, double blind study. Anesth Analg 89:711-716
14. Katz J, Clairoux M, Kavanagh BP et al (1994) Pre-emptive lumbar epidural anaesthesia reduces postoperative pain and patient-controlled morphine consumption after lower abdominal surgery. Pain 59:395-403
15. Bugedo GJ, Carcamo CR, Mertens RA et al (1990) Preoperative percutaneous ilioinguinal and iliohypogastric nerve block with 0.5% bupivacaine for post-herniorrhaphy pain management in adults. Reg Anesth 15:130-133
16. Richmond CE, Bromley LM, Woolf CJ (1993) Preoperative morphine pre-empts postoperative pain. Lancet 342:73-75
17. Campbell W, Kendrick R, Patterson C (1990) Intravenous diclofenac sodium. Does its administration before operation suppress postoperative pain? Anaesthesia 45:763-766
18. McQuay HJ, Carroll D, Moore RA (1988) Postoperative orthopedic pain – the effect of opiate premedication and local anaesthetic blocks. Pain 33:291-295
19. Campbell WI, Kendrick RW, Fee JP (1998) Balanced pre-emptive analgesia: does it work? A double blind, controlled study in bilaterally symmetrical oral surgery. Br J Anaesth 81: 727-730
20. Wilson RJ, Leith S, Jackson IJ et al (1994) Pre-emptive analgesia from intravenous administration of opioids. No effect with alfentanil. Anaesthesia 49:591-593
21. Eisenach JC (2000) Preemptive hyperalgesia, not analgesia? Anesthesiology 92:308-309
22. Celerier E, Rivat C, Jun Y et al (2000) Long-lasting hyperalgesia induced by fentanyl in rats: preventive effect of ketamine. Anesthesiology 92:465-472

23. Trujillo KA, Akil H (1991) Inhibition of morphine tolerance and dependence by the NMDA receptor antagonist MK-801. Science 251:85-87
24. Aida S, Yamakura T, Baba H et al (2000) Preemptive analgesia by intravenous low-dose ketamine and epidural morphine in gastrectomy. Anesthesiology 92:1624-1630
25. Gurman GM (1994) Assessment of depth of general anesthesia. Observation on processed EEG and spectral edge frequency. Int J Clin Monit Comput 11:185-189
26. Gurman GM, Gruzman I, Porath A (2000) Cortical electrical activity during anesthesia and its influence on pain level after laparoscopic cholecystectomy. In: Jordan C, Vaughan DJ, Newton DE (eds) Memory and awareness in anesthesia. Imperial College Press, London, p 339
27. Kissin I (1994) Preemptive analgesia: terminology and clinical relevance. Anesth Analg 79:809-810

PAEDIATRICS

Strategies to Maintain Homeostasis in Major-Risk Pediatric Surgery

R. Pagni, S. Avenali, I. Laganà

The appropriate definition of the term "perioperative risk" is still debated, mostly as far as the pediatric field is concerned. Since the 1950s, many reports have been published on the statistical data regarding pediatric perioperative mortality, aiming to establish standard criteria on which mortality, surely related to the anesthesia, could be based and to compare data from different sources. None of these studies has achieved the purpose, mostly due to the presence of several variables: 1) age of the patient; 2) ASA group; 3) type of disease to be treated; 4) type of surgical treatment; 5) concomitant diseases; 6) emergency or elective surgery; 7) standard of perioperative care available.

The improved outcome of the surgical patient [1], as reported in the past 10 years, has been ascribed mainly to sophisticated diagnostic and monitoring equipment, and the use of more-reliable drug dispensers. At the same time clinicians and researchers have identified a wide range of clinical conditions, frequently associated with perioperative sequelae, suggesting for each specific or possible problem one or more therapeutic solutions. Moreover, a large part of the anesthesiological training involves the acquisition of knowledge and practical experience on how to protect the patient from the negative effects of surgical treatment and from drug toxicity, especially patients with pre-existing diseases.

Late in 1941, the American Society of Anesthesiology introduced a scale to grade the risk in each single patient, which allows clinicians to give detailed information to the patient, to provide documentation in case of debate, to standardize the outcome data, and to contain costs. Subsequently other grading scales for surgical procedures have been reported, but the ASA-PS scale remains a good basis for the realistic prediction of perioperative morbidity [2], especially if supported by an evaluation of the surgical risk, graded on the basis of the tissual trauma and of the alteration of the homeostasis induced by the surgical procedure.

In our opinion the assigning a patient to a certain risk group, without performing any procedure to improve his clinical condition prior to surgery is a worthless exercise. Our feeling is that all the specialists in the field should address their efforts towards the creation of guidelines, in order to standardize the perioperative approach to the high-risk patient. At present, there is still a great variability in management with relevant differences in the patients outcome. The main goals are the realization of specific algorithms of treatment for the different risk factors, using a standardized language, the realization of specific and precautionary procedure protocols, and the introduction of computerized systems allowing the detection of carefully checked clinical information.

Determinant factors for perioperative risk

Age

Besides the significant decrease in the perioperative mortality rate reported in all pediatric studies, what remains unchanged is the incidence of mortality, complications, and sequelae in children younger than 1 year when compared to older children [3]. This can be explained by the peculiar anato-physiological arrangement that characterizes the child in his 1st year of life, making him completely different from both the adult and the older child. This is particularly true of the premature infant or ex premature, before the 50th postconceptional week, due to the respiratory and/or neurological outcomes that he can exhibit, and to the high risk of postoperative apnea episodes. The most-significant differences between a child and an adult can be listed as below.

Cardiovascular function

During the postnatal period the systemic vascular resistance increases and, as a consequence, the work of the left heart increases too, with its thickness doubling in the first 3 months of life. The lung vascular resistance decreases, as the work of the right ventricle, whose muscular growth is slower than the left. The circulating volume of the baby is greater than the adult compared to body weight (70-80 ml/kg) but numerically poor, so even small losses can produce a significant reduction of the circulating volume. At birth the cardiac output is very high compared to the weight (300 ml/kg per min) and the cardiac index is slightly higher than the adult (from 3 to 4.5 l/min per m^2 body surface). As the heart rate is high and the injection volume low (1.5 ml/kg), the cardiac output is directly proportional to the heart rate and tachycardia is a good means of increasing the output at any pediatric age.

It is very important to remember that the autonomic nervous system is not mature during the first weeks of life, norepinephrine is scarce, the response of the heart to exogenous cathecolamines is reduced, with a mature parasympathetic innervation with related vagal hypertone and bradycardia.

Lung function

At birth the control of respiratory activity by the central nervous system is already effective, since both central and peripheral chemoreceptors are present.

The airways are anatomically structured, but show several differences with the adult airways (minor volume, reduced muscular structure, reduced cartilaginous support). This is the reason why they collapse more easily in the presence of edema, hypersecretion, and spasm. The small diameter of the airways is responsible for the relevant increase of resistance when the diameter itself becomes smaller. In childhood, the closure volume is higher than in adult life, so that the child develops atelectasis and airtrapping more easily. The larynx is placed forward, the epiglottis is rigid, and intubation can be more difficult. The trachea is relatively short and the canalization of the right bronchus is facilitated. Due to the higher compliance of the thoracic chest, the maintenance of the residual functional capacity (RFC) is harder, with an increased respiratory work, also increased by the ribs horizontalization, by the lack of diaphragmatic fibers resistant to stress, and by the poor tonicity, resistance, and co-ordination of the respiratory muscles.

Any event that induces abdominal distension or reduces the compliance of the abdominal wall (gastric distension, peritonitis) the diaphragm being the prevalent muscle, complicates the ventilation.

Metabolic control and electrolytes

Renal function is not completely mature at birth, both in the perfusion and glomerular filtration processes. The kidney of the newborn produces urine at a low concentration due to low urea availability, reduced length of the tubule, and reduced sensibility to antidiuretic hormone. Moreover, the ability to handle high sodium loads is poor, as is the capacity to absorb bicarbonate and excrete acids.

Forty percent of the body weight is made up of extracellular fluids, with a high water/electrolytes turnover. The body surface/weight ratio is higher in the child than in the adult, and this is the reason why the child has greater insensible losses that, in addition to an accelerated metabolism, make the water need per kilogram higher.

Gastrointestinal function

The newborn has a slow gastric motility and gastroesophageal reflux is always present. Liver function is not mature from the enzymatic point of view and the synthesis of clotting factors is reduced. The newborn easily develops jaundice due to a reduced bilirubin conjugation in a period when the bilirubin production is increased, with poor re-uptake, liver conjugation, and excretion.

Thermoregulation

The larger body surface determines a greater heat loss, which increases when the baby is kept a low temperature. The baby is not able to shiver, and to start the thermogenesis he has to secret noradrenaline to induce brown-fat breakdown. This kind of thermogenesis requires a significant oxygen consumption.

Immunological differences

The newborn is particularly prone to infections. Passive immunity is due to antibodies crossing from the mother during pregnancy, and this is the reason why the premature baby is less protected toward infections. The newborn has a low number of neutrophils, which are also partially immature; his bone marrow produces few phagocytes and cell-forming antibodies.

Nociperception

Although the myelinization of the nervous fibers is poor in the newborn, it has been reported that the spino-thalamo pathways achieve a complete myelinization by the 30th week of gestation and the thalamo-cortical pathways by the 37th week. Substance P and endogenous opioids are present in the fetus, while inhibitory pathways are lacking. Although in the newborn the evaluation of pain is difficult, it should be borne in mind that pain has both hormonal and metabolic negative effects.

Pharmacokinetics

The pharmacokinetics in the newborn are closely related to the body water content, with reduced ability to establish binding protein, with reduced renal excretion, and slowed drug metabolism.

Elective/emergency surgery

The clinical conditions requiring immediate surgical treatment in the pediatric age group are few (intestinal obstruction, strangulated hernia, funicular torsion). Besides the rare cases of acute massive bleeding, all pediatric surgical emergencies can be postponed to allow a satisfactory evaluation of the patient and stabilization of his clinical conditions, minimizing the perioperative risk.

Invasive aspects of the surgical procedures

The duration and nature of the tissue trauma during the operation quantitatively and qualitatively influence the intraoperative fluid loss. Moreover, surgical intervention, both for the position the patient has to maintain and for the region to be treated, can interfere with the physiological mechanisms that control vital functions.

Standard of perioperative treatment

While low-risk surgery can be carried out in every structure, always bearing in mind the peculiar features of the child, major-risk surgery needs structures, equipment, and operators exclusively dedicated to the care of the pediatric patient.

Treatment strategy

The strategy for reducing the perioperative risk in major-risk surgery is mainly based on three fundamental concepts: 1) careful preoperative clinical observation and preparation; 2) accurate choice of the appropriate anesthesiological technique and intraoperative treatment; 3) appropriate intensive postoperative care.

Preoperative evaluation and preparation

Preoperative evaluation [4, 5] starts with obtaining the family history (previous events related to anesthesia, sudden deaths, congenital defects), the personal history, with particular attention to the pregnancy and delivery (gestational age, weight, Apgar index, perinatal respiratory distress), allergies, previous anesthesia, past and present pathological history. Particular attention should be addressed to specific diseases, such as congenital heart defects, asthma, cystic fibrosis, myelomeningocele, sicklecell anemia, and epilepsy.

Congenital heart diseases should be separated into complicated and non-complicated. For the former, it is mandatory to collect information about surgical correction and the relevance of the residual cardiopathy, with particular attention to the alterations of systemic and pulmonary flow; it is also very important to achieve the best hemodynamic compensation, evaluating the previous pharmacological treatment. In patients with non-complicated congenital heart defects, the most-relevant aspect to consider is the prophylaxis of bacterial endocarditis, according to universal protocols [6].

In subjects suffering from asthma and cystic fibrosis, the basal treatment has to be ensured and, in selected cases, a short-term therapy with steroids must be planned; the surgery has to be postponed in cases of inflammation of the upper airways, since asthmatic patients have an increased intraoperative incidence of bronchospasm from 0.2-8‰ to 8.4-71‰.

Patients with previous meningocele have to be treated with latex-free protocol. When sickle-cell anemia is present it is mandatory to give high-fluid support in the preoperative stage, to maintain the level of HbS lower than 40%. In patients with epilepsy, therapeutic ranges of drugs should be checked, and treatment should be continued.

In oncology patients under chemotherapy, it is important to know the kind of drugs used, since many influence cardiopulmonary function; in patients with a tumor of the anterior mediastinum there is a significant risk during the induction of anesthesia. In children with intracranial hypertension the procedures for the protection of the central nervous system have to be carried out.

The clinical examination of all apparatus and systems, nutritional evaluation have to be considered. Particular attention must be addressed to all congenital and acquired conditions that can lead to difficult intubation. The laboratory investigations, which are few in routine pediatric surgery, will be more complex in major-risk surgery, to find possible alterations that should be corrected in the preoperative period.

Choice of the anesthesiological technique and intraoperative treatment

Pharmacological premedication has an important role in major-risk pediatric surgery with the following goals: 1) sedation to reduce emotional stress due to parental separation; 2) synergism with the anesthetic and analgesic drugs; 3) prevention of vagal reflexes; 4) control of secretions.

The large number of reports in the literature confirms that the best pre-anesthetic technique is still under debate, as far as drugs and means of administration. Vagolytic drugs have not lost their importance, especially in infants; sedative drugs, together with a proper psychological training, are important in the 1- to 10-year age group, which is characterized by anxiety during unusual events. The best ways of administration seem to be the oral and the nasal routes. In the presence of an abnormal gastroenteral motility or in case of an emergency, the parenteral route is preferred.

Drugs most commonly used are:

1. Midazolam: p.o. 1 mg/kg (maximum 10 mg) nasal/sublingual 0.4 mg/kg
2. Ketamine: p.o. 4 mg/kg – i.m. 3 mg/kg
3. Droperidole: i.m. 0.3 mg/kg
4. Midazolam plus ketamine
5. Atropine: i.m. 10 g/kg
6. Ranitidine: p.o. 2.5 mg/kg – i.v. 2 mg/kg
7. Metoclopramide: p.o. or i.v. 0.2 mg/kg

The choice of anesthesiological method in major-risk surgery can be general anesthesia, with inhalation or parenteral administration, loco-regional anesthesia, or both. The choice has to be based on the age of the patient, on the pathology to be treated, and on associated diseases. Any anesthesiological technique has to ensure blocking of the body reaction toward the operation. It is common knowledge that surgical stress is responsible for a reaction bearing several neurohumoral phenomena, mediated by nociceptive reflexes, through nervous pathways or direct tissue trauma. If this reaction escapes control, it can lead to: 1) hyperdynamic cardiovascular activity; 2) hypercoagulability; 3) delayed wound healing; 4) depression of immunocompetence (particularly relevant in oncological surgery, in relation to the possible metastatic diffusion with a lack of immune surveillance).

Inhalation anesthetics can also be utilized in the newborn, since the MAC is a relative concept, and volatile anesthetics have to be tried in a dose-response curve, with the aim of velocity of induction but, especially, the prevention of cardiovascular depression. The newborn exhibits a higher alveolar ventilation and lower RFC than the adult, which is the basis of a faster wash-in and wash-out of the anesthetic. The smaller muscular volume endows the noble parenchyma with a higher flow. Accordingly, the alveolar pressure of the volatile agent increases faster in the child and the brain and heart become saturated more rapidly. A good practice is to administer a vagolytic premedication, the fluid volume should be maintained normal and the concentration of the anesthetic should be reduced when in controlled ventilation.

Sevorane is the inhalation anesthetic of choice in pediatrics due to the absence of evoked reflexes of upper airways during induction, and to its low blood and tissue solubility and its cardiovascular stability.

Intravenous anesthesia, preferred by the authors, offers the advantage of avoiding the upper airways reflexes and the cardiovascular depression, which can take place during the inhalation induction. The technique is rapid and has a good acceptance by the patient, mostly when the stress due to the venous puncture is under control. Several drugs can be used for the induction (midazolam, propofol); the morphine-like drugs are better utilized for the maintenance, due to the cardiocirculatory stability they confer. To gain advantage from these positive effects, it is important that their dosage is related to the hepatic clearance of the patient. Airways control is obtained by intubation, following muscle relaxant agent, paying attention to the proper size of the tracheal tube, to avoid postextubation reactions. A flowchart is mandatory to face a possible difficult intubation, together with all the instrumentation needed [7]. Muscle relaxants can also be used in the newborn, bearing in mind the following: 1) the higher water volume of the baby determines a higher distribution volume, with a lower amount of muscle relaxant reaching the neuromuscular junction; 2) the glomerular filtration rate is lower and the muscle relaxant action time is prolonged; 3) the neuromuscular junction immaturity influences the variability of the response to the muscle relaxant.

Depolarizing muscle relaxants do not enjoy great favor in pediatric anesthesiology due to a supposed activation of brady-arrhythmias and an increase of intraocular and endocranial pressure. Short, mean, and long-term depolarizing muscle relaxants are all in use. Locoregional anesthesia alone, or associated with general anesthesia, has the advantage of ensuring a good analgesia, both during and after surgery, and avoiding tracheal intubation in at-risk subjects that were premature. The availability of needles and catheters purposely created for pediatric patients, of local anesthetics with low toxicity, and of drugs enhancing the anesthetic block has widened the utilization of this technique.

Monitoring is the basis of the perioperative strategy in major-risk surgery [8]. Once the anesthesia is induced, in addition to the peripherally inserted catheter, a central venous catheter [9] is positioned, which allows: 1) rapid infusion of fluids, plasma-expanders, and blood; 2) safe administration of osmotic and inotropic agents and potassium; 3) detection of central venous pressure. The central vein will be chosen on the bases of surgical field.

An arterial catheter will allow the continuous monitoring of the systemic pressure and gas analysis. The urinary catheter will permit us to calculate the diuresis every hour, for fluid balance. Cardiovascular monitoring is achieved by electrocardiographic (ECG) tracing. The central venous and arterial catheters, through a PICCO device, allow less-invasive monitoring of cardiac output, index and systemic resistance, than the Swan-Ganz catheter. The monitoring of respiratory function is achieved by pulse oximetry, capnometry, end-tidal values of volatile anesthetics, and gas analysis data. The monitoring of body temperature is particularly important in the newborn, both to carry out all procedures to reduce the heat waste and to control the phase of re-heating, after operations requiring hypothermia. The monitoring of neuromuscular block is useful to avoid overdosing and to establish the proper extubation time. EEG monitoring, with or without non-invasive transcutaneous cerebral saturation and brainstem potentials, is used in surgical procedures, potentially damaging the brain, or in patients suffering from head trauma. Monitoring is completed by the biochemical monitoring of hemoglobin, glycemia, lactate, electrolytes, and clotting cascade.

The timely monitoring of these parameters and the careful evaluation of intraoperative losses are fundamental guides for pharmacological and fluid support, always taking in account the pathophysiology of the main and associated diseases.

Intraoperative fluids, during the 1st hour are administered at 25 ml/kg or 15 ml/kg, accordingly to age (age < or > 4 years), to replace the losses due to preoperative fasting; in the following hours the fluid delivery is 4 ml/kg of maintenance, plus 6 ml/kg to replace the losses due to tissue trauma and exposure. We have to consider that a body temperature increase of 1°C causes losses of 10%.

In the evaluation of hypovolemia, it is important to point out that clinical signs (skin, ocular globes, fontanel) often precede the alterations of blood pressure and heart rate, which can remain unchanged even for losses higher than 10%. As far as losses are concerned, it is necessary to quantify them both quantitatively and qualitatively. Vomit and cellular trauma are responsible of isotonic losses, while diarrhea and sweating give hypotonic losses. This difference influences the choice of replacement fluids, since the child has a higher volume of extracellular water, and electrolyte (especially sodium) and water turnover is higher. If isosmotic losses are replaced with hypotonic solutions, the kidney will excrete the extra water, losing sodium too. If 5% glucose is utilized there could be an osmotic diuresis with further water and sodium depletion. The possible outcome of both situations is brain edema, and, in this case, the drug of choice is 6% sodium bicarbonate (2 ml/kg) followed by administration of balanced electrolytic solution. When fluid demand is higher than 30 ml/kg per hour the utilization of plasma expanders has to be considered, paying attention to their molecular weight and the kidney ability to excrete them. The majority of authors agree that 5% protein solutions are most suitable in pediatrics. Great attention is, at the present time, addressed to blood transfusion, due to the risk of infectious diseases and to immunosuppression-related pathologies. Acute hemoglobin values ranging from 7 to 10 g/dl give time for clinical evaluation, based on arterial oxygenation, venous pO_2, systemic pressure, cardiac output, and lactate values. If hemoglobin is less than 7 g/dl (normally corresponding to losses higher than 20% of total circulating blood), replacement therapy is required, preferably using frozen red cells (lower incidence of viral infection transmission and immune adverse reactions, better preservation of 2,3-diphosphoglycerate, lower potassium and citrate content). Fast transfusions put the child at risk of hyperkalemia and hypocalcemia, hence these electrolytes have to be monitored together with coagulation parameters. Major-risk surgery is often characterized by the presence of cardiorespiratory distress, which is successfully treatable with several drugs [11]. The aim is to obtain an improvement in oxygen delivery, through the increase of the cardiac index and the vascular tone.

Nevertheless, drugs in use have side effects, which is why knowledge of their working process and proper dosage is necessary, in addition to careful monitoring of the efficacy and toxicity, since the pharmacokinetics and the cellular response varies with age, in pediatric patients. Dobutamine is used to treat the low cardiac syndrome with normal or high vascular resistance; since it stimulates β-receptors without the need for endogenous epinephrine supply, it is more effective than dopamine in infants. Its utilization is instead contraindicated in hyperdynamic shock with high cardiac output and low resistance. Dopamine is used in all pediatric age groups as inotropic and vasopressor, in case of reduced heart contractility with poor peripheral perfusion, without relevant hypotension. In case of altered myocardial function, with very severe hypotension epinephrine and norepinphrine are to be preferred.

Isoproterenol has a restricted use due to its enhancement of tachycardia. Pediatric data are scarce on the use of phosphodiesterase inhibitors, however they can find use postcardiosurgery. Their efficacy in septic shock has not been proved yet.

Vasodilatator drugs are used in pediatrics, even though the potential risk of increasing the intrapulmonary shunt in patients with significant alveolar damage has to be taken into account. Nitric oxide is used in the surgical correction of congenital diseases that determine pulmonary hypertension. Lastly it is important to underline the relevance of good analgesic intra-operative treatment to control stress-induced reactions.

Postoperative intensive care

Postoperative intensive care represents the direct continuation of the intra-operative treatment, both as far as monitoring and therapy are concerned. A very important aspect is the choice of timing for extubation, which has to take place when results of gas analysis are favorable, but in the presence of cardiocirculatory stability, and in the absence of fever, anemia, and abdominal distension.

In the child the so-called deep extubation is always preferred; it means a complete elimination of muscle relaxant agent, in the presence of analgesia and sedation to prevent the child from developing laryngospasm secondary to the extubation. The antibiotic therapy is important for the prevention of infections, both due to surgery and invasive monitoring; nevertheless, we believe that good nutrition is fundamental to guarantee immunocompetence and vital for the surgical wounds rapid healing. The choice between enteral or parenteral nutrition relies on the state of the intestine, on the presence of prior malnutrition, and on the need to continue mechanical ventilation.

The use of uncuffed tubes exposes the child to the risk of silent aspiration, and the sedation utilized for the adaptation to the ventilator slows down the gastric transit; abdominal distension makes weaning more difficult. Postoperative analgesia is very important to achieve hemodynamic stability and the recovery of good respiratory function.

Conclusions

The strategy to improve the safety and outcome of pediatric patients undergoing major-risk surgery finds its basis in the creation of guidelines based on knowledge of the anatomy and physiology of the child in every age group, and the availability of structures, technologies, and medical equipment exclusively dedicated to pediatric patients. Finally, in our opinion, a very important strategic element is a deep love and devotion to that unique and not inimitable creature that is the child.

References

1. Motoyama EK (1996) Safety and outcome in paediatric anaesthesia. In: Motoyama EK, Davis PJ (eds) Smith's anesthesia for infants and children. 6th edn. Mosby, Philadelphia, pp 897-907
2. Cohen MM, Cameron CB, Duncan PG (1990) Paediatric anaesthesia morbidity and mortality in the perioperative period. Anesth Analg 70:160-167
3. Morray JP, Geiduschek JM, Caplan RA et al (1993) A comparison of paediatric and adult anaesthesia closed malpractice claims. Anesthesiology 78:461-467
4. CAS guidelines for preoperative assessments - Canadian Anaesthesia Society, www.cas.ca/public
5. Pasternak RL (1996) Preoperative evaluation – a systematic approach. Annual ASA refresher course lecture
6. AHA (1990) Endocarditis prophylaxis guidelines. JAMA 264:22
7. Benumof JL (1991) Management of the difficult adult airway. Anesthesiology 75:1087-1110
8. American Society of Anaesthesiologist's Task Force on Management of the Difficult Airway (1993) Practice guidelines for the management of the difficult airway. Anesthesiology 78:597-602
9. American Academy of Paediatrics, Committee on Drugs (1992) Guidelines for monitoring and management of paediatric patients during and after sedation for diagnostic and therapeutic procedures. Pediatrics 89:1110-1115
10. Chameides L, Hazinski MF (1997) Vascular access. In: Elk Grove Village IL (ed) Paediatric advanced life support. American Heart Association/American Academy of Paediatrics, Dallas, Texas
11. Berry FA (1992) Perioperative fluid management for paediatric patients. Annual ASA refresher course lecture
12. Chameides L, Hazinski MF (1997) Fluid therapy and medications. In: Elk Grove Village IL (ed) Paediatric advanced life support. American Heart Association/American Academy of Paediatrics, Dallas, Texas

Useful Guide for Management of Postoperative Pain

P. Busoni

Children fear the prospect of severe pain following surgery. In designating a comprehensive plan for postoperative analgesia, the objectives need to be clearly defined for each patient. Decisions regarding postoperative pain need to be made with a complete understanding of the surgical procedure and expected convalescence. Postoperative pain management needs to promote recovery rather than delay a return to normal function. The surgical procedure and expected postoperative course guide the initial design of a postoperative analgesia plan. Pain management needs to be tailored to the location, extent, and invasiveness of the surgical procedure, as well as the expected severity of the postoperative pain. The effects of depression, anxiety, and fear contribute to the child's pain in the postoperative period. Also the postoperative environment plays a vital role in the pain management intervention.

After these general considerations on postoperative pain in children a question arises: is a guide for management of postoperative pain useful? As with any therapy, safety and effectiveness increase as physicians and nurses repeatedly employ an analgesic medication or technique. New medications and techniques occasionally offer important theoretical and practical advantages over older medications and techniques; yet, inexperience often dilutes these advantages. Timing of redosing, managing side effects, adjusting the size of a medication dose, or manipulating a new technique requires both knowledge and experience. Caretakers require education and close supervision prior to the introduction of new medications and techniques; without the appropriate understanding and knowledge of the operation and the analgesic intervention, effective pain management often fails to achieve appreciable results. Therefore guidelines are useful, but they must be personalized, i.e., tailored not only to the location, extent, and invasiveness of the surgical procedure, but also to the particular environment, the experience and the habits of caretakers. A guide useful for a particular surgical intervention could be inadequate for a different one. However, in general postoperative pain management techniques can be assigned to five broad areas: analgesia induced by opioids, local anesthetics, mechanical devices, anti-inflammatory agents, and psychological interventions.

Measures of pain

It is impossible to manage any clinical problem without having a measure on which to base treatment [1]. Measurement of pain is important, but it is also important to measure the sometimes associated sedation. Pain and sedation measurement scales should always be available in any surgical setting. Pain in children presents particular problems in measurement due to the wide age range, from the neonatal period to the adolescent. Many pain scales are described in the medical literature. A discussion on this issue is far beyond the scope of this manuscript, and the reader is referred to classic textbook about pediatric pain. However, for clinical purposes a simple four-point scale for pain (calm and tranquil, pain on movement, pain at rest, excruciating pain) and a three-point scale for sedation (awake, drowsy but arousable, not arousable) is sufficient. Nurses should measure pain and sedation every hour in the immediate postoperative period.

Particular problems in neonates

In neonates, despite the advances in pain assessment and management, prevention and treatment of unnecessary pain (e.g., postoperative pain) remain limited. According to the American Academy of Pediatrics, several important concepts must be recognized to provide adequate pain management for the preterm and term neonate [2]:

- neuroanatomical components and the neuroendocrine system are sufficiently developed to allow transmission of painful stimuli;
- exposure to prolonged or severe pain may increase neonatal morbidity;
- infants who have experienced pain during the neonatal period respond differently to subsequent painful events;
- severity of pain and effects of analgesia can be assessed in the neonate;
- neonates are not easily comforted when analgesia is needed;
- a lack of behavioral responses (including crying and movement) does not necessarily indicate a lack of pain.

It is therefore important to treat, or better to prevent, any acute pain during and after surgery or a painful procedure. Regional anesthesia, local infiltration anesthesia, opioids, and nonsteroidal anti-inflammatory drugs should be used in the neonate as in children and adults.

Treatment of pain

Pain can be treated by oral, parenteral, or regional analgesic. The operative anesthetic plan should always include a strategy for postoperative analgesia.

Frequently the postoperative analgesia is initiated during surgery. Local infiltration of the surgical wound is mandatory in any case, even when regional anesthesia has been used. Regional anesthesia is best administered under light general anesthesia, either before or after the surgical procedure. Intravenous narcotics may be given as a single dose early during surgery or in divided doses toward the end of surgery, to ensure that the patient wakes with analgesia present. Surgical procedures that are unlikely to cause postoperative pain may not require any intraoperative analgesic, but there should be a plan for careful assessment and treatment of pain postoperatively should it occur.

Pediatric outpatient

The pediatric outpatient has analgesic needs which are different from those of the pediatric inpatient. Outpatient procedures should not involve significant postoperative pain. Children need to eat, drink, urinate, and ambulate fairly soon after anesthesia for outpatient procedures. Regional analgesia is particularly useful in the outpatient setting because it allows normal mental and motor functioning. Opioids are avoided to minimize postoperative vomiting. Any further analgesia must be given orally or rectally by the parents at home.

Oral analgesic

Paracetamol can be used to treat mild postoperative pain. It is available in liquid and tablet preparations to suit children of various ages. Most parents and children are familiar with it. Aspirin should be avoided for treatment of postoperative pain in children because of bleeding caused by its antiplatelet activity and because of the association with Reye's syndrome. Other nonsteroidal anti-inflammatory drugs have not been widely used in children and are generally not indicated in the postoperative setting. The combination of paracetamol and codeine is useful for moderate pain. It is better administered via the rectal route, since codeine can cause gastrointestinal upset and vomiting.

Parenteral analgesia

Intravenous narcotic administration is the commonest means of providing relief of postoperative pain for children. Intramuscular injection of narcotic is more painful and is usually avoided. It is best to treat pain swiftly with repeated intravenous boluses of morphine sulfate in a dose of 0.05 - 0.10 mg/kg or fentanyl in a dose of 1 - 2 μg/kg. Multiple small doses of narcotics that are titrated to relieve pain do not depress respiration. Patient-controlled analgesia (PCA) is an excellent method of administering narcotics provided the children can understand the simple statement "press the button to kill the pain". Fentanyl may offer some advantage over morphine because of its rapid onset of analgesia, but morphine has the advantage of longer-lasting analgesia [3]. Concomitant use of opioids and benzodiazepines necessitates a decrease in the total dose of opioid and benzodiazepine. However, nonopioid medications should not be used in place of opioids, because they do not possess analgesic properties. Moreover, the risk of respiratory depression may be additive or synergistic. Meperidine is not recommended for prolonged administration owing to the possibility of accumulation of toxic metabolites capable of causing seizures [4].

When opioid or ions, such as benzodiazepines, are administered for a prolonged period, physical dependence and tolerance may develop, thus increasing the opioid or sedative requirements to maintain patient comfort [5]. When stress or pain medications are no longer deemed necessary, slow weaning of the patient from opioids and other sedatives over a long period may be required. Such weaning may be a gradual reduction in daily drug dosage, with frequent reassessment to ensure the patient is free of pain and withdrawal symptoms, or it may be a change to longer-acting oral medications, such as methadone, that can be tapered [6, 7].

Regional anesthesia

Sophisticated techniques of regional anesthesia administration are being used in children. Children are excellent candidates for regional procedures because their anatomy is rarely altered by bony abnormalities of the spine or by obesity. In addition, children whose parasympathetic tone is greater than their sympathetic tone rarely have hemodynamic instability following the sympathetic block induced by some forms of regional anesthesia. All regional blocks can be administered under general anesthesia, before or after surgery, so that co-operation of the child is unnecessary. Bupivacaine 0.25% without adrenaline provides 4 - 8 h of sensory block postoperatively without motor block or urinary retention. For thoracic or abdominal surgery, an indwelling lumbar epidural catheter for continuous infusion or boluses of narcotics or bupivacaine provides excellent analgesia [8]. Regional analgesia has the advantage over intravenous or oral narcotics of causing less nausea and vomiting.

Table 1. PCA-NCA infusion (patient-controlled analgesia - nurse-controlled analgesia) – morphine

Initial bolus	Dose PCA/NCA	Baseline infusion[a]	Dosage max/h	Lockout
0.02 mg/kg[b]	0.02 mg/kg	0.02 mg/kg per hour	0.1 mg/kg	3-5 min

[a] Baseline infusion should be used when the child is sleepy or when NCA is used
[b] 10 minutes increments until satisfactory pain control is achieved

Table 2. EPCA (epidural patient-controlled analgesia) – morphine[a]

Dose EPCA	Baseline infusion	Lockout
1.25 µg/kg	5 µg/kg per hour	15 min

[a] Bellamy CD, McDonnel FJ, Kolclough GW et al (1990) Anesth Analg 70:S19

Table 3. Rectus sheet continuous infusion

Anesthetic drug	% concentration	Infusion rate
Bupivacaine	0.25	0.1 mg/kg per hour

[a] Cornish P, Anderson B, Chambers C (1993) Pediatr Anesth 3:191-193

Table 4. Central blocks: Prolonged infusion (mg/kg per hour)

	Infants and children	Newborns
Lidocaine	1.5-2	1
Bupivacaine	0.4	0.2

References

1. Finley GA, McGrath PJ (1998) Introduction: the roles of measurement in pain management and research. In: Finley GA, McGrath PJ (eds) Measurement of pain in infants and children. IASP Press, Seattle, pp 1-4
2. American Academy of Pediatrics (2000) Prevention and management of pain and stress in the neonate. Pediatrics 105:454-461
3. Hug CC (1984) Pharmacokinetics and dynamics of narcotic analgesics. In: Prys-Roberts C, Hug CC Ir (eds) Pharmacokinetics of anaesthesia. Blackwell Scientific Publications, Oxford, p 199
4. Armstrong PJ, Bersten A (1986) Normeperidine toxicity. Anesth Analg 65:536-538
5. Bhatt-Mehta V (1996) Current guidelines for the treatment of acute pain in children. Drugs 51:760-776
6. Van Engelen BG, Gimbrere JS, Booy LH (1993) Benzodiazepine withdrawal reaction in two children following discontinuation of sedation with midazolam. Ann Pharmacother 27:579-581
7. Yaster M, Kost-Byerley S, Berde C et al (1996) The management of opioid and benzodiazepines dependence in infants, children and adolescents. Pediatrics 98:135-140
8. Dalens B, Tanguy A, Haberer J (1986) Lumbar epidural anesthesia for operative and postoperative pain relief in infants and young children. Anesth Analg 65:1069-1074

Recommendations on Paediatric Basic Life Support

A. SARTI

"...When Elisha reached the house, there was the boy lying dead on his couch. He went in, shut the door on the two of them and prayed to the Lord. Then he got on the bed and lay upon the boy, mouth to mouth, eyes to eyes, hands to hands. As he stretched himself out upon him, the boy's body grew warm. Elisha turned away and walked back and forth in the room and then got onto the bed and stretched out upon him once more. The boy sneezed seven times and opened his eyes...".

The Bible, 2 Kings 4:32-36

Unlike adult patients, infants and children usually suffer cardiac arrest as the terminal event in conditions resulting in progressive respiratory and circulatory failure. The cessation of respiratory efforts almost always precedes bradycardia and cessation of spontaneous circulation. The haemodynamic deterioration occurs in a context of arterial hypoxemia, myocardial ischaemia and profound acidosis (Fig. 1). On the contrary, the most frequent adult CPR recipient is an otherwise healthy individual with a primary ventricular dysrhythmia and there is normal oxygenation and circulation immediately prior to cardiac arrest. In paediatrics, respiratory and circulatory failure, resulting from a variety of medical diseases or injuries, leads to inadequate gas exchange with progressive hypoxemia, hypercarbia and acidosis and culminates in asystolic cardiac arrest. The commonest underlying cause of cardiac arrest in children is respiratory failure. The cessation of circulation is preceded by respiratory distress and may result from lung or airway diseases, such as pneumonia, pneumothorax, asthma, bronchiolitis, croup, epiglottis and thoracic trauma. Cardiac arrest preceded by respiratory depression is caused by prolonged convulsions, central nervous system trauma, raised in-

Abbreviations

Infant: a child in the first year of life
Child: from the end of the first year to 8 years of age
CPR: cardiopulmonary resuscitation
AHA: American Heart Association
ERC: European Resuscitation Council

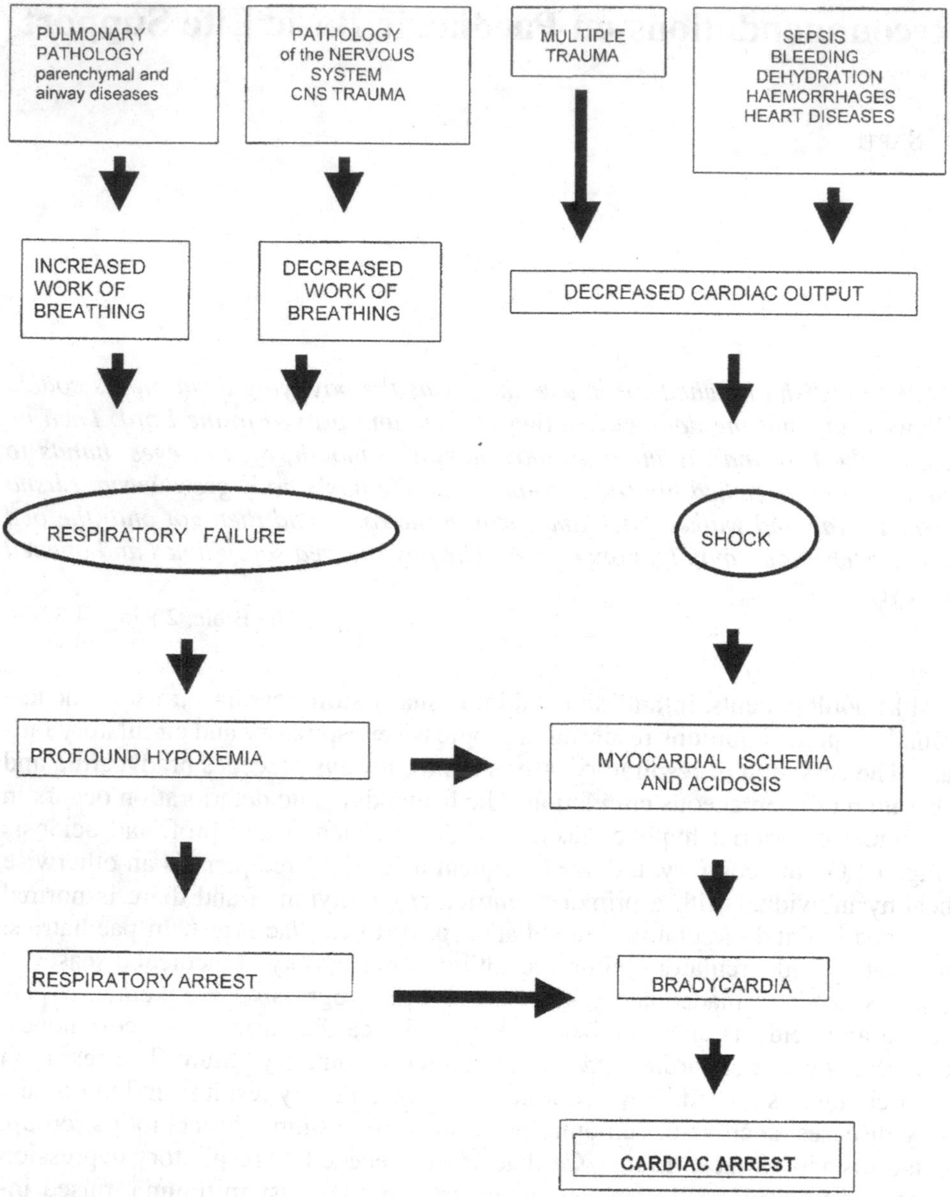

Fig. 1. Progression of acute pathology in paediatrics

tracranial pressure, neuromuscular pathology and poisoning. The second main pathway to cardiac arrest in children is through circulatory shock, caused most frequently by sepsis, haemorrhages, traumatic blood loss and fluid loss brought about by vomiting and/or diarrhoea (Fig. 1) [1, 2]. Cardiac arrest does not occur in paediatrics until the child's physiologic reserves are exhausted. Primary sudden cardiac arrest is very rare. Ventricular fibrillation has always been reported in less than 10% of children with pulseless arrest [1-3]. A recent study confirms that asystole was the most common presenting rhythm (83%), pulseless electric activity occurred in 12% and ventricular fibrillation in 4% [4]. Ventricular fibrillation and pump failure are more likely in children with complex congenital heart diseases and seen most frequently in the paediatric intensive care ward of a cardiothoracic unit. Neonates are less likely to develop ventricular tachyarrhythmias than older children, probably because of insufficient cardiac mass and different balance between α and β adrenergic receptors [5].

Overall, the outcome from cardiac arrest in children is worse than the outcome of cardiac arrest in adults [1, 2]. However, survival rate approaches 50% after resuscitation in children with respiratory arrest alone [6]. Outcome of paediatric cardiac arrest is usually poor, but it is difficult to be accurate since most studies are retrospective [5]. Moreover, different populations and locations of arrest are studied. Intuitively, outcome may be different if the cessation of circulation occurs out of hospital, in emergency rooms, or in hospitals, either in general wards or in intensive care units. In some studies, survival is less than 10% and the majority of those who are resuscitated suffer neurologic damage [5]. The survival rate for paediatric patients with out-of-hospital cardiac arrest is 8.4%, compared with 24% for paediatric inpatients, according to a recent review [7]. In the out-of-hospital setting, the outcome depends on several factors, including the provision of by-stander cardiopulmonary resuscitation, prompt activation of the emergency system, the presenting rhythm, and time to definitive treatment [8]. Children with cardiac arrest who were witnessed had a 19% survival rate, and those that received bystander resuscitation had an improved survival of 26%. Unfortunately, only 30% of paediatric patients with witnessed arrest received by-stander cardiopulmonary resuscitation [7]. Thus, neurologically intact survival from cardiac arrest in the paediatric age group depends on very early intervention. According to a recent world's literature review [7], the overall hospital discharge for pulseless paediatric patients is 13%, with 62% of the survivors having good neurologic outcome. A poor outcome is associated with traumatic arrest (4%) and even worse outcome (0.2%) is associated with sudden infant death syndrome [7, 9]. The presenting rhythm is important since the survival rate is 30% for ventricular fibrillation [10]. The poor outcome from many cardiac arrests can be understood by the appreciation of the severity and the duration of tissue hypoxemia and/or ischaemia which has to occur before the child's previously healthy heart succumbs. Respiratory arrest alone has a significantly better outcome because hypoxemia is not sufficiently maintained for the heart to stop. Thus, cardiac arrest is not sudden in paediatrics and can be anticipated in most cases. The progressive nature of acute pathology of infants and children offers a unique chance to prevent cardiac arrest by step by step intervention for interrupting the progression toward respiratory arrest and final haemodynamic deterioration (Fig. 1) [11]. Early diagnosis and aggressive treatment of respiratory and circulatory insufficiencies are the key to improving intact survival of seriously ill children. The paediatrician practitioner should be familiar with the use of emergency drugs and in a position to perform basic and at least some advanced techniques of life support. Institutional guidelines for paediatric emergencies must be fixed in every hospital and checked periodically. When at last, despite previous treatment, respiratory efforts and later circulation cease, outcome depends on prompt, adequate resuscitation. The most important action and prerequisites to any other forms of treatment in paediatric resuscitation are establishing a clear airway and ventilation. It should be emphasized that resuscitation must begin immediately, without awaiting the arrival of equipment, especially for in-hospital emergencies. Since respiratory or cardiac arrest may occur everywhere out of the hospitals, basic life support courses should be offered not only to medical students, doctors and nurses, which is mandatory, but also to parents, teachers, sports supervisors and day-care personnel. Parents of infants and children at high risk, discharged more and more frequently by the neonatal and paediatric intensive care units, and their surrogates should be particularly entitled to these courses. Definitely, much room for improvement exists in the vast area of public education in basic CPR for infants and children.

Basic life support is not only about CPR. It comprehends:

1. preventive strategies;
2. evaluation of the potential environmental risks at the scene;
3. recognition of an infant or child in distress;
4. determining responsiveness;
5. activation of the emergency medical system;
6. helping a choking child by performing appropriate manoeuvres for relieving a foreign body airway obstruction; and
7. cardiopulmonary resuscitation.

A summary scheme of paediatric basic life support manoeuvres is outlined in Figure 4.

Foreign body obstruction sequence

Choking and suffocation are common causes of preventable death in infants and young children. There is no doubt about the diagnosis if the aspiration is witnessed. Otherwise a complete obstruction due to a foreign body must be suspected after repeated attempts to open the airway and ventilate the unconscious child during the cardiopulmonary sequence. An airway obstruction in paediatrics causing acute distress may be due also to infections that cause upper airway swelling, most often epiglottis or croup. In these cases, prompt medical attention in a hospital's emergency department should be warranted without any delay. Children in distress will often position themselves to maintain patency of the partially obstructed airway and should be allowed to remain together with their parent, in the position most comfortable for them. A complete airway obstruction means that the child is unable to speak, cough or breathe. If the child is coughing the airway is only partially obstructed. Coughing is thus encouraged and no intervention is needed as long as gas exchange continues. Poor air exchange is evident by ineffective cough, stridor or high-pitched noises while inhaling, severe distress and later blueness of the lips. However, cyanosis is strictly haemoglobin-dependent and thus not easily found in anaemic infants, even in conditions of profound hypoxemia. Special measures to clear the obstructed airway must be undertaken only if the child is exhausted or not able to breathe or cough. The older child may use the so-called "universal distress signal of choking", that is clutching the neck between the thumb and index finger. First aid to victims of choking due to airway obstruction can be very effective, but is not always easy to learn and perform. A 60% fall in death from choking was followed after the introduction of the American Heart Association's guidelines in the USA [1]. In order to recall the manoeuvres and maintain one's skill it is necessary to refresh the techniques on manikins on a regular basis. As suggested by the European Resuscitation Council [2], five repetitions of each technique is easier to teach and recall. Since the child's larynx is cone-shaped, a foreign body may be expelled by increasing the pressure below it. It seems to be reasonable to arrange in an ordered sequence all the known techniques for dislodging the foreign body out of the airway by an artificial cough. The sequence should not be interrupted until advanced life support facilities are available. Abdominal thrusts are not recommended for infants because of the risk of lacerating the large infant's liver. Nevertheless, in the author's opinion, since death from choking is worse than the potential risk of a liver injury, abdominal thrusts should not be omitted under one year of age as a last resort if chest thrusts are repeatedly ineffective. Indeed, the only complication of the Heimlich manoeuvre reported in children is a pneumomediastinum in a three-year-old, without serious sequels [12]. The sequences for infants and children, according to the ERC guidelines, are reported in Figures 2-4.

CPR: general aspects

Since CPR of children remains a rare event, either out of the hospital or in the hospital, there is a lack of adequate power outcome or handicap studies of paediatric resuscitation. Concerns about the lack of standardisation led to the development and publication of the Utstein style for uniform reporting of data from out-of-hospital cardiac arrest [13]. Unlike adult patients, the paediatric guide-

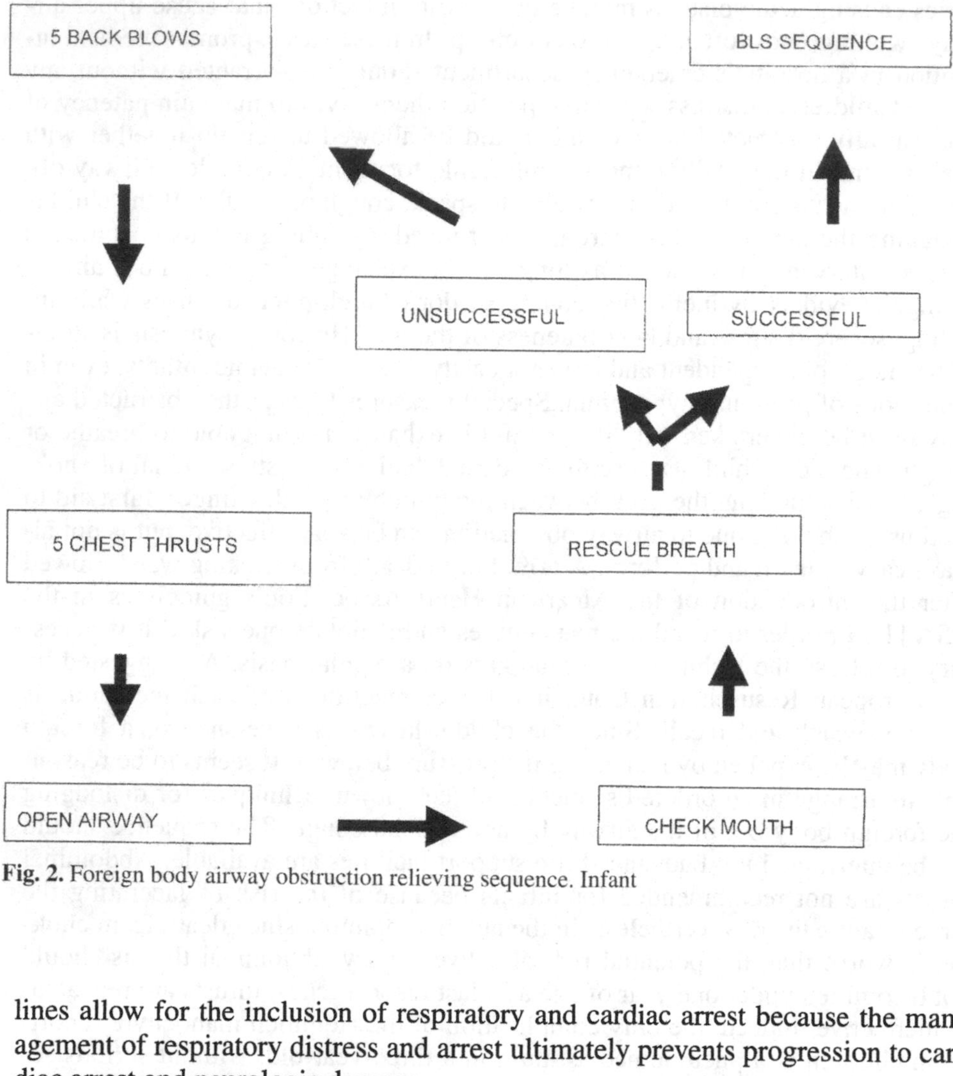

Fig. 2. Foreign body airway obstruction relieving sequence. Infant

lines allow for the inclusion of respiratory and cardiac arrest because the management of respiratory distress and arrest ultimately prevents progression to cardiac arrest and neurologic damage.

Children vary dramatically in size and maturity. We must make decisions in paediatric resuscitation based on extrapolation from young animal studies, such as piglets, puppies, lambs and kittens, adult human studies and scant paediatric data. Obviously, human volunteers do not exist. CPR is considered to be difficult in infants and young children, but can be very effective in many patients when optimally applied. Difficult successes may be won with strict adherence to all the details and taking advantage offered by circumstances. It is noteworthy that the first patient resuscitated with modern closed-chest CPR was a 5 year-old-boy in 1958 [14], just before the widespread introduction of closed-chest cardiac massage in 1960 [15].

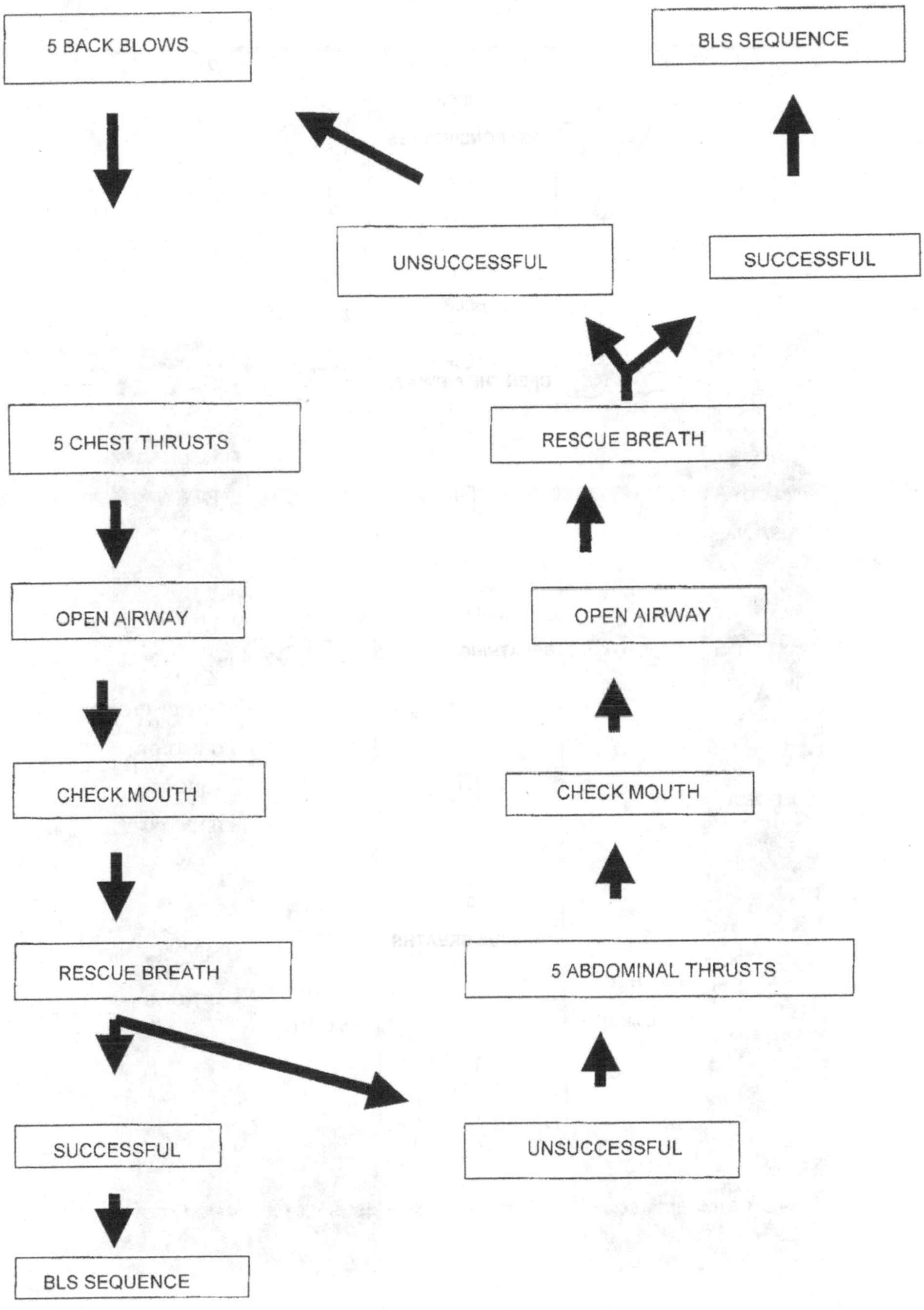

Fig. 3. Foreign body airway obstruction relieving sequence. Child

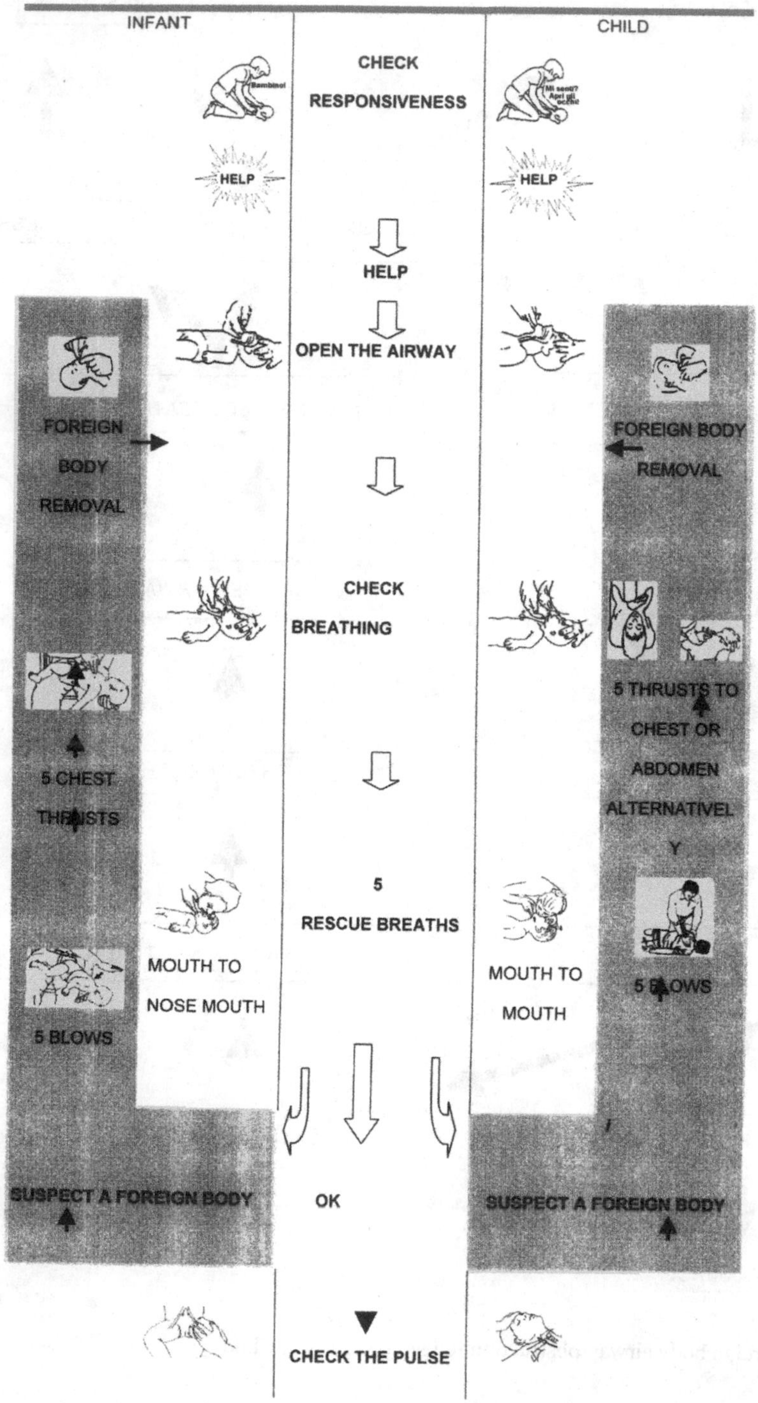

Fig. 4. Summary scheme of paediatric basic life support

Competence in performing CPR in children depends on the frequency of practice, since motor skills deteriorate rapidly [16]. Full retraining is recommended every 1 to 2 years, but occasional practice every now and then on manikins and reviewing of every real resuscitation episode step by step are paramount in order to retain the necessary skills. Another critical issue is the co-ordination of the rescue-team. The leader, the most experienced one, must ensure order and synchrony. Counting aloud may facilitate the interposition of ventilation and compressions.

Determining responsiveness and initiation of CPR

The level of responsiveness can be assessed first by speaking loudly to the child, then by tapping him or her gently [1, 2]. The child should not be shaken, but, in the author's opinion, if there is no response after gentle tapping, a painful stimulus such as pinch may help in determining whether the child is conscious and responsive to pain. If the child responds by movement it is better to leave the child in the position you found him or her and get help. If no response is elicited it is mandatory to shout for help and ask another rescuer or a nearby bystander to activate the emergency system. Movement of the child is mandatory only if the child is found in a dangerous location. The child should be always moved carefully, especially if there is evidence or suspicion of trauma. The head and trunk must be held and turned as a unit. If the rescuer is alone, one minute of effective CPR should be provided before spending some time to activate the emergency system, for instance for reaching the closest telephone. This is because oxygenation and perfusion are an absolute priority. After one minute of effective CPR, the alone rescuer may consider moving an infant close to a telephone while performing uninterrupted CPR.

Checking airway patency, breathing and pulses

The child's airway must be opened by head tilting and chin lifting. If neck injury is suspected, only the jaw thrust is applied, while the cervical spine is completely immobilised. Head extension should not be forced in infants since stretching and narrowing of the trachea and further obstruction may result. Also, care is needed to avoid pushing on the soft tissues under the chin. A generally gentle touch is mandatory in order to perform effective CPR manoeuvres on infants and young children. Then, keeping the airway open, the rescuer must check for breathing efforts by looking at the chest and abdomen – since an infant's breathing is mainly diaphragmatic – and feeling and listening for air flow.

Airway opening is essential in paediatrics because the simple manoeuvre of clearing the airway may be all that is required in the majority of children resuscitations. Relaxation of muscles and passive posterior displacement of the tongue resulting in complete airway obstruction is very frequent in young unconscious victims [17]. This easily occurs with central nervous system pathology, head trauma, an intoxication, a seizure attack or just after the intravenous administration of a sedative or anticonvulsant agent [11]. Opening the airway may well interrupt the vicious circle of hypoxemia, further central nervous system depression and subsequent muscle relaxation and thus prevent the progression to respiratory and cardiac arrest in many children [18].

Not only parents and other laypersons, but also nurses and doctors have difficulty in identifying pulses, especially in hypotensive children [19, 20]. Overdiagnosis of cardiac arrest is very probable. The palpation of the femoral pulse for infants [2] has been removed in the recent ERC guidelines [21]. The brachial artery pulse in infants is particularly difficult to palpate and even expert operating theatres nurses, surgeons and anaesthesiologists may have difficulties in the diagnosis of presence or absence of this pulse (personal unpublished data). In the author's experience, if no pulse is palpated on the inner aspect of the upper arm, it is still often possible to palpate a carotid pulse even in infants (personal unpublished observation). The AHA guidelines [1] suggest that the rescuer should spend only a few seconds attempting to locate a pulse, while the last version of the ERC guidelines [21] allows ten seconds for the diagnosis of no pulse in infants and suggest massaging the heart if there is no sign of circulation or the heart rate is very slow, less than one beat per second. This recommendation implies that external cardiac massage provides superior circulation in comparison to spontaneous low-rate circulation, but this is unproven and it appears that CPR can be harmful therapy for hypotension [3]. According to Goetting [3], in the author's opinion, all but the most feeble of spontaneous contraction may be better in producing a perfusion pressure than cardiac massage. However, a heart rate under 60 per minute is very transient in infants and either increases very rapidly if oxygenation is provided or as much rapidly deteriorates to extreme bradycardia or cardiac arrest without adequate intervention.

Rescue breathing

Since most paediatric emergencies are associated with airway and ventilatory compromise, five [2] rather than two [1] initial breaths (ERC guidelines versus AHA guidelines) are recommended to provide sufficient oxygenation of the child. Also, five repetitions allow a breath by breath self-improvement in the technique of airway opening and rescue ventilation. Moreover, all repetitions in paediatric resuscitation are performed five times for ease of teaching and recall [5]. An inspiratory time of one and half seconds is necessary to obtain better lung inflation and less gastric distension. Indeed, during CPR positive pressure ventilation may lead to gastric insufflation because of decreased lower oesophageal sphincter tone. Overinsufflation of infants and young children with consequent gastric distension is likely by unskilled rescuers and may result in severe ventilatory compromise [22] and regurgitation of gastric content with subsequent pulmonary aspiration [23]. A small tidal volume is better as this may provide reasonable ventilation while avoiding massive stomach inflation, especially if a bag and mask technique is used. A shallow movement of the child's chest and abdomen means adequate ventilation.

Since the nasal and not the oral airway is patent on inspiration in infants, the caregiver must place his/her mouth over the infant's mouth and nose to create a seal. It has been demonstrated that not all the mothers of a group of infants were able to cover with their mouths the nose plus mouth of their infant son or daughter [24]. As early as 3 to 6 months of age, many adult caregivers, especially female, may not be able to form a seal for mouth to nose and open-mouth infant rescue breathing, but almost 100% of caregivers should be able to seal their infant's nose and closed-mouth [25], thus the mouth should not be taught to be opened while performing rescue breaths, since this makes getting a seal more difficult and, in any case, air flows through the nasal airway.

Chest compression

Recent work has shown that the heart is directly compressed in paediatric CPR [26]. In infants and young children, the cardiac pump model seems to be more consistent than the thoracic pump model. Therefore, the precise position of the hand or fingers for compression is important. The heart lies under the lower third of the sternum in all ages [27], but the current method of locating finger position for chest compression in infants can cause pressure on the abdomen and it has been suggested changing the current method to locate fingers position – one finger's width below the intermammary line [1, 2] – to one using sternal anatomy [28]. Even medical personnel often fail to give adequate compressions in infants [5]. The two-thumb method was as adequate as the two-finger method in a recent study, although more compressions were measured as shallow with the two-finger method [29].

The chest should be compressed to depress the sternum approximately 1/3 to 1/2 of the depth of the victim's chest [2]. This is age-independent and much easier to recall and apply than a "precise" depth of 0.5 to 1 inch as suggested by the AHA guidelines for infants [1]. The compression rate should be at least 100 per minute [1, 2]. In the author's experience a rate of 120 to 140 is more difficult to maintain, but may generate a higher mean arterial pressure, as repeatedly observed during CPR of infants with invasive arterial pressure monitoring in paediatric intensive care units (personal unpublished observation). The compression should be smooth [1] and compression and relaxation should be of equal duration. The massage must not be a blow since this does not produce much flow. To achieve a 50% duty cycle, it is necessary to consciously sustain sternal depression before releasing it [3]. A recent study supports the use of a compression-ventilation ratio of 5:1 for both one-rescuer and two-rescuer in paediatric CPR [30].

Active compression-decompression CPR was developed after a case report of a man who was resuscitated by a household plunger. To date no studies have examined the use of this technique in children. Simultaneous chest compressions and rescue ventilation does not seem to be superior in CPR and may be dangerous, especially for non-intubated patients [31]. Interposed abdominal compression CPR is a technique that involves the application of pressure to the abdomen during the decompression phase of cardiac massage. Again, no paediatric studies have been performed on this technique.

Conclusions

Survival and neurologic outcome among paediatric patients may improve with strict adherence to specific principles of infant and child CPR. CPR can be remarkably effective in many children when optimally applied. Very poor neurologic outcome is to be expected with prolonged resuscitation efforts even after return of spontaneous circulation because the brain is much closer to the brink of irreversible damage at the moment of pulsenessness. Although more research is needed, most paediatric intensivists and emergency physicians are moving away from protracted efforts at resuscitation, with the exception of hypothermic children [8]. Improved survival rates among children who received bystander CPR implies that more public education in basic life support for children is absolutely necessary in order to offer the best chance of good recovery [32]. The strategy of "deferred consent" will soon produce more scientifically valid research in paediatric emergency medicine and resuscitation [8]. Unexpected death, especially in children is unacceptable and causes a great emotional strain even in the most experienced health care workers. By contrast, there is immense joy and relief when a child returns and fully recover from clinical death.

Children are the most vulnerable members of our society, but the best investment, from all points of view. They are entitled to extra protections.

References

1. American Heart Association (1992) Guidelines for cardiopulmonary resuscitation and emergency cardiac care. JAMA 268:2251-2261
2. European Resuscitation Council (1994) Guidelines for paediatric life support. Resuscitation 27:91-105
3. Goetting MG (1994) Mastering pediatric cardiopulmonary resuscitation. In: Orlowsky JP (ed) Pediatric Critical Care. Ped Clin North Am 41, Saunders Company, Philadelphia, pp 1147-1181
4. Sirbaugh PE, Pepe PE, Shook JE et al (1999) A prospective population-based study of the demographics, epidemiology, management, and outcome of out-of-hospital pediatric cardiopulmonary arrest. Ann Emerg Med 33:1-12
5. Richmond CE, Bingham RM (1995) Paediatric cardiopulmonary resuscitation. Paediatr Anaesth 5:11-27
6. Rourke PP (1986) Outcome of children who are apneic and pulseless in the emergency room. Crit Care Med 14:466-468
7. Zaritsky A, Nadkarni V, Gelson P et al (1987) CPR in children. Ann Emerg Med 16:1107-1111
8. Gausche M, Seidel JS (1999) Out-of-hospital care of pediatric patients. In: Emergency Medicine. Ped Clin North Am 46, Saunders Company, Philadelphia, pp 1305-1327
9. Fisher B, Worthen M (1999) Cardiac arrest induced by blunt trauma in children. Pediatr Emerg Care 15:274-276
10. Young KD, Seidel JS (1999) Pediatric cardiopulmonary resuscitation: A collective review. Ann Emerg Med 33:195-205
11. Sarti A (1997) Il bambino e l'emergenza. In: Sarti A, Busoni P (eds) Emergenze pediatriche. Pacini, Pisa, pp 7-16
12. Fink JA, Klein RL (1989) Complications of the Heimlich maneuver. J Ped Surg 24:486-487
13. Zaritsky A, Nadkarni V, Hazinsky MF et al (1995) Recommended guidelines for uniform reporting of pediatric advanced life support: The pediatric Utstein Style. Pediatrics 96:765-779
14. Knouwenhoven WB, Langworthy OR (1973) Cardiopulmonary resuscitation: An account of forty-five years of research. Hopkins Medical Journal 132:186
15. Knouwenhoven WB, Jude JR, Knickerbocker GC (1960). Closed chest cardiac massage. JAMA 173:1064-1067
16. Fossel M (1983) Retention of CPR skills by medical students. Journal Medical Education 58:568-572
17. The National Committee for Injury prevention and Control (1989) Traffic Injuries. Am J Prev Med 5:115-144
18. Sarti A (1999) Il pediatra di famiglia e l'emergenza. Primula Multimedia, Pisa, pp 15-34
19. Cavallaro DL, Melker RJ (1983) Comparison of two techniques for detecting cardiac activity in infants. Crit Care Med 11:189-193
20. Krongrad E (1986) Near miss sudden infant death syndrome episodes. A clinical correlation. Pediatrics 77:811-816
21. The 1998 European Resuscitation Council Guidelines for Paediatric Life Support (1998). Resuscitation 56:83-97
22. Berg MD, Idris AH, Berg RA (1998) Severe ventilatory compromise due to gastric distention during cardiopulmonary resuscitation. Resuscitation 36:71-73
23. Wenzel V, Idris AH, Banner MJ et al (1998) Influence of tidal volume on the distribution of gas between the lungs and the stomach in the nonintubated patient receiving positive pressure ventilation. Crit Care Med 26:364-368
24. Tonkin SL, Davis SL, Gunn TR (1995) Nasal route for infant resuscitation by mothers. The Lancet 345:1353-1354
25. Dembofsky CA, Gibson E, Nadkarni V et al (1999) Assessment of infant cardiopulmonary resuscitation rescue breathing technique: Relationship of infant and caregiver facial measurement. Pediatrics 103:E17

26. Goetting MG (1994) The mechanism of blood flow in pediatric CPR. Ann Emerg Med 34: 48-52
27. Phillips GWL, Zideman DA (1986) Relation of infant heart to sternum: Its significance in CPR. Lancet i, 1024-1025
28. Clements F, Mc Gowan J (2000) Finger position for chest compressions in cardiac arrest in infants. Resuscitation 44:43-46
29. Whitelaw CC, Slywka B, Goldsmith LJ (2000) Comparison of a two-finger versus two-thumb method for chest compressions by healthcare providers in an infant mechanical model. Resuscitation 43:213-216
30. Kinney SB, Tibbals J (2000) An analysis of the efficacy of bag-valve-mask ventilation and chest compression during different compression-ventilation ratios in manikin-simulated paediatric resuscitation. Resuscitation 43:115-120
31. Patterson MD (1999) Resuscitation update for the pediatrician. In: Emergency Medicine. Ped Clin North Am 46, Saunders Company, Philadelphia, pp 1285-1303
32. Sarti A, Magnani M, Balagna R et al (1998) The Italian Resuscitation Council Paediatric Activity: A three years' experience. Resuscitation 37:S32

What's New in Acute Respiratory Distress Syndrome in Infants and Children

G. Zobel, S. Rödl, H.M. Grubbauer, M. Trop

Acute respiratory distress syndrome (ARDS) was first described in 1967 by Asbough et al. as a clinical syndrome that occurs 24 to 48 hours after a direct or indirect lung injury [1]. It is characterised by dyspnea, tachypnea, hypoxemia refractory to oxygen therapy, decreased lung compliance, and diffuse alveolar infiltrates on chest X-ray. ARDS is a rare disorder in childhood. The incidence varies from 0.8 to 4.4% among all admissions to the paediatric ICU [2-8]. ARDS is a significant cause of morbidity in critically ill children. While therapeutic interventions remain supportive, the management of evolving acute lung injury is often a controversial issue in the paediatric ICU. There has been significant progress in our understanding of the pathophysiology of acute lung injury and in our understanding of how lung injury is often amplified in the course of mechanical support. This understanding has led to a strategic shift in ventilation style principally geared to optimally recruiting and then maintaining end-expiratory lung volume, preventing the traumatic cycle of derecruitment-recruitment, and finally, limiting alveolar stretching during tidal inflation.

Ventilator induced lung injury (VILI)

The negative impact of mechanical ventilation on the disease process in acute lung injury has been assumed for years, based on animal studies. These studies showed that ventilation with the use of large tidal volumes caused the disruption of pulmonary epithelium and endothelium, lung inflammation, atelectasis, hypoxemia, and the release of inflammatory mediators [9-13]. Thus the traditional approach to mechanical ventilation may exacerbate or perpetuate lung injury in patients with ARDS. Protecting the "normal" population of compliant alveoli within heterogeneous lung necessitates limiting transalveolar pressure to 30-35 cm H_2O. Beyond this limit, it is important to recognize the significance of the upper inflection point in the pressure/volume (P/V) curve. When endexpiratory lung volume is appropriately optimized, avoidance of the upper inflection point generally requires limiting volume-cycled breaths to 4-8 ml/kg. A similar tidal volume may be targeted when the transalveolar pressure excursion is limited by fixing end-expiratory and end-inspiratory pressures. This excursion should be in the general range of 20 cm H_2O.

Permissive hypercapnia (PHC)

In 1990 Hickling et al. introduced the concept of low volume pressure limited ventilation with permissive hypercapnia for patients with severe ARDS [14]. This ventilatory strategy avoided further ventilator induced lung damage while moderate or even severe hypercapnia was well tolerated by the critically ill patients. In this uncontrolled study in patients with severe ARDS Hickling showed that the hospital mortality rate was significantly lower than predicted by Apache II (16% versus 39.6%).

In a recent study on ARDS patients ventilation with lower tidal volumes (6 ml/kg) was compared with traditional tidal volumes (12 ml/kg) [15]. The primary outcome was death before a patient was discharged home and was breathing without assistance. The second primary outcome was the number of days without ventilator use from day 1 to day 28. The trial was stopped after enrolment of 861 patients because mortality was lower in the group treated with lower tidal volumes (31% vs. 39.8%, $p < 0.01$), and the number of days without ventilator use was greater in this group (12 ± 11 vs. 10 ± 11, $p < 0.01$). The authors concluded that in patients with acute lung injury and ARDS mechanical ventilation with lower tidal volume than is traditionally applied results in decreased mortality and increases the number of days without ventilator use.

There are only few reports on controlled hypoventilation in paediatric patients with ARDS [16-18]. A randomized trial of permissive hypercapnia in preterm infants showed that a ventilatory strategy of permissive hypercapnia is feasible, seems safe, and may reduce the duration of assisted ventilation [19]. There were no differences in mortality, air leaks, intraventricular haemorrhage, periventricular leukomalacia, retinopathy of prematurity, or patent ductus arteriosus.

We used this ventilatory strategy with tidal volumes of 8 ml/kg in 20 paediatric patients with ARDS or acute lung injury. This strategy resulted in $PaCO_2$ values between 60 and 80 mmHg associated with pH values between 7.25 and 7.35. The overall mortality in these 20 patients was 30%. Baro-volutrauma was observed in 6 patients. Additional therapies included NO inhalation ($n = 17$), surfactant therapy ($n = 11$), and ECMO support ($n = 5$).

Recruitment manoeuvres

There is now further evidence from experimental data that lung recruitment during small tidal volume ventilation allows ventilation on the deflation limb of the pressure-volume curve of the lungs at a PEEP < Pinflex [20]. This strategy minimizes lung injury and ensures a lower PEEP, which may minimize the detrimental consequences of high volume ventilation. These sustained inflation manoeuvres for alveolar recruitment are safe in adult patients with ARDS resulting in improved oxygenation [21]. In a recent abstract Gaudencio et al. reported that lung recruitment manoeuvres with PEEP values between 30 and 40 cm H_2O improved gas exchange in 4 paediatric patients with ARDS without negative haemodynamic effects [22].

High frequency oscillation (HFO)

This form of ventilatory support does not create normal bulk flow ventilatory patterns through changes in lung volume and delivered pressure, but rather maintains lung recruitment via a steady inflating pressure (generally 15 to 30 cm H_2O) around which high-frequency oscillations (range between 4 and 15 Hz with an amplitude of 20 to 60 cm H_2O) generate alveolar ventilation. Tidal volumes are smaller than anatomic deadspace resulting in lower peak alveolar pressures than observed during CMV. Mean airway pressure during HFO is most commonly set above closing pressure and lung volume is maintained steadily without deflation. During HFO lung volume will not travel along the deflation curve to the point of derecruitment. Therefore, the lung may be optimally protected from the stress of cyclic derecruitment that occurs during CMV.

HFO has been widely studied in animal models of acute lung injury [23-25]. It has been shown that HFO improves oxygenation, minimizes histopathologic alterations of acute lung injury when compared to CMV, reduces activated pulmonary neutrophils, and reduces important inflammatory mediators [26, 27]. There is evidence that HFO may be most effective when used early in the course of acute respiratory failure. An optimal lung volume is best achieved with an aggressive initial volume recruitment strategy with relatively high Paw values. There is an important gradient in both peak and mean Paw values from the ventilator to alveolus.

In 1994 Arnold et al. published their experience with high frequency oscillation and conventional mechanical ventilation in 58 paediatric patients with acute respiratory failure [28]. In their prospective, randomized study with crossover design they used a high volume HFO strategy to optimise lung recruitment. Although they used higher Paw during HFO than during CMV the barotrauma frequency was lower during HFO. Of 29 patients enrolled to the HFO group 17 patients (58%) showed a good response to HFO and one patient died. However, 11 patients (38%) crossed over to CMV and 9 (82%) subsequently died. The authors concluded that early institution of a high lung volume strategy using HFO would be the ideal ventilatory approach in paediatric patients with ARDS. Nonresponders to this ventilatory strategy should be considered for alternative approaches such as extracorporeal life support. We used HFO as a rescue therapy in 7 patients with ARDS when conventional respiratory support had failed. In this situation HFO with a high volume strategy improved gas exchange in only one patient. The use of HFO as a rescue strategy when all other therapeutic steps have failed might explain the disappointing results with HFO in our patients.

Partial liquid ventilation (PLV)

The rationale for mechanical ventilation in acute lung injury is to apply a PEEP to prevent end-expiratory collapse of collapsible alveoli and to select a tidal volume to limit overdistension of lung units [29]. Another therapeutic option would be to eliminate the increased forces acting at the air-liquid interface in the acutely damaged lung by filling the lungs with a perfluorochemical liquid [30].

Perfluorocarbon liquids are organic hydrogen molecules in which carbon-bound hydrogen atoms are replaced by fluorine atoms. They are biologically inert, non-biotransformable and immiscible in both aqueous and lipid media. Perfluorocarbon liquids are absorbed minimally by the respiratory epithelium, and are eliminated by evaporation through the lungs. Oxygenated perfluorocarbon liquids have the ability to lower surface tension in surfactant-deficient lungs, to increase functional residual capacity (FRC), and are able to dissolve large amounts of respiratory gases.

In 1991 Fuhrman et al. introduced the technique of perfluorocarbon-associated gas exchange or PLV [31]. This new technique combined liquid ventilation at functional residual capacity and tidal gas volume ventilation using a conventional ventilator. Meanwhile a number of experimental studies have shown that PLV significantly improves oxygenation, lung mechanics, decreases further alveolar damage and decreases serum tumour necrosis factor-a concentration in acute lung injury [32-38]. Most investigators filled up the lung with PFC-liquid at FRC level (30 mL/kg) and used volume-controlled mechanical ventilation with a tidal volume > 15 mL/kg and a PEEP level between 2 and 6 cm H_2O in both the PLV as well as the control groups.

Greenspan and colleagues reported on the first human liquid ventilation experience in preterm infants [39]. Meanwhile the technique of PLV has been studied in neonatal, paediatric, and adult patients [40-42]. Leach et al. reported that partial liquid ventilation resulted in significant improvement in oxygenation in 13 premature infants with RDS after conventional treatment, including surfactant therapy, had failed [40]. A paediatric study in children with ARDS was stopped at enrolment of 182 patients, due to design problems of the study. Series of case reports have shown that partial liquid ventilation in adults is well tolerated and has resulted in improvement in oxygenation. A phase 2 clinical study included 90 patients, 65 of whom were treated with partial liquid ventilation [43]. Overall, the results from this study demonstrated no statistical differences between the treated and control patients. A multicenter study on PLV in adults with ARDS is running involving centres in the USA, Canada, and Europe.

Extracorporeal membrane oxygenation (ECMO)

Rescue therapy with ECMO for patients with severe refractory hypoxia remains of unclear benefit outside the neonatal population. A recent retrospective review by Masiakos et al. showed an overall survival rate of 53% for non-neonatal acute respiratory failure and ECMO support [44]. ELSO registry from July 1999 reported similar survival data of paediatric patients with acute respiratory failure [45]. MOSF and longer time on mechanical ventilation before ECMO predicted worse outcome, whereas duration of ECMO did not influence outcome. In another recent publication from a single institution Swaniker et al. reported an overall lung recovery in paediatric patients with acute respiratory failure of 77% and a hospital survival rate of 71% [46]. Zahraa et al. reported that the outcome of paediatric patients with acute respiratory failure supported by veno-arterial or veno-venous extracorporeal lung support was comparable (survival rate: 55.8% vs. 60%) and that neurological complications were not different between patients supported by veno-arterial or venous-venous bypass [47].

In our series of 11 patients 8 were supported by the veno-venous technique, 1 by veno-arterial technique, and 2 patients switched from veno-venous to veno-arterial bypass. The overall survival rate was 55%.

ARDS-Adjuncts

Surfactant

ARDS is associated with a quantitative decrease in total lung surfactant, changes in phospholipid/surfactant protein ratios, and surfactant inhibition from pathologic events in the alveolar space. While surfactant replacement therapy is well established in preterm and term infants, this therapy remains unproven beyond the neonatal period [48, 49]. In 1999 Wilson et al. showed in a multi-institutional, prospective, randomised, controlled study in 42 children with acute hypoxemic respiratory failure that patients who received surfactant therapy demonstrated rapid improvement in oxygenation, and, on average, were extubated 4.2 days (32%) sooner and spent 5 fewer days (30%) in paediatric intensive care than the control patients [50]. There was no difference in mortality rate or overall hospital stay. In the surfactant group 2 patients were on HFO, one patient inhaled NO, and one patient was on ECMO support, whereas in the control group 6 patients were on HFO, 2 inhaled NO, and one patient was on ECMO support. The overall mortality rate in this study was 11.9%, and only one death was from progressive respiratory failure. In this study 8 of 21 patients received a single dose of surfactant, and 10 patients a second dose. After the second dose the patients did not improve acutely. This is in contrast to the neonatal experience, where multiple doses have been shown to be beneficial. However, this study was not designed to compare single versus multiple doses of surfactant.

Inhaled nitric oxide (NO)

Acute respiratory failure is often associated with severe pulmonary ventilation-perfusion mismatch and pulmonary hypertension. Conventional intravenous vasodilator therapy results in a reduction of both the pulmonary and systemic pressures and worsening of gas exchange caused by a nonselective vasodilation of pulmonary arteries. Inhaled NO is a selective pulmonary vasodilator without any systemic side effects [51]. Inhaled NO rapidly diffuses from the alveoli of ventilated regions to the surrounding tissue causing relaxation of vascular smooth muscle cells. In the blood stream NO is rapidly bound to haemoglobin forming methemoglobin. In 1993 Rossaint et al. reported that inhaled NO reduces the pulmonary artery pressure and increases arterial oxygenation by improving ventilation-perfusion mismatch without producing systemic vasodilation [52]. Abman et al. reported their experience with inhaled NO in 10 paediatric patients with ARDS and 7 with severe viral pneumonias [53]. Inhalation of 20 ppm NO increased PaO_2 levels within 30 minutes by approximately 50% in each group. In addition mean pulmonary artery pressure was lowered from 42 ± 6 mmHg to 31 ± 6 mmHg ($p < 0.01$) and intrapulmonary shunt fraction decreased from 39 ± 7% to 32 ± 7% ($p < 0.01$). However, the mortality rate of 50% in the 10 children with ARDS was quite high.

Despite acute physiologic effects, it remains uncertain whether improved oxygenation and pulmonary haemodynamics during iNO therapy are "cosmetic" or actually translate to significant benefits in long-term outcomes. Recent multicenter, randomized trials of iNO therapy have consistently demonstrated improved oxygenation in adults with ARDS, but have not shown a reduction in mortality or morbidity [54]. Recently a randomized multicenter study on iNO therapy in paediatric patients with acute hypoxemic respiratory failure was published by Dobyns et al. [55]. One hundred and eight patients were enrolled for the study. Patients were randomized to iNO (10 ppm) or placebo treatment groups throughout a 3 day study period. Treatment failure defined as OI > 25 for 6 hrs or OI > 40 for 3 hrs was the primary study endpoint. Progressive haemodynamic deterioration, metabolic acidosis, methemoglobinemia or high NO_2 levels were criteria to exit the study and to receive "rescue" therapy. Oxygenation improved over time in both groups, but the response was greater with iNO treatment at 4 and 12 hrs. The rate of treatment failure remained greater in the control group over the first 24 hours. Despite this acute response, the proportion of patients who met treatment failure criteria was not different over the 3-day study. Mortality was not different between both groups (43%), but since cross-over was allowed, this mortality was not an end point of this study. During prolonged therapy the failure rate was reduced in the iNO group patients. The authors concluded that iNO causes an acute improvement in oxygenation in children with severe acute hypoxemic respiratory failure. Two subgroups (immunocompromised and an entry OI > 25) appear to have a more sustained improvement in oxygenation, and the authors speculated that these subgroups may benefit from prolonged therapy.

In a recent paper Ream et al. showed that inhaled NO at doses < 5 ppm improved oxygenation and to a lesser extent ventilation of 62% of children with acute, hypoxic respiratory failure [56]. Mortality was not influenced by prolonged inhalation of NO at doses < 20 ppm. The unpredictable response of patients necessitates individualized dosing of inhaled NO, starting at concentrations of < 1 ppm.

We used inhaled NO in 17 paediatric patients with ARDS. As shown in Table 1 we observed an acute increase in arterial oxygen saturation in 59% of the patients. However, despite this initial improvement in oxygenation, there was no significant difference in duration of mechanical ventilation, ECMO-support, and mortality rate between initial iNO responders and nonresponders.

Table 1. Inhaled NO in pediatric patients with ARDS ($n = 17$)

	Responder	Nonresponder
No. of patients	10	7
Duration of MV(d)	22 ± 5	26 ± 11
iNO (ppm)	4 ± 0.8	9.5 ± 2.1 *
ΔSpO_2 (%)	9.2 ± 1.7	0.28 ± 0.89*
ARDS (n)		
Primary	5	5
Secondary	5	2
LIS	3.2 ± 0.15	3.3 ± 0.2
OI	29.4 ± 3.8	31.1 ± 5
VI	50.2 ± 5.5	45 ± 6.5
Immunosuppression (n)	2	3
ECMO-support (n)	4	2
Mortality rate (%)	40	43

Responder ($\Delta SpO_2 > 5\%$); Nonresponder ($\Delta SpO_2 < 5\%$); LIS = lung injury score; OI = oxygenation index (Paw * FiO_2 * 100/PaO_2); VI = ventilation index ($PaCO_2$ * PIP * RR/1000)

Prone position

There is now some evidence that turning a hypoxemic patient with ARDS from supine to prone position may improve oxygenation [57]. The proposed mechanisms for this improvement are an increase in FRC, change in regional diaphragm motion, redistribution of blood flow to less injured lung units and improved secretion clearance. Studies of experimental lung injury have shown that when turning to the prone position, preferential perfusion does not shift to the ventral part of the lung and that edema is more uniformly distributed along the gravitational axis. There was also no change in FRC or regional diaphragm movement. The explanation for the decreased shunting seen with prone position seems to be that the gravitational distribution of pleural pressure is much more uniform in the prone position [58]. In the supine position the gravitational forces result in pleural pressure becoming positive in the dependent lung regions and dorsal lung units are below closing volume. This finding suggests that transpulmonary pressure may not exceed airway pressure in this region, resulting in lung collapse. The gravitational pleural pressure differences in the thorax are much less in the prone position, resulting in less of the lung below closing volume and decreased shunt. Recently Curley et al. demonstrated in a prospective case series in paediatric patients with acute lung injury that oxygenation improved without serious iatrogenic injury after prone positioning [59]. On the basis of their clinical findings the authors proposed a prospective randomized study investigating the effect of early and repeated prone positioning on clinical outcomes in paediatric patients with acute lung injury.

Outcome in ARDS

ARDS is a syndrome with many different aetiologies and the outcome will be greatly influenced by the underlying cause. For instance, the mortality in ARDS associated with sepsis is higher than that associated with trauma or patients with single system lung disease without other organ dysfunction. In a published series of adult ARDS patients hypoxemia was the primary cause of death in only 16% of patients, the rest being sepsis and multiorgan failure. Therefore the ability to demonstrate improved oxygenation alone using a non-conventional approach would be unlikely to have a significant impact on outcome unless it could be shown that it either decreases the amount of lung injury or shortens the duration of ventilator support. There is now experimental data showing that lung overdistension results in the release of cytokines which may be responsible for multiorgan injury and dysfunction [60]. This provides a further rational for the use of ventilator strategies which prevent these events.

Most of the published data on ARDS in paediatric patients are small series reporting mortality rates between 40 and 70% [2-6, 8, 61]. A multicenter prospective study carried out on over 400 paediatric patients with acute respiratory failure, collected over a 1-year period, who required the combination of $FiO_2 > 0.5$ and PEEP > 6 cm H_2O for more than 12 hours, reported a mortality rate of 43% [62]. We treated 61 paediatric patients with ARDS over a time period of 16 years, 17 children between 1983 and 1990 with a conventional ventilatory approach and 44 children treated between 1991 and 2000 using a more lung protective approach. Mortality rate in patients treated before 1990 was 59% and the mortality in patients treated after 1990 was 27% (Fig. 1).

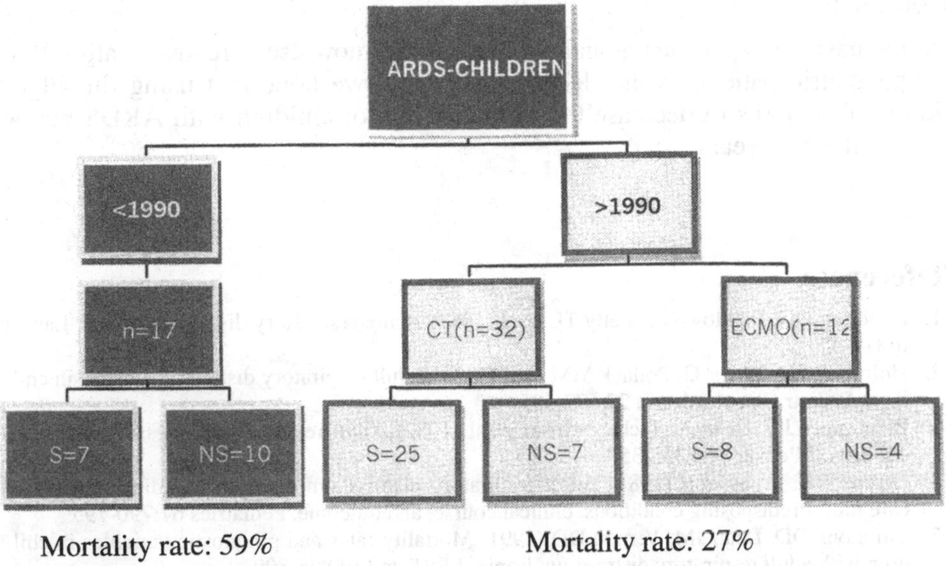

Fig. 1. Prognosis of ARDS in children under conventional mechanical ventilation and "lung protective" ventilation
CT: conventional therapy; ECMO: extracorporeal membrane oxygenation; S: responders; NS: nonresponders

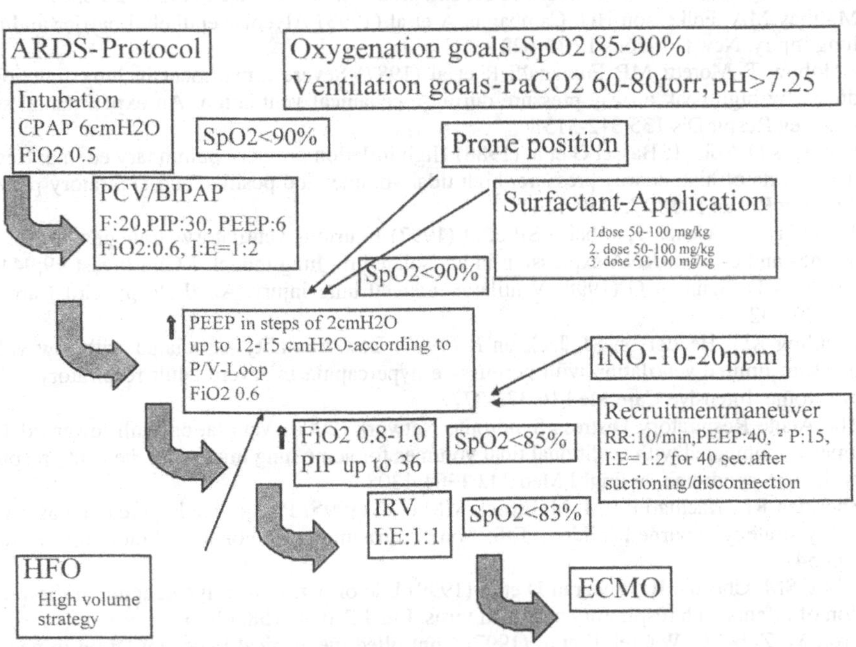

Fig. 2. Therapeutic algorithm for children with ARDS

Conclusion

On the basis of experimental and clinical data we now use a treatment algorithm for paediatric patients with ARDS (Fig. 2) and we hope that using this algorithm will help us to decrease the mortality rate of children with ARDS below 20% in the next years.

References

1. Asbough DG, Bigelow DB, Petty TL et al (1967) Acute respiratory distress in adults. Lancet ii:319-323
2. Holbrook PR, Taylor G, Pollack MM et al (1980) Adult respiratory distress syndrome in children. Pediatr Clin North Am 27:677-685
3. Pfenninger J, Gerber A, Tschappeler H et al (1982) Adult respiratory distress syndrome in children. J Pediatr 101:352-357
4. Lyrene RK, Truog WE (1981) Adult respiratory distress syndrome in a pediatric intensive care unit: Predisposing conditions, clinical course, and outcome. Pediatrics 67:790-795
5. Timmons OD, Dean JM, Vernon DD (1991) Mortality rates and prognostic variables in children with adult respiratory distress syndrome. J Pediatr 119:896-899
6. DeBruin W, Notterman DA, Magid M et al (1992) Acute hypoxemic respiratory failure in infants and children: Clinical and pathologic characteristics. Crit Care Med 20:1223-1234
7. Royall JA, Levin DL (1988) Adult respiratory distress syndrome in pediatric patients. I: Clinical aspects, pathophysiology, pathology and mechanisms of lung injury. J Pediatr 112: 169-180
8. Davis SL, Furman DP, Costarino AT et al (1993) Adult respiratory distress syndrome in children: Associated disease, clinical course, and predictors of death. J Pediatr 123:35-45
9. Matthay MA, Folkesson HG, Campagna A et al (1993) Alveolar epithelial barrier and acute lung injury. New Horizons 1:613-622
10. Kolobow T, Moretti MP, Fumagalli R et al (1987) Severe impairment in lung function induced by high peak airway pressure during mechanical ventilation. An experimental study. Am Rev Respir Dis 135:312-315
11. Dreyfuss D, Soler P, Basset G et al (1988) High inflation pressure pulmonary edema: Respective effects of high airway pressure, high tidal volume, and positive end-expiratory pressure. Am Rev Respir Dis 137:1159-1164
12. Tremblay L, Valenza F, Ribeiro SP et al (1997) Injurious ventilatory strategies increase cytokines and c-fos m-RNA expression in an isolated rat lung model. J Clin Invest 99:944-952
13. Dreyfuss D, Saumon G (1998) Ventilator-induced lung injury. Am J Respir Crit Care Med 157:294-323
14. Hickling KG, Henderson SJ, Jackson R (1990) Low mortality associated with low volume pressure limited ventilation with permissive hypercapnia in severe adult respiratory distress syndrome. Intensive Care Med 16:372-377
15. The Acute Respiratory Distress Syndrome Network (2000) Ventilation with lower tidal volumes as compared with traditional tidal volumes for acute lung injury and the acute respiratory distress syndrome. N Engl J Med 342:1301-1308
16. Sheridan RL, Kacmarek RM, McEttrick MM et al (1995) Permissive hypercapnia as a ventilatory strategy in burned children: Effect on barotrauma, pneumonia, and mortality. J Trauma 39:854-859
17. Tibby SM, Cheema IU, Sekaran D et al (1999) Use of permissive hypercapnia in the ventilation of infants with respiratory syncytial virus. Eur J Pediatr 158:42-45
18. Trop M, Zobel G, Waniek E et al (1997) Controlled mechanical hypoventilation in pediatric burn patients as treatment of acute respiratory distress syndrome. Burns 23:166-169

19. Mariani G, Cifuentes J, Carlo WA (1999) Randomized trial of permissive hypercapnia in preterm infants. Pediatrics 104:1082-1088
20. Rimensberger PC, Pristine G, Mullen BM et al (1999) Lung recruitment during small tidal volume ventilation allows minimal positive end-expiratory pressure without augmenting lung injury. Crit Care Med 27:1940-1945
21. Lapinsky SE, Aubin M, Mehta S et al (1999) Safety and efficacy of a sustained inflation for alveolar recruitment in adults with respiratory failure. Intensive Care Med 25:1297-1301
22. Gaudencio AMAS, Troster EJ, Faria LF et al (2000) Effects of a lung recruitment maneuver keeping PEEP before and after L-Pflex on gas exchange in chilled ARDS patients. Critical Care 4[Suppl 1]:S67
23. Hamilton PP, Onayemi A, Smith JA et al (1983) Comparison of conventional and high-frequency ventilation: Oxygenation and lung pathology. J Appl Physiol 55:131-138
24. DeLemos RA, Coalson JJ, Gerstmann DR et al (1987) Ventilatory management of infant baboons with hyaline membrane disease: The use of high frequency ventilation. Pediatr Res 21:594-602
25. McCulloch PR, Forkert PG, Froese AB (1988) Lung volume maintenance during HFO in surfactant deficient rabbits. Am rev Respir Dis 137:1185-1192
26. Sugiura M, McCulloch P, Wren S et al (1994) Ventilator pattern influences neutrophil influx and activation in atelectasis prone rabbit lung. J Appl Physiol 77:1355-1365
27. Imai Y, Kawano T, Miyasaka K et al (1994) Inflammatory chemical mediators during conventional and during high frequency oscillatory ventilation. Am J Respir Crit Care Med 150: 1550-1554
28. Arnold JH, Hanson JH, Toro-Figuero LO et al (1994) Prospective, randomized comparison of high-frequency oscillatory ventilation and conventional mechanical ventilation in pediatric respiratory failure. Crit Care Med 22:1530-1539
29. Lachmann B (1992) Open up the lung and keep the lung open. Intensive Care Med 18: 319-321
30. Lachmann B, Verbrugge S (1996) Liquid ventilation. Current Opinion in Critical Care 2: 60-66
31. Fuhrman BP, Paczan PR, DeFrancisis M (1991) Perfluorocarbon-associated gas exchange. Crit Care Med 19:712-722
32. Tütüncü AS, Faithfull NS, Lachmann BL (1993) Intratracheal perfluorocarbon administration combined with mechanical ventilation in experimental respiratory distress syndrome: Dose-dependent improvement of gas exchange. Crit Care Med 21:962-969
33. Tütüncü AS, Faithfull NS, Lachmann BL (1993) Comparison of ventilatory support with intratracheal perfluorocarbon administration and conventional mechanical ventilation in animals with acute respiratory failure. Am Rev Respir Dis 148:785-792
34. Leach CL, Fuhrman BP, Morin III FC et al (1993) Perfluorocarbon-associated gas exchange (partial liquid ventilation) in respiratory distress syndrome: A prospective, randomized, controlled study. Crit Care Med 21:1270-1278
35. Papo MC, Paczan PR, Fuhrman BP et al (1996) Perfluorocarbon-associated gas exchange improves oxygenation, lung mechanics, and survival in a model of adult respiratory distress syndrome. Crit Care Med 24:466-474
36. Hirschl RB, Tooley R, Parent AC et al (1996) Evaluation of gas exchange, pulmonary compliance, and lung injury during total and partial liquid ventilation in the acute respiratory distress syndrome. Crit Care Med 24:1001-1008
37. Quintel M, Heine M, Hirschl RB et al (1998) Effects of partial liquid ventilation on lung injury in a model of acute respiratory failure: A histologic and morphometric analysis. Crit Care Med 26:833-843
38. Rotta AT, Gunnarsson B, Hernan LJ et al (1999) Partial liquid ventilation influences pulmonary histopathology in an animal model of acute lung injury. J Crit Care 14:84-92
39. Greenspan JS, Wolfson MR, Rubinstein SD et al (1990) Liquid ventilation of human preterm neonates. J Pediatr 117:106-111

40. Leach CL, Greenspan JS, Rubinstein SD et al (1996) Partial liquid ventilation with perflubron in premature infants with severe respiratory distress syndrome. N Engl J Med 335:761-767
41. Gauger PG, Pranikoff T, Schreiner RJ et al (1996) Initial experience with partial liquid ventilation in pediatric patients with acute respiratory distress syndrome. Crit Care Med 24:16-22
42. Hirschl R, Pranikoff T, Wise C et al (1996) Initial experience with partial liquid ventilation in adult patients with acute respiratory distress syndrome. JAMA 275:383-389
43. Bartlett R, Croce M, Hirschl RB et al (1997) A phase II randomized, controlled trial of partial liquid ventilation in adult patients with acute hypoxemic respiratory failure. Crit Care Med 25:A135
44. Masiakos PT, Islam S, Doody DP et al (1999) Extracorporeal membrane oxygenation for nonneonatal respiratory failure. Arch Surg 134:375-379
45. ELSO report 1999, Ann Arbor, Michigan
46. Swaniker F, Kolla S, Moler F et al (2000) Extracorporeal life support for 128 pediatric patients with respiratory failure. J Pediatr Surg 35:197-202
47. Zahraa JN, Moler FW, Annich GM et al (2000) Venovenous versus venoarterial extracorporeal life support for pediatric respiratory failure: Are there differences in survival and acute complications? Crit Care Med 28:521-525
48. Long W, Corbet A, Cotton R et al (1991) A controlled trial of synthetic surfactant in infants weighing 1250 g or more with respiratory distress syndrome. The American Exosurf neonatal study group I, and the Canadian Exosurf neonatal study group. N Engl J Med 352:1696-1703
49. Auten RL, Notter RH, Kendig JW et al (1991) Surfactant treatment of full-term newborns with respiratory failure. Pediatrics 87:101-107
50. Wilson DF, Zaritsky A, Bauman LA et al (1999) Instillation of calf lung surfactant extract (calfactant) is beneficial in pediatric acute hypoxemic respiratory failure. Crit Care Med 27:188-195
51. Zapol WM, Hurford WE (1993) Inhaled nitric oxide in the adult respiratory distress syndrome and other lung diseases. New Horizons 1:638-650
52. Rossaint R, Falke KJ, Lopez F et al (1993) Inhaled nitric oxide in adult respiratory distress syndrome. N Engl J Med 328:399-405
53. Abman SH, Griebel JL, Parker DK et al (1994) Acute effects of inhaled nitric oxide in children with severe hypoxemic respiratory failure. J Pediatr 124:881-888
54. Dellinger RP, Zimmermann JL, Taylor RW et al (1998) Effects of inhaled NO in patients with ARDS: Results of a randomized phase II trial. Crit Care Med 26:15-23
55. Dobyns EL, Cornfield DN, Anas NG et al (1999) Multicenter randomized trial of the effects of inhaled NO therapy on gas exchange in children with acute hypoxemic respiratory failure. J Pediatr 134:406-412
56. Ream RS, Hauver JF, Lynch-RE et al (1999) Low-dose inhaled nitric oxide improves the oxygenation and ventilation of infants and children with acute, hypoxemic respiratory failure. Crit Care Med 27:989-996
57. Blanch L, Mancebo J, Perez M et al (1997) Short-term effects or prone position in critically ill patients with acute respiratory distress syndrome. Intensive Care Med 23:1033-1039
58. Lamm WJ, Graham MM, Albert RK (1994) Mechanism by which the prone position improves oxygenation in acute lung injury. Am J Respir Crit Care Med 150:184-193
59. Curley MA, Thompson JE, Arnold JH (2000) The effects of early and repeated prone positioning in pediatric patients with acute lung injury. Chest 118:156-163
60. Ranieri VM, Suter PM, Tortorella C et al (1999) Effect of mechanical ventilation on inflammatory mediators in patients with acute respiratory distress syndrome: A randomized controlled trial. JAMA 282:54-61
61. Zobel G, Kuttnig M, Trop M et al (1990) A respiratory severity index for children with ARDS. Clin Intensive Care 1:17-21
62. Timmons OD, Havens PL, Fackler FC et al (1995) Predicting death in pediatric patients with acute respiratory failure. Chest 108:789-797

OBSTETRICS

Heart Disease and Pregnancy

C. KESSIN, J.O.C. AULER JR

Due to the constant improvement in the preventive care of major obstetric problems such as hemorrhage, infection, and toxemia, maternal mortality and morbidity have declined dramatically over the past decades. This has resulted in a relative increase in maternal deaths from nonobstetric causes. Heart disease during pregnancy is uncommon, but remains the leading cause of maternal death due to pre-existing conditions. With advances in neonatology, cardiology, and cardiac surgery, more women are reaching childbearing age with congenital heart lesions, prosthetic heart valves, implanted permanent pacemakers, and pharmacologically treated ischemic or other heart diseases [1-5].

Incidence and prevalence of heart disease during pregnancy

The routine practice of performing a cardiovascular examination of all pregnant women during the first visit has been justified by reports on confidential inquiries into maternal deaths. The majority of pregnant patients have been found to have normal hearts, but there are more deaths attributed to heart disease in pregnancy than to direct causes of maternal mortality, such as thromboembolism or hypertension [5-8].

Practical aspects

Caring for a pregnant patient with heart disease requires a thorough understanding of the interaction between maternal and fetal physiology and the impact of pregnancy on the hemodynamic response to the patient's heart condition. Optimal care should begin before conception for many reasons. First, if the patient has not been examined until she becomes pregnant, the physician may underestimate the severity of the lesion. For example, the murmur of aortic insufficiency and mitral regurgitation decrease during pregnancy, presumably because of a decrease in systemic vascular resistance. Second, patients with prostethic valves may need a change in medication before conception. Third, in some cases it may be best to avoid pregnancy [1-8].

Preoperative evaluation

Functional status prior to and during pregnancy and the obstetrical risk are good predictors of maternal outcome, and help determine the need for invasive monitoring at the time of labor and delivery. However, functional status may deteriorate during pregnancy, especially when volume increases and cardiac output is maximal at 28-30 weeks' gestation, during labor, and immediately postpartum [9].

Table 1. New York Heart Association Classification [9]

Class I:	asymptomatic (Ib asymptomatic using pharmacological treatment)
Class II:	symptoms with greater than normal activity (IIb symptoms with greater than normal activity and using pharmacological treatment)
Class III:	symptoms with normal activity
Class IV:	symptoms at rest

Generally, patients in class I, Ib, II, and IIb have a good prognosis. Exceptions include patients with pulmonary hypertension, significant left ventricular dysfunction, and cases of Marfan syndrome (with aortic valve involvement). These lesions determine very high risk and may contraindicate pregnancy, regardless of their functional class. The type of heart lesion also influences maternal risk. A mortality of 25-50% is related in patients with pulmonary hypertension, coarctation of the aorta with valvular involvement, and Marfan syndrome with aorta involvement. A mortality of 5-15% can be expected in patients with mitral stenosis class III and IV or atrial fibrillation, aortic stenosis, coarctation of the aorta without valve involvement, uncorrected tetralogy of Fallot, previous myocardial infarction, and Marfan syndrome with a normal valve [1-5, 9, 10].

Normal physiological changes of pregnancy

Central and peripheral nervous system

The pregnant patient will be more sensitive to potent inhaled anesthetics, with reduced minimal alveolar concentrations in approximately 25-30%. At the same time the pregnant woman's nerves are more sensitive to local anesthetic agents as a result of hormonally related changes in diffusion barriers to local anesthetic and concurrent activation of central endogenous analgesic systems (their requirement is 30% less) [11].

Airway

Manipulation must be performed carefully to prevent trauma and bleeding to the highly vascular airway mucosa. Tracheal intubation can be difficult because of anatomical changes associated with weight gain (enlarged neck, breasts, and chest wall), impairing insertion of the laryngoscope and obstructing the visualization of the larynx [1-4].

Pulmonary

Oxygen consumption increases by approximately 20%, because of increased maternal metabolism and increased oxygen consumption by the uterus and placenta. Airway resistance decreases by 50%, because of the effects of progesterone on bronchial smooth muscle. Respiratory changes are summarized in Table 2 [1-4].

Table 2. Respiratory changes

Vital capacity (VC), inspiratory capacity (IC), closing capacity (CC)	↔
Functional residual capacity (FRC)	↓ 20%
Expiratory reserve volume (VER), Residual volume (RV)	↓ 20%
Minute ventilation (MV)	↑ 50%
Respiratory rate (RR)	↑ 15%
Tidal volume (TV)	↑ 40%
Anatomical dead space	↑ 40%
Alveolar ventilation	↑ 70%
Vd/Vt	↔

Hematological changes

The increase in volume averages almost 50%, reaching a maximum in the late third trimester and remaining fairly stable for the few weeks before delivery. The expansion begins in the first trimester, but it is much more rapid in the second trimester. Expansion then remains stable for 6-8 weeks before delivery. There is a diffuse hyperplasia of the hematopoietic system, and normal hemoglobin concentration at term of 12-13 g/dl. The total leukocyte count usually increases in pregnancy with a range of 10,000-14,000/ml. The white blood cell concentration can increase dramatically with the onset of labor, reaching 25,000/ml [1-4].

Hypercoagulability

Several factors involved in blood coagulation increase during pregnancy, most notably fibrinogen, which increases about 50% to a normal pregnant value of 450 mg/dl. The increase in coagulation factors accounts for the increased sedimentation rate seen in normal pregnancy. Other factors that increase include VII, VIII, IX, and X. Platelets do not change in concentration, morphology, or function during normal pregnancy. However, patients that require anticoagulation, have an increased need, with related risks (replace Coumadin with approximately 10,000U SQ heparin every 8 to 12 h, maintaining the activated partial thromboplastin time (aPTT) at twice control; if necessary heparin can be reversed with protamine intrapartum) [1-3, 7, 12].

Cardiovascular

The heart shifts leftward because of elevation of the diaphragm. The electrocardiogram changes that result may include benign arrhythmia, left axis deviation, down sloping ST segments, and T-wave inversion in lead III.

Hypotension may occur in the supine position because of aortocaval compression by the gravid uterus. Significant aorto-iliac artery compression occurs in 15-20% of pregnant women and vena cava compression in all pregnant women. Antepartum and intrapartum left uterine displacement and supplemental oxygen is recommended.

Cardiac output increases 30-50% above pre-pregnancy values by 20-24 weeks of gestation, declining slightly during the last 10 weeks of gestation; thus, disease that tends to limit cardiac output (mitral or aortic stenosis) may exert its maximal effects before the fetus is viable and may require extensive limitation of physical activity to lessen demands on cardiac reserves. Conditions that tend to decrease venous return (fever, hypoxia, and anemia) should be avoided. Cardiac output and heart rate increase during labor and volume shifts occur at delivery. Cardiac output increases maximally (80%) just after delivery, with the autotransfusion of blood from the uterus as it contracts completely. This increase in cardiac output and preload after delivery is so substantial that pregnant women with heart problems (such as mitral stenosis) may do well through pregnancy and labor, but have problems (congestive heart failure) in the postpartum period.

Because of the hyperdynamic state of pregnancy, the cardiac muscle thickens, chamber volume increases, and functional flow murmurs are common. Central venous pressure and pulmonary capillary wedge pressure remain unchanged despite increased blood volume, because this increased blood volume is received by a dilated pulmonary and peripheral vascularization that begins in early pregnancy. Women who have heart lesions that depend on a normal afterload for cardiac output (like subaortic stenosis) or for adequate oxygenation (like pulmonary hypertension) may experience a worsening of their clinical condition as the peripheral vascular resistance decreases (it causes more right to left shunting) [1-4, 6, 13-15].

Renal function

During pregnancy, renal blood flow (RBF) and the glomerular filtration rate (GFR) increase by approximately 60%. Tubular reabsorption of water and electrolytes also increases, and, consequently, electrolyte and fluid balance remain normal. With elevations in RBF and GFR, the normal values of blood urea nitrogen (BUN) and serum creatinine for pregnant women are approximately 50% of those for non-pregnant women (normal BUN 8-9 and normal serum creatinine 0.4-0.6) [1-4].

Gastrointestinal system

A pregnant woman's uterus displaces her stomach cephalic and anterior. It displaces the pylorus cephalic and posterior. Gastric pressure is increased and gastric reflux is common during gestation. Gastric plasma levels increase, increasing gastric acidity at term gestation. After delivery, a woman's gastric emptying remains slow and her gastric production remains high for at least 48 h postpartum (consider full stomach precautions from the 2nd trimester until at least 48 h after delivery!) [1-4].

Neuroanatomy, pharmacology, and labor pain

Type C fibers predominate in the first stage of labor; these are small fibers that are poorly myelinated, and their conduction velocity is quite slow. They tend to synapse widely after entry to the dorsal grey matter of the spinal cord. During the second stage of labor, type Aδ fibers dominate. These neurones are significantly larger in diameter and better myelinated, with more-rapid conduction velocity.

Muscarinic (cholinergic) receptors have also been found in the dorsal horn of the spinal cord. Application of α-adrenergic agonistic to the spinal cord increases the level of acetylcholine in spinal cord interstitial fluid at the same time as it produces analgesia.

Local anesthetics

The site of action of local anesthetics is the sodium channel of the neuronal cell membrane. The smaller and more poorly myelinated the neurone is, the more susceptible it is to local anesthetics. As sensation from the first stage is transmitted primarily via type C fiber, it is very easy to block these fibers and lessen labor pain with a very low concentration of local anesthetics. The Aδ fibers innervating the perineum require a slightly higher concentration for effective blockade, but both types can readily be blocked with concentrations of local anesthetics that should have a minimum effect on the large motor fibers to the lower extremities and to the musculature's pelvic floor. The sensation of "pressure" associated with contraction is carried mainly via Aβ fibers that are relatively resistant to blockade.

Opioids

Receptors are found in the substantia gelatinosa of the spinal cord and periaquaductal grey matter. Receptors are concentrated on the terminals of type C, but not Aδ neurones. Presynaptically, opioid antagonism results in a decreased release of neurotransmitters by the primary afferent neurone. Postsynaptically, receptor activation decreases excitability of the postsynaptic membrane [1-4].

Heart disease during pregnancy

Congenital heart disease

General care consists of antibiotic prophylaxis and a pediatrician present during labor in the delivery room to evaluate congenital hearts lesion in the neonate. Most of the lesions are corrected early in life (atrial septum defect, ventricular septum defect, patent ductus arteriosus, tetralogy of Fallot, and transposition of great vessels and tricuspid atresia). Occasionally, patients with no correction come to the obstetrical clinics with an uncorrected lesion or a lesion that has undergone partial correction [14, 16-20].

Left-to-right shunts

It may produce a minor degree of intracardiac shunting, which is well tolerated during pregnancy. Anesthetic management of patient with left-to-right shunt defect should include avoiding accidental intravenous infusion of air bubbles. Secondly, if epidural anesthesia is the technique of choice, for identification of the space saline should be used for the loss of resistance. Epidural injection of small amounts of air can result in systemic embolization. Thirdly, analgesia should start early in labor. Pain causes increased maternal concentration of catecholamines and increased maternal systemic vascular resistance. Therefore pain may increase the severity of left-to-right shunt which may result in pulmonary hypertension and right ventricular failure. Fourth, slow onset of epidural is advised to avoid rapid decrease in systemic vascular resistance that could result in reversal of shunt with maternal hypoxemia. Fifth, supplemental oxygen should be given and hemoglobin saturation monitored. Lastly, hypercarbia and acidosis, which may increase pulmonary vascular resistance, should be avoided [14, 16-20].

Tetralogy of Fallot

Tetralogy of Fallot comprises ventricle septum defect, right ventricular hypertrophy, pulmonary stenosis, and overriding aorta. The most-common congenital heart lesion is right-to-left shunt, typically with cyanosis. Most lesions are corrected early in childhood. Correction involves closure of the ventricle septum defect and widening of the pulmonary outflow tract. Symptoms depend on the residual ventricle septum defect, the magnitude of residual pulmonary stenosis, and the contractile performance of the right ventricle (echocardiography should be performed before and during early pregnancy). The anesthetic administration is the same as for most heart lesions. Avoid rapid decrease in systemic vascular resistance (risk of increase right-to-left shunt) and maintain an adequate intravascular volume and venous return. If the right ventricle is compromised, high filling pressure is needed to enhance right ventricle performance and ensure adequate pulmonary blood flow. Atrial and ventricular arrhythmia may be present due to surgical correction; 12-lead ECG should be performed and an ECG monitor must be present in the labor and delivery room [20].

Eisenmenger syndrome

Eisenmenger syndrome is defined as a pulmonary hypertension due to high pulmonary vascular resistance with reversed or bi-directional shunt at the aorto-pulmonary, ventricular, or atrial level. Management includes anticoagulation to decrease the risk of thromboembolic events and careful monitoring [20-24].

Aortic and mitral regurgitation

Both aortic and mitral regurgitation is characterized by left ventricular volume overload. Eccentric hypertrophy provides the extra left ventricle mass to return wall stress toward normal. Enlarged cavity size increases ventricular compliance, normalizing end-diastolic left ventricular pressure. Left ventricle ejection is usually above normal until myocardial contractility declines. With mitral regurgitation, left atrial enlargement increases atrial compliance but eventually leads to atrial fibrillation. Angina is rare. Tachycardia is preferable to bradycardia: the size of the left ventricular cavity at the end of diastole is increased with long diastolic times; mitral regurgitation is exacerbated in most patients. In aortic insufficiency the "backward" flow occurrs in diastole. The ventricle may also distend to the point of failure if heart rate is low. In both lesions the heart is volume loaded and an increased heart rate is beneficial to maintain forward flow [1, 2, 10, 13].

Mitral stenosis

The normal orifice of the mitral valve has a surface area of 4-6 cm^2. Symptoms typically develop when the size of the orifice is 2 cm^2 or less. A reduction to 1 cm^2 or less is considered severe and often requires intervention. Mitral stenosis prevents emptying of the left atrium, which results in increased left atrial and pulmonary arterial pressures. Symptoms of increased pulmonary hypertension include dyspnea, hemoptysis, and pulmonary edema. Tachycardia is not well tolerated and the use of β-blockers may be beneficial. Atrial fibrillation should be treated promptly with digoxin with or without β-blockers or cardioversion [8, 10, 11, 25, 26].

Aortic stenosis

Critical aortic stenosis (valve area is under 0.7 or 0.5 cm^2) is one major risk factor for perioperative event and death. Nonsurgical sudden death is usually, but not always, preceeded by symptoms of dyspnea, angina, or syncope. The valve narrows slowly over decades because of degenerative disease, rheumatic disease, or a congenitally bicuspid valve. The left ventricle has an elevated pressure load and massive concentric left ventricular hypertrophy is the usual result. The diastolic dysfunction precedes left ventricular systolic dysfunction. The stiffness of a hypertrophied left ventricle is often exacerbated by multiple episodes of subendocardial ischemia, micro-infarcts and scarring, even without coronary disease. Coronary perfusion pressure is reduced by elevated left ventricular and diastolic pressure in patients with a component of aortic insufficiency. Avoid afterload reduction and tachycardia, both are poorly tolerated due to the minimal coronary blood flow reserve. If ischemia does occur, the ventricle may have difficulty in managing the elevated systolic pressure required to overcome severe valvular obstruction. This may result in a rapid downward spiral of hypotension, ischemia decreased cardiac output, and further hypotension [10, 13, 15, 27].

Peripartum cardiomyopathy

Cardiac failure develops in the last trimester or more commonly within 6 months of delivery without etiology. In spite of careful management, the mortality rate of this entity remains at approximately 30%, and in patients surviving the initial episode of cardiac failure, nearly half have persistent left ventricular dysfunction [28-32].

Myocardial infarction - ischemic heart disease

This is a rare event, but it is associated with substantial maternal and fetal morbidity and mortality, especially during the third trimester. Prompt diagnosis and an immediate clinical and/or surgical intervention have been suggested for an uncomplicated antepartum, intrapartum, and postpartum course in pregnant patients with myocardial infarction [33-37].

Marfan syndrome

This is a hereditary disorder of collagen and elastin in which patients have long and slender extremities. Patients may develop dilatation of the ascending aorta, which may progress to dissecting aneurysm, aortic incompetence, and rupture of the aorta [38].

Aortic dissection

There is an increased incidence of aortic dissection during pregnancy and, when suspected, medical and surgical procedures should start immediately. Management includes aggressive control of blood pressure with a vasodilator, a β-blocker to decrease the force of ventricular ejection, and relief of pain. Patients with a known small, controlled aortic dissection may undergo labour and delivery with dense epidural anesthesia [39].

Infective endocarditis

This is a severe invasion and colonization of the cardiac valves, endocardium, and congenital or prosthetic cardiac tissue by an infectious pathogen (Staphylococcus aureus, enterococcus, Streptococcus viridans, and group B streptococcus). The major causes of death includes congestive heart failure, embolic cerebral infarction, arrhythmia, renal failure, septic emboli, and mycotic aneurysm formation with rupture. It seems prudent to avoid regional anesthesia in patients with sepsis or acute infective endocarditis [1-5, 10, 13, 26].

Table 3. Prophylactic antibiotic regimen [2]

Drug	Dosage
Ampicillin, gentamicin, and amoxicillin	Intravenous or intramuscular administration of ampicillin 2.0 g, plus gentamicin 1.5 mg/kg (not to exceed 80 mg) 30 min before the procedure; followed by amoxicillin 1.5 g orally, 6 h after the initial dose; or the parenteral regimen may be repeated once, 8 h after the initial dose
Ampicillin-, amoxicillin-, and penicillin-allergic regimen: vancomycin and gentamicin	Intravenous administration of vancomycin 1.0 g over 1 h, plus intravenous or intramuscular administration of gentamicin 1.5 mg/kg (not to exceed 80 mg) 1 h before the procedure; may be repeated once, 8 h after the initial dose
Alternative low-risk patient regimen: amoxicillin	2.0 g orally before the procedure; then 1.5 g 6 h after the initial dose

Dysrhythmia

Disturbances of the rhythm that affect hemodynamics may occur during labor and delivery, however electrical cardioversion is rarely necessary during gestation. Medications include digitalis and quinidina for atrial tachyarrhythmia. Procainamida is used for transplacental cardioversion of a fetal tachyarrhythmia (hypotension and widening of the QRS), disopyramide for atrial and ventricular tachyarrhythmia, and ß-blockers for atrial and ventricular tachyarrhythmia, as well as hypertension, mitral stenosis, and asymmetric septum hypertrophy. Verapamil is used for maternal tachyarrhythmia. Lidocaine is used for ectopic ventricular arrhythmia. Phenytoin is used for the treatment of digitalis toxicity or refractory ventricular arrhythmia, but more often is administered as an anticonvulsive. However, these women are at risk for fetal malformations. Amiodarona may be used for atrial and ventricular arrhythmia and also for fetal tachyarrhythmia when refractory arrhythmia is unresponsive to other agents. Adenosina is indicated for paroxysmal supraventricular tachycardia, which is the most-common arrhytyhmia in pregnant women. Symptomatic bradyarrhythmia is treated with placement of standard, ventricular permanent pacemakers. Cardioversion should be limited to patients with tachyarrhythmia who are unresponsive to medical therapy, or to those with hemodynamic instability [40, 41].

Chagas disease

This is a systemic infectious disease (Trypanosoma cruzi, identified 90 years ago, with a prevalence of 16-18 million in Latin America, in Brazil 3-4 million) occurring mostly at the forest fairway regions with a slow regression. Clinical manifestations include ventricular dysfunction, arrhythmia, and thromboembolism [10, 40].

Prosthetic valves, anticoagulation, and pregnancy

In women with a mechanical heart valve, atrial fibrillation, or thromboemboli in the presence of a porcine valve, anticoagulant therapy during pregnancy is essential. Warfarin readily crosses the placenta, is teratogenic, and predisposes to fetal bleeding. Warfarin is thus contraindicated in pregnancy, especially between the 6th and 12th week. In such situations, subcutaneous full-dose heparin should be given during the first trimester, warfarin should be given from the 13th to the 36th week, and anticoagulation with heparin should then be recommenced, being suspended at the time of onset of labor. The INR should be monitored frequently during warfarin administration in pregnancy, and both the aPTT and platelet count should be monitored during heparin administration [7, 12].

Monitoring

ECG should be undertaken when there are suspected arrhythmias and echocardiography when there are murmurs, diastolic and pansystolic murmurs, systolic murmurs of grade III (or greater) intensity, the presence of other abnormal signs (cardiomegaly), cyanosis, or symptoms that suggest progression or lead to severe restriction of normal activities [1-6, 8, 10, 13-17, 36].

Table 4. Categories of heart lesions

Categories	Lesion
Congenital heart disease	Prolapse of the mitral valve
	Ventricular septal defect
	Atrial septal defect
	Pulmonary stenosis
	Patent ductus arteriosus
	Fallot's tetralogy
	Bicuspid aortic valve
	Coarctation of aorta
	Transposition of great arteries
	Aortic stenosis
	Anomalous venous drainage
Acquired heart disease	Rheumatic heart disease
	Cardiomyopathy
	Previous endocarditis
	Previous rheumatic fever
	Hypertensive heart disease
	Ischemic heart disease
	Atrial myxoma
	Primary pulmonary hypertension
	Previous myocarditis
Physiological murmur	
Arrhythmia	

Intraoperative management

Labor, delivery, and postpartum periods are critical times for a patient with a heart condition. In general, because the hemodynamic changes that occur with caesarean delivery are more rapid and dramatic than those that occur with vaginal delivery, maternal heart disease is not a formal indication for caesarean delivery. Contractions are accompanied by a significant increase in cardiac output, and the presence of pain and anxiety accentuates these changes. In addition, bearing down in the second stage of labour diminishes venous return. In cases in which tachycardia is best avoided, epidural anesthesia is recommended. In patients with significant cardiac disease or who are high risk for cardiac failure during labor, many use invasive central monitoring with a Swan-Ganz catheter to allow minute-to-minute assessment of both right-sided and left-sided pressures. It is important tobe alert to the possible development of arrhythmia during labor, and continuous cardiac monitoring is highly recommended [1-4, 11, 14, 18, 22, 27, 31, 34, 40-43].

Induction of anesthesia

Any technique of anesthesia should be preceded by aspiration prophylaxis using a H_2-receptor antagonist, metoclopramide, and a nonparticulate antacid. Regional anesthesia is recommended for most conditions to minimize the fluctuation in cardiac output and heavy monitoring. However, a parturient with severely stenotic valvular lesions or right-to-left shunts (severe mitral or aortic stenosis, pulmonary hypertension, cyanotic congenital lesions) may not tolerate any decrease in systemic vascular resistance or any decrease in venous return to the right ventricle. Labor analgesia in these patients should be managed with intrathecal opioids, either single shot or through a continuous spinal catheter, or with intravenous controlled analgesia with opioid and a pudendal block for delivery. For patients on anticoagulation therapy, neuroaxial technique should not be performed if discontinuation is not planned in advance and/or aPTT is greater then 2, with the risk of epidural hematoma. Intravenous analgesia or anesthesia should be carried out with opioids. If general anesthesia is required a slow controlled induction using opioids and a rapid sequence induction technique should be performed [1-4, 11, 14, 18, 22, 27, 31, 34, 40-43].

Epidural

It is important to emphasize that the rich network of arteries and nerves in this space is increased during pregnancy. Epidural anesthesia is a very effective technique for decreasing cathecolamines and increasing uterine blood flow. It has minimal effects on, heart rate, blood pressure, and systemic vascular resistance, also on ventilatory cycles (hyper or hypoventilation) [1-4, 18, 31, 34, 41].

Combined spinal-epidural technique

Intrathecal opioid is given with or without a low dose of local anesthetic agent followed by slow epidural administration of a dilute solution of local anesthetic, with or without an opioid (e.g., 0.0625% or 0.125% with fentanyl 2 μg/ml) [1-4, 10, 11, 14, 25, 27, 41, 43, 44, 45].

Table 5. Side effects of some medication with hemodynamic consequences that maybe harmful for specific lesions

↑ HR	↓ HR	↑ PVR (if hypoxia and/or hypercarbia)	↑ SVR	↓ SVR
β-antagonist tocolytics	Fentanyl (large doses)	Methergine	Methergine	β-antagonist tocolytics
Meperidine		Butorfanol	PGF2-α	
		PGF2-α		Oxytocin (bolus)
		Parenteral opioids		Mg, RA, PGE-2, morphine

HR heart rate, *PVR* pulmonary vascular resistance, *SVR* systemic vascular resistance, *RA* regional anaesthesia, *Mg* magnesium

Cardiac surgery

Maternal mortality is comparable to the nonpregnant cardiac surgery patient, although fetal mortality maybe higher if preterm labor occurs. When it is really needed, cardiac surgery should be performed during the second trimester to decrease risks of teratogenicity or preterm labor. Use high pump flows and pressures to minimize uterine blood flow, and use fetal monitoring after 24 weeks' gestation to optimize the uterine environment. Cardioplegic solution should not be reabsorbed but aspirated in order to maintain potassium levels. The fetal mortality rate remains high (30-50%) [15, 26, 46-48].

Conclusion

Heart disease is a rare cause of maternal mortality. Heavy monitoring with pulmonary artery catheterization is rarely necessary in pregnant women with most forms of congenital heart disease, including Eisenmenger syndrome. However, it maybe useful for the patient with a recent myocardial infarction.

Intrathecal opioids have an excellent effect in patients who do not tolerate changes in systemic vascular resistance or decreased venous return. Only for a few cardiac lesions is regional anesthesia an absolute contraindication. Slow induction of epidural anesthesia is necessary for safe management of these patients and combined spinal-epidural anesthesia is an optimal choice in most cardiac patients for both labor analgesia and caesarean section. Cardiac surgery remains a challenge. Maternal mortality is higher then in nonpregnant patients and the fetal mortality rate remains high.

References

1. Mangano DT (1993) Anesthesia for the pregnant cardiac patient. In: Shnider SM, Levinson G (eds) Anaesthesia for obstetrics, 3rd edn. Williams and Wilkins, Baltimore, pp 485-523
2. Camann WR, Thornhill ML (1999) Cardiovascular disease. In: Chestnut DH (ed) Obstetric anaesthesia, 2nd edn. Mosby, St Louis, pp 776-808
3. McAnulty JH (1995) Heart and other circulatory diseases. In: Bonica JJ, McDonald JS (eds) Principles and practice of obstetric analgesia and anaesthesia, 2nd edn. Williams and Wilkins, Baltimore, pp 1013-1039
4. Dellazzana JEF, Petry FLF (1997) Anestesia em obstetricia. In: Manica JT (ed) Anestesiologia: princípios e técnicas (2 ed). Artes Médicas, Porto Alegre, pp 541-553
5. Tan J, de Swiet M (1998) Prevalence of heart disease diagnosed de novo in pregnancy in a West London population. Br J Obstet Gynaecol 105:1185-1188
6. Whitty JE, Cotton DB (1996) Obstetric emergencies in the patient with cardiac disease. In: Kvetan V, Dantzker DR (eds) The critically ill cardiac patient. Lippincott-Raven, Philadelphia, chapter 16
7. Ferraris VD, Klingman RR, Dunn L et al (1994) Home heparin therapy used in a pregnant patient with a mechanical heart valve prothesis. Ann Thorac Surg 58:1168-1170
8. Siu SC, Sermer M, Harison DA et al (1997) Risk and predictors for pregancy-realated complication in women with heart disease. Circulation 96:2789-2794
9. Smith TW (1992) Approach to the patient with cardiovascular disease. In: Wyngaarden JB, Smith Jr LH, Bennet JC (eds) Cecil textbook of medicine, 18th edn. Saunders, Philadelphia, pp 147-151
10. Carvalho JCA (1989) Anaesthetic management of the pregnant cardiac patient. ASA Refresher Course Lectures
11. Forster R, Joyce T 3rd (1989) Spinal opioids and the treatment of the obstetric patient with cardiac disease. Clin Perinatol 16:955-974
12. Chan WS, Anad S, Ginsberg JS (2000) Anticoagulation of pregnant women with mechanical heart valves a systematic review of the literature. Arch Intern Med 160:191-196
13. Thilén U, Olsson SB (1997) Pregnancy and heart disease: a review. Eur J Obstet Gynecol Reprod Biol 75:43-50
14. Lockhart EM, Penning DH, Olufolabi AJ et al (1999) SvO_2 monitoring during spinal anaesthesia and caesarean section in a parturient with severe cyanotic congenital heart disease. Anaesthesiology 90:1213-1215
15. Mul TF, van Herwerden LA, Cohen-Overbeek TE et al (1998) Hypoxic-ischemic fetal insult resulting from maternal aortic root replacement, with normal fetal heart rate at term. Am J Obstet Gynecol 179:825-827
16. Harkness CB, Serfas DH, Imseis HM (1999) L-Transposition of the great arteries presenting as severe preeclampsia. Obstet Gynecol 94:851
17. Buckland R, Pickett JA (2000) Pregnancy and the univentricular heart: case report and literature review. Int J Obstet Anesth 9:55-63
18. Groves ER, Groves JB (1995) Epidural analgesia for labour in a patient with Ebstein's anomaly. Can J Anaesth 42:77-79
19. Tahir H (1995) Pulmonary hypertension, cardiac disease and pregnancy. Int J Gynecol Obstet 51:109-113
20. Niwa K, Perloff JK, Kaplan S et al (1999) Eisenmenger syndrome in adults: ventricular septal defect, truncus arteriosus, and univentricular heart. J Am Coll Cardiol 34:223-232
21. Lust KM, Boots RJ, Dooris M et al (1999) Management of labour in Einsenmenger syndrome with inhaled nitric oxide. Am J Obstet Gynecol 181:419-423
22. Goodwin TM, Gherman RB, Hameed A et al (1999) Favorable response of Eisenmenger syndrome to inhaled nitric oxide during pregnancy. Am J Obstet Gynecol 180:64-67
23. Daliento L, Sommerville J, Presbitero P et al (1998) Eisenmenger syndrome: factors relating to deterioration and death. Eur Heart J 19:1845-1855

24. De Backer TL, De Buyzere ML, De Potter CR et al (1999) Primary pulmonary hypertension with fatal outcome in a young woman and review of the literature. Acta Cardiol 54:31-39
25. Kee WD, Shen J, Chiu AT et al (1999) Combined spinal-epidural analgesia in the management of labouring parturient with mitral stenosis. Anaesth Intensive Care 27:523-526
26. Birincioglu CL, Küçüker AS, Yapar et al (1999) Perinatal mitral valve interventions: a report of 10 cases. Ann Thorac Surg 67:1312-1314
27. Pittard A, Vusevic M (1998) Regional anaesthesia with a subaracnoid microcatheter for caesarean section in a parturient with aortic stenosis. Anaesthesia 53:169-191
28. Nishikawa K, Sato H (1999) Peripartum cardiomyopathy presenting after Caesarean section. Eur J Anaesth 16:130-132
29. Bolis C, Protti S, Piantanida S et al (1999) La cardiomiopatia dilatada peripartum. Messa a punto e descrizione di un caso clinico. Minerva Anestesiol 65:665-673
30. Ben Letaïfa D, Slama A, Khemakhem K et al (1999) Cardiomyopathie du péripartum. Série de cas cliniques. Ann Fr Anesth Reanim 18:677-682
31. Autore C, Brauneis S, Apponi F et al (1999) Epidural anesthesia for caesarean section in patient with hypertrophied cardiomiopathy: a report of three cases. Anesthesiology 90:1205-1207
32. Chan F, Ngan Kee WD (1999) Idiopathic dilated cardiomyopathy presenting in pregnancy. Can J Anesth 46:1146-1149
33. Patti G, Nass G et al (2000) Myocardial infarction during pregnancy and post partum: a review. G Ital Cardiol 29:333-338
34. Alam S, Sakura S, Kosaka Y (1995) Anaesthetic management for caesarean section in a patient with Kawasaki disease. Can J Anaesth 42:1024-1026
35. Webber MD, Hallinger RE, Schumacher JA (1997) Acute infarction, intracoronary thrombolysis, and primary PTCA in pregnancy. Cathet Cardiovasc Diagn 42:38-43
36. Mayr A, Lederer W, Mortl M et al (1999) Successful treatment of severe myocardial failure after postpartum haemorrhage with the use of an intra-aortic balloon pumps. Intensive Care Med 25:223-225
37. Tay SM, Ong BC, Tan AS (1999) Caesarean section in a mother with uncorrected congenital coronary to pulmonary artery fistula. Can J Anesth 46:368-371
38. Puebla G, Escudero MA, Perz-Cerda F et al (1996) Anastasia en tres casos de sindrome de Marfan. Rev Esp Anestesiol Reanim 43:30-33
39. Ecknauer E, Schmidlin D, Jenni R et al (1999) Emergency repair of incidentally diagnosed ascending aortic aneurysm immediately after caesarean section. Br J Anaesth 83:343-345
40. Esmail MM, Catling S et al (2000) Anaesthetic management of caesarean section in a patient with a permanent pacemaker and severe bilateral ventricular dilation. Int J Obstet Anesth 9:51-54
41. Hofstadler G, Tulzer G, Schmitt K et al (1998) Symptomatischer kongenitaler kompletter atrioventrikulärer Block - eine medizinische Herausforderung. Klin Padiatr 210:30-33
42. Abramovitz SE, Beilin Y (1999) Anaesthetic management of the parturient with protein s deficiency and ischemic heart disease. Anesth Analg 89:709-710
43. Ransom DM, Leicht CH (1995) Continuous spinal analgesia with sufentanil for labour and delivery in parturient with severe pulmonary stenosis. Anesth Analg 80:418-421
44. Rawal N, Van Zundert A, Holmstrom B et al (1997) Combined spinal-epidural technique. Reg Anesth 22:406-423
45. Mitterschiffthaler G (1996) Regional anaesthesia for the pregnant cardiac patient. Acta Anaesthesiol Scand [Suppl]109:180-184
46. Weiss BM, von Segesser LK, Alon E et al (1998) Outcome of cardiovascular surgery and pregnancy: a systematic review of the period 1984-1996. Am J Obstet Gynecol 179:1643-1653
47. Connolly HM, Grogan M, Warnes CA et al (1999) Pregnancy among women with congenitally corrected transposition of great arteries. J Am Coll Cardiol 33:1692-1695
48. Tripp HF, Stiegel RM, Coyle JP (1999) The use of pulsatile perfusion during aortic valve replacement in pregnancy. Ann Thorac Surg 67:1169-1171

[illegible]
[illegible] patient [illegible]
[illegible]

Risk Assessment for Obstetric Anesthesia

G. Capogna, R. Parpaglioni

In obstetrics there are two main objectives of antenatal assessment by the anesthesiologist. The first involves the assessment of the risk concerning a possible anesthesia or analgesia for labor, delivery or postpartum period. The second objective is to exchange information and to obtain an informed consent.

Ideally the anesthesiologist should see all the pregnant women at the end of their pregnancy and should not limit this service to those listed for elective procedures.

The basic idea is that any pregnant women may need a form of anesthesia or analgesia during her staying in the hospital and the antenatal assessment may effectively reduce the risks and anticipate the problems.

Anesthesia is a discipline that does not usually have an infrastructure for outpatient care and before an effective antenatal assessment can be routinely provided, a number of organizational problems must be resolved. However, the quality of an anesthetic service would be greatly improved if all the parturients underwent an individual consultation.

While we must accept that unpredictable emergencies are the nature of obstetric practice, might we also accept that knowledge of the parturient could reduce the incidence of anesthesia-related accidents? Ignorance of, for example, a serious allergy or a problem intubation during a previous general anesthetic, can have serious consequences. It seems logical that an opportune assessment of risk at a time when haste and anxiety do not feature, will permit a management plan with safety in mind.

The most important aims are to detect potential airway problems since the greatest hazard associated with obstetric anesthesia is failure to intubate; to identify contraindications, both relative and absolute, to regional anesthesia and analgesia, since epidural analgesia tends to be the most popular form of pain relief in labor; and to identify obstetric indications for urgent fetal delivery with a requirement for urgent anesthesia. Also worthwhile are assessments of risk factors for thromboembolism, postpartum hemorrhage and allergic reactions. Preexisting neurological conditions should be also documented, since their reappearance in the postpartum period could be confused with complications of epidural anesthesia.

Antenatal anesthetic assessment may reduce the risk to the parturient. For example, the early identification of high risk of an emergency cesarean section or difficult intubation allows the anesthetist to advocate epidural analgesia from the onset of labor. In this case the antenatal evaluation leads to a different management plan.

Evaluation of risk factors for emergency cesarean section may be correctly identified in 87% of cases and the use of "preventive" epidural analgesia in early labor may avoid general anesthesia in 90% of cases [1].

A large study [2] of outpatient obstetric anesthesia clinics reported that 10% of the clinic population had at least one predisposing factor for difficult intubation. These women were encouraged to have an early epidural catheter placement during labor. The study demonstrated that the percentage of patients requiring general anesthesia in case of emergency cesarean section was significantly lower when an epidural catheter was already in place and intubation failure occurred only in those without an epidural at the time of cesarean section.

When antenatal consultation allows evaluation of the "risk profile" of the parturient, this can subsequently be taken into account in the different situations for labor analgesia and for occasional emergency delivery.

At Fatebenefratelli Isola Tiberina Hospital the obstetric anesthesia staff offer the following services to all the parturients:

- antenatal classes
- self-rating questionnaire
- individual consultation
- inpatient consultation for difficult cases and obstetric pathology

Antenatal classes provide information on labor pain and pain relief. The information is given by the anesthesiologist himself. The class takes the form of a talk followed by a question and answer session. This has the advantage not only of allowing each women to ask her own questions but also for others to hear the answers. This provided also an opportunity for the primiparous woman to share the experience of those who have previously had an epidural analgesia (or other forms of analgesia). During the classes information about practical concerns may be given and the women may be also invited to fill out a self-rating questionnaire and to ask for an individual consultation.

A self rating questionnaire for anesthesia has several advantages. It has a low cost, it can be completed in a waiting room, and while tick boxes are very simple, they allow interrogation to an adequate level. We use it as a complementary tool to the individual consultation.

The traditional private one-to-one individual consultation enables detailed and personalized history to be taken. It allows also a physical examination. At least 5-20 minutes must be devoted to each parturient to allow enough time for the necessary exchanges and notation. It is more time consuming and more expensive, but it remains the most appropriate approach. The obstetric anesthesiologist team should discuss in advance the method and the contents of the risk assessment in obstetric anesthesia. Key questions must be clearly identified before the interview and these should be targeted at the three basic objectives: identifying the risks associated with general anesthesia, regional blockade and obstetric intervention. The opportunity to discuss the practical aspects of epidural analgesia, the pros and cons, the physiological effects and at the same time to correct the misinformation and half truths that abound in antenatal circles, will allow the women to participate in their own care in a reasoned and effective manner. This kind of discussion forms the basis for the written informed consent which is obtained at the end of consultation.

Our hospital guidelines establish that every inpatient parturient who did not have an antenatal consultation must have it at the time of the admission. In particular the anesthesiologist on duty must be informed every day of the admission to the obstetric ward of parturients with coexisting medical or obstetrical diseases. In addition, the anesthesia staff must be aware of all the parturients whose labors are likely to be induced because these parturients are particularly at risk of receiving some form of analgesia/anesthesia.

We believe that there are no acceptable reasons why parturients regularly seen by the obstetric team could not benefit from at least one anesthesia consultation at the end of their pregnancy. Anesthetic antenatal consultation can be accomplished efficiently in an outpatient context with promise of improved safety.

In this way the anesthesiologist is no longer seen as a technician but rather a physician managing both the pain of labor and delivery and the risks that may be associated with the pregnancy.

References

1. Morgan BM, Magny V, Goroszeniuk T (1990) Anaesthesia for emergency caesarean section. Br J Obstet Gynecol 97:420-424
2. Hamza J, Ducot B, Dupont X, Benhamou D (1995) Anaesthesia consultation can decrease the need for general anaesthesia for emergency caesarean section in parturients with difficult airway. Br J Anaesth 74:A353

Foetal Complications During Complicated Delivery

E. MARGARIA, G. SORTINO, E. GOLLO, R. SINIGAGLIA

Birth has always been, in the history of mankind, a wonderful but dramatic moment as regarding the consequences that can derive from it if, as may happen, all does not proceed physiologically.

Epidemiological data relative to maternal and perinatal mortality in the early years of the last century are alarming. The figures are very high and greatly exceed the morbidity and the mortality today in developing countries where, even though social conditions are very poor there is mobility of medical and technical means to follow the event, and we are now witnessing a progressive improvement of birth control.

The great social and technological changes that have taken place in the last 50 years have fortunately greatly reduced these figures, often making us forget how great the risks were that our grandmothers ran giving birth.

In order to be able to lower, or even to erase, these figures which are still too high for a civilised country, it is extremely important to understand the physiology of pregnancy and then any pathological processes which can occur altering both maternal homeostasis and, directly or indirectly, maternal-foetal exchanges.

In the experience of the Department of Anaesthesiology and ICU of S. Anna Hospital the admission of obstetric patients is unexpectedly high – young and healthy – (140 per year of 7,500 deliveries, equal to 1.86%) in comparison to gynecological patients – much older, mean age 67.5 years – (30 per year of 17,495 operations, equal to 0.17%).

The data show that a very high number of pregnant women need resuscitation therapies (2% of deliveries, among which mortality is at present equal to 0.0038% of all deliveries). The reasons are manifold and can be subject to further analyses. First and foremost it is necessary to emphasize that birth comes as an ordeal for any woman, compared by many authors to a very difficult strain.

Pregnancy is defined as **pathological** when for the mother and/or for the baby the outcome could be inauspicious, either as regards morbidity or mortality.

Maternal pathologies can be observed:

– before pregnancy

- occurring in pregnancy or at delivery
- peculiar to pregnancy
- puerperal

In preceding studies (E. Margaria et al., 1997) two categories of pathologies that result in maternal or fetal risk where it is possible, indeed essential, to intervene in order to lower maternal and foetal-neonatal morbidity and mortality, emerged.

The first group includes *causes which are independent of pregnancy pathologies*:

- advanced age
- poor cultural and socio-economic conditions
- obesity, anorexia
- incorrectly diagnosed pre-existing pathological conditions
- previously diagnosed pathological conditions in women who go against medical advice as regards becoming pregnant
- intercurrent or surfacing pathologies in pregnancy
- caesarean section, especially if in emergency
- inadequate assistance, inexperience on the part of staff (gynecologists, anaesthesiologists, surgeons)

The second group includes complications linked to *pregnancy's specific pathologies*:

- miscarriage
- ectopic pregnancy
- multiple pregnancy
- pregnancy jaundice
- hypertension, pre-eclampsia and its complications (eclampsia, DIC, HELLP, etc.)
- placental insertion pathologies
- pulmonary oedema
- haemorrhage
- thrombosis
- pulmonary embolism
- renal failure
- pathologies of the uterus (laceration, inversion, etc.)

The whole period of pregnancy is to be considered at risk, actually the most pathological events occur at the time of delivery or in the immediate post-partum period (85%), 75% after caesarean section.

All pre-existing pathologies can constitute a risk and can aggravate emergency situations. The principle step in order to recognise these pathologies early and thus to intervene successfully is to control and monitor pregnancy even when it appears to be physiological. While a healthy young patient may undergo an operation without any recent laboratory examinations, on the basis of an accurate pre-operative examination and of a good anamnesis, the pregnant patient must be monitored, especially those parameters which are physiologically modified. These modifications must be kept within well-defined ranges, under which or above which possible pathologies are to be suspected.

Pathologies preceding pregnancy are increasingly numerous since the present tendency is to allow patients who previously would have been advised against becoming pregnant to enjoy the wonder of maternity. It is important for women to understand and to know risks which can emerge. It would be prudent to involve at an early stage the anaesthetist-resuscitator, as recognising high risk pregnancies can lead to preliminary discussion about possible problems and result in a course of action to avoid catastrophes.

Even in patients who begin pregnancy in healthy condition, *pathologies which are specific to gestation* can arise.

The most common pathology is pre-eclampsia with its complications: eclampsia, DIC, HELLP, pulmonary oedema, cerebral haemorrhage, etc.

Even in normal pregnancies pre-eclampsia is the most frequent and life threatening pathology. If, however, it is recognised early and appropriately treated, this very specific condition need not affect negatively maternal and foetal outcome. However, we are now seeing an elevation of maternal and foetal risks as regarding mortality and morbidity.

There are many reasons for this phenomenon. Firstly, even women in poor health do not take advice against becoming pregnant. The age of first pregnancy and thus of first delivery has shifted by ten years (Fig. 1).

The mean age of patients who are admitted is 34 years (range 17-40 years). In only 40% of cases is there a wish for a second pregnancy, but rarely a third or a fourth pregnancy.

Advanced age is unanimously considered a risk factor, since the human organism starts to show a decrease in physical performance after 20 years. Furthermore, young women use contraceptives that can be directly or indirectly a source of pathologies (infections, thrombo-embolic pathologies, etc.). In these conditions, pregnancy is affected both by maternal risks, linked to social and economic status, and by foetal risk due to the direct effect of drugs, and the way of life of the pregnant mother (abuse of opiates, cigarettes, caffeine, malnutrition, sleep-wakening alteration rhythm, scarce attention to health advice, etc.).

The increase in maternal age is connected to the risk of miscarriage (Fig. 2) and to the low weight of the new-born (Fig. 3). The incidence of miscarriage is estimated to be between 5 and 20% of pregnancies clinically recognised.

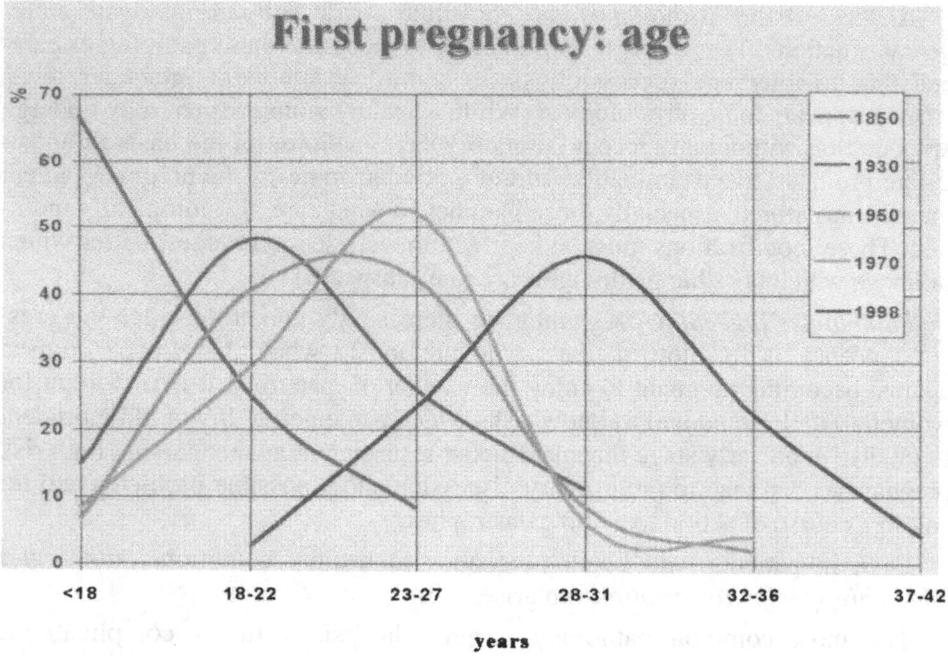

Fig. 1.

Women's social life, in the last 20 years, has greatly changed, leading to an incontestable better quality of life, which, however, involves their foregoing many things, and feeling guilty, especially considering the weight of work linked to psychological stress, which weighs heavily on their emotional life and health.

Obesity becomes a risk factor when BMI exceeds 30, for respiratory and cardio-circulatory difficulties. Weight, during pregnancy, has to be controlled weekly in order to verify foetal growth to be regular.

In vitro fertilization overcomes female sterility, even through hormonal and surgical manipulations with a frequent outcome of multiple pregnancies, whose percentage of pathological evolution is very high, as the data of admissions to intensive therapy demonstrate.

Other factors which contribute to the increase in complications are:
- increase in pathologies specific to pregnancy
- increase in pathologies such as autoimmune diseases and allergies
- immigration from countries with different cultures and religions
- great demand for invasive tests and diagnostic procedures

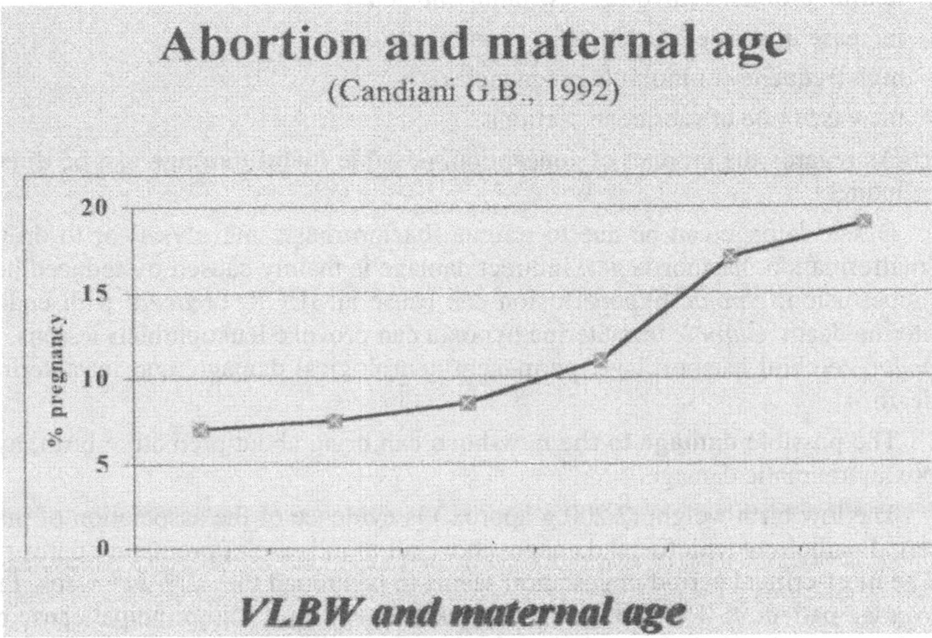
Abortion and maternal age
(Candiani G.B., 1992)
% pregnancy
20
15
10
5
0
VLBW and maternal age

Fig. 2.

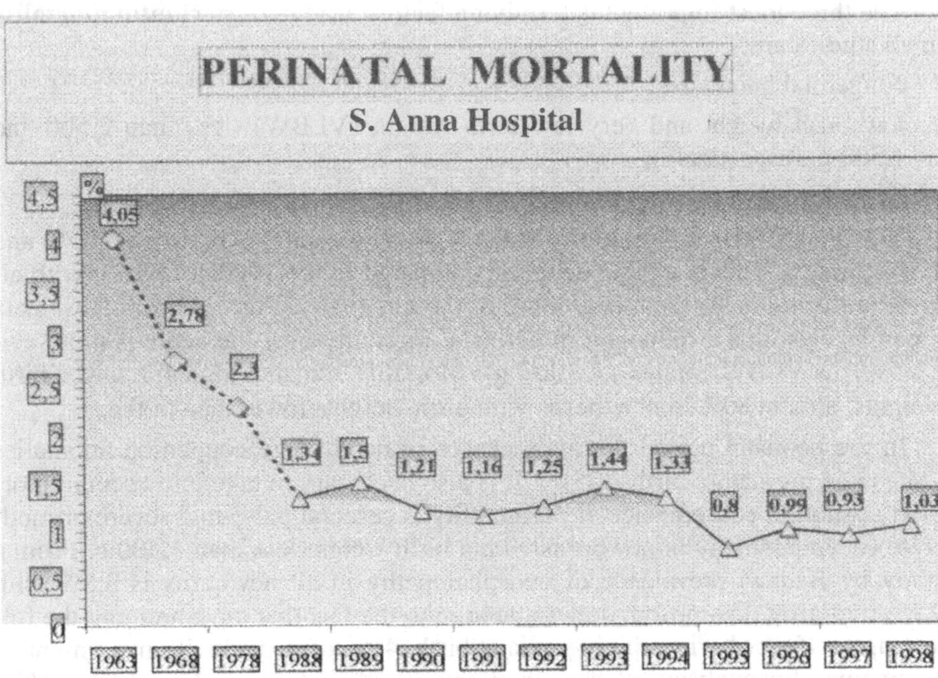
PERINATAL MORTALITY
S. Anna Hospital
%
4,5
4
3,5
3
2,5
2
1,5
1
0,5
0
4,05
2,78
2,3
1,34
1,5
1,21
1,16
1,25
1,44
1,33
0,8
0,99
0,93
1,03
1963
1968
1978
1988
1989
1990
1991
1992
1993
1994
1995
1996
1997
1998

Fig. 3.

- marital problems (divorce, new family nucleus)
- increase in accidents (domestic or on the road)
- high frequency of multiple pregnancies
- increased rate of caesarean sections

As regards the product of conception, possible **foetal damage** can be direct or indirect.

Direct damage can be due to trauma (haemorrhage, mazolysis) or to drugs (malformation, haemorrhage). Indirect damage is mainly caused by reduced hemoperfusion: *chronic* hypoperfusion can cause an IUGR, or *acute* with endouterine death. *Chronic* intrauterine hypoxia can provoke leukophthisis lesions, if *acute*, cerebral haemorrhage, permanent neurological damage, and intrauterine death.

The possible **damage to the new-born** can bring about premature birth, hypoxia, traumatic damage.

The low birth weight (2,200 g approx.) is evidence of the association of maternal pathology with foetal damage, above all in the case of premature delivery. The most-critical period in gestation seems to be around the 32nd-34th week, the average patient in ICU is in her 33rd week of pregnancy. The principal cause of premature delivery is not only low birth weight, despite the fact that this is a high risk factor, but intrauterine growth arrest as a result of hypoperfusion.

The three most-important determining factors as regards **perinatal mortality** in all studies are:

1. congenital anomalies;
2. low birth weight and very low birth weight (VLBW) (less than 2,500 and 1,500 g, respectively);
3. hypoxia.

The rate of perinatal mortality at the S. Anna Hospital is between 0.75% and 1.5% (Fig. 3). This is a great decrease compared to the 1960s (4.05%), with almost uniform results from beginning of the the 1990s (Fig. 3). From these data it can be seen that a reduction in perinatal mortality over the years is more evident all in VLBW infants (> 1000 g). Mortality remains high for lower birth weights, almost 80% in new-borns with birth weights lower than 500 g.

In the neonatal period the main causes of death were congenital anomalies (24%) and premature births (25%). It is also necessary to take into account morbidity. Another consequence of prematurity is cerebral palsy and severe or moderate encephalopathy in newborns with a birth weight less than 1,500 g. From a study by Badawi prevalence of encephalopathy in all newborns is 3.8% with 9.1% mortality. Thompson, draws attention to the fact that on examining the follow-up of 45 newborns with hypoxia at birth, 4 of these died within six months, 1 remained hospitalised; of the remaining 40, 58% developed normally, while 42% were affected by neurological sequelae. Besides, a study by Badawy states that only 10-15% of the cases of cerebral palsy are co-related to events which occurred during labour and delivery, therefore we most suppose that other causes can intervene during pregnancy.

Role of secondary and tertiary prophylaxis

The advancement in diagnostic techniques (ultrasonography, echodoppler, fetoscopy, etc.) and the improvement in resuscitation and neonatal assistance has brought about a remarkable and regular decrease in perinatal mortality since the 1960s, which is continuing throughout Europe.

It must be remembered that WHO has emphasized that the perinatal mortality rate is the most reliable and sensitive indication, not only of medical assistance but also of the socioeconomic changes that are taking place in a society (Zanetti et al., 1989).

As our knowledge has increased, we have become more and more aware that delivery is only the last of a series of events in which both foetus and mother participate. The necessity to make birth more humane and the requests for fewer drugs, which in western culture today is the case, have been tackled. The attempt to render delivery more "natural" depends on identifying with great precision those (mother and child) with a greater risk of morbidity and mortality. To this end, in the 1960s there was an attempt to create tables to quantify pregnancy risks, but this was abandoned by all, since it is extremely difficult to quantify risk.

Some maternal infections such as German measles, toxoplasmosis, or bacterial sepsis can be vertically transmitted and can be responsible for fetal malformation. A maternal disease can hinder fetal growth or, as in the case of diabetes, induce macrosomia. Defects like anomalous uterus conformation can impede normal placentation; cervix anomalies induce internal uterine orifice incompetence and premature delivery. Fibromas that can dislocate the uterus cause anomalies in the placentation process.

Life at a high altitude is one of the factors causing LBW. In a study conducted by Lubtchencho (Lubtchencho, 1993) approx. 30% of the babies delivered in Colorado above an altitude of 1,000 m were born with a LBW in comparison to the gestation period.

Other factors which can contribute to perinatal morbidity or mortality include exposure to environmental risks or risks in the work place, such as radiation or lead, and a poor level of maternal education.

Teratogenous agents and toxins can also play a role, even though somewhat minor, in perinatal damage in developed countries.

Meiotic and mitotic division errors can lead to chromosome anomalies and multiple pregnancies (especially caused by infertility treatment), both common in women over 30 years. Deaths due to lethal congenital malformation are now lower due to prenatal diagnosis, genetic advice and ensuing abortion.

Signs of neonatal risk, of maternal origin, in the peripartum

The placenta represents the only way of communication between mother and foetus and all the complex functions carried out through it are closely linked to the efficient function of the syncytiumtrophoblast, which is its active part.

Every factor, of endogenous or exogenous origin, which can alter the placental equilibrium leads irrevocably, during pregnancy, to a reduction in the maternal-fetal exchange area, with dramatic consequences for the fetus itself.

The placental blood flow can be influenced by different factors (cardiac output variations, contraction length, placental pathologies, etc.). The efficiency and stability of the maternal systolic pressure are essential for optimal placental perfusion. Every fall in blood pressure to below the minimum level necessary to guarantee adequate perfusion determines, inevitably, foetal asphyxia; if the hypotensive status is not rapidly corrected, it can lead to metabolic acidosis, with permanent damage, already evident at birth.

Signs of neonatal risk linked to drug administration during pregnancy

Drugs given to the mother can affect the fetus in two different ways:

- directly: with effects that appear after the drug passage though the placental barrier
- indirectly: by modifications which appear primitively in the maternal organism

Factors that regulate drug passage from mother to fetus are strictly dependent on Fick's law and particularly:

1. molecular liposolubility grade (the more liposoluble they are, the more easily they go through the placenta;
2. ionization grade (non-ionized drugs go through the placenta more rapidly);
3. concentration gradient (direct proportion between the drug concentration in the maternal circuit and the fetal circuit);
4. molecular weight (high molecular weight drugs go through the placenta with more difficulty).

Feto-neonatal effects of anesthesia

Fetal homeostasis and uterus-placental flux may be affected by any type of anesthesia or anesthetic agent, and effects also vary according to the dose and the way they are given. Fetal homeostasis conditions are of primary importance in anesthesiological evaluation, as hemodynamic modifications induced by even a short duration of drugs can, by modifying placental perfusion parameters, place a fetus already compromised by other causes at risk.

Most drugs used in anesthesia, including inhalation gas, pass through the placenta by simple diffusion. Inhalation agents, such as nitrous oxide, halothane, enflurane, and isoflurane, reach the fetal circuit by the same mechanism, but with different intensity of action, depending on their concentration. The cardiac and respiratory depressive effects on the newborn, even if moderate, can be of a high level.

Barbiturates, which fetal liver can not metabolize adequately, go through the placenta easily by lipidic diffusion. When fetal concentrations reach higher levels than in the mother (which is relatively frequent when intravenous thiobarbiturates are used) fetal resuscitation is often needed.

Also ketamine, even if its use in obstetric analgo-anesthesia is very rare, if given at a dosage higher than 1 mg/kg, can lead to neonatal respiratory depression and persistent crises of muscular rigidity.

The characteristic of opiates is that they depress respiratory function, and, although less, the cardio-circulatory function. The concentration of meperidine reaches higher levels in the fetus than in the mother after only 2 h, and common opiate antagonists are ineffective with meperidine. When the pattern is the result of the intense action of morphine-like drugs (fentanyl), however, the use of specific antagonists (naloxone) is efficacious.

Myorelaxant drugs, which have particular structural characteristics that delay passage through the placental barrier, atropine, neostygmine, and sedatives, if given at a correct, adequate dosage, do not have any important effects on the fetus.

The use of barbiturates as anesthetics, especially in high doses, can lead to a great drop in uterus blood flow, also interacting with the vasoactive agent response.

In the same way, inhalation agents like halothane can cause a significant reduction in uterine flux, lowering the vasoactive substance response, and thus induce fetal acidosis.

No significant data that can indicate compromises in fetal well-being and in placental perfusion have emerged from comparative studies (Cosmi EV) on the effects of thiopentone and propofol.

Regional anesthesia, both spinal and epidural, can induce a drop in maternal blood pressure and in uterine blood flux, causing fetal asphyxia. An adequate pre-hydration of the patient with an electrolytic solution and mechanical dislocation of the uterus can prevent maternal hypotension damage without having negative effects either on uterine placental flux or on maternal-fetal circulation, as demonstrated by the pulsatility index measured by uterus, umbilical and media cerebral artery level Doppler technique.

The use of *general anesthesia* is advisable in various conditions, like hypovolemia associated with hemorrhagic pathologies, situations of fetal stress, placenta previa, certain medical pathologies, and in all those situations that require rapid delivery. The most-appropriate technique must always depend on the condition of the mother and of the fetus; in addition, drugs which can interact with uterus-placental circulation must not be used.

In the choice of the type of anesthetic, it must be emphasized that there are serious complications that derive from the interaction between anesthetic agents and other drugs (myorelaxant, anti-inflammatory and anti-hypertensive drugs) and that it is necessary to be cautious so as to avoid unpleasant side-effects on the feto-placental unit.

References

Badawi N (1998) Intrapartum risk factors for newborn encephalopathy: the Western Australian case-control study. BMJ 317:1549

Margaria E (2000) La rianimazione primaria del neonato. Min. Anest. Atti 54° Congresso Nazionale SIAARTI, vol 66, n 9

Thompson CM (1997) The value of a scoring system for hypoxic ischaemic encephalopathy in predicting neurodevelopmental outcome. Acta Paedatr

Volpe JJ (1987) Brain injury in the premature infants. Anestesiology

LIVER, PANCREATITIS, COAGULATION

Function and Dysfunction of the Liver: An Overview

L.S. Crocè, I. Rigato, C. Tiribelli

The liver is a complex organ with many interrelated functions such as: 1) excretory and secretory function; 2) synthetic activity; 3) detoxification and drug metabolism; and 4) storage. Each function plays an important role in the overall homeostasis of the body, so that the partial or complete impairment of any of these is associated with important clinical entities.

Excretory and secretory function: bilirubin metabolism

Bilirubin, the principle pigment in bile, is derived from the breakdown of hemoglobin when aged red blood cells are phagocytosed by the reticuloendothelial system, primarily in the spleen, liver, and bone marrow. About 85% of bilirubin produced in the body daily is released from hemoglobin as a result of red blood cells destruction. The remaining 15% of bilirubin is produced from erythrocyte precursors destroyed in the bone marrow and from the catabolism of other heme-containing proteins, such as myoglobin, cytochromes, and peroxidases [1]. After it is produced in peripheral tissues, bilirubin is transported to the liver in association with albumin. Bilirubin is then taken up by hepatocytes across the sinusoidal membrane by a carrier-mediated, active transport process. Once inside the liver cells, bilirubin is conjugated with glucuronic acid (glucuronyl transferase) to produce bilirubin mono- and diglucuronide (conjugated bilirubin), which are then excreted into bile.

The impairment of any of these metabolic steps leads to a yellow coloration of the sclera and the skin, which has long been associated with liver dysfunction. The level of unconjugated bilirubin is rarely higher than 3.0 mg/dl, although a notable exception is newborn jaundice when bilirubin can reach 10-12 mg/dl. Although usually benign, newborn jaundice may complicate with the precipitation of bilirubin in certain portions of the brain (basal ganglia and cerebellum in particular) resulting in a severe and permanent neurological damage (kernicterus).

In contrast to unconjugated bilirubin, an increment in the level of conjugated bilirubin is more frequently encountered, and is usually associated with a parallel increment in the level of bile acids and lipids (cholesterol in particular) normally excreted in the bile. The conjugated bilirubin has been shown to be a prognostic indicator in conditions related to chronic cholestasis, such as primary biliary cirrhosis [2], and it has been used in the timing of liver transplantation in these patients.

Synthetic activity

Liver is capable of synthesis of proteins, carbohydrates, and lipids. Liver plays an important role in the synthesis of several plasma proteins, in particular albumin clotting factors, except factor VIII. This peculiar function of the liver has been used extensively in determining the degree of involvement in liver damage, both in acute and chronic conditions. In acute liver function, the serum level of albumin is of little diagnostic help, since the half life of this protein is relatively long (20 days). In these circumstances, the level of clotting factors, in particular prothombin and factor V [3], appears to be a good indicator of the extent of the damage and the possibility of recovery [4], and also indicates the need for liver transplantation [5]. In chronic liver disease, the prognostic utility of the clotting factors is greatly reduced and albumin has been demonstrated a better, more-reproducible and less-expensive marker of liver dysfunction. The value of the albumin determination has long been acknowledged by its inclusion in several scoring systems, such as the Child-Plough Score [6], used in clinical practice [7, 8].

Detoxification and drug metabolism

The liver plays a crucial and central role in the detoxification of several potentially harmful compounds, both endogenous and exogenous. Among the endogenous compounds, bilirubin is a key example of how conjugation of a water-insoluble molecule (unconjugated bilirubin) may result in a much more-soluble molecule, easily excreted by bile or urine (conjugated bilirubin). Among the most-important mechanisms in detoxification provided by the liver is the microsomal drug metabolizing system, where several different substances (drugs in particular) are converted to more-polar metabolites. It is important to take into account the possible reduction in metabolizing drugs when reduced liver function is present, since the administration of a standard dosage of drugs to these patients may result in several side effects due to their accumulation.

Storage

Liver is one of the major tanks of including the body, being metabolically equipped to store and release many substances, glucose, minerals (iron and copper), and vitamins. This explains why the accumulation of these substances, as in the case of glycogenosis or primary hemochromatosis, is closely related to damage of liver function. Conversely, the alteration of liver function by other causes (i.e., acute hepatitis) is associated with a decrease of glucose blood level that, in the case of acute liver injury, may have an important prognostic value.

Liver disease: how big is the problem?

Liver disease may occur for several reasons, although the two leading causes are viral infection and alcohol consumption. Both of these "toxic agents" may result in acute hepatic damage, although the vast majority of liver disorders are chronic. Thus, a better understanding of the number of liver disorders and their natural history is important to understand the need for specific treatments and preventive programs. Retrospective autopsy studies performed in Trieste indicated that the prevalence of cirrhosis is around 10% [9], and it is often associated with the development of hepatocellular carcinoma [10]. In Trieste, the large majority of deaths occur in hospital (80-90%) and more than 70% of these cases are autopsied, and thus, the autopsy samples provide a reliable picture of the various diseases in the population. Of not is the observation that when population screening studies are performed in the entire population, the percentage of clinically evident cirrhosis drops to 1.5% [11]. This indicates that in the vast majority (about 70%) of cases the presence of cirrhosis is an incidental finding at necroscopy, and the disease is symptom free. This is important since it indicates that chronic liver diseas is a major clinical and social problem, and that minor toxic damage (viral infection and/or administration of drugs) may acutely precipitate hepatic insufficiency if the liver is already damaged. It is not unusual in clinical practice for a severe reduction in liver function to be observed after standard treatments, questioning the role of the administered drug in hepatoxicitry.

Hepatitis C virus infection (HCV) is the most-common cause of chronic viral hepatitis in the Western world. Non-A, non-B (NANB) hepatitis, diagnosed before 1990, was revealed in the large majority of cases (roughly 70%) to be due to HCV [12], although the role of HCV infection in the development of chronic liver disease is still unclear. An increased incidence of NANB hepatitis was reported in the 1980s world wide [13, 14], which declined thereafter [15]. In contrast, the incidence of liver disease due to ethanol abuse was quite stable [16]. The natural history of HCV-related chronic liver disease is also still unknown, although it has been proposed that a period of three to four decades occurs from acute infection by blood transfusion [17, 18] or immunoglobulin administration

[19, 20] to the development of liver cirrhosis and hepatocellular carcinoma. To better understand the role of HCV in the development of cirrhosis, a retrospective study was recently perform in cirrhotic subjects who died between 1969 and 1994 to assess the presence of HCV infection. The overall HCV genome frequency was about 50%. Interestingly, the positivity was quite constant in the 1969-1979 period (35-38%), but sharply rose to 65 and 77% in 1984 and 1989, respectively to decrease to 50% in 1994 [21]. These findings indicate for the first time that a widespread HCV infection occurred around the late 1950s to early 1960s, thus supporting the hypothesis of a cohort effect.

It has been recognized for centuries that alcohol abuse is a major cause of both chronic and acute liver disease [22, 23]. A close correlation between the amount of alcohol consumed and the mortality from liver disease has been found [24]. In spite of intensive investigation, the exact molecular mechanism of alcoholic liver disease is still obscure. This is mainly due to the lack of a reliable animal model and to the difficulty in obtaining clinical series sufficiently large and homogeneous to draw sound conclusions. Many studies failed to clearly define the risk threshold dose of alcohol ingestion, and no clear information is available on the potential additional role of the type of alcoholic beverages and drinking habits. The Dionysos Study [11] provided hints on these clinically relevant questions. Multivariate analysis showed that the risk threshold for developing alcoholic liver damage was the ingestion of more than 30 g alcohol per day in both sexes. Using this threshold value, 21% of the population screened was at risk, although only 5.5% of these subjects showed persistent signs of liver damage [25]. This finding stresses that additional factors (most probably genetic) play an important role in determining the hepatic susceptibility to alcohol [26]. In those subjects drinking more than 30 g alcohol per day, the risk of developing liver damage increases with age and peaked after the age of 45 years. This study allowed the conclusion that a safe dose of alcohol exists, although it is rather small, being less that 30 g per day in both sexes equal to 3-4 glasses of wine, 2-3 pints of beer, or 2 drinks. Not only the amount but also the habit of drinking (consumption of alcohol with or outside meals) and the type of alcoholic beverage consumed are important factors in the development of alcohol-related liver damage.

Liver support and transplantation in liver failure

The need to support liver functions when the organ has been injured by acute damage has long been recognized, and is based on the observation that regeneration of liver cells may eventually overcome the insufficiency should the patient be given enough time for such an event. Several methods have been proposed, although to date the efficacy in reducing mortality and the need for transplantation has not been demonstrated.

Hemodialyisis has been suggested and is focussed on "blood detoxification". The removal of blood ammonia alone showed no improvement of survival, in spite of a significant improvement of mental status [27]. This technique is now almost abandoned. The same lack of efficacy was observed for hemofiltration [28], which is severely limited by thrombocytopenia, thus leading to bleeding in a patient with an already compromised clotting status. The use of exchange transfusion and plasmapheresis was also investigated [29, 30] but, in spite of a significant improvement in mental status, no effect on survival was observed. The same lack of clear beneficial effects was observed when blood was perfused on charcoal columns (charcoal hemoperfusion). Although an encouraging increase in survival rates of acute liver failure patients was reported [31], the lack of properly performed clinical trials prevents definitive conclusions.

Most recently, the use of hepatocytes isolated from pig [32] or human hepatoblastoma cell lines [33] has been proposed. These devices are grouped under the name of bioartificial liver (BAL). Although BAL seems to provide a more-rational approach to liver support in acute liver failure, present data are limited in term of efficacy and improved survival [34, 35]. This may be mainly attributable to the low hepatic mass of cells compared to normal liver, and to the lack of polarity of the cells. Thus BAL seems to have a possible indication as a "bridge to transplantation" rather than as the much more-desirable "bridge to regeneration". In the late 1970s a device was proposed in which a whole liver of baboon was used in cases with acute liver failure [36]. Although the first reports were encouraging, this technique has been abandoned for more that 25 years, but has reappeared recently [37]. This approach is more physiological and could provide an important means of reducing the need for liver transplantation, which is still the treatment of choice in cases of liver insufficiency [38].

References

1. Tiribelli C, Ostrow JD (1996) New concepts in bilirubin and jaundice: report of the Third International Bilirubin Workshop, April 6-8, 1995, Trieste, Italy. Hepatology 24:1296-1311
2. Murtaugh PA, Dickson ER, Van Dam GM et al (1994) Primary biliary cirrhosis: prediction of short-term survival based on repeated patient visits. Hepatology 20:126-134
3. Izumi S, Langley PG, Wendon J et al (1996) Coagulation factor V levels as a prognostic indicator in fulminant hepatic failure. Hepatology 23:1507-1511
4. Mitchell I, Bihari D, Chang R et al (1998) Earlier identification of patients at risk from acetaminophen-induced acute liver failure. Crit Care Med 26:279-284
5. O'Grady JG, Alexander GJ, Hayllar KM, Williams R (1989) Early indicators of prognosis in fulminant hepatic failure. Gastroenterology 97:439-445
6. Conn HO (1981) A peek at the Child-Turcotte classification. Hepatology 1:673-676
7. Shetty K, Rybicki L, Carey WD (1997) The Child-Pugh classification as a prognostic indicator for survival in primary sclerosing cholangitis. Hepatology 25:1049-1053
8. Propst A, Propst T, Zangerl G et al (1995) Prognosis and life expectancy in chronic liver disease. Dig Dis Sci 40:1805-1815

9. Giarelli L, Melato M, Laurino L et al (1991) Occurrence of liver cirrhosis among autopsies in Trieste. IARC Sci Publ 112:37-43
10. Tiribelli C, Melato M, Croce LS et al (1989) Prevalence of hepatocellular carcinoma and relation to cirrhosis: comparison of two different cities of the world. Trieste, Italy, and Chiba, Japan. Hepatology 10:998-1002
11. Bellentani S, Tiribelli C, Saccoccio G et al (1994) Prevalence of chronic liver disease in the general population of northern Italy: the Dionysos Study. Hepatology 20:1442-1449
12. Hoofnagle JH (1997) Hepatitis C: The clinical spectrum of disease. Hepatology 26:15S-20S
13. Seeff LB (1997) Natural history of hepatitis C. Hepatology 26:21S-28S
14. Alter MJ (1997) Epidemiology of hepatitis C. Hepatology 26:62S-65S
15. Margolis HS, Alter MJ, Hadler SC (1991) Hepatitis B: evolving epidemiology and implications for control. Semin Liver Dis 11:84-92
16. Corrao G, Ferrari P, Zambon A et al (1997) Trends of liver cirrhosis mortality in Europe, 1970-1989: Age-period- cohort analysis and changing alcohol consumption. Int J Epidemiol 26:100-109
17. Kiyosawa K, Sodeyama T, Tanaka E et al (1990) Interrelationship of blood transfusion, non-A, non-B hepatitis and hepatocellular carcinoma: analysis by detection of antibody to hepatitis C virus. Hepatology 12:671-675
18. Tong MJ, el Farra NS, Reikes AR, Co RL (1995) Clinical outcomes after transfusion-associated hepatitis C. N Engl J Med 332:1463-1466
19. Dittmann S, Roggendorf M, Durkop J et al (1991) Long-term persistence of hepatitis C virus antibodies in a single source outbreak. J Hepatol 13:323-327
20. Qu D, Li JS, Vitvitski L et al (1994) Hepatitis C virus genotypes in France: comparison of clinical features of patients infected with HCV type I and type II. J Hepatol 21:70-75
21. Stanta G, Croce LS, Bonin S et al (2000) Cohort effect of HCV infection in liver cirrhosis assessed by a 25 year study. J Clin Virol 17:51-56
22. Lieber CS (1994) Alcohol and the liver: 1994 update. Gastroenterology 106:1085-1105
23. Bouchier IA, Hislop WS, Prescott RJ (1992) A prospective study of alcoholic liver disease and mortality. J Hepatol 16:290-297
24. Grant BF, Dufour MC, Harford TC (1988) Epidemiology of alcoholic liver disease. Semin Liver Dis 8:12-25
25. Bellentani S, Saccoccio G, Costa G et al (1997) Drinking habits as cofactors of risk for alcohol induced liver damage. The Dionysos Study Group. Gut 41:845-850
26. Bellentani S, Saccoccio G, Masutti F et al (2000) Risk factors for alcoholic liver disease. Addiction Biol 5:261-268
27. Denis J, Opolon P, Nusinovici V et al (1978) Treatment of encephalopathy during fulminant hepatic failure by haemodialysis with high permeability membrane. Gut 19:787-793
28. Rakela J, Kurtz SB, McCarthy JT et al (1988) Postdilution hemofiltration in the management of acute hepatic failure: A pilot study. Mayo Clin Proc 63:113-118
29. Redeker AG, Yamahiro HS (1973) Controlled trial of exchange-transfusion therapy in fulminant hepatitis. Lancet 1:3-6
30. Matsubara S, Okabe K, Ouchi K et al (1990) Continuous removal of middle molecules by hemofiltration in patients with acute liver failure. Crit Care Med 18:1331-1338
31. O'Grady JG, Gimson AE, O'Brien CJ et al (1988) Controlled trials of charcoal hemoperfusion and prognostic factors in fulminant hepatic failure. Gastroenterology 94:1186-1192
32. Gerlach JC, Encke J, Hole O et al (1994) Hepatocyte culture between three dimensionally arranged biomatrix- coated independent artificial capillary systems and sinusoidal endothelial cell co-culture compartments. Int J Artif Organs 17:301-306
33. Ellis AJ, Hughes RD, Wendon JA et al (1996) Pilot-controlled trial of the extracorporeal liver assist device in acute liver failure. Hepatology 24:1446-1451
34. Riordan SM, Williams R (2000) Acute liver failure: targeted artificial and hepatocyte-based support of liver regeneration and reversal of multiorgan failure. J Hepatol 32:63-76

35. Shakil AO, Mazariegos GV, Kramer DJ (1999) Fulminant hepatic failure. Surg Clin North Am 79:77-108
36. Abouna GM, Cook JS, Fisher LM et al (1972) Treatment of acute hepatic coma by ex vivo baboon and human liver perfusions. Surgery 71:537-546
37. Abouna GM, Ganguly PK, Hamdy HM et al (1999) Extracorporeal liver perfusion system for successful hepatic support pending liver regeneration or liver transplantation: a pre-clinical controlled trial. Transplantation 67:1576-1583
38. Carithers R (2000) Liver Transplantation. Liver Transpl 6:122-135

Pathophysiology of Liver Dysfunction

N. Brienza

Hepatic involvement in the critical setting is chiefly secondary to shock states and/or multiple organ system failure. After severe shock, ischaemic hepatitis may ensue as a consequence of low oxygen delivery to the liver. Due to redistribution of flow to vital organs (heart, brain), during global DO_2 reduction splanchnic vasoconstriction is disproportionately greater than in other vascular beds, and this condition perpetuates even when normal systemic haemodynamics is reestabilished.

Liver receives 25-30% of total cardiac output from both the portal vein and the hepatic artery. As portal inflow and portal oxygen delivery are determined by intestinal flow and intestinal oxygen extraction, the liver can control its own flow only by modulating hepatic artery resistance and flow (usually supplying 75% of total hepatic oxygen delivery). When portal flow is reduced, such as during splanchnic vasocostriction, hepatic arterial resistance decreases and arterial flow increases, i.e. hepatic artery buffer response (HABR) [1]. Several experimental observations support the physiological role of HABR. During profound haemorrhage [2, 3] and hypoxia [4], the quantity of flow to each organ declines, but the fraction of cardiac output received by heart, brain and liver (through the hepatic artery) increases, while the fraction received by gut and kidney decreases. Nevertheless, in the setting of prolonged and marked shock states, liver hypoxia may ensue, striking centrolobular zones and causing ischaemic hepatitis with elevation of alanine and aspartate aminotransferases (ALT, AST). This process, even though it may predispose to subsequent liver dysfunction, is a self-limiting event and does not cause significant liver dysfunction.

More subtle is the other involvement of liver in critically ill patients, i.e. jaundice. Jaundice represents the classic hepatic alteration observed during multiple organ dysfunction in sepsis, and it is usually associated with high mortality. Differently from ischemic haepatitis, there is no marked alteration in plasmatic level of aminotransferase, i.e. there is no major liver damage. However, the absence of significant hepatocellular damage does not exclude the presence of liver dysfunction. Although classic liver failure is generally thought to be a late complication following pulmonary or renal failure [5], hepatic dysfunction, ranging from slight changes to frank hyperbilirubinaemia, is mild early after the onset of sepsis but is a progressive phenomenon [6]. Due to the major role in the metabolism and in the integration of the systemic response to inflammatory/septic stress, it is increasingly evident that the liver must be viewed as a critical determinant in the development of multiple organ failure. Therefore, it should be viewed not only as target of multiple organ dysfunction occurring during the septic process, but also as a co-factor in MODS pathogenesis.

Most experimental and clinical studies have demonstrated that during sepsis, the pronounced vasodilation of the hepatic artery without significant changes in portal flow allows global liver blood flow to be preserved or even increased. Nevertheless during sepsis, liver is characterized by a state of relative ischaemia, in that increased metabolic requirements are not matched by adequate increases in blood flow [7].

Even though global liver flow may be preserved, heterogeneity of microcirculation and of sinusoidal perfusion occurs. Sepsis increases portal and sinusoidal pressure, probably due to cell swelling and other sinusoidal alterations [8, 9] and, by endothelin-1 effects, activates Kupffer and Ito cells with sinusoidal obstruction. Most studies demonstrate that, independently from any change in global liver flow, sinusoidal perfusion is heterogeneous and this phenomenon is further magnified during stress condition with clear microcirculatory failure in some liver areas.

In experimental sepsis, liver dysfunction is depressed as early as 90 minutes after the onset of hyperdynamic state and persists during the late hypodynamic stage of sepsis [10]. This early dysfunction, as mentioned above, is not directly related to a significant decrease in absolute liver blood flow and cannot be corrected simply by increasing the volume of cristalloid resuscitation: even when cardiac output and hepatic microcirculation are significantly increased by volume resuscitation, depressed hepatocellular function is still occurring [11].

However, mainteinance of adequate blood inflow to liver is clinically relevant. Mainteinance of portal blood flow by dopexamine infusion during sepsis does not prevent structural destruction (as accounted for by increase in sinusoidal leukocytes, endothelial swelling and hepatocellular destruction) [12], but attenuates inflammatory reaction and ultrastructural changes when compared to placebo infusion [13].

Liver dysfunction during sepsis seems rather associated with increased plasma levels of inflammatory cytokines, such as TNF-α [10]. PMN activation by sepsis-related mediators may promote their adhesion to hepatic endothelium by intercellular adhesion molecules (ICAM-1), upregulated by cytokines and platelet activating factor. It is interesting to notice that circulating ICAM-1 levels in the early phase of septic shock are an early prognostic marker and facilitate identification of those patients with the highest risk of developing liver dysfunction, since they are higher in non-survivors than in survivors, and show a significant correlation with the highest serum bilirubin level observed in the 28 days following sepsis [14].

Diverse experimental evidence suggests that amplification of the above response activates expression of TNF-α mRNA in Kupffer cells, becoming a major source of inflammatory cytokine release. Kupffer cells, due to their position along the mainstream of splanchnic flow, receive a constant exposure to gut-derived mediators known to activate macrophages [15]. Among these mediators, the gut is a major source of norepinephrine release during sepsis, able to regulate Kupffer cell sensitivity by increasing TNF-α release [15]. Kupffer cell activation may promote production of oxygen free radicals, further cytokines, nitric oxide, and other mediators contributing to hepatic injury. Hepatocytes, when exposed to the effects of these mediators, will reduce cytochrome P-450-related drug metabolism [16] and specific hepatocyte metabolic pathways. As a matter of fact, endotoxin, interleukin-1, and TNF inhibit albumin synthesis and increase acute phase protein synthesis [17]. Moreover, liver dysfunction, when initiated, may perpetuate itself by promoting further hepatocyte injury due to increased bacterial translocation and Kuppfer cell phagocytic depression. Therefore, in absence of liver hepatocellular damage, hepatocellular dysfunction ensues.

Indocyanine-green (ICG) is cleared exclusively by hepatocytes in an energy-dependent membrane transport process [18]. The protein responsible for ICG transport is organic anion transporting protein-1 (OATP-1), whose levels are reduced following endotoxaemia [19]. When liver function is monitored by indocyanine green clearance, it becomes clear that it is depressed as early as 90 minutes after the onset of hyperdynamic sepsis. While ICG clearance explores the cholephilic organic anion transport function of hepatocytes, lidocaine clearance measures cytochrome P-450 enzyme system and represents another important monitoring tool of hepatocellular function.

Liver, mechanical ventilation and PEEP

During sepsis, ventilation may further produce liver alterations. Early studies reported that continuous positive-pressure ventilation decreased total hepatic blood flow mainly by reduction of portal venous flow. The splanchnic area is particularly sensitive to the effects of PEEP. Because of the combined effects of decreased cardiac output and increased outflow pressure. In addition, the effects of diaphragmatic swings may compress liver vasculature, futher compromising liver blood flow. It has been demonstrated that application of high PEEP levels reduces portal vein flow due to an increase in both backpressure to flow (related to increase in right atrial pressure) and resistance to flow [20]. While portal flow decreases, hepatic arterial resistance does not change, even though hepatic arterial buffer response is still active. The failure of hepatic arterial resistance to decrease in the presence of a decrease in portal flow means that HABR, during PEEP application, is counterbalanced by a constrictive action of PEEP on hepatic arterial bed [20]. Therefore, even though HABR is still active, a decrease in arterial flow is expected during PEEP ventilation, depriving the liver of richly oxygenated flow. This deprivation is further magnified by the occurrence of systemic hypoxia.

Hepatic dysfunction has been reported during mechanical ventilation with and without PEEP [21]. Low values of hepatic venous oxygen pressure and hepatic venous oxygen saturation have been observed during ventilation with PEEP 15 cm H_2O, suggesting liver hypoxia [22]. This was associated with a stimulated hepatic glucose production rate, a major determinant of hepatic oxygen consumption, accompanied by enhanced hepatic uptake and utilization of free fatty acids as fuel substrates [22]. However, Matuschak and Pinsky [23] showed that addition of PEEP did not influence indocyanin green clearance, postulating that increase in liver backpressure may counterbalance flow reduction by increasing trans-sinusoidal passage of diffusable substances and by enhancing their uptake. An increase of liver back pressure above a threshold value, instead of being beneficial, may be detrimental per se [24]. The effects reported by Matuschak and Pinsky may be different in the presence of lung injury. During lung injury states, a decrease in liver flow may be further enhanced by PEEP application with consequent alteration in lidocaine metabolism and hepatic function [25]. However, when total cardiac output is not decreased, PEEP by itself may not always have consistent effects on splanchnic blood flow and metabolism [26].

Liver dysfunction, a critical feature of ARDS, MODS, sepsis, and shock states [27], is initiated and propagated by a combination of both haemodynamic alterations and cellular dysfunction. Both are detrimental not only for the liver itself, but also for the overall integration of the global response to stress states [28].

References

1. Ayuse T, Brienza N, O'Donnell CP, Robotham JL (1994) Pressure-flow analysis of portal vein and hepatic artery interactions in porcine liver. Am J Physiol 267:H1233-H1242
2. Kaihara S, Rutherford RB, Schwentker EP, Wagner HN (1969) Distribution of cardiac output in experimental hemorrhagic shock in dogs. J Appl Physiol 27:218-222
3. Sapirstein LA, Sapirstein EH, Bredemeyer A (1960) Effect of hemorrhage on the cardiac output and its distribution in the rat. Circ Res 8:130-148
4. Adachi H, Strauss W, Ochi H, Wagner H (1976) The effect of hypoxia in the regional distribution of cardiac output in the dog. Circ Res 39:314-319
5. Fry DE, Pearlstein L, Fulton RL, Polk HC (1980) Multiple system organ failure: the role of uncontrolled infection. Arch Surg 115:136-140
6. Wang PA, Ba ZF, Chaudry IH (1997) Mechanism of hepatocellular dysfunction during early sepsis: key role of increased gene expression and release of proinflammatory cytokines tumor necrosis factor and interleukin-6. Arch Surg 132:364-370
7. Dahn M, Lange P, Lobdell K (1987) Splanchnic and total body oxygen consumption differences in septic and injured patients. Surgery 101:69-80
8. Brienza N, Ayuse T, Revelly JP et al (1995) Effects of endotoxin on isolated porcine liver: pressure-flow analysis. J Appl Physiol 78:784-792

9. Ayuse T, Brienza N, O'Donnell CP et al (1995) Alterations in liver hemodynamics in an intact porcine model of endotoxin shock. Am J Physiol 268:H1106-H1114
10. Wang PA, Chaudry H (1996) Mechanism of hepatocellular dysfunction during hyperdynamic sepsis. Am J Physiol 270:R927-R938
11. Wang P, Ba ZF, Ayala A, Chaudry IH (1992) Hepatocellular dysfunction persists during early sepsis despite increased volume of crystalloid resuscitation. J Trauma 32(3):389-396
12. Webb AR, Moss RF, Tighe D et al (1991) The effects of dobutamine, dopexamine and fluid on hepatic histological responses to porcine faecal peritonitis. Int Care Med 17(8):487-493
13. Tighe D, Moss R, Haywood G et al (1993) Dopexamine hydrocloride maintains portal blood flow and attenuates hepatic ultrastructural changes in a porcine peritonitis model of multiple system organ failure. Circ Shock 39(3):199-206
14. Weigand MA, Schmidt H, Pourmahmoud M et al (1999) Circulating intercellular adhesion molecule-1 as an early prognostic marker of hepatic failure in patients with septic shock. Crit Care Med 27(12):2656-2661
15. Koo DJ, Chaudry IH, Wang P (2000) Mechanism of hepatocellular dysfunction during sepsis: the role of gut-derived norepinephrine. Int J Mol Med 5(5):457-465
16. Ghezzi P, Saccardo B, Villa P et al (1986) Role of interleukin-1 in the depression of liver drug metabolism by endotoxin. Infect Immun 54:837-840
17. Hawker F (1991) Liver dysfunction in critical illness. Anaesth Intens Care 19:165-181
18. Chaudry IH, Schleck S, Clemens MG et al (1982) Altered hepatocellular active transport: an early change in peritonitis. Arch Surg 117:151-157
19. Lund M, Kang L, Tygstrup N et al (1999) Effects of LPS on transport of indocyanine green and alanine uptake in perfused rat liver. Am J Physiol 277:G91-G100
20. Brienza N, Revelly JP, Ayuse T, Robotham JL (1995) Effects of PEEP on liver arterial and venous blood flows. Am J Respir Crit Care Med 152:504-510
21. Hedley-Whyte J (1976) Effect of pattern of ventilation on hepatic, renal, and splanchnic function. In: Hedley-Whyte J (ed) Applied physiology of respiratory care. Little, Brown, Boston, pp 27-36
22. Schricker T, Kugler B, Schywalsky M et al (1995) Effects of PEEP ventilation on liver metabolism. Infusionsther-Transfusionsmed 22(3):168-174
23. Matuschak GM, Pinsky MR (1987) Effect of positive end expiratory pressure on hepatic blood flow and performance. J Appl Physiol 62:1377-1383
24. Higashiyama H, Yamaguchi M, Kumada K et al (1994) Functional deterioration of the liver by elevated inferior vena cava pressure: a proposed upper safety limit of pressure for maintaining liver viability in dogs. Int Care Med 20:124-129
25. Purcell PN, Branson RD, Schroeder TJ et al (1992) Monoethylglycinexylidide production parallels changes in hepatic blood flow and oxygen delivery in lung injury managed with positive end-expiratory pressure. J Trauma 33:482-486
26. Kiefer P, Nunes S, Kosonen P, Takala J (2000) Effect of positive end-expiratory pressure on splanchnic perfusion in acute lung injury. Int Care Med 26:376-383
27. Schwartz DB, Bone RC, Balk RA et al (1989) Hepatic dysfunction in the adult respiratory distress syndrome. Chest 95:871-875
28. Brienza N, Ayuse T, Revelly JP, Robotham JL (1998) Peripheral control of venous return in critical illness: role of the splanchnic vascular compartment. In: Dantzker DR, Scharf SM (eds) Cardiopulmonary critical care. WB Saunders, Philadelphia, pp 93-114

Acute Pancreatitis in the ICU

A.F. Hammerle, C. Tatschl

Acute pancreatitis in Western countries occurs with an estimated annual incidence of 10 new cases per 100 000 inhabitants [1]. A large variety of etiologic factors (including gallstones and other obstructive causes, alcohol, drugs, trauma, metabolic abnormalities, vascular abnormalities, infections, or inherited conditions) may initiate acute inflammation of the pancreas [2]. Whatever the cause, these conditions enter a final common pathway which results in the premature intracellular activation of trypsinogen and other digestive enzymes. In combination with reactive oxygen species, these enzymes damage the acinar cell. As a result cytokines and vasoactive mediators are released. Attraction of inflammatory cells and activation of the vascular endothelium result in perturbation of the pancreatic microcirculation. This in turn promotes the progression from edematous inflammation to necrotizing pancreatitis [3]. Although 80-90% of patients suffer from only mild disease, 10-20% progress to severe pancreatitis and have to be treated in an intensive care unit (ICU) [4].

Definitions

In September 1992, a group of 40 experts in the field of acute pancreatic inflammation were assembled at an international symposium in Atlanta in order to find a consensus regarding the terminology of acute pancreatitis and its complications. The results of this conference were published in 1993 [5].

Acute pancreatitis

Acute pancreatitis is an acute inflammatory process of the pancreas, with variable involvement of other regional tissues or remote organ systems. Clinically it is of rapid onset and is accompanied by upper abdominal pain. Acute pacreatitis is associated with variable abdominal findings, ranging from mild tenderness to rebound. It is often accompanied by vomiting, fever, tachycardia, leukocytosis, and elevated pancreatic enzyme levels in the blood and/or urine.

Mild pancreatitis

Mild pancreatitis is associated with minimal organ dysfunction and an uneventful recovery. It lacks the features defining severe acute pancreatitis (see below). The clinical course is uncomplicated in approximately 75% of cases. Patients with mild pancreatitis respond to appropriate fluid administration with prompt normalization of physical signs and laboratory values within 48-72 hours after the initiation of treatment.

Severe acute pancreatitis

Severe acute pancreatitis is associated with organ failure and/or local complications, such as necrosis, abscess, or pseudocyst. Severe acute pancreatitis is characterized by three or more Ranson criteria [6] or eight or more APACHE II (acute physiology and chronic health evaluation) points [7].

Organ failure is defined as shock (systolic blood pressure less than 90 mmHg), pulmonary insufficiency (PaO_2 60 mmHg or less), renal failure (creatinine level greater than 2 mg/dl after rehydration), or gastrointestinal bleeding (more than 500 ml/24 hours).

Acute fluid collections

Acute fluid collections occur early in the course of acute pancreatitis, are located in or near the pancreas, and always lack a wall of granulation or fibrous tissue. Acute fluid collections represent an earlier point in the development of acute pseudocysts or pancreatic abscess although most fluid collections regress.

Pancreatic necrosis

Pancreatic necrosis is a diffuse or focal area of nonviable pancreatic parenchyma, which is typically associated with peripancreatic fat necrosis. The onset of infection results in infected necrosis. Due to the differences in mortality and therapeutic consequences, the clinical distinction between infected and sterile necrosis is of importance.

Acute pseudocyst

A pseudocyst is a collection of pancreatic juice enclosed by a wall of fibrous or granulation tissue, which arises as a consequence of acute pancreatitis, pancreatic trauma, or chronic pancreatitis.

Pancreatic abscess

A pancreatic abscess is a circumscribed intra-abdominal collection of pus, usually in proximity to the pancreas, containing little or no pancreatic necrosis. It arises as a consequence of acute pancreatitis or pancreatic trauma.

General management of acute severe pancreatitis

Patients with severe acute pancreatitis should be managed in an intensive care unit with *full resuscitation* in order to prevent early deaths due to circulatory, respiratory and renal failures.

As a minimum, a peripheral venous access, a central venous line for fluid administration and CVP monitoring, a urinary catheter, and a nasogastric tube are recommended. A pulmonary artery catheter is required if cardiocirculatory compromise is a problem. Regular arterial blood gas analysis is necessary to detect hypoxia and acidosis. Radiological facilities should be available and dynamic computed tomography (CT) scanning should be performed in all patients with severe acute pancreatitis between 3 and 10 days of admission. Facilities to perform endoscopic retrograde cholangiopancreatography (ERCP) should be available [8].

Pain control is achieved with the injection of narcotic agents or by patient-controlled analgesia [9]. *Pharmacological treatments to put the pancreas at rest* (somatostatin, glucagon) or to oppose the action of proteases (aprotinin) are not recommended for the therapy of acute pancreatitis. It has been argued that such therapeutic approaches that directly interfere with the pathophysiologic process may always come too late due to the unavoidable lag between the onset of autodigestion and hospital admission. *Prevention of infection* of pancreatic necrosis is the most promising approach [10].

Infectious complications in acute pancreatitis

Relationship between extent of necrosis, infection and outcome

Infectious complications account for the majority of deaths resulting from acute pancreatitis. The organisms most frequently found to be the cause of pancreatic infection are *E. coli*, *Klebsiella*, *Enterococcus*, *Staphylococcus*, *Pseudomonas*, *Proteus*, aerobic *Streptococcus*, *Enterobacter*, and *Bacteroides*. Other organisms were less frequently detected [11]. It is believed that bacterial translocation from the colon is an important source for supervening infections in the course of acute pancreatitis [12].

The incidence of infection increases with duration of necrotizing pancreatitis with contamination rates of 25% after the first and 60% after the third week

[13]. Furthermore, other factors such as etiology seem to impact on the incidence and type of infection. Räty et al. [14] compared microbial isolates from patients with either biliary or alcoholic origin of acute pancreatitis. Pancreatic necrosis was more often infected in those patients with biliary pancreatitis than in the patients with alcoholic pancreatitis, even though the extent of necrosis did not differ. Gram-negative bacteria were rare in alcoholic pancreatitis but were frequently isolated in biliary pancreatitis. In patients suffering from alcoholic pancreatitis, Gram-positive bacteria were predominantly detected in necrotic material.

Isenmann and colleagues [15] evaluated the risk factors predisposing to organ failure in acute necrotizing pancreatitis in regard to the extent of organ destruction and the presence or absence of infection in 273 patients. Organ failure such as pulmonary insufficiency, sepsis/sepis-like syndrome or coagulopathy occured significantly more frequently if pancreatic infection was present. The incidence of infection significantly increased with the extent of necrosis. The overall incidence of organ failure increased with the extent of necrosis. However, the frequency of organ failure increased significantly with the extent of necrosis only in those patients with sterile necrosis. In the presence of infected necrosis the incidence of organ failure was high irrespective of the extent of necrosis. Patients with organ failure had a significantly higher mortality than those patients without.

The type of infection seems to be another important contributor to outcome. Luiten et al. [16] found that patients initially presenting with sterile necrosis had a 1.6-fold higher death rate if infection with *Gram-positive* organisms occured during the course of disease. However, if they acquired a *Gram-negative* pancreatic infection, mortality increased more than 14-fold. In patients with combined Gram-negative/Gram-positive infections, death rate was increased almost 16-fold. These results emphasize the hazards of Gram-negative infection in severe acute pancreatitis and give further rationale to the idea of antibiotic prophylaxis in these patients.

Clinical studies with prophylactic antibiotics in acute pancreatitis

For the use of antibiotics in the prevention of infection of necrotic tissue in acute pancreatitis, it is critical that the agent used covers the usual flora responsible. Furthermore, the agent has to penetrate into the pancreas in order to reach therapeutic levels.

The first study using such an antibiotic was performed by Pederzoli and colleagues [17]. In their study 74 patients were randomized to a control group or were given 0.5 g *imipenem* every 8 hours for 2 weeks. The prophylactic regimen reduced the incidence of pancreatic sepsis and sepsis of non-pancreatic origin significantly. However, this could not be translated into an improved outcome. The incidence of multiple organ failure, need for surgical intervention and mortality were not influenced by antibiotic prophylaxis.

Beneficial effects of *cefuroxime* in antibiotic prophylaxis were observed by Sainio and coworkers [18]. Patients in the antibiotic group received cefuroxime at a dose of 1.5 g three-times per day until clinical recovery and a fall of C-reactive protein concentrations to normal values. Patients were eligible if they had a C-reactive protein concentration above 120 mg/l within 48 hours of admission in addition to low enhancement of the pancreas on contrast-enhanced computed tomography. Control patients were given no antibiotics unless infection or a secondary rise in C-reactive protein occured. Significantly more infectious complications were observed in the non-antibiotic group than in patients on antibiotic prophylaxis. When infectious complications were analyzed according to the type of infection, only the difference in urinary-tract infection reached statistical significance. In addition, application of cefuroxime affected outcome in this study since it resulted in a significantly lower mortality in the treatment group.

Delcenserie et al. [19] evaluated antibiotic prophylaxis in patients with acute alcoholic pancreatitis in whom computed tomography demonstrated two or more fluid collections. Patients received either nonantibiotic treatment or *ceftazidime*, *amikacine*, and *metronidazole* as prophylactic antibiotics for 10 days. The incidence of pancreatic infection and septic shock was significantly higher in the group receiving no antibiotics. No infection occurred in patients who were given prophylactic antibiotics.

Ofloxacin and *metronidazole* were given as prophylactic antibiotics in the study by Schwarz et al. [20]. Thirteen patients with acute sterile necrotizing pancreatitis were assigned 200 mg ofloxacin and 500 mg metronidazole twice daily for two weeks. Antibiotics did not prevent bacterial infection of the necroses and no difference in the time to the occurrence of infection was observed. However, the clinical course differed significantly. APACHE II scores showed a significant improvement under antibiotic coverage, whereas the clinical course deteriorated significantly in the control group. No patient died under antibiotic treatment. By contrast, the mortality was 15% in controls.

Finally, Bassi and colleagues [21] compared the two antibiotics *perfloxacin* and *imipenem*. Patients with acute necrotizing pancreatitis with necrosis of at least 50% of the gland were given perfloxacin at a dose of 400 mg twice daily or were prescribed 500 mg imipenem three-times per day. Imipenem was significantly more effective in the prevention of infection but there was no difference in death rates between the two groups. However, the study was criticized because the antibiotic treatment regimen of 14 days might have been insufficient, given the severity of the necrosis (above 50%) [22].

Yet another approach was chosen by Luiten et al. [23]. This group evaluated the benefits of *selective decontamination* of the gut in patients with severe acute pancreatitis. Decontamination regimen consisted of oral and rectal administration of a combination of *colistin sulfate*, *amphotericin* and *norfloxacin*. However, the patients additionally were given a short-term systemic prophylaxis with cefotaxime until Gram-negative bacteria were eliminated from the oral cavity and rectum. Gut decontamination resulted in a significant decrease mainly in late mortality (i.e. after 2 weeks) which could be attributed to a significant decrease in Gram-negative infections. The use of systemic cefotaxime in this study has been a matter of criticism, because the clinical improvement might have been the consequence of the systemic antibiotic effect and not achieved by the agents used for the decontamination of the gut [24].

Although the results of clinical studies on the usage of antibiotic prophylaxis in severe acute pancreatitis are conflicting in terms of outcome, the reduction in infectious complications prompted a widespread acceptance of this therapeutic approach in the initial management of patients who are at risk of developing infection of the pancreatic necrosis. However, a substantial number of clinicians tend to apply antibiotics in all patients with acute pancreatitis, including those with mild disease who are not considered to benefit from this policy [25].

A frequently recommended regimen consists of imipenem or the combination of a quinolone and metronidazole. Antibiotics should be given until resolution or at least for two weeks [26].

Screening for infection

It is of critical importance not to miss the onset of infection in patients with severe acute pancreatitis. Infection of the gland changes therapy and requires surgical intervention [27]. *CT-guided percutaneus aspiration* and *Gram-stain* are helpful to establish the diagnosis of infection. A review of 377 patients who had undergone CT-guided percutaneous aspiration revealed that the method has a sensitivity of 96.2% and a specificity of 99.4% [28].

Recently Rau et al. [29] demonstrated that *procalcitonin* (PCT) might serve as a noninvasive early parameter for the detection of patients at risk of infected necrosis in whom further diagnostic work-up such as guided fine needle aspiration is mandated. In patients with infected necrosis, the overall PCT levels were significantly higher than in those with sterile necrosis, whereas C-reactive protein did not differentiate between the two conditions. Using a cut-off value for PCT concentration of 1.8 ng/ml, infected necrosis was predicted with a sensitivity of 95%, a specificity of 88%, and an accuracy of 90%.

Nutrition in acute pancreatitis

Much controversy exists concerning nutritional support in patients with acute pancreatitis. Patients with pancreatitis show metabolic alterations similar to those observed in septic patients [30]. The inflammatory response leads to increased resting energy requirements and loss of protein mass [31]. In addition, the nil per os status to rest the pancreas may lead to metabolic depletion. It is not clear, however, whether patients with acute pancreatitis profit from nutritional support, and if they do, which route of administration – i.e. total parenteral nutrition (TPN) or total enteral nutrition (TEN) – is to be prefered. In addition, there are no reliable data on when to reinstitute oral intake.

Total parenteral nutrition

Sitzman et al. [32] studied the role of TPN in 73 patients with acute severe pancreatitis. Of all the patients, 80% had abnormal nutritional indices, such as albumin, transferrin or total lymphocyte count, indicating that patients with acute severe pancreatitis represent a malnourished population. In addition, 80% of patients were able to achieve a positive nitrogen balance in two weeks with concurrent improvement in the parameters mentioned. In this study, patients who remained in negative nitrogen balance had a significantly (tenfold) increased mortality rate.

By contrast, Sax and collegues [33] found no benefit of parenteral nutrition in patients with mild disease. There was no difference in the number of days to oral intake, total hospital stay or number of complications between patients who were treated conventionally and those treated with parenteral support. Of note, the patients in the TPN group had a significantly higher rate of catheter-related sepsis when compared to contemporaneous patients without pancreatitis, who were on TPN.

Enteral or parenteral nutrition?

As previously mentioned, the colon is most likely the source of bacteria involved in the development of septic complications in patients with acute pancreatitis. Translocation of these organisms from the lumen of the gastrointestinal tract is the proposed mechanism. It has been demonstrated that TEN is superior to TPN in preserving the integrity of the gastrointestinal mucosal barrier [34], although it is clear that timing of initiation of enteral nutrition is critical in this context [35].

It is a particularity of acute pancreatitis that nutritional support should not stimulate the gland in order to prevent aggravation of the disease process. This problem may be overcome if enteral nutrition is applied via a nasojejunal tube that is placed below the level of the ligament of Treitz. This approach keeps the pancreas at rest as indicated by clinical experience. Patients who did not tolerate oral refeeding or those in whom the catheter is displaced into the stomach displayed resolution of symptoms and normalization of pancreatic enzymes when they were placed back on jejunal feeding or when the tube was replaced back into the jejunum [36].

Windsor et al. [37] randomized patients to receive either enteral or parenteral feeding. Following a 7-day period of *enteral nutrition*, there was a significant reduction in serum CRP and APACHE II scores, indicating conversion from severe to mild disease according to the Atlanta criteria. No such observations were made in the patients on parenteral nutrition. Furthermore, patients receiving parenteral nutrition exhibited an increase in anti-endotoxin antibodies and a fall in total antioxidant capacity, whereas enterally fed patients did not, indicating that parenterally fed patients had to face a higher degree of systemic exposure to endotoxin and experienced more oxidative stress. Of interest, these changes were not accompanied by changes of pancreatic injury on CT.

Kalfarentzos et al. [38] randomized patients with acute severe pancreatitis to receive enteral nutrition through a nasoenteric tube or to be treated with TPN. In this study enteral nutrition again was well tolerated. Patients with TPN experienced significantly more total complications and had a significantly increased risk of developing septic complications. Nutritional status was well maintained by enteral nutrition. Analysis of treatment costs revealed that TPN was associated with a 3-times higher financial burden.

Enteral nutrition versus conventional therapy

Although it seems likely that TEN is superior to TPN, data regarding the effectiveness of enteral nutrition per se are conflicting. In a study that is currently published only in abstract form, Powell and collegues [39] compared enteral nutrition to conventional therapy in patients with prognostically severe pancreatitis as evidenced by Glasgow [40] and APACHE II scores. In their study, enteral nutrition had no significant effect on serum anti-endotoxin core antibodies, serum interleukin 6 levels, serum soluble tumor necrosis factor receptor I, and serum C-reactive protein levels. No significant difference in organ dysfunction score was found between the groups. In addition, patients receiving enteral nutrition had worse intestinal function and tube dislodgement was common.

In contrast, in a preliminary report comparing enteral nutrition versus fluid administration in postoperative patients with acute pancreatitis, no difference in the pattern of bowel transit was found. Furthermore, patients in the fed group developed fewer complications and less patients died in this group [41].

In a recent article [42] reviewing the results of 100 clinical and experimental studies concerning the problem of nutritional support of patients with acute pancreatitis, the following conclusions were drawn:

- the diagnosis of acute pancreatitis is not itself an indication for the institution of artificial nutrition because there is no evidence that artificial nutritional support alters outcome unless the patient is malnourished;
- patients who are hypercatabolic and/or are unable to eat normally for more than 7-10 days should receive artificial nutritional support either parenterally or via the jejunum. In patients who are malnourished on admission, artificial nutrition should be introduced as soon as possible;
- unlike nasogastric or nasoduodenal feeding, parenteral nutrition and nasojejunal or jejunostomy feeds are well tolerated and do not stimulate pancreatic secretion.

When to start refeeding the patient?

Oral intake of nutrients may cause pain, nausea, vomiting and an increase in pancreatic enzymes. No data are currently available to indicate when the patient may receive oral nutrients without the hazard of recurrence of symptoms or aggravation of the disease process. The only study dealing with this clinical dilemma was published by Levy and colleagues [43]. The frequency of pain relapse during the refeeding period and the associated risk factors were investigated in 116 patients after a fasting period of at least 48 hours. The decision to start refeeding was left to the individual clinician responsible. Pain relapse occurred in one-fifth of the patients and mainly in those with long periods of pain, necrotic pancreatitis and elevated lipase concentrations just before refeeding. In these patients, the rate of recurrence of pain was found in almost 40%.

Therefore, the decision to reintroduce oral intake is mainly based on clinical judgement. The patient may be refed after relief of pain or abdominal tenderness and when bowel sounds have returned [9].

Conclusions

Acute severe pancreatitis is an indication for transfer to the ICU and requires a multidisciplinary approach. Due to aggressive use of ICU resources, mortality from cardiorespiratory deterioration is no longer the predominant problem in these patients. Rather, prevention of infection and septic complications is the main goal in modern therapy.

In this context prophylactic use of antibiotics and early nutritional support, especially using the jejunal route of administration, hold promise for the future to be added to the armamentarium to improve outcome.

However, it has to be stated that the data published so far are intriguing but not yet undisputedly convincing. Many clinicians feel that the rigorous use of potent antibiotics will further aggravate the appearance of microbial resistance, outweighing the potential benefit in patients with pancreatitis.

References

1. Secknus R, Mossner J (2000) Changes in incidence and prevalence of acute and chronic pancreatitis in Germany. Chirurg 71:249-252
2. Steinberg W, Tenner S (1994) Acute pancreatitis. N Engl J Med 330(17):1198-1210
3. Klar E, Werner J (2000) New pathophysiologic knowledge about acute pancreatitis. Chirurg 71:253-264
4. Uhl W, Isenmann R, Buchler MW (1998) Infections complicating pancreatitis: Diagnosing, treating, preventing. New Horiz 6[Suppl]:S72-79
5. Bradley EL 3rd (1993) A clinically based classification system for acute pancreatitis. Summary of the International Symposium on Acute Pancreatitis, Atlanta, Ga, September 11 through 13, 1992. Arch Surg 128:586-590

6. Ranson JH, Rifkind KM, Roses DF et al (1974) Prognostic signs and the role of operative management in acute pancreatitis. Surg Gynecol Obstet 139:69-81
7. Knaus WA, Draper EA, Wagner DP, Zimmerman JE (1985) APACHE II: A severity of disease classification system. Crit Care Med 13:818-829
8. – (1998) United Kingdom guidelines for the management of acute pancreatitis. British Society of Gastroenterology. Gut 42[Suppl 2]:S1-13
9. Banks PA (1997) Practice guidelines in acute pancreatitis. Am J Gastroenterol 92:377-386
10. Uhl W, Buchler MW, Malfertheiner P et al (1999) A randomised, double blind, multicentre trial of octreotide in moderate to severe acute pancreatitis. Gut 45:97-104
11. Lumsden A, Bradley EL 3rd (1990) Secondary pancreatic infections. Surg Gynecol Obstet 170:459-467
12. Marotta F, Geng TC, Wu CC, Barbi G (1996) Bacterial translocation in the course of acute pancreatitis: beneficial role of nonabsorbable antibiotics and lactitol enemas. Digestion 57:446-452
13. Beger HG, Rau B, Mayer J, Pralle U (1997) Natural course of acute pancreatitis. World J Surg 21:130-135
14. Raty S, Sand J, Nordback I (1998) Difference in microbes contaminating pancreatic necrosis in biliary and alcoholic pancreatitis. Int J Pancreatol 24:187-191
15. Isenmann R, Rau B, Beger HG (1999) Bacterial infection and extent of necrosis are determinants of organ failure in patients with acute necrotizing pancreatitis. Br J Surg 86:1020-1024
16. Luiten EJ, Hop WC, Lange JF, Bruining HA (1997) Differential prognosis of gram-negative versus gram-positive infected and sterile pancreatic necrosis: Results of a randomized trial in patients with severe acute pancreatitis treated with adjuvant selective decontamination. Clin Infect Dis 25:811-816
17. Pederzoli P, Bassi C, Vesentini S, Campedelli A (1993) A randomized multicenter clinical trial of antibiotic prophylaxis of septic complications in acute necrotizing pancreatitis with imipenem. Surg Gynecol Obstet 176:480-483
18. Sainio V, Kemppainen E, Puolakkainen P et al (1995) Early antibiotic treatment in acute necrotising pancreatitis. Lancet 346:663-667
19. Delcenserie R, Yzet T, Ducroix JP (1996) Prophylactic antibiotics in treatment of severe acute alcoholic pancreatitis. Pancreas 13:198-201
20. Schwarz M, Isenmann R, Meyer H, Beger HG (1997) Antibiotic use in necrotizing pancreatitis. Results of a controlled study. Dtsch Med Wochenschr 122:356-361
21. Bassi C, Falconi M, Talamini G et al (1998) Controlled clinical trial of pefloxacin versus imipenem in severe acute pancreatitis. Gastroenterology 115:1513-1517
22. Runzi M, Isenmann R (1999) News on antibiotic prophylaxis of necrosis infection in severe acute pancreatitis: The Italian viewpoint. Z Gastroenterol 37:765-767
23. Luiten EJ, Hop WC, Lange JF, Bruining HA (1995) Controlled clinical trial of selective decontamination for the treatment of severe acute pancreatitis. Ann Surg 222:57-65
24. Wyncoll DL (1999) The management of severe acute necrotising pancreatitis: An evidence-based review of the literature. Intens Care Med 25:146-156
25. Powell JJ, Campbell E, Johnson CD, Siriwardena AK (1999) Survey of antibiotic prophylaxis in acute pancreatitis in the UK and Ireland. Br J Surg 86:320-322
26. Laws HL, Kent RB 3rd (2000) Acute pancreatitis: Management of complicating infection. Am Surg 66:145-152
27. McFadden DW, Reber HA (1994) Indications for surgery in severe acute pancreatitis. Int J Pancreatol 15:83-90
28. Banks PA, Gerzof SG, Langevin RE et al (1995) CT-guided aspiration of suspected pancreatic infection: Bacteriology and clinical outcome. Int J Pancreatol 18:265-270
29. Rau R, Steinbach G, Baumgart K et al (2000) The clinical value of procalcitonin in the prediction of infected necrosis in acute pancreatitis. Intens Care Med 26: S159-164
30. Shaw JH, Wolfe RR (1986) Glucose, fatty acid, and urea kinetics in patients with severe pancreatitis. The response to substrate infusion and total parenteral nutrition. Ann Surg 204: 665-672

31. Havala T, Shronts E, Cerra F (1989) Nutritional support in acute pancreatitis. Gastroenterol Clin North Am 18:525-542
32. Sitzmann JV, Steinborn PA, Zinner MJ, Cameron JL (1989) Total parenteral nutrition and alternate energy substrates in treatment of severe acute pancreatitis. Surg Gynecol Obstet 168:311-317
33. Sax HC, Warner BW, Talamini MA et al (1987) Early total parenteral nutrition in acute pancreatitis: Lack of beneficial effects. Am J Surg 153:117-124
34. Hadfield RJ, Sinclair DG, Houldsworth PE, Evans TW (1995) Effects of enteral and parenteral nutrition on gut mucosal permeability in the critically ill. Am J Respir Crit Care Med 152:1545-1548
35. Kompan L, Kremzar B, Gadzijev E, Prosek M (1999) Effects of early enteral nutrition on intestinal permeability and the development of multiple organ failure after multiple injury. Intens Care Med 25:157-161
36. McClave SA, Greene LM, Snider HL et al (1997) Comparison of the safety of early enteral vs parenteral nutrition in mild acute pancreatitis. JPEN J Parenter Enteral Nutr 21:14-20
37. Windsor AC, Kanwar S, Li AG et al (1998) Compared with parenteral nutrition, enteral feeding attenuates the acute phase response and improves disease severity in acute pancreatitis. Gut 42:431-435
38. Kalfarentzos F, Kehagias J, Mead N et al (1997) Enteral nutrition is superior to parenteral nutrition in severe acute pancreatitis: Results of a randomized prospective trial. Br J Surg 84:1665-1669
39. Powell JJ, Hill G, Storey S et al (1999) Phase II randomised controlled trial of early enteral nutrition in predicted severe acute pancreatitis. Gastroenterology 116[Suppl]:A1342
40. Blamey SL, Imrie CW, O'Neill J et al (1984) Prognostic factors in acute pancreatitis. Gut 25:1340-1346
41. Pupelis G, Austrums E, Jansone A et al (2000) Randomised trial of safety and efficacy of postoperative enteral feeding in patients with severe pancreatitis: Preliminary report. Eur J Surg 166:383-387
42. Lobo DN, Memon MA, Allison SP, Rowlands BJ (2000) Evolution of nutritional support in acute pancreatitis. Br J Surg 87:695-707
43. Levy P, Heresbach D, Pariente EA et al (1997) Frequency and risk factors of recurrent pain during refeeding in patients with acute pancreatitis: A multivariate multicentre prospective study of 116 patients. Gut 40:262-266

Management of Consumption Coagulopathy

M. LEVI

A consumption coagulopathy is defined as a derangement of the coagulation system as a consequence of massive and systemic activation. Due to ongoing consumption and subsequent exhaustion of platelets and plasma coagulation proteins, thrombocytopenia and coagulation factor deficiencies occur, which may ultimately lead to bleeding. Hence, although bleeding may be the presenting symptom, a consumption coagulopathy is in fact the result of a prothrombotic state. Indeed, simultaneously with bleeding (or a bleeding tendency) widespread intravascular thrombotic obstruction of mid-size and small vessels occurs, which may contribute to organ failure. The appreciation of this mechanism is illustrated by synonyms for consumption coagulopathy, such as 'disseminated intravascular coagulation' (DIC) or 'systemic thrombo-hemorrhagic disorder' [1-3]. Obviously, the presentation of a simultaneously occurring thrombotic and bleeding problem in a patient can complicate proper treatment strategies.

Although there is no general consensus regarding the definition of consumption coagulopathy or DIC, the subcommittee on DIC of the International Society on Thrombosis and Hemostasis (ISTH) has proposed the use of the following definition: "DIC is an acquired syndrome characterized by the intravascular activation of coagulation with loss of localization of response arising from different causes. It can originate from and cause damage to the microvasculature, which if sufficiently severe, can produce organ dysfunction".

Clinical conditions associated with consumption coagulopathy

Consumption coagulopathy may complicate a variety of clinical disorders, of which the most important are the following. Bacterial *infection*, in particular severe sepsis, is the most-common entity associated with DIC [1, 3]. In addition, systemic infections with any other microorganism, such as viruses and parasites, may lead to the occurrence of DIC. A common pathogenetic feature of DIC as a result of severe infection is the generalized inflammatory response, characterized by the systemic release of cytokines [5].

Severe *trauma* is another clinical condition frequently associated with consumption coagulopathy [6, 7]. A combination of mechanisms, including release of tissue material in the circulation (fat, phospholipids), hemolysis, and endothelial damage, may contribute to the systemic activation of coagulation. In particular, in head trauma patients local and systemic coagulation activation is detectable, which may be understandable in view of the relatively large amount of tissue factor in the cerebral compartment.

Both *solid tumors and hematological malignancies* may be complicated by a consumption coagulopathy. The mechanism of the derangement of the coagulation system in this situation is poorly understood. However, most studies indicate that tissue factor, potentially expressed on the surface of tumor cells, is implicated [9]. A distinct form of DIC is frequently encountered in acute promyelocytic leukemia, which is characterized by a severe hyperfibrinolytic state on top of an activated coagulation system [10]. Although clinical bleeding predominates in this situation, disseminated thrombosis is found in a considerable number of patients with acute promyelocytic leukemia at autopsy.

An acute and classical form of consumption coagulopathy occurs in *obstetric emergencies* such as placental abruption and amniotic fluid emboli [13]. Amniotic fluid has been shown to be able to activate coagulation in vitro, and the degree of placental separation correlates with the extent of DIC, suggesting that leakage of thromboplastin-like material from the placental system is responsible for the occurrence of DIC. The most-common obstetric complication associated with activation of blood coagulation is eclampsia and the HELLP (hemolysis, elevated liver enzymes, and low platelets) syndrome [11]. This latter situation, however, is characterized by a microangiopathic hemolytic anemia with secondary changes in the coagulation system, a situation that is related to, but clearly distinct from DIC.

Vascular disorders, such as large aortic aneurysms or giant hemangiomas (Kasabach-Merrit syndrome), may result in local activation of coagulation [12]. Activated coagulation factors can ultimately "overflow" to the systemic circulation and cause a consumption coagulopathy, but more common is the systemic depletion of coagulation factors and platelets as a result of local consumption. This may result in a clinical condition that is hardly distinguishable from DIC.

Pathogenesis of consumption coagulopathy

In recent years the mechanisms involved in the pathological systemic fibrin deposition in DIC have become increasingly clear. Enhanced fibrin formation is caused by tissue factor-mediated thrombin generation and simultaneously occurring dysfunction of inhibitory mechanisms, such as the antithrombin system and the protein C and S system. In addition to enhanced fibrin formation, fibrin removal is impaired due to depression of the fibrinolytic system. This impairment of endogenous thrombolysis is mainly caused by high circulating levels of plasminogen activator inhibitor-1 (PAI-1). In a later stage of DIC, fibrinolytic activity may be increased and contribute to bleeding. The derangement of coag-

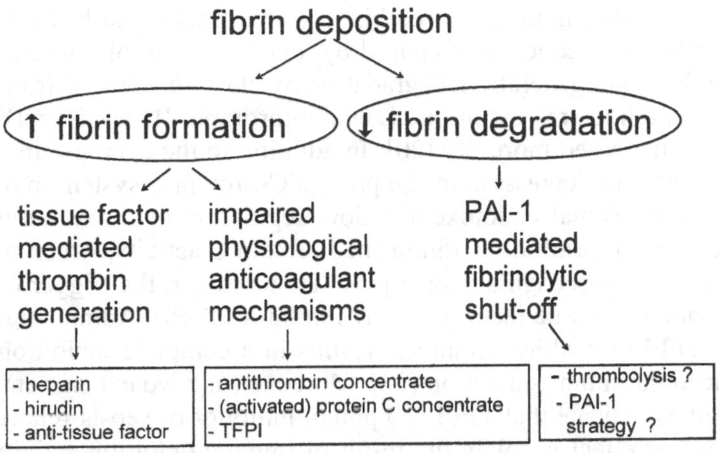

Fig. 1. Schematic representation of the pathogenesis of consumption coagulopathy and the currently available or future therapeutic options that may be used for each of these pathways (*PAI-1* plasminogen activator inhibitor-1)

ulation and fibrinolysis is mediated by several cytokines, in particular in the case of DIC associated with infectious disease, but probably also in most other clinical conditions associated with DIC.

Activation of blood coagulation in DIC

In all experimental models, thrombin generation is detectable at 3-5 h after the infusion of microorganisms or endotoxin [14, 15]. Several lines of evidence point to a pivotal role of the tissue factor/factor VIIa system in the initiation of thrombin generation. Firstly, experiments of human endotoxemia or in humans infused with the pro-inflammatory cytokine tumor necrosis factor (TNF) did not show any change in markers for activation of the contact system [16]. In line with this observation, inhibition of the contact system did not prevent activation of coagulation in bacteremic baboons [17]. Furthermore, abrogation of the tissue factor/factor VII(a) pathway by monoclonal antibodies specifically directed against tissue factor or factor VIIa activity resulted in a complete inhibition of thrombin generation in endotoxin-challenged chimpanzees and prevented the occurrence of DIC and mortality in baboons that were infused with Escherichia coli [18, 19].

Suppression of physiological anticoagulant pathways and impaired fibrinolysis

An impaired function of various natural regulating pathways of coagulation activation may contribute to the fibrin formation. Plasma levels of the most-important inhibitor of thrombin, antithrombin III, are usually markedly reduced in septic patients. This reduction is caused by a combination of consumption, due to ongoing thrombin generation, degradation by elastase released from activated neutrophils, and impaired synthesis. Low antithrombin III levels in DIC are associated with increased mortality [20]. In addition to the decrease in antithrombin III, a significant depression of the protein C-protein S system may occur. In models of experimental endotoxemia, downregulation of thrombomodulin has been demonstrated, resulting in diminished protein C activity, which may potentially enhance the procoagulant state [21]. Tissue factor, the trigger of coagulation, is inhibited by tissue factor pathway inhibitor (TFPI). Administration of recombinant TFPI to healthy volunteers results in a complete inhibition of endotoxin-induced thrombin generation [22]. Moreover, in vivo experiments in lethal baboon models indicate that TFPI is a potent inhibitor of sepsis-related mortality. Whether this effect is solely the result of impaired clotting activity remains uncertain. In contrast to other coagulation inhibitors, acquired deficiencies of TFPI have not been observed, and DIC is in general associated with only modestly reduced levels, or even increased concentrations of TFPI.

Experimental models indicate that at the time of maximal activation of coagulation, the fibrinolytic system is largely shut off. Experimental bacteremia and endotoxemia results in a rapidly occurring increase in fibrinolytic activity, most probably due to the release of plasminogen activators from endothelial cells. This pro-fibrinolytic response is almost immediately followed by a suppression of fibrinolytic activity, due to a sustained increase in plasma levels of PAI-1 [23].

Cytokines

The derangement of coagulation and fibrinolysis is mediated by several pro-inflammatory cytokines, such as TNF-α, interleukin-1 (IL-1), and IL-6 (IL-6). The principal mediator of coagulation activation in DIC appears to be IL-6 [24]. TNF-α indirectly influences the activation of coagulation, due to its effects on IL-6, and TNF-α is the pivotal mediator of the dysregulation of the physiological anticoagulant pathways and the fibrinolytic defect [25]. Anti-inflammatory cytokines, such as IL-10, may modulate the activation of coagulation, as it was shown that administration of recombinant IL-10 to humans was able to completely abrogate the endotoxin-induced effects on coagulation [26].

Diagnosis of consumption coagulopathy in routine clinical settings

There is no single test to accurately assess the diagnosis of DIC in an individual patient. However, a combination of a clinical condition that may be complicated by consumption coagulopathy with a number of laboratory results will establish the presence of DIC with an acceptable level of certainty. Some novel laboratory tests (such as assays for soluble fibrin) will become available soon and may be helpful in the diagnosis; however, most of the newer tests are presently available in specialized laboratories only. In these circumstances a diagnosis of consumption coagulopathy may be made by a combination of platelet count, measurement of global clotting times (activated partial thromboplastin time and prothrombin time), measurement of antithrombin III and/or 1 or 2 clotting factors, and a test for fibrin degradation products [2]. It should be emphasized that generally serial coagulation tests are more helpful than single laboratory results in establishing the diagnosis DIC. A reduction in the platelet count or a clear downward trend on subsequent measurements is a sensitive (though not specific) sign of DIC. The prolongation of global clotting times may reflect the consumption and depletion of various coagulation factors, which potentially may be further substantiated by the measurement of one or two selected coagulation factors. The accuracy of one-stage clotting assays in patients with consumption coagulopathy has, however, been contested.

Measurement of antithrombin III has the additional advantage of specifically assessing the consumption of the most-important inhibitor of thrombin. Measurement of fibrinogen has often been advocated, but is not very helpful in diagnosing DIC in most cases. Fibrinogen acts as an acute-phase reactant and, despite ongoing consumption, plasma levels can remain well within the normal range for a long period of time. In a consecutive series of patients, the sensitivity of a low fibrinogen level for the diagnosis of DIC was only 28% and hypofibrinogenemia was detected in very severe cases of DIC only. Tests for fibrin degradation products (such as FDPs or D-dimer) may be helpful to differentiate from other conditions that may be associated with a low platelet count and prolonged clotting times.

Current and future treatment of consumption coagulopathy

Several issues regarding the proper management of patients with consumption coagulopathy remain controversial. These controversies are based on the fact that due to the complexity of the clinical presentation of the syndrome, the variable and unpredictable course, and the either subtle or catastrophic clinical consequences of the presence of consumption coagulopathy, properly conducted clinical trials on consumption coagulopathy treatment are few. Besides, the clinical picture of a patient with widespread thrombotic deposition in small vessels of various organs on the one hand, and bleeding due to consumption and subsequent depletion of platelets and coagulation factors on the other hand, does not directly guide the physician to specific therapies for this condition. However, despite all these complicating circumstances, it is well established that the cornerstone of consumption coagulopathy treatment is the specific and vigorous treatment of the underlying disorder. In some cases, the DIC will completely resolve within hours after the resolution of the underlying condition (for example in cases of consumption coagulopathy induced by abruptio placentae and amniotic fluid embolism). However, in other cases, such as DIC in patients with sepsis and a systemic inflammatory response syndrome, DIC may be present for a number of days, even after proper treatment has been initiated. In these patients, supportive measures to manage the consumption coagulopathy may be necessary. Briefly, these interventions may consist of plasma and platelet substitution therapy, anticoagulant strategies, or administration of physiological coagulation inhibitors.

Plasma and platelet substitution therapy

Low levels of platelets and coagulation factors may increase the risk of bleeding. However, plasma or platelet substitution therapy should not be instituted on the basis of laboratory results alone, but is only indicated in patients with active bleeding and in those requiring an invasive procedure or otherwise at risk for bleeding complications [27]. The suggestion that administration of blood components might add "fuel to the fire" has, in fact, never been proven in clinical or experimental studies [1]. The efficacy of treatment with plasma or platelets has not been proven in randomized controlled trials, but appears to be a rational therapy in bleeding patients or in patients at risk for bleeding with a significant depletion of these elements.

Anticoagulants and improvement of fibrinolysis

Experimental studies have shown that *heparin* can at least partly inhibit the activation of coagulation in sepsis and other causes of DIC [28]. Uncontrolled case series in patients with consumption coagulopathy claimed to be successful. However, a beneficial effect of heparin on clinically important outcome events in patients with consumption coagulopathy has never been demonstrated in controlled clinical trials [29, 30]. Also, the safety of heparin treatment is debatable in consumption coagulopathy patients that are prone to bleeding. On the other hand, most patients with DIC should receive adequate prophylaxis to prevent venous thromboembolism [31], which may be achieved with low-dose heparin. In view of that, there is a case for administering subcutaneous heparin or maybe even intravenous low-dose heparin to patients with DIC. Higher doses of heparin should be reserved for patients with clinically overt thromboembolism or extensive fibrin deposition, like purpura fulminans or acral ischemia [30].

Theoretically, the most-logical anticoagulant agent to use in DIC is directed against tissue factor activity. Recently, a potent and specific inhibitor of the ternary complex between tissue factor/factor VIIa and factor Xa has been developed [33]. This agent (rNAPc2) is derived from the family of nematode anticoagulant proteins (NAPs), which originally have been isolated from hematophagous hookworm nematodes. At present, rNAPc2 is being investigated in phase II/III clinical studies, including a study in DIC patients.

Thrombolytic therapy may potentially overcome the suppression of the fibrinolytic system. However, the bleeding risk associated with these agents is very large, which seriously hampers their clinical application in patients with a consumption coagulopathy. Theoretically, inhibitors of PAI-1 may be a good therapeutic option; however, such agents are not yet available.

Coagulation inhibitor concentrates

Since antithrombin III is one of the most-important physiological inhibitors of coagulation and antithrombin III treatment showed promising results in animal models of DIC, the use of antithrombin III concentrates in patients with DIC has been studied relatively intensively. There are a number of controlled clinical trials on the use of antithrombin concentrates in DIC patients. Most of these trials concern patients with sepsis and/or septic shock. All trials show some beneficial effect in terms of improvement of a DIC score, shortening of the duration of DIC, or even improvement in organ function. In the more-recent clinical trials very high doses of antithrombin concentrate to attain supraphysiological plasma levels were used and the beneficial results in these trials seem to be more distinct. Some trials showed a modest reduction in mortality in antithrombin-treated patients, however, the effect did not reach statistical significance. If one, however, performs a meta-analysis on the effect of antithrombin III treatment on mortality in the trials [34-37], a statistically significant reduction in mortality (from 47% to 32%) is observed (odds ratio 0.59, 95% confidence interval 0.39-0.87). It is not clear from the literature which patients will benefit most from antithrombin III treatment in terms of clinically important outcomes (such as mortality or organ failure).

Depression of the protein C system may significantly contribute to the pathophysiology of consumption coagulopathy, and clinical observations suggest that this is associated with a fatal outcome. Hence, supplementation of *protein C* might potentially be of benefit in patients with DIC. A favorable effect of the administration of protein C concentrate in experimental animals with DIC lends support to this notion. There are some reports of successful treatment with protein C concentrates in patients with DIC, but adequately controlled clinical trials are not available. Finally, in view of the pivotal role of tissue factor in the initiation of thrombin generation in DIC, administration of (recombinant) *tissue factor pathway inhibitor (TFPI)* might prove to be of benefit [22].

Acknowledgements. This article is adapted from the paper "Disseminated Intravascular Coagulation: state-of-the-art", presented at the XIVth Congress of the International Society of Thrombosis and Hemostasis (ISTH), Washington 1999 (Thromb Haemostas 1999; 82:695-705) and "Disseminated Intravascular Coagulation: current concepts", N

Engl J Med 1999; 341:586-592. M.L. is an investigator of the Royal Dutch Academy of Arts and Sciences.

References

1. Marder VJ, Martin SE, Francis CW et al (1987) Consumptive thrombohemorrhagic disorders. In: Colman RW, Hirsh J, Marder VJ, Salzman EW (eds) Hemostasis and thrombosis. Basic principles and clinical practice. Lippincott, Philadelphia, pp 975-1015
2. Levi M, ten Cate H (1999) Disseminated intravascular coagulation: current concepts. N Engl J Med 341:586-592
3. Baglin T (1996) Disseminated intravascular coagulation: Diagnosis and treatment. BMJ 312: 683-687
4. Müller-Berghaus G, Madlener K, Blombäck M et al (eds) (1993) DIC. Pathogenesis, diagnosis and therapy of disseminated intravascular fibrin formation. Elsevier Science Publishers BV, Amsterdam
5. Levi M, van der Poll T, ten Cate H et al (1997) The cytokine-mediated imbalance between coagulant and anticoagulant mechanisms in sepsis and endotoxemia. Eur J Clin Invest 27:3-9
6. Bick RL (1992) Disseminated intravascular coagulation: a common complication of trauma and shock. In: Borris LC, Lassen MR, Bergqvist D (eds) The traumatized patient. Romer Grafik, pp 33-53
7. Gando S, Kameue T, Nanzaki S et al (1996) Disseminated intravascular coagulation is a frequent complication of systemic inflammatory response syndrome. Thromb Haemost 75: 224-228
8. Roumen JMH, Hendriks T, van der Ven J et al (1993) Cytokine patterns in patients after major vascular surgery, haemorrhagic shock, and severe blunt trauma. Ann Surg 6:769-776
9. Contrino J, Hair G, Kreutzer D et al (1996) In situ detection of expression of tissue factor in vascular endothelial cells: correlation with the malignant phenotype of human breast tissue. Nat Med 2:209-215
10. Falanga A, Consonni R, Marchetti M et al (1998) Cancer procoagulant and tissue factor are differently modulated by all-trans-retinoic acid in acute promyelocytic leukemia cells. Blood 92:143-151
11. Martin JN, Stedman CM (1991) Imitators of preeclampsia and HELLP syndrome. Obstet Gynecol Clin North Am 18:181-198
12. Gibney EJ, Bouchier-Hayes D (1990) Coagulopathy and abdominal aortic aneurysm. Eur J Vasc Surg 4:557-562
13. Ruggenenti P, Lutz J, Remuzzi G (1997) Pathogenesis and treatment of thrombotic microangiopathy. Kidney Int 58:S97-101
14. van Deventer SJH, Büller HR, Ten Cate JW et al (1990) Experimental endotoxemia in humans: analysis of cytokine release and coagulation, fibrinolytic, and complement pathways. Blood 76:2520-2526
15. Taylor FB Jr (1993) Role of tissue factor in the coagulant and inflammatory response to LD100 E. coli sepsis and in the early diagnosis of DIC in the baboon. In: Muller-Berghaus GM, Madlener K, Blomback M, ten Cate JW (eds) DIC. Pathogenesis, diagnosis and therapy of disseminated intravascular fibrin formation. Excerpta Medica, Amsterdam, pp 19-32
16. van der Poll T, Buller HR, ten Cate H et al (1990) Activation of coagulation after administration of tumor necrosis factor to normal subjects. N Engl J Med 322:1622-1627
17. Pixley RA, de la Cadena R, Page J et al (1993) The contact system contributes to hypotension but not disseminated intravascular coagulation in lethal bacteremia: in vivo use of a monclonal anti-factor XII antibody to block contact activation in baboons. J Clin Invest 92:61-68

18. Levi M, ten Cate H, Bauer KA et al (1994) Inhibiton of endotoxin-induced activation of coagulation and fibrinolysis by pentoxifylline or by a monoclonal anti-tissue factor antibody in a chimpanzee model. J Clin Invest 93:114-120
19. Biemond BJ, Levi M, ten Cate H et al (1995) Complete inhibition of endotoxin-induced coagulation activation in chimpanzees with a monclonal antibody to factor VII/VIIa. Thromb Haemost 73:223-228
20. Fourrier F, Chopin C, Goudemand J et al (1992) Septic shock, multiple organ failure, and disseminated intravascular coagulation. Compared patterns of antithrombin III, protein C, and protein S deficiencies. Chest 101:816-823
21. Conway EM, Rosenberg RD (1988) Tumor necrosis factor suppresses transcription of the thrombomodulin gene in endothelial cells. Mol Cell Biol 8:5588-5592
22. de Jonge E, Dekkers PEP, Creasey AA et al (1999) Tissue factor pathway inhibitor (TFPI) dose-dependently inhibits coagulation activation without influencing the fibrinolytic and cytokine response during human endotoxemia. Blood (in press)
23. Biemond BJ, Levi M, ten Cate H et al (1995) Endotoxin-induced activation and inhibition of the fibrinolytic system: effects of various interventions in the cytokine and coagulation cascades in experimental endotoxemia in chimpanzees. Clin Sci (Colch) 88:587-594
24. van der Poll T, Levi M, Hack CE et al (1994) Elimination of interleukin 6 attenuates coagulation activation in experimental endotoxemia in chimpanzees. J Exp Med 179:1253-1259
25. van der Poll T, Levi M, van Deventer SJH et al (1994) Differential effects of anti-tumor necrosis factor monoclonal antibodies on systemic inflammatory responses in experimental endotoxemia in chimpanzees. Blood 83:446-451
26. Pajkrt D, van der Poll T, Levi M et al (1997) Interleukin-10 inhibits activation of coagulation and fibrinolysis during human endotoxemia. Blood 89:2701-2705
27. Alving BM, Spivak JL, DeLoughery TG (1998) Consultative hematology: hemostasis and transfusion issues in surgery and critical care medicine. In: McArthur JR, Schechter GP, Schrier SL (eds) Hematology. The American Society of Hematology, pp 320-341
28. du Toit HJ, Coetzee AR, Chalton DO (1991) Heparin treatment in thrombin-induced disseminated intravascular coagulation in the baboon. Crit Care Med 19:1195-1200
29. Corrigan JJ Jr (1977) Heparin therapy in bacterial septicemia. J Pediatr 91:695-700
30. Feinstein DI (1982) Diagnosis and management of disseminated intravascular coagulation: the role of heparin therapy. Blood 60:284-287
31. Goldhaber SZ (1998) Venous thromboembolism in the intensive care unit: the last frontier. Chest 113:5-7
32. Audibert G, Lambert H, Toulemonde F et al (1987) Utilisation d'une heparine de bas poids moleculaire, la CY 222, dans le traitement des coagulopathies de consommation. J Mal Vasc 12[Suppl]:147-151
33. Bergum P, Cruikshank A, Maki S et al (1998) The potent, factor X(a)-dependent inhibition by rNAPc2 of factor VIIa/tissue factor involves the binding of its cofactor to a exosite on factor VII, followed by occupation of the active site. Blood 92[Suppl]:2760
34. Fourrier F, Chopin C, Huart JJ et al (1993) Double-blind, placebo-controlled trial of antithrombin III concentrates in septic shock with disseminated intravascular coagulation. Chest 104:882-888
35. Baudo F, Caimi TM, DeCataldo F et al (1998) Antithrombin III replacement therapy in patients with sepsis and/or postsurgical complications: a controlled double-blind, randomized, multicenter study. Intensive Care Med 24: 336-342
36. Eisele B, Lamy M, Thijs LG et al (1998) Antithrombin III in patients with severe sepsis. A randomized placebo-controlled, double-blind multicenter trial plus meta-analysis on all randomized, placebo-controlled, double-blind trials with antithrombin III in severe sepsis. Intensive Care Med 24:663-672
37. Schuster HP, Matthias FR (1995) Antithrombin III in severe sepsis. 15th International Symposium on Intensive Care and Emergency Medicine, Brussels, pp 21-24

TRANSPLANTATION

Liver Transplantation - Anesthesia and Intensive Care

H. HETZ, F. MANLIK, C.G. KRENN, H. STELTZER

In the General Hospital of Vienna, Austria, orthotopic liver transplantation (OLT) has been performed since about 18 years ago with a steadily increasing incidence to about 80 transplants a year. To date we are overviewing 800 OLT procedures in organ recipients. Indications for OLT are alcoholic liver cirrhosis, cirrhosis due to chronic hepatitis B or C, hepatocellulary carcinoma, primary biliary cirrhosis, sclerosing cholangitis, acute liver failure and rare cases of hereditary hemochromatosis, Morbus Wilson, Morbus Byler and Budd Chiari Syndrome.

We routinely perform OLT without venovenous bypass during the anhepatic period. In most cases we transplant complete cadaveric livers; however, we have increased the rate of split livers from cadaveric or living donors.

The same team of anaesthetists is in charge of recipient evaluation, anaesthesia and postoperative care in order to provide continuous treatment of the patient.

Anesthesia

Preoperative evaluation

Due to an institutional interdisciplinary agreement potential recipients have to consult the anaesthetist before being definitely placed on the waiting list. The aim of this examination is to detect severe co-existing diseases and strong contraindications for transplantation. For routinely preoperative investigations see Table 1. When indicated special check-ups like coronary angiogram, stress echocardiogram or myocardial scintigram are requested.

Anaesthetic considerations

Anaesthetic management during OLT is divided into two stages according to surgical procedure:

Table 1. Common problems associated with end-stage liver disease and tests

Organ	Pathology	Test
Lung	COPD	Pulmonary function tests
	Pleural effusion	X-Ray
	Decreased FRC	Arterial blood gas analysis
Heart	Coronary heart disease	Electrocardiogram
	Cardiomyopathy	Echocardiogram
Vessels	Carotis stenosis	Flow-Doppler
Kidney	Hepatorenal syndrome	Serum electrolytes, creatinine, body urea nitrogen
	Diuretics	Urine electrolytes
Blood	Anaemia	Blood counts
	Thrombocytopenia	
Coagulation	Coagulation disorders	International normalized ratio, partial thromboplastin time, fibrinogen, AT III, thrombelastogram
Metabolism	Hypoalbuminemia	Complete laboratory status
	Hyperammoniumemia	
	Metabolic acidosis	
Brain	Encephalopathy	
Gastrointestinum	Bleeding	Endoscopy
Immune System	Potential septic sources	Teeth status, ENT examination

FRC = functional residual capacity

1. Preanhepatic or preparation period: due to portosystemic shunts and former upper abdominal operations, surgical difficulties with consecutive increased blood loss and prolonged operation time can occur. Frequently bleeding is aggravated by poor coagulation, so we transfuse fresh frozen plasma and red blood cell units in a ratio of 1:1 right from the beginning. The preanhepatic period ends with cross-clamping of the portal vein and inferior caval vein in its sub- and suprahepatic segment. Before cutting the vessels we always carry out a "test clamping" to be on the safe side confirming that the patient will haemodynamically tolerate the anhepatic stage.
2. Anhepatic period: cross-clamping of the inferior vena cava reduces cardiac output and oxygen delivery by approximately one half [1]. Nevertheless oxygen delivery can remain adequate since cirrhotic patients usually have a supranormal cardiac output [2]. The anhepatic patient often presents as severe hypovolemic, but excessive fluid substitution should be avoided (see Fluid Management). Adequate blood pressure is maintained using vasopressors.

To prevent severe hyperpotassiumemia the donor liver is flushed with albumin to wash out the preservation solution. After finishing the venous anastomosis the clamps are removed and the graft is reperfused.

Reperfusion period

Unclamping of the major vessels and reperfusion of the graft can lead to hypotension, hypothermia, coagulopathy, lactic acidosis and electrolyte disturbances, commonly reported as postreperfusion syndrome (PRS). Cardiovascular collapse can occur due to decreased myocardial contractility by inflow of myocardial depressing substances, acute increased intracardial volume, increased pulmonary vascular resistance, loss of total peripheral resistance, severe air embolism or pulmonary thromboembolism.

Preparation for anaesthesia

Before the surgery the anaesthesiologists re-evaluate the patient and actual laboratory tests are checked. We inform our institutional blood bank to prepare erythrocyte concentrates, thrombocyte concentrates and fresh frozen plasma. For stress ulcer prophylaxis we administer omeprazole, for antibiotic prophylaxis cephalosporines and metronidazole. Fluid deficits are corrected with cristalloids through a peripheral venous access.

Induction and maintenance

In the operating room the patient is prone positioned with both arms abducted. In most cases we are performing crush induction because of the high regurgitation and aspiration risk. The routinely used drugs are listed in Table 2. We do not use nitric oxide because of its potential disadvantages in case of air embolism [3, 4], which is common during reperfusion of the transplanted liver and may be disastrous in case of an open foramen oval. For prevention of reperfusion damage of the new organ we routinely administer mannitol and antioxidants, although positive effects are still lacking, as reported in an institutional trial [5].

All central lines are inserted after induction under strictly aseptic conditions.

Intraoperative monitoring

Our standard monitoring includes ECG, pulse oximetry, end-tidal CO_2, arterial blood pressure (radial and femoral artery), central venous pressure (jugular and femoral vein), pulmonary artery and wedge pressure (jugular vein) continuous cardiac output, continuous mixed venous saturation, core temperature and urine output.

Transexophageal echocardiography (TEE) is an excellent monitoring technique in OLT, because it provides useful on-line information about preload and myocardial function during the rapidly changing loading conditions and intraoperative cardiac challenges [6]. Furthermore it is able to detect venous air embolism and thromboembolic events.

Table 2. Commonly used anaesthetics

Drug	Dosage	Indication
Midazolam	3-5 mg	Sedation
Natriumpentothal	5 mg/kg	Crush induction
Fentanyl	3-10 mcg/kg	Analgesia
Succinylcholine	100 mg	Crush induction
Cisatracurium	Relaxometry	Muscle relaxation
Pancouronium	Relaxometry	Muscle relaxation
Sevoflurane	1-3 vol %	Maintenance
Dopamine	2 mcg/kg/min	Diuresis
Norepinephrine	< 0.1 mcg/kg/min	Pressure support
Calcium chloride	5-10 mmol	Hypocalcemia, hyperkaliemia
THAM buffer	20-60 mmol	Acidosis, hyperkaliemia
Natrium bicarbonate	50-100 mmol	Acidosis, hyperkaliemia
Dexamethasone	40 mg	Immunosuppression
Furosemide	20 mg	Diuresis
Mannitol 20%	100 ml	Diuresis
Aprotinine	1 MU, 0.25 MU/hr	Hyperfibrinolysis
Vasopressine, DDAVP	30 mcg	Poor platelet function

MU = Mega unit

For "on-line" evaluation of the coagulation state we use a bed-side thrombelastograph [7, 8], so we can treat coagulopathies adapted to the patient's demand efficiently.

Additionally the transpulmonary double indicator dilution method can help to evaluate changes in lung function by measurement of extravascular lung water, intrathoracic blood volume and pulmonary blood volume [9]. Furthermore indocyanine green kinetics can intraoperatively predict postoperative graft function (unpublished institutional data).

Thermoregulation

In our experience and according to the literature, hypothermia is a common and severe problem in OLT. Decreased heat production of the cirrhotic liver, heat loss through the laparatomy, implantation of a cold organ, infusion of large cold fluid volumes and general anaesthesia contribute to hypothermia. Consecutive complications are a worsened coagulation, an increased blood loss, a potential higher postoperative wound infection incidence and a higher complication rate in the post-anaesthesia period. Concerning this we are cautious to avoid any heat loss, which is ensured by using 2 forced-air-warming devices for the upper and lower body, a fluid warming device for all intraoperative infusions and a Rapid Infusion System (RIS) for blood products [10, 11].

Fluid management

End-stage liver disease patients are often hypovolemic due to ascites and diuretic therapy. The hypovolemia can be severely aggravated in the preanhepatic period by intraabdominal fluid loss caused by suction and evaporation. So re-establishment of the euvolemic state has to be a priority of intraoperative management before the anhepatic stage. This ensures a stable haemodynamic profile, a sufficient compensation of reduced venous reflow and enough urinary output. On the other hand hyperinfusion of an anhepatic patient can result in pulmonary edema or, in the worst case, right heart failure after reperfusion. Another disadvantage of high venous filling pressures can be the congestion of the transplanted liver and impeded recovery from post-reperfusion edema [12].

Intensive care

Graft function

It is evident that initial function of the transplanted liver [13, 14] has influence on postoperative course and survival. Graft function is evaluated by serial determinations of transaminases, canalicular enzymes, bilirubin, bile production, coagulation parameters, lactate, glucose, Doppler ultrasound imaging and dynamic liver function tests, such as indocyanine green kinetics.

There are several classifications of graft function published in the literature [13, 15, 16]. According to [13], primary dysfunction (PDF) is defined on ALAT levels > 2000 U/l, prothrombin time > 16 sec and ammonia levels > 50 mmol/l within the first postoperative week. Primary non function (PNF) is the most serious form of PDF, and these patients die within one week without retransplantation. Recently published institutional data [17] showed that 65.6% of our patients had good function, 19.1% had fair function (84.7% immediate function), 8.7% had poor function, and 6.6% had primary non function (15.3% PDF). Common reasons for graft failure were septic complications and multiple organ failure (54%), viral infections (18%), bacterial infections (9%), and others. Risk factors for developing PDF are long duration of cold ischaemic and second warm ischaemic time, transfusion of more than 10 blood units, recipient's high age and high preoperative Child score, donor's body mass index and sodium level. It is remarkable that these data suggest a better long-term survival in early re-transplanted patients if primary dysfunction occurred.

Detection and differential diagnosis of severe graft dysfunction

Liver function can be altered by preservation injury, technical complications like hepatic artery or portal vein thrombosis and mechanical biliary obstruction, rejection, sepsis, relapse of hepatitis, cholestasis and secondary organ damages due to cardiovascular failure or drug side effects, and other rare cases [18].

It is fundamental to recognize surgical complications as early as possible to beware the allograft of secondary damage, if correction is delayed. Warning signs of primary non function are delayed recovery from anaesthesia, hypoglycemia and persistent hypothermia. In the presence of these symptoms doppler ultrasound imaging, computer tomography and/or selective angiography should immediately be performed. We also serially determine plasma disappearance rate of indocyanine green (PDRig) with the Pulsion COLD System® [19].

Acute rejection commonly occurs after the first postoperative week, but rare cases of earlier "hyperacute" rejections have been reported. The definite diagnosis of rejection has to be made by biopsy, because clinical signs and laboratory determinants are often inconclusive. Therapy of rejection includes increasing or switching immunosuppression or re-transplantation in intractable cases.

Pulmonary complications

Pleural effusions are common, especially in patients with ascites and low colloidosmotic pressure due to hypoalbuminemia. They are often accompanied by basal atelectasis preferring the right hemithorax [20]. Pulmonary edema secondary to increased capillary permeability or to drug-induced side-effects (OKT3) may occur. In case of infection signs and new pulmonary infiltrates aggressive evaluation of nosocomial pneumonia has to be performed. A specific entity is the hepatopulmonary syndrome characterized by arterial hypoxemia, intrapulmonary arterio-venous shunts and ventilation-perfusion mismatch due to a decreased hypoxic pulmonary vasoconstriction. It usually resolves after OLT [21], but can require prolonged mechanical ventilation.

Renal complications

The incidence of acute renal failure (ARF) after OLT is reported to range from 21 to 70% [22]. Increasing mortality up to 60% is reported in patients who need renal replacement therapy [23]. Hepatorenal syndrome, defined by serum creatinine > 1.5 mg/dl or creatinine clearance < 40 ml/min, proteinuria < 500 mg/dl, urine sodium < 10 mEq/l and absence of parenchymal renal disease, obstructive uropathy, shock, hypovolemia, infection and nephrotoxic substances [24], usually resolves postoperatively. Shock, sepsis, poor graft function and nephrotoxicity of immunosuppressant drugs seem to be frequent triggers of ARF. If volume substitution, restoration of adequate filling pressures and diuretic therapy fail, renal replacement therapy is the treatment of choice. We commonly perform continuous venous hemofiltration or -diafiltration.

Infectious complications

As mentioned above [17], infectious complications are the leading reasons for graft failure. In presence of specific immunosuppression nosocomial infections are frequent. We perform antibiograms as soon as possible to guide antibiotic, fungicide or antiviral therapy in co-operation with the department of infectiology.

References

1. Steltzer H, Tüchy G, Hiesmayr M, Zimpfer M (1993) Oxygen kinetics during liver transplantation: The relationship between delivery and consumption. Journal of Critical Care 8:12-16
2. St Amand M, Al-Sofayan M, Gent C, Wall WJ (1999) Liver transplantation. In: Sharpe MD, Gelb AW (eds) Anesthesia and transplantation. Butterworth-Heinemann, Boston, pp 171-200
3. Kutt JL, Gelb AW (1984) Air embolism during liver transplantation. Can Anaesth Soc J 31:713-715
4. Prager MC, Gregory GA, Ascher NL, Roberts JP (1990) Massive venous air embolism during orthoptic liver transplantation. Anesthesiology 72:198-200
5. Plochl W, Krenn CG, Pokorny H et al (2000) The use of the antioxidant tirilazad mesylate in human liver transplantation: Is there a therapeutic benefit? Intensive Care Med 25(6):616-619
6. Greher M, Huemer G, Krenn CG, Zimpfer M (2000) Liver transplantation: Transesophageal echocardiography in the perioperative period. In: Pasetto A, Colò F, Dal Pos L et al (eds) Liver anesthesia and intensive care, proceedings book. Forum, Editrice Universitaria Udinese, Udine, pp 49-55
7. Willschke H, Kozek S, Felfernig M, Zimpfer M (2000) Thrombelastography in liver transplantation. In: Pasetto A, Colò F, Dal Pos L et al (eds) Liver anesthesia and intensive care, proceedings book. Forum, Editrice Universitaria Udinese, Udine, pp 79-83
8. Kettner S, Schellongowski KN, Blaicher A et al (1998) Endogenous heparin-like substances significantly impair coagulation in patients undergoing orthotopic liver transplantation. Anesth Analg 86:691-695
9. Krenn CG, Plochl W, Nikolic A et al (2000) Intrathoracic fluid volumes and pulmonary function during orthotopic liver transplantation. Transplantation 69(11):2394-2400
10. Müller CM, Langenecker S, Andel H et al (1995) Forced-air warming maintains normothermia during orthotopic liver transplantation. Anaesthesia 50:229-232
11. Müller CM, Gabriel H, Langenecker S et al (1993) Effectiveness of rapid infusion and Bair hugger systems in maintaining normothermia during orthotopic liver transplantation. Transplant Proc 25(2):1833-1834
12. Krenn CG, Zimpfer M (1999) Management of marginal graft function: Is there a liver oriented support? In: Pasetto A, Colò F, Dal Pos L et al (eds) Liver anesthesia and intensive care, proceedings book. Forum, Editrice Universitaria Udinese, Udine, pp 49-55
13. Ploeg RJ, D'Alessandro AM, Knechtle SJ et al (1993) Risk factors for primary dysfunction after liver transplantation - a multivariate analysis. Transplantation 55(4):804-813
14. Strasberg SM, Howard TK, Molmenti EP, Hertl M (1994) Selecting the donor liver: Risk factors for poor function after orthotopic liver transplantation. Hepatology 20:829-838
15. Gruenberger T, Steininger R, Sautner T et al (1994) Influence of donor criteria on postoperative graft function after orthotopic liver transplantation. Transp Int 7[Suppl 1]:672-674
16. Deschêns M, Belle SH, Krom RAF et al (1998) Early graft dysfunction after liver transplantation. Clin Transpl 12:123-129
17. Pokorny H, Gruenberger T, Soliman T et al (2000) Organ survival after primary dysfunction of liver grafts in clinical orthotopic liver transplantation. Transpl Int 13[Suppl 1]:154-157

18. Plochl W, Spiss CK, Steltzer H (1999) Death after transplantation of a liver from a donor with unrecognized ornithine transcarbamylase deficiency. N Engl J Med 341(12):921-922
19. Krenn CG, Schafer B, Berlakovich GA et al (1998) Detection of graft nonfunction after liver transplantation by assessment of indocyanine green kinetics. Anesth Analg 87(1):34-36
20. Pinsky MR, Angus DC, Boujoukos AJ, Thomas E (1999) Intensive care unit management of transplantation - Related problems. In: Sharpe MD, Gelb AW (eds) Anesthesia and transplantation. Butterworth-Heinemann, Boston, pp 171-200
21. Scott V, Miro A, Kang Y et al (1993) Reversibility of the hepatopulmonary syndrome by orthotopic liver transplantation. Transplant Proc 25:1878-1888
22. De Gasperi A (1999) Livergraft malfunction and MODS: Managing fluid balance and renal failure? In: Pasetto A, Colò F, Dal Pos L et al (ed) Liver anesthesia and intensive care, proceedings book. Forum, Editrice Universitaria Udinese, Udine, pp 49-55
23. Bilbao I, Charco L, Balsells J et al (1998) Risk factors for acute renal failure requiring dialysis after liver transplantation. Clin Transpl 12:123-129
24. Arroyo V, Gines P, Gerbes AL et al (1996) Definition and diagnostic criteria of refractory ascites and hepatorenal syndrome in cirrhosis. International Ascites Club. Hepatology 23(1): 164-176

Challenges in Perioperative Care Transplantation: Heart Transplant

V. PIRIOU, O. BASTIEN, J. NEIDECKER, S. ESTANOVE, J.J. LEHOT

The first cardiac transplantation was performed by Barnard in 1966. A great improvement of prognosis is related to ciclosporine introduction in 1982.

After an initial increase, the number of heart transplants reached a peak in the 1990s and is now declining [1]. In France, 636 transplantations were performed in 1990 and only 370 in 1998 [2]. Major indications of heart transplantations are equally represented by ischaemic and dilated cardiomyopathies. Results are now acceptable: one year survival is 79% and 5 years 60%. The first year, mainly the first month, is characterised by a peak of mortality. For patients surviving after the first year, half-life is 11.5 years [1]. Mortality rate is higher in centres performing less than 9 transplants per year [3].

Heart transplantation criteria

Recipient evaluation includes routine biological chemistry, haematology, viral status (HIV, hepatitis, cytomegalovirus and Epstein Barr virus) and research of neoplasm (systematic cerebral tomodensitometry and thoracic tomodensitometry or coloscopy in case of previous history or age superior to 60).

Donor-recipient matching for ABO is mandatory. Donor-recipient matching for HLA antigen is not yet currently performed although HLA-A, B or DR mismatch is associated with a higher rate of rejection [4].

End stage of cardiomyopathy is confirmed by physical examination, functional status (NYHA = 4), echocardiography and right heart catheterisation. A peak of maximal oxygen consumption (max$\dot{V}O_2$) less than 10 ml/kg/min is a very sensitive index of poor prognosis [5], therefore heart transplantation is usually proposed when peak of oxygen consumption is less than 14 ml/kg/min [6].

Pulmonary hypertension is common in patients with end stage heart failure. Measurement of pulmonary vascular resistance is crucial. Depending on severity and duration of heart failure, pulmonary hypertension can be fixed or not. One of the challenges is to determine preoperatively the risk of developing right ventricular failure after transplantation because of high fixed pulmonary resistance. The right ventricle responds by inappropriate dilation to the abrupt increase of afterload after transplantation in case of pulmonary hypertension. Bourge et al. [7] suggested that after transplantation pulmonary pressure remains partially high because the fixed component is persisting. Exact value of pulmonary vascular resistance contraindicating heart transplantation is still debated. An indexed value of more than 6 Wood Units (480 dynes.$^{s-}$1.cm^{-5}.m^{-2}) is commonly admitted [8]. Transpulmonary gradient can also be used successfully to determine the risk after transplantation, with a threshold of 15 mmHg [9]. Pulmonary resistance greater than 3-4 Wood Units needs to be tested in terms of reversibility by pharmacological evaluation (inotropes or vasodilator) [10]. Preoperative sodium nitroprusside infusion test can be helpful to determine the prognosis after transplantation, but is currently replaced by dobutamine test. This test has to be reevaluated every 3-6 months. Chen et al. [11] studied 476 patients and showed a good predictive value of nitroprusside test; however, patients with high pulmonary artery resistance were excluded in this study. Caution must be exercised when using pulmonary vasodilators such as nitric oxide to test pulmonary resistance, because such agents can lead to left ventricular failure when a poor functional ventricle is protected by pulmonary hypertension.

We report retrospectively 93 transplanted patients with pulmonary resistance greater (n = 16) or smaller (n = 77) than 6 wood units without 5 years' survival difference (64 vs. 68% respectively). We showed that patients displaying a decrease in pulmonary resistance (> 20%) (n = 46) during dobutamine stress tended to have a better prognosis than patients displaying stable (–20 to +20%) (n = 27) or an increase (> 20%) (n = 20) in pulmonary resistance (5 year survival was 74, 67 and 55% respectively). In our institution, right heart catheterisation with a single pulmonary artery resistance measurement is no longer used as a formal contraindication to heart transplant. In case of severe pulmonary hypertension, all data are reanalysed and discussed.

Our institution usually requires a patient to be less than 60 years old, although we have carried out successfully transplantation in a 72-years-old patient. Diabetes mellitus without complication is no longer a formal contra-indication in our experience [12].

Mechanical circulatory support can be used as a bridge to transplantation in patients with acute end stage ventricular failure [13, 14].

During the last 5 years, in our institution, we experienced 47 biventricular supports bridged to transplantation. We used exclusively pneumatic bi-ventricular assistance (Thoratec). These patients were 45 ± 14 years old. Actuarial survival rate after heart transplantation was 56%. Waiting time before transplantation was 36 ± 36 days. The period since 1998 was characterised by an increasing number of indications of mechanical assistance, and an increase in the assistance duration (maximum of 9 months) together with an improvement of the patient's outcome (70% survival rate).

Perioperative care

Monitoring of patients includes invasive arterial pressure measurement, multilumen central venous catheter (placed on the left side preferentially to allow future endomyocardial biopsies) which will be used intra and postoperatively, measurement of urine output and central temperature. Insertion of radial artery catheter prior to anaesthetic induction is safer to diagnose and avoid severe hypotension. A Swan-Ganz catheter is commonly inserted. In our institution we are used to inserting a catheter with continuous oxygen venous saturation measurement and right ejection fraction calculation although calculation of right ejection fraction has been criticised after heart transplantation [15]. We find it useful to diagnose early right ventricular failure and to monitor the effects of treatment.

Anaesthetic induction adds to the problems of emergency (full stomach patient) in a patient with a very poor left ventricular function. Anaesthetic agents need to have few haemodynamic effects; etomidate, high doses of opioids and benzodiazepines can be used quite safely. Anaesthetic induced sympatholysis can lead to severe hypotension in such patients with high vascular systemic resistance; vasoconstrictive and inotropic agents can be useful to restore haemodynamic stability. End stage cardiac failure patients are administered frequently high doses of angiotensin converting enzyme inhibitors. Anaesthetic induction will be performed cautiously with optimal loading to avoid severe collapse. Patients receive frequently an anticoagulation therapy. 5 mg vitamin K and vitamin K-dependent coagulation factors are used if patients are taking coumadine or warfarin preoperatively.

Antibiotic prophylaxis will be continued during 48 hours.

Surgical procedure is now well standardised. Cannulation of bypass includes distal ascending aorta and both caval veins via the right atrium. Bicaval anastomosis decreases further requirement of pacing.

A perioperative hypervolaemia is often observed, mostly in case of dilated cardiomyopathy. In this case haemofiltration is often required during cardiopulmonary bypass. Withdrawal of 1500 to 2000 ml can avoid transfusion and readministration of a large volume of blood at the end of the bypass. Indeed, right ventricular failure can be triggered by high blood volume readministration at the end of the surgical procedure.

We report the case of a 50 year old transplanted patient who developed a right ventricular failure after readministration of 2.5 litres of blood in 5 hours at the end of the cardiopulmonary bypass. Although preoperative pulmonary vascular resistance was low (200 dynes.sec^{-1}.cm^{-5}) and weaning of CPB easy, pulmonary pressure increased from 39/20 (32) mmHg to 46/26 (42) mmHg with a concomitant decrease of urine output and decrease in right ejection fraction (from 0.23 to 0.18). Right ventricular failure was confirmed by transoesophageal echocardiography (TOE). Treatment included increase in diuretics and epinephrine doses, and nitric oxide inhalation. The outcome was favourable because pulmonary pressure decreased to 35/18 (27) mmHg and right ejection fraction increased to 0.22 on day 1.

At the end of surgery, lungs are reventilated and heart cavities are de-aired. Then, weaning of CPB can be started. An infusion of low doses of epinephrine and isoproterenol is almost systematically required to obtain inotropic and chronotropic effects. Indeed, inotropic sensitive myocardial stunning is often observed and a low ventricle frequency can lead to ventricular dilation and failure. A sinus bradycardia or an atrioventricular block are often observed. A rate of between 80 and 100 beats per min is usually required. If isoproterenol is insufficient to accelerate the heart rate, the heart needs to be paced, and definitive pacing is sometimes required.

Summary of aetiologies of graft dysfunction
Primary problem on the graft:
Donor heart disease: cardiomyopathy (dilated, ischaemic, toxic...)
Secondary to: brain death ("cathecholamine storm"), traumatic contusion...
Iatrogenic: poor quality of myocardial preservation
Recipient's disease:
Pulmonary hypertension
Volume overload
Mechanical problem:
Anastomotic surgical problem
Inadequacy of weight, size, gender...

At the end of the surgical procedure, TOE, right heart catheterisation data and visual aspect of the heart are useful to diagnose right ventricular dysfunction. Nitric oxide inhalation is commonly used to treat this complication. Because of its selective pulmonary vasodilator effect, this inhaled agent has been shown to be efficient and safe in adults [16-18].

We reported the first utilisation of nitric oxide after orthotopic heart transplantation [17]. A 61 year old man with preoperative hypertension had developed rapidly a pulmonary hypertension after transplantation. As shown in Figure 1, nitric oxide inhalation produced a decrease in pulmonary pressure and an increase in systemic arterial pressure secondary to an improvement of right ventricular function. However, this patient died 48 h later with a multi organ failure syndrome because this treatment may have started too late.

Inhaled prostacyclin (PG I_2) can be used alternatively to treat post operative right ventricular failure [19]. In case of nitric oxide-insensitive right ventricular failure resulting from pulmonary hypertension, a right ventricular mechanical support needs to be quickly inserted before right ventricular dilation.

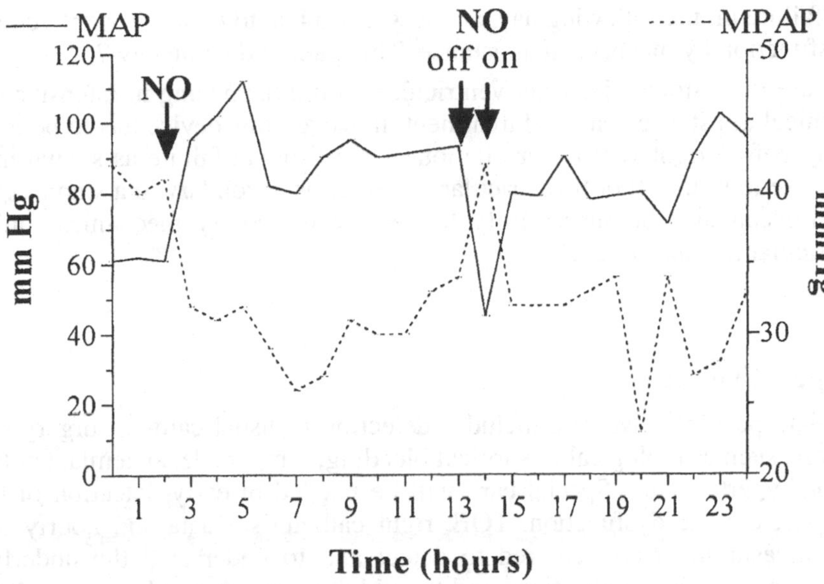

Fig. 1. MAP = mean arterial pressure; MPAP = mean pulmonary arterial pressure. After heart transplantation, inhaled nitric oxide administered with a concentration of 10 to 15 ppm decreased reversibly the pulmonary arterial pressure leading to an improvement of right ventricular function. Peak of pulmonary pressure and transient decrease in systemic pressure are due to the changing of nitric oxide container

A centrifugal assist device, such as a Bio-Medicus pump (cannula implanted in the right atrium and in the pulmonary artery) is commonly used in this indication [20-22].

We report the case of 3 transplanted patients with high preoperative pulmonary pressure (80/40, 74/40, 56/35 mmHg) and high pulmonary vascular resistance (1100, 700 and 820 dynes.s^{-1}.cm^{-5} respectively). Right ventricular assistance by centrifugal pump was used systematically (patient #1 and #3) or because of the impossibility of cardiopulmonary bypass weaning (patient #2). Weaning of Biomedicus pump happened between postoperative day 2 and 3 and extubation on postoperative day 3 to 5. In contrast, a 52 year old transplanted woman with preoperative pulmonary hypertension (pulmonary pressure was 70/27 mmHg and pulmonary vascular resistance 441 dynes.s^{-1}.cm^{-5}) presented with a postoperative right ventricular failure. Weaning of cardiopulmonary bypass was performed easily without adjunction of any pulmonary vasodilator. On the 6th postoperative hour, a right ventricular failure occurred with anuria, hypotension, decrease of right ventricular ejection fraction and echocardiographic right ventricular dilation. The patient was slightly improved by nitric oxide inhalation and inodilator milrinone infusion. However, she presented a multiple organ failure on the following day, and it was too late to treat this right ventricular dysfunction by mechanical assistance. This patient died on day 7.

In case of postoperative right ventricular failure happening in intensive care, mechanical assistance is a good treatment, however, this device has to be inserted early before right ventricular dilation or multi-organ failure as shown in the above case report. Left or biventricular dysfunction secondary to a stunning myocardium can also be successfully treated by temporary mechanical unit or biventricular assistance [23, 24].

Postoperative care

Immediate postoperative care includes detection of usual cardiac surgery complications such as biological or surgical bleeding, tamponade, anaemia, acidosis, hypo or hypertension... Special care will be needed in early detection of right and/or left cardiac dysfunction. TOE, right catheterism data and hourly urine output measurement are required to detect and to understand the underlying mechanism of such complications and to guide the treatment. Unexplained postoperative cardiac failure or arrhythmia can be symptomatic of acute rejection. In uncomplicated cases, ventilation weaning occurs within 24 postoperative hours. Endomyocardial biopsies are performed routinely at the end of the first week to detect a silent acute rejection. Patients are usually discharged from ICU after day 5 to 8 in our institution.

Criteria of suspected acute rejection
Right ventricular failure
Arrhythmia
Recent cardiomegalia
Decrease of summated electrocardiographic voltage (Shumway indice) (often missing in patients taking cyclosporine treatment)
Hepatomegalia
Fever
Echocardiography data:
Oedema of ventricular wall
Right ventricular dilation
Isovolumetric relaxation time less than 60 ms
Positive endomyocardial biopsy (cellular infiltration)

Immunosuppression

Immunosuppression is essential in postoperative treatment. Immunosuppressive protocols vary among the different centres, however, induction of immunosuppression is based on four drug regimes, followed by a triple therapy for maintenance (cyclosporine, azathioprine and steroids) [25].

Cyclosporine was introduced in the early 1980s. Cyclosporine inactivates calcineurin which prevents interleukin-2 production. However, cyclosporin has some side effects such as nephrotoxicity, hypertension, dyslipidaemia. To avoid toxicity, serum concentrations have to be monitored. The poor and variable oral absorption has contributed to the development of a new oral lipid microemulsion with a more consistent bioavailability, called neoral. Neoral is used at 6 mg/kg/day in two takes. Doses are adapted following serum concentrations measured by HPLC (therapeutic concentrations are 150-300 ng/ml). Therapeutic concentrations are usually obtained after 3 to 5 days. Intravenous treatment requires about a third of the oral dose. A new calcineurin inhibitor, the macrolide *tracolimus* (FK 506) is under investigation in heart transplantation.

Inhibitors of DNA synthesis immunosuppressive agents, such as *azathioprine*, have been available since the 1960s. *Mycophenolate mofetil* can be used as an alternative when a cyclosporine nephrotoxicity is observed, to decrease cyclosporine concentrations and prevent chronic rejection.

Corticosteroid, used at high concentration during the immunosuppressive induction period, acts as a non specific anti-inflammatory agent. Main side effects are glucose intolerance, infection, hypertension, dyslipidaemia, osteoporosis, etc.

Antilymphocyte antibodies are used to induce immunosuppression immediately after heart transplantation. Polyclonal antithymocytes globulin (ATG) and antilymphocytes globulin (ALG) from horse or rabbit are available. Rabbit antithymocyte globulin (RATG) is commonly used to induce the immunosuppression and to treat acute rejection. Mouse monoclonal antibody OKT3 is used as an alternative treatment. However, such treatment should be short (less than 10 days or after obtaining therapeutic cyclosporine concentrations) because it increases the incidence of lymphoma.

As an example, in our institution, the following immunosuppresssive protocol is used:

- Steroids: Methylprednisolone 10 mg/kg perioperatively, before aortic clamping. 250 mg on day 1, 120 mg on day 2 and 3 and 1 mg/kg thereafter;
- Cyclosporine: Initial oral treatment: Neoral started on day 3. First administration is 100 mg x 2 per day, adapted to cyclosporine level.

Initial intravenous treatment: cyclosporine, 50 mg per day increased on the following days until the achievement of a therapeutic concentration.

Concentrations (RIA on whole blood) have to be monitored daily; 200 to 300 µg/l are usually required.

- Azathioprine: This agent is started on day 1 with a dose of 2 mg/kg. Neutropenia and hepatic cytolysis lead to a transitory stop of treatment;

– Antilymphocyte antibodies are used to induce the immunosuppression during the first postoperative days. We use rabbit antilymphocyte antibodies started at the dose of 1 flask/10 kg (< 7 flasks) on day 1.

Other treatment includes stress ulcer prophylaxis with anti H_2, intra venous gancyclovir prophylaxis (5 mg/kg/day) in case of cytomegalovirus mismatch or acyclovir in the other case, and prevention of toxoplasmosis and pneumocystis related disease by sulfamethoxazole/trimethoprime (400 mg/day during the first year).

Conclusion

Orthotopic heart transplantations are now routinely performed. Great improvement of prognosis is due to using cyclosporine, trained surgical teams and improvement of perioperative care. Shortage of donors leads to a decrease of transplantations and to the use of "border line" donors. Development of definitive implantable devices is an alternative way to transplant, and the future of heart transplantation remains unknown.

References

1. Hosenpud JD, Bennett LE, Keck BM et al (1999) The Registry of the International Society for Heart and Lung Transplantation: Sixteenth official report - 1999. J Heart Lung Transplant 18:611-626
2. Rapport du conseil médical et scientifique de l'établissement des greffes (1998) Le prélèvement et la greffe en France, 1998, Paris
3. Hosenpud JD, Breen TJ, Edwards EB et al (1994) The effect of transplant center volume on cardiac transplant outcome. A report of the United Network for Organ Sharing Scientific Registry. JAMA 271:1844-1849
4. Opelz G, Wujciak T (1994) The influence of HLA compatibility on graft survival after heart transplantation. The Collaborative Transplant Study. N Engl J Med 330:816-819
5. Mancini DM, Eisen H, Kussmaul W et al (1991) Value of peak exercise oxygen consumption for optimal timing of cardiac transplantation in ambulatory patients with heart failure. Circulation 83:778-786
6. Pina IL (1995) Optimal candidates for heart transplantation: Is 14 the magic number? J Am Coll Cardiol 26:436-437
7. Bourge RC, Kirklin JK, Naftel DC et al (1991) Analysis and predictors of pulmonary vascular resistance after cardiac transplantation. J Thorac Cardiovasc Surg 101:432-444
8. Addonizio J, Gersony WM, Robbins RC (1976) Elevated pulmonary vascular resistance and cardiac transplantation. Circulation 76:V52-55
9. Murali S, Kormos RL, Uretsky BF et al (1993) Preoperative pulmonary hemodynamics and early mortality after orthotopic cardiac transplantation: The Pittsburgh experience. Am Heart J 126:896-904
10. Murali S, Uretsky BF, Reddy PS et al (1991) Reversibility of pulmonary hypertension in congestive heart failure patients evaluated for cardiac transplantation: Comparative effects of various pharmacologic agents. Am Heart J 122:1375-1381

11. Chen JM, Levin HR, Michler RE et al (1997) Reevaluating the significance of pulmonary hypertension before cardiac transplantation: Determination of optimal thresholds and quantification of the effect of reversibility on perioperative mortality. J Thorac Cardiovasc Surg 114:627-634
12. Rhenman MJ, Rhenman B, Icenogle T et al (1988) Diabetes and heart transplantation. J Heart Transplant 7:356-358
13. Park SJ, Nguyen DQ, Bank AJ et al (2000) Left ventricular assist device bridge therapy for acute myocardial infarction. Ann Thorac Surg 69:1146-1151
14. Keon WJ, Olsen DB (1996) Mechanical circulatory support as a bridge to transplantation: Past, present and future. Can J Cardiol 12:1017-1030
15. Starling RC, Binkley PF, Haas GJ et al (1992) Thermodilution measures of right ventricular ejection fraction and volumes in heart transplant recipients: A comparison with radionuclide angiography. J Heart Lung Transplant 11:1140-1146
16. Carrier M, Blaise G, Belisle S et al (1999) Nitric oxide inhalation in the treatment of primary graft failure following heart transplantation. J Heart Lung Transplant 18:664-667
17. Girard C, Durand PG, Vedrinne C et al (1993) Case 4-1993. Inhaled nitric oxide for right ventricular failure after heart transplantation. J Cardiothorac Vasc Anesth 7:481-485
18. Kieler-Jensen N, Lundin S, Ricksten SE (1995) Vasodilator therapy after heart transplantation: Effects of inhaled nitric oxide and intravenous prostacyclin, prostaglandin E1, and sodium nitroprusside. J Heart Lung Transplant 14:436-443
19. Haraldsson A, Kieler-Jensen N, Ricksten SE (1996) Inhaled prostacyclin for treatment of pulmonary hypertension after cardiac surgery or heart transplantation: A pharmacodynamic study. J Cardiothorac Vasc Anesth 10:864-868
20. Chen JM, Levin HR, Rose EA et al (1996) Experience with right ventricular assist devices for perioperative right-sided circulatory failure. Ann Thorac Surg 61:305-310
21. Fonger JD, Borkon AM, Baumgartner WA et al (1986) Acute right ventricular failure following heart transplantation: Improvement with prostaglandin E1 and right ventricular assist. J Heart Transplant 5:317-321
22. Odom NJ, Richens D, Glenville BE et al (1990) Successful use of mechanical assist device for right ventricular failure after orthotopic heart transplantation. J Heart Transplant 9: 652-653
23. Dureau G, Obadia JF, Ferrera R et al (1996) Complete recovery of posttransplant primary heart dysfunction by prolonged mechanical assistance: Report of two cases and arguments for a state of stunned myocardium. Transplant Proc 28:2871-2874
24. Obadia JF, Janier M, Dayoub G et al (1997) Posttransplant primary heart dysfunction and myocardial stunning. J Cardiothorac Vasc Anesth 11:880-882
25. Denton MD, Magee CC, Sayegh MH (1999) Immunosuppressive strategies in transplantation. Lancet 353:1083-1091

ANAESTHESIA AND CRITICAL CARE: TECHNOLOGY AND STANDARDS OF CARE

Challenge in Perioperative Care Transplantation: Lung Transplant

G. DELLA ROCCA, C. COCCIA, P. PIETROPAOLI

Lung transplantation (lung Tx) is the only therapeutic option for a selected group of patients with end-stage lung disease. In the last few years there have been new developments, including improved recipient selection, intraoperative techniques, and immunosuppressive drugs. Recipients are affected by end-stage respiratory failure with different degrees of chronic pulmonary hypertension and cor pulmonale. Conacher [1] described lung Tx as: "a pneumonectomy in a patient who, under normal circumstances, would be adjudged unfit for such an operation!".

Assessment of recipients involves clinical assessment of their pulmonary disease, including its likely progression: objective test of lung function such as FeV_1, FVC, and blood gas analysis, helps decisions on referral for transplantation. Cardiac assessment includes right heart catheterization to measure pulmonary artery pressure and cardiac output, transthoracic echocardiography to evaluate heart wall motion and valvular function, and in same cases coronary angiography to diagnose the presence of coronary artery disease.

All preoperative information is carefully considered, in particular respiratory evaluation and functional status of pulmonary circulation and of the right ventricle are the principal considerations governing the intraoperative management and the choice of pharmacological, ventilatory, and circulatory support strategies. During lung transplantation the problems concerning the patient's condition are associated with potential rapid and dramatic hemodynamic and respiratory deterioration occurring during the surgical procedure [2]. Extensive monitoring, starting before induction of anesthesia, is essential for the management of these changes during lung Tx [3] (Table 1). Introperative management focuses on: 1) appropriate hemodynamic management to avoid right heart failure; 2) appropriate ventilation techniques and oxygenation in patients with end-stage respiratory disease. Single lung transplantation and bilateral sequential double lung transplantation are performed with cardiopulmonary bypass (CPB) stand by. During the procedure there are four crucial points where hemodynamic or respiratory decompensation of the patient may occur and if treatment is unsuccessful, CPB is necessary (Fig. 1) [4].

Table 1. Monitoring required for anesthesia for lung transplantation

ECG, two-lead
Pulse oximeter
Radial and femoral arterial line for arterial pressure and sampling
Central venous catheter for drug infusion
Capnography
Urine ouput mesurament
Monitors of airway pressure, inspired-expired tidal volume and minute volume
In-ex inhalatory volatile anesthetic monitoring
Pulmonary artery catheter with continuous cardiac output and SvO_2 measurement
Volumetric assessment: PiCCO or COLD
Transesophageal echocardiography

ECG electrocardiography, SvO_2 venous oxygen saturation, *PiCCO*
COLD

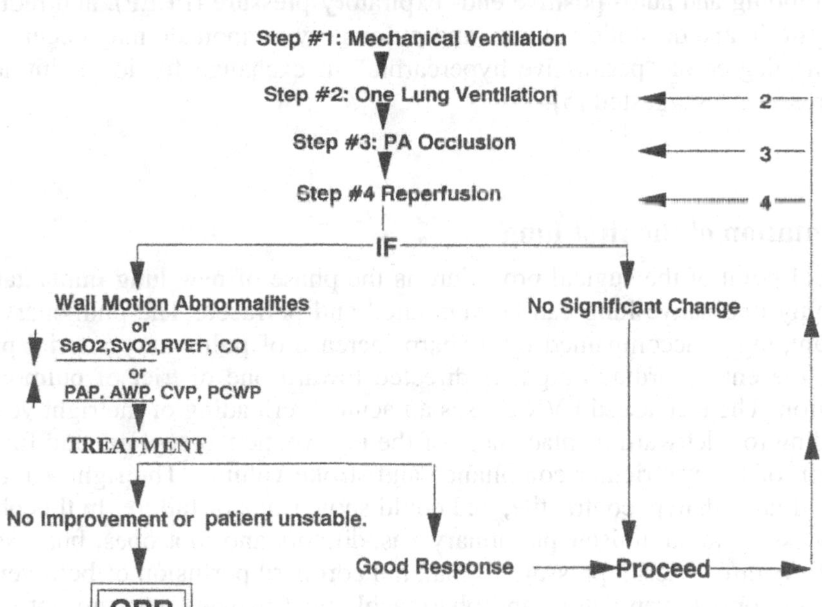

Fig 1. Main steps of intraoperative management during anesthesia for lung transplantation [4]

RVEF right ventricular ejection fraction, *CO* cardiac output, *PAP* pulmonary artery pressure, *AWP* airway pressure, *CVP* central venous pressure, *PAWP* pulmonary artery wedge pressure, *CPB* cardiopulmonary bypass

Induction of anesthesia and mechanical ventilation

Induction of anesthesia should be gradual and performed with care. It should include consideration of full stomach, sitting position to improve spontaneous ventilation, and increased endogenous cathecolamine "drive", induced by chronic hypoxia and hypercarbia, which could abruptly decrease if anesthetics are administered rapidly or in large doses, resulting in circulatory collapse [2]. It is preferable to administer anesthetic drugs slowly, on demand, rather than on a body weight basis.

The hemodynamic and respiratory condition can be compromised with the trasition from spontaneous to mechanical ventilation (Fig. 1). Adequate ventilation is necessary to avoid hypoxia, but intermittent positive pressure ventilation (IPPV) can lead to cardiocirculatory instability. Increased intrathoracic pressure and/or large tidal volume reduces venticular filling and stroke volume and increases pulmonary vascular resistance (PVR). In addition, particulary in patients with chronic obstructive pulmonary disease, insufficient expiration time increases air-trapping and auto- positive end- expiratory pressure (PEEP), and reduces heart systolic and diastolic volume, and pulmonary tamponade may occurr. Often some degree of "permissive hypercarbia" in exchange for lower intrathoracic pressure is suggested [5].

Implantation of the first lung

A critical point of the sugical procedure is the phase of new lung implantation when only one native lung can be ventilated and perfused. The pulmonary artery clamping is accompanied by a sharp increase of pulmonary arterial pressure as the entire cardiac output is directed toward one district of pulmonary circulation. The increasesd PVR causes an acute overloading of the right ventricle leading to a leftward displacement of the intraventicular septum, and further reduction of left ventricular compliance and stroke volume. The right ventricle appears dilatated, hypocontractile, and could show signs of failure. In this phase it is necessary to administer pulmonary vasodilators and inotropes, but also to support systemic arterial pressure to mantain coronary perfusion of both ventricles. If appropriate ventilatory and pharmacological management are not sufficient to maintain hemodynamic and oxygenation stability, CPB is necessary (Fig. 1) [4, 6]. Sodium nitroprusside, nytroglycerin, prostaglandin (PG) E_1, and prostacyclin administration have all been reported during lung transplantation to control pulmonary hypertension [2-4, 6]. PGs increases cardiac output by decreasing right ventricle afterload and postcapillary vasoconstriction in the lung, decreasing microvascular pressure and lung edema formation [7]. PGs inhibit the activation of platelets and inflammatory cells, playing a role in reducing the perpetuation of inflammation that occurrs in acute lung injury [8, 9]. PGE_1 causes a more-selective pulmonary vasodilation than PGI_2, because it is almost all deactivated (80-90%) during the first passage through pulmonary circulation [10]. However, all intravenously administered pulmonary vasodilators worsen oxygenation because of the increase of the intrapulmonary shunt, and lead to concomitant systemic hypotension [11]. Inhaled administration restricts the vasodilatore action to the perfusing pulmonary vessels in well-ventilated areas, decreasing pulmonary hypertension and reducing ventilation/perfusion mismatching [11, 12]. Inhaled nitric oxide (iNO) has been reported to obviate the need for CPB during lung transplantation [13, 14]. Myles describes its use to reduce pulmonary vascular resistance and to increase right ventricular performance, minimizing the requirement for intravenous vasodilators and inotropic support with a concomitant increase in tissue oxygen delivery [3]. Early institution of iNO therapy seems to moderate fluctations in pulmonary artery pressure [15]. It was confirmed in our previous report, in which we described the hemodynamic and oxygenation stability obtained during anesthesia for lung transplant with iNO administration [16]. The association of intravenous prostanoids with iNO seems to have the same beneficial effect [17, 18]. Kuhlen et al., in a combined treatment with iNO and intravenous PGI_2 of a patient with acute respiratory distress syndrome, observed a marked decrease of pulmonary artery pressure which was accompanied by an increase of cardiac output [17]. Even though the association of PGI_2 with iNO was accompanied by an improvement of oxygenation compared to baseline, a slight decrease in paO_2 and a mild worsening in intrapulmonary shunt were observed when compared to iNO alone. NO, PGE_1 and PGI_2 when inhaled are potent. They have a selective pulmonary vasodilating effect with improved arterial oxygenation. Inhaled areosolized prostacyclin (IAP) seems to be as effective as iNO in treating primary or secondary pulmonary hypertension, showing a similar beneficial effect on right ventricular performance [12, 19].

Reperfusion of the first lung

After implantation of the new lung, circulation and ventilation are restored. If there are no problems with the transplantated lung, most of the hemodynamic and ventilatory problems ameliorate (Fig. 1). Reperfusion syndrome is a complication that frequently manifests as pulmonary edema and elevated pulmonary artery pressure, with the resultant loss of lung compliance and poor oxygenation. The cause of this injury has been attribuited to either the postischemic process or the result of denervation and loss of lymphatic drainage. Because of the potential ischemic injury, concerns for free radical damage, oxygen toxicity, ventilatory setting, and low-pressure capillary leak should remain considerations in the anesthesiologist's clinical decision-making processes. Massive edema must raise the question of acute rejection. NO and PGs may play an important role in the maintenance of vascular homeostasis and microvascular permeability [21]. Whereas no adverse effects have been found with administration of IAP, the toxic effects of NO on lung function are controversial. Particularly during lung reperfusion, NO may react with the superoxide anion to form peroxynitrite, which is cytotoxic and responsible for surfactant damage, inducing lung injury [22]. Animal studies suggest that iNO significantly reduces lung ischemia-reperfusion injury with an effect that seems to be mediated by preventive action on development of endothelium injury and neutrophil adherence [23, 24]. In human lung allografts, iNO does improve gas exchange and pulmonary hemodynamics of early graft dysfunction [25, 26]. Because of the potential toxicity, it is not safe to use iNO in high concentration. Murakami [25] suggests administering iNO at a lower concentration than 30 ppm to achieve a protective effect on ischemia-reperfusion lung injury.

Double lung transplantation

During bilateral sequential single lung transplantation, after a period of stabilization, follows the implantation of the second lung. In this phase the only ventilated and perfused lung is the transplantated one. Because of different functional characteristics of the allograft exposed for many years to ischemic and cold preservation, changing of the ventilatory setting is necessary. Increased tidal volume, slower respiratory rate, and the use of PEEP may be more appropriate for better gas exchange [4]. After implantation follows the reperfusion, when all the transplanted lung are ventilated and perfused.

Cardiopulmonary bypass

Although for graft implantation in heart-lung and en-bloc double lung transplantation CPB is indispensible, it can be avoided in most cases during sequential double lung transplantation and single lung transplantation. CPB adds technical complexity, increases time of surgery and ischemia time, and is associated with prolonged postoperative ventilation [27]. The necessary volume loading and systemic anticoagulation may lead to perioperative hemodynamic instability or bleeding, with subsequent allograft compromise; this is particularly important for patients with a previous thoracic procedure or pleural adesions of other origin [28]. Patients requiring CPB had more complications. Circulating levels of vasoconstricting substances are increased with bypass. CPB is known to activate complement and neutrophils and to increase circulating levels of cytokines, such as endotoxin, interleukins, and tumor necrosis factor. The ischemic and reperfusion injuries incurred by the transplanted lung produce significant dysfunction of the mechanisms of pulmonary vasorelaxation. Fullerton et al. demonstrated that this vasomotor dysfunction is significantly exaggerated if CPB is used to perform the lung translant operation [29]. Hence impaired pulmonary vasorelaxation may result in increased PVR.

Conclusion

Lung transplantation is a procedure with increasing application and is likely to become more common; the main impediment to its use is the scarcity of suitable donor organs. The anesthesia for lung transplantation requires careful preoperative evaluation, significant operating room resources, special attention to aseptic technique, and preparation for aggressive cardiopulmonary manipulations. The recipient presents particular anesthetic problems, which are added to the desire to avoid CPB. Ventilation poses problems not encountered in the thoracic surgical population, and their solution may involve unusual strategies. The intraoperative management of lung transplantation is particularly challenging for anesthesiologists, requiring their constant attention and flexibility to manage the dynamic response of the respiratory and cardiovascular systems. Problems involve the choice of selective pulmonary vasodilators, fluid management during lung damage and capillary leak, and early or late extubation. Their solutions will improve anesthesiological management and results.

References

1. Conacher ID (1988) Isolated lung transplantation: a review of problems and guide to anaesthesia. Br J Anesth 61:468-474
2. Truman K (1997) Lung transplantation: historical perspective, current concepts and anesthetic considerations. J Cardiothorac Vasc Anesth 11:220-241
3. Myles PM, Weeks AM, Buckland MR et al (1997) Anesthesia for bilateral sequential lung transplantation: experience of 64 cases. J Cardiothorac Vasc Anesth 11:177-183
4. Triantafillou AN (1993) Anesthetic consideration of lung transplantation. Chest Surg Clin North Am 3:49-73
5. Quinlan JJ, Buffington CW (1993) Deliberate hypoventilation in a patient with air trapping during lung transplantation. Anesthesiology 78:1177-1181
6. Raffin L, Nichel-Cerqui M, Sperandio M et al (1992) Anesthesia for bilateral lung transplantation without cardiopulmonary bypass. J Cardiothorac Vasc Anesth 6:409-417
7. Zimmerman JL, Hanania NA (1998) Vasodilators in mechanical ventilation. Crit Care Clin 14:611-627
8. Moncada S, Vane JR (1979) Arachidonic acid metabolites and the interaction between platelets and blood vessels wall. N Engl J Med 300:1142
9. Fantone JC, Kunkel SL, Ward PA (1981) Suppression of human polymorphonuclear function after intravenous infusion of prostaglandin E_1. Prostaglandins Med 7:195
10. Heerdt PM, Weiss CI (1996) Prostaglandin E_1 and intrapulmonary shunt in cardiac surgical patients with pulmonary hypertension. Ann Thorac Surg 49:463-465
11. Triantafillou AN, Pohl MS, Okabayashi K et al (1995) Effect of inhaled nitric oxide and prostaglandin E_1 on hemodynamic and arterial oxygenation in patients following single lung transplantation. Anesth Analg 80:SCA40
12. Walmrath D, Schermuly R, Pilch J et al (1997) Effect of inhaled versus intravenous vasodilators in experimental pulmonary hypertension. Eur Respir J 10:1084-1092
13. Myles PS, Venema H (1995) Avoidance of cardipulmonary bypass during bilateral sequential lung transplantation using inhaled nitric oxide. J Cardiothorac Vasc Anesth 9:571-574
14. Della Rocca G, Pugliese F, Antonini M et al (1998) Inhaled nitric oxide during anesthesia for bilateral single lung transplantation. Minerva Anestesiol 64:297-301

15. Adatia I, Lillehei C, Arnold JC et al (1994) Inhaled nitric oxide in the treatment of postoperative graft dysfunction after lung transplantation. Ann Thorac Surg 57:1311-1318
16. Della Rocca G, Coccia C, Pugliese F et al (1997) Intraoperative inhaled nitric oxide during anesthesia for lung transplantation. Tranplant Proc 29:3362-3366
17. Kuhlen R, Walbert E, Frankel P et al (1999) Combination of inhaled nitric oxide and intravenous prostacyclin for successful treatment of severe pulmonary hypertension in a patient with acute respiratory distress syndrome. Intensive Care Med 25:752-754
18. Aranda M, Bradford KK, Pearl RG (1999) Combined therapy with inhaled nitric oxide and intravenous vasodilators during acute and chronic experimental pulmonary hypertension. Anesth Analg 89:152-158
19. Zwissler B, Welte M, Messmer K (1995) Effect of inhaled prostacyclin as compared with inhaled nitric oxide on right ventricular performance in hypoxic pulmonary vasoconstriction. J Cardiothorac Vasc Anesth 9:283-289
20. Lindberg L, Kimblad PO, Sjoberg T et al (1996) Inhaled nitric oxide reveals and attenuates endothelial dysfunction after lung transplantation. Ann Thorc Surg 62:1639-1643
21. Ignarro LJ (1989) Biological actions and properties of endothelin derived nitric oxide formed and released from artery and vein. Circ Res 65:1-12
22. Freeman B (1994) Free radicals chemistry of nitric oxide: looking at the dark side. Chest 334:930-933
23. Murakami S, Bacha EA, Herve P et al (1997) Prevention of reperfusion injury by inhaled nitric oxide in lung harvested from non heart beating donors. Ann Thorac Surg 62:1632-1638
24. Okabayashi K, Triantafillou AN, Yamashita M et al (1996) Inhaled nitric oxide improves lung allograft function after prolonged storage. J Thorac Cardiovasc Surg 112:293-296
25. Date H, Triantafillou AN, Trulock EP et al (1996) Inhaled nitric oxide reduces human lung allograft dysfunction. J Thorac Cardiovasc Surg 111:913-916
26. MacDonald P, Mundy J, Rogers P et al (1995) Successful treatment of life threatening acute reperfusion injury after lung transplantation with inhaled nitric oxide. J Thorac Cardiovasc Surg 110:861-863
27. De Hoyos A, Demajo W, Snell G et al (1993) Preoperative prediction for the use of cardiopulmonary bypass in lung transplantation. J Thorac Cardiovasc Surg 106:787-796
28. Triantafillou AN, Pasque MK, Huddleston CB (1994) Predictors, frequency and indications for cardiopulmonary bypass during lung transplantation in adults. Ann Thorac Surg 57:13-18
29. Fullerton DA, McIntyre RC Jr, Mitchell MB (1995) Lung transplantation with cardipulmonary bypass exaggerates pulmonary vasomotor dysfunction in the transplant ed lung. J Thorac Cardiovasc Surg 24:212-216

TRAUMA

Bad and Good News From the Emergency Department

P. Pietropaoli, F. Spinelli, C. Mattia

The emergency department (ED) is key in establishing hospital reputation; meeting patients expectations in the emergency setting is key for the hospital marketing. Traditionally, quality in healthcare has been measured by clinical indicators. However, increased competition, rising consumerism, growing public demand, and increased awareness of cost inefficiency have drawn attention to the customer's perspective on quality. Generally, patients are unable to evaluate the validity and efficacy of the technical care they received, the focus of their quality assessment is more often on the timing and on the effective aspects of how the care is delivered [1].

Currently there are two major competing visions for delivering emergency care:

1. bringing the patients to hospital-based ED, so that they may be provided a higher level of care (the American model); in the pre-hospital setting emergency care is initiated by physician extenders and continues into the ED, where the emergency physician provide definitive emergency care;
2. sending physicians and technology to the scene in the hope of providing a higher level of emergency care before the patient's arrival at the hospital (the European model).

The major difference is that the American system relies on specially trained hospital-based physicians to deliver a broad range of services for all patients presenting a separate ED. In contrast the European model focuses on delivering resuscitative care in the field; this care is usually provided by anesthesiologists, with subsequent triage of patients directly to specific speciality service of care [2]. Emergency medicine in Italy has developed largely along the lines of the European model, although EDs are currently in every hospital.

Recently the Italian law regarding emergency medicine has focused on the need for improvements in both pre- and in-hospital healthcare providers and equipment. Health care reform legislation in 1992 allocated additional funds for the development of emergency medicine systems (EMS), including the institution of 24-h dispatch centers and a common toll-free access number. Additionally, the roles of the ED and EMS were more clearly defined and a larger and multidisciplinary division was instituted, called the "Department of Emergency and Admittance" (DEA) [3]. The DEA deals with all aspects of emergency care delivery, and includes the ED, the medical surgical services of all disciplines and specializations, and a short-term observation area.

As a part of the healthcare transformation, traditional roles of patients and physicians have been changing. For much of medicine's long history, physicians practicing medicine have had absolute authority over the diagnosis and treatment of their patients. Patients were expected to comply with recommended tests and regimens and to accept the professional authority of the physician without question. Although many patients still interact with physicians in this manner, increasingly patients are demanding to be part of the decision-making process in terms of evaluation and treatment. Furthermore, the relationship between physicians and other members of the healthcare delivery system have also changed; the physician is a member of the care delivery team. To survive in such an environment, physicians must arm themselves with data that will help them better understand what their patients expect from the healthcare delivery system and how patients feel about the medical services they receive. Valid and reliable data are important tools that will enable physicians to take the lead in initiating needed improvements.

The study of the ED has been conducted using the most-important principles of healthcare quality. Total quality management (TQM), continuous quality improvement (CQI), and quality control are terms that are becoming very familiar to workers in the healthcare environment. In other environments, TQM has produced significant increases in productivity while increasing effectiveness. Its application to the healthcare environment is the provision of the best-possible care through continuously improving services to meet or exceed the needs and expectation of customers [4].

TQM is based on CQI, defined as continuous effort on the part of the organization to furnish products or services that meet or exceed the expectations of customers through an organized structure that identifies and improves an operating processes at the relief and administrative levels, and through a set of statistically analytical data available to the operators.

The CQI activity is based on the FOCUSPDCA models (find a process to be improved upon), organize (organize a team that knows the process), clarify (current knowledge of the process),understand (understand the causes), select (select the most-appropriate improvement), plan (map out an improvement plan and continuous gathering of data), do (carry out the improvement), check (study the results), act (operate in order to maintain the advantage) [5].

One of the best indicators of patients' satisfaction in the ED is waiting time, which seems to matter to same patients more than clinical expertise [6]. CQI program selects as a quality indicator the percentage of patients leaving without being seen (LWBS) because the primary reason for LWBS was dissatisfaction with waiting time [7]. So total ED lengths of stay (LOS) is as important as overall resources of efficiency. The relationship between LOS and LWSB are the reference to patients' satisfaction [8].

This paper describes quality measurement parameters in the old and in the new ED of the Policlinico Umberto I, University of Rome "La Sapienza". Two comparable periods of 2 weeks were retrospectively evaluated. A number of studies have focused on the link between customer expectations and customer satisfaction. Five caring behavior categories were considered to represent the patient perception of the service: timely care, responsive care, understandable care, humane care, professional care [1].

At the time of arrival at our ED, a patient is subjected to an examination of his health conditions and then classified on the basis of the seriousness of the pathology evidenced by triage. At the end of the examination, the patient is assigned with an emergency code with four different colours: red if in immediate danger of losing life; yellow if there is serious damage to any organ associated with the three vital functions (i.e., cardiocirculatory, respiratory, and nervous system); green if there are no serious conditions that require immediate attention and cure; white if patients require medical assistance with no emergency criteria that are generally provided by structures outside the hospital. Triage is carried out by paramedical staff trained and co-ordinated by medical staff.

Another very important indicator for defining the quality of ED is, therefore, the precision of the triage. Sometimes, a patient admitted with an emergency code may be reallocated, this phenomenon is defined as "change of priority" and can be due to an "under triage" when the pathology is underestimated, or "over triage" when the pathology is excessively appraised.

The old DEA of the "Policlinico Umberto I", which is the largest recipient of patients in Rome, was expanding horizontally in line with all the other sections of the hospital. In this framework, the reception for admittance was on the ground flour with a waiting room, three areas for medical pathology and two for surgical pathology, while on the basement floor, there was a waiting room, orthopedics department, and an X-ray area. Outside of this structure, but forming part of the DEA, were the traumatology, intensive care, coronary, computed tomography, and magnetic resonance imaging (MRI) units. Every additional structure entails an additional waiting time for the patient. In this setting the patients needed to wait for various laboratory and test results from various units, and for the movement and transportation of patients from one unit to the other after the emergency intervention. Because of the amount of time necessary for the different diagnostic and intervention procedures, discharge of patients was slow, influencing the waiting time after the triage [9, 10]. In the old DEA the increased waiting time was also determined by a shortage of paramedical staff during the periods of maximal access. Increase in "preload" with slow "afterload" causes one of the most-serious problems of the ED: overcrowding.

A negative impact on the quality of an ED is overcrowding because it causes an extension of access time to the DEA, discontent of the patients, incorrect use of the resources, risk of under triage. Overcrowding is evidenced at the waiting halls and along the corridors, with an accumulation of stretchers waiting for placement in various cubicles.

Owing to long waiting times and the poor impression of the ED, the patient remains unsatisfied. The extension of LOS was related to the increase of LWBS [11].

Analysis at admittance to the DEA yielded information on the: average admissions to the DEA on a daily and hourly basis; admissions to the major hospital sections [general surgery, specialist surgery; general medicine, specialist medicine; emergencies (neurosurgery, orthopedics, reanimation, emergency medicine); infant maternity, infectious disease]; result indicator (4e09) (number of admissions to DEA followed by hospitalized cases/ total number of admissions to DEA) [12].

Analysis of the state of patient flow yielded information on waiting time before a visit and time required to carry out complete treatment.

Based on the analysis of patient flow, we recorded two peaks of admission to the DEA: Monday between 8.00 and 12.00 a.m. and Saturday between 16.00 and 20.00 p.m. Monday was adequately covered by medical and paramedical staff, but for Saturday the need for healthcare deliverers was seriously underestimated (Figs. 1, 2).

To improve these factors the DEA of the "Policlinico Umberto I" has been completely reorganized, applying the most-important principles of CQI. Today, our DEA is located in front of the main entrance of the hospital and extends vertically. On the ground floor we have the reception for recording of patients' data; a waiting room with medical and paramedical staff for triage. Beside the triage there is the room for medical evaluation. On the same floor there are two areas for emergency patients (red code) with all the equipment for medical intervention and monitoring, three areas for surgical pathology, and six areas for medical pathology. On the same floor is the radiology, with all the diagnostic systems such as like X-ray, MRI, and echography.

In the basements are a large waiting room, orthopedics service with plaster section, and operating theaters for orthopedics, general emergency surgery, and neurotraumatology. On this same floor is the unit for subintensive therapy with 12 beds. These units are linked with real-time communication devices.

The logistics of this system focus on a better and easier discharge of patients from DEA and a reduction of "afterload". In addition, the medical staff has been strengthened at points of greater access to the ED, with the goal of reducing "preload". The causes of overcrowding have therefore been reduced, with a reduction of waiting time, reduction of LWBS, and greater satisfaction to the patient.

Triage is carried out discretely by nursing staff who are fully trained and kept up to date with refresher courses arranged by a competent physician in a position to furnish the latest guidelines to be followed. There is consequently a reduction in "priority changes" and the risk of under triage.

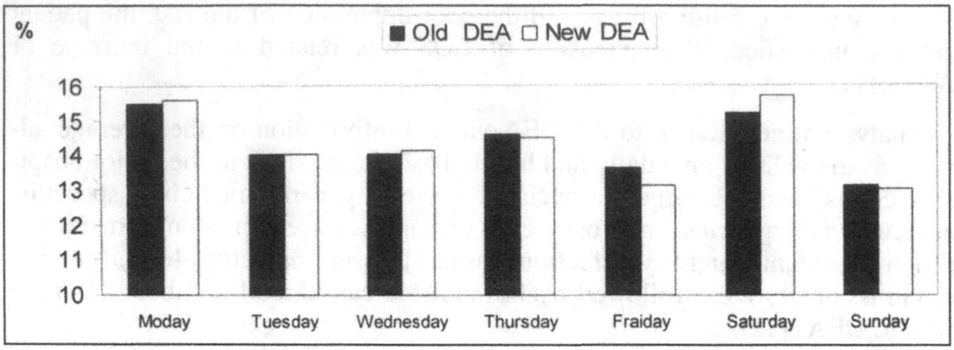

Fig.1. Weekly flux in old and new Department of Emergency and Admittance (*DEA*)

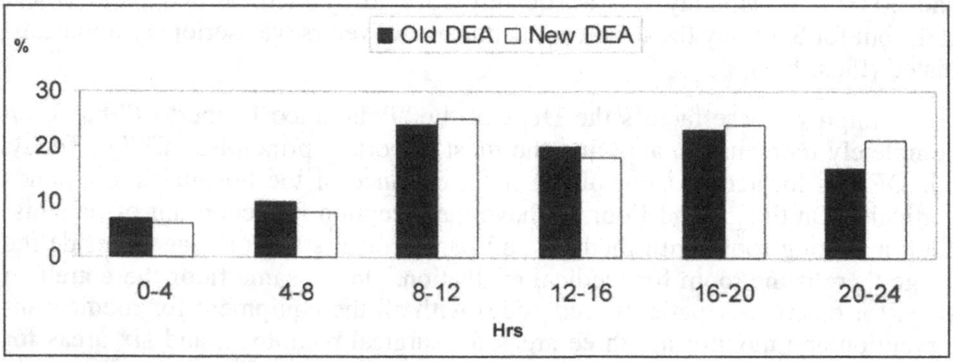

Fig. 2. Daily flux in old and in new DEA

In the old DEA, 20% of patients needed hospitalization after emergency evaluation (4e09 indicator); 1.5% were transferred to other hospitals, 8.5% refused hospitalization, 10.2% did not respond to calls and 59.6% did not need hospitalization (Table 1). The ratio between in-hospital patients and all observed patients (4e09 indicator) was at the upper limit of normal range (18-22%) [12]. Mean waiting time, calculated independently from triage code, was 60 min while mean total interventions time was 156 min. Waiting time was absent for the red code, 43 min for yellow, 62 min for the green, 200 min for the white code. Mean total intervention time was 225 min for patients with the red code, 200 min for the yellow, 143 min for the green, and 97 min for the white (Table 2). We have highlighted a " priority change" of 40% for red code, –13% for the yellow, –23% for the green, and 144% for the white.

Table 1. Patients flow in the old and new Department of Emergency and Admittance (*DEA*)

	Old DEA (%)	New DEA (%)
At home	59.6	52
Hospitalized	20.4	25*
Transfer	1.2	1.7
Non response	10.2	7.4*
Refusal to hospitalization	8.5	8.6
Death	0.1	0.1

Table 2. Mean waiting time and mean care time in the emergency department.* $p < 0.05$

Code	Old DEA		New DEA	
	Waiting time	Time to complete treatment	Waiting time	Time to complete treatment
	Average (min)	Average (min)	Average (min)	Average (min)
Red	–	225	–	200*
Yellow	43	200	33*	121*
Green	62	143	52*	130*
White	200	97	111*	76*
Indifferent	62	156	58	140

In the new ED the peak of admittance has remained constant with analogous hourly intervals as for important movements in units of general surgery and medicine.

Hospitalized patients were 25% after emergency evaluation, patients transferred to other hospitals were 1.7%; 8,6% refuse hospitalization, 7.4% did not respond to calls and 52% did not need hospitalization. The 4e09 indicator remains at 25%, which is reasonably high (Table 1).

Mean waiting time, calculated independently from triage code, was 58 min, while mean total intervention time was 140 min. Waiting time was zero for the red code, 33 min for yellow, 52 min for the green, and 111 for the white code. Mean total intervention time was 200 min for patients classified as red code, 121 min for the yellow, 130 for the green, and 76 for the white (Table 2). We have highlighted a "priority change" of 12% for red code, -2% for the yellow, -20% for the green, and 75% for the white.

"Undertriage", frequently seen in ischemic heart disease, the major case of death worldwide, is an unresolved question. The institution of a "chest unit" would be an answer. The evolution of cardiac care units has improved patient survival from myocardial infarctions, but requires a high-tech, very expensive treatment facility. Chest pain centers, located in ED, present an efficient alternative to triage patients with chest pain, providing prompt and accurate diagnosis, risk evaluation, and appropriate treatments.

Hospitals benefit from this cost-effective approach, .as resources are used more efficiently, and patients benefit from a supportive treatment facility that focuses on early intervention [13].

In conclusion, the clinical quality of care delivered by an ED is based on medical knowledge, team work, and the quality of medical equipment available. The distribution of heathcare providers based on the analysis of admittance flows and facilities engineered on the basis of dedicated design may improve customer satisfaction. Facilities dedicated to specific pathology like "chest pain unit" or "trauma center" may further improve the quality of health care provided [14, 15]. Therefore, the costs of low-quality healthcare in the ED is higher than the costs of healthcare delivery based on the principles of total quality management.

References

1. Seff LR (1995) Management of emergency department: service is quality standard in the emergency department 53:482-491
2. Thomas D (1998) Emergency medicine around the world. Ann Emerg Med 32:237-238
3. Joffrey L (1999) International emergency medicine and the recent development of emergency medicine worldwide. Ann Emerg Med 33:97-103
4. McDonald SC (1994) Total quality management in health care. J Can Diet Assoc 55:12-14
5. Zanetti M (1996) Il medico ed il managment. Accademia Nazionale di Medicina Genoa, pp 384-386
6. Bruce TA (1998) Factors that influence patient satisfaction in the emergency department. J Nurs Care Qual 13:31-37
7. Schwab RA, DelSorbo SM (1999) Using statistical process control to demonstrate the effect of operational interventions on quality indicators in the emergency department. J Health Qual 21:38-41
8. Kyriacou DN, Ricketts V (1999) A 5-year time study analysis of emergency department patient care efficiency. Ann Emerg Med 34:326-335
9. Cook S, Sinclair D (1997) Emergency department triage: a programme assessment using the tools of continuous quality improvement. J Emerg Med 15:889-894
10. Wilkinson RA (1999) Triage in accident and emergency. 1. An overview of the literature. Br J Nurs 10;8:86-88,101-102
11. Lynn SG (1995) Management of emergency department: service is quality standard in the emergency department. Mosby 18:173-178
12. Defta I, Bigioni M (1998) Analisi dell'attività di un servizio pronto soccorso. QA 9:135-144
13. Dudly P (2000) Chest pain centre: moving toward proactive acute coronary care. 72:101-120
14. Goodacre SW (2000) Should we establish chest pain observation units in the UK? A systematic review and critical appraisal of the literature. J Accid Emerg Med 17:1-6
15. West TD (1997) Improving quality while managing costs in emergency medicine. J Health Care Finance 27:17-29

Cerebral Blood Flow and Metabolism in Neurotrauma

F. DELLA CORTE, A. CARICATO, F. LA MURA

Primary neurological injury due to any kind of insult (traumatic, ischaemic, hypoxic, metabolic) can be followed by a chain of pathological events, that can worsen or perpetuate the primary lesion within minutes, hours or days. This group of derangements is traditionally defined as secondary damage, and its principal determinant, regardless of the producing cause, is ischaemia-anoxia.

The ischaemic-anoxic damage occurs every time there is an imbalance between delivery and oxygen and substrates requirements to meet cerebral metabolism.

This condition may happen when:
- delivery is diminished (because of reduced CBF or O_2 delivering capacity);
- requirements are increased (hypertermia, seizures, local metabolic activation);
- cellular O_2 and substrates utilization capacity is altered.

Mechanical or metabolic factors allow cerebral tissue to maintain blood flow adequate to its metabolic status.

Correlations between flow and metabolism in severe head injury

Following head injury, for reasons not known yet, autoregulation systems can be damaged. Therefore, perhaps, all the efforts to schematize cerebral blood flow (CBF) profiles following traumatic insults have always led to a wide variety of results, and so far it has never been possible to show a clear relationship between CBF and clinical state and prognosis. A major issue in these attempts is the complexity and the high cost of the equipment necessary to measure and to monitor CBF. For this reason there are few studies applied to this field of neurotraumatology.

Bouma et al. [1] supposed that the timing of measurement was a discriminating parameter for data interpretation.

They observed that the lowest CBFs, that in a third of cases were below the ischaemic value of 18 ml/100 g/min, were recorded within the sixth hour after trauma. These measurements were significantly correlated to the severity of the primary lesion assessed with GCS, and to the jugular artero-venous difference. Furthermore, it seemed that they could have a prognostic significance, since CBF values in patients who survived were significantly higher than in those who died.

This correlation was lost in the determinations taken after the sixth hour after trauma.

Gopinath et al. [2], using continuous monitoring of SjO_2 by fiberoptic catheter, came to the same results: they observed a higher incidence of jugular desaturation (SjO_2 < 50% for 5 min or longer) in the first hours after trauma, and a close correlation between the number of desaturations in each patient and a poor prognosis was found.

Twenty-four hours after trauma CBF profile is still uncertain. The incidence of ischaemic flow values is less, and most authors were unable to reveal any relationship with GCS or prognosis. However, Robertson et al. [3] in 102 patients detected that higher CBF values during the first 10 days after trauma were related to a better prognosis.

Kelly et al. [4] postulated a triphasic temporal profile of CBF after head injury. During the first phase, that occurs in the initial hours after trauma, blood flow is at its lowest, falling to less than 50% of normal. By as early as 12 hours post injury the second phase begins, marked by a rise in CBF that approaches or exceeds normal values and persists for the next 4 or 5 days. The third phase is characterized by a period of low CBF that lasts for up to 2 weeks post injury. In some patients, anyway, CBF remains depressed or elevated; they observed that patients who developed an increase of CBF after the first phase of hypoperfusion had a better prognosis than those who had a persistently depressed or elevated CBF. They moreover proposed a functional significance to this increase in CBF: using positron emission tomography by fluorodeoxyglucose they found an increase in the consumption of glucose following head trauma, and they particularly noted that the temporal profile of hyperglycolysis was the same as that of the hyperemia. So, the increase in CBF could represent a response to the higher requirement of glucose of brain tissue, accounting for a mechanism of compensation to the compromised oxidative metabolic pathways, demonstrated by the persistent reduction in cerebral oxygen consumption ($CMRO_2$) after trauma.

In our recent study [5], using a tomographic CBF measurement technique, Xe-SPECT, we have confirmed, as already found by Jaggi with non tomographic method [6], that the reduction of cerebral oxidative metabolism represents one of the most striking factors in the prognosis of severe head injury, and that it is closely linked to the initial clinical severity and to prognosis at six months.

Due to the inefficiency of anaerobic glycolysis as a source of energy, patients who are not able to develop hyperemic values of CBF might not satisfy the metabolic requirements of brain tissue, and might develop ischemia in the face of normal values of jugular artero-venous differences.

A similar profile has been revealed by Sakas et al. [7] in normal parenchymal regions near focal ischaemic lesions: if in the contusive zones shown by CT-scan there is a reduction of $CMRO_2$ and of local blood flow and an increase in vascular permeability, then local blood flow in the surrounding areas is higher for some days after trauma, and it is correlated to a better outcome. This event might be due to a mechanism of local metabolic activation mediated, perhaps, by H^+, ADP, and CO_2. They hence differentiated two forms of hyperemia: a "malignant" one, more common in young patients, associated with global loss of autoregolation, persistent intracranial hypertension, brain swelling and poor prognosis; a "benign" one, that is focal and it is not associated with the elevation of intracranial pressure and with alterations in CT- and NMR-scans. These two forms of hyperemia are not mutually exclusive: they can be shown in the same patient at different times, and they could represent two extremes of a unique spectrum of alterations where an increase of CBF is seen.

All these data could demonstrate, therefore, that the patient's ability to recover is strictly linked to the integrity of the autoregulation mechanisms. By the time they are altered, CBF is no longer regulated by the metabolic requirements of the parenchyma, but it is strictly dependent on the fluctuations in cerebral perfusion pressure (CPP). In this phase the prognosis of the patient is highly correlated with the possibility of continuously monitoring the efficiency of oxygen and substrates delivery to cerebral tissue.

Cerebral ischaemia detection techniques in head injury

Methods of CBF measurement such as the Kety-Schmidt technique with nitrous oxide, Xe washout or tomographic systems (Xe-Ct and SPECT) can yield accurate but intermittent estimates of CBF. Techniques now available to continuously monitor CBF are Laser-doppler flowmetry and thermal diffusion: they require, yet, a surgical positioning and only local flow values are obtained. The possibility of CBF measurements by double indicator dilution technique, using a catheter placed in jugular bulb and thoracic aorta, is extremely interesting. However, the accuracy of this method is still unclear [8].

Promising perspectives for continuous monitoring of cerebral metabolism can be recognized in microdialysis and in the measurement of tissular pO_2 (PtO_2).

Microdialysis is based on the introduction of a catheter in the cerebral parenchyma to analyze the composition of extracellular fluid. So far, knowledge of biochemical markers is drawn from non microdialytic methods, obtained by the analysis of blood, CSF or brain tissue homogenizer, without any interstitial cerebral fluid examination. Thus, comparison of data is difficult. Moreover technical artifacts may occur, since time is necessary for the equilibrium of the system and glial proliferation possibly occurs around the probe, after a long permanence period (more than 7 days). Several factors, such as transmembrane pressure, molecular weight of substances and temperature, may affect metabolites' diffusion over the dialysate. For this purpose measurement of concentrations' ratio is more accurate than the absolute value. Despite these limits, microdialysis is one of the few methods that enables us to investigate the biochemical function of brain tissue, to evidence the markers of the ischaemic damage (lactate, glutamate, aspartate, taurine, potassium, ratio of lactate to piruvate and lactate to glucose) and suggests hypothesis on alternative metabolic pathways developing in brain tissue after an injury.

Goodman et al. found that in 78% of patients in which an episode of jugular desaturation or a persistent increase of intracranial pressure above 20 mmHg for more than 10 minutes was observed, the concentration of extracellular lactate was increased, and this was often associated with elevated levels of glutamate, aspartate and taurine; barbiturate coma was able to lower the concentration of these excitatory aminoacids in the extracellular fluid [9]. Actually some authors observed that lactate levels were high in patients without any signs of ischemic injury too. Goodman et al. investigated the concentrations of lactate, PtO_2 and SjO_2 in 126 patients affected by head injury and found that lactate levels were elevated while PtO_2 and SjO_2 were within normal limits in 10 subjects [10]. Alessandri et al. suggested that, as already experimentally known, this phenomenon could be the effect of post-traumatic or post-hypoxic activation of alternative metabolic pathways; so the decrease of oxidative metabolism in neuronal tissue could be associated with an increase of glycolysis in astrocytes, led by glutamate, and the accumulating lactate could be processed on Krebs' cycle in neuronal mitochondria. High concentrations of glutamate in the very early phase after trauma, and the increase of lactate levels only after 12 hours from injury, provide experimental evidences *in vivo* of this hypothesis [11].

PtO_2 is measured by a polarographic catheter (Clark's electrode) which is introduced in the parenchyma, and left in place. It is still too early to give a complete evaluation of this technique; a system that analyzes the tissular oxygenation would be the "golden standard" of the monitoring, although the features of a microscopical determination could limit the clinical usefulness and reliability of this method.

The principal determinants of PtO_2 are PaO_2 and CPP.

PtO_2 increases with increasing PaO_2; Santbrink et al. [12] developed an index of reactivity to O_2 that is given by the percent variation of PtO_2 to the increase of PaO_2. They revealed a close correlation between these two parameters, that was more evident in the cases of lower PtO_2. Furthermore they observed that patients with a higher dependence of PtO_2 from PaO_2 had a worse prognosis, emphasizing a prognostic relevance of metabolic cerebral oxygen autoregulation. The correlation between PaO_2 and PtO_2 has been also investigated by Menzel et al. [13], who have observed an increase of PtO_2 from 100% to 500% in response to variations of FiO_2 from 30% to 100%. The pathophysiology of this correlation is not clear. It is known that the increase of FiO_2, above complete haemoglobin saturation, results in an increase of only the physiologically dissolved oxygen in plasma, which represents about 2-3% of the overall oxygen transport. It is possible that in cerebral capillaries non-haemoglobin oxygen transport may be more significant than formerly thought. In effect, associating PtO_2 measurements with lactate determinations by microdialysis, same authors found a significant reduction of lactate together with an increase of PaO_2, probably indicating a shift to aerobic metabolic status [13].

An insufficient CPP seems to be the most important factor responsible for the low values of PtO_2. It is difficult to find a threshold value above which rising CPP is not accompanied by an elevation in PtO_2. Bruzzone et al. [14] detected that at CPP values between 40 and 50 mmHg, mean values of PtO_2 were an average 10 mmHg lower than those found at CPPs more than 70 mmHg. These values, yet, still seem insufficient to warrant a $PtO_2 > 25$ mmHg in the zones of parenchyma with focal lesions. In fact dependence of PtO_2 from PPC is higher in these districts than in healthy parenchyma, because of increased cerebrovascular local resistance and/or regional alterations of autoregulation. This is the most important advancement of this monitoring system, that is the possibility of positioning the probe on vulnerable areas of parenchyma and evaluating their adequate oxygenation. The placement on healthy areas may provide probably similar results obtained by other global cerebral oxygenation indexes, such as SjO_2.

The correlation between PtO_2 and CO_2 variations is not completely understood. Meixensberger et al. observed a wide range of PtO_2 values in response to hyperventilation, without any correlation with the decrease of SjO_2 [15]. In order to measure the relationship between SjO_2, PtO_2 and CO_2 variations, Gupta et al. placed the probe in healthy and in CT scan hypodense zones [16]. The authors found that in normal cerebral tissue PtO_2 decreased in parallel to SjO_2 during hypocapnia. Despite SjO_2 reduction no changes were identified in the pathologic areas. It is maybe the effect of regional differences in the reactivity to CO_2. These data confirm that simultaneous monitoring of SjO_2 and PtO_2 may provide complementary results, thus allowing us to speculate a distinction between global and regional hypoxia, due to different lesion mechanisms and with need of different treatment and techniques of monitoring. Furthermore these experimental data seem to support the evidence that short-term hyperventilation may improve perfusion in zones of cerebral parenchyma at high risk of hypoxia.

Actually because of the intrinsic characteristics of the monitoring, it is very difficult to define what values can be considered normal for PtO_2, and if a "critical threshold" may exist for ischaemia. Hoffman et al. observed values of 37 mmHg ± 12 in healthy parenchyma of patients who underwent neurosurgical elective procedures [17]. Doppenberg et al. [18] demonstrated a close relationship between CBF and PtO_2 ($r = 0.78$, $p = 0.0001$), showing that the standard threshold of ischaemia of 18 ml/100 g/min corresponds to PtO_2 of 22 mmHg.

Van den Brink et al. evaluated the correlation between PtO_2 values and outcome of 101 patients. The authors observed PtO_2 values less than 15, 10 and 5 mmHg for measurements longer than 30, 45 and 60 minutes in the healthy zones of cerebral parenchyma, emphasizing that the severity and duration of hypoxia were independent factors for the impairment of prognosis [19].

In conclusion we think that PtO_2 measurement is one of the most important advancements in the monitoring of head trauma. The accurate information regarding global or local cerebral oxygenation may allow us to investigate trauma mechanisms and develop individual treatments.

Implications for therapy

In the last years most of the clinical trials involving the treatment of cerebral trauma focused on two different trends, in order to maintain an adequate perfusion pressure or to control intracranial hypertension. For this purpose fluid load and vasopressor drugs, on one side and hyperventilation the other side, were proposed. Recently Robertson et al. compared the efficacy of the two treatments, being not able to show difference on neurological outcome [20]. So far several suggestions concerning the best therapeutic management are controversial because of the different pathophysiology of the lesions, triggered by head injury. Thus, in order to compare clinical results, patients should be possibly divided into categories as homogeneous as possible, in relation to type of lesion and cerebral trauma response.

One of the most important parameters is the presence or absence of pressure autoregulation. The study of pressure autoregulation is difficult and based on time-related phenomenon that is not homogeneous in the cerebral parenchyma. However global changes of pressure autoregulation seem to be very important in the clinical practice; in fact several studies have observed a significant correlation between autoregulation and outcome [21]. It is reasonable that a treatment to support elevated perfusion pressure may have different results according to the presence or absence of autoregulation. In one case in fact the treatment may decrease CBV and the risk of ischaemia, while it may facilitate cerebral oedema and intracranial hypertension in the other.

Moreover after a trauma cerebral tissue reacts in different and time-related ways. As above mentioned, during the early traumatic phase CBF is reduced, and it is followed in the next days by hyperaemia or recovery of normal values. The risk of ischaemia is elevated within the first 24 h after an injury and thus hyperventilation has no advantages for the management of intracranial hypertension, without signs of cerebral herniation. Other treatments, such as administration of sedative, control of hypertermia and eventually moderate induced-hypotermia, in order to decrease cerebral metabolism seem therefore more appropriate.

In conclusion clinical and experimental data suggest that the treatment of intracranial hypertension should be targeted on the basis of prominent alterations in that patient and on the type of the lesion. Perhaps only the integration of clinical evidence with monitoring systems, providing information about district or global damage, physiopathology of lesion mechanisms and effects of injury, allow us a prompt recognition and treatment of secondary ischaemic lesions.

References

1. Bouma GJ, Muizelaar JP, Choi SC et al (1991) Cerebral circulation and metabolism after severe traumatic brain injury: the elusive role of ischemia. J Neurosurg 75:685-693
2. Gopinath SP, Robertson CS, Contant CF et al (1994) Jugular venous desaturation and outcome after head injury. J Neurol Neurosurg Psychiatry 57:717-723
3. Robertson CS, Contant CF, Gokaslan ZL et al (1992) Cerebral blood flow, arteriovenous oxygen difference, and outcome in head injured patients. J Neurol Neurosurg and Psychiatry 55: 594-603
4. Kelly DF, Martin NA, Kordestani R et al (1997) Cerebral blood flow as a predictor of outcome following traumatic brain injury. J Neurosurg 86:633-641
5. Della Corte F, Giordano A, Pennisi MA et al (1997) Quantitative cerebral blood flow and metabolism determination in the first 48 hours after severe head injury with a new dynamic spect device. Acta Neurochirurgica 139:636-642
6. Jaggi JL, Obrist WD, Gennarelli TA et al (1990) Relationship of early cerebral blood flow and metabolism to outcome in acute head injury. J Neurosurg 72:176-182
7. Sakas DE, Bullock MR, Patterson JP et al (1995) Focal cerebral hyperemia after focal head injury in humans: a benign phenomenon? J Neurosurg 83:277-284
8. Mielck F, Stephan H, Scholz M et al (1996) A new method for cerebral blood flow measurement. Br J Anesth 76:A12
9. Goodman JC, Gopinath SP, Valadka AB et al (1996) Lactic acid and aminoacid fluctuations measured using microdialysis reflect physiological derangements in head injury. Acta Neuroch [Suppl]67:37-39
10. Goodman JC, Valadka AB, Gopinath S et al (1999) Extracellular lactate and glucose alterations in the brain after head injury measured by microdialysis. Crit Care Med 27:1965-2064
11. Alessandri B, Doppenberg E, Zauner A et al (1999) Evidence for time-dependent glutamate-mediated glycolysis in head injured patients: a microdialysis study. Acta Neuroch [Suppl]75: 25-28
12. Santbrink H, Maas AIR, Avezaas CJJ (1996) Continuous monitoring of partial pressure of brain tissue oxygen in patients with severe head injury. Neurosurg 38:21-31
13. Menzel M, Doppenberg EMR, Zauner A et al (1999) Increased inspired oxygen concentration as a factor in improved brain tissue oxygenation and tissue lactate levels after severe human head injury. J Neurosurg 91:1-10
14. Bruzzone P, Bellinzona G, Imberti R et al (1998) Effects of cerebral perfusion pressure on brain tissue PO_2 in patients with severe head injury. Acta Neuroch [Suppl]71:111-113
15. Meixensberger J, Buchner K, Dings J et al (1998) Transcranial cerebral oximetry: non invasive monitoring of regional oxygen saturation after acute brain injury. Acta Neuroch [Suppl] 71:182-185
16. Gupta AK, Hutchinson PJ, Al-rawi P et al (1999) Measuring brain tissue oxygenation compared with jugular venous oxygen saturation for monitoring cerebral oxygenation after traumatic brain injury. Anesth Analg 88:549-553
17. Hoffman, WE, Charbel FT, Edelman G (1999) Brain tissue oxygen, carbon dioxide, and pH in neurosurgical patients at risk for ischemia. Anaesth Analg 82:582-586

18. Doppenberg E, Zauner A, Bullock MR et al (1998) Determination of the ischemic threshold for brain tissue oxygenation in the severely head injured patient. Acta Neuroch [Suppl]71: 166-169
19. Van den Brink WA, Santbrink H, Steyerberg EW et al (2000) Brain oxygen in severe head injury. Neurosurgery 46:868-878
20. Robertson C, Valadka A, Hannay J et al (1999) Prevention of secondary ischemic insults after severe head injury. Crit Care Med 27:2086-2095
21. Czosnyka M, Smielewski P, Kirkpatrick P et al (1996) Monitoring of cerebral autoregulation in head-injuried patients. Stroke 27:1829-1834

Neurotrauma: Monitoring and Management of Early and Late Complications

N. STOCCHETTI, S. ROSSI, V. VALERIANI

Early and late complications

Complications after head injury, and mainly after severe head injury, play a major role in both the clinical course and the final outcome. The first cause of severe damage after head injury is the increase of intracranial masses. The overall organization of rescue and transport, both outside and inside the hospital, is aimed at promptly identifying patients at risk of intracranial masses and at the fast transfer of such patients to trauma centers where surgery can be performed.

Early complications are not limited to neurosurgical problems. It has been estimated that the association of brain injury with other insults, capable of reducing cerebral blood flow, such as arterial hypotension, may increase the mortality rate three times [1, 2].

Arterial hypotension is more dangerous than hypoxia because the brain may compensate for reduction of oxygen content by increasing cerebral blood flow (under extreme circumstances it may increase up to four times the baseline value). This mechanism is not viable in cases of arterial hypotension, which itself reduces cerebral blood flow.

Early complications can be detected only when appropriate surveillance is established. Such surveillance is of course very difficult during rescue, for example at the accident scene, but may be performed in a very simple way by measuring arterial saturation, by pulse oximetry, and by carefully and repeatedly measuring arterial pressure. This regimen has proved capable of detecting important disturbances very early after injury [3].

There are many late complications that are capable of damaging the brain and they are indicated as insults. Table 1 summarizes both intra- and extracranial insults.

It should be noted that the brain after injury becomes more vulnerable to insults, so that any given level of insult may profoundly disturb cerebral physiology, even when it could be better tolerated under normal circumstances.

Table 1. Intra- or extracranial insults

Intracranial insults
Intracranial hypertension
Mass lesions
Edema
Hydrocephalus
Infections
Seizures
Alterations of regional and global flows
Damage caused by free radicals and excitotoxic substances
Extracranial insults
Arterial hypotension
Hypoxia
Anemia
Hyperthermia
Hyper/hypocapnia
Electrolyte anomalies (mainly hyponatremia)
Hypo/hyperglycemia
Alterations of the acid-base balance

How to identify insults and complications

The intracranial system is by definition quite difficult to explore. It may be studied by indirect methods, and careful neurological observation represents a very well-established way of exploring cerebral function. Unfortunately patients after head injury suffer profound reductions in all neurological responses and are less suitable for neurological examination. This suggests the necessity of intracranial monitoring. Intracranial monitoring was started in the late 1940s by intracranial pressure (ICP) measurement. In a recent European survey [4], the frequency of intracranial hypertension requiring treatment was assessed both in patients in whom ICP was directly measured and in patients who were not submitted to measurement. The participant physicians were asked to report on the occurrence of intracranial hypertension in patients admitted to prominent neurotrauma centers, and some 800 patients were investigated.

Only 12% of patients without ICP monitoring were suspected of having a ICP rise compared with 50% of patients with ICP monitoring. Since the two groups were comparable for other predictors of severity, it is likely that intracranial hypertension is undetected in 80% of head injury patients, who may suffer a ICP rise if ICP measurement is not applied.

ICP and cerebral perfusion pressure

ICP control is necessary for treating patients during intensive care after head injury. Intracranial hypertension has an impact on outcome after head injury, and it cannot be estimated without precise measurement. The indications for ICP monitoring are now well defined in adults with severe head injury, while they are less defined in other pathologies. Various guide lines [5, 6] have been published reporting the indication for ICP monitoring. Briefly, ICP should be monitored in all trauma patients who are comatose with the Glasgow coma scale ≤ 8 and who at computerized tomographic (CT) scan show pathological findings, and especially when the third ventricle and/or the basal cysterns are compressed [7]. The literature also reports intracranial hypertension in patients without CT scan alterations [8]. Finally, all cases in whom surgical evacuation of hematomas has been performed, are candidates for ICP monitoring.

ICP is a problem in itself, but is also a critical component of cerebral perfusion pressure, which is calculated as the difference between mean arterial pressure and mean ICP. A level of cerebral perfusion pressure below the capability of autoregulation determines a reduction of cerebral blood flow and, therefore, is the main cause of cerebral ischemia after head injury.

Jugular bulb saturation

The measurement of the arterial jugular difference of oxygen content is useful for estimating the relationship between cerebral blood flow and cerebral oxygen consumption. Jugular bulb saturation monitoring has limitations and recently the clinical usefulness of this measurement has been criticized [9]. It is our view that jugular bulb saturation gives useful hints for two main purposes: 1) for assessing the dangerous situation of desaturation (desaturation may contribute to worsening outcome); 2) for establishing the appropriate level of $PaCO_2$ during artificial ventilation. A drop in CO_2 may cause an acute reduction of cerebral blood flow, which may be dangerous. It is not unusual, for example, to discover jugular desaturation due to inappropriate hyperventilation during the first hours after injury.

Management of complications

Intensive care is not just a matter of monitoring, it is a matter of appropriate action undertaken on the basis of precise measurements. The main goal of intensive care after injury is to prevent, to limit, or to avoid further insults to the brain. The damage can only be prevented or limited at the moment of impact by preventive strategies. The secondary damage, however, is a process which starts after injury and may continue for hours or days. Therefore, it provides the best opportunity for effective interventions. Careful surveillance, appropriate management, and fast action based on physiological measures are probably the key points for providing patients with the best chances of good outcome after injury.

References

1. Piek J, Chesnut RM, Marshall LF et al (1992) Extracranial complications of severe head injury. J Neurosurg 77:901-907
2. Chesnut RM, Marshall LF, Klauber MR et al (1993) The role of secondary brain injury in determining outcome from severe head injury. J Trauma 34:216-222
3. Stocchetti N, Furlan A, Volta F (1996) Hypoxemia and arterial hypotension at the accident scene in head injury. J Trauma 40:764-767
4. Murray GD, Teasdale GM, Braakman R et al (1999) On behalf of the European Brain Injury Consortium: the European Brain Injury Consortium Survey of Head Injuries. Acta Neurochir 141:223-236
5. Bullock R, Chesnut R, Clifton G et al (1996) Guidelines for the management of severe head injury. J Neurotrauma 13:639-734
6. Procaccio F, Stocchetti N, Citerio G et al (1999) Raccomandazioni per il trattamento del grave traumatizzato cranico adulto. I. Valutazione iniziale, osservazione e trattamento preospedaliero, criteri attuali di ospedalizzazione, monitoraggio sistemico e cerebrale. Minerva Anestesiol 65:147-158
7. Narayan RK, Kishore PRS, Becker DP et al (1982) Intracranial pressure: to monitor or not to monitor? A review of our experience with severe head injury. J Neurosurg 56:650-659
8. O'Sullivan MG, Statham PF, Jones PA et al (1994) Role of intracranial pressure monitoring in severely head-injured patients without signs of intracranial hypertension on initial computerized tomography. J Neurosurg 80:46-50
9. Latronico N, Beindorf AE, Rasulo FA et al (2000) Limits of intermittent jugular bulb oxygen saturation monitoring in the management of severe head trauma patients. Neurosurgery 46: 1131-1139

Anaesthesia Management Problems in Trauma

A.J. SUTCLIFFE

Preventable deaths in injured patients are known to occur in the pre-hospital setting and in the emergency room [1]. These deaths are commonly attributed to failure to protect the airway, failure to replace blood loss adequately and failure to diagnose and treat life-threatening injuries. Much effort has been put into reducing the number of early preventable deaths. Detailed studies in one hospital have shown that, between 1984 and 1991, the overall incidence of preventable deaths has reduced from 23% to 7%. However, the pattern of preventable deaths has changed. Half of them now occur in the Intensive Care Unit. Many of these deaths are due to sepsis [2]. Sepsis is one of the causes of multiple organ failure which is still a feared complication after trauma. Multiple organ failure is probably caused by the systemic inflammatory response syndrome (SIRS). However, not all severely injured patients develop SIRS. Consequently the Two-Hit causation model has been proposed [3]. During the first hit, which may be due to direct tissue injury or ischaemic injury secondary to hypovolaemia, the neutrophils are primed. Then, a second insult (the second hit) activates neutrophils causing an autodestructive inflammatory response. Secondary insults include surgery, sepsis and probably other factors such as recurrent episodes of hypoxia and/or hypovolaemia.

There is far less information about preventable deaths in the operating room. A detailed study carried out in five American trauma centres found that different surgical management strategies may have prevented death in approximately 10% of patients [4]. Sadly the contribution of skilled anaesthetic management to the survival of patients was not considered by these authors.

Since 1956, it has been recognized that in a mixed group of patients presenting for urgent surgery, failure to provide adequate fluid resuscitation prior to induction of anaesthesia and inadequate care of the airway increases mortality [5]. Regrettably, similar errors continue to occur [6]. The contribution of anaesthesia to mortality and morbidity in injured patients has not been studied in detail. Commonsense, however, suggests that the lessons learned in the emergency room and Intensive Care Unit should be applied in the operating room. Whole textbooks have been written about trauma anaesthesia. In a chapter such as this, the discussion is inevitably brief and should not be regarded as a complete description of the anaesthetic management of the trauma patient. Rather, it is a collection of management problems that will be faced by many anaesthetists and for which there are recent publications which may have relevance now or in the future. Furthermore, the topics chosen reflect the personal concerns of the author. The discussion is most applicable to the severely injured patient but the principles apply equally to those patients with minor injuries. The problems discussed include the following:

- timing of anaesthesia and surgery
- the full stomach
- endotracheal intubation for patients with, or at risk of, unstable cervical spine injury
- preventing regurgitation of stomach contents during induction of anaesthesia and endotracheal intubation
- induction of anaesthesia
- fluid replacement during anaesthesia
- management of anaesthesia and surgery to minimize the risk of multiple organ failure
- postoperative pain relief

Timing of anaesthesia and surgery

It is important to strike a balance between the need for rapid anaesthesia and surgery and the need to resuscitate as completely as is sensible prior to anaesthesia. The need of the patient for emergency surgery to correct life threatening airway problems and uncontrollable, torrential haemorrhage is usually obvious. However, many anaesthetists will be faced with a group of patients who require urgent surgery but in whom some delay is acceptable as long as the time is used for resuscitative measures or other interventions which improve the patient's physiological condition. The essence of successful management is communication between the anaesthetist and the surgeon. In theory, the solution. The correct time for anaesthesia and surgery is when the risks of proceeding are less than the risks of delay. In practice, these decisions are often not simple and require the anaesthetist to be an integral and respected member of the trauma team.

The full stomach

Post mortem studies have shown that following injury, stomach emptying may be delayed for eight hours or more [7]. The injury itself, pain, and opiate analgesics are all thought to play a part. In the past, anxiety was often included in this list. It has now been shown not to delay stomach emptying [8]. Recently, the need for prolonged preoperative fasting has been questioned for many groups of patients [9] but trauma patients are still thought to be at risk of delayed gastric emptying [10]. In the U.K., personal experience suggests that many trauma victims have recently eaten a meal and that the contents of their stomachs are not acidic. Thus the greater risk of aspiration is due to mechanical obstruction due to solid stomach contents rather than chemical injury. There is no published evidence to support this view.

A survey of methods used by anaesthetists to identify trauma patients at risk of aspiration showed that most took note of the interval between eating and injury and the use of opioid analgesia. The authors comment that although trauma delays gastric emptying, there is little evidence to confirm that there is an increased risk of aspiration following trauma [11]. It is probable that reducing gastric volume and increasing gastric pH improve safety [12] but benefit from antacids, H2 receptor blockers, proton pump inhibitors or prokinetics is unproven for any population [12]. These findings might be explained if stomach contents are not acidic as suggested above.

Endotracheal intubation for patients with, or at risk of, unstable cervical spine injury

Ideally, unstable cervical spine injury should be excluded prior to endotracheal intubation. The entire upper spine down to and including T1 should be visualized on plain radiographs. If this is not possible, a CT scan is needed. Some centres are able to provide rapid Magnetic Resonance Imaging which is a better method of identifying soft tissue injury [13]. Many techniques are described for emergency airway maintenance in the emergency room [14], but in the operating room, endotracheal intubation is usually indicated. During intubation, a study on cadavers has shown that the predominant motion in the intact spine is extension. This changes to flexion following injury. Furthermore, for injuries below the atlantooccipital junction, none of the interventions commonly employed by anaesthetists to prevent spinal movement actually do so [15]. In the clinical setting however, oral intubation following rapid sequence induction with the application of cricoid pressure and manual in-line stabilization is not associated with neurological sequelae [16]. Of the techniques available, fibreoptic intubation appears to be the method of choice [17]. It is disappointing that the intubating laryngeal mask, used with or without a light wand, has not lived up to its early promise. Adjusting movements are required in 100% of patients to achieve a successful intubation [18].

For patients at risk of aspiration, preoxygenation, rapid sequence induction, and cricoid pressure are commonly recommended. The presence of a collar makes intubation difficult [19]. However, removal of the collar may also cause movement as may single handed cricoid pressure. If the patient is immobilized in a hard collar, the safest option is probably removal of the anterior part and single-handed cricoid pressure. In the absence of a collar, bimanual cricoid pressure should be used [20].

Induction of anaesthesia

Prior to induction, preoxygenation is recommended for patients in whom there is a risk of gastric aspiration. There is some debate about how long oxygen should be given for. For most purposes, one minute of breathing 100% oxygen through a tightly fitting mask allows three minutes of apnoea without significant peripheral desaturation. However, measurement of end-tidal oxygen is said to be more accurate. The physiology is complex. Despite the fact that end-tidal oxygen and oxygen saturation are not improved by three minutes of breathing 100% oxygen, the period of apnoea this allows is almost doubled [21]. This may be useful for trauma patients where intubation is likely to be difficult. Maintaining adequate oxygenation is important for all patients but is particularly important for head injured patients. It is well known that even a brief period of hypoxia during the resuscitation period worsens outcome after head injury and the effect is much worse if hypotension also occurs [22]. This is also true of hypoxia and hypotension occurring in the first 24 hours of ICU care (Fig. 1). Hypoxia should also be avoided in the operative period. This, and other chapters, lay much stress on the difficulties of intubating patients with a cervical spine injury. The association between head and spinal injury is well known. However, for the individual anaesthetist on the emergency rota, the probability of being asked to anaesthetize patients with an isolated head injury is much higher than the probability of being asked to anaesthetize a patient with both in-

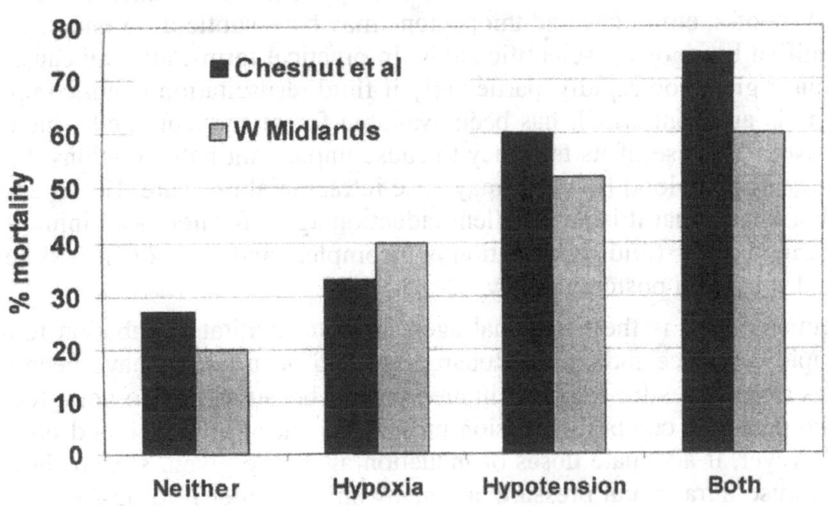

Fig. 1. Secondary ischaemic injury and mortality after head injury

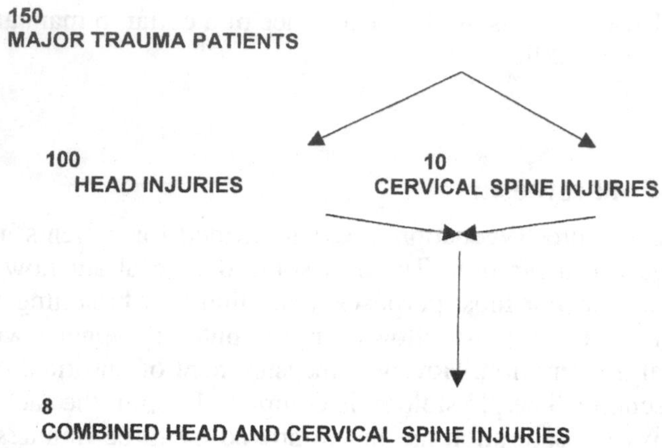

Fig. 2. Incidence of cervical spine injury in a major trauma population (personal data, 1991)

juries. Figure 2 illustrates this. Given that a significant proportion of unstable spinal injuries are diagnosed prior to induction of anaesthesia, it is important to keep a sense of proportion. When the possibility of a spinal cord injury cannot be excluded, it is still far more likely that a head injured patient will be damaged by allowing hypoxia to occur while struggling to intubate without moving the neck than it is that paralysis will occur secondary to neck movement. Furthermore, there is a lot of evidence to suggest that the greatest risk of spinal cord damage is from prolonged hypoperfusion with, or without, inappropriate positioning on the operating table [23].

The choice of induction agent for trauma patients is a matter of personal choice. Propofol, etomidate and thiopentone may have subtle differences, which are identified by rigorous scientific study. In practical terms, all may cause hypotension if given too rapidly, particularly if fluid resuscitation is not complete. Ketamine is an agent which has been available for many years and which fell out of favour because of its tendency to cause unpleasant hallucinations. It also increases cerebral blood flow and may raise intracranial pressure. However, it is the author's view that it is an excellent induction agent for non head injured patients particularly if fluid resuscitation is incomplete and the patient will be sedated and ventilated postoperatively.

Suxamethonium is the traditional agent used to facilitate intubation following a rapid sequence induction. Rocuronium and vecuronium have been suggested as alternatives for the head injured patient because they do not affect intracranial pressure, cerebral perfusion pressure or mean arterial blood pressure [24]. However, if adequate doses of induction agent are given, suxamethonium does not raise intracranial pressure and many still consider it to be the agent of choice [25].

There is increasing interest in the release of toxic cellular metabolites as a cause of organ damage following reperfusion. Myocardial reperfusion injury can be reduced by isoflurane and sevoflurane [26]. Although it is unwise to extrapolate from the myocardium to other organs, this should make us think about our choice of anaesthetic vapour in terms other than the immediate effects on key physiological parameters.

Fluid replacement during anaesthesia

In the past, there was extensive debate about the relative merits of crystalloid versus colloid solutions during the resuscitation of severely injured patients. However, no one disputes that blood should be given with crystalloid or colloid solutions. In older studies, the colloid used was albumin. In recent years, a number of synthetic colloidal solutions have become available. The chemical structure of these solutions influences their properties. Knowledge of these properties should help the anaesthetist to make a rational choice of fluid [27]. Starch solutions have attracted particular interest. Depending on the molecular weight and substitution rate of the starch, beneficial effects on platelet and leucocyte function, volume replacement and endothelial integrity can be demonstrated [28]. Higher molecular weight starches accumulate in the tissues and cause severe itching in some patients. Medium molecular weight starches have advantages [29]. The newest medium molecular weight starches with a low degree of substitution (6% hydroxyethyl starch 130/0.4) may prove to be useful.

Four years ago, work was published which showed excess mortality in trauma patients when a rapid infusion system was used [30]. The findings were widely quoted without qualification. Perusal of the original paper is enlightening. It is highly probable that some patients were overloaded because fluids could be given so quickly. During the study period, everyone was taught to be liberal with fluid and to resuscitate their patients fully. Prior to the introduction of rapid infusion systems it was difficult to keep up with rapid blood loss. This paper showed that too much fluid is as dangerous as too little and that fluid replacement must always be meticulously monitored. This said, we still do not know what the end-points of resuscitation should be. It has been suggested that in the future fluid resuscitation will be guided by non-invasive monitoring [31]. The 'correct' end points for resuscitation are still unclear. Hypotension is undoubtedly detrimental. As well as keeping up with blood loss while the surgeon controls bleeding, perhaps we should copy our cardiac and hepatology colleagues and use aprotinin more often [32].

Management of anaesthesia and surgery to minimize the risk of multiple organ failure

Multiple organ failure is a feared complication of severe injury. Improvements in resuscitation have reduced early mortality from injury. Hypoxia and hypovolaemia, however, have also been implicated in the late development of multiple organ failure. Thus, although there are little data to support the contention, it is probable that efforts to improve emergency room management have also reduced the incidence of multiple organ failure. Reperfusion injury caused by toxic metabolites increases capillary leakiness [33] and contributes to organ failure. It seems logical, therefore, to control haemorrhage as rapidly as possible and to try avoid prolonged periods of reduced tissue perfusion. Many trauma centres subject severely injured patients to prolonged operative procedures to control intra-cavity haemorrhage and to fix fractures. Despite the anaesthetist's best efforts, it is difficult to keep the patient well filled and warm for the duration of the procedure. Furthermore, access to the patient is limited and positioning may be other than supine. Consequently, the interpretation of monitoring results may be less easy than in the controlled environment of the intensive care unit. Some surgeons are advocating damage control surgery for the treatment of intra-abdominal haemorrhage [34]. During the first operative procedure, surgery is limited to that necessary to control haemorrhage. The patient is then nursed in the intensive care unit until such time as physiological stability is achieved. Particular attention is paid to correcting volume deficits, acid base status, clotting and hypothermia. Definitive surgery is then performed. A large study comparing damage control surgery with traditional surgery has not been undertaken. At present, therefore, this is only a promising technique.

Those anaesthetists who work in both the operating room and the intensive care unit will be aware that both oxygen and mechanical ventilation can cause lung damage and prevent the resolution of the adult respiratory distress syndrome [35]. Thus for intensive care patients we use the minimum amount of oxygen compatible with acceptable arterial oxygenation. We also limit both tidal volume and peak inspiratory pressure. In the operating room, if the patient is well oxygenated and arterial carbon dioxide is within normal limits, less attention is paid to ventilator settings. This is perhaps another area where the trauma anaesthetist could modify his practice and contribute to a better outcome for the patient.

Postoperative pain control

Many severely injured patients are ventilated postoperatively. In order to settle the patient on a ventilator sedation and analgesia are routinely prescribed. For the patient who is less severely injured and nursed on a ward, adequate pain control is a key issue. From time to time, I review papers where it is suggested that if the patient has a lower leg fracture, the ability to feel pain is essential so that compartment syndrome can be readily diagnosed [36]. Adequate pain relief is a basic human right. Guidelines have been specifically written about pain relief for trauma patients [37]. Pain relief can, and should, be provided. A variety of techniques are available [38] and are shown in Table 1.

Table 1. Methods of pain relief

Remove pain	Drug treatment	Regional analgesia	Physical methods	Psychological methods
Surgery	Opiods	Epidural	Physiotherapy	Relaxation
Splinting	NSAIDs	Nerve block	Manipulation	Hypnosis
	Paracetamol	Infiltration	TENS	
	Ketamine		Ice	
			Acupuncture	

Conclusions

The evidence base for most anaesthetic interventions is weak [39]. In this review, I have described current best practice and highlighted areas of concern which would benefit from detailed scientific study.

References

1. McDermott FT, Cordner SM, Tremayne A (1996) Evaluation of the medical management and preventability of death in 137 road traffic fatalities in Victoria, Australia: an overview. Consultative Committee on Road Traffic Fatalities in Victoria. J Trauma 40:520-533
2. Thoburn E, Norris P, Flores R et al (1993) System care improves trauma outcome: patient care errors dominate reduced preventable death rate. J Em Med 11:135-139
3. Moore FA, Moore EE (1995) Evolving concepts in the pathogenesis of postinjury multiple organ failure. Surg Clin N Amer 75:257-277
4. Hoyt DB, Bulger EM, Knudson MM et al (1994) Death in the operating room: an analysis of a multi-center experience. J Trauma 37:426-432
5. Edwards G, Morton HJV, Pask EA et al (1956) Deaths associated with anaesthesia. Anaesthesia 11:194-220
6. Webb RK, Van Der Walt JH, Runciman WB et al (1993) Which monitor? An analysis of 2000 incident reports. Anaesth Intens Care 21:529-542
7. Rose EF (1979) Factors influencing gastric emptying. J Forensic Sci 24:200-206
8. Lydon A, McGinley J, Cooke JT et al (1998) Effect of anxiety on the rate of gastric emptying of liquids. Br J Anaesth 81:522-525
9. Simini B (1999) Preoperative fasting. Lancet 353:862
10. Soreide E, Stromskag KE, Steen PA (1995) Statistical aspects in studies of preoperative fluid intake and gastric content. Acta Anaesthesiol Scand 39:738-743
11. Hardman JG, O'Connor PJ (1999) Predicting gastric contents following trauma: an evaluation of current practice. Eur J Anaesthesiol 16:404-409
12. Engelhardt T, Webster NR (1999) Pulmonary aspiration of gastric contents in anaesthesia. Br J Anaesth 83:453-460

13. Benzel EC, Hart BL, Ball PA et al (1996) Magnetic resonance imaging for the evaluation of patients with occult cervical spine injury. J Neurosurg 85:824-829
14. Thierbach AR, Lipp MDW (1999) Airway management in trauma patients. Anesthesiol Clin N Am 17(1):63-81
15. Lennarson PJ, Smith D, Todd MM et al (2000) Segmental cervical spine motion during orotracheal intubation of the intact and injured spine with and without external stabilization. J Neurosurg 92:S201-206
16. Criswell JC, Parr MJ, Nolan JP (1994) Emergency airway management in patients with cervical spine injuries. Anaesthesia 49:900-903
17. Fuchs G, Schwarz G, Baumgartner A et al (1999) Fibreoptic intubation in 327 neurosurgical patients with lesions of the cervical spine. J Neurosurg Anesthesiol 11:11-16
18. Kihara S, Wantanabe S, Taguchi N et al (2000) A comparison of blind and lightwand-guided tracheal intubation through the intubating laryngeal mask. Anaesthesia 55:427-431
19. Asai T, Barclay K, Power I et al (1994) Cricoid pressure impedes placement of the laryngeal mask airway and subsequent intubation through the mask. Br J Anaesth 72:47-51
20. Fletcher SN, McNeill JM (1998) Tracheal intubation in trauma. Br J Anaesth 80:270
21. Campbell IT, Beatty PCW (1994) Monitoring preoxygenation. Br J Anaesth 72:3-4
22. Chesnut RM, Marshall SB, Piek J et al (1993) Early and late systemic hypotension as a fundamental source of cerebral ischemia following severe brain injury in the Traumatic Coma Data Bank. Acta Neurochir 59[Suppl]:121-125
23. McLeod ADM, Calder I (2000) Spinal cord injury and direct laryngoscopy - the legend lives on. Br J Anaesth 84:705-709
24. Schramm WM, Strasser K, Bartunek A et al (1996) Effects of rocuronium and vecuronium on intracranial pressure, mean arterial pressure and heart rate in neurosurgical patients. Br J Anaesth 77:607-611
25. Brown MM, Parr MJA, Manara AR (1996) The effect of suxamethonium on intracranial pressure and cerebral perfusion pressure in patients with severe head injuries following blunt trauma. Eur J Anaesthesiol 13:474-477
26. Ross S, Foex P (1999) Protective effects of anaesthetics in reversible and irreversible ischaemia-reperfusion injury. Br J Anaesth 82:622-632
27. Traylor RJ, Pearl RG (1996) Crystalloid versus colloid: all colloids are not created equal. Anesth Analg 83:209-212
28. Vincent J-L (1991) Plugging the leaks? New insights into synthetic colloids. Crit Care Med 19:316-317
29. Prough S, Kramer G (1994) Medium starch, please. Anesth Analg 79:1034-1035
30. Hambly PR, Dutton RP (1996) Excess mortality associated with the use of a rapid infusion system at a level 1 trauma center. Resuscitation 31:127-133
31. Asensio JA, Demetriades D, Berne TY et al (1996) Invasive and noninvasive monitoring for early recognition and treatment of shock in high-risk trauma and surgical patients. Surg Clin N Amer 76(4):985-997
32. Schneider B (1976) Results of a field study on the therapeutic value of aprotinin in traumatic shock. Arzneimittelforshung 26:1606-1610
33. Zikria BA (ed) (1994) Reperfusion injuries and capillary leak syndrome. Futura Publishing Company Inc, New York
34. Rotondo MF, Zonies DH (1997) The damage control sequence and underlying logic. Surg Clin N Amer 77(4):761-777
35. Sutcliffe AJ (1999) ARDS: pathophysiology related to cardiorespiratory embarrassment. In: Alpar EK, Gosling P (eds) Trauma, a scientific basis for care. Arnold, London, pp 142-152
36. Sutcliffe AJ (2000) Annotation. Injury 31:359
37. Follin SL, Charland SL (1997) Acute pain management: operative or medical procedures and trauma. Am Pharmacother 31:1068-1076
38. McQuay H, Moore A, Justins D (1997) Treating acute pain in hospital. Br Med J, 314:1531-1535
39. Myles PS, Bain DL, Johnson F et al (1999) Is anaesthesia evidence-based? A survey of anaesthetic practice. Br J Anaesth 82:591-595

Imaging of Neurotrauma

R. Pozzi-Mucelli, M. Locatelli

Trauma is the leading cause of death in individuals under the age of 45 years, with head injury the major contributor to mortality in over half of these cases. Most craniocerebral trauma victims requiring hospitalized care are young (between the ages of 15 and 24 years). The etiology of craniocerebral trauma includes falls from heights, motor vehicle accidents, sports and recreational injuries, and acts of violence. In the countries of the European Union, motor vehicle accidents are by far the most-important etiological factor in head injuries. Motor vehicle accidents are responsible for approximately 65,000 deaths and 1,500,000 injuries per year. Mild trauma constitutes the majority of the injuries [1].

Mechanisms of traumatic brain injury

Traumatic brain injury can be divided into penetrating and non-penetrating injury. Non-penetrating traumas are most common. In non-penetrating trauma, the effects of a blow to the head are determined by the type, direction, and importance of the forces acting on the head and the structural characteristics of the scalp, skull, and the brain.

Brain tissue has two physical properties that are important in understanding the effects of trauma: it is non-compressible and it is susceptible to shearing forces. Therefore the brain damage following a blunt trauma arises from brain compression, torsion, and axonal shearing stresses. These mechanical stresses on brain tissue are induced by sudden deceleration or angular acceleration and rotation of the head. Both events may occur together.

The rotational injury produces mechanical trauma of the neuronal axons and blood vessels within the white matter. Shearing lesions, also known as diffuse axonal injuries, may be extensive and severe, are often multiple and bilateral, and can even occur when there is no direct impact to the head. Brain may be damaged adjacent to the site of trauma or at a distance due to the contrecoup impact of the brain with the skull or rigid dural membrane. This tears the delicate meninges and can result in subdural hematoma.

Clinical considerations

The outcome of patients admitted after craniocerebral trauma is related to a series of parameters, which can be categorized into four major groups:
- severity of the initial injury
- prior condition of the patient
- timing of therapeutic intervention
- quality of care and patient management

Severity of trauma

The Glasgow Coma Scale (GCS) is a standardized scale of responsiveness which is used in head trauma victims to assess the degree of brain impairment and to identify the seriousness of injury in relation to outcome. The GCS was first introduced in the 1970s, and is now widely used throughout the world. It provides a numerical expression of the clinical severity of head injury and predicting the victim's likelihood of recovery. The GCS calculates the severity of a patient's injury based on his/her ability to perform three major neurological functions: 1) eye opening, 2) verbal response, and 3) motor response. These determinants are evaluated separately according to a numerical value that indicates the level of consciousness and the degree of dysfunction. The total GCS score is the sum of the scores for the three individual components [2-4].

GCS scores run from a high of 15 to a low of 3; the more severe the injury, the lower the score on the scale, and the poorer the outcome prognosis. Patients with a GCS score of 13-15 are considered to have suffered a "mild" head injury. A score of 9-12 is considered to indicate a "moderate" brain injury and a score of 8 or less reflects a "severe" brain injury. A low score suggests a very severe injury and little likelihood of total recovery.

Prior condition of the patient

Patient outcome is determined to a large extent by pre-existing conditions. The most-important factor is the age of the patient. Patient age is inversely related to prognosis after head trauma. This can be explained by a number of factors:
- ageing of the brain results in cerebral atrophy, decreased cerebral plasticity, and decreased flexibility of blood vessels due to atherosclerosis. As the brain shrinks, its blood vessels become increasingly tethered, which enhances their vulnerability to trauma;
- older patients are at greater risk for cerebrovascular disease;
- older individuals have a higher risk of concurrent medical conditions (heart disease, obstructive lung disease, diabetes, obesity, etc.) which are correlated with a poor outcome.

Timing of therapeutic intervention

Favorable outcome is determined to a large extent by the time interval from injury to competent care in a specialized institution. Evaluation with computed tomography (CT) scanning should be performed as quickly as possible. However, if a patient's condition deteriorates rapidly, the CT examination should be shortened.

Quality of care

Patient outcome is related to the quality of care in the acute and subacute stages of craniocerebral trauma, although this factor is very difficult to quantify. Mortality rates for patients treated in specialized neuro-intensive care units or dedicated trauma centers appear to be lower than for patients treated in non-trauma centres.

Plain X-ray films

Routine skull radiographs are the most-basic and readily available imaging study, yet potentially the least informative [5-7]. Their use in head injury is currently highly controversial. Plain skull X-rays are primarily used for the detection of fractures; their use for diagnosing intracranical mass effect by showing a pineal shift has been superseded by CT scanning.

It is well known that the diagnostic yield of plain skull films is low. Less than 9% of skull radiographs reveal fractures. Moreover, a large proportion (up to 50%) of skull films obtained in emergency units are diagnostically unsatisfactory.

Moreover, there is little relationship between calvarial and intracranial injury. It is generally stated that only one-quarter to one-fifth of patients with skull fractures have intracranial injury. Conversely, of all the patients with intracranial injury, over half do not have skull fractures.

In many trauma centers, patients with head trauma are categorized into one of three groups:

- low-risk patients are asymptomatic or have limited symptoms and signs (headache, dizziness, or scalp hematoma, laceration, contusion, or abrasion);
- high-risk patients have obvious, severe open or closed head injury;
- the moderate-risk group includes all other patients.

Based on this algorithm for radiological evaluation of the head-injured patient, skull films are potentially useful in the moderate-risk group but they are not indicated when CT examination is to be performed.

Computed tomography

Since its introduction, CT scanning has revolutionized the management of head-injured patients [8]. It has become the imaging method of choice in patients with acute craniocerebral trauma and has largely supplanted conventional skull X-rays in most trauma centers. The availability of CT scanning has dramatically improved the survival of patients with epidural or subdural hematomas (survival of epidural hematoma patients 84.4 to 100%; mortality of subdural haematoma patients: 63-68% to 27-36%). The advantages of CT scanning are its rapidity, its accuracy for the diagnosis of surgically amenable lesions, and the relative ease of monitoring severely ill patients in a scanner. The contribution of CT to the management of head injuries includes both the diagnosis and the prognosis [9-11].

In a patient with craniocerebral trauma, the CT examination should start with a lateral scout view, also known as localizer image. This digitized image of the skull should be carefully inspected for the presence of fracture lines. When a linear skull fracture is oriented parallel to the plane of the axial sections, it can easily be missed on axial images, and will be visible only on the scout view. Moreover, the digital scout image is not only useful for the detection of fracture line, but also for demonstrating the presence of radio-opaque foreign bodies, maxillofacial injury, and intracranial air.

The diagnostic potential of a CT scan is related to its ability to demonstrate differences in attenuation value of different tissues. In trauma patients, this implies that axial images are best viewed with two window settings:

- brain parenchyma window (level = 40 HU, width = 80-120 HU); this window setting provides the best evaluation of intracranial soft tissues;
- bone window (level = 500 HU, width = 2000-4000); this is used for the detection of fractures and foreign objects. Recalculation of the image raw data with a specific "bone" or "edge" algorithm may be necessary for the detection of hairline fractures, which can be missed on "routine" bone windows of images obtained with a brain algorithm.

Initial head trauma studies do not require the use of intravenous contrast agents. They can even cause diagnostic difficulties by masking acute clotted blood. Contrast agents are only useful in the diagnosis of isodense extracerebral blood collections, but with the improved quality of scanners, this has become a rare occurrence.

Magnetic resonance imaging

Although magnetic resonance imaging (MRI) is the best imaging modality to image the brain, it has a limited role in acute craniocerebral trauma [12-14]. There are several disadvantages (compared to CT) most dealing with the general condition of the patient. These limitations are related to:

– relatively (compared to CT) long acquisition time. Although fast spin-echo MRI techniques have decreased the imaging time, they are relatively insensitive to the presence of hemorrhage. The role of the new echoplanar imaging techniques in the setting of acute craniocerebral traumas remains to be investigated. However, to date, echoplanar and, in general, ultrafast sequences are available only on a few machines.

Limitations of MRI include difficulty in bringing life support and traction equipment into the magnet room; relatively low sensitivity to acute subarachnoid blood; limited value in depicting osseous lesions of the skull; risk of dislodging metallic foreign bodies.

On the other hand MRI is the preferred technique for the evaluation of traumatic brain injury in the subacute and chronic traumatic stages (except for documentation of old skull fractures and detection of small bone fragments).

Imaging findings and outcome

Several studies have been dedicated to the correlation of the imaging findings (mainly on CT) and patient outcome [11, 15, 16]. In many studies a strong relationship between the CT scan appearance, mortality, and the frequency of elevated intracranial pressure has been demonstrated. Among the CT features the most important in order to predict the patient outcome are the existence of a mass lesion (> 15 ml, either intra- or extracerebral), midline shift (greater than 3 or 5 mm), compressed cisterns, compressed (small) ventricles, and subarachnoid hemorrhage [11].

It has been shown that CT findings indicating herniation, either transtentorial or subfalcian (particularly abnormal mesencephalic cisterns and midline shift), are strongly associated with the risk of elevated intracranial pressure and death. Normal CT scan as well as abnormal CT scans not demonstrating abnormal mesencephaalic cisterns, midline shift, or mass effect are associated with a low risk of elevated intracranial pressure and death.

Mass effect

An association has been reported between the presence of a mass lesion as seen on CT scans and poor outcome. However, the volume of a mass alone is not a particularly strong predictor of death.

Abnormal mesencephalic cisterns

The state of the mesencephalic cisterns predicts outcome following severe head injury and is considered the most-important CT predictor of outcome. If the mesencephalic cisterns are obliterated or compressed on the first CT scan, the outcome is much more likely to be poor.

Midline shift

Although there is not complete agreement, the midline shift is a very strong predictor of abnormal intracranial pressure. Furthermore, an association between the degree of midline shift and the risk of dying has also been demonstrated.

Size of the ventricles

Ventricular compression correlates with elevated intracranial pressure, although this finding has a low predictive value compared to previous findings. Asymmetrical ventricles have been shown to have a low predictive value with regard to elevated intracranial pressure.

Follow-up

CT is the main radiologic tool in diagnosing and localizing head injury lesions, but, at the same time, CT is an important tool for the follow-up of patients with head traumas [16-18]. The goal of follow-up CT scans is to detect any new and to monitor existing lesions. The timing for scanning a patient who has had an initially positive CT scan is not completely defined but, in general, follow-up CT scans are performed at 12-24 h and, eventually, at 72 h, 5-7 days, and 14 days (after the initial CT scan, on the basis of the severity of trauma and clinical indications). It is generally recognized that, following major head traumas, a follow-up CT scan within 24 h of the injury should detect the majority of new and worsening lesions. The percentage of radiographic worsening ranges from 28 to 43% of the patients with severe head injury. The most-common delayed lesions are intracerebral hemorrhage, contusion, and infarct.

Although CT is a useful modality in the follow-up, the patient's overall status, including the assessment of GCS, pupillary reactivity, level of consciousness, and intracranial pressure should give a fairly good indication whether a follow-up CT scan is needed. It had been demonstrated that a change in GCS alone has a statistically significant correlation with the change on follow-up CT scans, both for improvement and deterioration. Therefore, clinical deterioration warrants an emergent CT scan to elucidate the underlying pathology.

References

1. Gean AD (1993) Imaging of head trauma. Lippincot-Raven, New York
2. Hall KM, Hamilton BB, Gordon WA, Zasler ND (1993) Characteristics and comparison of functional assessment indices: disability rating scale, functional independence measure, and functional assessment measure. J Head Trauma Rehabil 8:60-74
3. Hra M, Kadowaki C, Watanabe H et al (1988) Necessity for ICP monitoring to supplement GCS in head trauma cases. Neurochirurgia (Stuttg) 31:39-44
4. Hennes H, Lee M, Smith D et al (1998) Clinical predictors of severe head trauma in children. Am J Dis Child 142:1045-1047
5. Ros SP, Cetta F (1992) Are skull radiographs useful in the evaluation of asymptomatic infants following minor head injury? Pediatr Emerg Care 8:328-330
6. Chan KH, Mann KS, Yue CP et al (1990) The significance of skull fracture in acute traumatic intracranial hematomas in adolescents: a prospective study. J Neurosurg 72:189-194
7. Gorman DF (1987) The utility of post-traumatic skull X-rays. Arch Emerg Med 4:141-150
8. Koo AH, La Roque RL (1981) Evaluation of head trauma by computed tomography. Radiology 123:345-350
9. Colquhoun IR, Burrows EH (1989) The prognostic significance of the third ventricle and basal cisterns in severe closed head injury. Clin Radiol 40:13-16
10. Dublin AB, French BN, Renick JM (1977) Computed tomography in head trauma. Radiology 122:365-369
11. Eisenberg HM, Gary HE, Aldrich EF et al (1990) Initial CT findings in 753 patients with severe head injury: a report from the NIH traumatic coma data bank. J Neurosurg 73:688-698
12. Gentry LR, Godersky JC, Thompson B (1988) MR imaging of head trauma: review of the distribution and radiopatholgic features of traumatic lesions. AJNR 9:101-110
13. Gentry LR, Godersky JC, Thompson B, Dunn VD (1988) Prospective comparative study of intermediate field MR and CT in the evaluation of closed head trauma. AJNR 9:91-100
14. Kelly AB, Zimmerman RD, Snow RB et al (1988) Head trauma: comparison of MR and CT – experience in 100 patients. AJNR 9:699-708
15. Kishore PRS (1981) Significance of CT in head injury: correlation with intracranial pressure. AJNR 2:307-311
16. Lee TT, Aldana PR, Kirton OC, Green BA (1997) Follow up CT scans in moderate and severe head injuries: correlation with Glasgow coma scores and complication rate. Acta Neurochir (Wien) 139:1042-1048
17. Stein SC, Spettel C, Young GS, Ross SE (1993) Delayed and progressive brain injury in closed head trauma: radiological demonstration. Neurosurgery 32:25-30
18. Stein SC, Young GS, Talucci RX et al (1992) Delayed brain injury after head trauma: significance of coagulopathy. Neurosurgery 30:160-165

INFECTIONS

Prevention and Reduction of Pneumonia Associated with Ventilation in Intensive Therapy

M.A. Pennisi, M. Antonelli, G. Conti, F. Cavaliere, A. Arcangeli

Ventilator-associated pneumonia (VAP) is usually a bacterial nosocomial pneumonia that develops in mechanically ventilated patients. The incidence of VAP ranges from as little as 3% to more than 52% [1]. Such large variation in incidence has been partly caused by different diagnostic criteria used, but probably mostly reflects variability in case mix and in infection control practices.

Crude mortality rates for patients with VAP depend on case mix and range from 20 to 50% [2]. Although not all deaths in patients with this form of pneumonia are directly attributable to infection, it has been shown to have an independent effect on mortality. Indeed, VAP attributable mortality estimated by case-control study ranges between 20 and 30% [3]. A clear understanding of the pathogenesis and risk factors may help to choose devices and strategies to reduce the incidence of VAP.

Aspiration of colonized or infected oropharyngeal or gastrointestinal content is probably the main cause of VAP. Most cases of VAP are caused by microorganisms residing in the adjacent oropharyngeal or upper gastrointestinal tract. In some cases heavily colonized gastric fluid appears to be a major source of pathogens. Factors allowing bacterial grow in the stomach and factors causing gastric content reflow are both involved. Bacterial growth occurs when acidity is lost (H_2 blockers, antiacids, tube feedings).

Several studies have suggested that prophylaxis with drugs without effects on gastric pH (sucralfate) may be associated with a lower incidence of VAP in comparison with anti H_2 receptor antagonist. [4-7]. Nevertheless, in 1998 a multicenter, randomized, blinded placebo-controlled trial comparing sucralfate and ranitidine for the prevention of upper gatrointestinal bleeding in patients requiring mechanical ventilation showed a non-significantly reduced incidence of VAP in the sucralfate group (19.1 vs. 16.2%), no difference in mortality and length of stay, and a statistically significant reduction of gastrointestinal bleeding in the ranitidine group [8]. In a multicenter natural history study of bleeding risk, the incidence of bleeding in the sucralfate group was 4%, equal to that observed in patients receiving no prophylaxis [9]. Potential mechanisms that contribute to reflux are: the use of drugs that impair esophageal motility (sedatives, adrenergic agonists, muscle relaxants) and impairment of lower esophageal sphincter due to nasogastric intubation.

Different strategies have been proposed to reduce the incidence of VAP by reducing the risk of colonization, minimizing the risk of aspiration, and preventing exogenous contamination. Hand washing associated with antiseptic products is a simple, but effective method to prevent colonization. In this regard, some antiseptics could be more effective than others. Doebelling et al. [10] conducted a randomized controlled trial involving 1894 adult patients in three intensive care units (ICUs), comparing chlorhexidine and isopropyl alcohol, for hand washing. When chlorhexidine was used there were significantly fewer nosocomial infections (152 versus 202).

The use of topical antibiotics delivered directly to the lower respiratory tract did affect mortality. This approach is believed to increase the risk of highly resistant pathogen infection. More interesting is the use of an infection prophylaxis regimen that employs topical and oral non-absorbable antibiotics to eradicate pathogenic microrganisms from the gastrointestinal tract.

The concept of selective decontamination of the digestive tract (SDD) was first introduced in 1983 [11]. The standard SDD regimen consists of two components: topical non-absorbed antibiotics polymixin E, tobramycin, and amphotericin B and intravenous cefotaxime until surveillance cultures demonstrate adequate decontamination of the gastrointestinal tract (usually 4 days). This combination is active against essentially all aerobic gram-negative bacteria and fungi, but is without effects on normal anaerobic flora.

Although SDD is widely used in intensive care units in Europe and few intensive care interventions have undergone as many clinical trials as SDD, it has not found favor in North America. The American Thoracic Society considered SDD as a regimen of unproven value. In 1998 D'Amico et al. [12] published a meta-analysis of 33 randomized controlled trials on SDD conducted from 1984 to 1996. Eligible trials were grouped in two categories on the basis of the type of antibiotic prophylaxis: 1) topical plus systemic antibiotics versus no treatment; 2) topical preparation with or without a systemic antibiotic versus a systemic agent or placebo.

Meta-analysis of aggregate data from 16 trials reported a strong significant reduction in infection [odds ratio 0.35, 95% confidence interval (CI) 0.29-0.41] and total mortality (OR 0.8, 95% CI 0.69-0.93) in association with SDD using topical plus systemic antibiotics. Similar analysis of 17 trials that tested only topical antibiotics demonstrated a clear reduction in infection (OR 0.56, 95% CI 0.46-0.68) but not in mortality.

A meta-analysis published by Nathens and Marshall [13] analyzed 11 prospective, randomized studies in surgical ICU patients and 10 in medical ICU patients. The results of this meta analysis showed that SDD could be of benefit in surgical patients, reducing nosocomial pneumonia rates, bacteremia, and nosocomial infections at remote sites. More important was the effect on mortality, with a statistically significant reduction in ICU mortality. In the same study a meta-analysis of SDD use in medical patients failed to demonstrate a statistically significant effect on mortality. The reasons proposed to explain the greater benefit of SDD in surgical patients were the higher frequency of nosocomial pneumonia in surgical patients and the greater mortality when it occurs. The authors concluded that further clinical trials were needed in homogeneous groups of patients at high risk of infection having as primary end point ICU mortality, and that detailed surveillance of the microbiological ecology of participating units would be needed to monitor the emergence of resistant microrganisms [13]. Indeed, the widespread use of prophylactic antibiotic agents can, theoretically, facilitate the emergence of multiple resistant microrganisms. Nevertheless, despite a large number of studies investigating SDD, there is a lack evidence of increased bacterial resistance other than that of coagulase-negative staphylococci to ciprofloxacin.

A different approach to the problem of VAP prevention is based on strategies for minimizing the risk of aspiration. Promising preventive modalities for reducing the risk of aspiration include: semirecumbent position and the use of endotracheal tubes that allow continuous aspiration of pharyngeal secretion. Both strategies are cheap and without collateral effects.

Body position affects the mechanism of gatroesophageal reflux and subsequent aspiration. Compared with the supine position, semirecumbent position appears to reduce the volume of aspirated secretion. In this regard, three randomized trials [14-16] in which patients were allocated to the supine or semirecumbent position have been conducted to evaluate the effect on scintigraphic evidence of aspiration. All trials documented a reduction in aspiration in the semirecumbent position. Torres et al. [14] compared samples taken simultaneously from gastric, pharyngeal, and endotracheal aspirates in 19 patients and observed the same microorganism in 68% of samples taken in the supine position and in 32% of samples taken while patients were semirecumbent. A trial by Drakulovic et al. [17] evaluated the influence of semirecumbency versus supine position on VAP incidence in 86 mechanically ventilated patients. The incidence of microbiologically confirmed pneumonia was 2 of 39 (5%) in the semirecumbent group versus 11 of 47 (23%) in the supine group (95% CI for the difference 4-33, $p = 0.018$). As a consequence of this evidences, the US Centers for Disease Control and Prevention (CDC) have recommended that patients on ICU be nursed in a semirecumbent position to minimize the likelihood of nosocomial infections. Nevertheless, despite experimental evidence that semirecumbent body position is a low-cost, easy-to-apply measure effective in reducing VAP, especially in patients receiving enteral nutrition and mechanical ventilation for more than 7 days [17], the percentage of patients without contraindications who are nursed in this position is still very low.

Another interesting strategy proposed to reduce the incidence of VAP is based on subglottic secretion drainage using endotracheal tubes that allow continuous aspiration of pharyngeal secretions. Cuffed endotracheal tubes are commonly thought to prevent aspiration, but secretion pooled above the cuff can cause pneumonia by passing through any leak between the cuff and tracheal wall. Mahul et al. [18] described the use of a modified endotracheal hourly aspiration of secretion in the subglottic space. In a randomized study of a total of 145 patients intubated for more than 3 days, subglottic secretion drainage treatment was associated with: 1) twice lower incidence of VAP (29.1% vs. 13%); 2) a prolonged time for onset of VAP (8.3 ± 5 days without versus 16.2 ± 11 with subglottic drainage).

A similar reduction in VAP incidence was demonstrated by Valles et al. [19] in a randomized, controlled, blinded study of 190 patients. Seventy-six patients were randomly allocated to receive continuous aspiration of subglottic space and 77 patients receive the usual care. The incidence rate of VAP was 19.9 episodes/1,000 ventilator days in patients receiving subglottic secretion drainage versus 39. 6 VAP/1,000 ventilator days in control patients. In this study subglottic drainage prevented early pneumonia caused by community bacteria gram-positive cocci and *Haemophilus influenzae*, but failed to control late pneumonia attributable to opportunistic aerobic gram-negative bacilli, such as *Pseudomonas aeruginosa* [19].

Probably, exogenous contamination from the ventilator circuit does not play a major role in VAP pathogenesis. The frequency of ventilatory circuit changes has little influence on the rate of VAP, but infrequent changes were associated with a small decrease of VAP incidence. Although the optimal circuit change schedule is still uncertain, a policy of no circuit changes is probably without risk and cost effective [20, 21].

Close suction systems are effective in reducing both the incidence of arterial desaturation during suctioning and the environmental contamination from respiratory organisms. However, studies comparing closed versus open suction systems did not find any difference in VAP rates, while the use of closed systems was even associated with increased tracheal colonization [22, 23].

A prospective randomized trial of 280 consecutive trauma patients comparing the effect of heat moisture exchange filter (HMEF) and heated wire humidifiers (HWH) on the incidence of VAP suggested that, compared to the conventional HWH circuit, the use of HMEF reduce late-onset VAP. HMEF protective effect can be explained by reduction in tubing condensate and colonization [24].

The use of endotracheal tubes and the duration of intubation have been associated with higher risk of VAP [25]. Endotracheal tubes compromise airway protective mechanisms (glottic closure, mucociliary clearance, and cough). Sedation, opioid analgesia, and muscle paralysis are frequently used in intubated patients and also depress the cough reflex. The endotracheal tube can harbor a large number of bacteria along its inner surface. Bacteria at this site will persist in the airway, free from the effect of antibiotic and host defenses. Hence, the management of the endotracheal tube plays a crucial role in preventing pneumonia. Routine intracuff pressure monitoring is essential [26]. Unplanned extubation increases the risk of VAP; therefore, appropriate securing of tracheal tubes and prevention of need for reintubation may reduce the risk of VAP [27]. If the procedure of intubation itself significantly increases the risk of VAP, avoiding endotracheal intubation is probably a correct target in preventing VAP.

Many studies have documented that non-invasive ventilation (NIV) is effective in correcting gas exchange abnormalities due to acute respiratory failure, reducing collateral effects of mechanical ventilation [28-31]. Randomized controlled trials and non-randomized studies showed that NIV reduces nosocomial pneumonia and nosocomial infections. In patients at elevated risk of developing nosocomial pneumonia, the use of NIV can be a very effective strategy for VAP prevention. In acute respiratory failure due to infectious complications of lung transplantation, when NIV is effective in avoiding endotracheal intubation, the incidence of bacterial pneumonia is extremely low [28]. Recently our group published a prospective randomized study comparing NIV versus standard treatment using supplemental oxygen administration to avoid endotracheal intubation in recipients of solid organ transplants. Compared with standard treatment, NIV had significantly lower rates of endotracheal intubation, septic complications, fatal complications, and ICU mortality [29].

In a prospective, non-randomized study, Nourdine investigated 761 patients undergoing mechanical ventilation for more than 48 h: 607 patients were intubated, 129 received non-invasive mechanical ventilation and 25 were treated with both methods. The incidence of VAP was significantly lower in the NIV group (4.4 vs. 13.2/1,000 patient-days) [30]. In a study published by Antonelli et al. [31] in 1998, 64 patients with acute respiratory failure were assigned in a randomized way to receive mechanical ventilation plus endotracheal intubation (32 patients) or NIV (32 patients). The incidence of pneumonia or sinusitis was significantly lower in the NIV group (3 versus 31%, $p = 0.003$).

Conclusions

In the prevention of nosocomial pneumonia, a major role can probably be played by simple, low-risk, and cost-effective interventions. Continuous aspiration of subglottic secretions, semirecumbent position, non-invasive mechanical ventilation are excellent examples of prevention strategies that should be implemented in all hospitals without collateral effects and significant impact on cost.

More-expensive strategies like SDD are controversial, but data showing a dramatic effect of SDD on mortality in surgical patients can support the use of SDD in those patients.

References

1. Craven DE, Steger KA (1996) Nosocomial pneumonia in mechanically ventilated adult patients: epidemiology and prevention. Semin Respir Infect 11:32-53
2. Gross PA (1999) Epidemiology of hospital acquired pneumonia. Semin Respir Infect 2:2-7
3. Heyland DK, Cook DJ, Griffith LE et al for the Canadian Critical Care Trials Group (1999) The attributable morbidity and mortality of ventilator-associated pneumonia in the critically ill patient. Am J Respir Crit Care Med 159:1249-1256
4. Dricks MR, Craven DE, Celli BR et al (1987) Nosocomial pneumonia in intubated patients given sucralfate as compared with antiacids or histamine type 2 blockers. N Engl J Med 26:1376-1382
5. Tryba M (1987) Risk of acute stress bleeding and nosocomial pneumonia in ventilated intensive care unit patients: sucralfate versus antiacids. Am J Med 83[Suppl 3B]:117-124
6. Prodhom G, Leuenberger P, Koerfer J et al (1994) Nosocomial pneumonia in mechanically ventilated patients receiving antiacid, ranitidine, or sucralfate as prophylaxis for stress ulcer: a randomized controlled trial. Ann Intern Med 120:653-662
7. Cook DJ, Reeve BK, Guyatt GH et al (1996) Stress ulcer prophylaxis in critically ill patients: resolving discordant meta-analyses. JAMA 275:308-314
8. Cook DJ, Guyatt GH, Marshall J et al for the Canadian Critical Care Trials Group (1998) A comparison of sucralfate and ranitidine for prevention of upper gastrointestinal bleeding in patients requiring mechanical ventilation. N Engl J Med 338:791-797
9. Cook DJ, Fuller H for the Canadian Critical Care Trials Group (1994) Risk factors for gatsrointestinal bleeding in critically ill patients. N Engl J Med 330:377-381
10. Doebelling BN, Gail MS, Stanley L et al (1992) Comparative efficacy of alternative handwashing agents in reducing nosocomial infections in intensive care units. N Engl J Med 327:88-93
11. Stoutenbeek CP, Van Saene HK, Miranda DR et al (1983) The effect of selective decontamination of the digestive tract on colonisation and infection rate in multiple trauma patients. Acta Anaesthesiol Belg 34:209-221
12. D'Amico R, Pifferi S, Leonetti C et al (1998) Effectiveness of antibiotic prophylaxis in critically ill adult patients: systematic review of randomised controlled trials. B M J 316:1275-1284
13. Nathens AB, Marshall JC (1984) Selective decontamination of the digestive tract in surgical patients. Arch Surg 134:170-176
14. Torres A, Serra Battes J, Ros E (1992) Pulmonary aspiration of gastric contents in patients receiving mechanical ventilation: the effect of body position. Ann Intern Med 116:540-543
15. Ibanez, Panafield A, Rurich JM (1992) Gastroesophageal reflux in intubated patients receiving enteral nutrition: effect of supine and semirecumbent positions. JPEN 16:419-422
16. Orozco-Levi M, Torres A, Ferrer M (1995) Semirecumbent position protects from pulmonary aspiration but not completely from gastroesophageal reflux in mechanically ventilated patients. Am J Resp Crit Care Med 152:1387-1390
17. Drakulovic MB, Torres A, Bauer TT et al (1999) Supine body position as a risk factor for nosocomial pneumonia in mechanically ventilated patients: a randomised trial. Lancet 354:1851-1858
18. Mahul C, Auboyer C, Jospe R et al (1992) Prevention of nosocomial pneumonia in intubated patients: respective role of mechanical subglottic secretions drainage and stress ulcer prophylaxis. Intensive Care Med 28:20-25
19. Valles J, Artigas A, Rello J et al (1995) Continuous aspiration of subglottic secretions in preventing ventilator associated pneumonia. Ann Intern Med 122:179-186
20. Dreyfuss D, Djedaini K, Weber P et al (1991) Prospective study of nosocomial pneumonia of patient and circuit colonization during mechanical ventilation with circuit changes every 48 hours versus no change. Am Rev Respir Dis 143:738-743
21. Kollef MH, Shapiro SD, Fraser VJ et al (1995) Mechanical ventilation with or without 7-days circuit changes. Ann Intern Med 123:168-174

22. Deppe SA, Kelley JW, Thoi LL et al (1990) Incidence of colonization, nosocomial pneumonia and mortality in critically il patients using Trach Care closed-suction system versus an open-suction system: a prospective, randomized study. Crit Care Med 18:1389-1393
23. Johnson KL, Kearney PA, Johnson SB et al (1994) Closed versus open endotracheal suctioning: costs and physiologic consequences. Crit Care Med 22:658-666
24. Kirton OC, DeHaven B, Morgan J et al (1997) A prospective, randomized comparison of an in line Heat Moisture Exchange Filter and Heated Wire Humidifiers. Chest 112:1055-1059
25. Cunnion KM, Weber DJ, Broadhead E et al (1996) Risk factors for nosocomial pneumonia: comparing adult critical care populations. Am J Respir Crit Care Med 153:158-162
26. Rello J, Sonora R, Jubert P et al (1996) Pneumonia in intubated patients: role of airway management. Am J Respir Crit Care Med 154:111-115
27. Torres A, Gatell JM, Aznar E et al (1995) Reintubation increases the risk of nosocomial pneumonia in patients needing mechanical ventilation. Am J Respir Crit Care Med 152:137-141
28. Ambrosino N, Rubini F, Callegari G et al (1994) Noninvasive mechanical ventilation in the treatment of acute respiratory failure due to infectious complications of lung transpalntation Monaldi Arch Chest Dis 49:311-314
29. Antonelli M, Conti G, Bufi M et al (2000) Non invasive ventilation for treatment of acute respiratory failure in patients undergoing solid organ transplantation. A randomized trial. JAMA 283:235-241
30. Nourdine K, Combes P, Carton MJ et al (1999) Does non invasive ventilation reduce the ICU nosocomial infection risk? Intensive Care Med 25:567-573
31. Antonelli M, Conti G, Rocco M et al (1998) A comparison of noninvasive positive pressure ventilation and conventional mechanical ventilation in patients with acute respiratory failure. N Engl J Med 339:429-435

New Perspectives in the Management of Gram-Positive Infections

A.R. De Gaudio, C. Adembri

In the 1970s and early 1980s, Gram-positive pathogens were of little concern and Gram-negative bacteria resistant to multiple antibiotics were the major issue in intensive care unit (ICU) nosocomial infections.

Over recent years, there have been significant changes in the causative microorganisms of nosocomial infections, with a shift to Gram-positive pathogens.

In the USA, data from the National Nosocomial Infection Survey (1990-1996) showed that Gram-positive bacteria were responsible for 39% of all nosocomial infections. Staphylococci were responsible for 47% of bloodstream infections, 34% of skin and soft tissue infections, and 21% of nosocomial pneumonia. Enterococci were responsible for 11% of overall infections and were the second most common isolates from nosocomial urinary tract infections [1]. Similar data have been obtained from the European Study Group on Nosocomial Infection: four out of the five most frequently isolated pathogens were *S. aureus* (15.1%), *S. epidermidis* (10.8%), other coagulase-negative species (CoNS) (7.0%) and *S. pneumoniae* (5.9%) [1]. The European Prevalence of Infection in Intensive Care Units (EPIC) study found that *S. aureus* was also the microorganism causing the largest proportion of cases of nosocomial pneumonia within the ICU [2].

This evolving problem of the emergence of Gram-positive microorganisms as major nosocomial pathogens is related to: a) changes in patient demographics, with increasing numbers of neutropenic and immunocompromised patients needing intensive care; b) the use of intravascular and other prosthetic devices and c) the large use of antimicrobial agents (i.e. cephalosporins) which are active against Gram-negative bacilli.

A shift from Gram-negative to Gram-positive bacteria as the predominant nosocomial pathogen would be of little concern if it were not for the increase in antimicrobial resistance among these Gram-positive strains [1].

By the end of the 1950s, at least 85% of *S. aureus* strains were resistant to penicillin. The introduction in 1959 of the new semisynthetic penicillins (methicillin and oxacillin), which are not inactivated by penicillinase, was expected to constitute breakthrough for the problem of resistance. Unfortunately, methicillin-resistant *Staphylococcus aureus* (MRSA) strains were detected in 1961 and in the last 30 years the percentage of MRSA has fluctuated in Europe from the initial 1-2% to the alarming current rate of 30-40% in Spain, France, and Italy [3].

Since 1988, vancomycin-resistant enterococci (VRE) have emerged as an increasingly important public health issue, especially in the USA where they have been responsible for almost 8% of all nosocomial enterococcal infections and almost 14% of infections in ICU [4].

In 1996, the first documented clinical infection due to *S. aureus* with intermediate resistance to vancomycin (glycopeptide-intermediate *Staphylococcus aureus*, GISA) was diagnosed in a patient in Japan [5] and in 1997 two infections due to *S. aureus* with reduced susceptibility to vancomycin were identified in the USA [6]. More recently, the emergence of vancomycin tolerance has been detected in *Streptococcus pneumoniae* [7].

Because of the increasing emergence of resistant strains, the need to find new antimicrobial drugs has increased.

Methicillin-resistant *S. aureus*

Some strains of MRSA are particularly capable of spreading within hospitals and, more recently, in nursing homes and in the community at large: they are defined as epidemic MRSA [1]. These epidemic MRSA have become endemic in many hospitals and other institutions. Among isolates of *S. aureus*, 40-50% are MRSA but the rates range widely among different geographical areas, among different hospitals in the same city, and even among different units of the same hospitals [1].

The main bacterial targets of the β-lactam antibiotics in *S. aureus* are the penicillin-binding proteins (PBPs), enzymes which have a key role in the biosynthesis of the bacterial cell wall through transpeptidase and carboxypeptidase activities. The antibacterial effect of β-lactams is primarily mediated by inactivation of PBP-1a and PBP-1b, or PBP2 and PBP3. The *S. aureus* strains that are resistant to methicillin produce an additional PBP-2a, encoded by the *mec* A gene, which is not targeted by β-lactam antibiotics and confers an intrinsic resistance on this class of drugs [3]. Furthermore, the gene that encodes methicillin-resistance in staphylococci is inside a transposon and contains a number of insertion sequences that allow multiple-resistance genes to accumulate within the same transposon [1]. In this way MR staphylococci (aureus and CoNS) are frequently resistant to other antibiotics.

The combination of a penicillinase-sensitive β-lactam with a penicillinase inhibitor has been studied against MRSA. Experimental studies have shown that the affinities of both amoxicillin and penicillin G for PBP-2a are more than tenfold greater than those of methicillin and oxacillin, and that amoxicillin combined with clavulanate, which protects amoxicillin from penicillinase inactivation, is at least as effective as vancomycin in the treatment of experimental MRSA endocarditis in rats [3]. Unfortunately, the in vitro efficacy of this combination has not to date been confirmed in the clinical setting. One of the probable limitations of the combination is that large doses of clavulanate would be required to be effective, which may be impossible to achieve clinically [3].

Because isolates of MRSA are also resistant to other antistaphylococcal agents (macrolides and fluoroquinolones), the treatment of MRSA infections is always limited to either vancomycin or teicoplanin. Vancomycin has a moderate extravascular diffusion and its slow time-dependent bactericidal effect may partly lower its effectiveness in vivo [8]. For this reason its continuous infusion seems necessary to obtain the best bactericidal effect [9]. On the other hand, teicoplanin seems to be more efficacious and well-tolerated, offering the advantage of a single daily dose [10].

Regarding the new antibiotics under investigation, the potential activity of new synthetic carbapenems, based on their high degree of affinity for PBP-2a, seems promising. Preliminary studies in experimental endocarditis have shown that these agents are at least as effective as vancomycin against MRSA [11].

Future fluoroquinolones with very high affinity for the mutated targets topoisomerase IV and gyrase might be able to overcome the observed resistance towards the current fluoroquinolone compounds [3].

The agents that are closest to being introduced into clinical practice are the first injectable streptogramin (quinupristin-dalfopristin) and linezolid, new classes of antimicrobial agents that inhibit onset of bacterial protein synthesis, and that have shown an interesting activity against MRSA both in vitro and in animal models [3, 12] (see below).

Vancomycin-resistant enterococcus

There is evidence for the presence in vancomycin-resistant enterococci (VRE) of two genes, harboured on a transposon, that are involved in an inducible mechanism of glycopeptide resistance [13]. The vanA and vanB phenotypes have mainly been described in *E. faecium* and *E. faecalis*. VanA is characterized by high-level resistance to vancomycin and teicoplanin, whereas vanB is associated with variable levels of resistance to vancomycin but remains susceptible to teicoplanin [3, 13]. The vanC phenotype produces resistance mostly in *E. gallinarium*, *E. casseliflavus* and *E. flavescens* and is characterized by a low-level vancomycin resistance but a persistent teicoplanin susceptibility [14].

The traditional treatment of systemic enterococcal infections is based on the bactericidal combination of a cell-wall-active antibiotic (β-lactam) plus an aminoglycoside. Triple combinations combining a β-lactam with a glycopeptide and gentamycin may be effective in vitro and in animal models of endocarditis against vanA strains that are resistant to amoxicillin but not to aminoglycosides even though the synergistic effect between β-lactams and glycopeptides is still controversial [3].

New semisynthetic glycopeptides, such as LY 333328, are also an interesting option for the future. Although their mechanism of action is still unknown, they have shown a 10-fold to 30-fold increased activity in vitro against VRE as compared with vancomycin.

Of the new fluoroquinolones, clinafloxacin and sparfloxacin seem to have the greatest activity against enterococci in vitro and they have yielded interesting results in experimental animals. Finally, glycylcyclines, which are related to tetracyclines, have shown a good in vitro activity against resistant enterococci [3].

According to Michel and Gutmann [3], a practical approach to VRE infection may be proposed as follows:

a) non-specific preventive measures and enteric eradication with oral bacitracin;
b) if the systemic infection is due to vanA type VRE, the level of resistance to amoxicillin must be considered and the combination amoxicillin plus aminoglycoside must be used. If the resistance to amoxicillin is intermediate, the triple combination of amoxicillin, teicoplanin and aminoglycoside could be effective;
c) if the level of resistance to amoxicillin is high, a possible triple combination is ceftriaxone plus teicoplanin plus gentamicin;
d) systemic infection due to vanB type VRE must be treated with amoxicillin plus aminoglycoside or in the case of a high resistance to amoxicillin, with teicoplanin combined with an aminoglycoside;
e) possible future approaches are: streptogramins (quinupristin-dalfopristin), linezolid, new glycopeptides, new fluoroquinolones (clinafloxacin, sparfloxacin) and glycylcyclines.

New perspectives

No clinically significant new classes of antibiotics were developed from the early 1980s until quite recently, when drugs like everninomycin, LY 333328, daptomycin, quinupristin/dalfopristin and linezolid have emerged.

Everninomycin has a good in vitro activity against all the resistant Gram-positive bacteria and the drug has entered into phase II trials. LY 333328 is a new glycopeptide with bactericidal activity against most of the important Gram-positive pathogens including VRE. It is still in the relatively early stages of clinical development [1]. Daptomycin is a bactericidal agent that produced dose-related muscular toxicity in early formulations. New formulations with low dosages are currently being evaluated in clinical trials.

Quinupristin/dalfopristin and linezolid are the only two new agents that seem to offer a promising alternative to glycopeptides and are closest to being introduced into clinical practice.

Quinupristin/dalfopristin

Quinupristin/dalfopristin (Q/D) belongs to the streptogramin family, a unique class of antibacterials in that each member consists of at least 2 structurally unrelated molecules: group A streptogramins (macrolactones) and group B streptogramins (cyclic hexadepsipeptides) [15, 16].

Group A and group B streptogramins inhibit protein synthesis by binding at two different sites of the 50S ribosomal subunit and act synergistically against many isolates. This synergism is why this class of antibiotics is also known as "synergitins" [15]. Their combination generates bactericidal activity and reduces the possibility of emergence of resistant strains. The mechanisms of acquired resistance to group B streptogramins are similar to those induced by erythromycin, but group A streptogramins remain unaffected by target modifications and active efflux [16].

The pharmacokinetic parameters of group A and group B streptogramins in the blood are quite similar. In addition, both the A and B groups penetrate and accumulate inside macrophages and in bacterial vegetations of experimental endocarditis. There are important biological differences between the streptogramins and the macrolides, the main differentiating ones being the rapid antibacterial killing of streptogramins and the rarity of cross-resistance between the 2 groups of antibiotics.

Most Gram-positive organisms are highly susceptible to the streptogramin quinupristin/dalfopristin [16]. Minimum inhibitory concentration for 90% of isolates (MIC_{90}) are $\leq$ 1 mg/l for *S. aureus*, *S. epidermidis*, *S. haemolyticus*, *Streptococcus pneumoniae*, *S. pyogenes* and *Listeria monocytogenes*.

Quinupristin/dalfopristin shows a similar activity against methicillin-susceptible and resistant strains of *S. aureus*, and against streptococci with benzylpenicillin (penicillin G)- or erythromycin-acquired resistance. Enterococci have a different susceptibility to Q/D, although most isolates tested are susceptible to the drug, including vancomycin-resistant and multiresistant *Enterococcus faecium*. Unfortunately, *E. faecalis* is generally the least susceptible.

Of the Gram-negative respiratory pathogens, *Moraxella catarrhalis* is susceptible and *Haemophilus influenzae* is moderately susceptible to Q/D; *Enterobacteriaceae*, *Pseudomonas aeruginosa* and *Acinetobacter* spp. are however resistant. The drug is active against the anaerobic organisms tested, including *Clostridium perfringens*, *Lactobacillus* spp., *Bacteroides fragilis* and *Peptostreptococcus*. Synergy of the combination vancomycin and Q/D has been demonstrated in vancomycin-resistant and multiresistant *E. faecium*, and in methicillin-sensitive and -resistant *S. aureus*.

Quinupristin/dalfopristin shows antibacterial activity in vivo in animal models of infection, including methicillin-sensitive and -resistant *S. aureus* infection in rabbits, *S. aureus* and *S. pneumoniae* in mice, and erythromycin-sensitive and -resistant viridans streptococci group infections in rats [16].

The drug is rapidly bactericidal against Gram-positive organisms (with the exception of enterococci and some MRSA MLSbc strains) at concentrations similar to or within 4-fold of the MIC, and it has a long postantibiotic effect both in vitro and in vivo.

Data regarding the clinical efficacy of this antimicrobial combination are so far limited. However, three phase III clinical trials, two in the treatment of skin and skin structure infections (SSSI), and one in nosocomial pneumonia (NP), have shown a favourable clinical response and the safety of intravenous (IV) administration [16].

The overall safety profile was similar for Q/D and reference molecules (gastrointestinal events were the most common adverse events reported in phase III clinical trials). Venous intolerance was more frequent in the Q/D group, when the peripheral IV route was used. The phase III studies demonstrated that the efficacy of Q/D is statistically equivalent to the control group (vancomycin, cefazolin or oxacillin) in the treated patients with nosocomial pneumonia or complicated skin and skin structure infections [17, 18].

The efficacy and safety of Q/D were also assessed in a non-comparative phase III study and in an emergency-use study [19]. The drug was generally well tolerated; the most frequently reported adverse events were venous intolerance, arthralgia, myalgia [19]. An increase in conjugated bilirubin and interactions with drugs metabolized by the cytochrome P 450 isoenzyme 3A4 (i.e. midazolam) have been reported [20]. These side effects were generally mild and transient and disappeared when the drug was discontinued.

At this moment in time, Q/D can be considered a valid therapeutic alternative to glycopeptides, especially in severely ill patients affected with multiresistant Gram-positive pathogens and/or in patients with renal failure.

Linezolid

Linezolid is a member of the oxazolidinone class of synthetic antibacterial agents that inhibit bacterial protein synthesis through a unique mechanism. In contrast to other inhibitors of protein synthesis, the oxazolidinones act early in translation by preventing the formation of a functional initiation complex. Consequently, linezolid is not expected to show cross-resistance with existing antibacterial agents [21, 22].

Linezolid is rapidly and completely absorbed after oral administration (600 mg), reaching peak plasma concentrations within 1-2 hours and having a mean absolute bioavailability of 103%. Linezolid has a steady-state volume of distribution of 50 l and is 31% bound to plasma proteins. After twice-daily intravenous administration, plasma concentrations remained above 4 mg/l for 9-10 hours of the 12-hour dose interval [22]. Tentative breakpoint criteria are MIC_{90} of < 4 mg/l for susceptibility and > 16 mg/l for resistance [22].

Dosage adjustment is unnecessary in individuals with mild to moderately impaired renal function, although supplementary doses may be necessary for those on haemodialysis [23].

The disposition of linezolid does not appear to be affected by mild to moderate hepatic impairment, while its pharmacokinetics have not been investigated in patients with severe hepatic impairment [22].

Linezolid is bacteriostatic against most susceptible organisms but displays bactericidal activity against some strains of pneumococci, *Bacteroides fragilis* and *C. perfrigens*. Linezolid has a wide-ranging bacteriostatic activity against Gram-positive organisms including methicillin-resistant staphylococci, penicillin-resistant pneumococci and vancomycin-resistant *Enterococcus faecalis* and *faecium*. Anaerobes such as *Clostridium difficile* and *Clostridium perfringens* are also susceptible to it.

Oral and intravenous administrations of linezolid have been evaluated in open label studies, in comparative studies and for compassionate use. In clinical trials involving hospitalized patients with skin and soft tissue infections (*S. aureus*), intravenous or oral linezolid produced clinical success in > 83% of patients. In patients with community-acquired pneumonia, success rates were > 94% [24, 25].

Preliminary clinical data also indicate that twice-daily intravenous or oral linezolid (600 mg) is as effective as intravenous vancomycin in the treatment of patients with hospital-acquired pneumonia and in those with infections caused by methicillin-resistant staphylococci. Moreover, it produced a positive effect in > 85% of patients infected by vancomycin-resistant enterococcal bacteria [22].

Linezolid is generally well tolerated and gastrointestinal disturbances are the most commonly occurring adverse events (nausea, diarrhoea, tongue discolouration, etc.).

In vitro studies have indicated that linezolid is a weak competitive inhibitor of human monoamine oxidase. However, no clinical evidence of adverse events due to monoamine oxidase inhibition has been reported during linezolid treatment [22, 26].

Conclusions

The emergence of multiple drug resistance among *S. aureus* and enterococci is a serious public health issue, especially in intensive care settings where Gram-positive bacteria are at present the most common nosocomial pathogens.

During the last few years much effort has been devoted to limiting the spread of MRSA, and to understanding the mechanisms of methicillin resistance in *S.*

aureus and the mechanisms of glycopeptide resistance in both *S. aureus* and enterococci. The transfer of enterococcal glycopeptide resistance to *S. aureus* is of the greatest concern because it has been demonstrated in vitro that vanA and vanB determinants are extremely mobile [3].

Since it is not possible to predict if and when acquisition of resistance to glycopeptides by MRSA will occur, strict enforcement of preventive measures together with the restricted use of glycopeptides (the relative advantage of one or the other being evaluated according to the specific circumstances) are the best currently applicable responses pending development of alternative antimicrobial strategies.

Since they are close to being approved for clinical use, quinupristin/dalfopristin and linezolid offer the most interesting alternative approaches of the new antimicrobial drugs.

References

1. Wood MJ (1999) Chemotherapy for Gram-positive nosocomial sepsis. J Chemother 6: 446-452
2. Spencer RC (1996) Predominant pathogens found in the European Prevalence of Infection in Intensive Care Study. Eur J Clin Microbiol Infect Dis 15:281-285
3. Michel M, Gutmann L (1997) Methicillin-resistant Staphylococus aureus and vancomycin-resistant enterococci: therapeutic realities and possibilities. Lancet 349:1901-1906
4. Centers for Disease Control and Prevention 1989-1993 (1993) Nosocomial enterococci resistant to vancomycin. MMWR 42:597-599
5. IIiramatsu K, Hanaki H, Ino T et al (1997) Methicillin-resistant Staphylococcus aureus clinical strain with reduced vancomycin susceptibility. J Antimicrob Chemother 40:135-136
6. Smith TL, Pearson ML, Wilcox KR et al (1999) Emergence of vancomycin resistence in Staphylococcus aureus. N Engl J Med 340:493-501
7. Novak R, Henriques B, Charpentier E et al (1999) Emergence of vancomycin tolerance in Streptococcus pneumoniae. Nature 399:590-593
8. Ackerman BH, Vannier AM, Eudy EB (1992) Analysis of vancomycin time-killing studies with Staphylococcus species by using stripping program to describe the relationship between concentration and pharmacodynamic response. Antimicr Agents Chemother 36:1766-1769
9. Di Filippo A, De Gaudio AR, Novelli A et al (1998) Continuous infusion of vancomycin in methicillin-resistant Staphylococcus infection. Chemotherapy 44:63-68
10. Charbonnau P, Harding I, Garaud JJ et al (1994) Teicoplanin: a well-tolerated and easily administered alternative to vancomycin for gram-positive infections in intensive care patients. Intens Care Med 20:S35-S42
11. Chambers HF (1995) In vitro and in vivo antistaphylococcal activities of L-695,256, a carbapenem with high affinity for the penicillin-binding protein PBP2a. Antimicr Agents Chemother 39:462-466
12. Ford CW, Hamel JC, Wilson DM et al (1996) In vivo activities of U-100592 and U-100766, novel oxazolidinone antimicrobial agents against experimental bacterial infections. Antimicr Agents Chemother 40:2820-2823
13. Arthur M, Reynolds P, Courvalin P (1996) Glycopeptide resistance in enterococci. Trends Microbiol 4:401-407
14. Woodford N, Johnson AP, Morrison D et al (1995) Current perspectives on glycopeptide resistance. Clin Microbiol Rev 8:585-615

15. Leclercq R, Courvalin P (1998) Streptogramins: an answer to antibiotic resistance in gram-positive bacteria. Lancet 352:591-592
16. Linden PK (1997) Quinupristin/Dalfopristin: a new therapeutic alternative for the treatment of vancomycin-resistant Enterococcus faecium and other serious Gram-positive infections. Today Therapeutic Trends 15:137-153
17. Nichols RL (1999) Optimal treatment of complicated skin and skin structure infections. J Antimicr Chemother 44:19-23
18. Fagon J, Patrick H, Haas DW et al (2000) Treatment of gram-positive nosocomial pneumonia. Prospective randomized comparison of quinupristin/dalfopristin versus vancomycin. Nosocomial Pneumonia Group. Am J Respir Crit Care Med 161:753-762
19. Moellering RC, Linden PK, Reinhardt J et al (1999) The efficacy and safety of quinupristin/dalfopristin for the treatment of infections caused by vancomycin-resistant Enterococcus faecium. J Antimicrob Chemother 144:251-261
20. Rubinstein E, Prokocimer P, Talbot GH (1999) Safety and tolerability of quinupristin/dalfopristin: administration guidelines. J Antimicrob Chemother 144:37-46
21. Shinabarger D (1999) Mechanism of action of the oxazolidinone antibacterial agents. Expert Opin Invest Drugs 8:1195-1202
22. Clemett D, Markkham A (2000) Linezolid. Drugs 59:815-827
23. Brier ME, Stalker DJ, Aronoff GR et al (1998) Pharmacokinetics of linezolid in subjects with varying degrees of renal function and on dialysis. J Invest Med 46:276A
24. Cammarata SK, Hafkin B, Demke DM (1999) Efficacy of linezolid in skin and soft tissue infections. Clin Microbiol Infect 5[Suppl 3]:133
25. Cammarata SK, Hafkin B, Todd WM (1999) Efficacy of linezolid in community-acquired S. pneumoniae pneumonia. Am J Respirar Crit Care Med 159[Suppl 2]:A844
26. Wilks NE, Mc Connell-Martin MA, Oliphant TH (1999) Safety and tolerance of linezolid in phase II trials. 39th Interscience Conference on Antimicrobial Agents and Chemotherapy, 24-27 September 1999, San Francisco, p 40

Focus on Peritonitis: Diagnostic Procedures

F. Pozzi-Mucelli

Effusions and collections that form in the peritoneal cavity and in the infra-peritoneal spaces are usually secondary to pathological processes of the intra-peritoneal organs and only rarely do they represent the extension of collections of juxta- and retroperitoneal compartments. They can be formed by transudates, exudates, blood, pus, bile, lymph, urine, pancreatic enzymes or food, and are caused by a wide range of inflammatory, vascular, traumatic, neoplastic or dysmetabolic processes, by hepatic, renal or cardiac failure, and by surgery.

In the peritoneal cavity, the collections may remain circumscribed in the recess where they formed or they may spread to all the compartments. Position, nature, composition and consistency of the collections are fundamental for their diffusion. Therefore, in the peritoneal cavity the transudates and the exudates (more fluid and less stimulating towards the peritoneum) can develop more quickly in the recesses and in the spaces, unlike the purulent hematic, biliary and urinary collections. Moreover, the peritoneum tries to form a protective wall.

Peritonitis is defined as the presence of an acute inflammatory process in the peritoneal cavity and in the infra-peritoneal spaces. Usually it is caused by diffusion for direct propagation, or by the lymphatic route, of inflammatory processes of abdominal organs (appendicitis, diverticulitis, cholecystitis, pancreatitis). In addition, they may develop from infections after abdomino-pelvic surgery or from anastomotic or suture leakage.

Less frequent causes of intraperitoneal inflammatory processes can be the breaking of bowel from trauma and perforation of the bowel wall from pathological (gastro-duodenal ulcers, bowel neoplasms) or iatrogenic (percutaneous transhepatic cholangiography, endoscopic procedures, etc.) causes. While appendicitis and ulcers were the most frequent causes of peritoneal abscess at the beginning of the last century, now they are the less frequent causes. Actually more than 70% of peritoneal abscesses are complications of surgery. Gastric, pancreatic and biliary surgery have a relatively high incidence of post-surgical abscesses [1, 2].

These inflammatory processes usually present with fever, abdominal pain, leucocytosis, abdominal wall defense. Sometimes the clinical findings have a subtle course: general indisposition, low fever, asthenia, and abdominal tenderness.

From the pathological point of view, these inflammatory processes show a wide range of alterations, from cellulitis with neutrophil accumulation in a tissue spread of bacteria with edematous and hyperemic suffusion, to the formation of phlegmons, abscessual collections, abscesses with central purulent collection besides which a barrier of highly vascular connective tissues forms. These processes may extend to other spaces, infra- or retroperitoneal, or to the peritoneal cavity, or evolve favorably until they resolve completely or leave remainders like fibrotic scars or little sack-like collections which sometimes cause the restarting of the infection.

The diagnosis of peritoneal collection has been a problem in the past, when only conventional radiology was available. Later, the introduction of ultrasound, and computed tomography (CT) has made possible this diagnosis in an elevated percentage of cases [3]. We will focus this paper on the possibilities of computed tomography and on the contribution of interventional radiology in this pathology [4, 5].

Computed tomography

Acute appendicitis

With CT the normal appendix shows a linear aspect, if collapsed, or tubular or anular, when it contains gas, fluid, feces or barium, with a thin wall (< 1 mm) and a sharp profile in the contiguous fatty tissue [6]. In an acute inflammatory process, the appendiceal wall becomes thick (2-3 mm) and shows a hyperdense pattern after contrast media. In its interior a mild quantity of liquids is frequently present and the typical calcified coprolith can also be seen.

The extension of the inflammatory process to the contiguous fat tissue causes a smooth increase of its density, at the beginning slender and then denser, and an increased thickness of the peritoneum that borders it. The phlegmon formation is characterized by the appearance of a small homogeneous mass that shows high density after contrast media, with smooth but badly defined margins.

The abscessual collections show the characteristic fluid density or moderately over-fluid, ill defined margins, surrounded by dense fat tissue while the mature abscesses are bordered by a thick and complete capsule. Within the collections, small gas bubbles can be seen; these represent the expression of an appendiceal perforation or of an infection by anaerobic microorganisms.

When the collections penetrate into the peritoneum, they tend to extend towards the right paracolic and overhanging perihepatic spaces or down in the Douglas cavity while the air goes below the diaphragm in the subphrenic recess.

The use of CT in acute appendicitis decreases the number of explorative laparatomies [7] and consents the setting of more appropriate therapy based on the pathological picture present:

- simple wide-spectrum antibiotic therapy in infection of only the appendix or infection complicated by small abscesses (< 3 cm) or phlegmon;
- percutaneous CT-guided drainage of the abscessual collection limited to the periappendiceal spaces [8, 9];
- surgical treatment, limited to only the patients with free diffused or multiloculated collections, or with perforation.

Acute diverticulitis

The typical CT findings are (Fig. 1):

- increased thickness and density of the bowel wall;
- increased density of the contiguous fat with dense lines;
- liquid or fluid-air collection located between bowel and thickened peritoneum;
- collections with air bubbles with intra- or retroperitoneum location in cases of perforation of a diverticulum.

The major limit of CT is due to the difficulties that may be encountered with a large bowel with thick wall, thin lumen, irregular external profile, paracolic or parasigmoid fat of increased density or with linear striations or nodes, in order to distinguish the inflammatory process from colic neoplasms extending outside

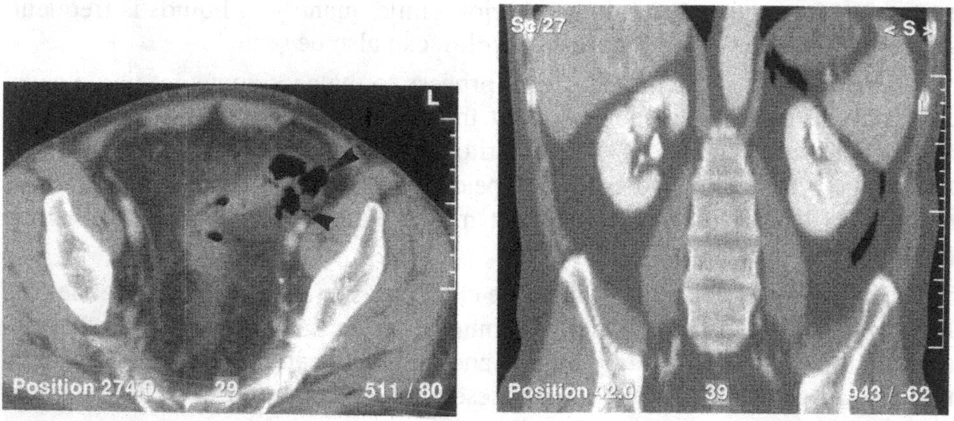

Fig. 1. Acute diverticulitis with retroperitoneal perforation: CT findings. A) Increased thickness of the wall of the sigma; a diverticula is visible; free air bubbles surrounds the sigma anteriorly (arrow-heads). B) Multiplanar coronal reconstruction clearly shows free air in the retroperitoneal spaces, around the left kidney

the wall and perforation. This occurs in 10% of the cases and a certain diagnosis is not possible [10].

Also in this pathology, CT is useful for choosing the therapeutic strategy that may to antibiotics in cases in which the inflammatory process is in the initial stage, while in the presence of a defined abscessual collection up to 3 cm in size, a CT-guided percutaneous drainage can be performed with recovery of almost all the cases [11].

Acute cholecystitis

Acute inflammatory processes of the gallbladder are usually related to the presence of stones that represents its principal etiologic factor. The inflammatory process causes an increased thickness of the wall with a hyperemic-edematous pattern that may evolve into suppuration to reach the external layers of the wall. Between the different layers of the wall, there may later form a liquid collection of exudate bile held from the peritoneum that covers the gallbladder. Enlarging, the inflammation may affect the soft tissue of the gastrohepatic, gastrocolic and hepatoduodenal ligaments both like hyperemic-edematous reaction and with the formation of collections that extend in the peritoneal cavity, causing a mixed purulent and biliary peritonitis that may become sack-like in the subhepatic space or may spread to all the peritoneum, but in particular to the recess of Morrison and to the Douglas cavity.

At CT examination [12, 13] (Fig. 2) the typical findings are in the first phase characterized by a thick wall, of at least 4 mm with elevated density after contrast media, sometimes with a hypodense intramural striation; the gallbladder frequently appears distended. When an abscessual evolution occurs, one or more small hypodense areas with a hyperdense rim in the interior of the wall can be seen at CT.

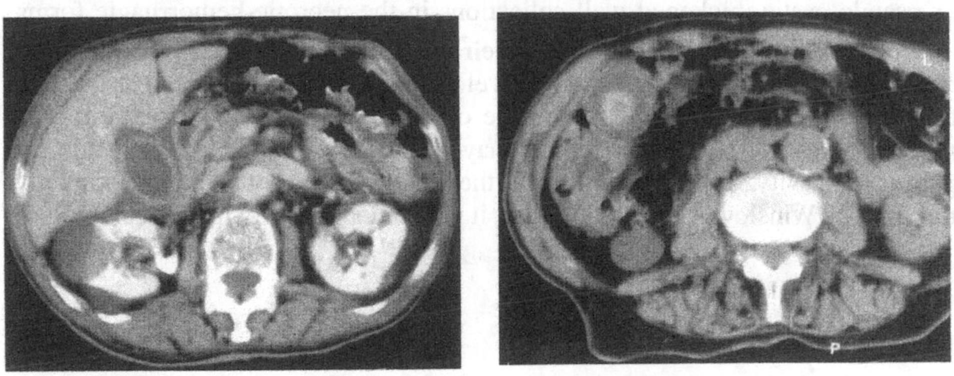

Fig. 2. Acute cholecystitis: CT findings. A, B) The gallbladder shows increased thickness of the wall and a calcified stone inside (B); free fluid surrounds the gallbladder

Acute pancreatitis

In acute pancreatitis the lytic action of pancreatic enzymes may lead to the formation of necrotic-hemorrhagic inflammatory collections that may spread from the pancreatic loggia to the anterior pararenal spaces, to infraperitoneal, mesocolic and mesenteric spaces. At the peritoneal cavity, peritonitis follows a predetermined way related to the disposition of the posterior peritoneum, of the mesocolon and of the mesentery and to the relations of contiguity and continuity that these structures have with the retroperitoneum. The anterior face of the pancreas is, in fact, in close contact with the posterior peritoneum which superiorly forms the posterior wall of the omental sac and inferiorly defines the mesenteric-colic cavities. Therefore, the diffusion of the collections from the pancreatic loggia will involve the epiploon cavity or the under-mesocolic cavities per solution of continuity of the peritoneum, while in the sub-peritoneal mesocolic or mesenteric spaces the diffusion will occur for simple detachment of the fat tissue between the peritoneal layers along the course of the vessels that from the retroperitoneum run in the mesenteriolum.

The collections occupy at first the peripancreatic fat tissue, for the most delimited anteriorly from the posterior peritoneum and posteriorly from the anterior renal fascia. Detaching then the fat tissue of the anterior pararenal, they may expand down until they reach the pelvis behind the sigmoid colon and the rectum and on the sides in the latero-conal spaces.

The CT evaluation of acute pancreatitis reveals the pathological characteristics (edematous or necrotico-hemorrhagic) and the characteristics of the collections in the various spaces. Therefore it is necessary for the choice of treatment, for the follow-up and for the eventual CT-guided drainage of the collections [14-16].

The involvement of the mesocolon and of the mesentery in acute pancreatitis shows up at CT with the simple increased density and striations of the subperitoneal fat tissue surrounding the middle colic vessels and at the collaterals of the superior mesenteric vessels in the edematous forms and with smoothly defined or pseudo-cystic thickened wall collections in the necrotic-hemorrhagic forms.

The appearance of gas bubbles in their interior suggests abscess formation in the collections or the presence of a bowel perforation. The extension at the peritoneal cavity happens frequently in the omental sac for the interruption of its posterior wall. The pancreatic fluid may penetrate sometimes also in the big peritoneal cavity, for direct lysis of the posterior peritoneum, or indirectly, through the Winslow foramen after that it penetrated in the epiploon cavity.

Interventional radiology

The use of diagnostic imaging and particularly CT have permitted the early and optimal individuation of abdominal fluid collections. The introduction of percutaneous drainage techniques has modified the therapeutic approach to consent a less invasive treatment that if initially was limited to simple unilocular collections, recently has been performed also for complex collections in the attempt to avoid reinterventions or at least to render it more comfortable, especially in the compromised patient. The positive results have led to the wide of this procedure also in multilocular collections or in cases complicated by connections with enteric fistulae due to appendicitis, pancreatitis and diverticulitis [17]. The choice of CT or ultrasound guidance depends on the skill of the interventional radiologist. CT guidance is preferred to ultrasound for the major precision of CT to localize the lesion (its accuracy is superior at 90%) [18], to identify the most secure way to follow in order to avoid the surrounding structures, and to control the correct positioning of the catheter. Even if CT requires a longer execution time and is more complex than ultrasound, it is more panoramic and it does not suffer from the guidance limits of ultrasound (bowel gas distension, wounds, dressings, drainages or scarce mobility of the patient).

Generally 90% of abdominal collections may be treated with a percutaneous approach. In a particular way, CT drainage (Fig. 3) represents the first approach because it is less invasive, repeatable, and low-risk due to general anesthesia [4, 19]. The surgical approach is reserved for cases in which valid results were not obtained with percutaneous drainage or when imaging did not precisely indicate the site and the characteristics of the abscess. Surgery is also indicated in cases of infected collections between the bowel loops, in cases of collections not

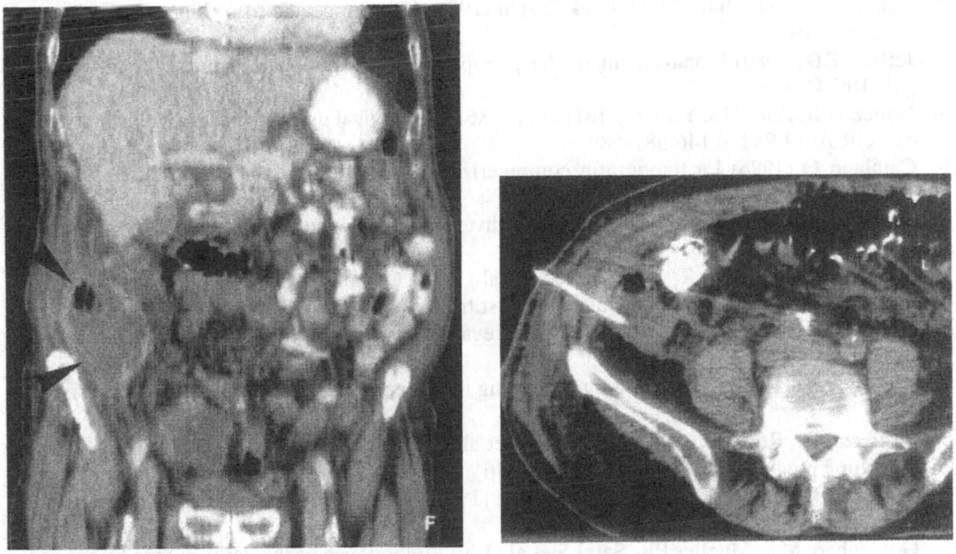

Fig. 3. Abdominal abscessual collection: CT findings and drainage. A) Multiplanar coronal reconstruction: abscessual cavity of the right flank (arrowheads) with some air bubbles inside. B) CT percutaneous drainage: a CT follow-up examinations shows decreased size of the collection

reachable with sureness with the radiological techniques and in the doubt of an underlying pathology.

The percentage of success of percutaneous drainage varies in the different series from 67 to 85.4% [20] and the failure rate varies from 14.6 to 31%.

Complications related to the percutaneous procedure are generally sepsis, hemorrhage and perforations of the bowel wall; such events cause a mortality of 14% [4] and a morbidity of about 10% [21]. Catheter-related problems such as bad positioning, dislodgment, and erosion into adjacent structures are also present [22].

References

1. Ghahremani GG, Gore RM (1989) CT diagnosis of postoperative abdominal complications. Radiol Clin North Am 27:787-804
2. Jasinski RW, Glazer GM, Francis IR (1987) CT and ultrasound in abscess detection at specific anatomic sites: a study of 189 patients. Comput Radiol 11:41-47
3. Lundstedt C, Hederstrom E, Holmin T et al (1983) Radiological diagnosis in proven intraabdominal abscess formation: a comparison between plain films of the abdomen, ultrasonography and computerized tomography. Gastroint Radiol 8:261-266
4. Lambiase RE, Deyoe L, Cronan JJ et al (1992) Percutaneous drainage of 355 consecutive abscesses: results of primary drainage with 1-year follow-up. Radiology 184:167-179
5. Mueller PR, van Sonnenberg E, Ferrucci JT Jr (1984) Percutaneous drainage of 250 abdominal abscesses and fluid collections. II. Current procedural concepts. Radiology 151:343-347
6. Balthazar EJ, Megibow AJ, Gordon RB et al (1989) Computed tomography of the abnormal appendix. J Comput Assist Tomogr 12:595-601
7. Balthazar EJ, Megibow AJ, Hulnick D et al (1986) CT of appendicitis. AJR Am J Roentgenol 147:705-710
8. Jeffrey RB (1989) Management of the periappendiceal inflammatory mass. Semin US CT MR 10:341-347
9. Nunez D Jr, Huber JS, Yrazarry JM et al (1986) Nonsurgical drainage of appendiceal abscesses. AJR Am J Radiol 146:587-589
10. Catalano O (1996) La tomografia computerizzata nello studio della diverticolite acuta del sigma. Radiol Med 92:588-593
11. Neff CC, van Sonnenberg E (1989) CT of diverticulitis: diagnosis and treatment. Radiol Clin North Am 27:743-752
12. Blankemberg F, Wirth R, Jeffrey RB Jr et al (1991) Computed tomography as an adjunct to ultrasound in the diagnosis of acute cholecystitis. Gastroint Radiol 16:149-153
13. Fidler J, Paulson EK, Layfield L (1995) CT evaluation of acute cholecystitis. AJR Am J Radiol 166:1085-1088
14. Balthazar EJ (1989) CT diagnosis and staging in acute pancreatitis. Radiol Clin North Am 27: 19-37
15. Balthazar EJ, Robinson DL, Megibow AJ et al (1990) Acute pancreatitis: value of CT in establishing prognosis. Radiology 174:331-336
16. Balthazar EJ, Freeny PC, van Sonnenberg E (1994) Imaging and intervention in acute pancreatitis. Radiology 193:297-306
17. Goldenberg MA, Mueller PR, Saini S et al (1991) Importance of the daily rounds by the radiologist after interventional procedure of the abdomen and chest. Radiology 180:767-771
18. Costello P, Gaa J (1993) Clinical assessment of an intervention CT table. Radiology 189: 284-285

19. Nunez D, Becerra JL, Martin LC (1994) Subhepatic collection complicating laparoscopic cholecystectomy: percutaneous management. Abdom Imaging 19:248-250
20. Bufalari A, Giustozzi G, Moggi L (1996) Postoperative intraabdominal abscesses: percutaneous versus surgical treatment. Acta Chir Belg 96:197-200
21. VanSonnemberg E, Mueller PR, Ferrucci JT Jr (1984) Percutaneous drainage of 250 abdominal abscesses and fluid collections. I. Results, failures and complications. Radiology 151: 337-341
22. Bertel CK, van Heerden JA, Sheedy PF II (1986) Treatment of pyogenic hepatic abscesses. Arch Surg 121:554-558

CARDIOPULMONARY RESUSCITATION

Early Defibrillation

T. Schneider, B. Wolcke

Electric countershock is the standard-of-care for patients with ventricular fibrillation (VF) and pulseless ventricular tachycardia (VT) (Fig. 1) [1, 2]. Simultaneous depolarization of all myocardial cells followed by a refractory phase aims at terminating the electric chaos which is characterized by an extremely high oxygen consumption despite the lack of any mechanical activities. Chances of survival decrease by 7-10% per minute of untreated VF [2]. Therefore all models of an ideal emergency medical services (EMS) system focus on early defibrillation [3]. Undoubtedly the early onset of Basic Life Support (BLS) warrants a minimal circulation with perfusion of heart, lungs, and brain. However, VF can be terminated by defibrillation only. As of today the gold standard for an effective EMS system is a discharge from hospital rate of 30% for patients found in VF [3]. Different prerequisites lead to the same results in different EMS systems, as demonstrated in Seattle and Mainz [3]. Whereas the rate of bystander BLS is high in Seattle, it is ashamingly low in Mainz, where, on the other hand, the full range of Advanced Life Support (ALS) and intensive care is available in a very short period of time. Although strengthening different ends of the chain of survival both systems have one thing in common: Defibrillation is available early, delivered by firefighters in Seattle, and by rescue assistants (RA) in Mainz.

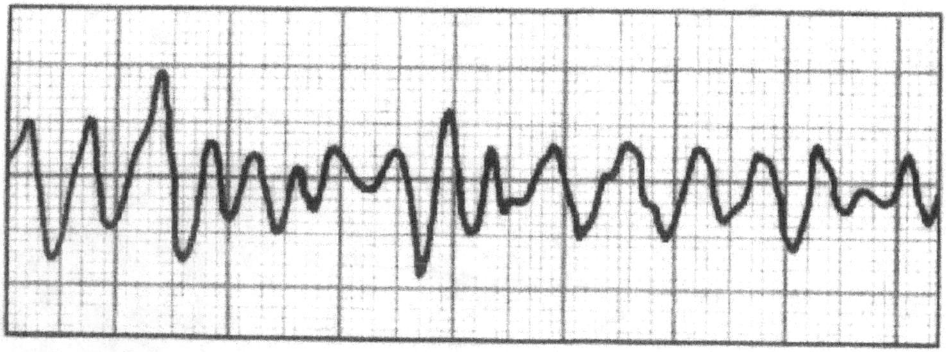

Fig. 1. ECG-strip showing ventricular fibrillation (VF)

Since the beginnings of cardiac electrical therapy efforts have aimed at 1) a further miniaturization and simplification of the devices in order to achieve a widespread distribution, and 2) an adjustment of the countershock to the individual needs of the patient. Besides a few anecdotes of resuscitation with the help of electric energy the first report on a successful defibrillation dates back to 1899 when VF was terminated in an open canine chest [4, 5]. The first open-chest defibrillation with alternating current (AC) in a human leading to a full recovery was published in 1947 [4, 6]. In the mid-fifties Zoll and Kouwenhoven developed the method of external defibrillation in an animal lab model. Following systematic research concerning electrode position, energy level, and impulse length, the method was applied to humans, and defibrillators for routine use were engineered [4, 7]. At that time the devices delivered AC shocks which made them extremely bulky and heavy. In the 1960s direct current (DC) defibrillation took over. Lown et al. demonstrated higher defibrillation and lower complication rates for DC as compared to AC [8]. With the development of portable DC devices defibrillation became available in out-of-hospital settings. Meanwhile defibrillation has become the most effective weapon in the fight against sudden death. As of today the standard of care has been the utmost early defibrillation with 200 J. In case VF persists, a second shock with the same amount of energy is delivered, followed by a third one with 360 J [1, 2]. In children the energy is adjusted to the individual body weight: 2 J/kg for the first and second, 4 J/kg for the third shock. In children and adults all further shocks are delivered with the energy level of the third shock [1, 2].

With regard to the rigid energy recommendations for adult patients new developments are under discussion, aiming to maximize the efficacy and minimize the complication rate. In the following sections 5 technological aspects will be discussed:

- Automated external defibrillators (AED)
- Defibrillation electrodes
- Automatic measurement of chest impedance
- Frequency analysis
- Biphasic waveforms

However, the method of defibrillation is optimized not only by technical developments. A crucial aspect for survival is the early availability of a defibrillator. Therefore 3 structural aspects will be discussed which aim at reducing the time from the onset of VF until the first defibrillation:

- Early defibrillation programmes
- First-responder projects
- Public access defibrillation

Technical aspects

Automated external defibrillators (AED)

Since the early 1980s AEDs have been used in the United States by Emergency Medical Technicians. Those devices are based upon the technology of implantable cardioverter-defibrillators (ICD) (Fig. 2). The device collects an ECG-signal via adhesive electrodes attached to the patient's bare chest. The signal is filtered and – provided it is recognized as a noise-free ECG – analyzed following an algorithm. Several algorithms are available on the market which basically analyse amplitude, rate, and slope of the signal for a few seconds (Fig. 3). In case VF or VT are detected the device charges up to a preselected energy level. Fully automated devices then deliver the shock right away. In semi-automated devices the user has to push a separate button, thus delivering the energy to the patient. In case of other rhythms than VF or VT the devices advise to check the patient's pulse and resume cardiopulmonary resuscitation (CPR), if necessary. The German Task Force on early defibrillation demands a sensitivity of more than 95% and a specificity of at least 98% in AEDs [9].

Defibrillation electrodes

In manual defibrillators energy is delivered via metal electrodes (paddles) which are pressed to the patient's chest with isolated handles. In order to reduce the amount of air in the lungs, thus reducing chest impedance, the paddles have to be applied firmly to the patient's chest after the contact plates have been covered with gel [1, 2]. With the introduction of AEDs self-adhesive electrodes became available. They consist of aluminum and an acrylic compound. Advantages over hand-held paddles are a safe distance of the rescuer from the patient during defibrillation, a constant contact surface, and a constant position of the electrodes during CPR. The lack of application pressure is compensated by an improved contact which leads to comparable impedance values in both hand-held and self-adhesive electrode types [10-12].

Automatic measurement of chest impedance

It is the electric current reaching the myocardium that is crucial for the success of defibrillation. This current depends on the level of energy and the impedance of the patient's chest [13, 14]. Impedance is influenced by the size of the chest, the contact between electrodes and skin, electrode position and size, the distance between the electrodes, and the volume of air in the lungs [13]. In humans impedance values range from 15 to 150 Ω with an average at 70 to 80 Ω [2]. In a high chest impedance the electric current reaching the myocardium is low. Therefore it seems to be promising to measure impedance and adjust the countershock accordingly. Different approaches are all based upon one principle: Measurement of chest impedance via self-adhesive electrodes at certain time-

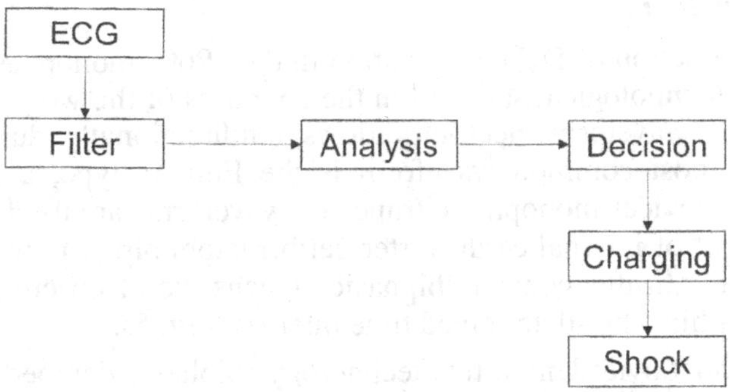

Fig. 2. Automated external defibrillator (AED): Sequence from signal uptake to shock delivery

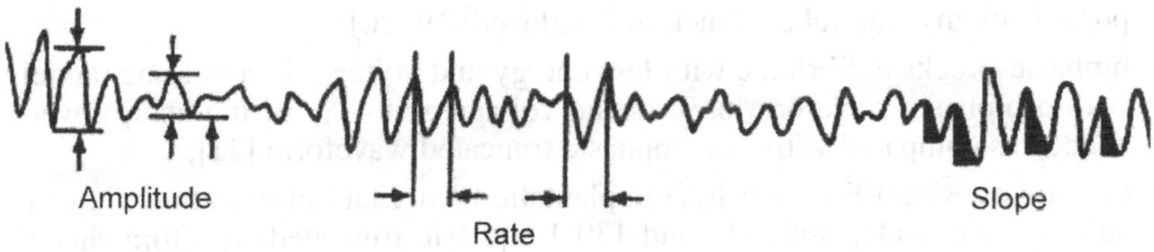

Fig. 3. Automated external defibrillator (AED): Algorithm analyzing amplitude, rate and slope of the ECG-signal

points with adjustment of either the energy-level or the current [10, 14-17]. Current-based defibrillation appears to be promising in patients with a high chest impedance. The optimal current of 30 to 40 A is reached with 200 J countershocks in patients with normal impedance values. With higher impedances current is reduced which also reduces the probability of a successful defibrillation. Therefore a pre-selection of the desired current with an automatic measurement of chest impedance, followed by an adjustment of the energy required by the micro-processor supported defibrillator seems to be ideal. In a prospective study in the electrophysiology-lab patients with VF of less than 15 seconds duration were defibrillated with 200-200-360 J, or 25-25-40 A, respectively, with continuous measurement of chest impedance in both groups. With the first shock efficacy being equal for both methods [81 vs. 79%], patients in the energy-based defibrillation group received 67% more energy and 38% higher currents than those in the current-based group [17].

Biphasic waveforms

Since the introduction of DC defibrillation in the 1960s monophasic waveforms have been the technological standard in the countries of the western hemisphere [18]. With this waveform electricity flows unidirectionally during discharge (Fig. 4). The most common waveform is the Edmark-type, a damped sinus wave. In a few devices monophasic truncated waveforms are used, instead. With the development of internal cardioverter-defibrillators biphasic waveforms have come into focus. In this context "biphasic" means the electricity flow changes its direction within a pre-determined time interval (Fig. 5).

In the former Soviet Union this technology (biphasic damped sinus wave = Gurvich type) has been the standard-of-care since the 1960s [18].

Studies in isolated myocadial cells, animal models, and in humans in electrophysiology-labs clearly demonstrate advantages of the biphasic over the monophasic waveforms, when applied internally and externally:

- post-shock myocardial dysfunction is reduced [19, 20];
- biphasic shocks defibrillate with less energy and voltage. In a porcine model, with a biphasic waveform 63% of the voltage and 41% of the energy were needed as compared with a monophasic truncated waveform [21];
- in patients with VF during ICD-implantation external defibrillation via self-adhesive electrodes with 115 and 130 J biphasic truncated wavefom shocks were equally as effective as 200 J monophasic damped sinus waveform shocks [22];
- higher conversion rates from VF were achieved with biphasic than with monophasic waveforms [23, 24]. In a randomized double-blind multi-centre study in patients with VF or VT in the electrophysiology lab either biphasic Gurvich shocks of 171 J or monophasic Edmark shocks of 215 J were delivered. The Edmark waveform terminated VF in 22 out of 28 patients with the first shock, whereas all 25 patients were successfully defibrillated with the first Gurvich type shock [23];
- biphasic waveforms reduce voltage and energy which leads to a further miniaturization of the devices which makes them smaller, lighter, and cheaper [18, 22, 23, 25];
- in a randomized pre-hospital multi-centre trial one biphasic waveform proved its superiority over monophasic waveforms: In 113 patients with VF occurring out of hospital the 150 J biphasic truncated exponential (BTE) waveform of the ForeRunner© defibrillator (Hewlett-Packard/Heartstream) terminated VF in 94% with the first shock (Fig. 5). With a series of up to 3 shocks with a constant energy level 98% of the patients were successfully defibrillated. With monophasic waveforms the first shock efficacy at 200 J was 58% ($p < 0.0001$), and three shocks with escalating energies (200-200-360 J) terminated VF in 67% ($p < 0.0001$). Significantly more patients achieved restoration of spontaneous circulation with 150 J BTE waveform shocks (76 vs. 55%, $p = 0.02$) [26].

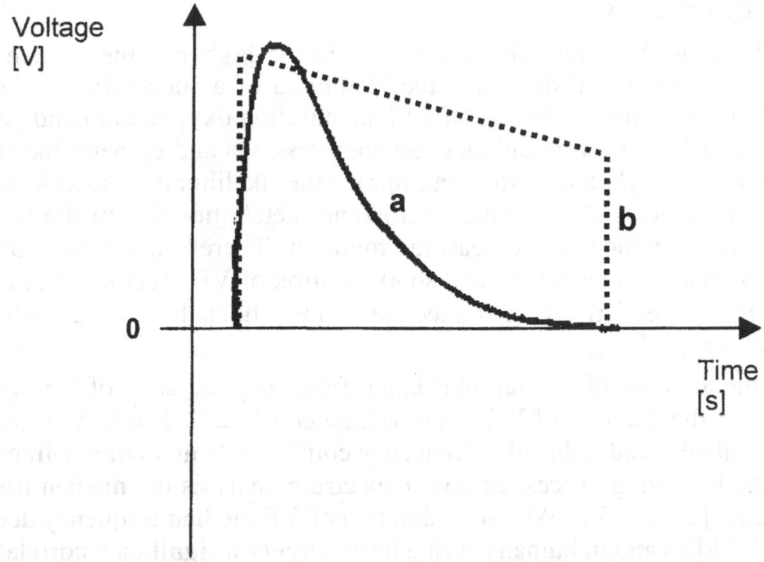

Fig. 4. Monophasic waveforms (a: Edmark-type damped sinus, b: truncated exponential)

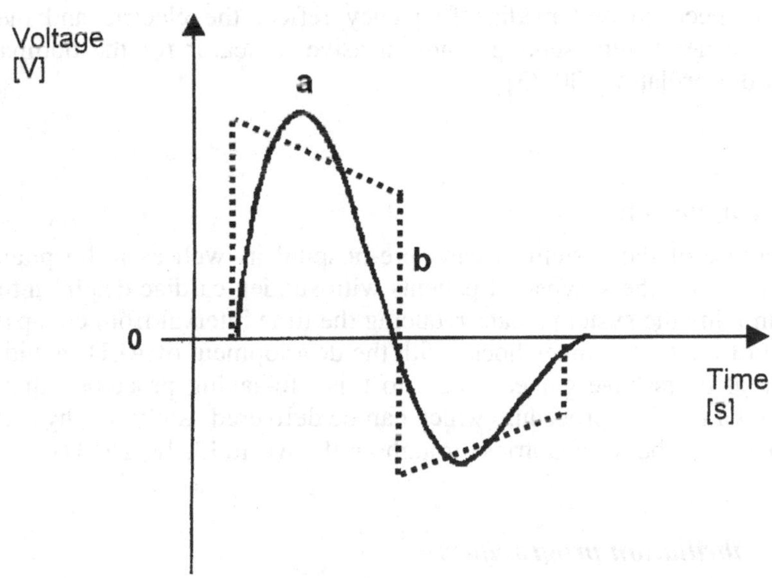

Fig. 5. Biphasic waveforms (a: Gurvich-type damped sinus, b: truncated exponential)

Frequency analysis

The earlier a defibrillatory shock is delivered the higher is the chance of survival. Persistence of VF decreases the likelihood of a successful defibrillation [2]. Study results suggest that in VF of long duration oxygenation and perfusion of the myocardium by ventilation, chest compressions and epinephrine administration prior to shock administration improve the likelihood of successful defibrillation. The crucial factor is the electric and metabolic state of the myocardium, a parameter which is not measured routinely. Therefore in praxi no distinction can be made between long and short duration of VF. According to all international recommendations an immediate countershock has to be delivered in case of VF or VT [1, 2].

With the analysis of median fibrillation frequency the state of the myocardium, and thus the duration of VF, can be estimated [27-29]. The ECG-signal is filtered, digitalized, and reduced to frequency components in a Fourier-transformation. In the following process of power spectrum analysis the median frequency is calculated [27, 28, 30]. With long duration of VF median frequency decreases. In animal studies and in humans during heart surgery a significant correlation between median frequency and defibrillation success could be demonstrated. Conversion rate decreased to 0% with a frequency of below 3 Hz, and rose to 100% with values above 5.5 Hz. High median frequencies were also correlated positively with the onset of a supraventricular post-shock rhythm [31].

Power spectrum and median frequency reflect the electric and metabolic state of the heart, representing a non-invasive indicator for the optimal timepoint for defibrillation [30-33].

Structural aspects

The structure of the system of care, pre-hospital as well as in-hospital, is the crucial factor for the survival of patients with sudden cardiac death. In this context optimizing the system means reducing the time interval from collapse to application of the first countershock. With the development of AEDs a wide range of potential users have gained access to this life-saving procedure that still is considered a medical procedure which can be delivered safely by physicians only in quite a number of countries throughout the world [3, 18, 25, 34].

Early defibrillation programmes

The International Liaison Committee on Resuscitation (ILCOR) recommends that resuscitation personnel be authorized, trained, equipped, and directed to operate a defibrillator if their professional responsibilities require them to respond to cardiac arrests. This includes all first-responding emergency personnel both in the hospital and out of hospital [35].

In early defibrillation programmes control systems should be set up that

- set written policies and guidelines based upon those developed by major resuscitation organizations;
- establish a training and quality management programme;
- place the programme under the direction and responsibility of a physician;
- use AEDs only;
- require that all defibrillators contain internal recording capabilities permitting documentation and review of all clinical uses of the device [35].

First responder projects

According to ILCOR a first responder is a trained individual acting independently with a medically controlled system. This may include

- police
- security personnel
- lifeguards
- airline cabin attendants
- railway station personnel
- volunteers who render first aid [35].

Training first responders in AED use is advisable in systems where those regarded as first responders are likely to be earlier at a patient's side than EMS personnel. In a pilot project in Rochester/Minnesota police officers were trained in BLS and AED use. The police vehicles were equipped with AEDs. A first analysis after defibrillation of 14 patients with VF by police officers demonstrated that the first shock was delivered in a mean time interval of 5.5 ± 1.2 minutes after reception of the emergency call at the dispatch centre. All of the 14 patients were defibrillated successfully, seven of them had a palpable pulse prior to arrival of the EMS, in seven spontaneous circulation was established with ALS by EMS personnel. All seven patients with an early ROSC and three of those with a late onset of ROSC were discharged alive from hospital [36].

ILCOR has considered the use of an AED to be within the domain of BLS [37]. Meanwhile BLS and AED use have become an integral part of the medical training for firefighters, cabin attendants of many airlines, and first aid providers in numerous organizations throughout the world.

Public access defibrillation

With the proven effects and safety of AEDs used by EMS personnel and first responders it seems to be promising to extend the AED concept to "Public Access Defibrillation". With a widespread distribution of AEDs that are simple to operate by minimally trained non-medical personnel many cases of cardiac arrests in public places could be treated prior to the arrival of medical personnel. Defibrillators for use in public access defibrillation programmes must be most simple to operate, utterly reliable and maintenance-free [18, 25].

Conclusion

Early defibrillation is the standard of care for patients with ventricular fibrillation (VF) and pulseless ventricular tachycardia (VT). Technical developments aim at further miniaturization and simplification of defibrillators as well as adaptation of energy requirements to the patient's needs. Implantable Cardioverter-Defibrillators (ICD) and automated external defibrillators (AED) are based upon the same technology. Both devices analyze the ECG-signal internally, followed by a "shock" or "no shock" decision. Use of automated devices is the prerequisite for defibrillation by non-physicians. Chest impedance measurements and use of alternative shock waveforms, such as biphasic, aim at adaptation of energy or current to the patient's individual needs and avoid application of unnecessarily high amounts of energy to the myocardium. Calculation of median frequency is a non-invasive method for analyzing the heart's metabolic and electrical state. It helps to determine the optimal moment for defibrillation during cardiopulmonary resuscitation (CPR). Developments concerning the structure of in-hospital emergency systems or pre-hospital emergency medical services (EMS) systems aim at further reductions in time from collapse of a patient until first defibrillation. Such developments include early defibrillation programmes for emergency medical technicians (EMT), nurses, fire- or police-department first responders as well as a wide distribution of easy-to-operate defibrillators to the public as discussed during the American Heart Association's (AHA) Public Access Defibrillation conferences. All programmes of that kind have to be organized and supervised by a physician who is responsible for training and supervision of the personnel involved.

References

1. Advanced Life Support Working Party of the European Resuscitation Council (1992) Guidelines for adult advanced cardiac life support. Resuscitation 24:111-121
2. American Heart Association (1994) Textbook of advanced cardiac life support. American Heart Association, Dallas
3. Cummins RO, Ornato JP, Thies WH et al (1991) Improving survival from sudden cardiac arrest: the "chain of survival" concept; a statement for health professionals from the advanced cardiac life support subcommittee and the emergency cardiac care committee, American Heart Association. Circulation 83:1832-1847
4. Kouwenhoven WB, Milnor WR, Knickerbocker GG et al (1957) Closed chest defibrillation of the heart. Surgery 42:550-561
5. Prevost JL, Batelli F (1899) La mort par les courants electriques-courants alternatifs à haute tension. J Physiol et Path Gen 1:427

6. Beck CS, Pritchard WH, Feil HS (1947) Ventricular fibrillation of long duration abolished by electric shock. JAMA 135:985
7. Zoll PM, Linenthal AJ, Gibson W et al (1956) Termination of ventricular fibrillation in man by externally applied electric countershock. N Engl J Med 254:726-732
8. Lown B, Neumann J, Amarasingham R et al (1962) Comparison of alternating current with direct current electroshock across the closed chest. Am J Cardiol 10:223-233
9. Arbeitsgemeinschaft Frühdefibrillation (1993) Empfehlungen zur Einführung eines Frühdefibrillationsprogrammes für qualifiziertes nichtärztliches Personal. Notfallmedizin 19: 229-231
10. Kerber RE (1984) External defibrillation: new technologies. Ann Emerg Med 13:794-797
11. Kerber RE, Martins JB, Ferguson DW (1985) Experimental evaluation and initial clinical application of new self-adhesive defibrillation electrodes. Int J Cardiol 8:57-66
12. Kerber RE, Martins J, Kelly KJ et al (1984) Self-adhesive preapplied electrode pads for defibrillation and cardioversion. J Am Coll Cardiol 3:815-820
13. Kenknight BH, Eyüboglu BM, Ideker RE (1995) Impedance to defibrillation countershock: does an optimal impedance exist? Pace 18:2068-2087
14. Kerber RE, Kouba C, Martins J et al (1984) Advance prediction of transthoracic impedance in human defibrillation and cardioversion: importance of impedance in determining the success of low energy shocks. Circulation 70:303-308
15. Kerber RE, Martins JB, Kienzle MG et al (1988) Energy, current and success in defibrillation and cardioversion: clinical studies using an impedance-based method of energy adjustment. Circulation 77:1038-1046
16. Kerber RE, McPherson D, Charbonnier F et al (1985) Automated impedance-based energy adjustment for defibrillation: experimental studies. Circulation 71:136-140
17. Lerman BB, DiMarco JP, Haines D (1988) Current-based versus energy-based ventricular defibrillation: a prospective study. J Am Coll Cardiol 12:1259-1264
18. Kerber RE, Becker LB, Bourland EE et al (1997) Automatic external defibrillators for public access defibrillation: recommendations for specifying and reporting arrhythmia analysis algorithm performance, incorporating new waveforms, and enhancing safety. A statement for health professionals from the American Heart Association task force on automatic external defibrillation, subcommittee on AED safety and efficacy. Circulation 95:1677-1682
19. Jones JL, Jones RE (1984) Decreased defibrillator-induced dysfunction with biphasic rectangular waveform. Am J Physiol 247:H792-H796
20. Jones JL, Jones RE (1983) Improved defibrillator waveform safety factor with biphasic waveforms. Am J Physiol 245:H60-H65
21. Gliner BE, Lyster TE, Dillon SM et al (1995) Transthoracic defibrillation of swine with monophasic and biphasic waveforms. Circulation 92:1634-1643
22. Bardy GH, Gliner BE, Kudenschuk PJ et al (1995) Truncated biphasic pulses for transthoracic defibrillation. Circulation 91:1768-1774
23. Greene HL, DiMarco JP, Kudenschuk PJ et al (1995) Comparison of monophasic and biphasic defibrillating pulse waveforms for transthoracic Cardioversion. Am J Cardiol 75:1135-1139
24. Schuder JC, McDaniel W, Stoeckle H (1984) Defibrillation of 100 kg calves with asymmetrical, bidirectional, rectangular pulses. Cardiovasc Res 18:419-426
25. Weisfeldt ML, Kerber RE, McGoldrick RP et al (1994) American Heart Association Report on the Public Access Defibrillation Conference December 8-10, 1994. Circulation 92:2740-2747
26. Schneider T, Martens P, Paschen H et al (1999) Randomized comparison of 150 J biphasic and 200-360 J monophasic AEDs in out-of-hospital cardiac arrest victims. Pacing and Clinical Electrophysiology 22:A146
27. Brown CG, Dzwonczyk R, Martin DR (1993) Physiologic measurement of the ventricular fibrillation ECG signal: estimating the duration of ventricular fibrillation. Ann Emerg Med 22:70-74

28. Brown CG, Dzwonczyk R, Werman HA et al (1989) Estimating the duration of ventricular fibrillation. Ann Emerg Med 18:1181-1185
29. Martin DR, Brown CG, Dzwonczyk R (1991) Frequency analysis of the human and swine electrocardiogram during ventricular fibrillation. Resuscitation 22:85-91
30. Brown CG, Griffith RF, Van Lighten P et al (1991) Median frequency - a new parameter for predicting defibrillation success rate. Ann Emerg Med 20:787-789
31. Strohmenger HU, Lindner KH, Lurie KG et al (1994) Frequency of ventricular fibrillations as a predictor of defibrillation success during cardiac surgery. Anesth Analg 79:434-438
32. Carlisle EJF, Allen JD, Kernohan WG et al (1990) Fourier analysis of ventricular fibrillation of varied aetiology. Europ Heart J 11:173-181
33. Strohmenger HU, Lindner KH, Prengel AW et al (1996) Effects of epinephrine and vasopressin on median fibrillation frequency and defibrillation success in a porcine model of cardiopulmonary resuscitation. Resuscitation 31:65-73
34. Schneider T, Mauer D, Diehl P et al (1994) Early defibrillation by emergency physicians or emergency technicians? A controlled, prospective multi-centre study. Resuscitation 27: 197-206
35. Kloeck W, Cummins RO, Chamberlain D et al (1997) ILCOR advisory statements: early defibrillation. Circulation 95:2183-2184
36. White RD, Vukov LF, Bugliosi TF (1994) Early defibrillation by police: initial experience with measurement of critical time intervals and patient outcome. Ann Emerg Med 23:1009-1013
37. Handley AJ, Becker LB, Allen M et al (1997) ILCOR advisory statements: single-rescuer adult basic life support. Circulation 95:2174-2179

Outcome and Cost-Effectiveness of Cardiopulmonary Resuscitation

J. NOLAN

Cardiac disease is the most common cause of death in the developed world. The incidence of sudden cardiac death in the United States is approximately 0.1% to 0.2% per year [1]. Although prompt cardiopulmonary resuscitation (CPR) has the potential to save a number of these victims of sudden cardiac death, the overall rate of survival remains depressingly low. The cost-effectiveness of cardiopulmonary resuscitation is linked inextricably to the survival rate; the cost per patient surviving to discharge increases exponentially as the rate of survival to discharge decreases [2]. This review will consider the available data on the outcome from CPR before then analysing the cost-effectiveness of this intervention.

Reporting of outcome from cardiopulmonary resuscitation

The outcome from CPR can be reported in a variety of ways but most clinicians would support the view that the ultimate goal is to return the patient to his or her prearrest level of neurological function. Guidelines for the reporting of outcomes from cardiac arrest were defined at the Utstein Consensus Conference [3]. Reported outcomes include return of spontaneous circulation, admission to the intensive care unit or ward, survival to discharge from hospital, and survival at one year. Ideally, the neurological recovery of the patient is reported according to the "best-ever achieved" Cerebral Performance Category (CPC) and Overall Performance Category (OPC). Unfortunately, a number of different denominators can be used when calculating the reported survival rates following cardiac arrest. Unless the denominator is defined precisely the reported survival rates can be difficult to interpret and compare with data from other studies. The Utstein Consensus Conference participants recommended reporting the number discharged alive divided by the number of persons with witnessed cardiac arrest, in ventricular fibrillation (VF), of cardiac aetiology [3]. In reality, this figure is rarely quoted explicitly.

Outcome after out-of-hospital cardiac arrest

The survival from out-of-hospital cardiac arrest varies substantially from one health care system to another. A recent review of defibrillator-capable emergency medical services (EMS), which included 33,124 patients, reported a median survival to hospital discharge rate of 6.4% with range of 0% to 20.7% (Table 1) [4]. The variation may be attributable to the proportion of victims receiving bystander CPR, the collapse to defibrillation interval, the characteristics of the population served, how the data are presented, or differences in the type of EMS system. There appears to be an inverse relationship between the incidence of cardiac arrest and survival (Table 2) [5]. This may be because some populations are older and/or sicker than others, or it may reflect differences in the criteria used to initiate CPR or declare death at the scene. There are often difficulties in obtaining accurate estimates of the population served by an individual EMS system.

Differences in the type of EMS system

There is considerable variation in the type of prehospital systems based on the personnel who deliver CPR. These can be single-tier or two-tier systems:

Single-tier

- Basic life support (BLS)
- BLS with defibrillation (BLS-D)
- Advanced life support (ALS)

Two-tier

- BLS + ALS
- BLS-D + ALS

Further variation is introduced by the fact that BLS and BLS-D may be performed by emergency medical technicians (EMTs) on ambulances or by fire fighters on pump vehicles, and that ALS may be provided by physicians or paramedics. In two-tier EMS systems, the BLS providers (first tier) usually arrive more quickly because there are normally more serving the community. About 75% of the American urban population are served by a two-tier rather than a one-tier system [10]. One metaanalysis has concluded that survival was 5.2% in a one-tier EMS system and 10.5% in a two-tier EMS system [10]. However, the data available for this analysis were thought to be suboptimal. It is possible that the type of EMS system influences survival primarily because of variation in the time to defibrillation. A recent metaanalysis, using robust data, has shown that use of a one-tier ALS system or two-tier BLS plus ALS or BLS-D plus ALS system was associated with greater survival than use of a one-tier BLS-D system (Table 3) [4]. Overall, mean survival was 6.3% within a one-tier EMS system and 10.8% within two-tier EMS systems. However, this study had insufficient power to demonstrate whether EMS systems that used ALS alone

Table 1. Rates of survival to hospital discharge and bystander CPR for EMS systems with defibrillator capabilities (adapted from Nichol G, Stiell IG, Laupacis A, De Maio VJ, Wells GA (1999). A cumulative metaanalysis of the effectiveness of defibrillator-capable emergency medical services for victims of out-of-hospital cardiac arrest. Ann Emerg Med 34:517-525)

City	Year	EMS System	Bystander CPR (%)	Survival to discharge (%)
Stockholm, Sweden	1987	BLS-D	15.0	3.6
Stockport, England	1987	BLS-D	38.0	0
Nottinghamshire, England	1987	BLS-D	44.7	10.9
Iowa, USA	1984	BLS-D	20.0	10.9
Milwaukee, USA	1989	BLS-D	49.0	6.4
Arrowhead, USA	1986	BLS-D	32.0	5.2
Brighton, England	1988	BLS-D	15.0	2.3
Rochester, USA	1990	BLS-D	35.0	6.0
Stockholm, Sweden	1990	BLS-D	27.0	1.9
Scotland	1996	BLS-D	37.0	6.7
Ipswich, Australia	1992	BLS-D	26.0	9.0
Odense, Denmark	1991	BLS-D	15.0	1.4
Ontario, Canada	1992	BLS-D	19.0	2.9
New Westminster, Canada	1978	ALS	-	8.5
Pittsburgh, USA	1984	ALS	21.0	9.6
Los Angeles, USA	1983	ALS	38.0	10.2
Lucas, Kent, Southfield, USA	1988	ALS	20.0	7.0
Vancouver, Canada	1983	ALS	14.0	11.5
Chicago, USA	1991	ALS	24.9	1.7
Torrance, USA	1977	ALS	0	13.4
West Yorkshire, England	1990	ALS	31.0	5.4
Cincinnati, USA	1978	ALS	-	15.0
St Louis, USA	1990	ALS	31.0	4.5
Royal Oak, USA	1989	ALS	-	9.1
South Glamorgan, Wales	1989	ALS	11.0	5.6
Milwaukee, USA	1989	BLS + ALS	-	12.6
Lincoln, USA	1974	BLS + ALS	-	20.7
Tucson, USA	1992	BLS + ALS	29.8	5.9
Seattle, USA	1988	BLS + ALS	22.4	8.6
Taipei, Taiwan	1994	BLS + ALS	5.8	1.3
Memphis, USA	1993	BLS + ALS	12.1	6.3
Minneapolis, USA	1977	BLS + ALS	15.0	16.1
King County, USA	1980	BLS + ALS	20.0	17.2
Tucson, USA	1990	BLS + ALS	28.9	8.4
Seattle, USA	1988	BLS-D + ALS	25.9	13.9
King County, USA	1987	BLS-D + ALS	61.0	12.8
Fresno, USA	1995	BLS-D + ALS	16.2	4.7
San Francisco, USA	1995	BLS-D + ALS	18.1	5.1
Memphis, USA	1993	BLS-D + ALS	13.4	8.9

were more effective than those that used BLS-D plus ALS. Other investigators have failed to show any benefit for ALS interventions over and above defibrillation [11-13].

Table 2. Survival ranked by the incidence of out-of-hospital cardiac arrest (updated from Becker LB, Smith DW, Rhodes KV (1993). Incidence of cardiac arrest: A neglected factor in evaluating survival rates. Ann Emerg Med 22:86-91)

Locality	Incidence rate*	Survival rate (%)
Arrowhead	128	3.3
Chicago	107	1.6
Stockholm	107	3.2
Manitoba	98	3.9
North-east Italy [6]	95	6.7
Milwaukee	79	8.3
South Glamorgan [7]	65.8	6.3
New York [8]	63.5	1.4
Kansas	61	16.8
Pittsburgh	60	9.6
Nova Scotia	57	7.0
Iceland	56	9.5
Michigan	55	7.1
California	50	9.3
Minneapolis	48	16.1
Finland	48	16.2
Portsmouth, UK [9]	47	5.6
Pennsylvania	47	6.4
Israel	46	6.6
North Carolina	45	8.7
Brighton, UK	40	11.2
King County	39	18.3
British Columbia	36	9.3
Nebraska	36	20.7

* Per 100,000 person-years

Table 3. Odds of survival with EMS systems compared with BLS-D (data from Nichol G, Stiell IG, Laupacis A, De Maio VJ, Wells GA (1999). A cumulative metaanalysis of the effectiveness of defibrillator-capable emergency medical services for victims of out-of-hospital cardiac arrest. Ann Emerg Med 34:517-525)

EMS	Odds of survival	95% CI	*p*
ALS	1.71	1.09-2.70	0.01
BLS plus ALS	1.47	0.89-2.42	0.07
BLS-D plus ALS	2.31	1.47-3.62	<0.01

Defibrillation response time

A reduction in defibrillation response time will increase survival from cardiac arrest [14]. Phase two of the Ontario Prehospital Advanced Life Support (OPALS) Study has shown the impact of reducing the defibrillator response interval (time from call received to arrival at scene of a vehicle equipped with a defibrillator) on an EMS system with a BLS-D level of care [15]. The local EMS system was optimised to achieve a rapid defibrillation time interval. This was achieved by a reduction of dispatch time intervals, more efficient deployment of existing ambulances, and by using fire-fighters to perform defibrillation. By increasing the proportion of cases meeting a defibrillator response interval of 8 minutes or less from 76.7% to 92.5%, the overall survival to hospital discharge for all rhythm groups combined improved from 3.9% to 5.2% ($p = 0.03$).

A metaanalysis of 39 EMS systems with defibrillator capability showed an overall mean response time interval of 6.1 minutes [4]. A 1-minute decrease in defibrillation response time interval was associated with an absolute increase of survival of 0.7% to 2.1%, depending on the type of EMS system. Despite this overwhelming evidence, one third of American EMS systems still do not provide first-responder defibrillation.

Cardiac arrest at public events

Major public events are generally supported well by medical, paramedical and first aid services. If these services are equipped with defibrillators, survival from cardiac arrest at these events may be surprisingly high. Over an eight-year period, the survival to hospital discharge was 71% amongst 28 cardiac arrest victims at the Melbourne Cricket Ground [16].

Public access defibrillation

Having determined that early defibrillation is the single most important intervention in cardiac arrest, a number of strategies are being adopted in an effort to reduce the time interval to defibrillation. One such strategy is to include defibrillation by minimally trained members of the public; this has been termed public access defibrillation (PAD) [17]. This may include non-traditional first-responder defibrillation by security personnel and airline flight attendants, etc., or minimally trained witness defibrillation. A PAD program was introduced into the Chicago Airport System in June 1999 [18]. Fifty-one automated external defibrillators were located on the walls of terminals, concourses and train stations. Up until April 2000, they had been applied to twelve adults in cardiac arrest. Eleven of these cases were in VF and 9 (82%) of them were resuscitated neurologically intact. Out of the eleven uses of the AEDs, 6 (58%) have been by Good Samaritans not associated or trained by the Chicago HeartSave Program.

These impressive survival figures have proven the validity of PAD. A cost analysis of this program is presented below.

Bystander CPR

Published figures for the proportion of bystander CPR varies from 5.8% in Taipei, Taiwan to 61% in King County, USA (Table 1). Bystander CPR does improve survival from cardiac arrest but reports on its precise impact are contradictory. The effect of bystander CPR will be confounded by factors such as witnessed arrests, response intervals and initial rhythm. The association between bystander CPR and survival in out-of-hospital cardiac arrest may also be confounded by CPR quality. In a large study from New York City, effective bystander CPR remained independently associated with improved survival (OR = 3.9; 95% CI 1.1 to 14.0; $p < 0.04$) after adjustment for witness status, initial rhythm, interval from collapse to CPR, and interval from collapse to ALS [19]. The mean proportion of bystander CPR across 39 EMS systems was 27.4% [4]. In this metaanalysis a 5% increment in bystander CPR was associated with an absolute increase in survival of 0.3% to 1.0% within any EMS system. A 5% increase in bystander CPR had less impact on survival than a 1-minute decrease in the defibrillation response time interval. This may be because bystander CPR is not as important as other factors or it may reflect a delay in calling the EMS when bystander CPR is undertaken (contrary to existing ERC and AHA guidelines).

Outcome for patients admitted to hospital after out-of-hospital cardiac arrest

Of those patients admitted to hospital after initially successful resuscitation from cardiac arrest out of hospital, approximately 40-54% will survive to hospital discharge [12, 20-22]. Of 494 patients admitted to hospital alive in the OPALS study, 268 (54%) survived to hospital discharge [12]. In a study of 1476 patients admitted to Scottish hospitals after out-of-hospital cardiac arrest 680 (46%) were discharged alive [21]. The median duration of hospital stay was 10 days in patients discharged alive and 1 day in those dying in hospital. Neurological status was moderately or severely impaired (including one comatose patient) in 71 patients, representing 10.5% of those discharged alive and 4.8% of those admitted to hospital. In this study patients were followed up for a median period of 25 (range 0-68) months. From these data the product limit estimate of overall survival in the patients was 84% at one year, 77% at two years, 73% at three years, and 68% at four years.

Outcome after in-hospital cardiac arrest

The reported survival from in-hospital cardiac arrest is also very variable. Most studies report rates of survival to hospital discharge after in-hospital cardiac arrest in the range of 14-24% [22, 23-28]. A metaanalysis of almost 20,000 in-hospital cardiac arrests revealed a survival to discharge rate of 15% [26]. Seventy-three percent of the deaths occurred within 72 hours of CPR and 1.6% of successfully resuscitated patients had permanent neurological impairment. In a survey of CPR in British hospitals (Bresus study) 541 out of 2648 (20.4%) of patients survived to hospital discharge [22]. In this study 45% of patients survived through the arrest and 32% survived for at least 24 hours.

The variable survival rates from in-hospital CPR probably reflect differences in casemix, difficulties in defining in-hospital cardiac arrest, and difficulties including all those patients in whom CPR is undertaken. In the Bresus study, 47% of in-hospital cardiac arrests took place in monitored areas. A very recent study of cardiac arrest in UK hospitals reports an overall survival to hospital discharge of 240/1368 (17.6%) [28]. In contrast to this UK study, investigators from Göteborg, Sweden, report a much higher survival to hospital discharge of 78/187 (41.7%) after in-hospital cardiac arrest [29]. However, 62% of these cardiac arrests occurred in monitored areas. In the recent UK study just 31.4% of the patients were reported as having an initial rhythm of VF or pulseless ventricular tachycardia (VT) compared with 64% in the Swedish study. Survival to hospital discharge after VF or pulseless VT was 42.2% in the UK study and 64.2% in the Swedish study. Many of these studies will capture only those cardiac arrests where a cardiac arrest is called. Patients going in to VF in a monitored area (e.g., coronary care unit or emergency department) may be defibrillated quickly by nursing or medical staff without triggering a cardiac arrest call and may evade inclusion in any study. The survival to discharge after in-hospital, early onset (< 4 hours) VF following acute myocardial infarction (AMI) has been reported to be as high as 93% [30]. The inclusion of these patients in outcome studies of in-hospital cardiac arrest would increase overall survival figures.

Preventing in-hospital cardiac arrest

The survival to discharge after in-hospital cardiac arrest from non-VF/VT rhythms is generally poor; 16% in the Swedish study and 6.2% in the UK study. This may reflect the late diagnosis of cardiac arrest with a delay in CPR or, more likely, it reflects the impact of significant non-cardiac co-morbidity [31]. In many cases it may have been inappropriate to attempt CPR. Fifty to eighty percent of patients have clear signs of clinical deterioration before in-hospital cardiac arrest [32, 33]. Identification of those patients at risk of cardiac arrest will allow intervention by a medical emergency team (MET) [34], or patient-at-risk team (PART) [35]. Early advice and active management should improve the patient's medical condition and/or may prompt a do not resuscitate (DNR) order [36]. These actions may reduce the incidence of in-hospital cardiac arrest and should reduce the number of inappropriate resuscitation attempts.

Duration of hospital stay after cardiac arrest

The duration of hospital stay, particularly the number of days spent in intensive care, will contribute greatly to the costs associated with CPR. Unfortunately, these data are reported only rarely. A study of CPR in a 576-bed community hospital in Virginia in 1989-1990 reported a mean length of stay after in-hospital cardiac arrest for initial survivors who died before discharge of 9.9 ± 2.6 days [37]. For those surviving to discharge the length of stay was 20.3 ± 3.3 days. Over half of the intensive care units (ICUs) in the UK send data on all ICU admissions to the Intensive Care National Audit & Research Centre (ICNARC) in London. In the UK, most patients (other than those with very short arrest times) surviving in- or out-of-hospital cardiac arrest will be admitted to an intensive care unit. In 1999 ICNARC reported on 1595 patients who had been admitted to ICU following a period of CPR and who had received mechanical ventilation in the first 24 hours in the unit [Data Analyses from the ICNARC Case Mix Programme Database, Issue 3 September 1999, Kathy Rowan]. The hospital mortality rate for these patients was 71.6%. The median length of stay in the ICU was 2 days (interquartile range 1-5 days) and the median length of hospital stay was 7 days (interquartile range 2-18) days. These data are likely to represent the worst case scenario after cardiac arrest, as those with very short arrest times would not be admitted to an ICU.

Prognostication after cardiac arrest

Minimising the duration of ICU stay should reduce costs associated with CPR. An accurate predictor of long term outcome for the patients admitted to the ICU comatose after cardiac arrest would be invaluable. This would allow the withdrawal of intensive care in those patients with no chance of survival to a quality of life that would be acceptable to them. In a metaanalysis of predictors of poor outcome in anoxic-ischaemic coma, the absence of pupillary light reflexes on day 3 and an absent motor response to pain on day 3 are both independently predictive of a poor outcome (death and vegetative state) with 100% specificity [38].

Quality of life for survivors of cardiac arrest

One of the factors that must be taken into consideration when undertaking a cost effectiveness analysis of CPR is the quality of life of the survivors. If quality of life in those patients surviving cardiac arrest is poor, then CPR may not be economically attractive. Investigators in Ontario, Canada, have studied the quality of life amongst 86 survivors of cardiac arrest (35 out-of-hospital arrest and 51 in-hospital arrest) at least 6 months after discharge from hospital [39]. Quality of life was assessed with the Health Utilities Index Mark 3, which describes functional ability on a scale from perfect health (equal to 1.0) to death (equal to 0). It assesses vision, hearing, speech, mobility, dexterity, emotion, cognition and pain. Most patients had no impairment or mild impairment in each of these attributes. The mean utility of the survivors interviewed at least six months after discharge was 0.72 (SD ± 0.22). Five (6%) had a utility score of 1.0; and 28 (33%) had a score of at least 0.9. The survivors of out-of-hospital cardiac arrest had a higher utility than those surviving in-hospital cardiac arrest (0.78 versus 0.69), but this difference was not statistically significant ($p = 0.07$).

Cost-effectiveness analysis

The evaluation of health care interventions involves five steps [40]:

1. demonstration of efficacy;
2. assessment of effectiveness;
3. efficiency or cost-effectiveness;
4. availability - matching the supply of services to locations where they are accessible to persons who require them;
5. distribution - an examination of who gains and who loses by choosing to allocate resources to one health care program instead of another.

Units of clinical outcome can be measured as life-years extended, termed "cost-effectiveness ratios". If the utility or quality of life is included, the analysis estimates "cost-utility ratios". By asking persons how much they would be willing to pay to receive a given health benefit it is possible to calculate a "cost-benefit ratio".

When undertaking a cost-utility study, the unit of measurement for the clinical outcome is usually quality-adjusted life years (QALYs). These take into account both the life expectancy and the quality of life after an intervention. Thus a life expectancy of 5 years with a utility of 0.7 gives 3.5 QALYs. Cost-utility ratios can be used to set health care priorities, but their use in this way may be limited by non-comparability of methods, inappropriate comparators, and non-generalisability of results [41]. Some analysts have suggested setting a threshold value for the cost per QALY that represents the willingness of society to pay for additional QALYs [42].

Cost-effectiveness of CPR

Cost-effectiveness analysis of a health care intervention requires a comparison of that intervention with alternative methods of dealing with the patient. The options for managing a cardiac arrest may appear limited to instituting CPR versus not attempting CPR. However, the different interventions that make up a resuscitation attempt will have a variable impact on outcome and can be subjected to separate cost-analyses. Determining the cost-effectiveness of CPR is extremely complex and requires different approaches for in-hospital CPR and out-of-hospital CPR [43]. Of the two settings, the costs associated with in-hospital are easier to define.

Cost-effectiveness of in-hospital CPR

An in depth cost analysis associated with in-hospital cardiac arrests in a 576-bed community hospital was undertaken over a 21-month period in 1989-90 [37]. There were 432 resuscitation attempts on 336 adults and 39 (11.6%) survived to hospital discharge. The total cost was approximately $60,000 per survivor or $7,000 per resuscitation attempt, and $2,352,771 for the whole CPR program over 21 months. This calculation included the following components:

Mean length of stay @ $957 per day:
- died before discharge = 9.9 days
- survived to discharge = 20.3 days

Average "crash cart" consumables = $75

Mean resuscitation time = 25 minutes

Average resuscitation team:
- 4.1 house staff
- 4.5 nursing staff
- 2.0 respiratory therapists
- 0.9 CRNAs
- 1.0 chaplain

Mean cost of personnel attending arrest = $96.50 per arrest

Cost of life support courses for personnel over 21 months = $307,000

Cost of resuscitation committee meetings

Vrtis pointed out, rather astutely, that it might be more cost-effective to focus training on prevention of in-hospital cardiac arrest ("Avoid-a-Code" programs) [37]. This advice is now being realised in the form of METs and PARTs. However, as yet no studies have assessed the cost-effectiveness of strategies to prevent in-hospital cardiac arrest [43].

Ebell estimated the cost of CPR after in-hospital cardiac arrest using a model that describes the CPR process as a series of decision points [44]. This model did not include the costs of initiating and maintaining a CPR program but did include the costs of nursing dependent patients after hospital discharge. The median survival following hospital discharge was estimated to be 3 years and a utility figure of 0.60 was applied. The estimated cost per patient surviving to discharge was $117,000 for a rate of survival to discharge of 10%. On this basis, the cost per QALY was $65,000 (adjusted to 1991 dollars). In comparison, the adjusted cost per QALY for coronary artery bypass surgery in patients with single vessel disease and moderate angina was $64,000. An attempt has been made to update these figures; estimates of the cost-effectiveness of CPR programs for all 6-month survivors from the Brain Resuscitation Clinical Trial study group were $406,000 per life saved and 225,000 per QALY [43].

Cost-effectiveness of out-of-hospital CPR

Cost-analyses of out-of-hospital CPR are limited by the fact that the EMS have a number of roles and it is very difficult to quantify the proportion of their time devoted to treating patients in cardiac arrest. Nonetheless, such analyses are important since the only medical problem for which prehospital intervention has been demonstrated to save lives is in resuscitation from cardiac arrest [45]. It may be more helpful to consider the incremental cost-effectiveness of modifications to the EMS. Nichol and colleagues have undertaken an extensive cost-effectiveness analysis of potential improvements to EMS systems based on outcome data from 41 series of out-of-hospital cardiac arrest [46]. Costs for the various aspects of the EMS systems were derived from Ontario. The fixed costs associated with a one-tier EMS system (operating a universal emergency telephone number, ambulance communication centre, ambulance bases) were common to all EMS systems so they had no effect on the incremental cost-effectiveness ratios. The variable costs of vehicles, equipment, wages, benefits, and education were converted to a cost per unit hour. One-tier systems were costed as ALS providers on ambulances. For the two-tier EMS systems, the initial component was costed as BLS-D fire fighters on pump vehicles. Thirteen percent of the firefighters' wages were allocated to the provision of emergency cardiac care. Hospital costs were derived from 42 patients admitted after out-of-hospital cardiac arrest in Ottawa. Estimates were made for the cost of training 1000 people (0.23% of the population of Hamilton). The costs of EMS components were estimated as:

– ALS providers	$75.60 per hour
– BLS-D providers, pump vehicles	$19.26 per hour
– BLS-D providers, ambulances	$66.51 per hour
– Fixed costs of first tier in two tier EMS	$651,129
– Costs of training 1000 to provide bystander CPR	$29,855
– Cost of hospitalisation, patient discharged alive	$21,745
– Cost of hospitalisation, patient died	$5,428

Expected survival after discharge from hospital alive was estimated to be 5.61 years and the mean utility was estimated at 0.84 (higher than the figure derived by the same authors in a later study). It was calculated that the addition of 40,000 more unit hours would improve the mean response time by 48 seconds. The incremental cost-effectiveness ratio of the options for making this change are given in Table 4. The two most cost effective options both involved increasing the use of BLS-D providers in pump vehicles. This theory was put into clinical practice in the OPALS study [15]. The addition of BLS-D firefighters to an existing BLS-D ambulance system contributed to a reduction in the defibrillator response time. The proportion of cases in which the interval between the call and arrival of the vehicle equipped with a defibrillator was 8 minutes or less improved from 76.7% to 92.5%; the survival to hospital discharge improved from 3.9% to 5.2% ($p = 0.03$). The costs were estimated to be $46,900 per life saved for establishing the rapid defibrillation program and $2,400 per life saved annually for maintaining the program. This study has highlighted the importance of optimising defibrillation response intervals and has shown that the use of professional first responder schemes is highly cost-effective.

Table 4. Incremental cost-effectiveness ratios of improvements in response to out-of-hospital cardiac arrest (adapted from Nichol G, Laupacis A, Stiell IG, O'Rourke K, Anis A, Bolley H, Detsky AS (1996). Cost-effectiveness analysis of potential improvements to the emergency medical services for victims of out-of-hospital cardiac arrest. Ann Emerg Med 27:711-720)

Parameters	**Cost per QALY (US 1993 Dollars/QALY)**
Improvement in response time in a one-tier EMS system by the addition of more EMS providers in ambulances	368,000
Improvement in response time in a two-tier EMS system by the addition of more BLS/BLS-D providers in pump vehicles to the first tier	53,000
Improvement in response time in a two-tier EMS system by the addition of more BLS/BLS-D providers in ambulances to the first tier	159,000
Change from a one-tier to a two-tier EMS system by the addition of BLS/BLS-D providers in pump vehicles as the first tier	40,000
Change from a one-tier to a two-tier EMS system by the addition of BLS/BLS-D providers in ambulances as the first tier	94,000

Cost-effectiveness of public access defibrillation

An extension of the OPALS study is to reduce time to defibrillation by using non-traditional responders (police or lay people) with AEDs. The cost-effectiveness of PAD has been estimated although, with one or two exceptions, there are insufficient outcome data from these programs to allow robust conclusions. Assuming a baseline survival to discharge rate of 8%, a standard EMS system had a median cost of $5900 per cardiac arrest patient [47]. In this model, implementation of PAD by lay responders was associated with a median incremental survival of 0.7% and a cost of $44,000 per additional QALY. In the same model, implementation of PAD by police was associated with a median cost of $27,200 per additional QALY. When only the immediate costs of defibrillation by police were considered (i.e., excluding hospital costs etc.), implementation of PAD was associated with a median cost of $6500 per additional QALY. The net cost of a police defibrillation program has been estimated to be $223 per cardiac arrest [47].

The costs associated with the introduction of the PAD program at Chicago Airport System can be estimated with some accuracy (Becker L, personal communication). Forty-two AEDs were installed at a unit cost of $3000. Assuming they last 4 years, this represents a total of $32,000 per year. Two thousand targeted responders were trained at a cost of $50 each, representing $100,000. They will need to be re-trained every 2 years, giving an annual cost of $50,000. The AEDs were hard-wired into the airport security system at a cost of $100,000; this is estimated to last 10 years so that the cost per year is $10,000. Thus, the total cost in the first year is $142,000. Nine lives have been saved in the first 10 months. This represents a cost of $13,100 per life saved in the first year and $8,500 per life saved in subsequent years. This system is likely to represent the ideal PAD program; nonetheless these cost-effectiveness data are impressive. In reality, it is likely that most PAD programs will be driven by liability insurance issues rather than by cost-effectiveness.

Conclusion

The cost-effectiveness of CPR is linked inextricably with the survival rate. After out-of-hospital cardiac arrest, the median survival rate to hospital discharge is 6.4%. A 5% increase in bystander CPR has less impact on survival than a 1-minute decrease in the defibrillation response time interval. Survival to hospital discharge after in-hospital cardiac arrest is approximately 15%. The cost of in-hospital CPR is $60-100,000 per survivor (1990 figures). The baseline costs for out-of-hospital CPR are difficult to quantify but the most cost-effective incremental enhancement is to reduce the defibrillator response time using BLS-D personnel.

References

1. Myerburg RJ, Kessler KM, Castellanos A (1993) Sudden cardiac death: Epidemiology, transient risk and interventional assessment. Ann Intern Med 119:1187-1197
2. Ebell MH, Kruse JA (1994) A proposed model for the cost of cardiopulmonary resuscitation. Med Care 32:640-649
3. Cummins RO, Chamberlain DA (1991) Recommended guidelines for uniform reporting of data from out-of-hospital cardiac arrest: The Utstein Style. Circulation 84:960-975
4. Nichol G, Stiell IG, Laupacis A et al (1999) A cumulative meta-analysis of the effectiveness of defibrillator-capable emergency medical services for victims of out-of-hospital cardiac arrest. Ann Emerg Med 34:517-525
5. Becker LB, Smith DW, Rhodes KV (1993) Incidence of cardiac arrest: A neglected factor in evaluating survival rates. Ann Emerg Med 22:86-91
6. Kette F, Sbrojavacca R, Rellini G et al (1998) Epidemiology and survival rate of out-of-hospital cardiac arrest in north-east Italy. The FACS study. Resuscitation 36:153-159
7. Weston CFM, Jones SD, Wilson RJ (1997) Outcome of out-of-hospital cardiorespiratory arrest in South Glamorgan. Resuscitation 34:227-233
8. Lombardi G, Gallagher J, Gennis P (1994) Outcome of out-of-hospital cardiac arrest in New York City. The pre-hospital arrest survival evaluation (PHASE) study. JAMA 271:678-683
9. Nolan JP, Smith G, Evans R et al (1998) The United Kingdom prehospital study of active compression-decompression resuscitation (ACD-CPR). Resuscitation 37:119-125
10. Nichol G, Detsky AS, Stiell IG et al (1996) Effectiveness of emergency medical services for victims of out-of-hospital cardiac arrest: A metaanalysis. Ann Emerg Med 27:700-710
11. Callaham M, Madsen CD (1996) Relationship of timeliness of paramedic advanced life support interventions to outcome in out-of-hospital cardiac arrest treated by first responders with defibrillators. Ann Emerg Med 27:638-648
12. Guly UM, Mitchell RG, Cook R et al (1995) Paramedics and technicians are equally successful at managing cardiac arrest outside hospital. BMJ 310:1091-1094
13. Mitchell RG, Guly UM, Rainer TH, Robertson CE (2000) Paramedic activities, drug administration and survival from out-of-hospital cardiac arrest. Resuscitation 43:95-100
14. Eisenberg MS, Horwood BT, Cummins RO et al (1990) Cardiac arrest and resuscitation: A tale of 29 cities. Ann Emerg Med 19:179-186
15. Steill IG, Wells GA, Field BJ et al (1999) Improved out-of-hospital cardiac arrest survival through the inexpensive optimisation of an existing defibrillation program. JAMA 281:1175-1181
16. Wassertheil J, Keane G, Fisher N, Leditschke JF (2000) Cardiac arrest outcomes at the Melbourne Cricket Ground and Shrine of Remembrance using a tiered response strategy - a forerunner to public access defibrillation. Resuscitation 44:97-104
17. Nichol G, Hallstrom AP, Kerber R et al (1998) American Heart Association Report on the Second Public access Defibrillation Conference, April 17-19, 1997. Circulation 97:1309-1314
18. Caffrey S (2000) Chicago HeartSave Program. Resuscitation 45:S26
19. Gallagher EJ, Lombardi G, Gennis P (1995) Effectiveness of bystander cardiopulmonary resuscitation and survival following out-of-hospital cardiac arrest. JAMA 274:1922-1925
20. Grubb NR, Elton RA, Fox KAA (1995) In-hospital mortality after out-of-hospital cardiac arrest. Lancet 346:417-421
21. Cobbe SM, Dalziel K, Ford I, Marsden AK (1996) Survival of 1476 patients initially resuscitated from out of hospital cardiac arrest. BMJ 312:1633-1637
22. Tunstall-Pedoe H, Bailey L, Chamberlain DA et al (1992) Survey of 3765 cardiopulmonary resuscitations in British hospitals (the BRESUS study): Methods and overall results. BMJ 304:1347-1351
23. Bedell SE, Delbanco TL, Cook EF, Epstein FH (1983) Survival after cardiopulmonary resuscitation in the hospital. N Engl J Med 309:569-576

24. Rozenbaum EA, Shenkman L (1988) Predicting outcome of in-hospital cardiopulmonary resuscitation. Crit Care Med 16:583-586
25. Hendrick JM, Pijls NH, van der Werf T, Crul JF (1990) Cardiopulmonary resuscitation on the general ward: No category of patients should be excluded in advance. Resuscitation 20: 163-171
26. Schneider AP 2nd, Nelson DJ, Brown DD (1993) In-hospital cardiopulmonary resuscitation: A 30-year review. J Am Board Fam Pract 6:91-101
27. George AL Jr, Folk BP 3rd, Crecelius PL, Campbell WB (1989) Pre-arrest morbidity and other correlates of survival after in-hospital cardiopulmonary arrest. Am J Med 87:28-34
28. Gwinnutt CL, Columb M, Harris R (2000) Outcome after cardiac arrest in UK hospital: Effect of the 1997 guidelines. Resuscitation (in press)
29. Andréasson A, Herlitz J, Bång A et al (1998) Characteristics and outcome among patients with a suspected in-hospital cardiac arrest. Resuscitation 39:23-31
30. Volpi A, Cavalli A, Santoro L, Negri E (1998) Incidence and prognosis of early primary ventricular fibrillation in acute myocardial infarction - results of the Gruppo Italiano per lo Studio della Sopravvivenza nell'Infarto Miocardico (GISSI-2) database. Am J Cardiol 82: 265-271
31. De Vos R, Koster RW, Haan RJ et al (1999) In-hospital cardiopulmonary resuscitation. Arch Intern Med 159:845-850
32. Smith AF, Wood J (1998) Can some in-hospital cardio-respiratory arrest be prevented? A prospective survey. Resuscitation 37:133-137
33. Schein RMH, Hazday N, Pena M et al (1990) Clinical antecedents to in-hospital cardiopulmonary arrest. Chest 98:1388-1392
34. Lee A, Bishop G, Hillman KM (1995) The Medical Emergency Team. Anaesth Int Care 23:183-186
35. Goldhill DR, Worthington L, Mulcahy A et al (1999) The patient-at-risk team: Identifying and managing seriously ill ward patients. Anaesthesia 54:853-860
36. Lawler PG (1999) The do-not-attempt-resuscitation order: A lever to improve outcome and deliver preventative care. Anaesthesia 54:923-925
37. Vrtis MC (1992) Cost/benefit analysis of cardiopulmonary resuscitation: A comprehensive study - Part II. Nursing Management 23(5):44-51
38. Zandbergen EGJ, de Hann RJ, Soutenbeek CP et al (1998) Systematic review of early prediction of poor outcome in anoxic-ischaemic coma. Lancet 352:1808-1812
39. Nichol G, Stiell IG, Hebert P et al (1999) What is the quality of life for survivors of cardiac arrest? A prospective study. Academic Emergency Medicine 6:95-102
40. Detsky AS, Naglie G (1990) A clinician's guide to cost-effectiveness analysis. Ann Intern Med 113:147-154
41. Mason J, Drummond M, Torrance G (1993) Some guidelines on the use of cost-effectiveness league tables. BMJ 306:570-572
42. Briggs A, Gray A (2000) Using cost effectiveness information. BMJ 320:246
43. Lee KH, Angus DC, Abramson NS (1996) Cardiopulmonary resuscitation: What cost to cheat death? Crit Care Med 24:2046-2052
44. Ebell MH, Kruse JA (1994) A proposed model for the cost of cardiopulmonary resuscitation. Med Care 32:640-649
45. Valenzuela TD, Criss EA, Spaite D et al (1990) Cost-effectiveness analysis of paramedic emergency medical services in the treatment of prehospital cardiopulmonary arrest. Ann Emerg Med 19:1407-1411
46. Nichol G, Laupacis A, Stiell IG et al (1996) Cost-effectiveness analysis of potential improvements to the emergency medical services for victims of out-of-hospital cardiac arrest. Ann Emerg Med 27:711-720
47. Nichol G, Hallstrom AP, Ornato JP et al (1998) Potential cost-effectiveness of public access defibrillation in the United States. Circulation 97:1315-1320

NEUROLOGY

Epidemiology of Epilepsy

G. Savettieri, P. Ragonese, G. Salemi

The term epilepsy identifies a group of disorders characterized by the recurrence of two or more epileptic seizures, unprovoked by any immediate identified cause [1]. An epileptic seizure is the clinical manifestation due to an abnormal and excessive discharge of a set of neurons in the brain [1]. The clinical manifestations consist of sudden and transitory abnormal phenomena, which may include alterations of consciousness, motor, sensory, autonomic, or psychic events perceived by the patient or an observer [1]. A seizure can be of partial or generalized onset, according to its clinical manifestation, and provoked or unprovoked, according to the temporal proximity to a precipitating event.

Despite the ancient identification of epilepsy, demonstrated by the pamphlet "Morbus saucer" written in 400 BC, and attributed to Hippocrates [2], and in spite of the high number of epidemiological studies on the disease [3, 4], the epidemiological data available are only partially comparable. The polymorphism of clinical epileptic manifestations and the use of different classifications or different case-finding strategies are among the main reasons for this difficulty. Moreover, different and changing degrees of disease denial, arising from religious belief and impinging upon educational, vocational, and marital opportunities, might justify differences in the ascertainment of cases among various countries, and among different time periods in the same country [5].

Descriptive epidemiology

Both incidence and prevalence studies indicate that epilepsy is one of the most-frequent neurological disorders [3, 4]. Incidence cohorts are preferred to prevalence cohorts because the potential loss of patient subgroups with a poor prognosis is avoided, and because incidence cohorts are useful for etiological studies. However, some pitfalls of incidence studies on epilepsy must be considered. Some studies on the incidence of epilepsy include patients who experienced an isolated unprovoked seizure. This could explain different frequencies observed in different studies. Moreover, incidence studies have been performed mainly in Western countries; consequently, a less-exhaustive pattern of epilepsy worldwide is achievable from incidence than prevalence studies. Studies performed in

Europe and in North America report annual incidence values varying from 24 to 53 per 100,000 person-years (Table 1). Comparable values are reported in some Asian countries, while slightly higher incidence values were found in some rural Ethiopian villages [6], and much higher incidence values in South America (113 new epileptics per year in Chile and 122 new epileptics per year in Ecuador) [4]. Such distribution is similar to that observed in prevalence studies. Age-specific incidence ratios indicate that epilepsy is a disease with onset at the extreme ages of life; gender-specific incidence ratios reveal that males have a high risk than females.

Table 1. Incidence ratios (cases/100,000 person-years) of epilepsy and first seizures

Population source	Incidence	Sex (M:F)
A. *Epilepsy*		
Rochester, USA, 1935-1967 [3]	48.7	1.1
Rochester, USA, 1935-1984 [7]	44	1.2
Rochester, USA, 1980-1984 [10]	52.3	1.1
Houston, Texas, USA, 1988-1994 [12]	35.5	NA
Andean region, Ecuador, 1986-1987 [4]	122	0.8
El Salvador, Chile, 1984-1988 [4]	113	1.2
Northern Norway, 1983-1984 [3]	33	NA
Faroes, Denmark, 1983-1985 [8]	42	NA
Copparo, Italy, 1964-1978 [9]	33.1	1.4
Carlisle, England, 195-1961 [3]	30.3	NA
Kent, England, 1.1.93-31.12.93 [13]	23	NA
Gironde, France [11]	24.5	NA
Rural South India, 1.4.90-31.3.91 [3]	49.3	NA
Six cities, China, 1982 [4]	35	1.7
Meskan and Mareko district, Ethiopia, 1990 [6]	64	1.3
Rural Iceland, 1995 [14]	47	NA
B. *First unprovoked seizure and epilepsy*		
Rochester, USA, 1935-1984 [7]	61	1.2
Martinique, 1.5.1994-30.4.1995 [15]	64.1	NA
Houston, Texas, USA 1988-1994 [12]	50.9	NA
Geneva, Switzerland, 1.6.90-31.5.91 [16]	45.6	1.6
Kent, England, 1.1.93-31.12.93 [13]	40	NA
Gironde, France [11]	42	NA

A small number of studies addressed the distribution of epilepsy per seizure type. Both in Rochester, USA (seizure description alone) [7] and in the Faroes (seizure description and electroencephalographic findings) [8] more than 50% of incident cases were classified as partial seizures. This contrasts with the finding of Granieri et al. [9], in Copparo, Italy. In this study, based on seizure description alone, only 32% of cases were considered partial. The incidence of epileptic syndromes is emphasized by clinicians, but the epidemiological approach is arduous. Two studies performed in Western countries addressed this issue, reporting comparable results (Table 2).

Table 2. Incidence ratios (cases/100,000 person-years) of epileptic syndromes

Epileptic syndrome	**Gironde** [11]	**Rochester** [10]
Localization-related epilepsies		34.9
– Idiopathic	1.7	0.2
– Symptomatic	13.6	17.2
– Cryptogenetic		17.5
Generalized epilepsies and syndromes		7.7
– Idiopathic	5.6	3.7
– Symptomatic	1.1	2.3
– Cryptogenetic		1.7
Epilepsies undetermined	1.9	9.7

Prevalence studies provide information regarding current burden of illness, and their primary use is for health planning. As measures of prevalence, studies on epilepsy generally report lifetime and active prevalence ratios. "Active" prevalence is defined as the number of individuals in the population who have had a recent seizure or who have been recently prescribed antiepileptic medication. A different span of years used to determine active epilepsy could yield incomparable prevalence ratios. Another source of bias is the use of case-ascertainment protocols that have shown a different accuracy. Bearing in mind these limitations, abundant information is available on the prevalence of epilepsy across countries (Table 3).

The reported prevalence of active epilepsy, measured as the rate per 1,000 population, varies widely from 2.5 to more than 40. In Western countries the prevalence ranges from 4 to 8 per 1,000 population [3, 4, 8, 9, 21, 22]. Comparable values have been observed in Asian countries, irrespective of the urban or rural origin of the investigated population [4, 25]. Higher prevalence ratios, ranging from 8 to 57 per 1,000 population, have been reported in Central and South America [17-20] and in Africa [23, 24]. Endemic conditions of *Taenia solium taeniasis* in Central and South America and by various parasites in Central Africa have been attributed as responsible for these higher frequencies of epilepsy [17]. However, the possibility that these high values may reflect different methods of investigation cannot be excluded. Most of these studies were performed using a protocol formulated by the World Health Organization whose case-verification methodology is not stringent. A study performed in Ecuador using a more-accurate protocol found a prevalence of 8 cases per 1,000 population [18].

Table 3. Prevalence ratios (cases/1,000 population) of active or lifetime epilepsy in population-based surveys

Population source	Prevalence	Year	Case ascertainment	Definition of epilepsy	Definition of active (year)	Sex (M:F)	Gen-partial (%)
Rochester, USA, UP [4]	5.4	1935-1967	RLS	RAS	5	1	40-60
Copiah County, USA, UP [4]	6.8	1.1.78	DD, ME, WHO modified	RAS	3	1.5	75-25
A rural village, Mexico, RP [17]	8	1988	DD, ME	RAS	5	NA	NA
Bocas del Toro, Panama, RP [17]	57	1988	DD, ME	RAS	2	NA	64-31
Bogotà, Colombia, UP [17] *	19.5	1975	DD, ME	RAS	NAP	NAV	73-27
Ecuador, RP [17]	17.1	1983	DD, ME, WHO	RAS	2	NAV	67-30
Andean region, Ecuador, RP [18]	8	10.3.87	DD, ME, ICBERG	RAS	1	0.7	52-46
Paluguillo, Ecuador, RP [19]	22.6	1994	DD, ME	RAS	25	NA	NA
Cordillera Province, Bolivia, RP [20]	11.1	1.11.94	DD, ME, WHO modified	RAS	5	0.9	47-53
El Salvador, Chile, U-RP [17]	17.7	30.6.88	RR	RAS	5	1	41-63
Faroes, N = [8] *	7.6	1983-1985	RR	RAS	NAP	NA	45-55
Iceland [4]	3.4	31.12.64	RR	RAS	1	1.2	60-40
Carlisle, England [3] *	5.5	1966	RR	RAS	NAP	NA	NA
Rural Iceland, RP [21]	4.8	31.12.93	RR	RAS	1	1.2	63-35
Copparo, Italy, RP [9]	6.2	31.12.78	RR	RAS	5	1.4	68-32
Vecchiano, Italy, RP [4]	5.1	1985	RR, DC	RAS	5	1.2	35-65
Riposto, Italy, RP [22]	2.7	1.11.87	DD, ME, WHO modified	RAS	5	0.9	78-22
Nigeria, 1935-1979, N = RP [23]	37	1985	DD, ME, WHO	RAS	5	NA	NA
Igbo-Ora, Nigeria, UP [24]	5.3	15.2.82	DD, ME, WHO	RAS	5	0.9	26-55
Daisen Town, Japan, UP [25] *	4.4	1.10.91	MQ, ME	RAS	NAP	NAV	NAV
Bombay, India, UP [4]	3.6	1.3.85	DD, ME, WHO	RAS	5	2.3	45-55
Kashmir, India, RP [4]	2.5	1986	DD, ME, WHO	RAS	5	1.4	79-11
Six cities, China, UP [4] *	4.4	1.1.83	DD, ME, WHO	RAS	NAP	1.3	81-19
Silivri, Turkey, UP [26]	10.2	1.10.94	DD, ME, WHO	RAS	5	1	41-53
Ankara, Turkey, UP [27]	4.5	1.2.87	DD, ME, ICBERG	RAS	5	NA	65-35
Elmadag and Kutludugun, Turkey, RP [27]	8.8	1.2.87	DD, ME, ICBERG	RAS	5	NA	80-20
Karachi, Pakistan, UP [27]	7.4	1.2.87	DD, ME, ICBERG	RAS	5	NA	
Mirpur Sakro, Pakistan, RP [27]	14.8	1.2.87	DD, ME, ICBERG	RAS	5	NA	

* Lifetime prevalence (*UP* urban population, *RP* rural population, *RLS* record-linkage system, *DD* door-to-door, *MQ* mail questionnaire, *ME* medical examination, *RR* record review, *DC* drug consumption, *WHO* World Health Organization protocol, *ICBERG* International Community-Based Epilepsy Research protocol, *RAS* recurrent afebrile seizures, *NAP* not applicable, *NAV* not available)

Higher prevalence values have been observed in rural areas in comparison with urban areas in Ecuador [18], Nigeria [23, 24], Turkey [27], and Pakistan [27]. These findings could support a role of endemic parasite infections for epilepsy in rural areas of less-developed populations. Age-specific prevalence increases from childhood to adulthood, and remains stable or increases slightly in the elderly. Most studies report a higher prevalence in men compared to women. Different from incidence, the frequency of seizure type is less definite: some studies report that the majority of patients have partial seizures, other studies show an opposite pattern. This discrepancy seems mainly to depend on methodology reasons.

Prognosis of epilepsy is at present excellent for most people, in terms of expected seizure control, remission, and medication withdrawal. The most-consistent and powerful risk factor for seizure recurrence is a history of an antecedent brain insult. Seizure type, abnormal electroencephalogram (EEG), history of epilepsy in the sibling, prior acute seizure, including febrile seizures, the occurrence of status epilepticus, or the presence of a Todd's paralysis after a seizure are also associated with an increased likelihood of having a second seizure [28]. Most individuals with epilepsy (70 - 80%) will ultimately become seizurefree and most can expect to discontinue antiepileptic medication [29].

Many papers indicate that mortality is increased in patients with epilepsy [3, 30]. The excess risk is greater in men than in women, irrespective of age, and is greater in individuals with remote-symptomatic epilepsy. In younger age groups, the excess mortality is associated with mental retardation, cerebral palsy, or congenital malformations of the brain. In older age groups, brain tumor and cerebrovascular diseases are the underlying pathological conditions. Thus, the excess mortality is in all likelihood related to the underlying cause of the epilepsy, rather than to the epilepsy per se. However, when the analysis is limited to cases of idiopathic epilepsy, an increased risk of mortality is also evident. However, if the analysis is restricted to those with idiopathic epilepsy with onset under 20 years of age, no increased risk is found. Mortality is higher in generalized tonic-clonic and myoclonic seizures. Higher seizure frequency is associated with increased mortality [31]. Among the specific causes of death, patients with epilepsy may commit suicide more frequently than controls [32]. Another important cause of death is sudden unexplained death in epilepsy (SUDEP). SUDEP probably depends on the presence of a heart disease [33], and is associated with a higher number of seizures per year, with earlyonset epilepsy, and with treatment with several antiepileptic drugs [34]. *Status epilecticus* (SE) is another cause of death in epileptics. SE is a pathological condition characterized by repeated and/or prolonged epileptic seizures. It is a medical emergency that requires prompt and appropriate therapy. Any type of epileptic seizure can develop into SE, but the syndrome most commonly associated with SE is the convulsive generalized form. The incidence of first SE is 20 per 100,000 per year [35], while more than 40 patients per 100,000 population present an episode of SE per year [36]. Recurrence rate of SE is > 13% [37].

Mortality rates of SE are 15 - 20% in adults and 3 - 15% in children. Acute complications result from hyperthermia, pulmunary edema, cardiac arrhythmias, and cardiovascular failure [37].

Analytic epidemiology

Various factors, either individual or environmental, have been proposed as risk factors for epilepsy. The strength of association is high for some factors, lower and less definite for others [3]. Table 4 lists most of the proposed risk factors.

History of head trauma is clearly associated with the development of epilepsy. The severity of consciousness alteration, the presence of early onset seizures, single brain computed tomographic lesion, and the development of an EEG focus 1 month after the trauma are associated with the development of epilepsy [38, 39]. Among central nervous system infections, viral encephalitis is more strongly associated with epilepsy than bacterial meningitis [3]. Cysticercosis infection is associated with epilepsy in South America [17].

Table 4. Risk factors for epilepsy

Factors associated with an evident brain lesion
Directly associated
Certain risk factor
Severe craniocerebral trauma
Cerebrovascular disease
Infections
Brain tumors
Degenerative disease of CNS *
Autoimmune disease of CNS *
Probable risk factor
Prenatal events
Perinatal events
Vaccine exposure
Independent outcomes of a common antecedent event
Febrile seizure
Mental retardation
Cerebral palsy
Factors not associated with an evident brain lesion
Familiarity
Sex
Socioeconomic status
Hypertension
Depressive illness
Alcohol consumption
Recreational drug abuse

* *CNS* central nervous system

Heavy drinkers not only have an increased risk for seizures with abrupt reduction or discontinuation of alcohol ingestion (withdrawal seizures), they also have a threefoldincreased risk for epilepsy [3]. Familial aggregation of epilepsy is consistent with a genetic tendency for epilepsy [3].

Febrile convulsions (FC) are associated with an increased risk for epilepsy. Generally, FC and epilepsy should be considered as independent outcomes of a common antecedent [3]. Pre-existing cerebral palsy or mental retardation, atypical features of the FC, high recurrence of FC, duration of febrile seizure for 10 min or more, predisposition for FC or epilepsy, and abnormalities on EEG are the major risk factors for epilepsy. When the type of epilepsy is assessed (e.g., generalized versus partial onset), different predictors emerge. Genetic factors are the major predictors of increased risk for generalized-onset epilepsy after FC. Evidence of localized brain dysfunction at the time of the first febrile seizure exists for partial epilepsy following FC.

Conclusions

Some recent statements of the International League Against Epilepsy are useful to conclude this review on the epidemiology of epilepsy [40]. The use of a common definition of epilepsy and of comparable methodologies is to be encouraged. The number of prevalence studies is exhaustive. If further studies are envisaged, they should be directed at specific epileptic syndromes. In contrast, well-conducted incidence studies, particularly in the developing countries, are necessary. Prospective population-based outcome studies of people with specific epileptic syndromes, and mortality studies in developing countries, are to be encouraged. Finally, epilepsy-related mortality, such as SUDEP, should be clarified, with special attention to the identification of causes or risk factors.

References

1. Commission of Epidemiology and Prognosis (1993) Guidelines for epidemiological studies on epilepsy. Epilepsia 34:592-596
2. Ippocrate (1976) Male sacro. In: Opere. Utet, Turin, Italy
3. Hauser WA (1994) Epidemiology of epilepsy. In: Gorelick PB, Alter M (eds) Handbook of neuroepidemiology. Dekker, New York, pp 315-355
4. Sander JWAS, Shorvon SD (1996) Epidemiology of the epilepsies. J Neurol Neurosurg Psychiatry 61:433-443
5. Jilek-Aall L (1999) Morbus sacer in Africa: some religious aspects of epilepsy in traditional cultures. Epilepsia 40:382-386
6. Tekle-Haimanot R, Forsgren L, Ekstedt J (1997) Incidence of epilepsy in rural central Ethiopia. Epilepsia 38:541-546
7. Hauser WA, Annegers JF, Kurland LT (1993) The incidence of epilepsy and unprovoked seizures in Rochester, Minnesota 1935-84. Epilepsia 34:453-468

8. Joensen P (1986) Prevalence, incidence and classification of epilepsy in the Faroes. Acta Neurol Scand 74:150-155
9. Granieri E, Rosati G, Tola R et al (1983) A descriptive study of epilepsy in the district of Copparo, Italy 1964-78. Epilepsia 24:502-514
10. Zarrelli MM, Beghi E, Rocca WA, Hauser WA (1999) Incidence of epileptic syndromes in Rochester, Minnesota 1980-1984. Epilepsia 40:1708-1714
11. Loiseau J, Loiseau P, Guyot M et al (1990) Survey of seizure disorders in the French southwest. I. Incidence of epileptic syndromes. Epilepsia 31:391-396
12. Annegers JF, Dubinsky S, Coan SP et al (1999) The incidence of epilepsy and unprovoked seizures in multiethnic Urban Health Maintenance Organizations. Epilepsia 40:502-506
13. Cockerell OC, Goodridge DMG, Brodie D et al (1996) Neurological disease in a defined population: the result of a pilot study in two general practices. Neuroepidemiology 15:73-82
14. Olafsson E, Hauser WA, Ludvigsson P, Gudmundsson G (1996) Incidence of epilepsy in rural Iceland: a population-based study. Epilepsia 37:951-955
15. Jallon P, Smadja D, Cabre P et al (1999) EPIMART: prospective incidence study of epileptic seizures in newly referred patients in a French Carribean island (Martinique). Epilepsia 40:1103-1109
16. Jallon P, Goumaz M, Haenggeli C, Morabia A (1997) Incidence of first epileptic seizures in the canton of Geneva, Switzerland. Epilepsia 38:547-552
17. De Bittencourt PRM, Adamolekum B, Bharucha N et al (1996) Epilepsy in the tropics. I. Epidemiology, socioeconomic risk factors, and etiology. Epilepsia 37:1121-1127
18. Placencia M, Shorvon SD, Paredes V et al (1992) Epileptic seizures in an Andean region of Ecuador: incidence and prevalence and regional variation. Brain 115:771-782
19. Basch EM, Cruz ME, Tapia D, Cruz A (1997) Prevalence of epilepsy in a migrant population near Quito, Ecuador. Neuroepidemiology 16:94-98
20. Nicoletti A, Reggio A, Bartoloni A et al (1999) Prevalence of epilepsy in rural Bolivia. A door-to-door survey. Neurology 53:2064-2069
21. Olafsson E, Hauser WA (1999) Prevalence of epilepsy in rural Iceland: a population-based study. Epilepsia 40:1529-1534
22. Reggio A, Failla G, Patti F et al (1996) Prevalence of epilepsy. A door-to-door survey in the Sicilian community of Riposto. Ital J Neurol Sci 17:147-151
23. Osuntokun BO, Adeuja AOG, Nottidge VA et al (1987) Prevalence of the epilepsies in Nigerian Africans: a community-based study. Epilepsia 28:272-279
24. Osuntokun BO, Adeuja AOG, Nottidge VA et al (1982) Research protocol for measuring the prevalence of neurological disorders in developing countries. Results of a pilot study in Nigeria. Neuroepidemiology 1:143-153
25. Nakashima K, Yokoyama Y, Shimoyama R et al (1996) Prevalence of neurological disorders in a Japanese town. Neuroepidemiology 15:208-213
26. Karaagac N, Yeni SN, Senocak M et al (1999) Prevalence of epilepsy in Siliviri, a rural area of Turkey. Epilepsia 40:637-642
27. Aziz H, Guvener A, Akhtar SW, Hasan KZ (1997) Comparative epidemiology of epilepsy in Pakistan and Turkey: population-based studies using identical protocols. Epilepsia 38: 716-722
28. Berg AT, Shinnar S (1991) The risk of seizure recurrence following a first unprovoked seizure: a quantitative review. Neurology 41:965-972
29. Shafer SQ, Hauser WA, Annegers JF, Klass DW (1988) EEG and other early predictors of epilepsy remission: a community study. Epilepsia 29:590-600
30. Shackleton DP, Westendorp RGJ, Kastelejin-Nolst Trenité DGA, Vandenbroucke JP (1999) Mortality in patients with epilepsy: 40 years of follow-up in a Dutch cohort study. J Neurol Neurosurg Psychiatry 66:636-640
31. Sperling MR, Feldman H, Kinman J et al (1999) Seizure control and mortality in epilepsy. Ann Neurol 46:45-50
32. Barraclough BM (1987) The suicide rate in epilepsy. Acta Psychiatr Scand 76:339-345

33. Natelson BH, Suarez RV, Terrence CF, Turizo R (1998) Patients with epilepsy who die suddenly have cardiac disease. Arch Neurol 55:857-860
34. Nilsson L, Farahmand BY, Persson PG et al (1999) Risk factors for sudden unexpected death in epilepsy: a case-control study. Lancet 13:888-893
35. Hersdorffer DC, Logroscino G, Cascino G et al (1998) Incidence of status epilepticus in Rochester, Minnesota, 1965-1984. Neurology 50:735-741
36. Waterhouse EJ, Garnett LK, Towne AR et al (1999) Prospective population-based study of intermittent and continuous convulsive status epilepticus in Richmond, Virginia. Epilepsia 40:752-758
37. Fountain NB (2000) Status epilepticus: risk factors and complications. Epilepsia 2:S23-S30
38. Angeleri F, Majkowski J, Cacchiò G et al (1999) Posttraumatic epilepsy risk factors: one year prospective study after head injury. Epilepsia 40:1222-1230
39. Annegers JF, Hauser WA, Coan SP, Rocca WA (1998) A population-based study of seizures after traumatic injuries. N Engl J Med 1:20-24
40. ILAE Commission Report (1997) The epidemiology of the epilepsies: future directions. Epilepsia 38:614-618

COMPUTERING

Local Area Network Videoconferencing for Continuous Anesthesia Quality Improvement

V. LANZA, L. GUGLIELMO

Education, training, research, and quality improvement are essential components of a quality anesthetic department. A new reality is emerging as cost limits are set for healthcare, and healthcare quality is becoming a major concern to taxpayers and patients [1]. Anesthesiology departments and healthcare organizations able to implement continuous quality improvement and to deliver effective health care will be more successful in the marketplace [2]. To be effective, a continuous quality improvement (CQI) program must collect data about techniques that may be utilized to define performance, track and validate indicators thought intuitively to impact outcome, and recognize problems in treatment and practice management processes [3]. Improvement is assessed through follow-up monitoring. CQI is certainly an effective mechanism to add value to our practice.

A basic instrument to carry out a CQI plan is continuing professional development [4], i.e., the process by which health professionals constantly update their knowledge to meet the needs of patients, the health service, and their own professional growth.

Videoconferencing may become a remarkably useful tool to improve professionalism, as it can increase the number of people participating in internal updating meetings. One important fact to be considered is that such meetings are usually attended by no more than 30-40% of the staff. Common reasons for this are staff members' absence from the hospital (going off duty after night shifts, on vacation, etc.) and the fact that even those who are at the hospital are required to be physically present in premises away from the conference room, so that although their duties would allow them to attend the meeting, they cannot desert their assigned place [recovery room, intensive care unit (ICU), etc.]. Videoconferencing solves both problems: recorded meetings can be viewed by absent personnel at a later time, while by showing live events in other hospital premises through a net, all staff present at the time of the meetings are enabled to attend. Commonly used videoconferencing systems are costly and require complex management or connections to other facilities. In other words, they are intended for large hospitals or universities, whereas they could represent a very valuable means to promote personnel updating, and therefore quality improvement, in smaller facilities whose staff is usually left out of the vocational education circuit.

Below is a description of Internet videoconferencing techniques and results achieved through their use in the field of anesthesiology updating in the Buccheri La Ferla Fatebenefratelli Hospital (Palermo) within a CQI program.

Videoconferencing

Image and sound transmission has always played an important role in critical area medicine. Voice and video communications, however, have traditionally been a privilege of large organizations, due to the huge expenditure involved in the use of television equipment. The technologies now available, developed in connection with Internet use, allow the use of reasonably priced, PC-based image transmission methods. Computer-based videoconferencing has truly represented a leap forward in telemedicine, i.e., image and voice transmission enabling a resuscitator, for example, to support first aid procedures at great distance. Another especially interesting application is the technique known as "telecommuting", which allows participants to take over control of the computer with which the users are connected. Through the use of programs that enable "telecommuting" the user can operate programs located on the remote computer, as well as transmit and receive videos from that equipment [5]. Videoconferencing participants can therefore work simultaneously on the same document, making it unnecessary to transmit files.

Computer videoconferencing

The rate required to transmit quality films from one computer to another is approximately 200 kilobytes/s, in order for image definition and motion speed to be satisfactory – this makes it difficult to conceive that films may be transmitted via computers and telephone lines at considerably lower rates. Table 1 shows transmission rates attainable through normal telephone lines.

As the values in Table 1 clearly show, only by reducing frames or using compression techniques would it be possible to transmit images via telephone connection. Voice transmission also requires compression techniques – in fact, a few minutes' conversation recorded in the form of audio file (.wav) take up many megabytes of space. In general, therefore, video and audio compression techniques are generally used in videoconferencing.

Video compression

Video techniques use programs able to compress film size, based mainly on three parameters: number of frames per second, size of video, number of colors, in addition to using compression algorithms similar to those applied in file zipping.

Table 1. Transmissions rates attainable through usual telephone lines

Type of data	File length	28.8 KBPS Modem	ISDN - 128 KBPS	DSL - 384 KBPS	DSL - 1.5 MBPS
A 20-s video	8 Mb	37 min	8.5 min	2.75 min	43 s

KBPS kilobytes/s, *MBPS* megabytes/s

Frame number

For a film to produce a satisfactory impression of motion its speed should be around 15-20 frames per second. The speed of videoconferencing films transmitted via computer is usually between 3 and 10 frames per second, which explains the slow-motion effect we often notice while watching them.

Video size

The size of images shown on computer screens involves the transmission of a greater or smaller number of Pixels (light units on a computer screen). Screens are generally set at a resolution of 640 pixels horizontally and 480 pixels vertically. An image transmitted in videoconferencing such as the one shown in Figure 1, with 16 million colors (24 bit), measuring 97x73 pixel, takes up 41.6 kilobytes on disk. If shown at 640x480, the same image will take up 1.7 megabytes. This enormous difference explains why the size of images sent is usually quite small.

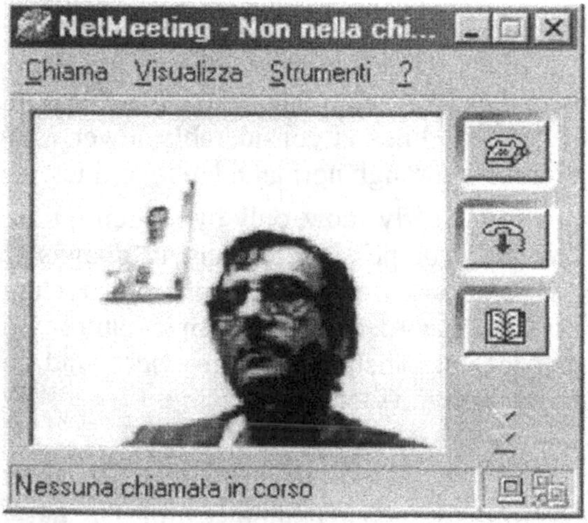

Fig. 1. A typical image transmitted in videoconferencing: 16 million colors (24 bit), 97x73 pixel, 41.6 kilobytes of disk space

Number of colors

Like size, the number of colors is important when trying to reduce the amount of data. By reducing colors to 256 in the image examined above, its size decreases to a 14 kilobytes. However, for the satisfactory transmission of such images as X-rays, shots of events etc., the required video resolution is 65,536 colors (16 bit).

Audio compression

Voice transmission is not as complex a problem, although a compression algorithm is also used for conversation. The best-known, and probably the most efficient, is GSM (Global System for Mobile Telecommunications) [6], in the recently released 6.10 version. This algorithm is used on the GSM telephone network, which transmits at a rate of 9600 bits per second. A recent update of this technology, based on a standard transmission protocol called H323 and adopted by several programs, enables videoconferencing among users operating with different programs. By using this or a similar sound compression technique, it is possible to transmit voice of acceptable quality even at fairly low rates.

Equipment required for videoconferencing via computer

Computer

In view of the extensive use of "compression" in videoconferencing programs, the PC should be equipped, at the very least, with a Pentium II 300 MHz microprocessor and 64-MB RAM, as the mathematical work required of the microprocessor is considerable. Another important component is the video card, which should feature a high-quality graphics accelerator and at least 8-MB RAM. Any higher values would not enable significantly better performances, as image transmission usually occurs through telephone lines, with the limitations described above.

Audio card

The audio card is very important, especially as regards features enabling the use of compression software and "Full Duplex" transmission, i.e., the possibility to route "voice in" on a different channel from "voice out". In this way, the two participants can speak at the same time. Single-channel transmission, where each participant can either speak or listen in turn, is called "Half Duplex". Last-generation audio cards feature "Full Duplex" software.

Camera

Video is what requires the most resources in videoconferencing. Viable solutions should include video cameras, so as not to impose an excessive image digitizing workload on the computer. Two types of video cameras can be used: analogic or digital.

Analogic cameras

Any amateur video camera can be used for videoconferencing, provided an analogic-digital conversion card is installed in the computer. In this way, films stored in the computer can be converted to the analogic format and recorded on videotapes. It is therefore possible to transfer digitized or CD-recorded films onto videotapes. The use of an analogic video camera is obviously a more-expensive option; it is, however, the one that ensures the best quality. Lastly, it should be pointed out that analogic cameras can also be used with laptop computers, due to PCMCIA credit-card size cards now available.

Digital cameras

These are the most commonly used in videoconferencing, due to their compact size (Fig. 2) and the small amount of microprocessor resources they require, since the images they send to the computer are already digitized. These cameras are marketed in multimedia kits that include audio cards and an appropriate microphone, or as stand-alone items (one example is Connectix famous Quickcam, currently produced by Logitech [7]). The most widely used versions of these cameras require no independent power supply and can be powered either through the keyboard or the computer's USB port. The former type (keyboard power supply) sends images through the parallel port (printer port), while in the USB version this port is the channel through which images are sent to the computer and power is supplied to the camera. Image quality is not as good as in traditional analogic cameras, but definitely satisfactory in videoconferencing. Digital video cameras cost around US$ 100 and are perfect for laptop computers.

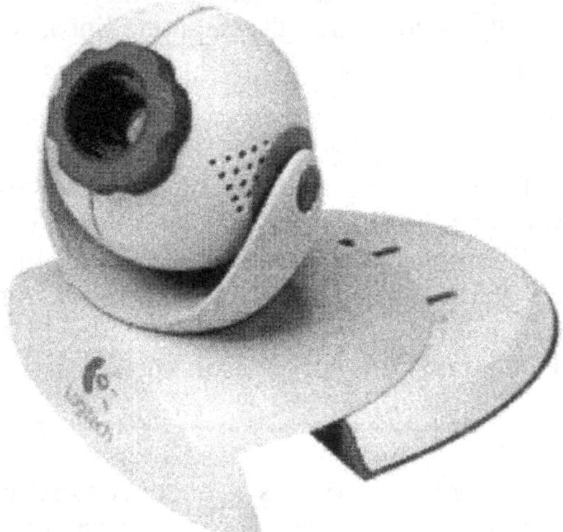

Fig. 2. USB digital camera

Programs

The programs utilized in videoconferencing are widely used by the Internet community. A distinction that can be made is between programs enabling users to interact, i.e., a mode where users can connect to each other, with characteristics similar to a video telephone, and another group enabling several users to connect to a videoconference as passive spectators. For the sake of simplicity, we will call the former "interactive programs" and the latter "videoconference servers".

Interactive videoconference programs

MULTI-POINT PROGRAMS

These programs enable several users to take part in the same conference. A server computer acting as "reflector" receives data from several users and is able to re-transmit them to those users. When this mode is used, each user connects to the "reflector", which contains the list and images of users connected at any given time, and is allowed to select one or more participants with whom to initiate a videoconference (Fig. 3). One example of this videoconferencing mode is the program called "CU-SeeMe". The program is called Meeting Point Conference Server [8].

POINT-TO-POINT PROGRAMS

Two users can establish a direct connection between two computers and transmit images and sounds. Many of the programs available in the Internet can be used to set up a "point-to-point" videoconference; the most popular are Microsoft Netmeeting and CU-SeeMe.

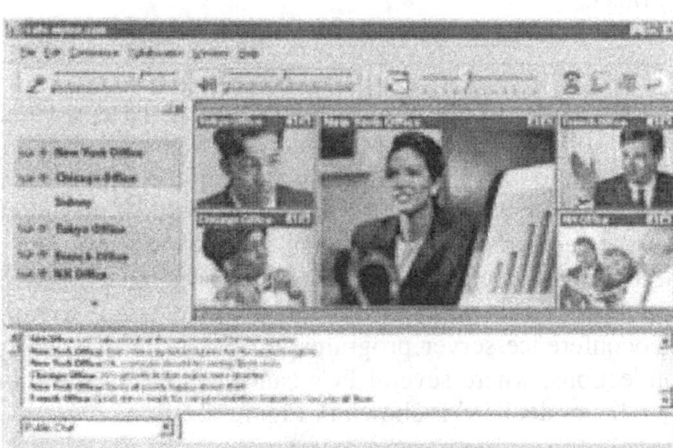

Fig. 3. White Pine CU-SeeMe (CU): a multi-party conference software; 100% reliability is achieved by using a fast communication line such as an Intranet

Microsoft Netmeeting

Microsoft Netmeeting (MN) is an Internet Explorer component. It can be downloaded free of charge from Microsoft's website [9]. The program features videoconference functions limited to two participants at the same time, and "telecommuting" function. In other words, it makes it possible to share programs (e.g., co-author a document) during the videoconference. These functions are very important for videoconference presentations: we can display a presentation, prepared using our habitual graphics program, on the other participant's monitor, and at the same time comment it. The other participant may also act on our computer to re-examine a past slide or draw something on our screen. This type of interactive videoconference is largely used in the corporate world. The program's limitation is the impossibility to show more than one participant at a time. As far as the Internet is concerned, this is actually a minor problem, since – at the kind of rate available to private users – it is difficult to set up a conference with more than two participants.

White Pine CU-SeeMe

White Pine CU-SeeMe (CU) is one of the first videoconferencing programs ever designed (Fig. 3). Although CU offers the possibility to set up a multi-party conference, 100% reliability can only be achieved by using a fast communication line such as an Intranet. At any rate, even in two-party videoconferences CU provides high-quality images and sounds. The CU "PRO" version features the same "telecommuting" characteristics as MN, with a component called "whiteboard", which can be used to write or draw graphs during the videoconference. White Pine has also developed another program, called "Class-Point" which includes many of MN's "telecommuting" features, extended for use in multi-party conference. The program was originally designed for teaching through an Intranet.

Videoconference servers

It is not always necessary for users to interact. In many cases a videoconference consists of a speaker's presentation with many participants attending, but without the need for them to interact with the orator until the end, when typically the audience can ask questions. Such is the case with medical presentations, where interaction between lecturer and participants is restricted to a few questions at the end of the presentation. In these cases, however, a top priority is to have as many participants as possible attending, so as to avoid having to repeat the presentation. Videoconference server programs are based on the same model used for online connections, where several PCs can receive data from a single computer (server). The model used is shown in Figure 4.

The speaker uses a computer equipped with a camera and an audio card. A program is started on the same computer to capture images and sound, and start a compression encoding procedure (ENCODER). The processed file is subse-

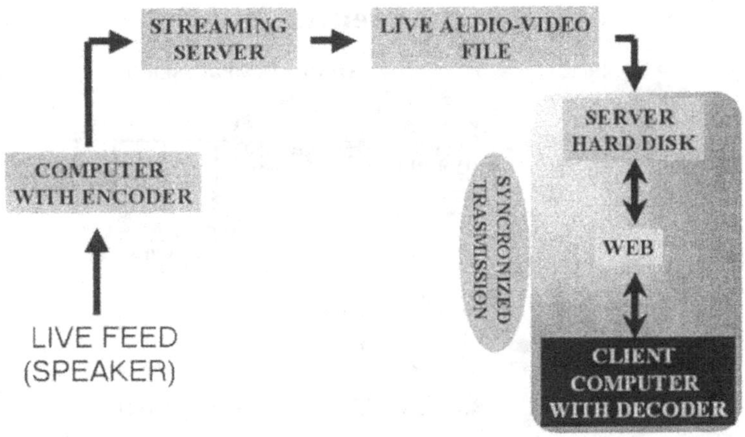

Fig. 4. Use of a videoconferencing server

quently sent in continuously flowing, synchronized form (streaming) to another computer on which the videoconference server program is running. This program produces a file containing video and voice, stored in the computer's hard disk. Participants connect to the videoconferencing server using a program (called DECODER) to read the streaming file continuously produced on the server. As in any other connection between server and client computers, file reading is synchronized according to the computers' respective rates, so as to prevent any interruption in data transfer which, in this case, would disrupt videoconference viewing.

The most-popular Internet-based programs are Microsoft Windows Media Tools, and RealNetworks Tools; free versions of both programs are downloadable online.

Microsoft Windows Media Tools (Fig. 5)

Microsoft's videoconference suite is composed of three programs [10].

Windows Encoder

This program is controlled from the lecturer's computer, and runs on Microsoft Windows 98. It supports various analogic-digital cards, for use with analogic as well as digital cameras on the USB port. In order to use this program, however, it is recommended that the computer be equipped with its own image-capturing card, since a great deal of the computer resources are used up by the ENCODER, and therefore it is best to have a video capturing card with its own microprocessor take care of image processing. Files produced are in the .mpeg format.

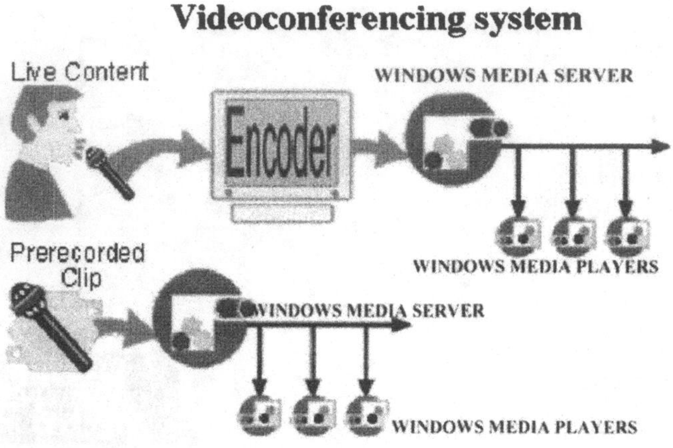

Fig. 5. Microsoft Windows Media Tools software

Windows Media Server

The server component runs on Windows NT 4.0 or Windows 2000. The server program receives files encoded by the ENCODER, stores them in a hard disk directory selected by the user, and enables the creation of a traditional Internet HTM file; a shortcut to the videoconference is inserted within the context of this file. The client user uploads the HTM page through a browser and accesses the videoconference by clicking the shortcut.

Windows Media Player

This component, installed in the client computer, enables viewing of the videoconference. There are two types of possible connection modes.

Via Browser

If an HTM page has been set up in the server, entering the address of this page will cause it to be displayed by the browser. The page may contain a description of the event, the time it will take place, etc. A click on the shortcut will actually activate Windows Media Server, which will connect directly with Windows Media Player on the client computer, thus enabling the viewing of the videoconference.

Direct use of Player

Windows Media Player can be used directly to view the videoconference. In this case, the user selects the file menu and enters the complete address of the film, which will be displayed without having to open the browser. The videoconference can also be recorded on an .mpeg-compressed AVI file and replayed offline. Space required is approximately 2 megabytes per film minute, with the following characteristics:

- size: 240x180 pixels
- colours: 24 bit (16 million)
- rate: 10 frames per second
- audio: 11Hz 8 bit mono.

ENCODER and server can be used on the same computer; minimum requirements, in this case, are 128 MB RAM, Pentium III 450 processor, and Windows NT or 2000 operating system.

REALNETWORKS TOOLS (Fig. 6) [11]

Real Producer

This program encodes conference images and sounds. It is installed in the speaker's computer and runs on Windows 98. It supports several analogic-digital cards for the use of analogic as well as digital cameras on the USB port. It produces compressed files in a RealNetworks proprietary format.

Real Server

Different versions of the Server component are available for the various operating systems, including Windows 98, so that the program can be used also in computers that have no specific network server characteristics. The same computer can host both "producer" and "server". In this case, however, minimum requirements include a Pentium II 300 processor and 128 MB RAM. Server features include the option to follow the event online or to record it for offline

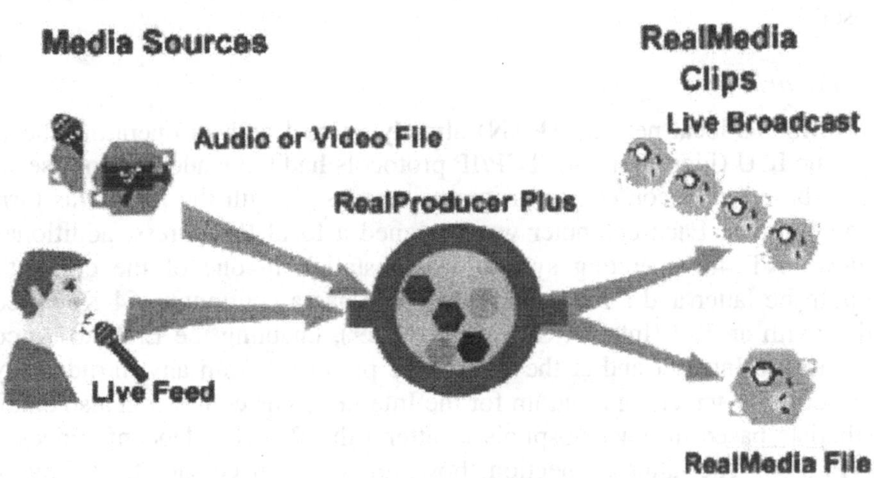

Fig. 6. Videoconferencing tools from RealNetworks company

viewing. The program's basic version, enabling connection of up to 25 users, is offered as freeware. A shortcut to the videoconference can be included in an HTM page, to view the conference via Internet browser, or the event can be played directly by the Real Player viewing program. Files produced for offline viewing are in the .rm format and their size is approximately 1.1 megabytes per min, when stored as explained above (paragraph Microsoft Windows Media Tools).

Real Player

This is the program used for videoconference viewing. It operates similarly to Windows Media Player.

Creation of a videoconference centre within an anesthesiology department, and operating methods

The Internet-based videoconferencing programs described above are inexpensive and require quite ordinary hardware - by equipping an anesthesiology department network it is possible to set up an easy-to-use, economical videoconference center. We will describe the system used and results obtained by applying these programs for the anesthesiology updating program of the Palermo Buccheri La Ferla Fatebenefratelli Hospital (BLFH).

Equipment

The hardware used in creating an internal videoconference center includes a set of low-cost tools, such as normally constitute the equipment of any private PC user.

The network

A 100 Mbits/s local network (LAN) already existed both in operating theaters and in the ICU (Figs. 7 and 8). TCP/IP protocols had to be adopted for use with Internet-based videoconference programs, and as a result the LAN was turned into an Intranet. Each computer was assigned a local IP address; additionally, Windows NT 4.0 operating system was installed in one of the computers. Through the latter and a router the LAN also has a continuous 64-Kbit/s connection with an ISP (Internet Service Provider), enabling the LAN to be connected to the Internet and at the same time protected from any intruders by a proxy server (a screening program for the Internet). The connection also enables anesthetists based in other hospitals to attend the BLFH videoconferences online (Fig. 9). The latter connection, however, is not necessary to the internal videoconferencing system.

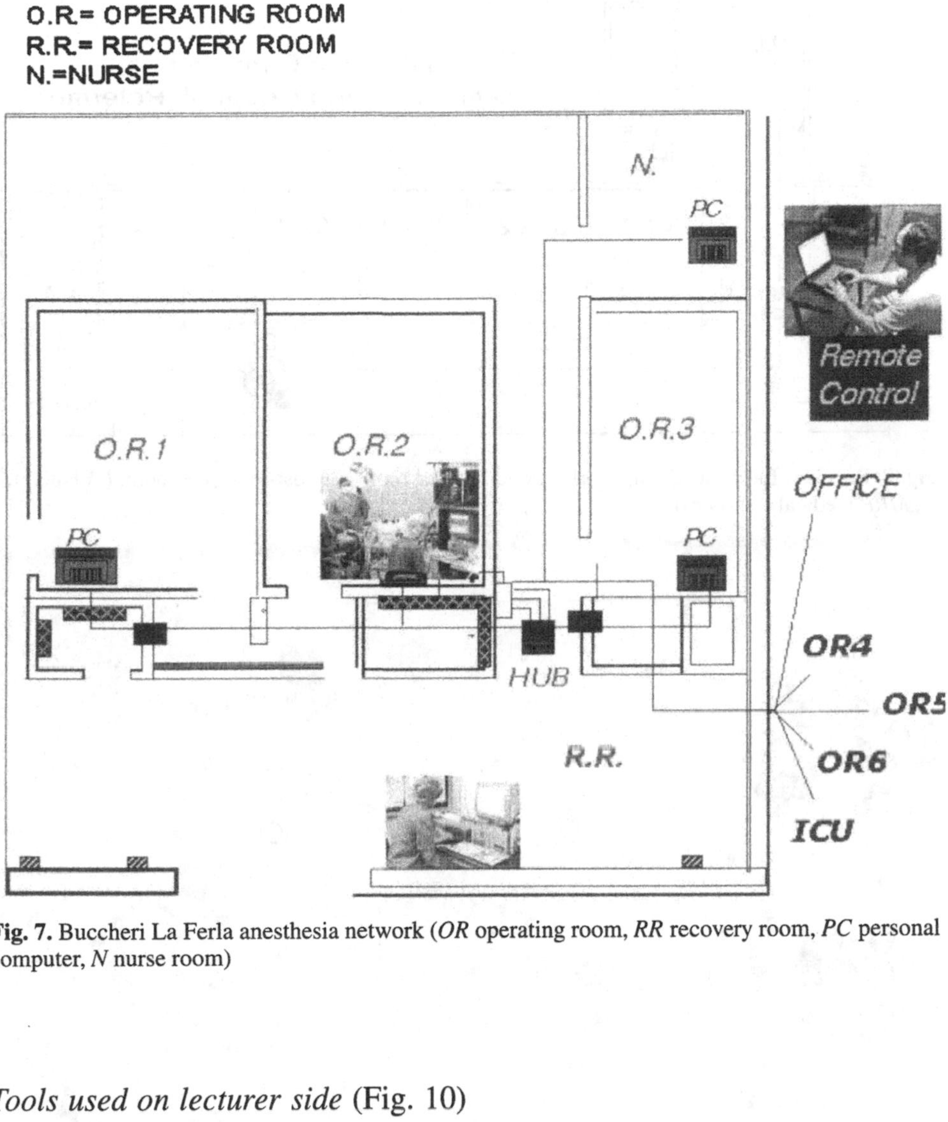

Fig. 7. Buccheri La Ferla anesthesia network (*OR* operating room, *RR* recovery room, *PC* personal computer, *N* nurse room)

Tools used on lecturer side (Fig. 10)

The computer located in the room where the videoconference is being held (Pentium II 350 MHz, 128 MB RAM, 15 gigabytes hard disk capacity) is equipped with an audio card and a Matrox Mistique video capture card. The computer video output is connected with a Polaroid video projector which projects it onto a large screen for the benefit of physically present participants. Background noise is blocked out by directing the lecturer's voice to the computer through a unidirectional microphone; images are captured by a Sony DCR trv9e camera connected to the Matrox card's RGB input.

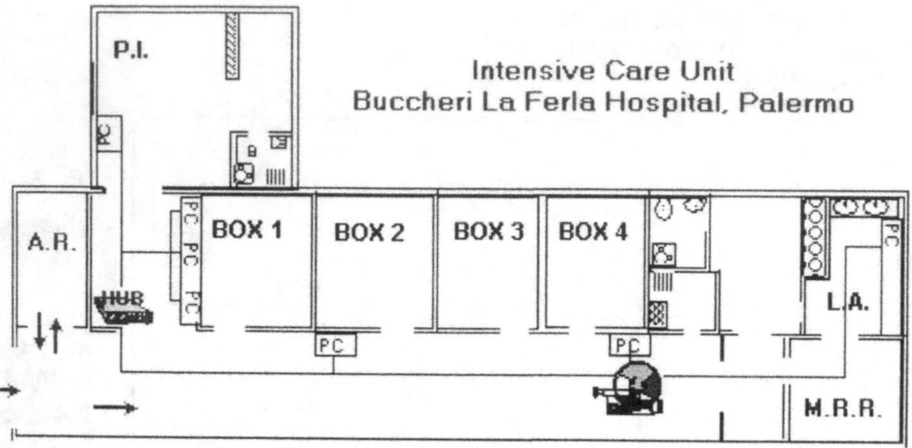

Fig. 8. Buccheri La Ferla ICU network (*AR* admittance room, *PI* post-intensive room, *LA* laboratory, *MRR* medical rest room)

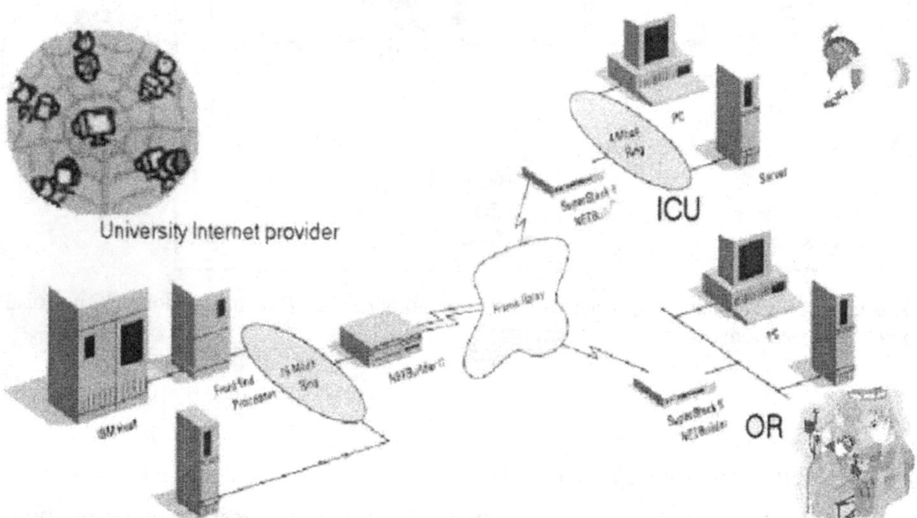

Fig. 9. The BLFH ICU and anesthesia networks are connected via a 64 Kbit/s connection to the Internet Service Provider of the Palermo University. The videoconferencing INTRANET system is also accessed from the INTERNET

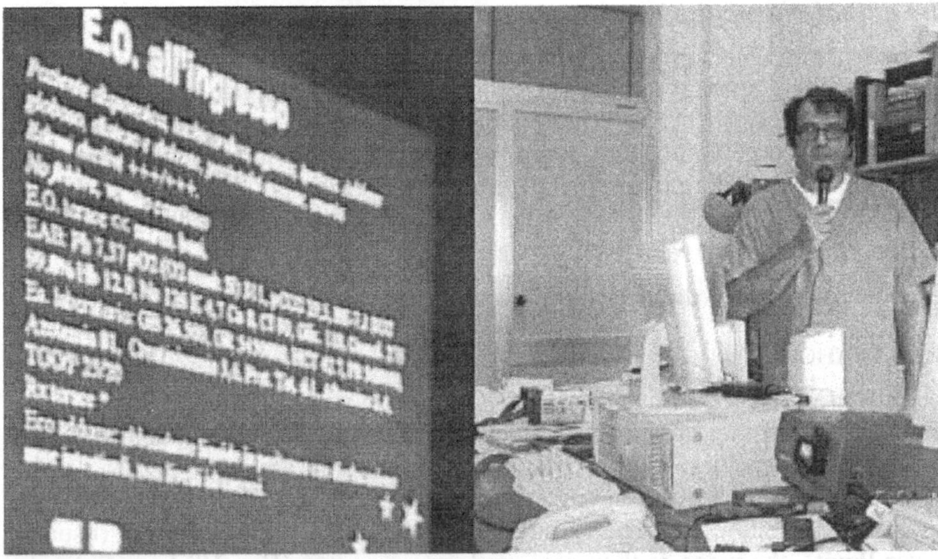

Fig. 10. Videoconferencing tools used from the speaker

Tools used on remote participants side

The computer used by remote participants is the same model as the one used by the speaker, but is equipped with an audio card only. Voice is captured by a unidirectional microphone; the image capturing tool is a Logitech digital Quickcam connected to the USB port on the computer.

Software

Microsoft Windows Media Encoder, installed on the speaker's computer, runs on Windows 98. The program enables image capture, encoding, and transmission to the server. Microsoft Windows Media Server, installed on the latter, runs on Windows NT server 4.0; this program processes the images it receives into a film which is stored in the hard disk as well as streamed (i.e., sent synchronously) to computers of participants who connect to the server. Connection procedures are the same as those used for the net: through a browser, users connect to the server and upload an HTM page showing a shortcut to the file of the videoconference being processed by the server. The conference is shown on participants' computers through Microsoft Windows Media Player. In addition, Microsoft Netmeeting, available to both speaker and participants, is used for discussions at the end of the presentation. Slides are prepared with either Microsoft Power Point or Microsoft Internet Explorer. All of the software used, except the operating systems and Microsoft Power Point, are free of charge and downloadable from the Microsoft website.

The actual videoconference

The videoconference circuit is composed of one station in the videoconference room, including speaker equipment, 20 seats in the conference room, and 3 remote stations located in the general surgery recovery room, in the ICU, and in the obstetric surgery recovery room, respectively. Videoconferences are held once a month according to a schedule drawn up every 6 months (Table 2).

Videoconference procedures

Videoconferences are divided into two parts: presentation and discussion.

Presentation

Lectures are prepared in turn by all physicians (15 persons) and by some of the nurses (5 of 30) that compose the anesthetic service. Lecturers acquire familiarity with presentation tools 1-2 days in advance and are requested to follow the instructions shown in Table 3. Average time of videoconferencing system use is approximately 2 h. The lecturers open the presentation program (usually Power Point), the video is then projected onto a screen (Fig. 10) by a Polaroid

Table 2. Example of the content of a videoconferences cycle

Walking-anesthesia in obstetrics
Effects of thoracic epidural analgesia on pulmonary function
Caudal block in children
Cost-effectiveness of peripheral nerve blocks for postoperative pain
Guidelines for preoperative testing for coronary artery disease
Perioperative management of the patient with non-ischemic cardiac disease
Preoperative data management
Difficult airway management algorithm
Total parenteral nutrition in acute pancreatitis
Pathophysiological changes in morbidly obese
Hemofiltration in ICU: indication and strategies
Quality assurance in anesthesia and intensive care
Infraclavicular brachial plexus block
Lower extremity blocks

Table 3. Suggestions to the speaker

Leam the videoconferencing system
Speak in a strong, clear voice
Move and gesture slowly and smoothly
Maintain enthusiasm toward the technology and the subject matter
Speak in simple scientific language

projector, so that participants in the room may view presentation images. At the same time, by activating Windows Media Encoder, videoconference images captured by the video camera and voice conveyed through a unidirectional microphone are sent to the server computer (active program: Windows Media Server). Thus, the three remote participants may download an HTM page from the server onto their computers, select the shortcut and follow the conference using Windows Media Player. The videoconference is also stored in the server's hard disk as an "ASF" file for viewing at a later time, by accessing the same HTM page and selecting the conference one wishes to watch. On average, a conference lasts for about 45 min and each of them takes up approximately 80 megabytes disk space.

Discussion

At the end of the presentation, Media Encoder is shut down, and both lecturer and remote participants launch Netmeeting, so that the audience may ask questions.

Costs

Costs can be summarized as follows:

1. speaker's station, including a good camera, e.g., Sony, and voice equipment: around US$ 2,500;
2. projector: approximately US$ 2,000;
3. each remote station with digital camera: approximately US$ 1,000;
4. server computer: approximately US$ 1,000;
5. computer network cards and hub to connect them: approximately US$ 250.

Therefore, total costs for a three-remote station system can be estimated at around US$ 11,750.

How videoconferences enhance knowledge

Assessment method

Videoconference effects on CQI has been assessed by examining a 12-month sample period of videoconferences. Of the 20 meetings that took place in the said period, 10 were carried out in the traditional fashion (TC), while 10 were videoconferences (VC). During each event, an independent observer noted the number of attending and remote participants, number of questions, and length of presentations. Knowledge acquired through the two techniques was assessed by means of a multiple choice questionnaire containing 20 questions on the topics dealt with in the presentations. The questionnaire shown in Table 4 was used to assess VC performance from a technical point of view. Participants were requested to assign a score from 1 to 5 for each question.

Table 4. The questionnaire used to assess videoconferences. Participants were requested to assign a score from 1 to 5 for each question

Please rate the **audio** quality of this presentation
Please rate the **visual** quality of this presentation
How well do you feel you now **understand** the topic as a result of this presentation?
Please rate the **participation** quality at this presentation
How would you classify the **environment** in which you followed the videoconference?

Results

Number of participants was 9 ± 0.94 in the TC group and 13.20 ± 1.32 in the VC group ($p < 0.05$) (Fig. 11). Length of events was 63 ± 9.49 min in the TC group and 82.50 ± 9.20 min in the VC group ($p < 0.05$) (Fig. 12). Number of participants' questions was 2 ± 0.94 in TC and 4.1 ± 1.20 in VC ($p < 0.05$) (Fig. 13). Percentage of correct answers to the questionnaire was 66.5% ± 10.29 in TC and 80 ± 8.16 in VC. Average score obtained in the technical performance assessment was 3.6 ± 1.07 (Fig. 14).

Discussion

Quality in health care is hard to define. Is it patient satisfaction, success of treatment, or length of stay for a particular illness? Each practice and health care organization can devise its own definition. Quality requires that we measure it, train our staff, and undertake research to improve our product and service delivery. Most quality and outcome measures represent the performance of the system rather than any one individual or group [12]. As a result of new technology, performance and quality information will become more and more widespread. Several health care organizations are already providing this information on the

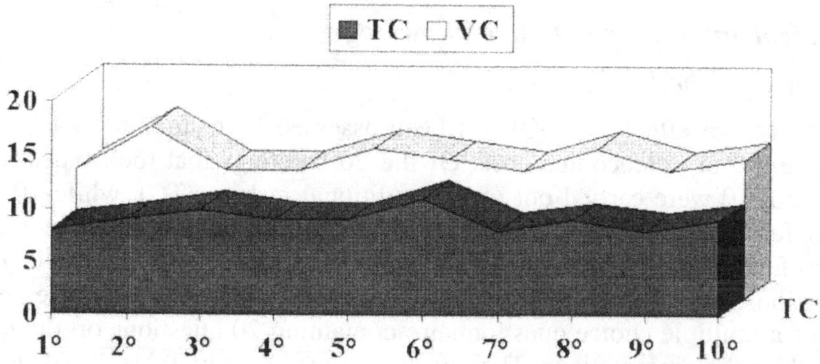

Fig. 11. Number of participants (Y axis) increases in VC group ($p < 0.05$) (*TC* traditional conference, *VC* videoconference)

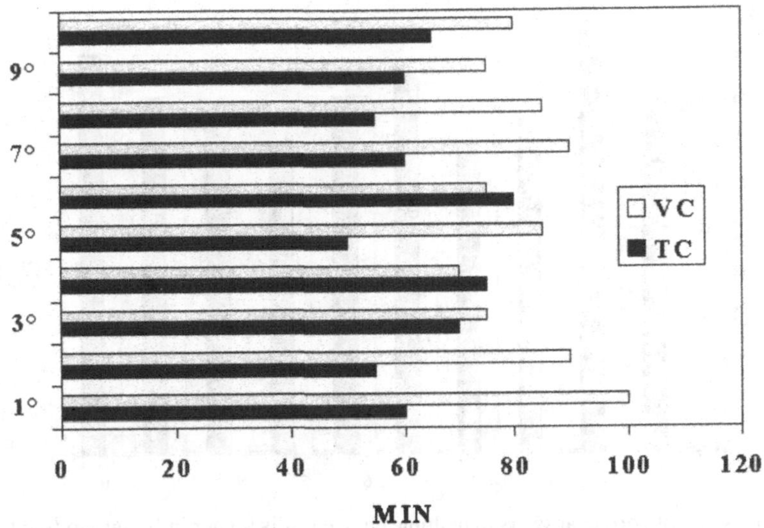

Fig. 12. The duration of the conference (presentation plus discussion) is higher in VC group ($p < 0.05$)

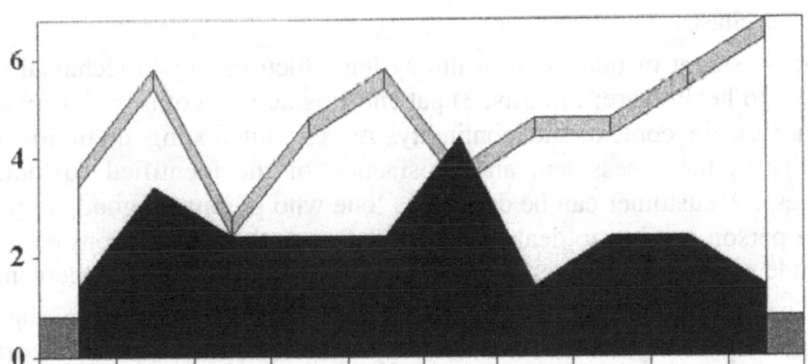

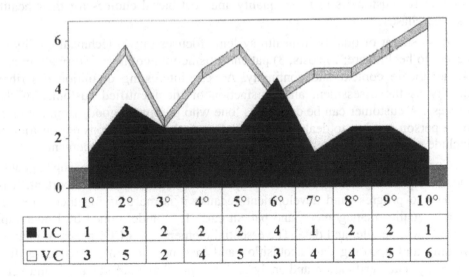

	1°	2°	3°	4°	5°	6°	7°	8°	9°	10°
■ TC	1	3	2	2	2	4	1	2	2	1
□ VC	3	5	2	4	5	3	4	4	5	6

Fig. 13. Interventions at the end of the exposition increase in the VC group ($p < 0.05$)

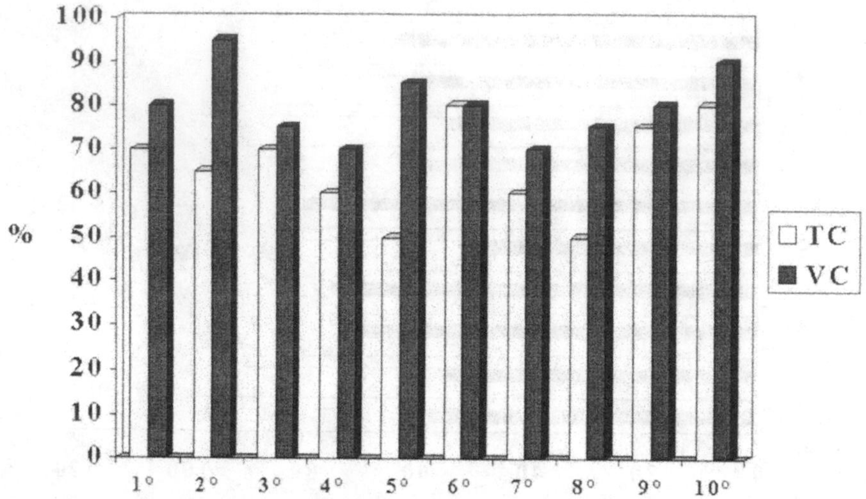

Fig. 14. Rate score of correct answers to multiple choice test is higher in VC group ($p < 0.05$)

Internet for customers to make quality and cost-based choices for their health care purchases.

Assessment of quality in health systems focuses on: 1) technical quality of access to health care; 2) costs; 3) patient satisfaction, comfort, information; and 4) healthcare context and continuity. A very interesting definition describes quality as the assessment and satisfaction of the identified customer of the process. A customer can be defined as 'one who purchases goods from another' or 'a person one has to deal with'. According to these definitions our customers include patients, surgeons, and other staff, and the hospital management.

Customer focus may seem an inappropriate direction for a sophisticated medical speciality such as anesthesia, yet it could not be more important. It is the key to progress and development because it is the unifying theme for research, quality management, and patient care. It is underpinned by leadership, consistency, people, and data. The essential elements of a CQI program include training and updating data acquisition and incorporation into a database, followed by data verification and analysis. Once problems are identified and verified, they lead to the development of plans whereby the system and processes can be modified and improved.

Processes can be improved by working on three factors: workmanship (clinical practice guidelines, care maps, and analysis of variance from expected care); performance quality indicators (predetermined measures that quantify aspects of care); technology and human resources (training, communication, participation, learning).

The international quality strategy for the new National Health Systems highlights lifelong learning as a way of improving healthcare [13]. Team learning is vital because it is largely through teams that organizations achieve their objectives. For an organization to be striving for excellence, the individuals within that organization must be constantly improving their own personal proficiencies. However, separate learning by the different professions in healthcare may be detrimental because individual virtuosity is insufficient: it is teams that deliver healthcare. Development of the whole team rather than learning within single professions is essential.

Knowledge dissemination has always aroused harsh debate in critical medicine. On the one hand, it is too costly to have at hand personnel able to cope with infrequent emergencies such as chemical disasters, aeroplane crashes, and so on, but, faced with this kind of emergency the professional abilities of critical area personnel prove to be inadequate, with obvious consequences on patient care. It is now widely acknowledged that internal updating meetings are an effective means to increase knowledge within hospitals and promote improvement in patient care. However, meetings can hardly involve all personnel, as clearly patient care must continue while meetings are being held, which means that personnel engaged in patient care are prevented from attending meetings. The possibility to hold meeting during breaks has traditionally given poor results. With the development of telemedicine, large facilities have tried to deal with the problems described above by offering support during emergencies [14] and to increase knowledge available to personnel through videoconferencing. This method offers an effective way to reach personnel on duty, who have the time to follow a lecture but are unable to be physically present in the room where it is held because they cannot leave their place (staff assigned to the recovery room, ICU, etc.). Projects pursued to date, however, have been based on the use of such equipment as shown in Figure 15 [15], which could only be implemented by applying the kind of resources available to large facilities. Such projects present three types of problems:

1. high price. The cost of a three- to four-station videoconferencing system is in the order of tens of millions, and can only be used for videoconferences;
2. need to hire an administrator. Traditional videoconferencing systems require technicians whose fees represent an additional cost;
3. difficulties in replaying videoconferences. In traditional systems videoconferences are recorded on videotapes, the viewing of which requires a VCR and TV set, not easily available in the workplace.

The system we have implemented at the Buccheri La Ferla Hospital provides solutions to the problems described above, in that:

1. it is inexpensive. The cost estimate for a system such as the one described herein is affordable by any healthcare facility. An additional advantage to be considered is the fact that these computers are not dedicated to videoconferences, but can be utilized for other purposes (to write reports, medical files,

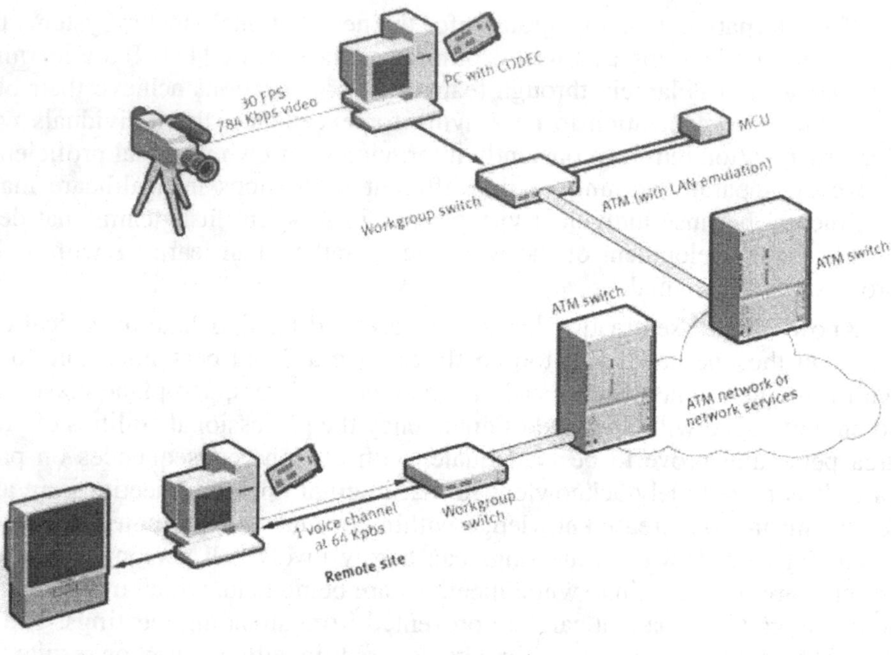

Fig. 15. Structure of an industrial videoconferencing system

and so on); moreover, ordinary PCs can be constantly upgraded due to the continuous developments;

2. it does not require dedicated technicians – any staff member can set up a videoconference;
3. it allows videoconferences to be replayed on computers, which are easily available in the workplace.

As far as knowledge improvement is concerned, our project has produced significant results. Video transmission is satisfactory, and the speaker's voice is clearly audible. Some anesthetists who normally feel daunted by the presence of other people in the room and refrain from asking questions felt at ease in front of a computer and took part in the discussion, as shown by the higher number of questions asked by the VC group compared to traditional meetings. The number of participants has also increased: in the case of anesthetists, up to 90% of the whole staff. Answers to multiple choice questionnaires evidence an improvement in meeting effectiveness, with more knowledge acquired, which can only have beneficial effects on treatment quality. Another positive result achieved by videoconferences was to force lecturers to adopt clear, concise topic delivery techniques, which is essential when using this type of equipment, but is also good training for congress presentations.

Conclusions

The use of Intranet videoconference allows the dissemination of live updating meetings and helps create an internal library always available to personnel at a later time for their professional development. Other material, such as updating courses on electronic media or documents downloaded from the Internet, can be added, so as to form, in time, an electronic library accessible from every anesthetist's desk.

References

1. Hinkle AJ (1996) What you need to know about total Quality Management techniques. ASA refresher courses 24:111-126
2. Lubarky DA (1997) Using an anesthesia information management system as a cost containment tool. Anesthesiology 86:1161-1169
3. Nolan TW, Provost LP (1990) Understanding variation. Quality progress, pp 70-78
4. Grant J, Stanton F (1998) The effectiveness of continuing professional development. Joint centre for education in medicine, pp 21-24
5. Remote Computing White Papers
6. GSM (Global System for Mobile Telecommunications)
7. Digital cameras
8. Videoconferencing software "Cu-seeme"
9. Videoconferencing software "Netmeeting"
10. Microsoft Windows Media Tools
11. RealNetworkss Tools
12. Bierstein K (1997) Setting Up a Quality Improvement Program. Asa News Letters 08
13. Davies TO, Nutley SM (2000) Developing learning organisations in the new NHS. BMJ 320:998-1001
14. Chemics96 Simulation Of Chemical Accident In Telepresence And Teleconsultation
15. Distributed Training for the Modern Enterprise

COST-EFFECTIVENESS IN ANAESTHESIA AND CRITICAL CARE

Monitoring of Performance in Anaesthesia and Intensive Care

Q. PIACEVOLI, E. FERRARI BALIVIERA, F. CACCAMO

The institutional task of those who work in the health-care sector is to meet the health needs of the population by providing suitable treatment, and to monitor performance in order to assess whether the objectives set have been achieved.

Monitoring performance in anaesthesia and intensive care means understanding what is and what is not clinically effective and assessing the results of the work from both the clinical and economic points of view. In order to achieve this objective targets have to be set for the use of resources: those pathologies which can really benefit from a given treatment have to be identified and the quality of service optimised keeping in mind the needs of the various parties involved (patients, health-care operators, public institutions, etc.). These concepts are the fundamental steps of an organisational process of clinical practice defined as benchmarking. What is benchmarking? According to economists it is a process that identifies and studies the best way to achieve the best performance of a system. More precisely the term benchmarking, imported from economics, refers to a whole set of marketing techniques and strategies which have long been used by the world's major companies. Over the last few years, a new figure has appeared in the Italian health-care system: the doctor-manager, who is responsible for the proper allocation of economic resources required to provide a top-quality service, and not merely with the solution of clinical problems. The result of this process is best practice which, in terms of the end product, is beneficial to the parties using a given service, in particular patients and health-care operators.

For the creation of a model of best practice, objectives regarding the clinical sector in question have to be identified:

1. identifying the state of the art in that sector (in the form of an evidence table);
2. analysing current treatment patterns;
3. developing strategies to optimise treatment.

In order to achieve these objectives three analytical strategies can be adopted:

1. comprehensive reading of review/meta-analysis;

2. the method known as giant regression, which consists of identifying large-scale administrative data representing the current variations of health-care treatment (sometimes linked with clinical data such as drugs records and retrospective chart audits) and producing a multi-variate regressive analysis to identify the real costs of the various treatments;
3. the development of a comprehensive model where major data are entered in the most suitable way.

A good model is a useful decision-making instrument when it is exhaustive and capable of undergoing reliable procedures [1]. An exhaustive model is one "whose form and content are sufficient to solve a particular problem" [1].

The use of these decision-making instruments is very controversial, above all because they are very likely to be misunderstood. At present, there are no guidelines capable of guaranteeing the reliability and quality of the models in question. There are, however, criteria which can help doctors choose between good and bad models. A good model has to have the following characteristics:

1. summarising the most important management features (simplifying but not too much);
2. using the best data available as inputs;
3. having been tested;
4. documenting its most important features (inputs, algorithms and assumptions) in a clear way.

A decision-making model which does not meet these requirements has to be regarded with suspicion.

The focus of the range of interest has moved from the single patient, which is what clinical operators and in particular anaesthetists-intensive care operators were used to concentrating on, to the functionality and well-being of all the users of a given service and those who work in it. A completely new vocabulary, which only few people have encountered in their scientific training, has to become familiar. The opinion of the senior and expert doctor is no longer considered sufficient to establish which treatment is best for a certain pathology. It is the sum of the opinions of the international medical community which is sought and assessed. The result of this new approach is evidence based medicine and evidence based decision making, the techniques which should guide today's doctors so as to guarantee a higher quality of their work.

Quality and quality monitoring in medicine

For some years now there has been a reawakening of interest for quality in medicine. The real problem is defining the term quality with a single adjective. At present, the term quality, which traditionally refers to an intrinsic characteristic of a product, is increasingly used to describe a service.

In 1980, Donabedian formulated a definition of quality in the medical sector which has become a classic [2]: "... the type of treatment which is believed to optimise the patient's well-being after expected benefits and costs which accompany the treatment in its entirety have been assessed".

Hence, in the health-care sector quality means: "the chances to obtain the desired outcome in a given health-care context, in line with current technical and professional knowledge" [3, 4].

Quality does not exist in itself. It requires multidimensional and multiskills components. Technical and organisational quality have to be guaranteed in any structure.

In the health-care sector there is technical, social (relations between users and patients, including their comfort and expectations) and economic quality.

Without precise parameters quality is also relatively subjective: the final judgement can change according to the observer. In order to remedy this disadvantage, quality indicators have been identified.

The following quality indicators are accepted in the health-care sector:

- accessibility
- acceptability
- adequacy
- effectiveness
- efficiency
- safety
- user satisfaction
- promptness [5].

According to whether the quality of the structure, the process or the results are being assessed, these quality indicators are given real "names" and are measured with suitable units: for example the evaluation of the promptness of an intervention in an emergency unit is assessed as the time interval within which a doctor has to see the patient.

According to Donabedian's theories, achieving total quality implies a three-tier intervention: on the structure in which one works, clinical processes or procedures and results achieved (outcome). Different instruments are recommended to assess and monitor quality in each sector.

In order to plan, achieve and ensure structural quality it is necessary to establish which quality standard has to be met. Meeting standards is the fundamental requirement to achieve good quality in an intensive care unit or operating theatre. Even in good structures, however, processes are not necessarily optimal and results obtained sufficient [6].

The quality of a health-care process is ensured if procedure guidelines are formulated, followed by operators and strengthened. Medical audits, that is the creation of large-scale data banks including information on diagnoses, demography, seriousness of pathologies, resources used and results obtained, are another important and effective means to improve and monitor the quality of processes. The setting up of the Intensive Care National Audit Research Center (ICNARC) and the Scottish Intensive Care Society Audit Group are an example of that [7]. There are also specific indicators which are of great help in measuring the quality process and assessing its result (Table 1).

Table 1. Relationships between the fields of action and the management instruments and their importance

	Standard	Guidelines	Indicators
Structures	XXX	X	X
Clinical procedures	XX	XXX	XX
Results	X	XX	XXX

The global quality of clinical procedure is the sum of all the measures taken and not taken during the patient's treatment, such as activity timing, accidents, delays, misunderstandings and unpredicted events. Other elements to consider are the expectations of patients and their relatives, their satisfaction and the accessibility of the intensive care unit and operating theatre. The quality of clinical procedures and results add to the global performance of the unit where one works [8]. It is common belief that the high costs of anaesthesia and intensive care are reflected by the high quality of the service provided. In fact, high costs do not necessarily ensure high quality and quality improvement is by no means linked to a parallel increase in costs.

Quality is an attribute of the structures where one works, the process carried out and the outcome obtained. It is not static but in constant evolution as a result of the interaction of many human and instrumental variables and can always be perfected (continuous quality improvement theory, CQI).

CQI is a continuous effort by the health-care organisation to provide services which meet or even exceed expectations, through a systematic procedure and consecutive training steps, provision of work material, consultation, training and stimulation of operators involved in the service, in order to achieve the scheduled improvement of the service while keeping costs low [9].

The continuous monitoring of performance and results obtained is fundamental in this system.

Quality monitoring in anaesthesia

The need to assess and improve the quality of the service is also felt in anaesthesia. What is meant by quality of anaesthesia?

The first variable to be analysed regards indicators.

As yet there are no common lists of universally applicable quality indicators for anaesthesia. Talking about quality is a luxury that takes for granted the high safety margin of anaesthesiological procedures.

At least two groups of quality indicators can be identified in anaesthesia:

- objective indicators
- subjective indicators

Objective indicators are identified by anaesthetists and regard the various steps of anaesthesia.

The ones most studied are those connected to some of the anaesthetists' specific behaviours, such as recording the preoperative examination and the anaesthesia itself on the anaesthesia card, and those concerning the occurrence of undesired effects and accidents (of varying seriousness).

Posner and Freund [9] identify the following 5 elements as quality indicators for anaesthesia provided to the users of their hospital:

1. percentage of *accidents* in the operating theatre (index calculated every month), where an accident is an undesired event which, however, does not produce an undesired outcome, such as the patient's death or serious injury, an escalation of treatment in the post-operative phase or an inefficiency of the operating block. An example of accident is a very short break down of the mechanical ventilator which is immediately identified without repercussions for the patient;
2. percentage of *serious injury* of patients connected to anaesthesia: any injury that modifies the physical state permanently;
3. percentage of cases where there is an *escalation of treatment* compared to the planned anaesthesia programme: for example when it is necessary to pass from local to total anaesthesia;
4. percentage of *inefficiency of the operating block*: for example postponement or cancellation of operations;
5. percentage of *human errors*.

The frequency percentages of these events are calculated on the basis of data provided in reports specially designed by the hospital under the continuous quality improvement programme and filled in by the doctors themselves.

These indicators attribute a value to the quality of anaesthesia which is inversely proportional to their frequency: the lower the frequency the higher the quality level.

These markers are selective and mainly focus on patients' safety and the functioning of the operating theatre.

As anaesthesia facilitates the surgical treatment of an illness but does not produce direct effects on health, with reference to Donabedian's quality definition [3], it is fundamental to try to avoid the occurrence of accidents or undesired effects due to anaesthesia, in order to ensure its quality. According to the authors, this can be done with a continuous and constant control of undesired effects, discussing the causes and factors which facilitate their occurrence and, if necessary, elaborating guidelines for each specific problem. All the anaesthetists of a hospital have to participate in this common development.

In addition to that, an anaesthesia with fewer complications will also lead to shorter post-operative stays in hospital and lower costs at the end of the treatment, translating into an important saving factor.

It is interesting to note that all the authors stress the importance of collecting data to evaluate the quality of the process and carry out the necessary corrections [10].

The quality of anaesthesia cards are also discussed [11] with surprising results. Their quality appears low (they are incomplete and illegible) and some plead for automated data recording during anaesthesia [12].

Subjective indicators are linked with the patient: the importance of patient/user satisfaction with the treatment received is taking root [13]. For our purposes it does not matter that the patient is technically incapable of understanding an anaesthesia, but rather to what extent he/she appreciated his/her anaesthesia. Of course, it is only possible to talk about satisfaction after waking up from an anaesthesia and in the immediate post-operative phase, as the patient is not aware of what happens during the operation (apart from unfortunate cases of patients waking up during an operation).

The QoR (quality of recovery) indicator attributes a numeric value to the quality the patient ascribes to the anaesthesia care received: the higher the figure, the more appreciated the treatment. There are various QoRs processed by the same authors [14, 15]. In any case, the patients answer a series of simple questions on the occurrence of any problem, even mild ones, with answers like "never, sometimes, almost always". By doing so they attribute a value to the quality of their recovery (example of question: "in the last few hours, after the operation, have you experienced nausea?").

There are many factors that contribute to patient satisfaction, including accessible and cheap services, pleasant structures and competence of the staff, beside their expectations and preferences. Most people expect anaesthesia without complications, even though the awakening is often accompanied by residual sedation, pain, nausea and vomit. These are the things patients complain the most about and which reduce their appreciation of the treatment received. Analysis and monitoring of these indicators also provide valuable indications for a cost/benefit assessment of some economic choices. For example, the preventive use of anti-nausea drugs, which may seem a superfluous expense (from the point of view of cost control), could turn out to be an investment capable of increasing the perceived quality of the service provided, with favourable long-term repercussions on the system's economy (increase of users and productivity).

Quality monitoring in intensive care

The experts in the sector propose the following quality indicators for intensive care [6]:

- *Guidelines.* The formulation of guidelines is considered a fundamental element in the organisation of the service. Anybody who is responsible for intensive-care units should revise the guidelines used in their unit regularly, introduce new ones regarding not clearly defined or out-of-date procedures and remember that the highest impact on daily life is the product of rules developed within the unit, especially if external guidelines are adopted (for example those deriving from the state of the art).
- *Global quality indicators of the clinical service.* Any unit director should select a set number of clinical procedures which together can represent the quality of all the clinical procedures carried out in the unit. Examples of clinical procedures to be analysed are: the time elapsed from admission to intensive care to the beginning of thrombolitic treatment after acute myocardial infarct, mechanical ventilation (number of days of autonomous breathing, re-intubation rate, etc.), success rate in cardiopulmonary reanimation procedures, rate of readmission in intensive care for pathologies not adequately diagnosed or treated during the previous hospital stay, claim management, periodic accident reports and hospital infections monitoring.
- *Timing of services.* Two of the most used time-dependent indicators are the time of weaning from mechanical ventilation and the "door-to-needle-time", that is the time passed between admission and injection of the thrombolitic drug.
- *Accidents.* The clinical situations in which the worst rules are applied, or the best are not applied, should not be labelled as mistakes but, more properly, accidents or undesired events. Accident reports drawn up on special forms, the same for all operators, can become excellent means to monitor and improve the quality of clinical procedures.
- *User satisfaction.* According to most studies, it is very difficult to assess the satisfaction expressed by the patients of an intensive-care unit given the peculiarities of people admitted to this unit. The assessment of the service appreciation by relatives is equally difficult [6].
- *Unit performance.* There are no definitions which can exhaustively explain what is understood by intensive care. A model unit, however, distinguishes itself by its capacity to admit patients rapidly, treat them efficiently and discharge them in a reasonably short time. Good interpersonal relationships, ac-

tive communication and a multidisciplinary aptitude are necessary to reach this goal.

As was said earlier, ensuring a good performance of intensive-care units requires a proper allocation or resources and improving the quality of the service offered.

One of the instruments the specialist can use for a proper allocation of resources is scoring systems [16] which should make it possible to obtain a prior estimate of the result of any intensive treatment. In other words, these systems should help assess which patients can benefit the most from this type of treatment. Despite the fact that experiments and controlled trials are the gold standard for the assessment of existing and new treatments, it is not always possible to carry them out in intensive care. For example, it is not morally acceptable to admit, at random, patients in very serious conditions to intensive care or internal medicine units. The alternative is simply to observe the results of treatment carried out in intensive care and try to reach some conclusions.

Scoring systems take into account different parameters such as age, seriousness of pathology, natural history of the disease, any emergency operation prior to admission in intensive care - all recognised as factors which determine a mortality increase [17]. The scores obtained using scoring systems are interpreted as an estimate of the result in terms of probability of death before leaving the hospital. One scoring system model is APACHE II (acute physiology and chronic health evaluation) devised by William Knaus in the 1970s, which gives a 1 to 4 score to each of the 12 physiological variables considered, calculating the worst anomalous value observed in the first 24 h of treatment [18]. In addition, a score is assigned to other parameters, such as age, seriousness of the pathology, etc. The score varies between 0 and 71 and the highest values correspond to the most serious clinical condition.

It is also believed that the condition which caused admission to intensive care influences the outcome. Most intensive care units do not have a sufficient number of patients in comparable clinical conditions. For that reason, mathematical equations have been elaborated to give an estimate of the survival probability of several thousands of patients coming from various intensive care units, using a general database.

Scoring systems can be useful for different operations, including *comparative audit*, that is the comparison between expected and achieved results which on one hand gives a quality measure of the various intensive care units, and on the other can provide an explanation for the reasons why unexpected results have been obtained, reasons which can be sought within a single unit. Another operation is *assessment research* which, with the use of accurate estimates of expected hospital mortality rates, can provide useful information in the search for those components of the intensive care structure which ensure better results and can be used for stratification in randomised clinical trials. Lastly, *clinical management* of single patients, which makes it possible to use a clinical shortcut, that is obtaining rapidly a wide range of information on each patient. In agreement with this last concept, scoring systems could be used as guidelines in the treatment of patients, and more specifically, help the doctor decide when the therapy is to be considered ineffective or the patient can be discharged. This proposal, of course, has given rise to many discussions, even though scoring systems have shown a predictive capacity comparable to that of clinical operators [16].

There are different scoring systems for intensive care [16, 17] which can be classified as: specific and generic (the former address a particular type of patient and the latter are used to assess all, or almost all, patients); anatomical and physiological (the former assess the extent of the injury and the latter the functional alteration caused by the injury). The most common scoring systems used in intensive care include Glasgow coma scale and APACHE II.

Possible roles of scoring systems
Comparative audit
Assessment research
Clinical management of patients

The problem of costs

As previously mentioned, the need to improve the quality of health-care services provided while controlling the costs involved is increasingly strongly felt. In some respects, the introduction of new forms of hospital management has led to an increase of competition among hospitals. Hence the effort to apply principles based on models used in economics, as already happens in other countries.

The most used economic analysis techniques are:

1. *Cost-minimisation*: it implies the comparison of costs, irrespective of results or side effects [19].
2. *Cost-benefit analysis*: it implies the comparison between costs and benefits translated into money terms [20].
3. *Cost-effectiveness analysis*: it expresses the cost of an intervention per unit of success or result (cost per patient without post-operative complications). It is often used instead of cost-benefit analysis owing to the difficulty of translating the results obtained into pure monetary values [21].
4. *Cost-utility analysis*: it is similar to cost-effectiveness analysis, but also assesses patients' preference and satisfaction with the quality of life achieved after treatment, expressing a result in terms of quality of future life (QALY = quality of adjusted life years) [22].

In health economy there are various types of costs and they include materials and structures used, staff and time dedicated to carrying out a certain task. What exactly is meant by cost?

In economics *cost* is the "sacrifice" measured as the price to pay for the irreversible use of a resource (of any type).

Costs and costs monitoring in anaesthesia

The search for the best outcome of a treatment at the reasonably lowest cost has now become a duty in anaesthesia: this is called value-based anaesthesia care.

The treatment will have the highest value by either achieving the same outcome with a lower expense or a better outcome at the same or higher cost.

From an economic point of view, the highest costs in clinical anaesthesia are those connected with medical and non-medical staff (salaries) [23]. The most expensive materials include blood and blood substitutes, medical products, drugs, in particular myorelaxants and inhaling halogenated anaesthetics. The cost of the anaesthesia staff is 5-15% and material 2-10% of the total perioperative costs. Despite the relatively low percentage value, the pressure to reduce the costs of anaesthesia, in particular those connected with drugs and equipment is continuous and high.

The various techniques of health-care economic analysis are often used in studies which intend to demonstrate the savings generated by the use or non-use of a certain product: the conclusions are often of no clinical utility, if not wrong.

They have demonstrated how it pays to use the low-flow ventilation technique, which brings about remarkable savings in drugs and money, without making anaesthesia lighter [24]. This information is very useful but the studies which produced it only took into account the cost aspect and nothing else connected to the use of techniques.

Using cost-benefit analysis, according to Roizen et al. [25] the installation of capnographers and pulse oxymeters in all operating theatres of a hospital was a positive factor from an economic point of view, as the saving resulting from the lower number of blood gas measurements carried out during operations was higher than the cost of purchasing the machines, and there was an improvement of the operating block performance. By definition, the most effective treatments on the basis of cost-effective analysis are not necessarily the cheapest. A very expensive treatment can be the most effective for a given pathology, if associated with a lower incidence of side effects, determining a better performance of the service provided.

For example, propofol seems more "effective" for day-hospital anaesthesia than thiopentone and forane: recovery from propofol is more rapid and with fewer side effects [26].

On the basis of the same analysis, the most effective technique for post-operative analgesia is the epidural, rather than oral or intramuscular administration of morphine, even though on the whole it is more expensive [27].

A correct economic analysis requires an in-depth monitoring of the side effects of the drug or of the treatment under examination.

Cost-utility analysis is difficult to apply to anaesthesia. As yet there are no data available on patients' preferences regarding anaesthesia, and the QALY index is difficult to apply to the outcome of an anaesthesia (or its undesired effects).

Costs and cost monitoring in intensive care

Intensive care involves high costs. According to some English authors [7], over 60% of the high daily cost per bed depends on staff salaries and the rest on the use of drugs and equipment.

Rather than being considered a unit with direct access and specialised multidisciplinary approach operating in a range of action going from diagnosis to therapy, intensive care is seen as a "consulting" service. For this reason, it is still difficult to allocate the right budget to a service which still lacks an independent role. For example, in the United Kingdom it is not uncommon for an intensive care unit to depend economically on the Anaesthesia or Surgery Unit, though larger units can receive their own budget.

Designing programmes to promote the development of intensive care as a multidisciplinary specialisation may change the current situation [28]. However, the increasing competition among hospital management teams might lead to the imposition of cost thresholds which would hinder the expansion and regionalisation of intensive care. A good starting point is certainly the optimisation of service performance, in terms of both results (shorter recovery time, lower incidence of hospital infections, etc.) and cost containment. In this respect mention has to be made of a Canadian study describing an audit system used in a Canadian intensive care unit [29]. This system emphasises the integration of data acquisition (database function) with the use and analysis of these data (decision function). The system inputs include demographic information on the patients, diagnoses, complications, procedures applied, seriousness of the disease (APACHE II), therapies (TISS) and nurses' workload GRASP e TISS. The outputs of the system were evaluated by survival, duration of stay and ability to return home.

The annual operational costs were US$ 7,333 for 277 patients staying in the intensive-care unit above. Costs increased by US$ 58,261, including development programmes and costs for IT instruments. The unit's non-survivors were mainly those patients with a high APACHE II score on admission and/or those with longer recovery times. The workload of nurses (from the first to the last day of stay) was higher for non-survivors. The limitations of this system were the delay between admission into intensive care and data input, and the lack of a documented cause/effect relation between interventions and complications. This system proved more useful to management than in ensuring a higher quality of the service provided. Cost monitoring through these audit systems, proposed by the various authors in different forms (for example control of hospital infections, duration of stays, use of drugs, etc.), seems to be one of the most important instruments for the management of an economically autonomous and multidisciplinary intensive care unit (not simply a service).

Performance evaluation

Most proposals for the reform of some foreign health-care systems require both a direct and indirect evaluation of performance in health-care. Indirect evaluation is the judgement expressed by users and their families on the service received. Though it may not seem so, the intensive care unit can be an appropriate place for users (relatives, friends) to evaluate results, minimal though they may be, given the particular difficulty of the work, often due to the simultaneous presence of different combinations of serious diseases, the need for extremely rapid treatment and diagnosis and the very limited contact between operators and patients.

The most interesting investigation techniques include report cards, even though according to various authors they cannot bring about considerable quality improvements such as an increase in compliance with guidelines [30]. Despite that, similar industrial models are taking root in the medical field. In general, the fundamental element which brings about a quality increase is collaboration among the various health institutes, in terms of willingness to discuss possible interventions, exchanging decision-making protocols and trying to identify the reasons for a poor performance.

Research carried out by single hospitals has shown that a continuous improvement in quality is unanimously considered to produce an improvement of the treatment provided [8]. Unfortunately, not much information is available regarding hospitals which are collaborating in this respect [31, 32]. Recently, the collaboration between some thoracic surgery centres, whose efforts have successfully contributed to the decrease of post-operative mortality, has been made public [33]. Another example of collaboration between health facilities is that which took place among five hospitals associated to Harvard University [30]; from February 1993 to May 1995 they collected report cards filled in on a voluntary basis by various patients and used them to provide the medical staff with guidelines and evaluate compliance. This study evaluates patients' perceptions of the system's performance.

The objective of this type of approach is the identification of indicators to measure the quality of the service provided. The main indicators include: *com-*

munication, that is the willingness to put patients at ease and clarify any doubt regarding their disease using a comprehensible language; *treatment and follow-up management*, that is the ability to provide any information requested regarding the type of therapy chosen, administering methods and possible risks and behaviour to adopt outside the hospital (Table 2).

In short, the whole of all these interventions make up what is known as best practice, which is the result of clinical trials, group studies, administrative data collection and, lastly, the indication of preference and/or criticism by patients, who constitute are the actual target of best practice. For this reason, the development of data-driven benchmarking is a fundamental step to create a sort of archive containing above mentioned data.

Table 2. Problems reported by patients during the study carried out at Harvard [30]

Communication
Incapable of reporting in a suitable way to relatives/friends
Did not specify how long patient would have to wait to be examined
No linguistic assistance when asked for
Patient did not understand the causes of his/her disease
Treatment management
Patient did not understand the methods of treatment
Patient did not understand the treatment side effects
Patient did not take the drugs prescribed on leaving the hospital
Diagnostic exams
Patient did not understand the reason for the tests he/she underwent
Patient did not understand the results of the tests
Follow-up
Patient did not understand when to return to hospital
Patient did not understand the signs/symptoms which entailed a return to hospital
Patient did not understand when he/she could resume normal activities
Patient did not understand when he/she could return to work

Conclusions

The ideal working procedure should:

1. apply best practice whenever possible taking into account what is likely to take place in every-day practice;
2. use best evidence medicine whenever necessary;
3. consider patients' needs;
4. use resources adequately;
5. record data on the highest number of possible variables in intensive care and anaesthesia in order to create a real archive to collect as much information as possible on our activity.

Monitoring the global activity of a service (intensive care and anaesthesia), that is to say its performance, requires the identification of suitable parameters in the various clinical situations which can express performance in the conduct of activity.

These are quality indicators (some of which have already been discussed) of the system, which enable us to use figures for the simple expression of an otherwise complex judgement.

Though it may seem reductive and incomplete to express the performance of an anaesthesia and intensive care service with numerical indices, it is the complexity of the work carried out by doctors, in particular anaesthetists and intensive care operators, which makes it difficult effectively to monitor activities carried out. Hitherto, indicators seem the most realistic and reliable way to monitor the performance of such delicate and complex work.

References

1. Matchar DB, Samsa GP (1999) Using outcomes data to identify best medical practice: the role of policy models. Hepatology 29[Suppl 6]:36s-39s
2. Donabedian A (1980) Explorations in quality assessment and monitoring. Vol I: the definition of quality and approaches to its assessment. Ann Arbor: Health Admin Pr
3. Donabedian A (1988) The quality of care. How can it be assessed? JAMA 260:1743-1748
4. Lohr KN, Donaldson MS, Harris-Wehling J (1992) Medicare: a strategy for quality assurance. Qual Rev Bull 18:120-126
5. Zanetti M et al (1996) Il medico e il management
6. Frutiger A (1997) Process quality in intensive care unit. Acta Anaesthesiol Scand [Suppl] 111:14-16
7. Bennett D, Bion J (1999) ABC of intensive care: organisation of intensive care. BMJ 318:1468-1470
8. Rubenstein L, Fink A, Yano EM (1995) Increasing the impact of quality improvement in health: an expert panel method for setting institutional priorities. Jt Comm J Qual Improv 21:420-432
9. Posner KL, Freund PR (1999) Trends in quality of anesthesia care associated with changing staffing patterns, productivity and concurrency of case supervision in a teaching hospital. Anesthesiology 91:839-847
10. Bothner U, Georgieff M, Schwilk B (1999) The impact of minor perioperative anesthesia-related incidents, events and complications on postanesthesia care unit utilization. Anesth Analg 89:506-513
11. Falcon D, Francois P, Jacquot XYZ et al (1999) Evaluating the quality of anesthetic records. Ann Fr Anesth Reanim 18:360-367
12. Heinrichs W, Monk S, Eberle B (1997) Automated anesthesia record system. Anaesthesist 46:574-582
13. Myles PS, Williams DL, Hendrata M et al (2000) Patient satisfaction after anesthesia and surgery: results of a prospective survey of 10811 patients. Br J Anaesth 84:6-10
14. Myles PS, Hunt JO, Nightingale CE et al (1999) Development and psychometric testing of a quality of recovery score after general anesthesia and surgery in adults. Anesth Analg 88: 83-90
15. Myles PS, Weitkamp B, Jones K et al (2000) Validity and reliability of a postoperative quality of recovery score: the QoR-40. Br J Anaesth 84:11-15

16. Gunning K, Rowan K (1999) ABC of intensive care: outcome data and scoring systems. BMJ 319:241-244
17. Metnitz GH, Passler C, Vesely H et al (1997) Medical documentation: the value of scoring systems and database in intensive care medicine. Acta Anaesthesiol Scand [Suppl]111:11-12
18. Campbell NN, Tooley MA, Willats SM (1994) APACHE II scoring system on a general intensive care unit: audit of daily APACHE II scores and 6-month survival of 691 patients admitted to a general intensive care unit between May 1990 and December 1991. J R Soc Med 87:73-77
19. Eisemberg JM (1989) Clinical economics: a guide to the economic analysis of clinical practices. JAMA 262:2879-2886
20. Robinson R (1993) Cost benefit analysis. BMJ 307:924-926
21. Robinson R (1993) Cost effectiveness analysis. BMJ 307:793-795
22. Robinson R (1993) Cost-utility analysis. BMJ 307:859-862
23. Bach A, Schmidt H, Bottiger BW et al (1998) Economic aspects of anesthesia II. Cost control in clinical anesthesia. Anaesthesiol Intensivmed Notfallmed Schmerzther 33:210-231
24. Cotter SM, Petros AJ, Dore CJ et al (1991) Low flow anesthesia. Practice, cost implication and acceptability. Anaesthesia 46:1009-1012
25. Roizen MF, Schreider B, Austin W et al (1993) Pulse oxymetry, capnography and blood gas measurements: reducing cost and improving the quality of care with technology. J Clin Monit 9:237-240
26. Sung YF, Reiss N, Tillette T (1991) The differential cost of anesthesia and recovery with propofol-nitrous oxide anesthesia versus thiopental sodium-isofluorane-nitrous oxide anesthesia. J Clin Anesth 3:391-394
27. Cohen SE, Subak LL, Brose WG (1991) Analgesia after cesarean delivery: patient evaluations and costs of five opioid techniques. Reg Anesth 16:141-149
28. Bion J (1994) Cost containment: Europe. The United Kingdom. New Horiz 2:341-344
29. Byrick RJ, Caskennette GM (1992) Audit of critical care: aims, uses, costs and limitations of a Canadian system. Can J Anaesth 39:260-269
30. Burstin HR, Conn A, Setnik G (1999) Benchmarking and quality improvement: the Harvard emergency department quality study. Am J Med 107:437-449
31. Institute for Health Care Improvement (1996) Breakthrough series report
32. Shortell SM, Bennett CL, Byck GR (1998) Assess the impact of continuous quality improvement on clinical practice. What will it take to accelerate progress? Millbank Quarterly 76:593-627
33. O'Connor GT, Plume SK, Olmstead EM (1996) A regional intervention to improve the hospital mortality associated with coronary artery by-pass surgery. JAMA 275:841-846

Albumin in Critical Care – Use, Abuse, or Misuse

F. Mercuriali, G. Inghilleri

Albumin is a small highly symmetric, slightly heterogeneous protein weighing 67,000 daltons with a high cysteine content, composed of a single chain of 584 amino acids with a quaternary helix-like structure. The center of the molecule is made up of hydrophobic radicals, which are binding sites for many ligands. The outer part of the molecule is composed of hydrophilic radicals. Albumin is a relatively small protein in terms of space, but its size is sufficient to prevent it from crossing the capillary membrane [1].

Albumin contains a large amount of aspartic and glutamic acids and few leucine and tryptophan. This structure explains the high stability of the protein with respect to physicochemical influences. Albumin's overall charge is negative under physiological conditions and it presents the best solubility characteristics of any plasma protein. At the pH of blood (pH 7.4), the net charge on the albumin molecule, calculated from its amino acid composition, is –15.

Albumin is the most-important plasma protein in quantitative terms and accounts for the biggest percentage of plasma protein (60%), the plasma concentration being 3.5 – 5g/dl. Its synthesis takes place exclusively in the liver, normally at a rate that is controlled largely by the osmotic pressure of the interstitial fluid. However, other factors such as the nutritional status, some cytokines, and several hormones including insulin, glucagon, cortisol, and thyroid hormones, may regulate its production. The synthesis of albumin, which represents about 10% of the liver's protein synthesis, is rapid but the hepatic reserves are small [2]. About 15 g of albumin (about 5%) is metabolized and synthesized daily in the normal steady state. Besides the small amount lost in the gut, the removal by circulation occurs in various organs but healthy kidneys. The median half life is about 18 days.

Total body stores in adults approximate 4.5 g/kg of body weight, about 60% of which is extravascular and 40% intravascular. Half of the extravascular albumin is concentrated close to the skin, which explains the rapid and dramatic protein losses occurring after burns. Generally the various extravascular pools equilibrate rapidly with the intravascular pool. These pools are part of a complex regulatory process of fluid exchange involving hydrostatic and osmotic forces. Albumin is a dynamic protein and in an hour about 5% of albumin leaves the circulation and, after tissue passage, returns through the lymphatic system. In 1 day the entire albumin pool is recycled. The exchange of albumin molecules between the intravascular and extravascular pools occurs by two general processes: endocytosis and a receptor-mediated transcytotic pathway by which molecules are transported through the endothelial cell to the target cell [2, 3].

Functions

The study of albumin reveals a complex picture of this molecule, which serves probably more functions than supposed to date. Albumin has a high water binding capacity of approximately 18 ml/g. This property, together with the rapidity with which the extravascular and intravascular pools equilibrate, determines the physiological importance of albumin in the regulation of water and volume distribution between intravascular and interstitial space. At the normal serum concentration, albumin accounts for a colloid osmotic pressure (COP) of 16-18 mmHg, that is from 60 to 70% of the total oncotic pressure at 26-28 mmHg.

Beside the major contribution to the COP in plasma, albumin exerts other biological functions, although in patients with hereditary abscncc of albumin the clinical picture is not seriously compromised and the disease allows the attainment old age [4].

Another important function of the albumin molecule, mainly due to the high negative charge, relates to the binding and transport of a large number of compounds, including drugs. Albumin is very effective in binding small molecules of many types and for this property is considered a sponge of the circulation. Both cations and anions can be reversibly bound by the albumin molecule. Trace metals, fatty acids, hormones, enzymes, and pharmaceutical products are transported and neutralized in this manner, and also metabolic products such as bilirubin. Albumin also binds foreign proteins, such as protein G of streptococcal cell wall [5]. This property of microbial proteins binding to albumin may contribute to microbial virulence, as this association prevents the identification and the elimination of the microbial agents by specific antibodies and complement.

Albumin products

Albumin solutions for therapeutic use have been available since the middle of the last century after the development of the cold alcohol fractionation technique (usually referred as Cohn alcohol extraction method) which, allows extraction of highly purified albumin protein from human plasma. The Cohn process is still the basis for the large-scale production of albumin today; however the quality of albumin preparations has definitely improved over the last 10 years, which should be kept in mind when reviewing results of earlier trials. The great advantage of the fractionation method lies in its proven safety. The Cohn fractionation process efficiently inactivates human immunodeficiency virus. Moreover, albumin products withstand virus inactivation by heat (pasteurization) [6, 7].

Three albumin products are currently manufactured: the albumin (human) 25%, albumin (human) 5%, and plasma protein fraction (PPF). To be designated albumin, > 96% of the protein content must be albumin. PPF is an albumin product of lower purity, obtained by co-precipitating fraction IV-4 with fraction V. The total protein in PPF must be 83% albumin, with 17% globulins, and 1% γ-globulin. PPF is more economical to produce than albumin. However, this product is less safe as the rapid infusion of PPF has been associated with hypotensive episodes.

Albumin 5% is an iso-oncotic infusion solution with normal plasma, which increases blood volume by the quantity actually administered. The use of 5% albumin solutions improves the microcirculation by reducing the viscosity of the circulating blood or blood plasma as a result hemodilution. This increases cardiac output.

Albumin 20% is a hyperoncotic infusion solution which creates a volume effect equivalent to approximately 3 or 4 times the quantity administered. This volume effect results in the withdrawal of liquid from the extravascular space. In case of volume deficiency, it must be administered together with another suitable fluid. Albumin 20% is ideally suited for treating hypoalbuminemia, as the volume load remains low.

Clinical use of albumin products

Albumin solutions were adopted with enthusiasm by the medical community with the hope that recipients would benefit from the many physiological roles of albumin, and because of the sense of security provided by pasteurization, and the perceived advantage of a human protein versus artificial colloids prone to provoke life-threatening allergic reactions [8]. In contrast to artificial colloids, albumin solutions have no maximal doses and have a sustained effect on volemia. One of the reasons that promoted the widespread use of albumin solution in the clinical setting was the observation that in patients with acute and chronic illness the serum albumin concentration is inversely related to the risk of death. A systematic review of cohort studies meeting specific criteria calculated that for each 2.5 g/l reduction in serum albumin concentration the risk of death increases by between 24% and 56% [9].

Thus, although albumin was first introduced as a plasma volume expander, albumin administration was proposed and widely utilized in all clinical conditions associated with hypoalbuminaemia, even if there was little or no supporting evidence of a benefit [10, 11]. In the last 2 decades concerns on the high cost and the limited supply of the drug led to a number of efforts to define appropriate and inappropriate uses of this product [2, 12, 13].

Currently licensed indications for human albumin solutions are the emergency treatment of shock and other conditions in which restoration of blood volume is urgent, the acute management of burns, and acute clinical situations associated with hypoproteinemia in intensive care patients. However, the administration of albumin in these clinical settings continues to be controversial, as a number of studies have questioned the efficacy of albumin supplementation.

In 1985, Grundmann and Heistermann [14] published the results of a prospective, randomized study investigating the relationship between the COP and the postoperative course of 220 patients. The patients were randomized into two groups, with patients in each group receiving albumin when their COP dropped below a defined limit, which was 24 cm H_2O for group 1 and 29 cm H_2O for group 2. There were no differences in length of stay, recorded complications, or need for artificial ventilation. Other studies have since shown the feasibility of managing patients at lower COP levels, sometimes below 15 mmHg [10].

Similar results have been obtained by Foley et al. [15], who compared treatment with 25% human albumin in order to keep serum albumin concentrations above 25 g/l versus no treatment in 40 consecutive randomly assigned adult patients referred to the nutrition support service in a major north-American hospital. Albumin administration was effective in correcting hypoalbuminemia and maintaining serum albumin concentration at target levels. However, no significant differences could be found in terms of mortality (7/18 treated patients, versus 6/22 untreated) or major complications (16/18 treated versus 17/22 untreated). Lengths of hospital and intensive care unit (ICU) stay, and duration of artificial ventilation were shorter in the untreated group, but these differences failed to reach statistical significance. It is interesting to note that serum albumin levels rose spontaneously in the group of patients receiving no albumin, as their underlying condition improved.

The authors have been criticised for having used questionable allocation procedures (patients were randomized according to their medical record number). Nevertheless, their study has been instrumental in showing that, while hypoalbuminemia remains an ominous sign in many pathologies, correcting this symptom with albumin transfusions will not improve outcome.

Albumin administration has also been found ineffective in improving morbidity and mortality in ICU patients in a very large study published by Stockwell et al. in 1992 [16]. In this study, 475 consecutive adult patients admitted to an ICU were randomized to receive either a 4.5% human albumin solution or a synthetic colloid (polygelin), whenever volume replacement was considered, based on clinical status or invasive pressure measurements [16]. All patients received crystalloid solutions and enferal/parnteral nutrition to satisfy their basic fluid and nutritional requirements. Despite an older age (64 versus 60 years) and a slightly higher APACHE II score (14 versus 12) in the polygelin group, the mortality was exactly the same with both regimens (20%), and so was the length of ICU stay (3 days). Subpopulation analyses of patients starting with more-severe clinical conditions (e.g., APACHE II > 10) or staying longer than 5 days in the ICU yielded similar results. In an associated paper, the same authors focused on the influence of treatment allocation on serum albumin concentrations [17]. In the albumin group, non-survivors showed a tendency for serum albumin to decrease below 25 g/l. However, in the polygelin group serum albumin concentrations rapidly decreased below 22 g/l in all patients, survivors and non-survivors alike. These findings indicate that a low serum albumin concentration per se was not a direct cause of poor outcome, although failure to maintain near normal serum albumin concentrations despite albumin infusions heralded a poor outcome. Among patients who stayed more than 5 days in the ICU, slightly more patients developed renal failure (10 versus 4%) pulmonary edema (15 versus 11%), or both (8 versus 6%) in the polygelin group, but these differences failed to reach statistical significance. Unfortunately, these issues are somewhat confounded because 4 patients in the albumin group and 13 in the polygelin group also received concentrated albumin to treat peripheral or pulmonary edema, mostly in association with dialysis. Besides confirmation of Foley's conclusions, the main value of this study for the clinician (and the manager) is its demonstration on a large scale that replacing expensive albumin solutions with polygelin solutions as first-line volume replacement in an ICU will not result in measurable changes in outcome.

Moreover, a recent meta-analysis performed by the Cochrane group of available randomized controlled trials comparing the administration of albumin solutions with standard therapies found very negative results with the use of albumin as a volume expander [18]. Thirty trials, published between 1975 and 1997, involving 1,495 patients were included and were subdivided according to the main indication for albumin administration: hypovolemia (20 trials, 790 patients), burn (3 trials, 163 patients), and hypoalbuminemia (9 trials, 542 patients). For all three main indications, the Cochrane analysis found an excess mortality in the albumin (or high-albumin) patients.

The relative risk of dying when allocated to receive albumin was 1.46 when the indication was hypovolemia, 1.69 for hypoalbuminemia, and 2.40 for burns. The overall excess mortality was 6.8%, or about 6 additional deaths for every 100 patients treated with albumin. The conclusion of the study was that "[...] the use of human albumin in the management of critically ill patients should be reviewed. A strong argument could be made that human albumin should not be used outside the context of a properly concealed and otherwise rigorously conducted randomized controlled trial with mortality as the end point".

Many critics have voiced concern of the selection of trial, the pooling of neonatal and adult populations, or the inclusion of studies conducted with old solutions of albumin prepared before the advent of modern purification techniques. It is indeed possible that some of the oldest trials heavily influenced the reported excess mortality. Reassessing the data to answer such critics could reduce the calculated excess mortality, but never reverse it. The major conclusion of the Cochrane analysis remains therefore unchallenged, namely that the administration of albumin solutions to a wide variety of acutely ill patients provides no proven benefit over crystalloids.

As a result of the debate on the efficacy of albumin solution, the utilization of albumin for the treatment of post burn shock has also dramatically changed over the last decade. Current guidelines favor the exclusive use of crystalloids during the 1st h post burn and propose the introduction of artificial colloids and human albumin solutions after the 8 h post burn [19, 20]. At this stage, colloids could have a positive effect by reclaiming water from edematous non-burned tissues when they regain a normal endothelial permeability. No attempt should be made to normalize serum albumin levels: it has been shown that concentrations as low as 15 g/l can be tolerated without deleterious consequences [21]. Furthermore, improving circulating volume may not improve renal function [22]. Therapy should be guided by the hemodynamic status, as assessed by urine output, cardiac echography, or more-invasive pressure and output measurements, rather than by serum albumin concentrations.

Albumin solutions are still considered the fluid of choice for fluid resuscitation in infants and neonates who present specific features as regards their circulating proteinic fluid balance. First, their plasmatic volume is relatively large compared to adults. Second, their endothelial permeability is greater than that of adults. third, their serum albumin concentration varies over time: it is low at birth but increases with age. Albumin plays a vital role during the first days of life because it transports and neutralizes unconjugated bilirubin, preventing this toxic metabolite from reaching the intracranial grey matter and protecting against the feared “kernicterus”. Fourth, maternal immunoglobulins contribute to the colloid osmotic pressure. Their concentration is lower in premature children and decreases after the 3rd month of life. For all these reasons, newborns, and especially premature babies, are at high risk of significant fluid shifts from the intravascular to the extravascular compartment, with subsequent hypovolemia and circulatory failure. Mild to moderate hypovolemia can be treated with 0.9% normal saline or lactated Ringer’s solutions, but fluid resuscitation should quickly resort to human albumin solutions because of the specific transport capacity of this protein. Artificial colloids are therefore not recommended in infants.

Conclusions

Increase of albumin use has been facilitated by the availability and the producers promoted uses for which there was little or no supporting evidence of a benefit. However, the high cost of albumin relative to less-expensive alternatives, such as non-protein colloid (e.g., hetastarch, dextran) and crystalloid solutions (e.g., lactated Ringer's solution, various sodium chloride solutions), has intensified clinical use of resuscitation fluids. In response to the controversy, a number of consensus conferences were held about the use of albumin in many countries [23, 24].

Their main conclusions are similar: there is no scientifically documented minimal albumin plasma concentration above which a specific treatment must be instituted; there is no obvious indication for using human albumin solutions to treat hypovolemia in emergency or intensive care situations; human albumin solutions are not first-line treatments for perioperative hypovolemia; human albumin is justified only when artificial colloids are contraindicated in case of severe hypoproteinemia (< 35 g/l) unrelated to dilution during resuscitation.

Residual indications concern mainly neonatology, end-stage medical conditions, adjuvant therapy for infrequent techniques such as plasma exchange, some transplantation surgeries, and burns (with some controversy). Almost nothing remains apart from its main usage as ideal volume replacement for the surgical or critically ill patient. Many questions remain unanswered concerning, for example, the pharmacological interactions of albumin transfusion. The place in modern pharmacopeia of this colloid with both a long intravascular half-life and a remarkable absence of toxicity remains to be defined. Despite so many years of clinical use, there is still a definite need for properly conducted prospective randomized trials.

References

1. Peters Jr (1985) The serum albumin. Adv Protein Chem 37:161-245
2. Sgouris JT, Rene A eds (1976) Proceedings of the workshop on albumin, 1975. National Heart and Lung Institute, US Dept of Heath, Education, and Welfare Publication NIH, Bethesda, Maryland, pp 876-925
3. Tullis JL (1977) Albumin. Background and use. JAMA 237:355-360
4. Watkins S, Madison J, Galliano M et al (1994) Analbuminemia: three cases resulting from different point mutations in the albumin gene. Proc Natl Acad Sci U S A 91:9417-9421
5. Falkenberg C, Bjork L, Akerstrom B (1992) Localization of the binding site for streptococcal proteins G on human serum albumin. Identification of a 5.5-kilodalton protein G binding albumin fragment. Biochemistry 31:14551-14557
6. Kistler P, Nitschmenn HS (1962) Large-scale production of human plasma fractions. Vox Sang 7:414-424
7. Burnouf T, Huart JJ (1994) Human albumin: toxicological and viral safety. Arch Public Health 52:331-345
8. Laxenaere MC, Charpentier C, Feldman L (1994) Anaphylactoid reactions to colloid plasma substitutes: incidence, risk factors mechanisms. A French multicenter prospective study. Ann Fr Anesth Reanim 13:301-310
9. Goldwasser P, Feldman J (1997) Association of serum albumin and mortality risk. J Clin Epidemiol 50:693-703

10. Grootendorst AF, vanWilgenburg MG, de Laat PH et al (1988) Albumin abuse in intensive care medicine. Intensive Care Med 14:554-557
11. James WPT, Hay AM (1988) Albumin metabolism: effect of albumin supplementation during parenteral nutrition on hospital morbidity. Crit Care Med 16:1177-182
12. Erstad BL, Gales B, Rappaport WD (1991) The use of albumin in clinical practice. Arch Intern Med 151:901-911
13. Swisher SN (ed) (1980) Report of Panel 6 on Safety and Efficacy of Blood and Blood Derivatives. Bureau of Biologics, Food and Drug Administration. The Federal Register
14. Grundmann R, Heistermann S (1985) Postoperative albumin infusion therapy based on colloid osmotic pressure. Arch Surg 120:911-915
15. Foley EF, Borlase BC, Dzik WH et al (1990) Albumin supplementation in the critically ill. Arch Surg 125:739-742
16. Stockwell MA, Soni N, Riley B (1992) Colloid solutions in the critically ill: a randomised comparison of albumin and polygeline. 1. Outcome and duration of stay in the intensive care unit. Anaesthesia 47:3-6
17. Stockwell MA, Scott A, Day A et al (1992) Colloid solutions in the critically ill. A randomized comparison of albumin and polygeline. 2. Serum albumin concentration and incidences of pulmonary oedema and acute renal failure. Anaesthesia 47:7-9
18. Cochrane Injuries Group Albumin Reviewers (1998) Human albumin administration in critically ill patients: systematic review of randomised controlled trials. B M J 317:235-239
19. Monafo WW (1996) Initial management of burns. N Engl J Med 335:1581-1586
20. Warden GD (1996) Fluid resuscitation and early management. Total Burn Care 53-60
21. Schlagintweit S, Snelling CGT, German E et al (1990) Major burns managed without blood or blood products. J Burn Care Rehabil 11:214
22. Gore DC, Dalton JM, Gehr TW (1996) Colloid infusions reduce glomerular filtration in resuscitated burn victims. J Trauma 40:356-360
23. Vermeulen LC, Ratko TA, Erstad BL et al (1995) A paradigm for consensus. The university hospital consortium guidelines for the use of albumin, nonprotein colloid and crystalloid solutions. Arch Intern Med 155:373-379
24. Yim JM, Vermeulen LV, Erstad BI et al (1995) Albumin and non protein colloid solution use in US academic health centers. Arch Intern Med 155:2450-2455

Real-Time Monitoring of the Process of Care

D. REIS MIRANDA, R. NAP

Monitoring in the intensive care unit

Monitoring is perhaps the most-important activity in the intensive care unit (ICU). In every indication for admission to the unit, the monitoring of one or more vital functions is always listed as a primary objective. Given the requirements for specialized staff and equipment, the monitoring of the critically ill patient in the hospital usually takes place in the ICU.

In general, the monitoring in the ICU fulfils three functions: 1) to complement the clinical information leading to meaningful diagnoses; 2) to objectively assess clinical changes of illness with time; 3) to detect the onset of life-threatening conditions occurring during the course of illness.

The nursing staff is responsible for the large part of monitoring. The monitoring of the critically ill is integrated in a cycle of professional actions depicted in Fig. 1, and usually called the 'cycle of titrated therapy': the registration of the values of the physiologic a parameters measured is regularly assessed, in the view of the objectives indicated in the previous paragraph.

It is fair to say that, for a substantial number of patient-days in the ICU, the monitoring performed is mainly associated with standards of quality of care in the unit. In other words, quite often, monitoring does not lead to particular action. In these cases, the monitoring registers are carefully observed, before the next policies of care are formalized.

In the ICU, the monitoring can be continuous (e.g., heart rate, blood pressure, oxygen saturation, and diuresis) or discontinuous (e.g., laboratory analysis). The type of, and methods used in the monitoring are almost standard in all ICUs around the world. The reason for this is that the design and the technical specifications of the equipment for monitoring (particularly continuous monitoring) are determined by the industrial enterprises involved in their complex manufacture. In the last 2 decades, much resources have been invested in the development of sophisticated features of monitoring. For example, the retrospective construction of trends of physiological variables with time and the generation of alarms when the variables fall outside a preset range of values. One may argue that some of those features are provided because they are technically possible. It would be however unfair to omit, that usually the industry performs these devel-

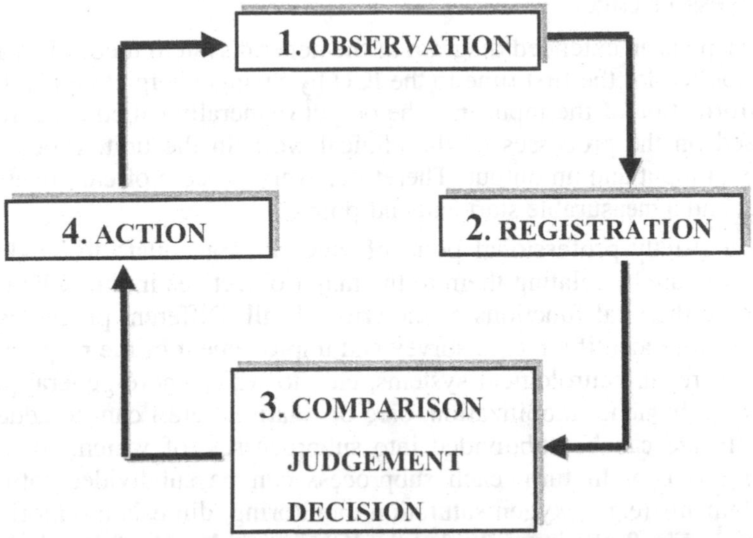

Fig. 1. Monitoring of the critically ill patient is integrated in a cycle of professional actions. With permission of Frice

opments in close collaboration with the medical and nursing professionals. The majority of the features included in the monitoring equipment purchased by the ICUs was suggested by those working in the field. The use of this equipment is recommended in the official guidelines available for ICUs [1, 2].

The purchase cost of this equipment is high (about 100,000 Euros per ICU bed). The exploitation costs of the monitoring can also be high, in those cases where specific disposals (catheters, tubings, etc.) are required. Besides the direct cost of the equipment, the cost incurred by the use of ICUstaff is much higher: the nurses spent about 20% of their time with the monitoring activities (Reis Miranda et al., in preparation).

In summary, there is a strong consensus among professionals about the importance of monitoring in the ICU, and about the parameters to be monitored; the performance of monitoring is perhaps the single most-expensive activity in the unit.

However, recent publications cast doubts on the value of the monitoring practised in the ICU [3-6]. The clinical value of the often-sophisticated alarm systems has particularly come under scrutiny [7]: the percentage of alarms not leading to clinical action (and therefore called false alarms) was high (33%), whereas only 6% of the alarms required the presence of a clinician.

The process of care

Figure 2 depicts an extended diagram of the general system theory [8]. This theory was applied for the first time to the ICU by Spangenberg et al. [9]. In Fig. 2, the transformation of the input into the output (generally called the throughput) is focussed on the processes of the clinical work in the unit. Processes have therefore an input and an output. Therefore, every process of care does have an objective, and a measurable start and end-point.

From a strictly professional point of view, it is adequate to subdivide the processes of care by relating them to the major objectives in the ICU: to survey and improve the vital functions of the critically ill. Different processes of care can be therefore identified, e.g., survey and improvement of the respiratory, cardiovascular, renal, neurological systems, etc., to which more-general processes of care (e.g., hygiene, mobilization, care of relatives, etc.) can be added. Each process of care can be subdivided into subprocesses, of which, for example, monitoring is one. In turn, each subprocess can be subdivided into smaller processelements (e.g., oxygen saturation monitoring, diuresis monitoring, etc.), and so on. In Fig. 2, the input is what the ICU gets to be transformed; the output will express both the objective of the transformation process, and the result of the transformation itself (allowing for the analysis of the effectiveness of the process). After the inventory of the processes of care in the ICU have been performed, all elements of every process are identified and understood in a dynamic manner.

In Fig. 2, decision making occupies a prominent position. Given the admitted case-mix, and the stated objectives of care, decision making is necessary regarding both the activities in the involved processes of care (e.g., guidelines, protocols, instructions in specific cases, etc.) and the related allocation/use of resources.

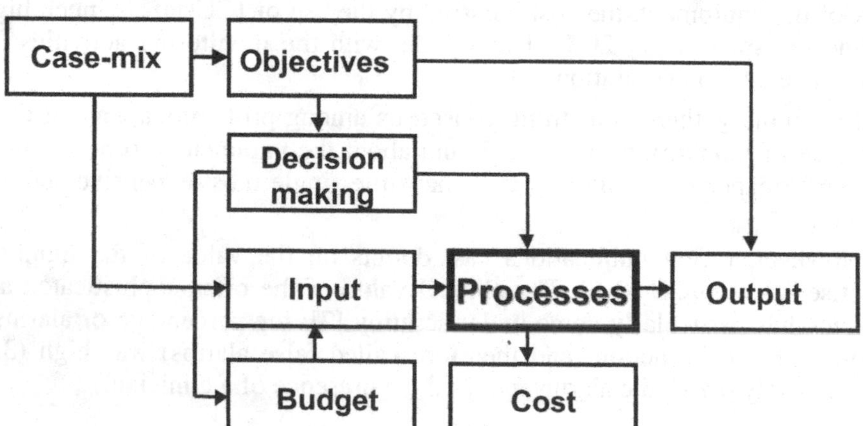

Fig. 2. General system theory. With permission of Frice

Results of the Euricus-II study

The Euricus-II study, or "the effect of harmonizing and standardizing the nursing tasks in the ICUs of the European Community", was a concerted action included in the Biomed-2 research program of the European Commission (Contract: BMH4-CT96-0817). This 3-year study (1996-1999) was implemented in 41 European ICUs by the Foundation for Research on Intensive Care in Europe (FRICE). Recently ended, the results of this study will be presented in different publications that are in preparation. The interested reader is recommended to visit the web site www.frice.nl, for further information.

The survey of the incidence and the duration of real-time alarm conditions, concerning the activity of monitoring in the ICUs, was an important part of the study. The physiological parameters assessed in the study were those commonly monitored in ICUs in a continuous manner: systolic blood pressure (BP), heart rate (HR), oxygen saturation ($SatO_2$), and urinary output. The nurses were instructed to register, on special study-forms, each time the values of the physiological parameters were out of the ranges set every day by the physicians. Ranges of normality/acceptance, developed by a panel of ICUprofessionals, were suggested to the leadership of the ICUs (so that a common baseline was created in the survey). The ICUs were, however, allowed to deviate from the suggested values, in case of need (e.g., chronic obstructive pulmonary disease, anuria, etc.). The recommended ranges were: 90-180 mmHg for BP, $\geq$ 90% for $SatO_2$, 60-120 beats per min for HR, and $\geq$ 30 ml/h for urine output.

In order to avoid alarms due to technical error, the 'out-of-rangemeasurements' (ORM, or deviance of range of acceptance) were registered only when the 'alarm' persisted for at least (about) 10 min. Two types of ORMs were defined: 1) "event" (Ev). The ORM lasted for more than 10 min and for less than 1 h (1 h or more in the case of urine output); 2) "critical event" (CrEv). The ORM lasted for more than 1 h (2 h or more in the case of urine output).

During the 10-month field research at the ICUs, data from 20,000 patients and 100,000 patient-days were collected. During this period, 300,000 ORMs were registered. At least 1 ORM was observed in three-quarters of all the patients. The incidence of Evs and CrEvs, indexed to the number of patient-days (overall and divided into survivors and non-survivors) is shown in Table 1. The incidence of Ev in the group of non-survivors was at least 3 times higher than in the group of survivors. Taking the example of BP, the patients who survived had on average one event every 2nd day; whereas those who died had, on average, almost two BP events every day. The mean duration of each CrEv was also significantly longer in the group of non-survivors (Table 1). The mean duration of a BP CrEv, for example, was about 2 h and a half in the survivors, and almost 4 h in the non-survivors.

A more-detailed analysis of the data (Silva et al., in preparation) has shown:

1. the incidence and the duration of ORMs is associated with mortality after controlling for (SAPS) (simple acute physiological score) and for age;

Table 1. Incidence of out-of-range measurements (ORM)

	Incidence of ORM		
Ev	Overall	Survivors	Non-survivors
BP	0.67 ± 1.33	0.50 ± 1.04	1.73 ± 2.16
HR	0.47 ± 1.21	0.36 ± 0.99	1.19 ± 1.96
$SatO_2$	0.27 ± 0.90	0.18 ± 0.70	0.79 ± 1.57
Urine output	0.72 ± 1.64	0.57 ± 1.33	1.66 ± 2.69
CrEv			
BP	0.25 ± 0.44	0.18 ± 0.36	0.68 ± 0.60
HR	0.17 ± 0.35	0.12 ± 0.29	0.47 ± 0.51
$SatO_2$	0.09 ± 0.26	0.05 ± 0.19	0.32 ± 0.47
Urine output	0.29 ± 0.50	0.23 ± 0.45	0.68 ± 0.64
CrEv duration (h)			
BP	2.97 ± 2.40	2.58 ± 1.99	3.95 ± 2.98
HR	3.60 ± 3.00	3.40 ± 2.80	4.05 ± 3.33
$SatO_2$	2.90 ± 2.69	2.55 ± 2.43	3.48 ± 2.99
Urine output	3.80 ± 3.47	3.03 ± 2.57	5.94 ± 4.57

Ev event, *CrEv* critical event, *BP* blood pressure, *HR* heart rate, $SatO_2$ oxygen saturation

2. the same is true for the association of ORMs with organ system failure;
3. the incidence and the duration of ORMs are better predictors of mortality than SAPS;
4. the incidence and the duration of ORMs the day before discharge to the ward are good predictors of after ICUdischarge mortality [10-12].

Real-time monitoring

During the last 2 decades, we have assisted with the impressive development of the science of predicting outcomes. As a consequence, the attention of the clinicians has been focussed on the outcomes of illness. In this scientific domain, the work of the research groups led by Knaus, Lemeshow, and Le Gall is sufficiently well known and will not be discussed here. After describing some relevant characteristics of the illnesses admitted to the ICU, these authors constructed scoring systems that are able to predict the outcome of patients, according to the observed combination of characteristics. Comparison of the predicted and observed outcomes has been advocated as a measure of the effectiveness of the ICU involved. In the last few years, however, the hope and enthusiasm surrounding these measurements has weakened. The expected precision of prediction was impaired by problems related to the methodologies used in the development of the scoring systems [13]. It has also became clear that the focus on the outcomes of illness does not provide information about the processes of transformation that lead to the outcomes under analysis. In other words, if one wants to influence the outcome of illness, one has to be able to influence the course of illness, by controlling the relevant processes of care.

The lack of expected success from the use of the severity of illness scoring systems focussed attention on the processes of care. To be more precise, however, the increasing focus on the processes of care in the ICU is due to an important change in the approach of health care systems in the last decade: the effectiveness and the efficiency of health care can only be mastered if one knows (and does!) what has to be done. The importance of this approach, is that it offers a more-rational organizational framework to care [14].

In the context of the above, the monitoring of the processes of care in the ICU should (will!) regain the attention of the critical care practitioners. It is a reliable guide in the timely support of vital functions and can be used for auditing the quality of care.

References

1. Task Force of Critical Care Medicine (1998) Recommendations for services and personnel for delivery of in a care critical care setting. Crit Care Med 16:809-811
2. Task Force of the European Society of Intensive Care Medicine (1997) Recommendations on minimal requirements for Intensive Care Departments. Intensive Care Med 23:226-232
3. Koski EM, Makivirta A, Sukuvaara T et al (1990) Frequency and reliability of alarms in the monitoring of cardiac postoperative patients. J Clin Monit Comput 7:129-133
4. Meredith C, Edworthy J (1995) Are there too many alarms in the intensive care unit? An overview of the problems. J Adv Nurs 2:15-20
5. Tsien CL, Fackler JC (1997) Poor prognosis for existing monitors in the intensive care. Crit Care Med 25:614-619
6. Friesdorf W, Buss B, Gobel M (1999) Monitoring alarms – the key to patient safety in the ICU? Intensive Care Med 25:1350-1352
7. Chambrin MC, Ravaux P, Calvelo-Aros D et al (1999) Multicentric study of monitoring alarms in the adult intensive care unit (ICU): a descriptive analysis. Intensive Care Med 25: 1360-1366
8. Hitchins DK (1992) Putting systems to work. Wiley, Chichester
9. Spangenberg JFA, van der Poel JHR, Iapichino G (1990) Management control in the ICU. In: Reis Miranda D, Williams A, Loirat P (eds) Management of intensive care: guidelines for better use of resources. Kluwer, Dordrecht, pp 103-123
10. Silva AM, Nap RE, Reis Miranda D (1999) Monitoring adverse events in the ICU and patient outcome. Intensive Care Med 25[Suppl 1]S166
11. Silva AM, Nap RE, Reis Miranda D (1999) Monitoring adverse events and organ dysfunction. Intensive Care Med 25[Suppl 1]S167
12. Silva AM, Nap RE, Reis Miranda D (2000) Last day monitoring in the intensive care and mortality after discharge. Intensive Care Med 26[Suppl]
13. Reis Miranda D, Moreno R (1997) Intensive care unit models and their role in management and utilization programs. Curr Opin Crit Care 3:183-187
14. Reis Miranda D, Ryan DW, Schaufeli WB, Fidler V (eds) (1998) Organisation and management of intensive care; a prospective study in 12 European countries. Springer, Berlin Heidelberg New York

EDUCATION

Anesthesia Residency Education in America

B. Mets

This review will be based on the available information defined in the references quoted as well as serve as a practical example of how a residency program is run based on my experience as Residency Director for Anesthesiology for the last 7 years. The Columbia Department of Anesthesiology has 47 residents and 15 fellows in training and comprises 70 academic faculty all of whom practise clinical anesthesiology. We practise all aspects of anesthesia and are a major heart, liver, lung and kidney transplant center. Our department has a major research component and more than 2 million dollars in NIH research funding annually.

Goals set by the American Board of Anesthesiology for anesthesia residency training in the USA

In 1941, the Advisory Board for medical specialities approved the establishment of the American Board of Anesthesiology as a separate primary Board [1].

The American Board of Anesthesiology (ABA) certifies specialists in Anesthesia, and controls the training of anesthesiologists by setting the goals for training, and determining the length as well as the structure of this training. In turn, the Board informs the Accreditation Council for Graduate Medical Education (ACGME) as to the training required of individuals seeking certification.

In the USA, residency program requirements (what constitutes an adequate program) are certified by the ACGME (Accreditation Council of Graduate Medical Education) [2]. Residency programs are inspected 5 yearly by this body to ensure this. The ABA (American Board of Anesthesiology) sets the standard and requirements that an individual must meet to be allowed to sit the examination to be certified as a Diplomat of the ABA. The clinical and professional component of this requirement is that after one year of an internship (designated PGY1; for postgraduate year one) a candidate completes three years of clinical anesthesia training (designated CA1, CA2 and CA3 years) in a program certified by the ACGME. Residency program directors have to submit, 6 monthly, a standard report to the ABA of satisfactory clinical competence for each resident trainee [1].

The categories that have to be designated as satisfactory vs unsatisfactory on a form are:

Table 1

Essential attributes

1. Is honest and ethical
2. Is reliable, conscientious and responsible
3. Learns from experience
4. Reacts to stressful situations in an appropriate manner
5. Has no documented abuse of alcohol or drugs in the last 6 month period. Has no cognitive, physical, sensory or motor impairment that precludes individual responsibility for any aspect of anesthesiology care

If any one of the above attributes is graded unsatisfactory the resident cannot get credit for the 6-month period

Acquired character skills

Knowledge

Judgement

i) General medicine appropriate for the practise of anesthesiology
ii) Preoperative preparation
iii) Intra-operative management
iv) Postoperative care

Clinical skills

i) General preparation
ii) General anesthesia
iii) Regional anesthesia
iv) Acute and chronic pain management
v) Special procedures

Overall clinical competence

If the overall clinical competence is regarded as unsatisfactory, the residency director must note on the form supplied for this purpose what the most serious deficiencies are [1]

In addition to this the resident, through the offices of the Residency Program, must submit yearly, the number of different procedures/anesthetics, defined by categories, on a standardized form, (now computerized) to the ACGME [2].

The ACGME has mandated the minimal experience in terms of what a resident must perform as indicated here (Table 2). It is expected that this experience be achieved within the first two clinical anesthesia years (i.e., the CA1 and CA2 years).

Thus in order to be eligible for entrance into the ABA examination system, a resident must complete an internship (clinical base year) in the USA and successfully complete 3 years of anesthesia residency. This is known as the continuum of education in anesthesia.

Table 2. ACGME clinical experience requirements [2]

Obstetrics
- 40 anesthetics for vaginal delivery
- 20 anesthetics for cesarean section

Pediatrics
- 100 children < 12 years
- Including 15 infants < 1 year
- Including infants < 45 weeks postconceptual age

Cardiacs
- Anesthesia for 20 surgeries with CPB
- 20 intrathoracic procedures
- 20 other major vascular cases

Neuro
- 20 open cranium operations
- Including intracerebral vascular procedures

General
- 50 epidurals for surgery or C-section
- 50 spinals for surgical procedures
- 40 peripheral nerve blocks for surgical procedures

Orthoepaedics
- 40 peripheral nerve blocks

Pain
- 25 nerve blocks for acute or chronic cancer or pain procedures
- Documented involvement in acute post-op pain, PCA, and other pain control modalities

Preop
- Documented involvement in systematic process of the preoperative management of the patient

Recovery room
- 2 continuous weeks

Significant experience with fiber-optic intubation, PAC placement, central catheterization, evoked potentials, EEG. "The patient's medical record should contain evidence of preoperative and postoperative anesthesia assessment"

American Board of Anesthesiology examination

The examination consists of a written part and an oral part. The written part is taken immediately after completion of the CA3 year and is designed to test the candidate's knowledge of basic and clinical sciences as they apply to anesthesia. It is taken on a (usually hot) Saturday in July and must be passed in order to qualify for the oral examination, which is taken at least 6 months after the written examination, in April and October of the following year [1]. Thus *board eligible anesthetists* will practise as consultants after their training before passing the final oral examination. The oral examination is designed to assess the candidate's ability to manage patients presented in clinical scenarios, with particular reference to the scientific and clinical rationale that supports the management [1]. The cost of this examination is $ 1,600. Upon passing the examination the anesthesiologist will become a *board certified anesthesiologist*.

The structure of residency training

General

The academic year starts in July when new (CA1) residents descend on residency programs en mass and are then teamed up with consultants in the operating theater for a month. They spend two weeks training with one consultant in the operating room and then two weeks with another, one of whom will usually be their faculty advisor for the duration of the three-year training period. Residents have early morning lectures (breakfast briefings) in our program for the duration of this month and have defined objectives that they must fulfil by the end of July. His or her "one-on-one" consultant evaluates each resident and this information is used to determine whether they are fit to be less stringently supervised. Residents then cover all subspecialties including at least 2 months of intensive care training (required by the ABA) over the next three years with cardiac, pediatric, pain, and obstetric anesthesia rotations usually starting after completion of the first year. These should all be one month rotations [2].

Subspecialty rotations

Although many programs do not have defined subspecialty rotations this is increasingly required by the ACGME. In addition a requirement is that there is an increasing gradation of difficulty and complexity of cases as the resident progresses through his/her clinical training. In order to ascertain this we have set up at Columbia University what I like to call "expectation based OR rotations". This program ensures that a defined set of goals and objectives, in written form, is given to each resident starting a subspecialty rotation. These pertain only to the particular rotation and would be different for their second or third rotation through that subspecialty. During the course of the month, faculty evaluate the residents (using the form shown in the appendix) and at the end of the month the resident is then tested on these expectations either via an oral or written or multiple choice test. In turn the resident (anonymously) evaluates all the faculty they have come in contact with by means of a standard form and also evaluates the rotation using a second form. The resident evaluation of faculty information is processed and in a batched form is returned to the concerned faculty biannually, as well as to the chairman of the department. Thus the residents not only have narrowly defined goals but also have definite input into the quality of their education by direct feedback to faculty as well as the chairman.

Resident work allocation

Residents are on call, but there are now strictly defined rules as to the number of hours that residents may work. Also there are guidelines from the ACGME that state that residents should not unduly be involved in non-educational activities. This behoves the institution to ensure that there are sufficient anesthesia technicians or phlebotomists for residents specializing in internal medicine.

According to the ABA, residents may not be away from the program for more than 20 working days in one year. A further 5 working days are allowed for meeting time.

Supervision

At all times in anesthesia training written guidelines have to be followed with respect to the level of supervision of residents by faculty. Thus in the initial training period (first month), we document that residents have satisfactorily completed 10 preanesthetic evaluations, 15 i.v. placements, 15 general anesthetics and 5 regional anesthetics. Indeed for billing purposes faculty have to sign and attest that they were present at key events of the anesthetic period i.e. induction, intubation and extubation, etc. In addition, for each year of training (CA1-CA3) guidelines for supervision are drawn up. In essence this means that residents never give a total anesthetic without the presence of a consultant at some time during the case. In addition the level of supervision may not be substantially different at any time of day or day of the week.

The curriculum that a resident might follow in training in America

While the ACGME specifies that most of the didactics for residents must be conducted by faculty who are appropriately qualified and learned as well as published in the field of anesthesiology, it is the ABA that provides a content guideline from which curriculum for residency programs may be set.

This "content outline" comprehensively covers the range of subject matter that residents in training need to study and associate examiners for the ABA examination are specifically charged with setting examination multiple choice questions from prescribed sections of this content outline booklet [3]. Thus it is left up to the residency program to decide how they want to develop a curriculum of anesthesia.

However, the ACGME has now specified that in addition to knowledge of anesthesia related topics, residents must specifically receive lectures on: operating room management, types of practice and job acquisition, financial planning, contract negotiation and billing arrangements as well as issues of professional liability and medical ethics [2]. Results of the yearly intraining examination (see evaluation section below) are furnished to programs with a break down of the results for each individual test taker as well as a summary for the whole program of those key areas (known as keywords) in which the program as a whole was deficient. This information can be used as a guide to structure the residency curriculum. At Columbia we incorporate the curriculum on many fronts, in a didactic lecture series run by faculty or invited speakers, in "keyword programs" researched and presented by residents under the keen eye of a faculty member as well as by faculty run problem based learning discussions (PBLDs). We also have a visiting guest lecture series and regular case conferences from each area of specialty as part of our weekly "grand rounds". Further, individual subspecialty rotations have their own didactic sessions either through "morning reports" before the start of the day, or noontime lectures in the ICU or after hours. In addition journal clubs are held for different subspecialties and interests.

A special series of lectures called "breakfast briefings" is held every morning for the first month of the residents' training (July) in order that the basics of anesthesia can be covered. Then during the course of the first year a lecture series entitled the "basic principles course" is held to cover the basics of anesthesia knowledge.

Resident evaluation, remediation and feedback as it pertains to USA residents

The strength of an anesthesia training program is based on its system of evaluation. This section will describe the available literature and also the philosophy and methods used at Columbia University in our department.

In 124 anesthesia programs surveyed between 1995-1996 evaluations of clinical competency were performed daily (21%), weekly (2.4%) or monthly (50.4%), some by computer entry but the vast majority by paper entry [4]. Most programs (65%) use as their basis for evaluation the above-enumerated ABA criteria and use a combined rating and narrative system (89%) [4]. Our program at Columbia University is no exception (see appendix).

Clinical competency committees are mandated to convene at least 6 monthly but on average meet 5 times per year in the USA [4]. The clinical competence committees are usually chaired by someone other than the head of department as is mandated by the ABA. They are comprised of faculty, and at times residents and will hear oral, and written testimony to assess the progress of resident trainees.

Establishing competencies

Appropriate evaluation of anesthetic trainees must be based on clear objectives. In the absence of these, evaluation can at best be arbitrary. We evaluate residents in three major categories, *academic*, *clinical* and *professional* competency.

Academic competency can be assessed by knowledge based tests, either as part of the rotation through subspecialties, from oral interrogation in the operating theatre (not a very accurate way of assessing knowledge) or from standardized tests. These tests can be set by the department internally, or can be set by an external body.

In the USA (Fig. 1) every resident takes the ABA inservice training examination (ABA-ITE) every year in July. These are scored and through complex for-

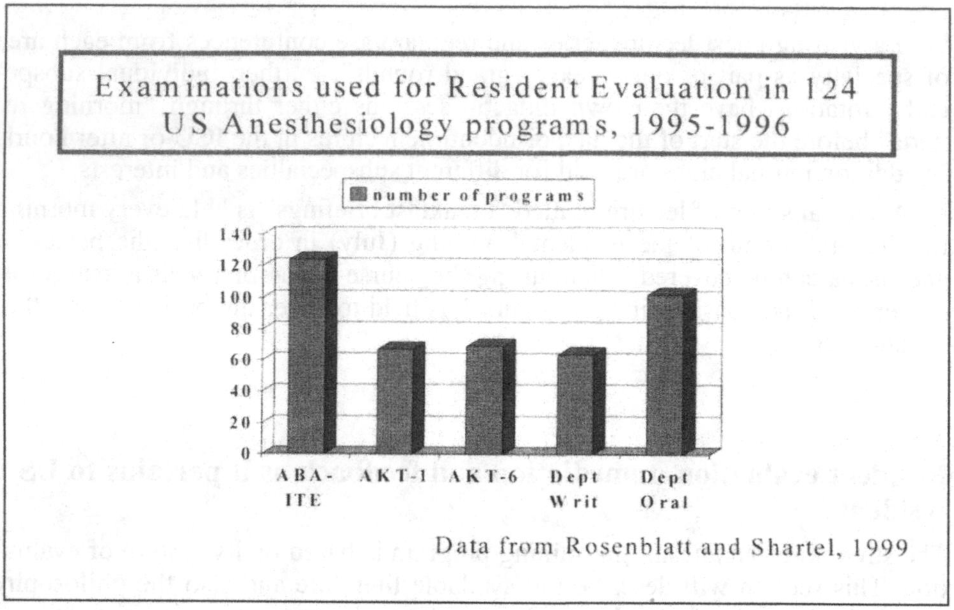

Fig. 1.

mulas are assigned the "scaled score" which can be used to establish the percentile ranking of a particular resident's score in relation to the scores of all American medical graduates taking the examination.

In addition another multiple choice test is prepared and provided (at a cost) to residency programs which is known as the anesthesia knowledge test (AKT). This is taken on arrival as a CA1 (Day1) (AKT-1), as well as at 6 months of training (AKT-6). Again one can establish the percentile ranking of a particular individual in relation to all test takers for this exam. Thus we have the potential to use objective test criteria to evaluate the knowledge of residents.

Clinical competency must by its very nature be assessed in a somewhat subjective way by performance in the OR, ICU or other location. However clear goals for competence can be established. Karen Madsen published a summary of the criteria set for her program in Wisconsin [5], which we have adapted for our program and now serves as the objectives that should be reached by residents at different stages of their training and as a basis for evaluation.

Professional competency. This category encompasses the ABA defined "essential attributes" described above. It can be summarized as "attitude". Beyond the objectives stated, this is a complex area of evaluation which, however may be a powerful tool to shape an appropriate culture for an anesthesia training program.

Maintaining academic and clinical standards

Expectations (the higher the better)

What follows is a practical application of the earlier mentioned principles.

CA-1 residents on the first day of their residency are apprized verbally and in written form of both the *academic*, *clinical* and *professional competency* requirements expected of them.

Academic competency

Residents (CA-1) are informed that they must achieve a certain score in the 6 month anesthesia knowledge test (AKT) examination. This can be arbitrarily set to be above the 25th percentile for all the candidates taking this examination in the country. Similarly, residents taking their CA-1 or CA-2 In service training examination (ITE, Fig. 1) are expected to achieve a specified percentile ranking. Again this might be set at greater than 25%.

Clinical competency

The expectations of clinical ability at the end of one month (after a one on one period) and after 6 months, as well as after the first, second and third year need to be clearly delineated. These can be based on "criteria for defining clinical competency of anesthesiology residents", Madsen et al. [5]. This excellent summary can be used as a guideline and adapted to suit the particular program. This may serve not only as a yardstick for the resident but can be referred to when deliberating on the progress of a particular resident during a clinical competency meeting.

Professional competency

The residents are informed that the objective of the program is to become a consultant in anesthesiology and thus they will be held to the "essential attributes" of the ABA and appropriate behavior within the norms of the department.

Evaluation

The co-ordination of evaluation is arranged by the residency program. Evaluation forms (see appendix) are sent to the subspecialty heads who in turn send these to the faculty in their area and they are then returned, to the sub specialty head, collated into one final evaluation form per subspecialty rotation, and subsequently returned to the residency director who sees all of them for entry into the resident's file. If poor evaluations are noted, these are immediately acted upon (see below).

The principle of evaluation is that when a resident performs poorly in one of the central competencies this provokes a closer inspection of the other competencies. If it is found that two competencies are impaired this may become ground for dismissal from the program.

Quarterly, or more often if needed, the clinical competency committee meets to assess the progress of residents and to make decisions as to whether residents need to go on remediation. In the past we have found in committee that establishing consensus as to the necessary plan for a failing resident can be very difficult. Thus we have established *remediation policies* with clear evaluation criteria that are known both to the resident as well as the faculty to guide our deliberations.

Remediation policies

Academic

Failure to achieve the stated criteria should result in the resident and their faculty advisor (FA) being notified (the resident in writing). An attempt should be made to ascertain why the resident's academic performance is impaired. An academic history needs to be taken, grade point average, scoring at medical school, etc. The resident's study habits need to be reviewed and emotional stability ascertained while possible disease, hypothyroidism/hyperthyroidism or substance abuse need to be excluded. Attention deficit disorders may also become a problem that manifests for the first time during residency training. A program of study for the resident then needs to be established. This may take the form of one on one tutorials. Alternatively, reading assignments followed by written (essay or MCQ) or oral testing at predefined intervals can be instituted. Many residents claim that they are poor test takers. Essay questions usually then establish what they really know. Upon achieving a score sufficient to surpass the 25th percentile in the next examination the candidate is relieved from being on remediation.

Clinical competency

The program should establish a written policy defining when a resident should be put on remediation. Clear criteria based on whatever mechanism is used for clinical evaluation of residents should be used. For example, the number of unsatisfactory evaluations needed or the evaluation score that could prompt clinical remediation needs to be established and agreed to by the clinical competency committee in advance. In our program the remediation policy is implemented when, based on faculty evaluations, residents receive an aggregate evaluation (from faculty in a rotation) or from two individual preceptors of *marginal* or *unsatisfactory* for any evaluation category (see appendix). The resident should then be counseled by the residency director and his faculty adviser and a remediation plan established with the resident. The discussion and plan should be documented in a letter to the resident who is then asked to countersign this. In our program the remediation plan is then implemented and the resident is more intensively evaluated and may not achieve two *unsatisfactory* evaluation or 3 *marginals* in a period of 6 months or risk dismissal. Thus it is important that part of the remediation policy addresses what criteria can be used as grounds for dismissal.

Issues relating to termination of a resident in a legal and fair way

An issue that is being critically addressed in US institutions is fair evaluation and if need be termination of residents by implementing the necessary steps of due process.

What does fair and equitable treatment entail?

"Courts will not over turn academic determinations when faculty members have exercised honest (non-capricious or arbitrary) professional judgement in the context of a resident's entire file". Faculty members may treat students differentially, evaluate residents in trouble in greater depth, notify faculty to enhance scrutiny, dismiss even if not done so in the past, *but must guard against treating students in similar circumstances disparately* [6].

What is due process for academic dismissals?

The resident should receive: notice of deficiencies and the consequences thereof if not remediated, an opportunity to review evaluations as well as an opportunity to respond. The resident should be able to present his or her view to decision makers but a full adversarial hearing (with lawyers) is not required at any stage as long as this is not an institutional requirement [6].

How much documentation is required for dismissal?

As much as possible. Written evaluations should relate to performance (as opposed to personality), be descriptive and observation should be separated from interpretation. In addition oral communications from faculty should be drafted as file memoranda by residency directors and sent to faculty. Professional judgement is key and will not be overridden by a court of law [6].

In general "courts have rather consistently sustained the rights and responsibilities of faculty to evaluate and to dismiss a resident based on academic performance" [7].

Suggestions for establishing a legally sound resident evaluation system [8]

1. Inform (verbally and in writing) each resident that he/she will be evaluated repeatedly, and that these evaluations are available for him/her to review or

contest at any time. Have the residents sign and date file each time they review it;
2. inform (verbally and in writing) each resident that occasionally someone is terminated from the program for failure to meet the department's minimum standard of clinical competence;
3. notify (verbally and in writing) every resident who has received an unsatisfactory rating in an evaluation and offer assistance to correct the problem;
4. make evaluation forms as objective as possible. Make documentation as specific as possible (time, date, place). Encourage (or insist) that a faculty member writing an "unsatisfactory" evaluation discuss the problem with the resident before filing the report. Whether or not the resident was informed of the unsatisfactory evaluation should be part of the written evaluation;
5. evaluate residents as early as possible and aim at terminating trainees of low aptitude or ability after no more than one year of training;
6. if a legal struggle seems possible contact the hospital attorney early;
7. encourage faculty to write full honest evaluations. If the evaluations are negative and turn out to be incorrect, they won't haunt or hinder the resident and the legal liability is very low. If the evaluations are correct they may prevent many problems and much unhappiness as well as unnecessary danger to future patients.

Conclusion

This has been a brief summary of current issues surrounding resident education in anesthesia in the USA.

But of course this is by no means an exhaustive summary. I have drawn on my own practical experience in describing certain aspects of dealing with residents in the hope that this will prove useful to the reader.

Appendix. Resident evaluation form

Columbia University - NY Presbyterian Hospital
Department of Anesthesiology

Resident's Name: ....

Evaluation Period: ....
Rotation

Evaluator: ....
Please Print & Sign Name
This evaluation is a summary of the opinions of the Core Attendings' Evaluations of the above-named resident

Evaluation scale:
Based upon your expectations for level of training, this resident was consistently:

O = Outstanding
AA = Above Average
S = Satisfactory
M = Marginal
U = Unsatisfactory

PREOP AND POSTOP EVALUATION OF PATIENTS:

a) Did resident communicate with attending about patients the day before surgery?

[O] [AA] [S] [M] [U]

b) Could resident give a structured account and pertinent summary of the anesthetic concerns related to the patient?

[O] [AA] [S] [M] [U]

c) Could the resident prioritize and plan anesthesia management?

[O] [AA] [S] [M] [U]

d) Did the resident visit/telephone the patient postoperatively?

[O] [AA] [S] [M] [U]

Comments: ....

CHARACTER SKILLS:

Comment on: reliability, honesty, responsibility, cooperation, conscientiousness, punctuality, communication skills, adaptability, flexibility, appropriate independence, reaction to criticism, initiative, and self-confidence

Comments: ....

Grade: (X)

[O] [AA] [S] [M] [U]

KNOWLEDGE:

Comment on: basic and clinical information: consider study habits, knowledge of medical literature. Teaching ability. Knowledge appropriate to cases managed

Comments: ....

Grade: (X)

[O] [AA] [S] [M] [U]

JUDGEMENT:

Consider: preoperative data collection and evaluation, decision making and problem solving ability; planning anesthetic management; evaluation of airway, fluid status, depth of anesthesia, etc., reaction to crisis and ability to set priorities

Comments: ....

Grade: (X)

[O] [AA] [S] [M] [U]

CLINICAL AND TECHNICAL SKILLS:

Consider: thoroughness, and expedition to set-up machine, equipment, monitors and syringes; airway management, line insertion, regional techniques; overall dexterity and ability to work with appropriate speed. Comment on quality of record keeping

Grade: (X)

Comments: ....

Grade: (X)

[O] [AA] [S] [M] [U]

OVERALL IMPRESSION:

Comment on: strengths and weaknesses – areas that need attention and improvement

Comments: ....

[O] [AA] [S] [M] [U]

NOTE: **If a "marginal" or "unsatisfactory" has been accorded in any category, please discuss with resident and document this below**:

Discussed with Resident: Yes ( ) No ( )

References

1. Information Booklet (2000) The American Board of Anesthesiology, Raleigh
2. Association AM (2000) Program requirements for residency education in anesthesiology. ACGME 2000-2001:44-50
3. Content Outline (1998) Joint council on intraining examinations. 520N. Northwest Highway, Parkridge, IL 60068-2573
4. Rosenblatt MA, Shartel SA (1999) Evaluation, feedback, and remediation in anesthesiology residency training: A survey of 124 United States programs. J Clin Anesth 1:519-527
5. Madsen K, Woehlck H, Cheng E et al (1994) Criteria for defining clinical competence of anesthesiology residents. Anesthesiology 80:663-665
6. Irby D, Milam S (1989) The legal context for evaluating and dismissing medical students and residents. Acad Med 64:639-643
7. Helms L, Helms C (1991) Forty years of litigation involving residents and their training: 1. General programmatic issues. Academic Medicine 66:649-655
8. Rosen D, Viets J, Sarnquist F (2000) Resident evaluation handbook

Education in Intensive Care

T. JACQUES

Postgraduate education in Intensive Care differs around the world. In many countries it has become the responsibility of distinct specialist colleges and trainees seek specific qualifications in the specialty of Intensive Care Medicine. In 1976 the world's first college based training and examination system was introduced in Australia. Good clinical leadership and mentorship rather than didactic, knowledge based training programmes foster thoroughness, discernment and the humanist qualities important to the development of an intensive care specialist. Knowledge and skills in managing conditions that are potentially life threatening are important but often neglected at an undergraduate level [1].

Undergraduate education: All new medical graduates should be equipped to recognise and begin treatment of those conditions posing an immediate threat to life. Critical care covers the knowledge and skills required for this and includes our specialty, Intensive Care Medicine. In a survey of the perceptions of final year medical students of their knowledge and skills for managing critical illness we reported a worrying deficit in competence in simple airway management and defibrillation [2]. Their experience in critical care procedures is outlined in Table 1. With early defibrillation being one of the few positive determinants of outcome in cardiac arrest this should be a mandatory skill. The students reported more confidence in their ability to manage symptoms of the domains of surgery and medicine (e.g. abdominal pain and chest pain). Our survey served as a quality audit of education at one particular university but also highlights the need to assess undergraduate teaching in medical emergencies and potential deficits in undergraduate education in critical care. This was reinforced by a survey of recent graduates from many universities reported in the same paper. Table 2 details their degree of confidence in managing common critical care scenarios. As a result of our study recommendations were implemented to introduce a formal undergraduate curriculum in critical care.

Given the expertise that exists in recognition and resuscitation of the critically ill and the understanding of the principles of monitoring among those involved in the specialty of Intensive Care Medicine and related specialties (Anaesthesia, Emergency Medicine, Trauma Care) it is appropriate that we are involved in undergraduate education of critical care. Indeed the teaching of critical care is an opportunity to bring together an undergraduate programme tradi-

Table 1. Undergraduate (final year medical student) experience with procedure ($n = 101$)

	Performed procedure %	Witnessed the procedure only %	Neither witnessed nor performed %
Venipuncture	99.0	1.0	–
IV cannula	98.0	2.0	–
Skin suturing	85.2	12.9	2.0
Basic CPR *	76.0	19.0	5.0
Bag-mask ventilation *	75.3	20.8	4.0
Male bladder catheter	74.0	23.0	3.0
Arterial puncture	71.3	17.8	10.9
Female bladder catheter	67.3	26.7	5.9
Tracheal intubation	52.5	27.7	19.8
12 lead ECG	51.0	37.0	10.0
Nasogastric tube	47.5	46.5	5.9
Pressure dressing	38.6	36.6	24.7
Blood transfusion	13.8	61.4	24.8
Defibrillation *	12.0	59.0	29.0
Intercostal catheter	10.9	51.5	37.6
Arterial cannula	9.0	41.0	50.0
Peritoneal lavage	8.9	40.6	50.5
Central venous catheter	6.9	70.3	22.8
Put patient on ventilator	6.9	37.6	55.5
Pulmonary artery catheter insertion	1.0	21.8	77.2

Reproduced from reference number 2
* Essential resuscitation skills

tionally fragmented into subspecialty areas. These specialties can also provide expertise in ethics, palliative care and care of the dying patient. Whether a traditional discipline-oriented medical curriculum (basic science first then clinical subspecialties) or organ module based (combining basic sciences with clinical sciences system by system), a curriculum inclusive of critical care provides opportunity to apply basic science knowledge to pathological processes affecting many organ systems and maintain a ‘whole patient’ approach to illness. Recognition and initial treatment of potentially life-threatening conditions are essential skills regardless of the specialties medical graduates pursue. Undergraduate core knowledge and skills in critical care should be defined and assessed for all medical undergraduate programmes.

Table 2. Junior doctor perceptions regarding their confidence, at the beginning of their intern year, in undertaking the management of critically ill patients ($n = 81$)

	Very confident %	Fairly confident %	Not confident %
Management of patient on mechanical ventilator	0	7	93
Use of capnograph	4	12	79
Resuscitation of a patient with severe trauma	4	23	73
Treatment of acid-base balance	4	32	64
Performance of advanced life support	6	31	64
Assessment of a patient in shock in the ICU	1	34	62
Decision on when to stop CPR in cardiac arrest	5	35	60
Interpretation of central venous pressure	5	43	52
Performance of external defibrillation	11	40	49
Management of life-threatening hypertension	7	49	44
Diagnosis of the cause of coma	7	52	41
Reversal of acute hyperkalaemia	19	53	28
Performance of a 12-lead ECG	28	46	26
Treatment of hypoxia of unknown aetiology	2	77	21
Correction of fluid or electrolyte disturbance	18	65	17
Performance of basic life support	30	61	9

Reproduced from reference number 2

Postgraduate non-vocational education

Reports have suggested delayed recognition and lack of an organised approach to critically ill patients prior to admission to Intensive Care [3]. More recently we recorded in a study of antecedent events and outcome of cardiac arrest across three hospitals that 36% and 34% of arrested patients had abnormal physiology 0-8 hours and 8-48 hours prior to cardiac arrest. The commonest abnormalities were hypotension (systolic blood pressure < 90 mmHg) and tachypnea (respiratory rate > 35 breaths per minute) [4]. With these abnormalities being recorded at prolonged intervals prior to arrest it is important to educate our junior medical staff to recognise and initiate treatment prior to arrest. This also serves to promote early ICU consultation.

To improve training in surgical critical care for junior doctors the Royal College of Surgeons of England commissioned a working party of intensive care specialists, anaesthetists and surgeons. They developed the "Care of the Critically Ill Surgical Patient" (CCrISP) course. This is to equip junior medical staff to recognise and initiate treatment in the critically ill surgical patient. It also emphasizes prevention of organ failure. Communication and organisational skills modules are included. The CCrISP course has been adopted by the Royal Australasian College of Surgeons. This is a useful model for hospital orientation programmes for junior medical staff. Intensive care specialists can provide expertise in such education. As a specialty we are also involved in Advanced Cardiac Life Support, Early Management of Severe Trauma (EMST), Advanced Paediatric Life Support (APLS), and other structured modular programmes. Within hospitals, having a formal orientation and education programme ensures important aspects of critical care including basic and advanced life support are covered in a systematic manner. An ad hoc "see one, do one, teach one" approach often applied to procedural education is being superseded by these more formal approaches. In Britain the intercollegiate board for training in intensive care medicine, supported by the medical, surgical and anaesthetic colleges, has defined goals for knowledge and skills in critical care required for physicians, surgeons and anaesthetists not undertaking vocational training in intensive care.

Vocational training in Intensive Care: Is Intensive Care Medicine a subspecialty, specialty or supra-specialty?

Around the world variation exists in intensive care training ranging from no recognition as a specialty, through multiple training bodies to a single specialist college [5]. About 60% of Australasian ICUs have a full time medical director and 60% of these have recognised qualifications in Intensive Care [6]. In Australia, the two traditional arms of training for Intensive Care through the Australian and New Zealand College of Anaesthetists (ANZCA) and Royal Australasian College of Physicians (RACP) have joined to form a joint specialist advisory committee. However, qualifying through the Faculty of Intensive Care, ANZCA, involves an exit exam, qualifying via RACP does not. Both colleges publish training objectives and appoint clinical supervisors to oversee trainees.

There is debate as to whether vocational training should involve an examination process. Most colleges maintain a general entrance examination although the relevance of an anaesthetic based entrance examination for those pursuing intensive care training via the anaesthetic colleges must be questioned. The examination process including preparation provides an objective, focused, and goal directed training programme. A broad knowledge base can be assessed in a way unlikely to be prejudiced by personal opinion or personality differences. In order to assess appropriate humanistic qualities or moral and ethical behaviour objective structured clinical examinations (OSCE) using actors to role play ethical scenarios can be used. OSCE can also be used to assess clinical judgement.

Many vocational training programmes require completion of a formal project. While this encourages research endeavour, only a basic knowledge of research methodology and statistics is required for trainees planning a clinical career. Mandatory projects should serve to promulgate research that contributes to our understanding and management of critical illness. Quality research is preferable to quantity.

When surveyed, Australian intensive care specialists have indicated their desire for an independent and unifying College of Intensive Care Medicine. Recently the pathways for training have been broadened to allow trainees in surgery, medicine, anaesthesia and emergency medicine to pursue specialisation in intensive care through the Faculty of Intensive Care, ANZCA. This way it is possible to acknowledge the varied background of clinicians seeking to work in Intensive Care but also endorse the maturity the specialty has achieved. Evidence is emerging in the literature for the positive benefit to patient outcome of having specialist Intensive Care directors and clinicians [7].

Post-graduate vocational training must involve an accreditation process of training units to ensure an appropriate standard of training environment. Accreditation by the training college implies adequate supervision and teaching of trainees, adequate volume and case mix of patients to provide broad ICU experience, and adequate staffing and equipment [5]. Supervisors should also ideally undertake training in adult education techniques and counselling. Ensuring good mentorship in a training programme is essential.

Simulation in intensive care education

One of the newer ways of providing training and assessing competency is by sophisticated, interactive simulator based scenarios. Application of aviation training methods has led to the use of simulators in Anaesthesia training for some time. Documented adverse incidents collated through the Australian Incident Monitoring Study for Intensive Care are incorporated into scenarios set up using a life size mannikin that responds to interventions. It is possible to simulate real adverse events in intensive care and transport of the critically ill [8, 9]. ICU teams including trainees and nursing staff are assessed in their dealing with these realistic events. Videotaping and debriefing are used. Emphasis is placed on "the learning environment" rather than the stress of passing or failing an exam. Simulator based education has now been accepted for CME accreditation. It is likely that this form of education will become more widespread in its use.

From slavery to shift worker: effects of work practice on education

The excess hours worked by junior doctors has been reported in many countries. In Britain in the 1980s major changes were proposed to reduce rostered hours. Subsequent concerns have also been raised in the European Union.

In consideration of occupational health and safety and patient safety obligations in Australia, national guidelines have been published for junior hospital staff including ICU trainees [10]. Therefore a reduction in rostered hours has been mandated. This brings trainee rosters in line with other industry sectors. As the previous longer hours were consumed in clinical service provision the effect on education opportunity with reduced hours is unmeasured. However, length of training programmes has been extended to ensure adequate clinical exposure. With reduced hours and budget constraints allocation of time for education is often difficult. Is this cost the domain of the health system or that of the individual trainee? In my experience it is a cost rarely acknowledged.

Australian Intensive Care specialists worked an average of 57.7 hours per week compared to an average of 42.7 hours for all medical specialists [5]. The principles governing the changes in junior medical staff rostering have yet to flow on to senior staff and again the allocation and cost of teaching time are rarely considered.

Funding for medical education varies from country to country. Undergraduate education is often a specific national budget item. Postgraduate education undertaken by specialist colleges is supported by levies on college members and trainees. With pressure to reduce costs the managed care system in the United States has placed financial pressures on graduate medical education. Clinical educators find their time consumed in clinical practice and documentation. There are many examples in the USA of contraction of teaching programmes [11]. On a positive note trainees are expected to understand "best practice", provide evidence for their clinical approach and responsibly apply finite medical resources. Regardless of the funding method, a costing allocation for staff education should be provided.

Continuing education

The need to continue education throughout one's career as an Intensive Care specialist has been acknowledged as requiring a formal approach. Either an overseeing body (e.g. the Accreditation Council for Continuing Medical Education or ACCME in America) or individual specialist colleges (e.g. Faculty of Intensive Care, ANZCA in Australia) supervise Continuing Medical Education (CME) or Maintenance of Professional Standards (MOPS) programmes. ACCME has defined CME as educational activities that serve to maintain or increase the knowledge, skills, professional performance and relationships that a physician uses to provide services for patients, the public or the profession. They focus on clinician knowledge base rather than performance or patient outcomes but cover a broad range of activities. Meetings, research, publications, quality assurance activities are all usually included. Self-directed learning is promoted by accrediting teaching, reading articles, and personal clinical audits including mortality review. It is important that more isolated practitioners are catered for. Results from a recent questionnaire study in Israel of primary care physicians suggests the opportunity for CME and professional updating reduces job stress and enhances job satisfaction [12]. More detailed practice review and re-certification are being introduced in many countries in an effort to improve physician performance and health outcomes. This has arisen as a result of external pressures, often political and medico-legal. However, to date, evidence for CME effectiveness is mixed [13]. Thus CME programmes should be subject to review, looking at their relevance and efficacy in ICU clinical practice.

Gaps in the system

Relying only on a knowledge of the scientific and technical aspects of modern Intensive Care is insufficient. Trainees, caught up in acquiring vast amounts of scientific knowledge enthusiastically talk of a case of 'this disease' or an X-ray of 'that pathophysiology' and focus on organ or system directed treatments. They need to be able to consider the implications of the disease, prognosis and treatment choices to each individual patient and communicate this information to patients and relatives. There is a changing doctor-patient (or relative) relationship, with patients taking part in clinical decision making and having increasingly greater expectations of outcomes [14]. This places a unique burden in the Intensive Care environment. The critical illness is often unexpected, there is loss of patient autonomy and the ability to communicate. Interaction with families under extreme stress who are dealing with their relationships with the critically ill patient and each other is challenging. With the move from open to closed intensive care units good communication between the ICU team and referring specialist teams is also important. Training in communication, ethics, and palliative care are all important but often neglected areas.

Other non-clinical aspects of ICU management are also being incorporated into vocational training programmes, e.g. knowledge of ICU costs, outcome measurement, staff management including crisis management and counselling and care of the staff. Courses for vocational trainees and the examination process for vocational training in Australia now involve use of actors to role play ethical and managerial scenarios to assess competency in these areas.

The challenge of balancing scientific and technological education with the development of humanistic qualities and appropriate ethical behaviour cannot rely on an examination process. How do you define and foster a 'well-rounded' Intensive Care specialist, knowledgeable in science and technology, a team leader, an accountant, a thorough, discerning and humanistic doctor? A continuum of education must occur throughout the trainee's working day with some of the most rewarding classroom interactions being our relationships with our colleagues, medical, nursing, allied health people on the ICU team and our patients and their families.

References

1. Buchman TG, Dellinger RP, Raphaely RC et al (1992) Undergraduate education in Critical Care Medicine. Crit Care Medicine 20:1595-1603
2. Harrison GA, Hillman KM, Fulde GWO, Jacques T (1999) The need for Undergraduate Education. In: Critical Care (Results of a questionnaire to Year 6 medical undergraduates, University of New South Wales and recommendations on a curriculum in Critical Care). Anaesth and Intens Care 27:53-58
3. McQuillan P, Pilkington S, Alan A et al (1998) Confidential enquiry into quality of care before admission to intensive care. BMJ 316:1853-1858
4. Jacques T, Bristow P, Hillman K et al (2000) Antecedent events and outcome from in-hospital cardiac arrest. Abstract for the 25th Australian and New Zealand Scientific meeting in Intensive Care, Canberra
5. Clarke GM, Harrison GA (1993) The training/examination programme in intensive care, Australian and New Zealand College of Anaesthetists 1. Training. Anaesth Intens Care 21: 848-853
6. Anderson T, Hart G (2000) ANZICS Intensive Care Survey 1998: An overview of Australian and New Zealand Critical Care resources. ANZICS Research Centre for Critical Care Resources, Melbourne
7. Pronovost et al (1999) Organisational Characteristics of Intensive Care Units Related to Outcomes of Abdominal Aortic Surgery. JAMA 281:1310-1131
8. Beckmann U, Gillies DM, Durie M (1999) Incidents relating to transportation of intensive care patients: An analysis of 5,500 reports submitted to the Australian Incident Monitoring Study (AIMS-ICU). Abstract in the 24th Australian and New Zealand Annual Scientific Meeting on Intensive Care
9. Watterson L, Flanagan B, Donovan B, Robinson B (2000) Anaesthetic simulators-training for the broader health care profession. Australian and New Zealand J. of Surgery (in press)
10. Draft National Code of Practice - Hours of Work, Shiftwork and Rostering for Hospital Doctors (1998) Australian Medical Association, Kingston
11. Kuttner R (1999) Managed Care and Medical Education. N Eng J Med 341:1092-1096
12. Kushnir T, Cohen AH, Kitae E (2000) Continuing medical education and primary physicians' job stress, burnout and dissatisfaction. Medical Education 34:430-436
13. Davis DA, Thomson MA, Oxman AD, Haynes B (1992) Evidence for the effectiveness of CME: A review of 50 randomised controlled trials. JAMA 268:1111-1117
14. Cassell, Eric J (1991) The Nature of Suffering and the Goals of Medicine. Oxford University Press, New York

Errors in the Intensive Care Unit

G.J. Dobb

Modern healthcare delivery is a highly complex process. In any episode of care, several healthcare practitioners, devices, procedures, and medications are commonly involved, compounding the potential for error. The landmark Harvard Medical Practice Study [1] reviewed over 30,000 hospital records of patients in the United States. Adverse events, defined as injuries directly arising from healthcare, occurred in 3.7% of hospital admissions. Over half were judged to be preventable and 13.6% led to death. A more-recent study from Australia [2] found 16.6% of hospital admissions were associated with iatrogenic patient injury, half being highly preventable. Nearly 1 in 20 resulted in death. Other estimates of the proportion of hospital admissions associated with errors causing adverse outcomes have been as high as 17% [3] and recent reports from the United States [4] Department of Veterans Affairs and also the Institute of Medicine suggest the medical error rate in American hospitals remains high. This latter report estimated that medical errors may kill 44,000-98,000 people each year in American hospitals. Medical errors attract considerable public and media interest and although this promotes a degree of sensationalism and exaggeration – as reflected by the headline for the Institute of Medicine report, "Medical errors kill almost 100,000 Americans a year" [5] – concern and action are needed.

The cost of medical errors is high in financial as well as human terms. A review of 14,732 randomly selected hospital discharges in Utah and Colorado [6] found 459 adverse events of which 265 were preventable. The total cost of these events was in 1996 nearly US$ 662 million with direct healthcare costs accounting for US$ 348 million, or 4.8% of healthcare expenditure in these states. It has been estimated that medical errors in Australia cost over Australian$ 800 million for the extra days spent in hospital alone [7]. The other important, but often underestimated, cost is the psychological stress to doctors and other healthcare workers associated with inquiries, litigation, or the guilt of "cover ups".

Defining "medical error"

The taxonomy of error is complex. Much of the conceptual framework is borrowed from other areas, including industry and aviation [8]. Expressions used for hospital errors have included [9]: "adverse occurrences", "iatrogenic complications", "human errors", "adverse events", and "incidents". These terms have not always been defined, and when they have been defined (Table 1) the definitions have often excluded errors that have occurred without evidence of an adverse event. An adverse event can be defined [10] as, "an injury or complication which resulted in disability or prolongation of hospital stay and was caused by the healthcare received rather than the disease from which the patient suffered".

It is important for a system focussing on errors to be able to detect, review, and take corrective action over all events, and not just those causing adverse outcomes. Only then is the true frequency evident and the lessons from "near misses" can be as important as those from the adverse outcomes, offering an opportunity for corrective action before actual harm occurs. Importantly there is no clear relationship between the subjective magnitude of the error and the consequences for the patient [8], making a consequence-related approach inappropriate. Anonymous reporting may facilitate collection of such information.

Simple classifications of error, for example into errors of commission and omission, have been unhelpful in addressing problems. Reason [11] views errors in two ways: the person approach and system approach, each giving rise to a different philosophy of error management. The person approach is dominant in medicine, focussing on errors and procedural violations that arise from lapses or variation in human behavior. Countermeasures include disciplinary action, litigation, retraining, and allocation of blame. Such an approach provides incentives to "cover up" or shift the blame and by concentrating on individuals it isolates unsafe acts from their system context.

The system approach assumes that humans are fallible and errors should be expected. The "causes" may be found in the organizational processes that give rise to them and countermeasures therefore address the safeguards within the system. Errors occur because of active failures and latent conditions, with nearly all adverse events involving elements of both. The active failures are mistakes by those in direct contact with the patient and have a direct but usually short-lived effect. As the proximal event they are more easy to identify. Latent conditions are the "accidents waiting to happen" - error-provoking conditions in the workplace (e.g., time pressure, understaffing, inadequate equipment) or weaknesses in the checks and safeguards (inadequate alarms, poor systems for checking of medications, unit design that makes close observation of more than one patient difficult).

The "system approach" can facilitate improved healthcare and holistic management of errors as they occur. This can be further assisted by analyzing and classifying the cause of errors as proposed for example by Wilson et al. [10] (Table 2). In the Quality in Australian Health Care Study (QAHCS) the human error categories accounted for over 6 times the number of adverse events that were associated with the delay or treatment categories and nearly 12 times the number in the investigative category. Over a third of the human errors were complications of, or failure in, the technical performance of a procedure or op-

Table 1. Proposed definitions for medical or healthcare error (*ICU* intensive care unit) *

An unintended injury that was caused by medical management and that resulted in measurable disability
An adverse event, occurring during ICU stay, that was independent of the patient's underlying disease
A deviation from standard conduct, as well as addition or omission of actions relating to standard operational instructions of the unit
Any event that could have reduced, or did reduce, the safety margin for the patient
All events when treatment or observation differed from a planned one, and when this was not a part of the natural course of the disease
An act of commission or admission that caused or contributed to the cause of unintended injury

* From information in [9, 10]

Table 2. Classification system for the cause of errors *

Human error categories
– complications of, or failure in, the technical performance of an indicated procedure/operation
– failure to synthesize, decide, and/or act on available information
– failure to request or arrange investigation, procedure, or consultation
– lack of care or attention, failure to attend
– misapplication of, or failure to apply, a rule; or use of a bad or inadequate rule
– violation of a protocol or rule
– acting on insufficient information
– slips and lapses, errors due to "absentmindedness" in activities in which the operator is skilled
– failure to continue established management
– lack of knowledge
– electively practicing outside area of expertise
– other
– unable to code
Delay categories
– diagnostic
– treatment
– administrative
Treatment categories
– no or inadequate treatment
– wrong/inappropriate treatment
– no or inadequate prophylaxis
– missed treatment
– treatment unclassified
Investigation category
– investigation not performed
– investigation not acted on
– investigation inappropriate
– investigation unclassified

* Modified from [10]

eration, but less than half were judged to be “highly preventable”. Failure to synthesize, decide, and/or act on available information accounted for 16%, failure to request or arrange an investigation, procedure, or consultation 12%, and lack of care or attention or failure to attend 11%. In total the top five categories accounted for over 80% of all the errors. Only 3% could not be classified and 3% were included under “other” categories of concern. Between 75 and 90% of the errors in the second to fifth most-frequent categories were judged to be “highly preventable”. Although the QAHCS was not specific to intensive care, the principles have general application. In particular, they can provide insights to help develop prevention strategies to reduce the frequency and severity of errors.

The greatest source of error is human error, but human error is inevitable. Leape [12] identified that safer practice comes from acknowledging the potential for error and applying error reduction strategies at every stage of clinical practice. Examples of high reliability organizations include nuclear aircraft carriers, air traffic control systems, and nuclear power plants [11]. Although seemingly remote from clinical practice, they have characteristics in common with intensive care, including management of complex technologies and a need to maintain the capacity to meet periods of very high peak demand that might occur unexpectedly and at any time. The characteristics of the example high reliability organizations are [11]:

- they are complex, dynamic, and intermittently intensely interactive;
- they perform exacting tasks under considerable time pressure;
- they carry out these demanding activities with low incident rates.

This is achieved by anticipating the worst and equipping themselves to deal with it. In medicine there have been recent constructive initiatives in many countries to improve patient safety [13, 14], drawing on approaches from industry and aviation.

The intensive care unit

The intensive care unit (ICU) is an extremely complex organization. Features that make it a high-risk environment are common. These include:

- complex, high-technology equipment;
- poor integration of monitoring and alarm systems;
- interaction between different hierarchies (medical, nursing, etc.);
- high staff turnover;
- long working hours (24 h/day);
- dependence on staff in training;
- dependence on external services;

- suboptimal environment, e.g., noise, dim lighting at night;
- multiple infusions, multiple medications.

Little information is available on the comparative frequency of errors between ICUs and general hospital wards. In pediatric practise, medication errors were found to be seven times more likely in the ICU [15], with doctors being responsible for nearly three-quarters of the errors. Prescription errors doubled when new doctors joined the rotation.

The effect of errors is likely to be compounded by the limited physiological reserve of critically ill patients, magnifying the effect of errors, so they are reflected by serious adverse events. ICUs also become involved in the care of patients who have suffered adverse events related to care outside the unit. A constructive, non-accusatory approach facilitates early referral of such patients. Over 10% of ICU admissions may be caused by iatrogenic disease [16], more than half of the events being preventable. The risk factors, causes, and consequences appear to have changed little over the last 20 years [16].

Error detection and reporting

The traditional methods of error detection and reporting have included autopsy, peer review, and audit. More-recent approaches have included critical incident reporting, other anonymous reporting and debriefing systems, and capture of clinical performance indicators.

Autopsy

Investigations into the correlation between the clinical diagnosis of the underlying disease in patients dying in ICUs and autopsy findings suggest the diagnosis is correct in only approximately two-thirds of the patients [17]. This is, of course, a highly selected sample and should not be extrapolated to suggest the overall diagnostic error rate is as high. In nearly a quarter of the adult patients who died in a Brazilian ICU [17], the correct diagnosis would have altered patient management in a way that may have altered the outcome. In other studies the rate of errors that might have affected outcome has been similar [18] or lower [19]. The relationship to duration of ICU stay has been variable, with missed diagnoses – mainly infections – being more common in patients with a prolonged stay in a surgical ICU [18], but no significant relationship being found in a more-general ICU population [19].

The disadvantages of autopsy as a method of error detection are that it is selective:

- errors in patients who survive are not detected;

- in most jurisdictions only a minority of patients who die have an autopsy;
- only a minority of errors may cause changes that can be detected at autopsy.

Peer review

Formal and informal peer review provide important opportunities for error detection and reporting. The inevitable sharing of care between specialist intensive care staff to provide 24-h cover, rostering arrangements for junior medical staff, and scrutiny of patient care by referring medical and surgical teams ensure a high level of informal peer review of patients needing intensive care. More formal review, for example morbidity and mortality meetings, is common.

The main disadvantages of formal peer review are that it tends to be selective, depending on the choice of cases for detailed review, and while it is not focussed primarily on error detection, the forums available may not be the best suited to evaluation of errors. Formal peer review can also suffer from being retrospective rather than contemporary. Peer review has a large subjective component and, even when two physicians jointly review an event, the agreement with other reviewers can be poor [20]. Standardized computer software may improve the quality and value of the review [21].

Audit

Is an extremely useful tool to determine the frequency of errors. Prospective audit should always be preferred to retrospective chart review. Audits carried out in ICUs have provided information on errors that have more than local significance and have the potential to guide error reduction strategies more widely. Examples include:

- audit of medication errors [15, 22], highlighting sources of recurrent errors leading to change in policies and training;
- severe trauma [23, 24], identifying a high frequency of management deficiencies and a significant number of system inadequacies;
- accidental removal of endotracheal tubes, nasogastric tubes, and intravascular catheters, providing benchmarks for the frequency of these adverse events and recommendations for their reduction [25];
- "stat" laboratory results [26], emphasizing the importance of quality control;
- positioning of nasogastric tubes [27], providing evidence for the value of chest radiography to confirm positioning after insertion.

An audit should be inclusive, focussed on specific questions and provide feedback to reduce the future frequency of the errors detected. The disadvantages are that it can be resource intensive and, although all patients may be included, only specific areas are addressed. Errors occurring outside the area of interest may be neither detected nor reported.

Critical incident reporting

Methods of error detection have traditionally relied on detecting adverse events. However, the "near misses" can be as relevant as those that lead to harm. Importantly, identifying systematic errors causing "near misses" may prevent a patient actually coming to harm. The Australian Incident Monitoring Study [28] is a national anonymous voluntary incident reporting system. Local unit review of reports provides an effective forum for constructive discussion of errors amongst a wide group of ICU staff. Participants are encouraged to suggest preventative strategies, the outcome of incidents can be reported, and national study findings relating to similar incidents can be explored. A similar approach has been used elsewhere, including Hong Kong [29] and Saudi Arabia [30], confirming its value as a technique to highlight problems previously undetected by quality assurance programs. A large national database makes it possible to identify common issues, for example, complications associated with arterial cannulation [31] or the contribution of nursing staff shortages to critical incidents [32].

The main weakness of this approach is that it provides no indication of the true frequency of errors or critical incidents. A unit-based anonymous reporting system in Norway recorded only 87 reports over 13 months [9]. In another study that used an independent observer it was found that staff reported only 50% of the actual errors [33]. An evaluation of adverse incident reporting in obstetrics [34] found staff reported less than a quarter of the adverse incidents and risk managers could identify a further 22%, but 55% of the total adverse events were only found by retrospective chart review. This may, of course, still underestimate the true total. Nearly half the serious incidents were reported by staff, but far fewer of the moderate or minor incidents. The main reasons for not reporting [35] were fears that junior staff would be blamed and high workload. Others have suggested errors and "near misses" are under-reported by a factor of 10 [36]. Nevertheless, a strong case can be made in favor of voluntary and anonymous reporting systems, rather than mandatory reporting programs [37]. Reducing the barriers to voluntary reporting should provide more-useful and complete information about errors and their causes, whereas fault-based mandatory reporting is a deterrent to reporting, and the reports are less likely to contain detailed information because self protection can be an overriding concern, rather than helping others avoid the same problem.

Confidential reporting and debriefing

The attributes of confidential voluntary reporting have been outlined. Additional approaches seeking to build on this concept include:

- "failure analysis" [38], which has the goal of making apparent system faults that are otherwise obscured. Analyses are directed to answering the questions, "What characteristics of the system failed to prevent a slip, mistake, or rule violation from evolving into an accident?" and "What system changes

might have offset, or prevented, the active error from contributing to the sequence of events culminating in injury?";
- "human factors engineering", which was originally applied to the design of military aircraft cockpits with specialists from the area now assisting the healthcare industry in identifying causes of significant errors [39];
- investigation of "sentinel events" through root cause analysis [40].

Although the names differ, the approaches all offer a structured analytical method for examining medical errors or potential errors and producing outcomes aimed at reducing the chance of repetition.

Clinical indicators

Events thought to be related to errors may be chosen as clinical indicators. Examples currently used in Australian intensive care include the frequency of pneumothorax after central venous catheterization, the frequency of inadvertent extubation, and the readmission rate to the ICU within 48 h of discharge. The clinical indicators are intended as measures of quality in healthcare delivery, but can correlate poorly with other ICU performance indicators [41]. The collection of clinical indicators can be mandatory, but unless other systems are in place, any errors or adverse events detected are not necessarily subject to investigation or analysis.

Prevention

Much has been learnt about the psychology of human error, especially from aviation [42, 43]. Human error is inevitable and to accept error as normal is a prerequisite to establishing the systems and approaches to minimize risk. Understanding the cause enables prevention. Recommendations for prevention should then flow from the systems for error detection, reporting, and analysis outlined above. Programs should remove obstacles that will predictably be encountered when looking for personal causes for error – being shamed, feeling fear and inadequacy – and encourage staff to make constructive changes in their own behavior [44]. This must be combined with a systems approach to maintain a balance with the personal responsibility model of managing errors in medicine.

Fatigue, stress, and a lack of teamwork are predictive of performance and recognized error-inducing conditions. In a recent survey [45] intensive care staff were less likely than surgeons to deny the effects of fatigue on performance and are more likely than surgeons to reject steep hierarchies in which senior team members are not open to input from junior colleagues. However, they remain much less self-critical of factors likely to affect performance than pilots, and seem particularly prone to play down the effects of stress.

Factors that have been repeatedly shown to be associated with an increased risk of error include [42, 43]:

- inexperience [46], for example, anesthetists with less than 1 year's experience make significantly more errors [47], although even experienced anesthetists make errors in both diagnosis and treatment when stressed by an emergency. Repetitive practice of drills and procedures, and simulator training can reduce the frequency of errors in these situations [42];
- ergonomic design failures; these should be minimized by incorporating human factors into the design of medical devices [48];
- fatigue;
- lack of teamwork, this has been shown to be an important contributor to emergency department malpractice incidents [49];
- environmental factors, noise, light, discomfort.

Attention to these issues should reduce errors. Other systematic measures include the availability of computerized protocols and bedside decision support [50], and inclusion of a pharmacist in the ICU team to reduce medication errors [51].

Effects of errors on ICU staff

Even when the investigation of errors is constructive and systems based or reporting confidential, the recognition of an error is to admit fallibility. Although patients are the first and obvious victims of medical mistakes, doctors are the second victims [52]. Traditionally, medicine has lacked processes that allow physicians to come to terms with their errors. The stress involved can be compounded by long drawn-out medical negligence litigation. The adversarial approach of the courts can inflict further stress and psychological disturbance that need careful management to prevent dysfunctional responses. Perhaps the greatest need is that of changing the cultural attitude in medicine to admission of error.

A teaching program to impart a tolerance of error to undergraduate medical students has been advocated [53]. Because acceptance of error is essential for accurate reporting as a prerequisite to analysis and prevention, a curriculum on medical error could help medical students cope with future mistakes and reduce their frequency.

Disclosure of error to patients

A survey of members of the European Intensive Care Society [54] found that only 32% would give a patient complete details of an iatrogenic accident, although 70% felt they should. Disclosure of medical errors allows patients to understand what has occurred. Offering an apology for harming a patient might be considered one of the ethical responsibilities of the medical profession [55]. Honest communication implies respect for the patient and is consistent with the trust patients expect from their physicians. In the ICU such communication may have to be with the patient's family. Their perceived duty to act as advocates for the patient may be particularly challenging, but can still be used to build a relationship of trust and respect.

Conclusion

Error recognition and prevention are still in their infancy in intensive care. Considerable work is needed to integrate our monitoring and alarm systems so information is presented more clearly. Other latent errors created by staff shortages, inexperience, and lack of training need to be addressed, and further information is needed on ICU design features that promote patient safety. A constructive and analytical approach to errors that do occur in a culture that does not have the allocation of "blame" as it primary goal allows us to learn from the errors of the past. Attention to patient safety and error reduction might do as much to improve outcomes from intensive care as any new drug or device likely to become available in the future.

References

1. Brennan TA, Leape LL, Laird NM et al (1991) Incidence of adverse events and negligence in hospitalized patients: results of the Harvard Medical Practice Study. N Engl J Med 324: 370-376
2. Wilson RM, Runciman WB, Gibbard RW et al (1995) The Quality in Australian Health Care Study. Med J Aust 163:458-471
3. Andrews LB, Stocking C, Krizek T et al (1997) An alternative strategy for studying adverse events in medical care. Lancet 349:309-313
4. Anonymous (2000) Hospital errors an important cause of patient fatalities, studies show. Crit Care Int 10:1-4
5. Charatan F (1999) News. Medical errors kill almost 100,000 Americans a year. BMJ 319:1519
6. Thomas EJ, Studdert DM, Newhouse JP et al (1999) Costs of medical injuries in Utah and Colorado. Inquiry 36:255-264
7. The Final Report of the Taskforce on Quality in Australian Health Care. Appendix 7. Canberra: AGPS, June 1996
8. Vincent C, Taylor-Adams S, Stanhope N (1998) Framework for analysing risk and safety in clinical medicine. BMJ 316:1154-1157
9. Flaatten H, Hevroy O (1999) Errors in the intensive care unit (ICU). Experiences with an anonymous registration. Acta Anaesthesiol Scand 43:614-617
10. Wilson RM, Harrison BT, Gibberd RW, Hamilton JD (1999) An analysis of the causes of adverse events from the Quality in Australian Health Care Study. Med J Aust 170:411-415

11. Reason J (2000) Human error: models and management. BMJ 320:768-770
12. Leape LL (1994) Error in medicine. JAMA 272:1851-1867
13. Leape LL, Woods DD, Hatlie MJ et al (1998) Promoting patient safety by preventing medical error. JAMA 280:1444-1447
14. Berwick DM, Leape LL (1999) Reducing errors in medicine. BMJ 319:136-137
15. Wilson DG, McArtney RG, Newcombe RG et al (1998) Medication errors in paediatric practice: insights from a continuous quality improvement approach. Eur J Pediatr 157:769-774
16. Darchy B, Le Miere E, Figueredo B et al (1999) Iatrogenic diseases as a reason for admission to the intensive care unit: incidence, causes and consequences. Arch Intern Med 159:71-78
17. Gut AL, Ferreira AL, Montenegro MR (1999) Autopsy: quality assurance in the ICU. Intensive Care Med 25:360-363
18. Mort TC, Yeston NS (1999) The relationship of pre mortem diagnoses and post mortem findings in a surgical intensive care unit. Crit Care Med 27:299-303
19. Berlot G, Dezzoni R, Viviani M et al (1999) Does the length of stay in the intensive care unit influence the diagnostic accuracy? A clinical pathological study. Eur J Emerg Med 6:227-231
20. Hofer TP, Bernstein SJ, De Monner S, Hayward RA (2000) Discussion between reviewers does not improve reliability of peer review of hospital quality. Med Care 38:152-161
21. Samuels L, Gordon JN (1997) Utility of a software assistant in critical care case review. Am J Emerg Med 15:43-48
22. Tissot E, Cornette C, Demoly P et al (1999) Medication errors at the administration stage in an intensive care unit. Intensive Care Med 25:353-359
23. Duke GJ, Morley PT, Cooper DJ et al (1999) Management of severe trauma in intensive care units and surgical wards. Med J Aust 170:416-419
24. McDermott FT, Cordner SM, Tremayne AB (1997) Management deficiencies and death preventability in 120 Victorian road fatalities (1993-1994). The Consultative Committee on Road Traffic Fatalities in Victoria. Aust NZ J Surg 67:611-618
25. Carrion MI, Ayuso D, Marcos M et al (2000) Accidental removal of endotracheal and nasogastric tubes and intravascular catheters. Crit Care Med 28:63-66
26. Plebani M, Carraro P (1997) Mistakes in a state laboratory: types and frequency. Clin Chem 43:1348-1351
27. Bankier AA, Wiesmayr MN, Henk C et al (1997) Radiographic detection of intrabronchial malpositions of nasogastric tubes and subsequent complications in intensive care unit patients. Intensive Care Med 23:406-410
28. Baldwin I, Beckman U, Shaw L, Morrison A (1998) Australian Incident Monitoring Study in intensive care: local unit review meetings and report management. Anaesth Intensive Care 26:294-297
29. Buckley TA, Short TG, Rowbottom YM, Oh TE (1997) Critical incident reporting in the intensive care unit. Anaesthesia 52:403-409
30. Qadir N, Takrouri MS, Seraj MA et al (1998) Critical incident reports. Middle East J Anesthesiol 14:425-432
31. Baldwin I, Beckman U, Carless R, Durie M (1999) Incidents relating to arterial line usage in intensive care: an analysis of 4000 reports submitted to the Australian Incident Monitoring Study (AIMS-ICU) (abstract). Anaesth Intensive Care 27:95
32. Beckman U, Baldwin I, Durie M et al (1998) Problems associated with nursing staff shortage: an analysis of the first 3600 incident reports submitted to the Australian Incident Monitoring Study (AIMS-ICU). Anaesth Intensive Care 26:396-400
33. Donchin Y, Gopher D, Olin M et al (1995) A look into the nature and causes of human errors in the intensive care unit. Crit Care Med 23:294-300
34. Stanhope N, Crowley-Murphy M, Vincent C et al (1999) An evaluation of adverse incident reporting. J Evaluation Clin Pract 5:5-12
35. Vincent C, Stanhope N, Crowley-Murphy M (1999) Reasons for not reporting adverse incidents: An empirical study. J Evaluation Clin Practice 5:13-21
36. Cullen DJ, Bates DW, Small SD et al (1995) The incident reporting system does not detect adverse drug events: a problem for quality improvement. Jt Comm J Qual Improv 21:541-548

37. Cohen MR (2000) Why error reporting systems should be voluntary. BMJ 320:728-729
38. Feldman SE, Roblin DW (1997) Medical accidents in hospital care: applications of failure analysis to hospital quality appraisal. Jt Comm J Qual Improv 23:567-580
39. Welch DL (1997) Human error and human factors engineering in health care. Biomed Instrum Technol 31:627-631
40. Anonymous (1998) Sentinel events: approaches to error reduction and prevention. Jt Comm J Qual Improv 24:175-186
41. Cooper GS, Sirio CA, Rotondi AJ et al (1999) Are readmissions to the intensive care unit a useful measure of hospital performance? Med Care 37:399-408
42. Green R (1999) The psychology of human error. Eur J Anaesthesiol 16:148-155
43. Arnstein F (1997) Catalogue of human error. Br J Anaesth 79:645-656
44. Casarett D, Helms C (1999) Systems errors versus physicians' errors: finding the balance in medical education. Acad Med 74:19-22
45. Sexton JB, Thomas EJ, Helmreich RL (2000) Error, stress and teamwork in medicine and aviation: cross sectional surveys. BMJ 320:745-749
46. Gwynne A, Barber P, Tavener F (1997) A review of 105 negligence claims against accident and emergency departments. J Accid Emerg Med 14:243-245
47. Byrne AJ, Jones JG (1997) Responses to simulated anaesthetic emergencies by anaesthetists with different durations of clinical experience. Br J Anaesth 78:553-556
48. Weinger MB, Pantiskas C, Wiklund ME, Carstensen P (1998) Incorporating human factors into the design of medical devices (letter). JAMA 280:1484
49. Risser DT, Rice MM, Salisbury ML et al (1999) The potential for improved teamwork to reduce medical errors in the emergency department. The MedTeams Research Consortium. Ann Emerg Med 34:373-383
50. Morris AH (1999) Computerized protocols and bedside decision support. Crit Care Clin 15:523-545
51. Leape LL, Cullen DJ, Clapp MD et al (1999) Pharmacist participation on physician rounds and adverse drug events in the intensive care unit. JAMA 282:267-270
52. Wu AW (2000) Medical error: the second victim. BMJ 320:726-727
53. Pilpel D, Schor R, Benbassat J (1998) Barriers to acceptance of medical error: the case for a teaching program. Med Educ 21:3-7
54. Vincent JL (1998) Information in the ICU: are we being honest with our patients? The results of a European questionnaire. Intensive Care Med 24:1251-1256
55. Finkelstein D, Wu AW, Holtzman NA, Smith MK (1997) When a physician harms a patient by a medical error: ethical, legal and risk management considerations. J Clin Ethics 8: 330-335

Error Prevention in Anesthesia and Critical Care Medicine

P.D. LUMB

"Health care is a decade or more behind other high-risk industries in its attention to assuring basic safety" [1]. This statement, in association with the published fact that "at least 44 000 Americans die each year as a result of medical errors" [2], focused public attention on an area of medical practice that previously had been the province of professional jurisprudence. Unfortunately, the report implied that organized medicine not only had allowed an unsafe situation to develop but also had minimal interest in rectifying an unsatisfactory condition. This is in direct contrast to the actual situation that exists in medical training and the outcome results for a number of high-risk procedures. The continued decrease in morbidity and mortality following cardiac surgical procedures demonstrates that improved surgical and anesthetic techniques partnered with technologic advances have successfully combined to create a situation in which the public confidence in intervention is warranted. Medical training emphasizes commitment to details, systematic thinking and personal intolerance of failure. This approach has created an enviable safety record in high-profile procedures, but there is a hidden concern in this success that may benefit from increased scrutiny and a re-evaluation of the traditional resolution of medical misadventure – individual physician blame. Similar to aviation's pilot error, this is an emotional subject, but unlike in the aviation industry, medicine has failed to create an environment in which alternative explanations for failure can be explored easily. The concept of a safe haven in which mistakes cannot only be analyzed but also become the basis for improvement has not been adopted in medicine. The reverse is true in other high-risk industries, and many safety advances derive from frank discussion of "near misses" caused by readily admitted human error. In contrast, the physician's cultural and training-imposed reliance on personal faultless performance excellence imposes an unreasonable expectation and an intellectual isolation not felt in other professions. As a result, useful information and improvement opportunity are lost. However, to blame this situation on an overly self-protective medical profession is unfair and ignores the legal environment in which physicians practice. Also, despite the legitimate concern over personal imperfection and desire to reduce unnecessary harm, liability concerns surrounding error or complication self-reporting have limited opportunities to capitalize on this stratagem. Finally, the 50% reduction in error rate called for in the Institute of Medicine (IOM) report is an unreasonable expectation given the overall low complication rate in most routine procedures; the perceived medical analogy to scheduled airline travel. Is this a reasonable comparison? It is important to differentiate between the environments in which anesthesiologists and other high-risk professionals work. Anesthesiologists and critical care physicians never "enter" the patient's situation, but the environment in which they work may contribute to procedural errors and ultimate adverse patient outcomes. Performance is likely dependent upon the interaction and communication between various professionals, and any delay, degradation or disruption in information transfer may thwart the best intentions and therapeutic strategies. Also, and more insidiously, recent changes in reimbursement have altered longstanding treatment strategies without analysis of consequence. In contrast, airline crews work in a structured environment in which roles are not only important, but also scripted and practiced in numerous training exercises. Advanced Cardiac Life Support courses attempt to replicate this preparation, but despite the hospital privileging requirement of successful completion, practical performance of basic airway and resuscitation techniques remains poor in many institutions. The disparity between theory and performance is more likely due to poor teamwork, role delegation and therapeutic prioritization at the point of care rather than inability to perform the techniques or remember the appropriate algorithm. It is unlikely that this level of discord would be tolerated in the airline or nuclear power industries. Before assuming an overly critical attitude towards physicians, it must be remembered that the performance standards required by current training programs and certifying examinations accentuate individual responsibility and action, and that medical systems and hospital environments may be more the culprit in causing medical error. It is this concern that is the focus of the following discussion.

The March 18 issue of the *British Medical Journal* was focused on safety in health care; the following excerpt is abstracted from the editorial by the issue's guest editors.

All physicians, after all, have had the unwelcome experience of becoming what Wu calls "the second victim", being involved in an error or patient injury and feeling the attendant sense of guilt or remorse as responsible professionals [3]. Familiar, too, are Helmreich's findings that doctors, like pilots, tend to overestimate their ability to function flawlessly under adverse conditions, such as under the pressure of time, fatigue, or high anxiety [4]… The necessary changes [to minimize error] are as much cultural as technical. Creating a culture of safety requires attention not only to the design of our tasks and processes, but to the conditions under which we work – hours, schedules and workloads –; how we interact with one another; and, perhaps most importantly, how we train every member of the healthcare team to participate in the quest for safer patient care… We have already learnt a great deal from the early experiences of error reduction in healthcare organisations. Firstly, we have discovered an immense reservoir of creativity and motivation among healthcare workers of all kinds…

Secondly… leadership is an essential ingredient of success in the search for safety… major systems changes require direction and support from the top… Thirdly, we have learnt that the problem of medical error is not fundamentally due to lack of knowledge… Health care alone refuses to accept what other hazardous industries recognised long ago: safe performance cannot be expected from workers who are sleep deprived [A current US television advertisement for Sealy Posturepedic mattresses claims that 68 million Americans are sleep deprived], who work double or triple shifts, or whose job designs involve multiple competing urgent priorities. Based on currently available knowledge, constructive, effective changes to improve patient care can begin at once… no other hazardous industry has achieved safety without substantial external pressure. Safe industries are, by and large, highly regulated… As we enter the new century, a key lesson from the old is that everyone benefits from transparency. Both the safety of our patients and the satisfaction of our workers require an open and non-punitive environment where information is freely shared and responsibility broadly accepted… Are we ready to change? Or will we procrastinate and dissemble – to lament later when the inevitable regulatory backlash occurs? It may seem to some that the race to patient safety has just begun, but the patience of the public we serve is already wearing thin. They are asking us to promise something reasonable, but more than we have ever promised before: that they will not be harmed by the care that is supposed to help them. We owe them nothing less, and that debt is now due" [5].

These sentiments are shared across the spectrum of health care professions and professionals as indicated by increased interest in the medication error rate in hospitals worldwide. "For the most part, patients or consumers have believed that when they enter the healthcare system, they are safe and protected from harm. The IOM report serves as a reminder that while not every mediation error will result in harm to the patient, many will, and clearly enough data exist to suggest a serious concern for patient safety" [6]. "… Medical errors can cause pain – pain suffered by patients, by relatives and, in different ways, by clinicians too –. Medical errors, by definition are unintentional, their causes usually multifactorial. Will chastisement, 'naming and shaming', or 'recertification' decrease current levels of medical error? If we are to make progress in this emotive area, profession and public alike will need to acknowledge that most errors do not amount to negligence; they stem more from systemic organizational failures rather than from the isolated failure of individuals" [7]. It is interesting to note the increased interest in the role delivery system design and environmental features play in causing medical error, either by commission or omission. Unfortunately, the public has, to a large extent, misinterpreted the results of the reports and believes that hospitals are increasingly dangerous, that physicians and administrators are aware of but unresponsive to the problem, and that errors are most likely attributable to individual malfeasance. This is a dangerous attitude for the medical profession in that it may delay necessary reform and support inappropriate behaviors among physicians who are unlikely to embrace the attitudinal, behavioral and educational changes that will be necessary to address the situation. Indeed, the reality is that medical care is safer, largely due to the work of physicians and other health care professionals, but that safety comes at a cost that is increasingly difficult to sustain with continued downward pressure on reimbursement. Indeed, headlines continue to support the continued difficulty encountered by HMOs: "HMO is pulling out on seniors; HealthAmerica to ax its midstate Medicare plan. Officials said the health plans are withdrawing for the same reason that Keystone Health Plan Central, HealthGuard of Lancaster, HealthCentral and Aetna U.S. HealthCare have withdrawn or otherwise changed their plans – the cost of running the programs is greater than the revenue the programs generate –" [8]. The medical profession must maintain the prerogative for directing change because the public has a misperception of medicine's safety and inability to perform accurate procedural risk assessments on complex medical interventions. New York State's publication of hospital- and surgeon-specific cardiac surgery outcome data caused significant initial confusion but did little to alter patient referral patterns (physician-based prerogative) or patient acceptance of treatment facility (patient prerogative that could be altered by reported data). The conclusions are that both consumer and provider need to understand the altered environment and that new approaches to error reduction must be developed.

Lessons may be learned from the aircraft industry. Early attention was placed on pilot training and simulation, and although intuitively attractive, simulation training has not been shown conclusively to either reduce accident rates or be an effective replacement for live "hands on" experience. Indeed, recent reports indicate that simulated takeoff and landing training does not prevent mistakes as noted on a recent flight outbound from Los Angeles to Japan that encountered flight difficulty following rollout that was inappropriately managed by the copilot responsible. Subsequently, minimum numbers of live takeoffs and landings were suggested to maintain competency. Despite this incident, there can be little doubt that planning and practicing for emergencies and/or unusual events makes sense and is beneficial. The concept of using a virtual hospital, case-based learning and standardized patients is gaining popularity in medical education, and in anesthesia, the use of full patient simulators is increasing in training and recertification programs amidst research designed to evaluate the effectiveness of the experience. Trainees who have learned to set up the anesthesia machine and associated patient monitoring technology and to manage a simple anesthetic from induction through emergence in the simulator are more comfortable in the patient care setting and are able to appreciate clinical teaching more easily (unpublished observations, Department of Anesthesia, PennState University College of Medicine). However, as in aviation there is no belief that simulation can match patient/procedure-based experience, but unlike aviation, medicine is behind in evolving the simulation experience from individual performance to team-based activities. This change has been noted in industry as altered focus from personal prerequisites to system requirements, and airline training has progressed from Crisis through Cockpit to the current Crew Resource Management strategies. The implication and practice recognize the fact that despite the announcement “Your Chicago-based flight crew would like to…”, the likelihood of the flight crew knowing one another is low to non-existent. Many crews meet for the first time at the aircraft door, and their ability to provide comprehensive and coordinated service is based not only on the involved individuals understanding the job descriptions and roles to which they are assigned but also performing them flawlessly, in routine and crisis situations. It is likely that this type of training will become commonplace in medicine as greater attention is paid to the work environment and cultural and behavioral integration of the members of the various care teams in a hospital. As previously noted, cardiac life support training under the auspices of the American Heart Association has become a gold standard for emergency response planning and training in US and European hospitals, and the protocols have been extended to off-site responders. At accident sites in which single or multiple victims and transports are encountered, emergency medical personnel can be predicted to perform similar tasks and prepare patients following standard protocols. At the referral center, patient handling is facilitated and comprehensive information transfer is expedited. Unfortunately, the elective surgical schedule and operating room environment in most institutions is less well organized and role definition is poorly understood, never practiced and often changes depending upon the personalities involved. To complicate matters, the equipment is not standardized, location of routine and emergency may be department-specific and personnel are often assigned to a new location without orientation or equipment familiarization. It is unlikely that the aircraft industry would intentionally alter the cockpit or galley controls of an MD-80 without specific requests from the customer and extensive notification that modifications had been performed. Despite the inappropriate public perception of unlicensed individuals performing medical care and procedures, the availability of manufacturer's representatives being available to detail new equipment in the clinical setting is beneficial. It must be remembered that no matter how robust simulation becomes in the near term, medicine will be “practiced live”. The profession's responsibility is to insure a physical and mental environment in which individual participants can perform at peak efficiency.

Following his overwhelming victory at the US Open golf tournament, Tiger Woods commented that he needed to improve his game and work on his swing. This followed extensive practice with his coach prior to the tournament, and an unending pursuit of personal excellence demanding exquisite attention to coordination and self-analysis. Professional athletes work on the physical aspects of their respective performances and hire professional coaches and fitness trainers to help them succeed in the task. Perhaps because their improvement target is obvious, victory and premier ranking, they are willing to accept the necessity for sometimes dramatic change in their approach or outlook. Similar traits are characteristic of successful performers in other publicly acclaimed specialties e.g. music, ballet. Physicians must aspire to similar standards of excellence, and in most cases appear to fulfill their obligations admirably. The significant difference between the other examples and the medical profession appears to be that the environment in which medical performance is judged is unequal to the responsibility of insuring the best possible outcome. The orchestra's rules are quite rigid, and although the soloist has personal prerogative, the audience's musical experience is dependent on the interaction between soloist and orchestra, adjudicated by the conductor in full view of critical reportage. Similar statements hold for most other professions; medicine is alone in its acceptance of individual peculiarity despite industrial models indicating that standardization is better for performance improvement and outcome enhancement. Robust outcome studies of individual performance are rare and in open peer review settings, most physicians are familiar with the "in my hands" phenomenon that exculpates any inadequacy. In defense, physicians are faced with a litigious society in which open reporting of potential error is fraught with the likelihood of personal legal retribution by the plaintiff's attorney's working on a contingency basis. Error reporting in aviation and other industries and in the Australian incident reporting systems is not only encouraged but also protected from undue legal intrusion. In order for meaningful change to occur in the prevailing reporting climate, general awareness and recognition of a problem of significant magnitude to warrant attention must prevail. Correction will require: behavioral modification at individual and team levels; encouragement of near miss reporting to analyze underlying, systematic causes; work environment changes with emphasis placed on team construction; and public information regarding appropriate perception of risks and realistic outcome expectation. Deviation from routine is unnerving, and any change to familiar conditions is likely to invoke employee discomfort and unease. Careful support and example must come from key institutional leaders, and change management should be addressed as a continuing project rather than for short-term political gain and false expectation of a uniformly supported activity.

The culture of undergraduate medical education needs to be one in which tomorrow's doctors are sensitized to the importance of error recognition, enumeration, and investigation. The 'bravado' culture identified in some medical schools almost certainly hinders recognition and investigation of clinical error and discourages the necessary sharing of emotions after error has been detected [9, 10]. The phenomenon of clinical error thereby continues to occupy a shadowy and barely acknowledged territory in medicine; a crucial aim must be to bring it forth to a more civic cultural position, open to scrutiny that is not necessarily driven by blame [7].

Anesthesiology has successfully reduced anesthesia mortality rates from two deaths per 10 000 anesthetics administered to one death per 200 000-300 000 anesthetics administered. This success was accomplished through a combination of:

- technological changes (new monitoring equipment, standardization of existing equipment);

- information-based strategies, including the development and adoption of guidelines and standards;
- application of human factors to improve performance, such as the use of simulators for training;
- formation of the Anesthesia Patient Safety Foundation to bring together stakeholders from different disciplines (physicians, nurses, manufacturers) to create a focus for action; and
- having a leader who could serve as a champion for the cause [11].

Although anesthesia has been a leader in making necessary adaptations to equipment and technology in order to promote patient safety, and the Anesthesia Patient Safety Foundation has been at the forefront of professional acceptance of responsibility in promulgating safety research and education, this example has not been adopted by other disciplines. Unfortunately, no organization covers the multiple professions represented in the medical environment, and to date error reduction efforts tend to be specialty related. Despite the value of these initiatives, it is unlikely that the root cause of certain problems will be ascertained, especially if it relates to interdisciplinary, environmental issues. The Institute of Medicine sponsored a multi-professional (pharmacy, nursing, and medicine) workshop to explore ways in which professional societies could work together to improve patient safety. "Four broad roles were identified that could be employed, individually or in combination, to create a culture of safety. These roles are: 1) defining standards of practice; 2) convening and collaborating among society members and with other groups; 3) encouraging research, training and education opportunities; and 4) advocating for change" [12]. Other organizations have devoted significant attention to patient safety, and the American Society of Health Care Pharmacists, the American Society of Anesthesiologists, the Society of Critical Care Medicine and the American Academy of Pediatrics to name a few have published practice guidelines for their members. Some of these are available through the National Guidelines Clearing House Web site or directly from the society [13]. Initiatives are underway to produce collaborative guidelines, and the Society of Critical Care Medicine is currently working with the Association of Health Care Pharmacists to publish collaborative patient care guidelines on the use of sedatives, analgesics and muscle relaxants in critical care medicine. To accomplish this goal, two multiprofessional task forces are working simultaneously; one is dealing with muscle relaxants and the other with analgesics and sedatives. Because of the frequent co-prescription of these agents, a common facilitator is coordinating the evidence-based task force activities. The College of Critical Care Medicine is sponsoring the task force activities and will champion the work product and coordinate its simultaneous publication following peer review by both sponsoring organizations. Although complex, this description supports the concept of drawing together multiple professionals in order to collaborate on safety improvement through publishing evidence-based prescription guidelines. More multidisciplinary collaboration of this nature is required to support the Institute of Medicine's recommendations.

It has been suggested that advances in medical technology have outpaced the advances in delivery systems and that a "chassis gap" exists; specifically, advanced therapeutic interventions are performed in an environment that is underpowered (e.g. lacking responsive information technology and reporting systems) for the requirements imposed upon it. Supermarkets and other marginal profit entities could not exist with similar constraints, yet physicians, nurses, pharmacists and other patient care advocates are forced to work with substandard information systems and available electronic safeguards. "Human factors is defined as the study of the interrelationships between humans, the tools they use, and the environment in which they live and work" [14]. The object of the research is to improve the conditions in which people work by studying the interface between person, machine and work environment or process. "This might include simplifying and standardizing procedures, building in redundancy to provide backup and opportunities for recovery, improving communications and coordination within teams, or redesigning equipment to improve the human-machine interface" [15]. The approaches used in analyzing human factors interfaces are either an analysis of critical incidents or by examining the manner in which individuals make decisions in their specific work environment. In order to expand the likelihood that practitioners will identify and report critical incidents for analysis, it will be necessary to minimize the current legal liability inherent in admitting potential fault. Although analysis may support a non-supportive system, nonetheless, the recognition that 82% of preventable incidents involved human error [16] and a litigious society stultifies self-reporting in the United States. "We don't talk much about errors because deep down we believe that individual diligence should prevent errors, and so the very existence of errors damages our professional image" [17].

Perrow has characterized systems according to two important dimensions: complexity and tight or loose coupling [18]. Further analysis of systems identifies those that may be more likely to be error prone. Complex systems are defined as those in which one component of the system can interact with multiple other components, often in unexpected fashion. Coupling comes from mechanics and identifies a system in which two items interact directly with no buffer or slack between them. Patient care systems tend to be large and tightly coupled with numerous examples of one process following another in a time-dependent fashion. Certainly, there is little slack at the point of care, and once the system begins to break down, retrieval is difficult and accidents are increasingly likely. Because of complexity and coupling, small failures can grow into large accidents [19]. Nolan has summarized a number of tactics to reduce errors and adverse events: 1) reduce complexity; 2) optimize information processing; 3) automate wisely; 4) use constraints; and 5) mitigate the unwanted side effects of change [20]. It is interesting to note that despite these insights, most medical systems have not encouraged the multidisciplinary cooperation necessary to effect necessary change. It may behoove medicine to recognize Bob Dylan's wisdom in that "the loser for now will be later to win, for the times they are a-changin" [21]. Simulation attempts to train team leaders to prioritize available medical information and to delegate tasks where appropriate. The distribution of workload is an important component of leadership responsibility, but it is important to understand the responsibility of the trained team in following appropriate directions. Equally, the team is responsible to provide feedback and avoid cognitive dysfunction and development of tunnel vision with inappropriate unitary focus on failing remedies. The concept of teamwork permeates industrial models of process improvement, and this must become one of the foci of medical change in the future.

Cognitive failures involve mismatch between intentions and actions, or, more specifically, the action result. No physician or health care professional wants or deserves a situation in which a patient is harmed or a medical decision or therapeutic outcome is judged unsatisfactory. Anesthesiologists and critical care physicians are well positioned to lead future innovation in healthcare quality initiatives. Although ambulatory sites will benefit, the inpatient and hospital environments are those in which the likelihood of error secondary to inefficient or inadequate systems designs are most likely to occur. Cognitive skills are taught efficiently in specialty training programs and proficiency is routinely assessed. Seldom are team skills developed; indeed, most medical training programs accentuate individual responsibility and independence. These are essential characteristics for successful physicians, but societal and institutional responsibilities are equally important and never assessed. This is an untenable situation if industrial models of error reduction are applicable to medicine. Physicians must develop a system of performance self-analysis and audit predicated on creating a non-threatening environment in which the aim is to improve the quality of medical care rendered. In order to do this effectively, observed performance must be compared with agreed upon and published criteria. The system should be formal, systematic, and peer reviewed, and the results of all inquiries must be published and made available to all participants in the relevant process or system. The review provides continuous information about the discrepancy between the expected and achieved outcomes and should indicate specific ways in which the deviation can be corrected. Constant vigilance must be tempered by wisdom and sensitivity to the personal nuances inherent in any complex series of human interactions. A standardized approach that has been developed through consensus strategies involving all team members is the most effective manner in which to not only create the best current situation but also to anticipate future advances and adjust processes expectantly to maximize team participation and innovation.

"Deaths due to medical errors are exaggerated in Institute of Medicine Report" [22] state McDonald et al. in a recent article published in the controversies section of the *Journal of the American Medical Association*. Not so retorts Leape in an accompanying counterpoint [23]. Certainly, it is unwise to adopt change without investigating the source material from which opinions and suggested behavioral change are taken. For this, McDonald et al. are to be congratulated. However, Leape summarizes the somewhat controversial task facing the medical profession as follows:

The IOM report has galvanized a national movement to improve patient safety. It is about time. Although the initial impact of the IOM report is in part due to the shocking figures (which, unfortunately, are not exaggerated), its long-term impact will result from the validity of its message that errors can be prevented by redesigning medical work. Rather than attempting to assuage guilt or outrage about errors by punishing, discounting or self-flagellation, physicians need to look to preventing recurrence of errors. Errors and "excess" mortality can be eliminated, but only if concern and attention is shifted away from individuals and toward the error prone systems in which clinicians work. That is the IOM message, and it is a hopeful one. Physicians should embrace this message with enthusiasm and vigor [24].

Anesthesia and critical care medicine depend on smooth interactions between numerous individuals, some obvious and others hidden. Irrespective of the difficulty, the challenge and responsibility are clear. Techniques exist to improve on our current performance, both as individuals and as team members and despite requisite behavioral changes, our patients, colleagues and society demands that we succeed.

References

1. Gaba D, Cooper J (1999-2000) Landmark report published on patient safety. Anesthesia Patient Safety Foundation Newsletter 14(4):37-52
2. Kohn LT, Corrigan JM, Donaldson MS (1999) To err is human. Building a safer health system. National Academy Press, Washington, DC
3. Joint Commission Accreditation statement. http://www.jcaho.org/whoweare_frm.html
4. Wu A (2000) Medical error: the second victim. BMJ 320:726-727
5. Helmreich RL (2000) On error management: lessons from aviation. BMJ 320:781-785
6. Leape LL, Berwick DM (2000) Safe health care: are we up to it? We have to be. BMJ 320: 725-726
7. Briceland LL (2000) Medication errors: an expose of the problem. Medscape Pharmacists, http://www.medscape.com?Medscape?pharmacists/journal/2000/v01.n03/mph0530.bric/mph0530.bric-01.1
8. Sheikh A, Hurwitz B (1999) A national database of medical error. J R Soc Med 92:554-555
9. McGaw J (2000) HMO is pulling out on seniors. The Patriot News (Harrisburg, PA), July 8, 159;161:1
10. Styles WM (1999) Stress in undergraduate medical education: 'the mask of relaxed brilliance'. Br J Gen Pract 43:46-47
11. – (1995) Review of guidance on doctors' performance. Maintaining medical excellence. Department of Health, London
12. Pierce EC (1996) The 34th Rovenstine Lecture, 40 years behind the mask: safety revisited. Anesthesiology 87(4):965-967
13. Kohn LT, Corrigan JM, Donaldson MS (1999) To err is human. Building a safer health system. National Academy Press, Washington, DC, p 125
14. – (1999) ASA Standards, Guidelines and Statements. American Society of Anesthesiologists, Park Ridge

15. Weinger MB, Pantiskas C, Wiklund M, Carstensen P (1998) Incorporating human factors into the design of medical devices. JAMA 280(17):1484
16. Reason J (1990) Human error. University Press, Cambridge
17. Kohn LT, Corrigan JM, Donaldson MS (1999) To err is human. Building a safer health system. National Academy Press, Washington, DC, p 54
18. Reinersten JL (2000) Let's talk about error: leaders should take responsibility for error. BMJ 320:730
19. Perrow C (1984) Normal accidents. Basic Books, New York
20. Kohn LT, Corrigan JM, Donaldson MS (1999) To err is human. Building a safer health system. National Academy Press, Washington, DC, p 50
21. Nolan TW (2000) System changes to improve patient safety. BMJ 320:771-773
22. Dylan B (2000) The times they are a-changin (recording)
23. McDonald CJ, Weiner M, Hui SL (2000) Deaths due to medical errors are exaggerated in Institute of Medicine report. JAMA 284:93-95
24. Leape LL (2000) Institute of Medicine medical error figures are not exaggerated. JAMA 284:95-97

Evidence-Based Medicine: An Effective Guide to Intelligent Physician

A. BRIENZA, N. BRIENZA, N. D'ONGHIA

The overwhelming growth of biomedical literature in the past 20 years, financial crisis of healthcare systems, traditional clinical practice characterized by medical actions not supported by valid scientific basis, and the development of the Internet and biomedical databases have all fostered the birth of evidence-based medicine (EBM), supported in the last 30 years by Archi Cochrane.

EBM must be viewed as a powerful self-learning process in which patient care is based on clinically relevant information concerning diagnosis, prognosis, and therapy, such that physicians should base their clinical decisions on the results of the best-available scientific literature.

All EBM working groups should address their activity to plan and produce only the best evidence-based studies (Table 1).

Table 1. Strength of evidence based on scientific literature about proposed treatment (*CI* confidence interval)[a]

Level I	Randomized trials with low false-positive and low false-negative errors (i.e., small 95% CI)
Level II	Randomized trials with high false-positive and/or high false-negative errors, i.e., trial with a not statistically significant trend about a treatment (i.e., with very large 95% CI). Pooling of data of two small level II trials by meta-analysis may result in overall level I evidence
Level III	Evidence from well-designed trials without randomization: single group pre-post, cohort, time series or matched case-controlled studies
Level IV	Evidence from well-designed non-experimental studies from more than one research center
Level V	Opinions of respected authorities based on clinical evidence, descriptive studies or reports of expert committees
Level VI	Someone once told me

[a] Modified from CLIB training guide

The basic aim is to restrict the huge field of clinical practice not supported by valid scientific basis (gray zones) and still characterized by personal opinion and/or school tradition [1].

On the other side, one of the most-dangerous EBM-related troubles is to consider scientific data as absolute dogma. Scientific data should be considered as the gold standard, but clinical decision-making must be the result of integrating scientific information and clinical experience.

Randomized controlled trial (RCT) is the best scientific study when comparing new and standard treatments, but clinical trials are often inhomogeneous when considering quality, aim of the study, sample, methods, and so on. Metaing-analysis is a powerful tool for collecting results of different trials concerning the same clinical problem.

Do meta-analysis conclusions always correspond to RCT conclusions? Very often, but not always!!! In the following table, results from meta-analysis and RCT about stress ulcer prophylaxis in the intensive care unit (ICU) are shown, as published by Brazzi et al. [2] (Table 2).

Table 2. Incidence of complications and stress ulcer prophylaxis

Confidence interval (95%)	**Multicenter trial** [3] **(Relative risk) Ranitidine vs. sucralfate**	**Meta-analysis** [4] **(Odds ratio) Sucralfate vs. ranitidine**
Gastrointestinal bleeding	0.44	0.95
Incidence of pneumonia	1.18	0.78
Mortality	1.03	0.83

Why do results differ? Inclusion criteria in RCT collected by meta-analysis may not take into account dangerous biases, such as sample and outcome inhomogeneity. It is a common belief that the power of meta-analysis relies on the ability to produce conclusions from studies with different sample size and characteristics. However, statistical conclusions may differ from clinical reality, and on a methodological basis, it is correct only to reach conclusions from experimentally overlapping studies. In the following pages, we will review some of the most clinically relevant questions in the field of intensive care on the basis of EBM.

Blood transfusion

Red cell transfusions are a key treatment in the critical care setting. However, some questions arise when considering the risk/benefit ratio of transfusions.

In the 1999 the *New England Journal of Medicine* published a multicenter RCT (first level of evidence) by Hebert et al. [5] evaluating the effects on mortality of two different transfusion strategies. Euvolemic critically ill patients were randomized to receive red cell transfusions at a hemoglobin level < 7 g/dl (restrictive strategy, 418 patients – maintenance hemoglobin level ranging from 7 to 9 g/dl) or < 10 g/dl (liberal strategy, 420 patients – maintenance hemoglobin level ranging from 10 to 12 g/dl). Although global ICU mortality was not different between the two groups, the study showed that mortality was significantly lower in less severely ill patients (APACHE II score < 20) and younger patients (< 55 years of age) of the restrictive strategy group when compared to the liberal strategy group. No difference was found between cardiac patients (acute myocardial infarction/unstable angina) of the two groups.

Mechanical ventilation

In patients with acute lung injury/acute respiratory distress syndrome (ALI/ARDS) the primary goal has always been to normalize gas exchange. In 1990, for example, respiratory acidosis from hypercarbia due to low tidal volumes (TVs) would have hardly been accepted. Nowadays, in ALI/ARDS patients, it is appreciated that ventilation must be as harmless as possible, and less traumatic mechanical ventilation has been proposed. The ARDS network has recently published a large multicenter RCT comparing low TV ventilation with high TV ventilation in ALI/ARDS patients [6]. Low TV patients were ventilated in the first 3 days with a mean TV of 6.2 ± 0.8 ml/kg, which was significantly lower than TV in the control group, averaging in the same period 11.8 ± 0.8 ml/kg. Similarly, mean plateau pressure was significantly lower in the low TV group (25 ± 6 cm H_2O) when compared to the high TV group (33 ± 8 cm H_2O). In low TV group, mortality was significantly lower than in the high TV group (31% vs. 39.8%, $p = 0.007$).

Thus, although three recent trials [7-9] have failed to demonstrate any significant benefit of low TV ventilation (probably due to inadequate differences in the ventilatory setting of the control group), other trials [6, 10] clearly demonstrated mortality and weaning time advantages when low TV ventilation strategy was compared to traditional TV ventilation.

Supranormal oxygen delivery

In 1988, Shoemaker et al. [11] published a randomized, controlled, prospective study in high-risk surgical patients. In the first group, hemodynamic treatment was guided by central venous pressure (control group), in the second group a Swan Ganz catheter was used to normalize hemodynamic status and oxygen delivery (Swan Ganz control group), and in the third group a Swan Ganz catheter was used in order to reach supranormal values of cardiac index, oxygen delivery, and oxygen consumption (CI > 4.5 l/min per m^2, DO_2 > 600 ml/min per m^2, $\dot{V}O_2$ > 170 ml/min per m^2) as therapeutic goals (Swan-Ganz supranormal group). Hospital mortality was 38, 23, and 4% in the three groups, respectively ($p < 0.05$), suggesting that maximizing hemodynamic values contributed to prevent oxygen debt and improved mortality. A subsequent study by Boyd et al. [12] confirmed Shoemaker's results; 28-day mortality was lower in high-risk patients treated on the basis of increasing DO_2 compared with control group mortality (6% vs. 22%). In 1994, Hayes et al. [13] performed a new randomized, prospective, controlled trial on elevation of oxygen delivery in critically ill patients. In the group treated according to Shoemaker's hemodynamic goals, mortality was significantly higher compared to control group (48% vs. 30%). More recently, an Italian multicenter, randomized, controlled trial [14] has shown no difference in mortality among patients randomized to reach cardiac index between 2.5 and 3.5 l/min per m^2, cardiac index > 4.5 l/min per m^2, or SvO_2 > 70%.

Where is the truth? Recent meta-analysis dealing with most of the above quoted studies has tried to clarify the issue of maximizing oxygen delivery [15]. The conclusion was that patients treated to reach supranormal values of cardiac index, oxygen delivery and oxygen consumption show an in significant trend towards mortality reduction. Relative risk (RR) averages 0.86 (95% CI ± 0.24), i.e., there is a slight, in significant benefit when supranormal values are reached. However, when treatment is begun in the preoperative phase, RR is only 0.2 (all patients have a RR < 1), while when treatment is begun after the onset of disease RR rises to 0.98.

Tracheostomy

Nowadays, tracheostomy may be performed by percutaneous (PTC) or surgical (STC) technique. In 1999, Dulguerov et al. [16] published a meta-analysis dealing with the comparison between STC and PTC. All studies published from 1960 to 1996 and addressing peri- and postoperative complications were included. STC studies were divided according to publication year into a 1960-1984 group and a 1985-1996 group. All PTC studies were published after 1985. Results of this meta-analysis include: 1) less-recent STC studies (1960-1984) present the highest complication rate both in the peri- and postoperative phase (8.5 and 33%, respectively); 2) when comparing contemporary STC and PTC studies, perioperative complications are higher in the PTC group (10% vs. 3%), while postoperative complications are more frequent in the STC group (10% vs. 7%).

Subsequent studies have restricted comparison to STC and Ciaglia PCT. Muttini et al. [17] do not report any significant difference in the perioperative complication rate between STC and Ciaglia PCT. However, the postoperative complication rate is higher in STC when compared with Ciaglia PTC.

Similar results are reported in the recent RCT by Hekkinen et al. [18]. Moreover, this study analyzes economical issue and shows a significantly better benefit/cost ratio in the Ciaglia PTC group when compared with the ST group.

Thus, although in past years there has been a progressive, marked improvement of the STC technique, PCT when performed with endoscopic control is an easy, safe and cost-effective procedure with a very low postoperative complication rate.

Crystalloid versus colloid solutions

Different colloid solutions are widely used in fluid resuscitation of critically ill patients, but there is ongoing debate about the relative effectiveness of these colloids compared to crystalloid fluids. Therefore a Cochrane review of RCTs has recently been performed [19]. The main results are as follows:

1. albumin or plasma protein fraction vs. crystalloids:
   - 18 trials including a total of 641 patients;
   - the pooled RR was 1.52 (95% CI);
   - the risk of death in the albumin-treated group was 6% higher than in the crystalloid group. When poor quality trials were excluded, the RR decreased to 1.34 (0.95 - 1.89);
2. hydroxyethylstarch (HES) vs. crystalloids:
   - seven trials including a total of 197 patients were included in the meta-analysis;
   - the RR was 1.16 (0.68 - 1.96);
   - there was no difference between HES and crystalloyd solutions;
3. modified gelatin and crystalloids:
   - four trials including a total of 95 patients;
   - the RR was 0.5 (0.08 - 3.03);
   - modified gelatin seems better, but CI is too large;
4. dextran vs. crystalloids:
   - eight trials including a total of 668 patients;
   - the RR was 1.24 (0.94 - 1.65);
   - small differences exist between the two fluids;
5. colloids in hypertonic crystalloids vs. crystalloids alone:
   - eight trials including 1,283 patients;
   - the RR was 0.88 (0.74 - 1.05);
   - small differences have been reported between these two solutions.

Therefore, there is no evidence from RCTs that volume replacement with colloids reduces the risk of death when compared with crystalloids in burn, trauma, and postsurgical patients.

Colloids are more expensive than crystalloids and are not associated with an improvement in survival. Thus, it is difficult to justify their continued use outside the context of RCTs.

Conclusions

Although it has strengthened health care, EBM should not become the new millennium myth. When dealing with "evidence" we should remember that evidence must not be viewed as undisputable. Clinical trials try to rebuild a clinical "hic et nunc" frame that does not always mirror individual clinical situations. Sometimes, EBM provides opposite messages. In 1998, in *New England Journal of Medicine* an editorial was published [20] comparing two similar randomized, controlled trials [21, 22] dealing with *Helicobacter pylori* eradication by antibiotic therapy. In each RCT, *H. pylori* was eradicated in 79% of patients receiving omeprazole and antibiotics, but only in a few patients receiving omeprazole alone. Dyspepsia resolved in more than 20% of patients receiving both drugs. However, while in the multicenter study of Blum et al. [21], dyspepsia resolved in a similar percentage oc patients treated with omeprazole alone, in the study of McColl et al. [22], dyspepsia resolved in only 7% of patients receiving omeprazole alone. Therefore, the two studies provide opposite conclusions regarding the effectiveness of antibiotics and of *H. pylori* eradication in resolving dyspepsia. Certainly it's a borderline case, but which evidence should be accepted?

An accurate clinical interpretation of the patient depends upon the physician's intelligence, expertise, and critical ability.

References

1. Cook DJ, Sibbald WJ, Vincent JL, Cerra FB for the Evidence Based Medicine in Critical Care Group (1996) Evidence based critical care medicine: what is it and what can it do for us? Crit Care Med 24:334-337
2. Brazzi L, Bertolini G, Minelli C (2000) Meta-analysis versus randomised controlled trials in intensive care medicine. Intensive Care Med 26:239-241
3. Cook D, Guyatt G, Marshall J et al (1998) A comparison of sucralfate and ranitidine for the prevention of upper gastrointestinal bleeding in patients requiring mechanical ventilation. N Engl J Med 338:791-797
4. Cook DJ, Reeve BK, Guyatt GH et al (1996) Stress ulcer prophylaxis in critically ill patients: resolving discordant meta-analysis. JAMA 275:308-314
5. Hebert PC, Wells G et al and the Transfusion Requirements in Critical Care Investigators for the Canadian Critical Care Trials Group (1999) A multicenter, randomized, controlled clinical trial of transfusion requirements in critical care (TRICC study). N Engl J Med 340:409-417
6. The Acute Respiratory Distress Syndrome Network (2000) Ventilation with lower volumes as compared with traditional tidal volumes for acute lung injury and the acute respiratory distress syndrome. N Engl J Med 342:1301-1308
7. Stewart TE, Meade MO, Cook DJ et al (1998) Evaluation of a ventilation strategy to prevent barotrauma in patients at high risk for acute respiratory distress syndrome. N Engl J Med 338:355-361
8. Brochard L, Roudot-Thoraval F, Roupie E et al (1998) Tidal volume reduction for prevention of ventilator-induced lung injury in acute respiratory distress syndrome. Am J Respir Crit Care Med 158:1831-1838
9. Brower RG, Shanholtz CB, Fessler HE et al (1999) Prospective, randomized, controlled clinical trial comparing traditional versus reduced tidal volume ventilation in acute respiratory distress syndrome patients. Crit Care Med 27:1492-1498
10. Amato MBP, Barbas CSV, Medeiros DM et al (1998) Effect of a protective-ventilation strategy on mortality in the acute respiratory distress syndrome. N Engl J Med 338:347-354
11. Shoemaker W, Appel P, Kram H et al (1988) Prospective trial of supranormal O_2 values as therapeutic goals in high risk surgical patients. Chest 94:1176-1186
12. Boyd O, Grounds RM, Bennett ED (1993) A randomized clinical trial of the effect of deliberate perioperative increase of oxygen delivery on mortality in high risk surgical patients. JAMA 270:2699-2707
13. Hayes MA, Timmins AC, Yau EHS et al (1994) Elevation of systemic oxygen delivery in the treatment of critically ill patients. N Engl J Med 330:1717-1722
14. Gattinoni L, Brazzi L, Pelosi P et al (1995) A trial of goal-oriented hemodynamic therapy in critically ill patients. N Engl J Med 333:1025-1032
15. Heyland DK, Cook DJ, King D et al (1996) Maximizing oxygen delivery in critically ill patients: a methodological reappraisal of the evidence. Crit Care Med 24:517-524
16. Dulguerov P, Gysin C, Perneger TV et al (1999) Percutaneous or surgical tracheostomy: a meta-analysis. Crit Care Med 27:1617-1625
17. Muttini S, Melloni G, Gemma M et al (1999) A prospective, randomized evaluation of early and late complications after either percutaneous or surgical tracheostomy. Minerva Anestesiol 65:521-527
18. Heikkinen M, Aarnio P, Hannukainen J (2000) Percutaneous dilational tracheostomy or conventional surgical tracheostomy? Crit Care Med 28:1399-1402
19. Anderson P, Schierhout G, Roberts I, Bunn F (2000) Colloids versus crystalloids for fluid resuscitation in critical patients. Cochrane Database Syst Rev CD000567
20. Friedman LS (1998) Helicobacter pylori and nonulcer dyspepsia. N Engl J Med 24:1928-3190
21. Blum AL, Talley NJ, O'Morain C et al (1998) Lack of effect of treating Helicobacter pylori infection in patients with nonulcer dyspepsia. N Engl J Med 339:1875-1881
22. McColl K, Murray L, El-Omar E et al (1998) Symptomatic benefit from eradicating Helicobacter pylori infection in patients with nonulcer dyspepsia. N Engl J Med 339:1869-1874

Long-Term Outcome of Intensive Care: How Well Are the Survivors?

P. Nair, T. Jacques

Severity of illness on admission to the intensive care unit (ICU), as measured by commonly used scoring systems, e.g., the Acute Physiological and Chronic Health Evaluation scoring system (APACHE 2) and the Simple Acute Physiological Score (SAPS 2), has been shown to correlate with short-term mortality in groups of patients [1-5].

Mortality statistics are commonly used to evaluate the performance of individual units, in quality management programmes, or to justify staffing or funding [6-8]. However, death is not the only undesirable outcome of treatment in intensive care. The ultimate goal of intensive care treatment should be to return a patient to society with what the patient perceives as a satisfactory quality of life (QOL). QOL has many facets, including health-related QOL or QOL as determined by such things as relationships and employment status. Our focus has been to study health-related QOL and the long-term outcome of intensive care. We have used three general (i.e., not disease-specific) published health-related QOL instruments that look at both physical and psychosocial dimensions of QOL to determine the long-term outcome of patients who survive a critical illness. In doing so we evaluated which of these instruments is most applicable to ICU patients.

The Sickness Impact Profile (SIP) was developed by Dr. Marilyn Bergner as a multi-dimensional profile of health-related QOL [9]. It consists of 136 items to which the respondent replies ‘yes’ or ‘no’. It has 12 scales, which make up two dimensions (physical and psychosocial). The scales of ambulation, mobility, body care, and movement make up the physical dimension. Communication, alertness behavior, emotional behavior, and social interaction form the psychosocial dimension. Independent scales are sleep, rest, eating, work, home management, and recreation and pastimes. The SIP was designed for use in longitudinal studies of subsets of the community, such as our group of ICU patients. The higher the SIP score, the worse the health status. This tool has been used internationally in a number of ICU outcome studies, including a large validation study by Tian and Reis Miranda on 6,247 ICU patients [10].

The Sydney Quality of Life Index (SQOL) was developed at the ICU of a teaching hospital in Sydney [11]. It is a subjective assessment of health, life domains, and satisfaction. It attempts to address the issue of the patient's perspective of QOL. There are 69 items on an 11-point bipolar scale. The SQOL scales are symptom problems, pain, mobility and activity, self-maintenance, general satisfaction, emotional strengths, positive affect, anxious depression, suicidal depression, personal appearance, and social appearance. All scales range from 0 to 10. The higher the SQOL score, the better the health status. Community normal values were established using a random telephone book sample. It is not designed to combine scales into the two domains of physical and psychosocial function as with the SIP.

The Short Form 36 (SF36) also looks at physical and psychosocial aspects of QOL [12, 13]. It is used worldwide and has been used for many diseases and outpatient health assessment in Australia. It is referred to as a generic measure because it assesses health concepts that represent basic human values that are relevant to everyone's functional status and wellbeing. The measures are not age, disease, or treatment specific. Questions can be altered to suit different cultures. The SF36 includes 36 questions, which make up the two dimensions of physical and psychosocial aspects of health-related QOL. The eight scales of the two dimensions included in the SF36 include physical function (PF), physical role (RP), bodily pain (BP), general health (GH), vitality (VT), social function (SF), role emotional (RE), and mental health (MH). The content of each of these scales is detailed in Table 1. Of particular value is the availability of Australian, American, and British normative data and the availability of data for individual co-morbidities such as diabetes. The higher the SF36 score, the better the health status.

Table 1. The eight scales of life examined in the SF36 questionnaire

Scale	Definitions
Physical function (PF)	Extent to which health limits daily physical activities
Role-functioning-physical (RP)	Extent to which physical health interferes with work or other daily activities
Body pain (BP)	Severity of pain and effect on normal activities
General health (GH)	Personal evaluation of health including current health and health outlook (i.e., getting worse or better)
Vitality (VT)	Feeling energetic versus feeling tired and worn out
Social functioning (SF)	Extent to which physical and emotional health interfere with normal social activities
Role functioning-emotional (RE)	Extent to which emotional problems interfere with work and other daily activities
Mental health (MH)	General mental health including depression, anxiety, happiness, and general positive affect

Long-term outcome studies

In three separate prospective longitudinal studies we aimed to document and describe health outcomes of all patients admitted to our ICU in terms of long-term mortality, and the physical and psychosocial status of survivors. The setting was a general ICU in a Sydney teaching hospital.

Study 1

The first cohort included all ICU admissions from 1 February 1994 to 31 July 1994. Individual demographic data and mortality statistics were collected (Table 2). QOL at 3 and 6 months following ICU discharge was studied in the survivors using the SIP and the SQOL. All patients above 18 years were asked to participate. A number of strategies were used to ensure participants completed all sections of the questionnaire, including appropriate interpreters, telephone calls, or personal home visits; 3- and 6-month scores were compared using chi square test for categorical data and Student's two-sample test and analysis of variance (ANOVA) for continuous data. To ascertain determinants of functional status and QOL as measured by the respective scores, regression analysis was performed using the multiple variables.

Table 2. Cohort 1 – mortality statistics

Total admissions = 303	**Number**	**Percentage of admissions**
Died in ICU	52	17.2%
Died in hospital ward	20	8.0%
Died at home < 3 months	6	2.6%
Died at home > 3 months	8	3.6%
Overall 6-month mortality	86	31.4%

Sample characteristics

Three hundred and three patients were admitted to the ICU over the study period. Mean length of ICU stay was 4.5 days. Overall mean APACHE 2 score was 17.1. One hundred and twenty-three patients completed the 3-month questionnaire; 4 of these died before the 6 months; 113 completed the questionnaire at 6 months; 98 completed the questionnaires at both intervals. Participation rate was 62.5% of survivors at 3 months, 60% at 6 months, and 52% at both intervals.

There was no significant difference in sex, APACHE 2 scores, ICU or hospital length of stay, ventilator days, or diagnostic categories between participants and non-participants. Non-participants were significantly younger (51.6 versus

61 years, $p = 0.002$). Therefore our participant sample was reasonably representative of all survivors.

Outcome measures

The mean total SIP score was not significantly different over the study period (15.8 at 3 months and 14.4 at 6 months). These scores are much worse than the normal community (score < 4). There was a non-significant trend to improvement in the total SIP score, and the physical and psychosocial dimensions over time (Fig. 1).

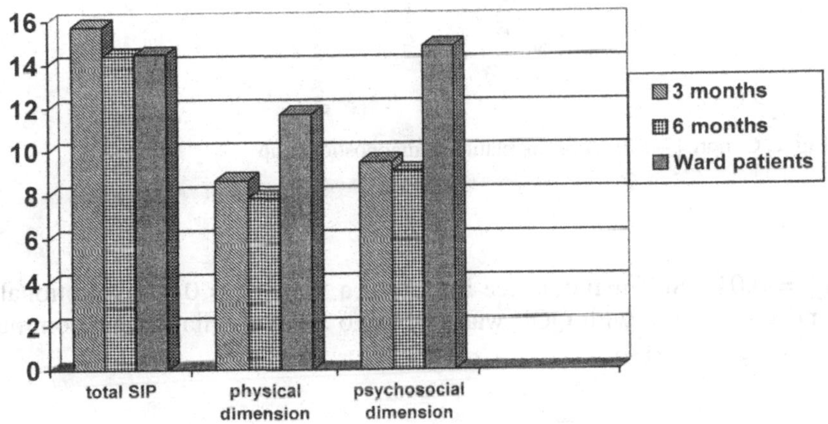

Fig. 1. Cohort 1 – SIP scores at 3 and 6 months compared with a cohort of general ward patients [note: higher Sickness Impact Profile (SIP), poorer quality of life (QOL)]

Both the physical and psychosocial dimensions of SIP were adversely affected by a critical illness. Of the individual SIP scales, work was most affected (mean score = 24.5). There was no difference between medical, elective surgical, and emergency surgical patients (Fig. 2). Multiple linear regression to look for predictors of SIP score, and hence long-term outcome and QOL, showed no correlation with sex, ICU admission diagnosis, and ICU or hospital length of stay. Severity of illness in ICU as measured by the APACHE 2 score correlated poorly with the SIP score ($r = 0.05$, $p = 0.68$). However there was a correlation between age and physical disability as measured by the SIP physical dimension ($r = 0.29$, $p = 0.003$). The correlation between age and the SIP psychosocial dimension was less marked ($r = 0.23$, $p = 0.04$).

There was no significant difference between 3- and 6-month scores of any of the SQOL dimensions. However, there was a trend to improvement in mobility ($p = 0.02$) and with this increase in mobility, a tendency for pain to increase

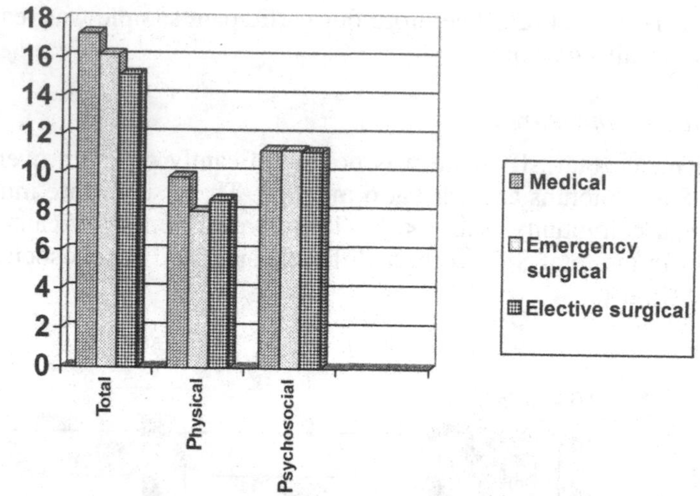

Fig. 2. Cohort 1 – SIP scores in relation to diagnostic group

($p = 0.01$). Self-maintenance improved a little ($p = 0.06$). Emotional strengths and satisfaction with QOL was similar to an Australian urban community sample (Figs. 3 and 4).

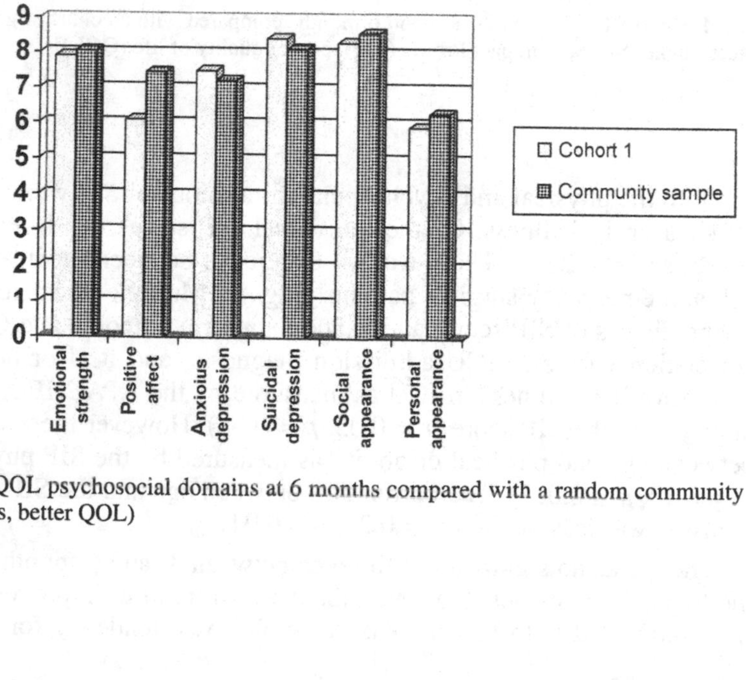

Fig. 3. Cohort 1 – SQOL psychosocial domains at 6 months compared with a random community sample (higher scores, better QOL)

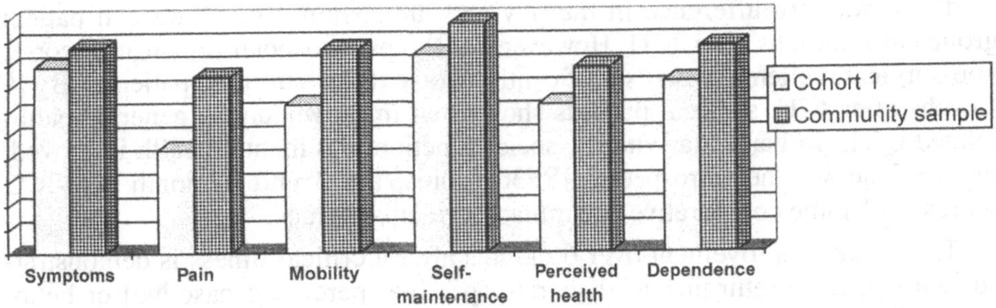

Fig. 4. Cohort 1 – SQOL physical domains at 6 months compared with a random community sample (higher scores, better QOL)

Study 2

The second cohort included all ICU admissions between 1 July 1995 and 31 December 1995. QOL was studied in all consenting survivors 3 and 6 months after discharge from ICU using the SIP and the SF36. In addition, a retrospective or baseline SF36 form was completed by the patients prior to hospital discharge. For this, patients were asked to recall their health prior to the critical illness that brought them to intensive care.

Sample characteristics

There were 388 ICU admissions in this study period and 105 (27%) deaths over the 6-month study period. The mean APACHE 2 score of this cohort was 17.04 (± 9.74). One hundred and twenty-six patients refused to fill out the questionnaires or remained uncontactable. This gave a participation rate of 65.7% of survivors. The non-survivors were older ($p < 0.001$), had higher APACHE II scores (26.2 ± 8.96) and risk of death ($p < 0.001$), had a longer stay in ICU ($p < 0.032$) and were ventilated longer ($p < 0.01$) than patients who participated in the study [6]. For the above variables, survivors who participated in the study did not differ from survivors who refused. Surgical patients were more likely to consent and had a lower mortality than non-surgical patients.

Outcome measures

For the physical and psychosocial dimensions of the SF36, there was no difference between the retrospective or baseline QOL and 3-month post-ICU QOL. Both the SIP and the SF36 tracked an improvement in health-related QOL from 3 to 6 months after ICU. While the overall QOL as measured by the SIP and SF36 remained below the community, the psychosocial dimension of the SF36 approached community values by 6 months.

There was no difference in the physical dimension scores between patient groups at 6 months after ICU. However, for the psychosocial dimension scores, non-surgical patients were significantly worse than surgical patients. By 6 months after ICU, surgical patients showed an improvement in general health-related QOL. In particular vitality, social function and mental health improved. Figure 5 shows the retrospective SF36 scores, the 3 and 6 month post-ICU scores, and some comparative Australian normative values.

The steady improvement over 6 months after a critical illness is demonstrated, with patients returning to their retrospective (perceived baseline) or better health (Fig. 5).

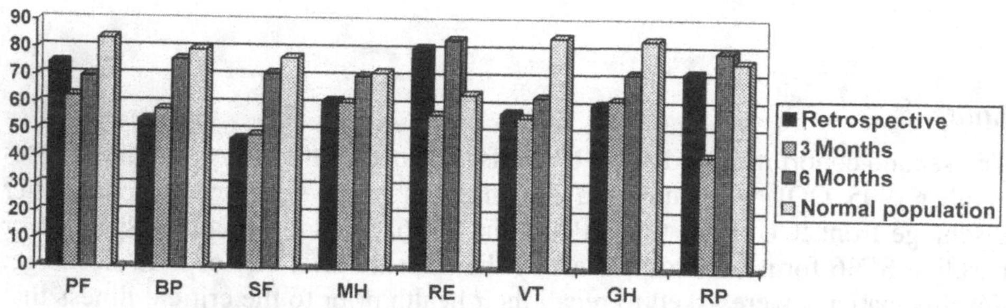

Fig. 5. Cohort 2 – SF36 scores for each scale – retrospective, 3 and 6 months post ICU, and comparison with Australian norms (higher score, better function) (*PF* physical function, *BP* bodily pain, *SF* social function, *MH* mental health, *RE* role emotional, *VT* vitality, *GH* general health,*RP* physical role)

Study 3

The third cohort of patients was one that was particularly ill, with a form of multiple organ failure known to have a very high mortality, i.e., severe combined acute respiratory and renal failure (SCARRF). This group was defined by the simultaneous requirement for respiratory support (mechanical ventilation) and renal support [continuous renal replacement therapy (CRRT)]. Such patients were identified between January 1993 and July 1996.

Sample characteristics

Demographic data and APACHE 2 scores are displayed in Table 3.

Table 3. Cohort 3 – characteristics of patients with severe combined acute respiratory and renal failure (SCARRF) compared with a general ICU population

Characteristic	76 SCARRF patients	2,287 other ICU patients
Age in yrs (SD)	61 ± 17	58.8 ± 19
APACHE II score (SD)	28 ± 7.7	17 ± 10
AP II ROD (SD)	56 ± 17%	28 ± 27%
Mortality	64%	21%
SMR (95% CI)	1.1 (0.81-1.47)	0.7 (0.68-0.81)
ICU stay in days (SD)	14 ± 12	4 ± 8
Patients ventilated (%)	100% (76)	67.5% (1545)
Patients vasopressors (%)	85% (65)	20% (458)
PA catheters	67% (51)	8% (201)

Outcome measures

QOL in the survivors was assessed using the SF36 at a given point in time, the minimum being 6 months after hospital discharge. Results were compared to Cohort two, the general ICU population studied 6 months after discharge and presented above. We excluded patients with SCARRF from that general cohort. In the SCARRF group, scores in the individual SF36 dimensions were plotted against age to look for an association with increasing age.

Over the 43 month study period, 76 patients (3.4%) developed SCARRF. Their mean APACHE 2 score was 28 ± 7.7 which was significantly higher than that of the control group (17 ± 10). The hospital mortality of the SCARRF group was 64% compared to the control group mortality of 21%. The treatment of these SCARRF patients (3.4% of ICU population) utilised 10.3% of total ICU days.

29 SCARRF patients (38%) survived to leave hospital. A further 8 (28%) died within 12 months of discharge giving a one-year mortality rate of 72%. Of the 21 survivors, 17 (81% of survivors) completed the SF36 questionnaire. Figure 6 shows the comparison between the SCARRF group, the control ICU population and the Australian population norms for all dimensions of the SF36 score. Patients with SCARRF scored significantly worse in all dimensions, particularly the physical ones, when compared to the normal Australian population. The scores, however, were not significantly lower than those of the control ICU population. No correlation was found with age in the individual SF36 dimensions. Survivors from SCARRF, like the general ICU survivors, while demon-

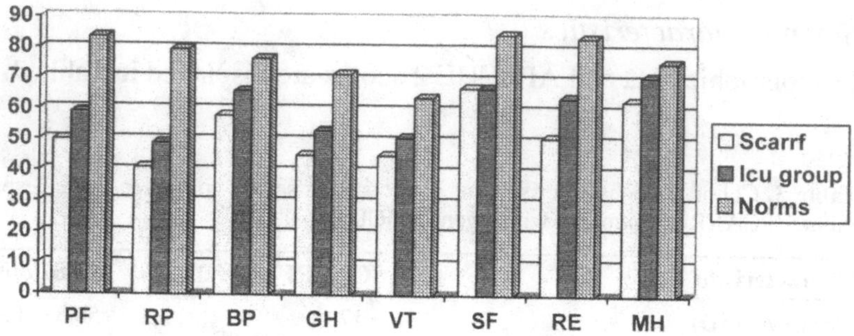

Fig. 6. Cohort 3 - SF36 scores of SCARRF patients as compared to those of a general ICU population and the Australian norms

strating continued physical impairment at 6 months adjust to these limitations. This is shown by their Mental Health and Social Function scores mirroring the general ICU group and approaching age matched normal values.

Discussion

There has been disagreement about the appropriate time to follow up ICU patients. Two important issues are when the post-hospital discharge mortality rate stabilises to that of the general population matched for age and chronic health and when the maximum level of improvement in health status and QOL has been reached. At some stage the continued mortality and decline in QOL is likely to be due to chronic medical conditions or a new condition as opposed to a consequence of their ICU stay.

Our participation rate of contactable survivors (50-60%) is comparable to other similar studies [13-15]. About 7% declined because they felt too unwell. So our 3 cohorts are reasonably representative of our patient population. Our studies showed that both the physical and the psychosocial dimensions of the SIP and SF36 showed a trend to improvement over the 6 month study period, suggesting that follow up before six months after discharge is not a good representation of long term QOL. The information we have gathered enables us to give patients and their families a more realistic expectation of time to recovery, i.e. far beyond their ICU stay, thereby preventing frustration and the negative impact on psychosocial wellbeing caused by unrealistic expectations of rate of recovery. This applies to all patient subgroups including those having elective surgery. This sort of information would aid patients, their families as well as admitting medical teams to make informed decisions on the level and extent of ICU therapy that it is appropriate to undertake. It also facilitates long term discharge planning and home support programmes.

QOL as measured by the three instruments we used, however, still remain worse than the general community [11]. The main improvements over time are seen in the psychosocial domains. This indicates that patients are adjusting to their limitations or perhaps they are recovering in a similar way to a grieving process or recovering from a depressive illness. Interestingly ICU patients at 6 months, score similar to a group of general ward patients (Fig. 1). This is probably the point where chronic co-morbid conditions dictate health-related quality of life. We studied a subgroup of patients in cohort 2 by asking them to complete a simple questionnaire on co-morbid illness. This was their subjective impression of their own chronic health. Of the 109 patients who completed the questionnaire 45% had hypertension and 44% had arthritis. 35% had asthma. 27% had diabetes. 17.4% had chronic headaches. Patients with arthritis and diabetes scored significantly worse in the physical dimensions of the SIP and SF 36 at 6 months ($p < 0.001$). Those with headaches had poorer mental health status ($p = 0.005$).

Acute severity of illness as measured by APACHE 2 remains a predictor of mortality for groups of ICU patients. However it did not predict long term impairment, nor was there a difference between elective surgical patients and others. In fact the only measured benefit of a surgical procedure 6 months after ICU was that surgical patients' mental health status improved!

In our third cohort of patients, we looked at the QOL in survivors from SCARRF. The reason we chose to study this form of MOF was its ease to define by bedside criteria, namely the requirement for mechanical ventilation and CRRT. This is unlike other forms of organ system failure, the definitions of which are controversial. This is a form of multiple organ failure (MOF) that has an especially high mortality [16-20].

The SCARRF patients had a significantly higher mortality in the first year following hospital discharge compared with general ICU population suggesting that many of the survivors, in fact, leave hospital in poor health, with a high risk of early death. In the survivors, the QOL was found to be significantly poorer in all 8 dimensions of the SF36 score when compared with the normal Australian population. However, when compared to the QOL of a general ICU population studied 6 months after discharge, the surviving SCARRF patients were no worse off. This suggests that if there was a more reliable way of predicting one year survivors in patients with SCARRF, they are a group worth treating aggressively, as the QOL of survivors appears to be no worse than that of their general ICU counterparts. In all 3 of our study cohorts mortality stabilised by 6-12 months.

A number of review articles on Outcomes research and QOL assessment have discussed the various methodologies and instruments available [21-24]. There are many allusions to the confusion of definitions and measurement in individual studies. We have focused on health-related QOL and used 3 different instruments. In cohorts 1 and 2 two different questionnaires were administered simultaneously, allowing comparison. The SIP was not intended to allow individual scales to be analysed separately. The SF36 allows separation of each of the scales to allow a more detailed analysis of different aspects of QOL. The SQOL does not use the standard physical and psychosocial dimensions. The SIP has been used internationally for ICU patients. In our experience it is complex and patient feedback suggested its length and complexity led to withdrawal from the study. In addition no Australian normative data is available. The SF36 had broad patient acceptance. It is short and simple and has been widely tested over many disease groups. Australian normative data is available. We were concerned that it would be too simple for the critically ill. For a general ICU a QOL instrument should have broad application. Both the SIP and SF36 have this. For ICU populations (i.e. a sick community group) the instrument should be responsive to small changes in QOL. In cohort 1 and 2 the SIP was less responsive than the SF36 over 6 months. Internal consistency and construct validity are important. Each scale should measure something different but the scales looking at physical function should go together as should the psychosocial scales to give us 2 clear dimensions of health- related QOL. In our second cohort the physical and psychosocial dimensions of the SF36 correlated with all the scales of the SIP. There was strong correlation between the SIP psychosocial and physical dimensions. Correlation between physical and psychosocial dimensions at 6 months for each instrument was: SIP $r = 0.7$, SF36 $r = 0.25$. This suggests that SIP scales are mixed concepts containing both physical and psychological aspects. Thus the SF36 is a more robust QOL instrument for ICU patients.

Conclusion

We have focused on health-related QOL and long term mortality. We recommend studying ICU survivors after at least 6 months. Mortality stabilises to community age-matched levels by 6-12 months. Remembering the ultimate goal of intensive care treatment should be to return a patient to society with *what the patient perceives* as a satisfactory QOL, our studies show patients adjust to their health status by 6 months. They reach community values for the psychosocial dimension of QOL. Our preferred instrument for long term follow-up is the SF36. A better way of identifying and quantifying chronic conditions such as diabetes, cardiac failure and chronic lung disease is required for incorporation into the study of the long term outcome of Intensive Care.

Acknowledgement. We would like to thank Glenyce McIlveen, Kris Southan and Sue Lee for their contribution in following up the ICU patients and data collection, and Robert Brooks for his advice with QOL instruments, in particular SQOL, and data analysis.

References

1. Rowan KM, Kerr JH, Major E et al (1993) Intensive Care Society's comparisons of intensive care units after adjustment for case mix by the American APACHE II method. BMJ 307:977-981
2. Beck DH, Taylor BL, Millar B et al (1997) Prediction of outcome from intensive care: A prospective cohort study comparing APACHE II & III prognostic systems in a United Kingdom intensive care unit. Critical Care Medicine 25: 9-15
3. Wong DT, Crofts SL, Gomez M et al (1995) Evaluation of predictive ability of APACHE II system and hospital outcome in Canadian intensive care patients. Critical Care Medicine 23:1177-1183
4. Le Gall JR, Lemeshow S, Saulnier F (1993) Development of a new scoring system, the SAPS II, from a European/North American multicentre study. JAMA 270: 2478-2486
5. Nair P, Southan K, Jacques T et al (1997) Outcome from severe combined acute respiratory and renal failure. Proceedings, Australia and NZ College of Anaesthetists and Faculty of Intensive Care, Christchurch 127
6. Knaus WA, Draper EA, Wagner DP et al (1985) APACHE 11: a severity of disease classification system. Crit Care Med 13: 818-829
7. Sirio C, Tajimi K, Tase C et al (1992) "An Initial Comparison of Intensive Care in Japan and the United States." Crit Care Med 20:1207-1215
8. Parikh CR, Karnad DR. (1999) Quality, cost and outcome of Intensive Care in a public hospital in Bombay, India. Crit Care Med 27:1754-1759
9. Bergner M, Bobbit RA, Kressel S (1981) The sickness impact profile: development and final revision of a health status measure. Med Care 19: 787-805
10. Tian ZM, Reis Miranda D (1995) Quality of life after intensive care with the sickness impact profile. Int Care Med 21:422-428
11. Brooks R, Kerridge R, Hillman K et al (1997) Quality of life outcomes after intensive care - comparison with a community group. Int. Care Med 23:581-586
12. Ware J. (1993) SF36 health survey, manual and interpretation guide. Boston: Medical Outcomes trust
13. Ware J, Kosinski M, Bayliss M et al (1995) Comparison of Methods for scoring and statistical analysis of SF-36 profile and summary measures: Summary of results from the medical outcomes study. Med Care 33:AS264-AS279
14. Sage WM, Rosenthal MH, Silverman JF. (1986) Is intensive care worth it - An assessment of input and outcome for the critically ill. Critical Care Medicine 14:777-782
15. Niskanen M, Ruokonen E, Takala J et al (1999) Quality of life after prolonged intensive care. Critical Care Medicine 27:1132-1139
16. Levy EM, Viscole CM, Horwitz RI. (1996) The effect of acute renal failure on mortality: a cohort analysis. JAMA 275:1489-1494
17. McCarthy JT (1996) Prognosis of patients with acute renal failure in the intensive care unit: a tale of two eras. Mayo Clin Proc 71:117-126
18. Brivet FG, Kleinknecht DJ, Loirat P et al on behalf of the French Study Group on Acute renal failure (1996) Acute Renal Failure in intensive care units - causes, outcomes and prognostic factors of hospital mortality: a prospective multicentre study. Crit Care Med 24:453-462
19. Turney JH (1990) Why is mortality persistently high in acute renal failure? Lancet 335:971
20. Jacobs CS, Van der Vlieb JA, Van RoozendaalMT et al (1988) Mortality and Quality of Life after intensive care for critical illness. Int Care Med 14:217-220
21. Heyland DK, Guyatt G, Cook DJ et al (1998) Frequency and rigor of quality-of-life assessments in critical care literature. Crit Care Med 26:591-598
22. Rubenfeld GD, Angus DC, Pinsky MR et al (1999) Outcomes research in Critical Care - results of the ATS Critical Care assembly on outcomes research. Am J Respir Crit Care Med 160:358-367
23. Fernandez RR, Sanchez Cruz JJ, Vazquez Mata G (1996) Validation of a quality of life questionnaire for critically ill patients. Intensive Care Med 22:1034-1042
24. Sanders C, Egger M, Donovan J et al (1998) Reporting on quality of life in randomised controlled trials: bibliographic study. BMJ 317:1191-1194

INDEX